IMMUNOLOGY OF HIV INFECTION

IMMUNOLOGY OF HIV INFECTION

Edited by

Sudhir Gupta, M.D., Ph.D.
University of California
Irvine, California

SPRINGER SCIENCE+BUSINESS MEDIA, LLC

Library of Congress Cataloging-in-Publication Data

On file

DOI 10.1007/978-1-4899-0191-0

Originally published by Plenum Publishing Corporation, New York in 1996
MyCopy version of the original edition 1996
10 9 8 7 6 5 4 3 2 1

CONTRIBUTORS

Henri Atlan • Human Biology Research Center/Department of Biophysics, Hadassah University Hospital, Jerusalem, Israel, and Medical Center Broussais-Hôtel Dieu, University of Paris VI, Paris, France; *present address*: Service de Biophysique, Hôpital de l'Hôtel Dieu, 75014 Paris, France

Brigitte Autran • Laboratoire d'Immunologie Cellulaire, URA CNRS 625–Hôpital Pitié-Salpêtrière, 75013 Paris, France

Ewa Björling • Microbiology and Tumorbiology Center, Karolinska Institute, S-171 77 Stockholm, Sweden

Dani P. Bolognesi • Center for AIDS Research, Duke University Medical Center, Durham, North Carolina 27708

Benjamin Bonavida • Department of Microbiology and Immunology, University of California School of Medicine, Los Angeles, California 90095

Christopher B. Buck • Department of Medicine, Johns Hopkins University School of Medicine, Baltimore, Maryland 21205

Ying-Hua Chen • Institute for Hygiene, Leopold-Franzens University, and Ludwig-Boltzmann Institute for AIDS Research, A-6010 Innsbruck, Austria

Mario Clerici • Cattedra di Immunologica, Università degli Studi di Milano, Milan, Italy

Irun R. Cohen • Department of Immunology, Weizmann Institute of Sciences, Rehovot, Israel

Manfred P. Dierich • Institute for Hygiene, Leopold-Franzens University, and Ludwig-Boltzmann Institute for AIDS Research, A-6010 Innsbruck, Austria

Anthony S. Fauci • Laboratory of Immunoregulation, National Institute of Allergy and Infectious Diseases, National Institutes of Health, Bethesda, Maryland 20892

Gwendolyn Anne Fyfe • Chiron Corporation, Emeryville, California 94608

Robert C. Gallo • Institute of Human Virology, Medical Biotechnology Center, University of Maryland, Baltimore, Maryland 21201

Enrico Garaci • Department of Experimental Medicine and Biochemical Sciences, University of Rome "Tor Vergata," 00173 Rome, Italy

Janis V. Giorgi • Department of Medicine, Jonsson Comprehensive Cancer Center, UCLA AIDS Institute and the Multicenter AIDS Cohort Study, UCLA Schools of Medicine and Public Health, Los Angeles, California 90095

David W. Golde • Memorial Sloan-Kettering Cancer Center, New York, New York, and Cornell University Medical College, New York, New York 10021

Allan L. Goldstein • Department of Biochemistry and Molecular Biology, The George Washington University Medical Center, Washington, D.C. 20037

Sudhir Gupta • Division of Basic and Clinical Immunology, University of California, Irvine, California 92697

John W. Hadden • Department of Internal Medicine, Division of Immunopharmacology, University of South Florida Medical College, Tampa, Florida 33612

Laura P. Hale • Department of Pathology, Duke University Medical Center, Durham, North Carolina 27710

Barton F. Haynes • Departments of Medicine and Immunology, and Center for AIDS Research, Duke University Medical Center, Durham, North Carolina 27710

Harry R. Hill • Divisions of Clinical Pathology and Clinical Immunology and Allergy, Departments of Pathology and Pediatrics, University of Utah School of Medicine, Salt Lake City, Utah 84132

Anahid Jewett • Department of Microbiology and Immunology, University of California School of Medicine, Los Angeles, California 90095

Stella C. Knight • Imperial College School of Medicine, Antigen Presentation Research Group, Northwick Park Institute for Medical Research, Harrow HA1 3UJ, United Kingdom

Prasad Koka • Division of Hematology–Oncology, Department of Medicine, University of California, Los Angeles, California 90095

H. Clifford Lane • National Institutes of Health, National Institute for Allergy and Infectious Diseases, Bethesda, Maryland 20892

Jeffrey A. Ledbetter • Bristol-Myers Squibb Pharmaceutical Research Institute, Seattle, Washington 98121

Linda B. Ludwig • Department of Medicine, State University of New York at Buffalo, Buffalo General Hospital, Buffalo, New York 14203

Jerry R. McGhee • Immunobiology Vaccine Center, Department of Microbiology, University of Alabama at Birmingham, Birmingham, Alabama 35294

Michael S. McGrath • Departments of Laboratory Medicine, Medicine, and Pathology, University of California, San Francisco, and San Francisco General Hospital, San Francisco, California 94110

Jean E. Merrill • Department of Immunology, Berlex Biosciences, Richmond, California 94804

Richard Morgan • Clinical Gene Therapy Branch, National Center for Human Genome Research, National Institutes of Health, Bethesda, Maryland 20892

Madhavan P. N. Nair • Department of Medicine, State University of New York at Buffalo, Buffalo General Hospital, Buffalo, New York 14203

Peter L. Nara • Laboratory of Tumor Cell Biology, Division of Basic Sciences, National Cancer Institute, National Institutes of Health, Frederick, Maryland 21702

Valerie L. Ng • Departments of Laboratory Medicine and Medicine, University of California, San Francisco, and San Francisco General Hospital, San Francisco, California 94110

Erling Norrby • Microbiology and Tumorbiology Center, Karolinska Institute, S-171 77 Stockholm, Sweden

Jan M. Orenstein • Department of Pathology, George Washington University Medical Center, Washington, D.C. 20037

Naoki Oyaizu • Department of Pediatrics, North Shore University Hospital–Cornell University Medical College, Manhasset, New York 11030

Savita Pahwa • Department of Pediatrics, North Shore University Hospital–Cornell University Medical College, Manhasset, New York 11030

Dhavalkumar D. Patel • Departments of Medicine and Immunology, and Center for AIDS Research, Duke University Medical Center, Durham, North Carolina 27710

Guido Poli • AIDS Immunopathogenesis Unit, DIBIT, San Raffaele Scientific Institute, 20127 Milan, Italy

Lee Ratner • Division of Molecular Oncology, Departments of Medicine, Pathology, and Molecular Microbiology, Washington University, St. Louis, Missouri 63110

Felipe Samaniego • Institute of Human Virology, Medical Biotechnology Center, University of Maryland, Baltimore, Maryland 21201

Prem S. Sarin • Department of Biochemistry and Molecular Biology, The George Washington University Medical Center, Washington, D.C. 20037

Arif R. Sarwari • Division of Infectious Diseases, University of Maryland School of Medicine, Baltimore, Maryland 21201

David T. Scadden • Massachusetts General Hospital and Harvard Medical School, Boston, Massachusetts 02114

Stanley A. Schwartz • Department of Medicine, State University of New York at Buffalo, Buffalo General Hospital, Buffalo, New York 14203

Gene M. Shearer • Experimental Immunology Branch, National Cancer Institute, National Institutes of Health, Bethesda, Maryland 20892

Shyh-Dar Shyur • Department of Pediatrics, Mackay Memorial Hospital, Taipei, Taiwan, Republic of China

Robert F. Siliciano • Department of Medicine, Johns Hopkins University School of Medicine, Baltimore, Maryland 21205

Phillip D. Smith • Department of Medicine, University of Alabama, School of Medicine, Birmingham, Alabama 35294

Herman F. Staats • Department of Medicine and Center for AIDS Research, Duke University Medical Center, Durham, North Carolina 27710

Heribert Stoiber • Institute for Hygiene, Leopold-Franzens University, and Ludwig-Boltzmann Institute for AIDS Research, A-6010 Innsbruck, Austria

Charles S. Via • Research Service, Baltimore VA Medical Center, and Division of Rheumatology and Clinical Immunology, University of Maryland School of Medicine, Baltimore, Maryland 21201

Sharon M. Wahl • Cellular Immunology, National Institute of Dental Research, National Institutes of Health, Bethesda, Maryland 20892

FOREWORD

The emergence of HIV as a major human pathogen and the recognition of AIDS, the terrible disease that it causes, have had enormous consequences for the health and well-being of individuals throughout the world. HIV has now penetrated virtually every region of the globe. In some areas, its impact has already been enormous; other regions are in great danger of public health calamities. The response to this epidemic requires the very best scientific and public health measures that world society can bring to bear.

AIDS is fundamentally a disorder of the immune system. The infection of the principal immunological regulatory cells and their gradual loss over time is responsible for many of the most crippling aspects of the disease. The need to develop strategies to prevent the disease, on the one hand, and to successfully treat those infected, on the other, requires a sophisticated understanding of the immune response to HIV and of the immunopathogenesis of AIDS.

While there can be little doubt that scientists have rallied to the study of HIV and of the means through which it causes AIDS, many in the immunological community have not fully realized the great medical and scientific challenges posed by the infection and the enormous need for a concerted immunological attack on the virus. In part, this has stemmed from the difficulty of studying a disease that has no adequate small animal model. However, an uncertainty on the part of many as to the approaches that would most likely provide the key insights needed for real progress to be made in the development of vaccines and of strategies to control the virus has been a major factor in their reluctance to devote their research to this crucial problem.

In *Immunology of HIV Infection*, Sudhir Gupta has assembled a remarkable set of experts to deal in detail with the critical immunological aspects of HIV infection and AIDS. Their efforts promise to go far to provide the springboard for the deeper involvement of immunologists in research on this critical problem. The book is organized so that it progresses from fundamental aspects of immunity to HIV to a detailed consideration of the mechanisms underlying the immunopathogenesis of the disease. It concludes with a consideration of approaches for vaccine design and for the treatment of established infection with agents whose principal targets are the restoration of immune function.

The publication of this book is particularly timely as it coincides with a renewed commitment among AIDS researchers toward a deeper analysis of the immunological mechanisms underlying the disease and toward the development of new approaches for the design of vaccines. It should be of great value both to those within the field, for whom it represents a synthesis of the diverse aspects of immunology of HIV infection, and to those who are preparing to enter the field. For the latter, the availability of the key information on the immunological aspects of HIV infection and AIDS in a single volume will be of particular value. Sudhir Gupta and his colleagues are to be congratulated for the efforts that have led to this important volume.

William E. Paul

Bethesda, Maryland

PREFACE

The immune system is the primary target of HIV. The clinical consequences are the results of immune dysfunction and depletion. In the past five years, major progress has been made in understanding the immunopathogenesis of HIV infection. This information is scattered throughout various journals, and most of the books on HIV infection have devoted one or two chapters to the immunology of HIV infection. The purpose of this book is to present the most comprehensive and up-to-date information regarding the immunology of HIV infection, contributed by a group of experts.

The book is divided into three sections. Section I deals with the basic mechanisms. New information has been reviewed regarding the role of HIV genes, especially the *nef* gene, in the biology of HIV infection; B- and T-cell epitopes in HIV glycoproteins; and the role of coreceptors in signaling of lymphocytes. Section II is comprised of 19 chapters regarding immunopathogenesis of HIV infection. These include a description of changes in and the role of specific immunity (cell- and antibody-mediated immunity) and nonspecific immunity (complement, polymorphonuclear leukocytes, and NK cells) in HIV infection. The roles of cytokines and cytotoxic T lymphocytes are discussed in detail. There is an increasing understanding of the important role of macrophages and dendritic cells in HIV pathogenesis. A chapter is included that reviews HIV in lymph nodes and thymus, and two major lymphoid tissues, as a target for HIV infection. Recent data on the effect of HIV envelope glycoproteins on the signaling pathway and their role in programmed cell death and neuropathology have been reviewed. A special chapter is devoted to mucosal immunity in HIV infection. New information regarding immunopathogenesis of lymphoma and Kaposi's sarcoma associated with HIV infection has been included. Section III focuses on immune-based therapy. In this section, immunopharmacotherapy, biological response modifiers, and the role of growth factors in treatment and their effects on the biology of HIV are discussed. The subjects of vaccine therapy and gene therapy are presented.

This volume should serve as a text on the immunology of HIV for basic scientists and clinical researchers, including internists, pediatricians, immunologists, and infectious disease specialists, interested in the area of HIV infection.

I thank all of the authors for providing their most updated contributions in a most timely manner, and to Dr. William Paul for writing the Foreword for the book. Last but not least, I wish to thank my Administrative Assistant, Nancy J. Doman, for her tireless efforts in preparing this volume.

Sudhir Gupta

CONTENTS

Section I. Basic Mechanisms

Chapter 1

GENETIC ORGANIZATION OF HIV

Lee Ratner

Chapter 2

T-CELL EPITOPES OF HIV-1 ENVELOPE GLYCOPROTEIN

Christopher B. Buck and Robert F. Siliciano

Section II. Immunopathogenesis

CHAPTER 5

HIV IN LYMPH NODE AND THYMUS

DHAVALKUMAR D. PATEL, LAURA P. HALE, AND BARTON F. HAYNES

CHAPTER 6

EFFECTS OF HIV-1 AND HIV-1 ENVELOPE GLYCOPROTEINS ON SIGNALING PATHWAYS IN HUMAN T LYMPHOCYTES

SUDHIR GUPTA

CHAPTER 7

LYMPHOCYTE APOPTOSIS IN HIV INFECTION

NAOKI OYAIZU AND SAVITA PAHWA

CHAPTER 10

CYTOTOXIC T-LYMPHOCYTE RESPONSES TO HIV: FROM PRIMARY INFECTION TO AIDS

BRIGITTE AUTRAN

CHAPTER 11

TYPE 1 AND TYPE 2 RESPONSES IN HIV INFECTION AND EXPOSURE

GENE M. SHEARER AND MARIO CLERICI

CHAPTER 12

HUMORAL IMMUNITY TO HIV-1: LETHAL FORCE OR TROJAN HORSE?

PETER L. NARA

Chapter 13

AUTOIMMUNITY IN HIV

Charles S. Via and Arif R. Sarwari

Chapter 14

CYTOKINE CASCADES IN HIV INFECTION

Guido Poli and Anthony S. Fauci

Chapter 15

MACROPHAGE FUNCTIONS IN HIV-1 INFECTION

Sharon M. Wahl, Jan M. Orenstein, and Phillip D. Smith

CHAPTER 18

HIV AND COMPLEMENT

MANFRED P. DIERICH, HERIBERT STOIBER, AND YING-HUA CHEN

CHAPTER 19

POLYMORPHONUCLEAR LEUKOCYTE FUNCTION IN HIV

SHYH-DAR SHYUR AND HARRY R. HILL

CHAPTER 20

MUCOSAL IMMUNITY IN HIV INFECTION

HERMAN F. STAATS AND JERRY R. MCGHEE

CHAPTER 21

THE PUTATIVE ROLE OF HIV-1 ENVELOPE PROTEINS IN THE NEUROIMMUNOLOGY AND NEUROPATHOLOGY OF CNS AIDS

PRASAD KOKA AND JEAN E. MERRILL

CHAPTER 22

IMMUNOPATHOGENESIS OF KAPOSI'S SARCOMA

FELIPE SAMANIEGO AND ROBERT C. GALLO

CHAPTER 30

GENE THERAPY

RICHARD A. MORGAN

SECTION I

BASIC MECHANISMS

CHAPTER 1

GENETIC ORGANIZATION OF HIV

LEE RATNER

HIV-1 is a member of the primate lentivirus subgroup of retroviruses (Weiss *et al.*, 1982), and is a close relative to HIV-2 and simian immunodeficiency viruses (SIV). More distantly related retroviruses infect sheep (visna virus), horses (equine infectious anemia virus), cats (feline immunodeficiency virus), and cattle (bovine immunodeficiency virus). These viruses are distinguished from murine and avian retroviruses in their vast array of regulatory and accessory gene products, in addition to the structural and enzymatic gene products common to all retroviruses. This chapter describes our current understanding of HIV-1 genes, their products, and functions. Rather than provide a lengthy list of references, this chapter refers to several excellent, recent reviews, and a selected group of more recent scientific papers.

1. GENETIC ORGANIZATION OF HIV-1

The HIV-1 particle includes two identical (+)-strand RNA copies of the viral genome (Weiss *et al.*, 1982). Upon infection of a susceptible host cell, the RNA genome is reverse transcribed into DNA, designated the *provirus*. The genetic elements of the HIV-1 provirus are shown in Fig. 1. The 5′ and 3′ ends of the provirus include long terminal repeat (LTR) structures of 634 nucleotides. The 5′-LTR regulates the initiation of RNA transcription, whereas the 3′-LTR regulates RNA termination and polyadenylation. Structural proteins of the virus particle are encoded by the *gag* and *env* genes. Gag proteins are viral core proteins. Envelope proteins, embedded in the lipid bilayer, mediate receptor binding and membrane fusion required for virus entry. The *pol* gene encodes for the viral protease, reverse transcriptase, ribonuclease H activity, and integrase. Regulatory proteins with a potent influence on HIV-1 replication are encoded by *tat* and *rev*. Tat, a transcriptional *trans*-activator protein, mediates its effects by the Tat-response (TAR) element. Rev, a post-

LEE RATNER • Division of Molecular Oncology, Departments of Medicine, Pathology, and Molecular Microbiology, Washington University, St. Louis, Missouri 63110.

Immunology of HIV Infection, edited by Sudhir Gupta. Plenum Press, New York, 1996.

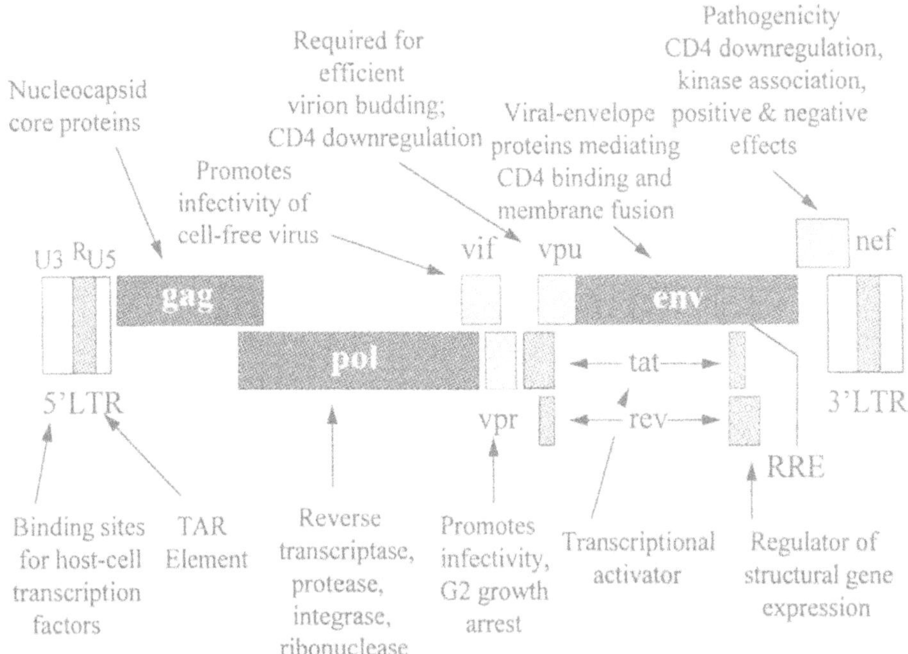

FIGURE 1. HIV-1 genome. The relative sizes and locations of each gene are shown together with the presumed functions.

transcriptional *trans*-activator, enhances structural gene expression by promoting transfer of incompletely spliced viral RNAs from the nucleus to the cytoplasm, mediated by the Rev response element (RRE) in the viral RNA. Accessory proteins which are at least partially dispensable for virus replication *in vitro* are encoded by *vif*, *vpr*, *vpu*, and *nef*. Vif, a virion infectivity factor, promotes infectivity of virus particles but is not packaged to a significant extent in the virus particle. Vpr, viral protein R, is homologous to Vpx, viral protein X, of HIV-2 and SIVs, and is packaged into the virus particle, but its function is incompletely described. Vpu, viral protein U, is required for efficient virus budding and CD4 downregulation. Nef, negative factor, has multiple effects on virus replication and T-cell activation.

2. HIV-1 REPLICATION CYCLE

The replication cycle provides a foundation on which to decipher the functions of individual viral components (Fig. 2). The infectious HIV-1 particle binds to a receptor on a susceptible host cell. The predominant receptor is CD4 (Maddon *et al.*, 1986), though other receptors have been proposed, such as galactosyl ceramide (Yahi *et al.*, 1995). CD4 is not sufficient for virus entry, which is mediated by additional cellular factors, which for the purpose of this chapter are designated *cell infectivity factor* (CIF). Human cells engineered to express CD4 are permissive to HIV-1 infection, whereas rodent cells expressing human CD4 bind HIV-1, but are blocked in virus entry (Maddon *et al.*, 1986), suggesting that CIF is expressed on human but not rodent cells. Fusion of rodent cells bearing human CD4, with

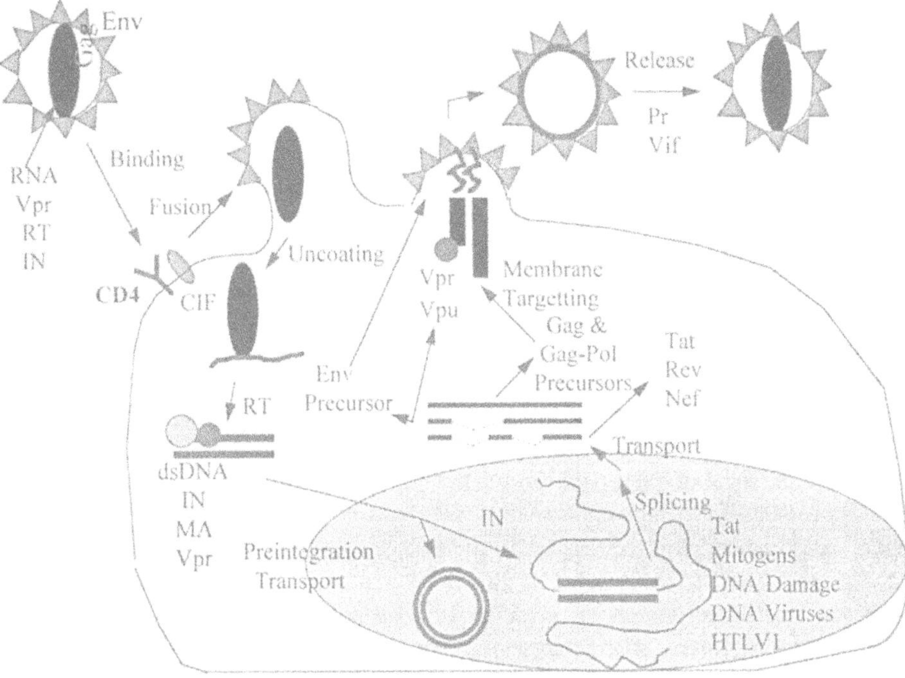

FIGURE 2. HIV-1 replication cycle.

human cells restores virus entry (Broder *et al.*, 1993). CIF may be a coreceptor that assists in virus interaction with the host cell, or it may be an enzyme that modifies a viral component after binding (Clements *et al.*, 1991). CIF is not well characterized, and many potential candidates have been proposed (CD44, CD26; Dukes *et al.*, 1995; Wang *et al.*, 1995); the most convincing data suggests that CIF is the chemokine receptor-related protein, fusin (Feng *et al.*, 1996).

After the fusion event, the virus capsid is partially uncoated, in a poorly understood manner, to form a ribonucleoprotein complex capable of reverse transcription. Reverse transcription, synthesis of DNA from an RNA template, is a critical event in the retrovirus life cycle, and a process for which retroviruses have received their designation since the normal flow of genetic information in the cell is from DNA into RNA (Weiss *et al.*, 1982). This process is mediated by the reverse transcriptase (RT), a component of the virion. Although reverse transcription is initiated in the virus particle prior to infection (Trono, 1992), complete reverse transcription only occurs after infection and uncoating. Reverse transcription is inefficient in quiescent cells, suggesting the involvement of host components in this process (Zack *et al.*, 1990).

The complex resulting from reverse transcription includes linear double-stranded DNA, the Gag matrix (MA) protein, the accessory Vpr protein, and the viral integrase (IN) (Heinzinger *et al.*, 1994). The protein components are all derived from the infecting virus, and no new protein synthesis is required. This nucleoprotein complex, the *preintegration complex*, is transported into the nucleus. Whereas onco-retroviruses require dissolution of the nuclear membrane with mitosis for preintegration transport, the HIV-1 preintegration complex can bypass this requirement, through independent nuclear targeting mechanisms of the MA and Vpr proteins.

In the nucleus, IN mediates a complex series of enzymatic steps, including exonuclease trimming of the linear double-stranded DNA, staggered endonucleolytic cleavage of host chromosomal DNA, and concerted ligation of the free viral and host chromosomal DNA termini (Katz and Skalka, 1994). Integration occurs at a large number of cellular loci, with preference to areas with an *open* chromatin structure. It has been suggested that integration is required for virus replication, but evidence for or against this hypothesis is not firm (Weiss *et al.*, 1982; Ansari-Lari *et al.*, 1995). A portion of the viral DNA fails to integrate, and is capable of circularizing into forms containing one or two LTR circles, as a result of the activity of cellular DNA ligases (Heinzinger *et al.*, 1994). Circular DNAs are a dead end for virus replication; nevertheless, they provide a useful marker to indicate that the preintegration complex has been transported into the nucleus.

In many cells, the provirus is not expressed and is considered *latent*. A large number of viral, cellular, and exogenous stimuli can activate transcription of the provirus from latency, or increase the level of expression from a low basal level. The viral transcriptional *trans* activator protein, Tat, which binds to the TAR element in all viral RNAs (Fig. 3; Gaynor, 1995), can stimulate virus expression. In addition, transcription is stimulated by mitogens, DNA damage such as that induced by ultraviolet irradiation, and mitomycin c. Transcriptional *trans*-activator proteins of a variety of DNA viruses (e.g., herpesviruses, adenoviruses, hepadnaviruses, papovaviruses) and another retrovirus, human T-cell leukemia virus type 1 (HTLV-1), that are found as coinfecting viruses in AIDS patients (Zack *et al.*,

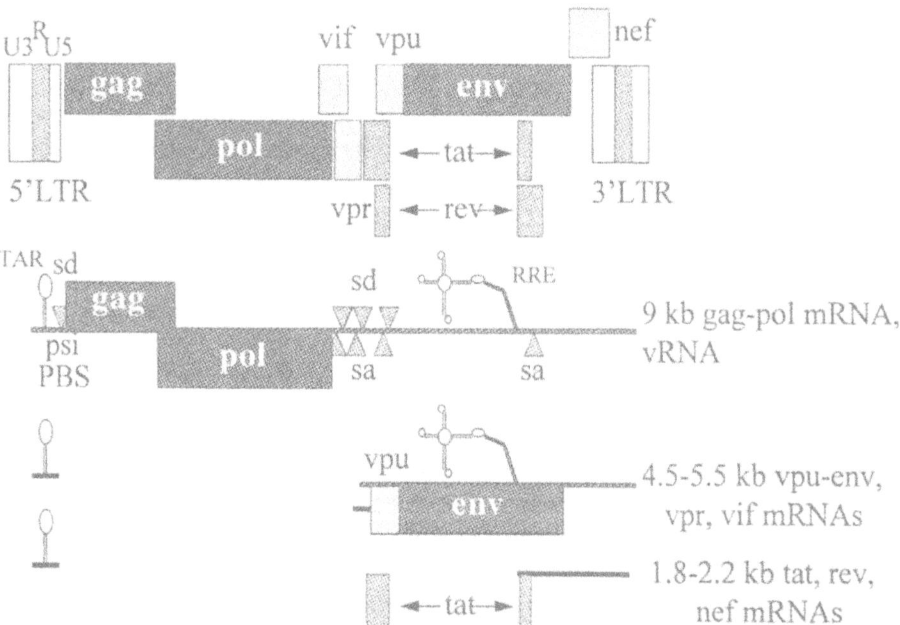

FIGURE 3. Viral RNAs. Elements present in unspliced (9 kb), single-spliced (4.5–5.5 kb), and multiple-spliced (1.8–2.2 kb) viral RNAs are shown. One member of each of the latter two classes of viral transcripts is illustrated. A schematic diagram of the proviral DNA is shown at the top.

1988; Stein *et al.*, 1989; Walker *et al.*, 1992), are also able to enhance the expression of HIV genes.

The full-length viral RNA species is 9 kb (Fig. 3). It is initiated from within the 5′-LTR at a point designated the U3–R boundary, and is terminated within the 3′-LTR at a point designated the R–U5 boundary (Weiss *et al.*, 1982). This RNA has a variety of different fates. It may serve as a substrate for the splicesome complex, giving rise to smaller spliced viral RNAs, resulting from utilization of the many different combinations of splice donor (sd) and splice acceptor (sa) sites (Schwartz *et al.*, 1990). Alternatively, this RNA may be transported to the cytoplasm to serve as the mRNA for synthesis of Gag and Gag–Pol precursor proteins, or it may be transported to the plasma membrane to serve as viral genomic RNA to be incorporated into the virus particle.

The group of single-spliced RNA species are 4.5–5.5 kb in size, and include mRNAs for Vpr, Vif, or a bicistronic mRNA for Vpu and Env (Fig. 3; Schwartz *et al.*, 1990). The group of multiple-spliced RNA species are 1.8–2.2 kb in size, and include mRNAs for Tat, Rev, and Nef. The level of unspliced and single-spliced mRNAs in the cytoplasm is increased by Rev, whose activity is mediated by the RRE found in these transcripts.

The envelope precursor protein is proteolytically processed in the secretory pathway of the cell, whereas the Gag and Gag–Pol precursors are processed incompletely in the cell and are assembled into virus particles at the plasma membrane (Fig. 2; Ratner, 1992; Wills and Craven, 1991). The process of virus assembly at the plasma membrane is enhanced by the Vpu protein (Jabbar, 1995). The components of the virus particle, Gag and Gag–Pol precursor proteins, processed envelope proteins, viral RNA, and the Vpr protein interact at the cell surface, and bud from the cell to form an immature noninfectious virus particle. Maturation of the free virus particle is mediated by the viral protease (Pr), resulting in proteolytic processing of the Gag and Gag–Pol precursor proteins, and infectious virus particles (Wills and Craven, 1991).

3. VIRAL RNAs

Virion RNA is initiated from a site in the 5′-LTR downstream of a TATA sequence and binding sites for transcriptional factors Spl and nuclear factor B (reviewed by Jones and Peterlin, 1994; Fig. 3). This RNA species includes the TAR element and the RRE that mediate Tat and Rev activities, respectively. This RNA species also includes the packaging signal, *psi*, required for virion incorporation (Carriere *et al.*, 1995). The psi signal interacts with the Gag precursor protein as well as the proteolytic Gag product, nucleocapsid (NC) (Luban and Goff, 1994). A molecule of $tRNA_3^{lys}$ is annealed to the 5′ end of this RNA at the primer binding site (PBS), which serves as the primer for (−)-strand DNA synthesis by RT (Weiss *et al.*, 1982). The 9-kb mRNA also serves as the mRNA for synthesis of the Gag and Gag–Pol precursor proteins. The Gag–Pol precursor protein is the product of a ribosomal frameshift event that occurs within the segment of the RNA containing the overlap of *gag* and *pol* genes (Jacks *et al.*, 1988). Frameshifting occurs during the translation of approximately 5% of these transcripts. The frameshifting signal includes a *slippery* uridine-rich sequence, followed by a pseudoknot structure that induces a pause in translation.

Multiple different splice sites are utilized to produce a large family of single- and multiple-spliced transcripts. Several different *cis*-acting sequences in the RNA can modulate the efficiency of splicing (Amendt *et al.*, 1995; Staffa and Cochrane, 1995). The Rev protein modulates the relative levels of unspliced and single-spliced transcripts through a direct effect on the splicesome and/or the nuclear–cytoplasmic RNA transport machinery (Hope and Pomerantz, 1995).

4. STRUCTURAL PROTEINS

4.1. Gag

The Gag precursor protein, Pr55^{gag}, is 55 kDa, and is the critical component for assembly of the virion (Spearman *et al.*, 1994; reviewed by Wills and Craven, 1991). It is cotranslationally modified by attachment of a 14-carbon saturated fatty acid, myristic acid, at its N-terminus (Fig. 4). Fatty acid attachment is mediated by the activity of a methionine amino peptidase that removes the initiator methionine, and by an *N*-myristyl transferase that is responsible for covalent attachment of the fatty acid to the amino group

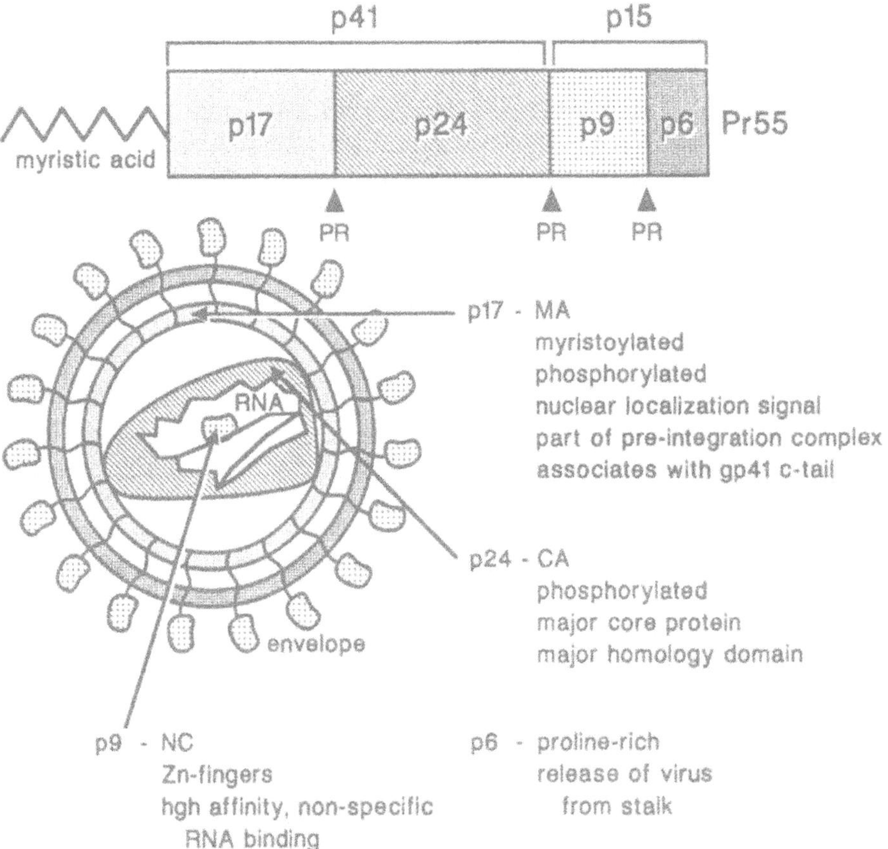

FIGURE 4. HIV-1 Gag proteins. The Pr55^{gag} precursor protein and its proteolytic products, location in virus particle, and functions are shown.

of the N-terminal glycine residue (Bryant and Ratner, 1990). Myristylation is important for targeting $Pr55^{gag}$ to the plasma membrane and assembly of virus particles at the cell surface. The critical role of myristylation has been demonstrated by inhibition of extracellular virus release by mutation of the N-terminal glycine residue or treatment of infected cells with myristic acid analogues (Bryant *et al.*, 1989; Bryant and Ratner, 1990).

$Pr55^{gag}$ is proteolytically processed by the viral protease to proteins of 17, 24, 9, and 6 kDa. The p17 protein is the matrix, MA, protein. In the mature virus particle, MA is situated between the nucleocapsid and the C-terminal tail of the transmembrane envelope protein, gp41 (Mammano *et al.*, 1995). The structure of this protein has been solved by nuclear magnetic resonance and X-ray crystallography, demonstrating several α-helical domains at the N-terminus, and a β-pleated sheet structure (Massiah *et al.*, 1994). A cluster of basic residues in the α-helical N-terminal 31 amino acids has been shown to be important for both targeting $Pr55^{gag}$ to the plasma membrane, as well as targeting MA to the nucleus as a component of the preintegration complex (Heinzinger *et al.*, 1994; Zhou *et al.*, 1994). The nuclear targeting function is disrupted by phosphorylation of the C-terminal tyrosine residue (Gallay *et al.*, 1995). Several serine residues of MA can also be phosphorylated. Serine 111 is phosphorylated by protein kinase C, resulting in enhanced plasma membrane association of this protein (Yu *et al.*, 1995). Domains of MA in addition to the myristic acid anchor are important for targeting $Pr55^{gag}$ to the plasma membrane (Spearman *et al.*, 1994). Mutations in several different domains of MA also result in virus particles lacking envelope proteins. Gag–Env interactions may also be important in determining the site on the plasma membrane for virus budding (Owens *et al.*, 1991).

The p24 capsid (CA) protein is the major structural component of the virion. It contains a sequence that is highly conserved among retroviral capsids, designated the *major homology domain* (Craven *et al.*, 1995). CA also includes several serine residues that are phosphorylated by protein kinases, but the effect of phosphorylation on CA function has not been explored (Veronese *et al.*, 1988). CA interacts with immunophilins, in particular cyclophilin A, directing its incorporation into virus particles, which increases the specific infectivity of the virus particle (Francke *et al.*, 1994; Thali *et al.*, 1994).

The p9 nucleocapsid (NC) protein is an RNA binding protein. This activity is mediated at least partially by a cluster of cysteine residues that form two zinc-fingers (Gorelick *et al.*, 1993). A stretch of basic residues in the N-terminus of this domain within $Pr55^{gag}$ may serve as a membrane targeting signal (Platt and Haffar, 1994).

The p6 protein of HIV-1 has no counterpart in avian or murine retroviral Gag proteins. The HIV-1 p6 protein mediates the incorporation of Vpr into the virus particle (Lu *et al.*, 1995), whereas the HIV-2 p6 protein mediates the incorporation of Vpx into the virus particle (Wu *et al.*, 1994). A proline-rich domain in the N-terminal portion of p6, in certain cellular contexts, regulates the release of virus particles from the cell surface (Gottlinger *et al.*, 1991).

4.2. Envelope

The viral envelope protein is synthesized as a 160-kDa precursor protein, gp160, on membrane-associated ribosomes, due to the presence of a hydrophobic signal sequence at the N-terminus (reviewed by Ratner, 1992). Transfer of the nascent envelope protein into the endoplasmic reticulum is halted by a hydrophobic *stop transfer* sequence 151 residues from the C-terminus. Oligosaccharide addition occurs on 30–36 asparagine residues of the envelope protein within the endoplasmic reticulum. Glycosylation is important for proper folding of the envelope precursor protein, proteolytic processing, high-affinity interactions with CD4, and presentation of neutralizing epitopes. During transport through the endoplasmic reticulum and Golgi apparatus to the plasma membrane, gp160 oligomerizes, and it is cleaved to gp120 surface (SU) and gp41 transmembrane (TM) proteins by Kex, furinlike cellular proteases. In addition, some of the N-linked oligosaccharides undergo modification from a high-mannose form to a complex-type oligosaccharide. After reaching the cell surface, the envelope protein complex may remain on the surface of the cell or it may be incorporated into a newly formed virus particle. Expression of the envelope protein on the cell or virion surface can result in interactions with the viral receptor, CD4. Some of the gp120 protein is spontaneously shed from gp41, or shedding is induced by CD4 interactions and conformational changes within the envelope protein complex. Released gp120 protein *in vivo* may bind to uninfected $CD4^+$ cells, making them targets for various immune effectors.

The gp120 SU protein is subdivided into five variable (V) loops that manifest the highest degree of sequence variation among HIV-1 strains (quasispecies; Starcich *et al.*, 1986). Four of these loops have been shown to be bounded by disulfide-linked cysteine residues (Fig. 5; Leonard *et al.*, 1990). The intervening domains are designated constant (C) domains. The V1 and V2 loops regulate the efficiency of virus entry and cell tropism (Shioda *et al.*, 1991; Koito *et al.*, 1995). The V3 loop is the major determinant of tropism of HIV-1 for T-cell lines or macrophages. Tropism characteristics of HIV-1 strains are often measured on the MT4 T-cell line, and HIV-1 isolates are designated as synctium-inducing (SI) or non-synctium-inducing strains (NSI). The V3 domain is also a primary target for neutralizing antibodies and cytotoxic T-cell responses (Wu *et al.*, 1995b). A region of gp120, including the V2 loop and the C4 domain, is involved in CD4 interactions and forms another epitope for neutralizing antibodies (Olshevsky *et al.*, 1990). The N- and C-termini of gp120, as well as portions of the C4 region, are involved in hydrophobic and ionic interactions between gp120 and gp41 (Helseth *et al.*, 1991).

The gp41 TM protein includes an *ectodomain*, exterior to the lipid bilayer, a membrane-spanning hydrophobic domain, and the C-terminal domain, interior to the lipid bilayer. The ectodomain includes a hydrophobic N-terminal sequence that mediates the fusion event, presumably by insertion into lipid bilayers when exposed after CD4 binding (Dedera and Ratner, 1991). Also present in the ectodomain is a leucine heptad repeat sequence that also regulates fusion. In addition, a disulfide-bounded cysteine loop of six amino acids is present, which is critical for proper folding and transport of the envelope protein in the secretory pathway of the cell (Dedera *et al.*, 1992). The membrane-spanning region includes two hydrophilic residues that are proposed to form a salt bridge in the lipid bilayer with adjacent gp41 subunits (Gabuzda *et al.*, 1991). The C-terminal domain of gp41 includes two amphipathic helices that may contribute to the cytopathic effects of the virus by binding and modulating calmodulin activity (Tencza *et al.*, 1995).

5. ENZYMATIC PROTEINS

The enzymatic proteins of HIV-1 are derived from the *pol* gene, expressed from a *gag–pol* mRNA as a result of a ribosome frameshifting event. The 180-kDa Gag–Pol precursor

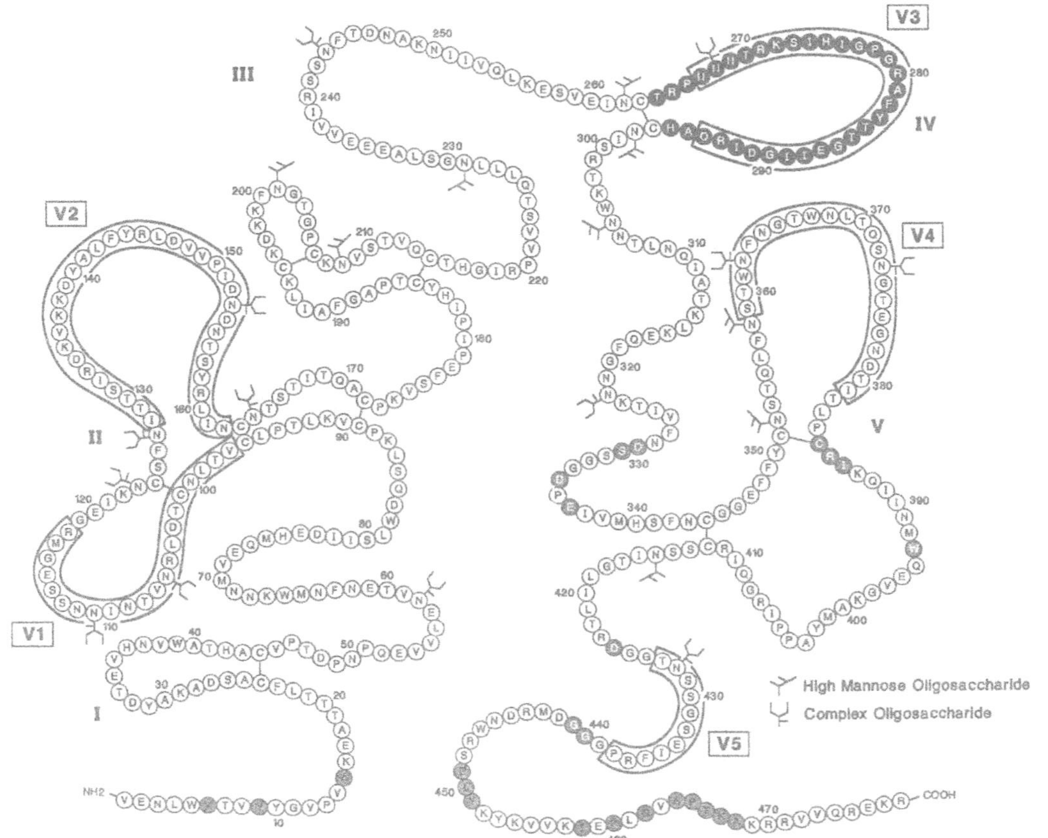

FIGURE 5. HIV-1 surface envelope protein. Sequences of the HIV-1 strain ADA are shown with disulfide-bonded cysteine residues, and oligosaccharide-modified asparagines. Black shading is shown for the V3 loop that is critical in regulating HIV-1 cell-specific tropism. Dark shading is shown for residues that mediate CD4 binding. Lighter shading is shown for residues at either end of gp120 that mediate interactions with TM.

protein is proteolytically processed within the virus particle by the viral protease, which is autocatalytically cleaved from this protein. Remarkable progress has occurred in research on the enzymatic proteins of HIV-1, including their structural definition by X-ray crystallography (Fig. 6). They are a target for specific inhibitory agents (reviewed by Katz and Skalka, 1994).

5.1. Protease

The protease is a homodimer of two 10-kDa, 99-amino-acid-long monomers, arranged in an antiparallel configuration. The protease is activated under conditions in which high concentrations of Gag–Pol precursor proteins are attained, resulting in their dimerization. Normally, the protease is activated in the immature virus particle, but premature protease activation may result in intracellular Gag and Gag–Pol precursor processing, and cytopathic effects. This enzyme is an aspartyl protease, with a highly conserved aspartate–threonine–glycine triplet at the catalytic site. The substrate is held within the catalytic site by two flaps (Fig. 6A). The cleavage sites for the protease are not unique, but some amino acids occur repeatedly at cleavage sites and are generally hydrophobic and located in extended, flexible regions of the precursor proteins. The protease can be inhibited by reduced amides, hydroxyethylene-containing compounds, hydroxyethylamino-containing molecules, statine-containing compounds (e.g., pepstatin), cyclic urea-containing compounds, and several other nonpeptidyl analogues (Wlodawer and Erickson, 1993). Mutants resistant to protease inhibitors have arisen in culture and show amino acid changes at residues 8, 31, and 82, whose side chains interact with the active site and substrate-binding subsites.

5.2. Reverse Transcriptase

The discovery of reverse transcriptase activity by Temin and Mizutani and by Baltimore was a seminal finding for biotechnology, as well as revealing a novel pathway of cellular DNA transposition. The reverse transcriptase (RT) of HIV-1 is a heterodimer of 66- and 51-kDa subunits, having a common N-terminus but different C-termini. The p66 and p51 subunits have distinct roles in the heterodimeric enzyme. The p66 subunit is primarily responsible for enzymatic activity, whereas the p51 subunit is primarily a structural component. The enzyme has three activities, including an RNA-dependent DNA polymerase, a ribonuclease H, and a DNA-dependent DNA polymerase. The initial event is the binding of the template-primer to RT, followed by binding of the dNTP substrate. The

→

FIGURE 6. Structures of HIV-1 enzymes: (A) protease and (B) reverse transcriptase. (A) The light lines indicate the carbon backbone of the protease with an empty substrate site, and the heavy lines the carbon backbone with an inhibitor-complexed protease to show the extensive movements, particularly in the *flap* region with substrate binding. (B) A linear map of RT is shown with the most highly conserved residues which are components of the active sites indicated by filled circles. Hatched areas indicate regions of homology among different retroviral enzymes. Filled areas indicate regions of homology with other polymerases or ribonucleases H. Below is an outline of the structure of RT with filled circles corresponding to the active-site residues. The RNA template–DNA product is shown lying in the cleft. Reprinted with permission from Katz and Skalka (1994).

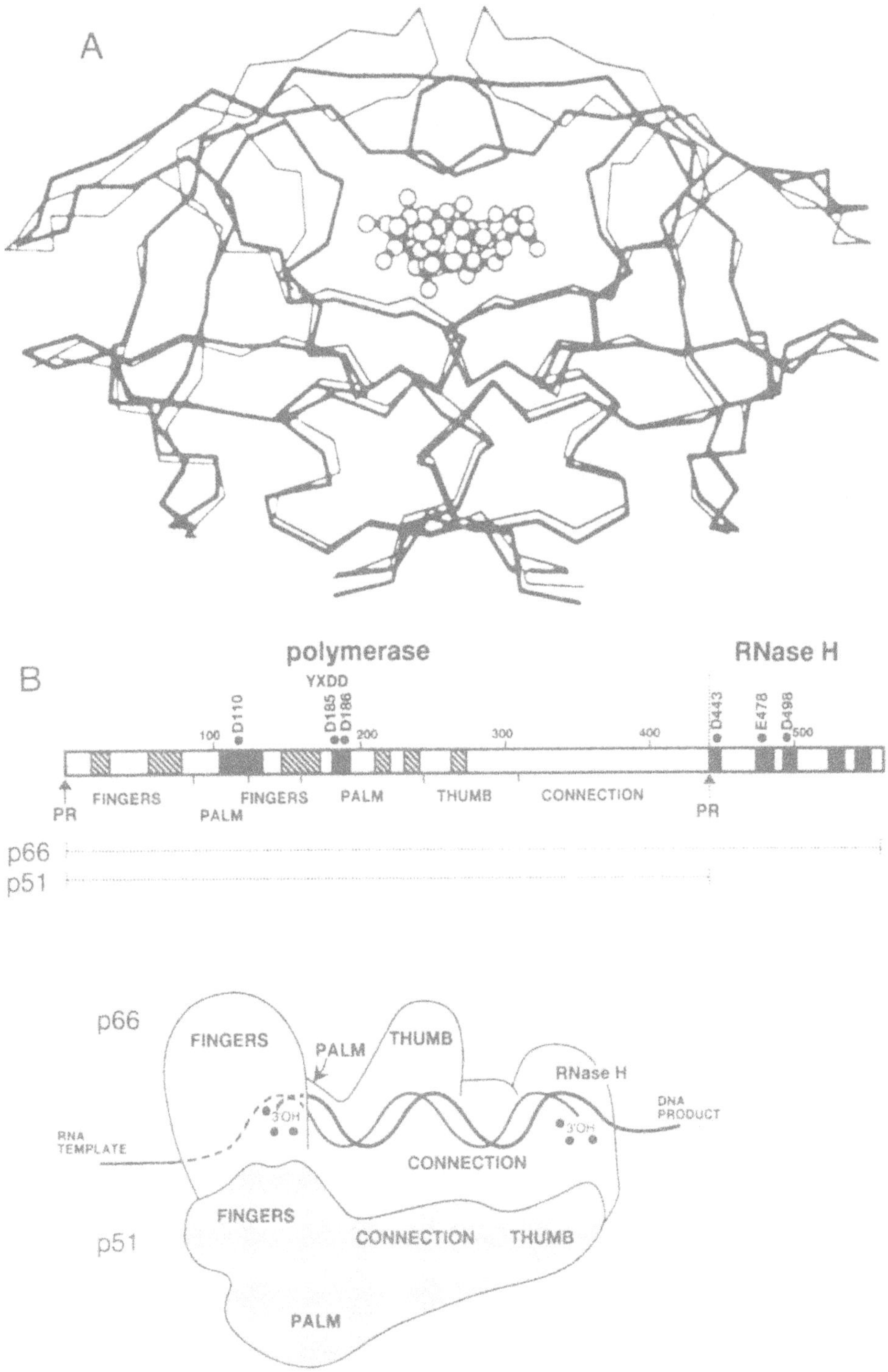

A

B

polymerase RNase H

YXDD

100 D110 D185 D186 200 300 400 D443 E478 D498 500

PR FINGERS PALM FINGERS PALM THUMB CONNECTION PR

p66

p51

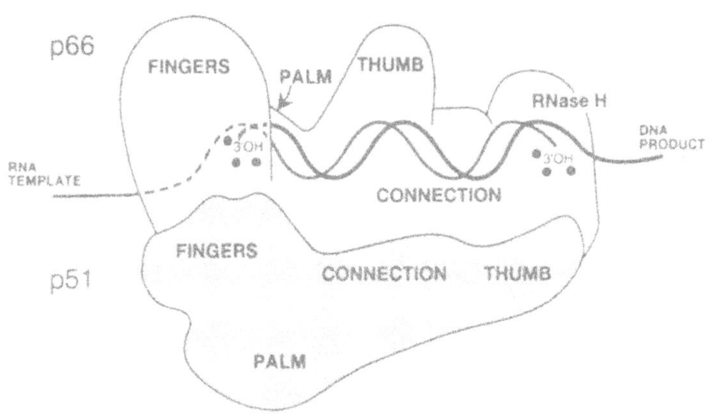

elongation rate of RT is similar to that of other eukaryotic DNA polymerases, but its processivity is low. During reverse transcription, two *jumps* occur between templates, which are essential for retrovirus replication.

The enzyme is divided into four subdomains denoted *finger*, *palm*, *thumb*, and *connection* (Fig. 6B). In p66, the *finger*, *palm*, and *thumb* form a *hand* which serves as a cleft for the template-primer. The RNase H subdomain, a p15 subunit at the C-terminus of the molecule, is attached via the *connection* subdomain. The highly conserved polymerase signature motif, tyrosine–X–aspartic acid–aspartic acid (YXDD), is found at residues 183–186, and is critical for RT activity. The polymerase and RNase H activities are interdependent, with the RNase H playing critical roles in removal of the RNA template strand to prepare for plus-strand DNA synthesis, and for providing specific cleavages involved in formation and removal of RNA primers.

Numerous errors occur during reverse transcription, and these are retained in the resulting DNA sequences because of the lack of an editing function. RT errors include misinsertions and rearrangements. Misinsertions include direct misincorporation resulting from nontemplated addition of a nucleoside, as well as *dislocation-mediated* substitution, where temporary base-pair slipping within homopolymeric runs extrudes a base on the template strand. Rearrangements are the result of the loose association of RT with the template, a necessity for jumping. One consequence of the error-prone nature of reverse transcription is the high rate of mutations and the generation of *quasispecies*. These include mutations that confer drug resistance. For example, mutations at codons 41, 67, 70, 215, and 219 mediate resistance to AZT, whereas mutations that result in resistance to nonnucleoside compounds arise frequently at tyrosines 181 and 188 which flank the YXDD motif.

5.3. Integrase

The integrase is a tetramer of 32-kDa monomeric subunits derived from the C-terminus of the Gag–Pol precursor protein (reviewed by Brown, 1990; Goff, 1990; Grandgenett and Mumm, 1990; Katz and Skalka, 1994). The N-terminal portion of the protein forms a zinc-finger-like structure that binds DNA, whereas residues 61–159 are part of the catalytic site. The structure of the catalytic core has been defined (Dyda *et al.*, 1994). It includes three acidic residues critical for the catalytic activity of integrase. The integration reaction is highly coordinated in that two linear viral DNA termini, separated by 10 kb, are brought in proximity with a host target site. Though most aspects of the integration reaction can be reproduced in a cell-free reaction with purified integrase protein and DNA, concerted insertions of both ends of HIV-1 DNA have not yet been observed under these conditions. Cellular proteins may interact with the integrase (Kalpana *et al.*, 1994). The reverse reaction, *disintegration*, can be mediated by integrase, but probably does not occur to a significant extent *in vivo*. The integration reaction results in a 5-bp duplication of host DNA sequences situated at either end of the viral DNA. Few integrase inhibitors have been described thus far.

6. REGULATORY PROTEINS

The regulatory proteins are potent positive regulators of virus gene expression that have been intensively studied.

6.1. Tat

Tat is a 16-kDa, 86-amino-acid protein (reviewed by Gaynor, 1995). Residues 2–11 are acidic and proline-rich, residues 22–37 compose a cysteine-rich domain capable of binding cadmium and zinc, residues 37–48 are designated the *core* domain, and residues 48–57 consist of basic residues required for nuclear and nucleolar targeting and RNA binding. Residues 57–72 augment Tat activity, and residues 72–86 contain sequences shown to be important for the binding of Tat to fibronectin and enhancing proliferation of Kaposi sarcoma cells. Tat binds to the TAR element at nucleotides 19–44. TAR consists of a stem, bulge, and a loop (Fig. 3). The upper portion of the stem and the bulge in TAR, and the basic residues in Tat are critical for their interaction. The TAR loop binds several cellular factors that are important for Tat-mediated transcriptional *trans*-activation. At least one of these cellular factors is not expressed in rodent cells, accounting for the defect in Tat activity in these cells. This activity is reconstituted in human–hamster somatic cell hybrid clones containing human chromosome 12. Tat appears to enhance the processivity of RNA polymerase II, reducing premature transcriptional termination, via interactions with TATA-binding proteins (Wu-Baer *et al.*, 1995). Though Tat is a potent enhancer of virus replication, it is not absolutely required for virus replication. Tat also appears to promote expression of cellular genes, including IL-1 and IL-6, as well as the promoter of the JC virus, responsible for progressive multifocal leukoencephalopathy which occurs as a complication of AIDS. A retrovirus vector expressing multiple copies of TAR, designated *TAR decoy*, can deplete Tat activity in tissue culture. A benzodiazepine inhibitor of Tat activity in tissue culture had no effect on virus load in one clinical study (Cupelli and Hsu, 1995).

6.2. Rev

The Rev protein is a 13-kDa phosphoprotein, 114 amino acids in length (reviewed by Hope and Pomerantz, 1995). It consists of a domain of amino acids 14–75 required for nucleolar localization, oligomerization, and binding to RRE. Residues 73–84 are leucine-rich and designated the *effector* domain, and a mutation in this region results in a *trans* dominant inhibitory form of Rev. This domain mediates Rev activity by binding to a nuclear pore-associated protein that is critical for RNA export (Bogerd *et al.*, 1995; Fischer *et al.*, 1995; Stutz *et al.*, 1995; Wen *et al.*, 1995). An RNA element from Mason–Pfizer monkey virus can potentially replace RRE activity. The aminoglycoside neomycin B can bind Rev and inhibit late virus gene expression.

7. ACCESSORY PROTEINS

The accessory proteins are dispensable for virus replication in tissue culture, but are believed to have important roles *in vivo*.

7.1. Vif

The *vif* gene is found in all lentiviruses except equine infectious anemia virus (reviewed by Volsky *et al.*, 1995). Vif is a 23-kDa protein, 192 amino acids in length. It is localized in infected cells to the cytoplasm and membranes, and approximately 10 molecules are found in each virion. Vif plays a role in the infected cells in altering the structure of the virus particle to increase its specific infectivity. One possible explanation of its activity is that Vif is required for efficient proteolytic cleavage of the Gag and Gag–Pol precursor proteins, but it is unclear whether this is a direct or indirect effect.

7.2. Vpu

The *vpu* gene is present in HIV-1 and chimpanzee SIV, but not HIV-2 or other SIVs (reviewed by Jabbar, 1995). Vpu is an 18-kDa, 81-amino-acid, homo-oligomeric, type II integral membrane protein. The N-terminal 27 amino acids are hydrophobic and serve as an anchor domain in the lipid bilayer. The remainder of the protein is situated interior to the lipid bilayer, and includes two α helices separated by an acidic domain. The latter domain includes serine residues 52 and 56 which are phosphorylated by casein kinase II.

Vpu has two distinct functions (Table I). The first function is to mediate CD4 downregulation, as a result of an interaction at the endoplasmic reticulum, markedly decreasing the stability of CD4. This activity requires the phosphorylation of Vpu serines 52 and 56, and is thought to be mediated by Vpu binding to the C-terminal cytoplasmic tail of CD4. The consequence of this activity is that there is less CD4 available for interaction with the gp160 precursor envelope protein in the endoplasmic reticulum, thus promoting envelope protein processing and transport to the cell surface.

The second function of Vpu is to enhance virus particle release at the plasma membrane. This activity is mediated at least partially by the anchor domain of Vpu which forms an ion channel (Schubert *et al.*, 1996). This activity is analogous to the structurally similar M2 influenza protein. Vpu enhances the release of HIV-1 particles, as well as a wide range of different retroviral particles.

7.3. Vpr and Vpx

The *vpr* gene is found in HIV-1, HIV-2, and most SIVs, whereas the *vpx* gene is found only in HIV-2 and SIVs derived from macaques, sooty mangabeys, mandrils, and African green monkeys (Table II; reviewed by Levy *et al.*, 1995; Kappes, 1995). The Vpr and Vpx proteins share 27–35% amino acid sequence homology, suggesting a common evolutionary origin. Vpr is a 16-kDa protein 96–105 amino acids in length, whereas Vpx is a 16-kDa protein that is 111–112 amino acids long. Vpr and Vpx both have an amphipathic helix in the

TABLE I. Vpu Activities

	CD4 downregulation	Enhanced virus release
Characteristics	Mediated by LSEKKT residues in C-terminal cytoplasmic tail of CD4	Not specific for HIV-1 Gag
Phosphorylation	Vpu phosphorylation-dependent	Vpu phosphorylation-independent
Responsible domain of Vpu	C-terminal half of Vpu and membrane anchor	Membrane anchor
Cellular location	Endoplasmic reticulum	Post-endoplasmic reticulum (? plasma membrane)
Proposed mechanism	CD4 binding and degradation	Related to ion channel activity

TABLE II. Comparison of Vpr and Vpx

	Vpr	Vpx
Expressed by HIV/SIV	All HIVs/SIVs except SIVagm	HIV-2, SIVmac,sm,agm,mn
Size	14 kDa, 96–105 amino acids	16 kDa, 112–113 amino acids
Cellular location	Nucleus	Cytoplasm
Determinant for virion packaging	Gag p6	Gag p6
Effect on cell proliferation	G2 arrest	?
Effect on virus replication	Enhanced replication in macrophages	Enhanced replication in primary T cells

N-terminal half of the molecule. Residues 60–80 of HIV-1 Vpr are rich in leucine, and have been suggested to be important for interaction with cellular proteins (Zhao *et al.*, 1994a). The C-terminus of HIV-1 Vpr is highly basic. Residues 73–89 of HIV-2 Vpx are cysteine-rich, and residues 101–112 are proline-rich. Vpr is primarily a nuclear protein (Lu *et al.*, 1993), mediating transport of the preintegration complex from the cytoplasm to the nucleus (Heinzinger *et al.*, 1994). In contrast, Vpx is primarily a cytoplasmic protein, whose function is not well defined. Both Vpr and Vpx are packaged into virions in quantities similar to that of Gag proteins. In both cases, the major determinant for packaging is within the C-terminal p6 domain of $Pr55^{gag}$ (Lu *et al.*, 1995; X. Wu *et al.*, 1995a). The amphipathic helix of Vpr is important for virion incorporation, and this domain has been used to target heterologous proteins into virions (Mahalingam *et al.*, 1995; X. Wu *et al.*, 1995). HIV-1 Vpr has been shown to inhibit cell proliferation, resulting in an arrest in the G2 phase of the cycle and the failure to establish chronic infections in tissue culture (Rogel *et al.*, 1995; Macreadie *et al.*, 1995). In contrast, SIV Vpr and Vpx have limited, if any, ability to arrest cell proliferation. Vpr has also been shown to interact with at least two different cellular proteins, one of which may be an intermediate in the glucocorticoid-response pathway (Zhao *et al.*, 1994a; Refaeli *et al.*, 1995). The interrelationship of these activities and the mechanisms involved in regulation of virus replication *in vivo* remain to be deciphered.

7.4. Nef

The *nef* gene is found in all species of HIV and SIV (Table III; reviewed by Ratner and Niederman, 1995). The Nef protein is 27–34 kDa and 206–265 amino acids in length. It is modified by myristic acid attachment to the N-terminal glycine, after removal of the initiator methionine. A proline-rich domain is found at residues 69–81 that mediates interactions with SH2 domains of tyrosine kinases. Residues 95–99 have homology to those present in

TABLE III. Characteristics of Nef

Size	206–265 amino acids long
Cellular localization	Membranes, cytosol, cytoskeleton, nucleus
Modifications	Myristylation, phosphorylation
Activities	CD4 downregulation
	Alteration of T-cell activation
	Effects on virus infection and replication

nucleotide-binding proteins. Nef has been localized within the cytoplasm, plasma membrane, and cytoskeleton, as well as a portion of Nef protein found in the nucleus.

Several different biological activities have been described for Nef, some of which remain controversial. The first activity of Nef is its ability to downregulate CD4 from the cell surface (Salghetti *et al.*, 1995). Residues in the C-terminal tail of CD4 are required for this activity, and include residues that interact with the tyrosine kinase, Lck. It is unclear whether this effect of Nef is related to direct or indirect interactions with CD4 or Lck (Ratner and Niederman, 1995; Greenway *et al.*, 1995). However, Nef does appear to bind directly to several different serine protein kinases, and studies in SIV suggest that binding to at least one such kinase may be important for virus replication *in vivo*.

The second activity of Nef is its ability to alter T-cell activation (Greenway *et al.*, 1995; Ratner and Niederman, 1995). Nef appears to depress NF κB and AP-1 activation, resulting in depressed transcription of the IL-2 gene. These functions may be mediated primarily by a cytoplasmic form of Nef, whereas a plasma membrane-associated form of Nef may enhance T-cell activation.

The third activity of Nef is its ability to perturb virus infection and/or replication. The most potent form of this activity is a positive effect of Nef on virus infection of quiescent T cells (Miller *et al.*, 1995). This effect appears to be mediated by a postentry effect on viral DNA synthesis, or subsequent early steps in virus replication (Aiken and Trono, 1995).

Nef appears to be important in mediating the pathogenicity of SIV in rhesus macaque models. SIV with a deletion in *nef* is incapable of generating a high virus load in adult macaques or causing immunodepletion, though pathogenic effects may still occur in newborn macaques (Baba *et al.*, 1995; Ratner and Niederman, 1995). A variant *nef* converts SIV from a virus inducing subacute or chronic immunodeficiency to a virus that induces an acutely lethal infection (Du *et al.*, 1995).

8. SUMMARY

The complexities of the HIV-1 genome and its replication strategy provide a highly adaptive interaction with the host. The error-prone nature of the reverse transcriptase and the high frequency of recombination during replication generate mutations at a rapid rate (Coffin, 1995). This provides a wide range of quasispecies of the virus allowing selection of the fittest progeny virus to evade immune and therapeutic restrictions. The complexity of the virus also provides many possibilities for antiviral development, and synergistic applications of treatments, disrupting distinct targets.

ACKNOWLEDGMENTS. I thank Ms. Holemon, Ms. Lu, Ms. Deora, and Mr. Hung for critical comments on the manuscript. Support was provided by grants from the Public Health Service and the American Foundation for AIDS Research.

REFERENCES

Aiken, C., and Trono, D., 1995, Nef stimulates human immunodeficiency virus type 1 proviral DNA synthesis, *J. Virol.* **69:**5048–5056.

Ansari-Lari, M. A., Donehower, L. A., and Gibbs, R. A., 1995, Analysis of human immunodeficiency virus type 1 integrase mutants, *Virology* **211:**332–335.

Amendt, B. A., Si, Z.-H., and Stoltzfus, M., 1995, Presence of exon splicing silencers within human immunodeficiency virus type 1 tat exon 2 and tat-rev exon 3: Evidence for inhibition mediated by cellular factors, *Mol. Cell. Biol.* **15:**4606–4615.

Baba, T. W., Jeong, Y. S., Penninck, D., Bronson, R., Greene, M. F., and Ruprecht, R. M., 1995, Pathogenicity of live, attenuated SIV after mucosal infection of neonatal macaques, *Science* **267:**1820–1824.

Bogerd, H. P., Fridell, R. A., Madore, S., and Cullen, B. R., 1995, Identification of a novel cellular cofactor for the Rev/Rex class of retroviral regulatory proteins, *Cell* **82:**485–494.

Broder, C. C., Dimitrov, D. S., Blumenthal, R., and Berger, E. A., 1993, The block to HIV-1 envelope glycoprotein-mediated membrane fusion in animal cells expressing human CD4 can be overcome by a human cell component(s), *Virology* **193:**483–491.

Brown, P. O., 1990, Integration of retroviral DNA, *Curr. Top. Microbiol. Immunol.* **157:**19–48.

Bryant, M. L., and Ratner, L., 1990, Myristoylation-dependent replication and assembly of HIV-1, *Proc. Natl. Acad. Sci. USA* **87:**523–527.

Bryant, M. L., Heuckeroth, R. O., Kimata, J. T., Ratner, L., and Gordon, J. I., 1989, Replication of human immunodeficiency virus 1 and Moloney murine leukemia virus is inhibited by different heteroatom-containing analogs of myristic acid, *Proc. Natl. Acad. Sci. USA* **86:**8655–8659.

Carriere, C., Gay, B., Chazal, N., Morin, N., and Boulanger, P., 1995, Sequence requirements for encapsidation of deletion mutants and chimeras of human immunodeficiency virus type 1 Gag precursor into retrovirus-like particles, *J. Virol.* **69:**2366–2377.

Clements, G. J., Price-Jones, M. J., Stephens, P. E., Sutton, C., Schulz, T. F., Clapham, P. R., McKeating, J. A., McClure, M. O., Thomson, S., Marsh, M., Kay, J., Weiss, R. A., and Moore, J. P., 1991, The V3 loops of the HIV-1 and HIV-2 surface glycoproteins contain proteolytic cleavage sites: A possible function in viral fusion? *AIDS Res. Hum. Retrovir.* **7:**3–16.

Coffin, J. M., 1995, HIV population dynamics *in vivo*: Implications for genetic variation, pathogenesis, and therapy, *Science* **267:**483–489.

Craven, R. C., Leure-duPree, A. E., Weldon, R. A., and Wills, J. W., 1995, Genetic analysis of the major homology region of Rous sarcoma virus gag protein, *J. Virol.* **69:**4213–4227.

Cupelli, L. A., and Hsu, M.-C., 1995, The human immunodeficiency virus type 1 tat antagonist, Ro 5-3335, predominantly inhibits transcription initiation from the viral promoter, *J. Virol.* **69:**2640–2643.

Dedera, D., and Ratner, L., 1991, Demonstration of two distinct cytopathic effects with syncytia-defective HIV-1 mutants, *J. Virol.* **65:**6129–6136.

Dedera, D., Gu, R., and Ratner, L., 1992, Conserved cysteine residues in the HIV-1 transmembrane envelope protein are essential to precursor envelope cleavage, *J. Virol.* **66:**1207–1209.

Du, Z., Lang, S. M., Sasseville, V. G., Lackner, A. A., Ilyinskii, P. O., Daniel, M. D., Jung, J. U., and Desrosiers, R. C., 1995, Identification of a Nef allele that causes lymphocyte activation and acute disease in macaque monkeys, *Cell* **82:**665–674.

Dukes, C. S., Yu, Y., Rivadeneira, E. D., Sauls, D. L., Liao, H.-X., Haynes, B. F., and Weinberg, J. B., 1995, Cellular CD44S as a determinant of human immunodeficiency virus type 1 infection and cellular tropism, *J. Virol.* **69:**4000–4005.

Dyda, F., Hickman, A. B., Jenkins, T. M., Engelman, A., Craigie, R., and Davies, D. R., 1994, Crystal structure of the catalytic domain of HIV-1 integrase: Similarity to other polynucleotidyl transferases, *Science* **266:**1981–1986.

Feng, Y., Broder, C. C., Kennedy, P. E., and Berger, E. A., 1996, HIV-1 entry cofactor: Functional cDNA cloning of a seven transmembrane, G protein-coupled receptor, *Science* **272:**872–877.

Fischer, U., Huber, J., Boelens, W. C., Mattaj, I. W., and Luhrmann, R., 1995, The HIV-1 Rev activation domain is a nuclear export signal that accesses an export pathway used by specific cellular RNAs, *Cell* **82:**475–484.

Francke, E. K., Yuah, H. E. H., and Luban, J., 1994, Specific incorporation of cyclophilin A into HIV-1 virions, *Nature* **372:**359–362.

Gabuzda, D., Olshevsky, U., Bertaini, P., Haseltine, W. A., and Sodroski, J., 1991, Identification of membrane anchorage domains of the HIV-1 gp160 envelope glycoprotein precursor, *J. Acq. Immune Defic. Syndr.* **4:** 34–40.

Gallay, P., Swingler, S., Aiken, C., and Trono, D., 1995, HIV-1 infection of nondividing cells: C-terminal tyrosine phosphorylation of the viral matrix protein is a key regulator, *Cell* **80:**379–388.

Gaynor, R. B., 1995, Regulation of human immunodeficiency virus type 1 gene expression by the transactivator protein Tat, in: *Transacting Functions of Human Retroviruses, Current Topics in Microbiology and Immunology*, Volume 193 (I. S. Y. Chen, H. Koprowski, A. Srinivasan, and P. K. Vogt, eds.), Springer-Verlag, Berlin, pp. 51–78.

Goff, S. P., 1990, Integration of retroviral DNA into the genome of the infected cell, *Cancer Cells* **2:**172–178.

Gorelick, R. J., Chabot, D. J., Rein, A., Henderson, L. E., and Arthur, L. O., 1993, The two zinc fingers in the human immunodeficiency virus type 1 nucleocapsid protein are not functionally equivalent, *J. Virol.* **67:**4027–4036.

Gottlinger, H. G., Dorfman, T., Sodroski, J. G., and Haseltine, W. A., 1991, Effect of mutations affecting the p6 gag protein on human immunodeficiency virus particle release, *Proc. Natl. Acad. Sci. USA* **88:**3195–3199.

Grandgenett, D. P., and Mumm, S. R., 1990, Unraveling retrovirus integration, *Cell* **60:**3–4.

Greenway, A., Azad, A., and McPhee, D., 1995, Human immunodeficiency virus type 1 Nef protein inhibits activation pathways in peripheral blood mononuclear cells and T-cell lines, *J. Virol.* **69:**1842–1850.

Heinzinger, N. K., Bukrinsky, M. I., Haggerty, S. A., Ragland, A. M., Kewalramani, V., Lee, M.-A., Gendelman, H. E., Ratner, L., Strevenson, M., and Emerman, M., 1994, The Vpr protein of human immunodeficiency virus type 1 influences nuclear localization of viral nucleic acids in nondividing host cells, *Proc. Natl. Acad. Sci. USA* **91:**7311–7315.

Helseth, E., Olshevsky, U., Furman, C., and Sodroski, J., 1991, Human immunodeficiency virus type 1 gp120 envelope glycoprotein regions important for association with the gp41 transmembrane glycoprotein, *J. Virol.* **65:**2119–2123.

Hope, T., and Pomerantz, R. J., 1995, The human immunodeficiency virus type 1 Rev protein: A pivotal protein in the viral life cycle, in: *Transacting Functions of Human Retroviruses, Current Topics in Microbiology and Immunology*, Volume 193 (I. S. Y. Chen, H. Koprowski, A. Srinivasan, and P. K. Vogt, eds.), Springer-Verlag, Berlin, pp. 91–106.

Jabbar, M. A., 1995, The human immunodeficiency virus type 1 Vpu protein: Roles in virus release and CD4 downregulation, in: *Transacting Functions of Human Retroviruses, Current Topics in Microbiology and Immunology*, Volume 193 (I. S. Y. Chen, H. Koprowski, A. Srinivasan, and P. K. Vogt, eds.), Springer-Verlag, Berlin, pp. 107–120.

Jacks, T., Power, M. D., Masiarz, F. R., Luciw, P. A., Barr, P. J., and Varmus, H. E., 1988, Characterization of ribosomal frameshifting in HIV-1 gag-pol expression, *Nature* **331:**280–283.

Jones, K. A., and Peterlin, B. M., 1994, Control of RNA initiation and elongation at the HIV-1 promoter, *Annu. Rev. Biochem.* **63:**717–743.

Kalpana, G. V., Marmon, S., Wang, W., Crabtree, G. R., and Goff, S. P., 1994, Binding and stimulation of HIV integrase to transcription factor SNF5, *Science* **266:**2002–2006.

Kappes, J. C., 1995, Viral protein X, in: *Transacting Functions of Human Retroviruses, Current Topics in Microbiology and Immunology*, Volume 193 (I. S. Y. Chen, H. Koprowski, A. Srinivasan, and P. K. Vogt, eds.), Springer-Verlag, Berlin, pp. 121–132.

Katz, R. A., and Skalka, A. M., 1994, The retroviral enzymes, *Annu. Rev. Biochem.* **63:**133–173.

Koito, A., Stamatatos, L., and Cheng-Mayer, C., 1995, Small amino acid sequence changes within the V2 domain can affect the function of a T-cell line-tropic human immunodeficiency virus type 1 envelope gp120, *Virology* **206:**878–884.

Leonard, C. K., Spellman, M. W., Riddle, L., Harris, R. J., Thomas, J. N., and Gregory, T. J., 1990, Assignment of intrachain disulfide bonds and characterization of potential glycosylation sites of the type 1 recombinant human immunodeficiency virus envelope glycoprotein (gp120) expressed in Chinese hamster ovary cells, *J. Biol. Chem.* **265:**10373–10382.

Levy, D. N., Refaeli, Y., and Weiner, D. B., 1995, The *vpr* regulatory gene of human immunodeficiency virus, in: *Transacting Functions of Human Retroviruses, Current Topics in Microbiology and Immunology*, Volume 193 (I. S. Y. Chen, H. Koprowski, A. Srinivasan, and P. K. Vogt, eds.), Springer-Verlag, Berlin, pp. 209–238.

Lu, Y.-L., Spearman, P., and Ratner, L., 1993, HIV-1 viral protein R localization in infected cells and virion, *J. Virol.* **67:**6542–6550.

Lu, Y.-L., Bennett, R., Wills, J., Gorelick, R., and Ratner, L., 1995, A leucine-triplet repeat sequence in Gag p6 required for HIV-1 Vpr incorporation, *J. Virol.* **69:**6873–6879.

Luban, J., and Goff, S. P., 1994, Mutational analysis of cis-acting packaging signals in human immunodeficiency virus type 1 RNA, *J. Virol.* **68:**3784–3793.

Macreadie, I. G., Castelli, L. A., Hewish, D. R., Kirkpatrick, A., Ward, A. C., and Azad, A. A., 1995, A domain of human immunodeficiency virus type 1 Vpr containing repeated H(S/F)RIG amino acid motifs causes cell growth arrest and structural defects, *Proc. Natl. Acad. Sci. USA* **92:**2770–2774.

Maddon, P. J., Dalgleish, A. G., McDougal, J. S., Clapham, P. R., Weiss, R. A., and Axel, R., 1986, The T4 gene encodes the AIDS virus receptor and is expressed in the immune system and the brain, *Cell* **47:**333–348.

Mahalingam, S., Khan, S. A., Murali, R., Jabbar, M. A., Monken, C. E., Collman, R. G., and Srinivasan, A., 1995, Mutagenesis of the putative alpha-helical domain of the Vpr protein of human immunodeficiency virus type 1: Effect on stability and virion incorporation, *Proc. Natl. Acad. Sci. USA* **92:**3794–3798.

Mammano, F., Kondo, E., Sodroski, J., Bukovsky, A., and Gottlinger, H. G., 1995, Rescue of human immunodeficiency virus type 1 matrix protein mutants by envelope glycoproteins with short cytoplasmic domains, *J. Virol.* **69:**3824–3830.

Massiah, M. A., Starich, M. R., Paschall, C., Summers, M. F., Christensen, A. M., and Sundquist, W. I., 1994, Three-dimensional structure of the human immunodeficiency virus type 1 matrix protein, *J. Mol. Biol.* **244:** 198–223.

Miller, M. D., Warmerdam, M. T., Page, K. A., Feinberg, M. B., and Greene, W. C., 1995, Expression of the human immunodeficiency virus type 1 (HIV-1) *nef* gene during HIV-1 production increases progeny particle infectivity independently of gp160 or viral entry, *J. Virol.* **69:**579–584.

Olshevsky, U., Helseth, E., Furman, C., Li, J., Haseltine, W., and Sodroski, J., 1990, Identification of individual human immunodeficiency virus type 1 gp120 amino acids important for CD4 receptor binding, *J. Virol.* **64:** 5701–5707.

Owens, R. J., Dubay, J. W., Hunter, E., and Compans, R. W., 1991, Human immunodeficiency virus envelope protein determines the site of virus release in polarized epithelial cells, *Proc. Natl. Acad. Sci. USA* **88:**3987–3991.

Platt, E. J., and Haffar, O. K., 1994, Characterization of human immunodeficiency virus type 1 $Pr55^{gag}$ membrane association in a cell-free system, *Proc. Natl. Acad. Sci. USA* **91:**4594–4598.

Ratner, L., 1992, Glucosidase inhibitors for treatment of HIV-1 infection, *AIDS Res. Hum. Retrovir.* **8:**165–173.

Ratner, L., and Niederman, T. M. J., 1995, Nef, in: *Transacting Functions of Human Retroviruses, Current Topics in Microbiology and Immunology*, Volume 193 (I. S. Y. Chen, H. Koprowski, A. Srinivasan, and P. K. Vogt, eds.), Springer-Verlag, Berlin, pp. 169–208.

Refaeli, Y., Levy, D. N., and Weiner, D. B., 1995, The glucocorticoid receptor type II complex is a target of the HIV-1 vpr gene product, *Proc. Natl. Acad. Sci. USA* **92:**3621–3625.

Rogel, M. E., Wu, L. I., and Emerman, M., 1995, The human immunodeficiency virus type 1 *vpr* gene prevents cell proliferation during chronic infection, *J. Virol.* **69:**882–888.

Salghetti, S., Mariani, R., and Skowronski, J., 1995, Human immunodeficiency virus type 1 Nef and $p56^{lck}$ protein-tyrosine kinase interact with a common element in CD4 cytoplasmic tail, *Proc. Natl. Acad. Sci. USA* **92:** 349–353.

Schubert, U., Bour, S., Ferrer-Montiel, A. V., Montal, M., Maldarelli, F., and Strebel, K., 1996, The two biological activities of human immunodeficiency virus type 1 Vpu protein involve two separable structural domains, *J. Virol.* **70:**809–819.

Schwartz, S. B., Felber, B. K., Benko, D. M., Fenyo, E.-M., and Pavlakis, G. N., 1990, Cloning and functional analysis of multiply spliced mRNA species of human immunodeficiency virus type 1, *J. Virol.* **64:**2519–2529.

Shioda, T., Levy, J. A., and Cheng-Mayer, C., 1991, Macrophage and T cell-line tropisms of HIV-1 are determined by specific regions of the envelop gp120 gene, *Nature* **349:**167–169.

Spearman, P., Wang, J.-J., Vander Heyden, N., and Ratner, L., 1994, Identification of human immunodeficiency virus type 1 Gag protein domains essential to membrane binding and particle assembly, *J. Virol.* **68:**3232–3242.

Staffa, A., and Cochrane, A., 1995, Identification of positive and negative splicing regulatory elements with the terminal tat-rev exon of human immunodeficiency virus type 1, *Mol. Cell. Biol.* **15:**4597–4605.

Starcich, B. R., Hahn, B. H., Shaw, G. M., McNeely, R. D., Morrow, S., Wolf, H., Parks, E. S., Parks, W. P., Josephs, S. F., and Gallo, R. C., 1986, Identification and characterization of conserved and variable regions in the envelope gene of HTLV-III/LAV, the retrovirus of AIDS, *Cell* **45:**637–648.

Stein, B., Kramer, M., Rahmsdorf, H. J., Ponta, H., and Herrlich, P., 1989, UV induced transcription from the human immunodeficiency virus type 1 (HIV-1) long terminal repeat and UV induced secretion of an extracellular factor that induces HIV-1 transcription in nonirradiated cells, *J. Virol.* **63:**4540–4544.

Stutz, F., Neville, M., and Rosbash, M., 1995, Identification of a novel nuclear pore-associated protein as a functional target of the HIV-1 Rev protein in yeast, *Cell* **82:**495–506.

Tencza, S. B., Miller, M. A., Islam, K., Mietzner, T. A., and Montelaro, R. C., 1995, Effect of amino acid substitutions on calmodulin binding and cytolytic properties of the LLP-1 peptide segment of human immunodeficiency virus type 1 transmembrane protein, *J. Virol.* **69:**5199–5202.

Thali, M., Bukovsky, A., Kondo, E., Rosenwirth, B., Walsh, C. T., Sodroski, J., and Gottlinger, H. G., 1994, Functional association of cyclophilin A with HIV-1 virions, *Nature* **372:**363–365.

Trono, D., 1992, Partial reverse transcripts in virions from human immunodeficiency and murine leukemia viruses, *J. Virol.* **66:**4893–4900.

Veronese, F. D., Copeland, T. D., Oroszlan, S., Gallo, R. C., and Sarngadharan, M. G., 1988, Biochemical and immunological analysis of human immunodeficiency virus gag gene products p17 and p24, *J. Virol.* **62:** 795–801.

Volsky, D. J., Potash, M. J., Simm, M., Sova, P., Ma, X.-Y., Chao, W., and Shahabuddin, M., 1995, The human immunodeficiency virus type 1 *vif* gene: The road from an accessory to an essential role in human immunodeficiency virus type 1 replication, in: *Transacting Functions of Human Retroviruses, Current Topics in Microbiology and Immunology*, Volume 193 (I. S. Y. Chen, H. Koprowski, A. Srinivasan, and P. K. Vogt, eds.), Springer-Verlag, Berlin, pp. 157–168.

Walker, S., Hagemeier, C., Sissons, J. G., and Sinclair, J. H., 1992, A 10-base pair element of the human immunodeficiency virus type 1 long terminal repeat (LTR) is an absolute requirement for transactivation by the human cytomegalovirus 72-kilodalton IE1 protein but can be compensated for by other LTR regions in transactivation by the 80-kilodalton IE2 protein, *J. Virol.* **66:**1543–1550.

Wang, Y.-H., Davies, A. H., and Jones, I. M., 1995, Expression and purification of glutathione S-transferase-tagged HIV-1 gp120: No evidence of an interaction with CD26, *Virology* **208:**142–146.

Weiss, R. A., Teich, N., Varmus, H. E., and Coffin, J. M., eds., 1982, *RNA Tumor Viruses*, Volume 1, Cold Spring Harbor Laboratory Press, Cold Spring Harbor, NY.

Wen, W., Meinkoth, J. L., Tsien, R. Y., and Taylor, S. S., 1995, Identification of a signal for rapid export of proteins from the nucleus, *Cell* **82:**463–474.

Wills, J., and Craven, R., 1991, Form, function, and use of retroviral gag proteins, *AIDS* **5:**639–654.

Wlodawer, A., and Erickson, J. W., 1993, Structure-based inhibitors of HIV-1 protease, *Annu. Rev. Biochem.* **62:**543–585.

Wu, X., Conway, J. A., Kim, J., and Kappes, J. C., 1994, Localization of the vpx packaging signal with type gag precursor protein, *J. Virol.* **68:**6161–6169.

Wu, X., Liu, H., Ziao, H., Kim, J., Seshaiah, P., Natsoulis, G., Boeke, J. D., Hahn, B. H., and Kappes, J. C., 1995a, Targeting fusion proteins to human immunodeficiency virus particles via fusion with Vpr and Vpx, *J. Virol.* **69:**3389–3398.

Wu, Z., Kayman, S. C., Honnen, W., Revesz, K., Chen, H., Vijh-Warrier, S., Tilley, S. A., McKeating, J., Shotton, C., and Pinter, A., 1995b, Characterization of neutralization epitopes in the V2 region of human immunodeficiency virus type 1 gp 120: Role of glycosylation in the correct folding of the V1/V2 domain, *J. Virol.* **69:**2271–2278.

Wu-Baer, F., Sigman, D., and Gaynor, R. B., 1995, Specific binding of RNA polymerase II to the human immunodeficiency virus trans-activating region RNA is regulated by cellular cofactors and Tat, *Proc. Natl. Acad. Sci. USA* **92:**7253–7257.

Yahi, N., Fantini, J., Baghdiguian, S., Mabrouk, K., Tamalet, C., Rochat, H., van Rietschoten, J., and Sabatier, J.-M., 1995, SPC3, a synthetic peptide derived from the V3 domain of human immunodeficiency virus type 1 (HIV-1) gp120, inhibits HIV-1 entry into CD4+ and CD4− cells by two distinct mechanisms, *Proc. Natl. Acad. Sci. USA* **92:**4867–4871.

Yu, G., Shen, F. S., Sturch, S., Aquino, A., Glazer, R. I., and Felsted, R. L., 1995, Regulation of HIV-1 gag protein subcellular targeting by protein kinase c, *J. Biol. Chem.* **270:**4792–4796.

Zack, J. A., Cann, A. J., Lugo, J. P., and Chen, I. S. Y., 1988, HIV-1 production from infected peripheral blood T cells after HTLV-I induced mitogenic stimulation, *Science* **240:**1026–1029.

Zack, J. A., Arrigo, S. J., Weitsman, S. R., Go, A. S., Haislip, A., and Chen, I. S. Y., 1990, HIV-1 entry into quiescent primary lymphocytes: Molecular analysis reveals a labile, latent viral structure, *Cell* **61:**213–222.

Zhao, L.-J., Mukherjee, S., and Narayan, O., 1994a, Biochemical mechanism of HIV-1 Vpr function. Specific interaction with a cellular protein, *J. Biol. Chem.* **269:**15577–15582.

Zhao, L.-J., Wang, L., Mukherjee, S., and Narayan, O., 1994b, Biochemical mechanism of HIV-1 Vpr function. Oligomerization mediated by the N-terminal domain, *J. Biol. Chem.* **269:**32131–32137.

Zhou, W., Parent, L. J., Wills, J. W., and Resh, M. D., 1994. Identification of a membrane-binding domain within the amino-terminal region of human immunodeficiency virus type 1 Gag protein which interacts with acidic phospholipids, *J. Virol.* **68:**2556–2569.

CHAPTER 2

T-CELL EPITOPES OF HIV-1 ENVELOPE GLYCOPROTEIN

CHRISTOPHER B. BUCK and ROBERT F. SILICIANO

1. INTRODUCTION

The presentation of viral proteins to T cells is a critical early step in the immune response to HIV-1. From the initial surge of cytotoxic T-lymphocyte (CTL) activity observed during the resolution of the acute viremia of early HIV-1 infection (Yasutomi *et al.*, 1993b; Koup *et al.*, 1994), to the T-helper-cell (T_h)-driven production of HIV-1-specific antibodies, immune responses to HIV-1 are critically dependent on the activities of T cells. It is thus important to understand how HIV-1 proteins are processed for T-cell recognition, and which regions (or epitopes) of these proteins are recognized in T-cell responses to the virus. The delineation of the HIV-1 epitopes presented to T cells has opened new avenues for exploration of host defense against virus infection and for the design of potential vaccines and therapeutic strategies.

Analysis of T-cell responses to the envelope (env) protein of HIV-1 is of particular interest because the env protein is the principal candidate antigen for an HIV-1 vaccine. The env protein is the major virus-encoded target of neutralizing antibodies and has been used in a number of vaccine strategies, including those involving recombinant protein (Dolin *et al.*, 1991; Redfield *et al.*, 1991), live viral vectors (Cooney *et al.*, 1991, 1993; Hammond *et al.*, 1992; Egan *et al.*, 1995), and naked DNA (animal models only) (Wang, 1995). Analysis of T-cell recognition of HIV-1 env epitopes has been an important readout in many of these trials. Delineation of the epitopes recognized by vaccine-induced T cells has provided insight into the likelihood that such T cells would be capable of recognizing diverse HIV-1 strains. In addition, analysis of env epitopes has yielded new information regarding the processing of HIV-1 proteins. Many studies of T-cell epitopes in the env protein and other HIV-1 proteins have been motivated by the notion that synthetic peptides containing critical

CHRISTOPHER B. BUCK and ROBERT F. SILICIANO • Department of Medicine, Johns Hopkins University School of Medicine, Baltimore, Maryland 21205.
Immunology of HIV Infection, edited by Sudhir Gupta. Plenum Press, New York, 1996.

immunogenic epitopes may represent a cost-effective and safe alternative to recombinant protein and live vector-based vaccine strategies.

The env protein is also a major target of CTL responses in infected individuals. The first evidence that CTL were involved in the immune response to HIV-1 during natural infection came from studies of env-specific CTL (Plata *et al.*, 1987; Walker *et al.*, 1987; Koenig *et al.*, 1988). Remarkably, for some infected individuals CTL responses to the env protein could be detected in assays on freshly isolated PBMC from some infected individuals without any *in vitro* stimulation (Walker *et al.*, 1987). Subsequent studies have shown that CTL specific for env, gag, and other HIV-1 gene products are an important element of the host response to HIV-1 (for reviews see Kalams and Walker, 1994; Bollinger *et al.*, 1996). Analysis of epitopes recognized by env-specific CTL has been useful in evaluating a number of issues, including the potential emergence of escape mutants that are no longer recognized by T cells in the host. $CD4^+$ T-cell responses to the env protein have also been used in the evaluation of immune status of infected individuals, particularly with respect to cytokine production (Clerici *et al.*, 1989). The importance of understanding the immune response to HIV-1 is the motivation for the present chapter, which summarizes current information regarding T-cell epitopes in the HIV-1 env protein.

2. THE HIV-1 ENVELOPE PROTEIN

In an HIV-1-infected cell, the env protein is translated on the rough endoplasmic reticulum (ER) as an 861-amino-acid precursor, gp160. This precursor, a type 1 transmembrane glycoprotein, is cleaved in the Golgi to form gp41, an integral membrane protein, and gp120, which remains noncovalently associated with gp41 (Allan *et al.*, 1985; Robey *et al.*, 1985; Willey *et al.*, 1988; Stein and Engleman, 1990; Earl *et al.*, 1991). Both subunits are heavily glycosylated, with as much as half of the apparent molecular mass of gp120 contributed by glycosylation of the polypeptide core (Lasky *et al.*, 1987). Following translocation into the ER, gp160 oligomerizes to form dimers and higher-order structures, probably tetramers. Oligomerization occurs in the ER and precedes cleavage of gp160 into gp120 and gp41, which occurs during transit through the Golgi. Oligomerization is a typical feature of the fusion and receptor binding proteins of many enveloped viruses (Earl *et al.*, 1990). These gp120/gp41 tetramer complexes form the spikes observed on newly released HIV-1 virions (Gelderblom *et al.*, 1987). Since the association between gp120 and gp41 is noncovalent, free gp120 can be released from the surface of virions and infected cells (Gelderblom *et al.*, 1985). The release of gp120 may be facilitated by binding to CD4, the viral receptor (Moore *et al.*, 1990).

As a result of the low fidelity of HIV-1 reverse transcriptase, mutations are introduced into the HIV-1 genome frequently during replication. Additional selective pressures operate on this substrate of mutation to generate a high level of sequence variability. Of the open reading frames in the HIV-1 genome, the sequence encoding the gp120 subunit of the env protein shows the highest level of nonsilent substitutions. Comparison of sequenced isolates has led to the identification of five hypervariable domains in gp120. Sequence heterogeneity in these hypervariable domains results in up to 25% overall variability between gp120 molecules of different viral isolates (Willey *et al.*, 1986; Modrow *et al.*, 1987). Since a single amino acid change within a T-cell epitope can result in loss of immune recognition, it is possible that this high variability may permit the virus to escape immune destruction (see below).

3. MECHANISMS OF ANTIGEN PRESENTATION TO T CELLS

Analysis of T-cell epitopes in HIV-1 proteins requires an understanding of the complex mechanisms by which viral antigens are processed and presented to T cells. All T cells express a somatically rearranged heterodimeric T-cell receptor (TCR), which recognizes specific peptide antigens presented on MHC class I or class II surface proteins. Mature T cells also express one of the MHC coreceptors, CD8 or CD4, which have affinity for MHC I or MHC II, respectively. T cells can also be subdivided into functional subsets including CTL, which have the ability to kill cells presenting the appropriate MHC/antigen complex, and "helper" T cells (T_h), which secrete cytokines that help mediate immune responses. T_h activities include activation of B-cell maturation and antibody production, and the clonal expansion of CTL. Generally speaking, CTL are $CD8^+$, whereas T_h are $CD4^+$, although exceptions are well documented. Interestingly, most $CD8^+$ T cells, including HIV-1-specific CTL, release cytokines following antigen-driven activation (Bollinger *et al.*, 1993; Jassoy *et al.*, 1993). In addition, some $CD4^+$ T cells are cytolytic. For example, a significant fraction of the vaccine-induced $CD4^+$ T cells specific for the HIV-1 env protein are cytolytic (Orentas *et al.*, 1990; Hammond, 1992; Stanhope *et al.*, 1993a,b; Miskovsky *et al.*, 1994).

The functional dichotomy in T-cell subsets is part of a larger dichotomy in antigen recognition that reflects the need to deal with different types of antigens. The class I and class II MHC molecules present different types of peptide antigens (Fig. 1). MHC class I

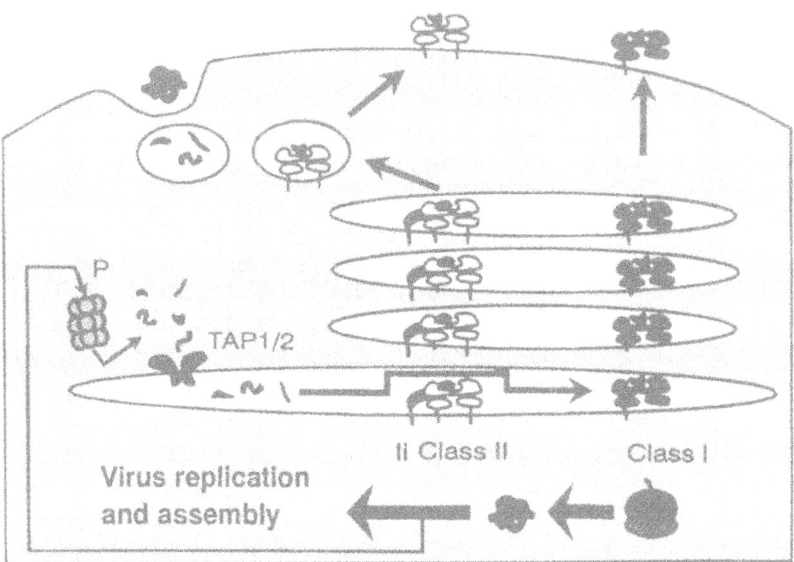

FIGURE 1. Antigen processing pathways. Viral proteins synthesized in infected cells are processed for association with class I MHC molecules. The proteins are degraded in the cytosol, probably by the proteasome (P), and the resulting peptides are translocated into the ER by the TAP-1/2 transporter. In the ER, the peptides associate with class I molecules. Both classes of MHC molecules are synthesized in the ER. Class II molecules do not bind peptides in the ER because they associate with another protein, the invariant chain (Ii), which prevents peptide binding. During export to the cell surface, class II molecules are diverted into a specialized compartment that intersects the endocytic pathway. In this compartment, the Ii chain is proteolyzed and proteins internalized from the extracellular environment are degraded into peptides that can bind the class II molecules. Special mechanisms for processing of the HIV-1 env protein are discussed in the text.

molecules typically present peptides derived from the degradation of cytoplasmic or nuclear proteins, including viral proteins present within the infected cell. Processing of class I epitopes is thought to begin when cytoplasmic proteins are degraded into short peptides in the cytoplasm by the 26 S proteasome complex, possibly with the participation of the proteasome subunits LMP-2 and -7. LMP-2 and -7 are encoded within the MHC, and can be induced to replace constitutive proteasome subunits by the cytokine interferon-γ (Akiyama *et al.*, 1994; Belich *et al.*, 1994; Fruh *et al.*, 1994).

Processed peptides are next transported from the cytoplasm into the ER by a unique transporter complex composed of the TAP (transporter associated with antigen processing) proteins, TAP-1 and TAP-2, which are encoded within the MHC, and which have homology to the ATP-binding cassette (ABC) family of transporters (Morrison *et al.*, 1986; Townsend *et al.*, 1986; Moore *et al.*, 1988; Yewdell *et al.*, 1988; Monaco *et al.*, 1990; Spies *et al.*, 1990; Trowsdale *et al.*, 1990; Powis *et al.*, 1991; Spies and DeMars, 1991; Attaya *et al.*, 1992; Kelly *et al.*, 1992; Kleijmeer *et al.*, 1992; Van *et al.*, 1992; Shepherd *et al.*, 1993). TAP-1 and TAP-2 form a heterodimer localized to the ER membrane and the *cis*-Golgi. The TAP-1/2 heterodimer selectively transports cytoplasmically processed peptides into the ER, where the peptides associate with newly synthesized class I molecules, a process facilitated by the fact that MHC I molecules associate noncovalently with the TAP-1/2 complex (Ortmann *et al.*, 1994; Suh *et al.*, 1994). It remains unclear whether peptides are presented exactly as processed in the cytosol, or whether further trimming occurs within the ER (reviewed in Heemels and Ploegh, 1995; Howard, 1995). Although longer peptides can be recovered from MHC I molecules under special circumstances (Collins *et al.*, 1994) minimal MHC I-restricted epitopes are generally 8–10 amino acids (aa) long. From the ER, peptide-loaded MHC I molecules move through the Golgi to the cell surface, where the peptide–MHC I complexes can be recognized by $CD8^+$ T cells. In general, activated $CD8^+$ CTL react by killing cells presenting nonself epitopes in association with class I MHC molecules. The class I-restricted antigen processing pathway likely evolved as a means for allowing the immune system to detect and eradicate cells infected with otherwise undetectable intracellular parasites such as viruses.

Unlike class I MHC molecules, which are expressed on almost all cell types, class II MHC molecules are found only on specialized antigen-presenting cells (APC), such as B cells, macrophages, and dendritic cells. In humans, activated $CD4^+$ T cells also express class II MHC molecules for reasons that are not clear. The primary function of class II MHC molecules is to present peptides derived from extracellular proteins that have been taken up by endocytosis and degraded in endocytotic compartments of APC. Peptides are loaded onto class II molecules in a specialized compartment which has endosomal and lysosomal characteristics (Guagliardi *et al.*, 1990; Amigorena *et al.*, 1994; Tulp *et al.*, 1994). The peptide–MHC II complexes are then transported to the cell surface, where they can be recognized by $CD4^+$ T cells. The structure of class II molecules generally allows presentation of longer peptides, 12–25 aa in length (reviewed by Rammensee, 1995).

Endocytosis of proteins destined for presentation on class II MHC molecules can occur in a variety of ways. In the case of B cells, the uptake of extracellular proteins is mediated by the binding of the relevant protein to surface immunoglobulin on B cells of the appropriate specificity. Other specialized APC, such as macrophages or dendritic cells, take up antigens for class II-restricted processing using high-affinity receptors such as the Fcγ or C3b receptors, or through other low-affinity nonspecific mechanisms.

In addition to these pathways for processing exogenous antigens, cells expressing class II MHC molecules can present the extracellular portions of endogenously synthesized proteins, including the HIV-1 env protein (Orentas *et al.*, 1990; Polydefkis *et al.*, 1990). This process can involve endocytosis of endogenously synthesized transmembrane proteins from the cell surface, or internal transport of newly synthesized proteins from the *trans*-Golgi directly to endosomal/lysosomal compartments (Rowell *et al.*, 1995a,b). These pathways for the processing of endogenously synthesized proteins for association with class II molecules may be particularly important in HIV-1 infection since most cell types that can be productively infected express class II molecules. Thus, HIV-1-infected cells can directly present env epitopes to env-specific $CD4^+$ T cells.

An additional pathway allows presentation of free gp120 released either from infected cells or from free virions. Free gp120 can be taken up and processed for MHC class II-restricted presentation by a unique pathway dependent on its high affinity for CD4. CD4 is expressed predominantly on a subset of T cells, but also at low levels on macrophages and some dendritic cells. The interaction between CD4 and free gp120 allows the uptake of gp120 by macrophages and activated $CD4^+$ T cells for class II-restricted antigen processing. Surface CD4 with bound gp120 is presumed to be endocytosed and transported to an MHC class II processing compartment, where the bound gp120 can be degraded for class II-restricted presentation (Siliciano *et al.*, 1989). This pathway may be important for understanding the immunogenicity of gp120 both in the vaccine setting and in the context of natural infection.

This pathway for presentation of gp120 also provides a potential mechanism for the destruction of noninfected $CD4^+$ T cells in infected individuals. Because activated $CD4^+$ T cells can take up and process shed gp120, they can be recognized by gp120-specific $CD4^+$ T cells. If the relevant gp120-specific cells are cytolytic, as many vaccine-induced gp120-specific $CD4^+$ T cells are, then the result is the lysis of the noninfected $CD4^+$ T cells that are presenting passively acquired gp120. Thus, uninfected "innocent bystander" $CD4^+$ cells might be destroyed *in vivo* during HIV-1 infection by this mechanism. It is not yet clear whether gp120-specific $CD4^+$ CTL are induced in natural infection to a sufficient extent to contribute to CD4 depletion through this mechanism.

4. THE ROLE OF THE PRESENTING MHC MOLECULE

Several interacting cellular systems determine which epitopes of a protein can be presented to T cells. Perhaps the most stringent determinant is whether the epitope can successfully bind an appropriate MHC molecule. X-ray crystallography of class I (Bjorkman *et al.*, 1987) and class II (Brown *et al.*, 1993; Stern *et al.*, 1994) molecules has revealed an antigen-binding cleft formed by two α helices and a β-pleated sheet "floor." Class I and class II molecules both bind peptide antigens in a peptide-extended conformation through interactions between amino acid side chains within the cleft and preferred "anchor" residues at specific positions in the bound peptide. In addition, class I molecules interact with the amino- and carboxy-termini of bound peptides. Thus, unlike class II molecules, which allow peptide ends to extend out from the cleft, class I molecules have a short, highly stringent peptide size preference (8–10 amino acids).

The MHC molecules are among the most allelically variant proteins found in humans. Each allele is expressed in only a small fraction of the population. The functional effect of this allelic polymorphism is a dramatic difference in the ability of different MHC alleles to present a given peptide to T cells. That is to say, a peptide that can be successfully presented to T cells in the context of one MHC allele is generally not presented by other allelic variants of the same MHC molecule. Thus, while it is clearly important to identify individual T-cell epitopes in HIV-1 proteins, such information is directly applicable only to a limited segment of the population—those who express the relevant MHC molecule.

Analysis of antigen recognition by T cells can be done with T-cell clones. In general, T-cell clones demonstrate a high degree of specificity not only for the antigenic peptide, but also for the presenting MHC molecule. The inability of allelic variants of MHC molecules to present a given peptide to a particular T-cell clone can be the result of either: (1) inability of the variant MHC molecule to bind the peptide, (2) induction of a peptide conformation unable to engage the TCR, or (3) polymorphism of MHC molecule residues which interact directly with the TCR. Even minor MHC sequence differences not detected by conventional serological HLA typing can influence the recognition process. Conventional HLA typing relies on panels of antibodies (80 or more) which are specific for various MHC alleles. However, even within a serologically defined allele there are subtypes which may differ only slightly in sequence (a few amino acids) but significantly in antigen presentation properties. For example, Olson and colleagues (Olson *et al.*, 1994) used a human $CD4^+$ CTL clone (Siliciano *et al.*, 1988) specific for an epitope in HIV-1 gp120 (amino acids 410–429) to analyze the effects of allelic variation on T-cell recognition of the epitope. The clone recognized the epitope in the context of a rare subtype of the class II molecule DR4 (DR4 Dw10) carried by the donor from whom the clone was derived. The clone also recognized the epitope in the context of the Dw13 subtype, but not in the context of subtypes Dw4, Dw14, or Dw15. Interestingly, it appears that the peptide can bind all of these alleles, suggesting that, in the particular case of the clone studied, the problem was at the level of interaction between the TCR and the MHC/peptide complex. The results also demonstrated that TCR engagement could be abrogated either by alteration of DR4 residues predicted to be oriented toward the bound peptide, or oriented toward the TCR. The negative effect of subtype variation on T-cell recognition has also been demonstrated in an analogous set of experiments involving presentation of a gp41 epitope in the context of the class II subtypes DPw4.1, DPw4.2, and DPw2.1 (Hammond *et al.*, 1991).

It is important to note that allelic variants that fail to present a particular epitope to a given T-cell clone in *in vitro* experiments may nevertheless be able to present the epitope to other T-cell clones. Individuals expressing the variant alleles will have a repertoire of T cells capable of recognizing peptides presented by that allele. As long as the variant allele can bind the relevant peptide, recognition is possible. The somatic rearrangement which produces the TCR can produce a highly diverse range of potential binding specificities. Because of this huge range of potential specificities, the functional limits to potential T-cell recognition of a given epitope are at the levels of epitope processing and MHC binding. Thus, although one T-cell clone might recognize a given epitope only in the context of a particular MHC allele, it is entirely possible that another T cell with a different TCR rearrangement could recognize the same epitope presented in the context of a different MHC allele. For example, an MHC I A31-restricted T-cell clone characterized by Safrit and colleagues (Safrit *et al.*, 1994b) recognizes the same epitope, 775-RLRDLLLIVTR-785, as an A3.1-restricted clone described by Takahashi and colleagues (Takahashi *et al.*, 1991).

5. THE PROBLEM OF HIV-1 SEQUENCE VARIABILITY

HIV-1 exhibits a high degree of genetic diversity. Even within a single infected individual, multiple distinct but related "quasispecies" can be found (Hahn *et al.*, 1986;

Fisher *et al.*, 1988; Saag *et al.*, 1988). Analysis of T-cell epitopes in the env protein of HIV-1 has been particularly useful for evaluating the effects of sequence variability on T-cell recognition of viral proteins. This is, of course, a critical issue in vaccine development and may also be important in understanding the course of the disease. There is considerable current interest in the issue of whether or not the naturally occurring genetic variation of HIV-1 contributes to the pathogenesis of AIDS by permitting the *in vivo* selection of variant viral clones that can escape recognition by existing neutralizing antibodies or virus-specific CTL. While there is good evidence for the selection of escape mutants by neutralizing antibodies (Hahn *et al.*, 1985; Shaw *et al.*, 1988), the question of CTL escape mutants in HIV-1 infection remains largely unresolved.

An interesting series of experiments by Safrit and colleagues address this question using CTL clones isolated from HIV-1-infected individuals during the acute phase of the infection (Safrit *et al.*, 1994b). Such CTL clones were found to be capable of recognizing all observed variant forms of their cognate epitopes found in naturally occurring autologous virus sequences up to 15 weeks after isolation of the clone. This suggests that, at least during this relatively short window of time, such CTL did not drive selection of HIV-1 escape mutants. These data are consistent with findings in SIV-infected rhesus monkeys (Chen *et al.*, 1992). Additionally, two of the clones that recognized the same 11-aa epitope (775-RLRDLLLIVTR-785), differed in their ability to recognize the HIV-1 RF strain sequence of their cognate epitope, implying that the clones are the result of two different TCR gene rearrangement events. This suggests that, during acute viremia, the CTL response to a given epitope is redundant and involves T cells expressing different receptors. The lack of variation in CTL epitopes observed in the studies cited above is somewhat at odds with earlier work involving the HIV-1 gag protein (Phillips *et al.*, 1991). Thus, additional studies are needed to help elucidate the complex interplay between viral variation and host CTL response.

6. THE DELINEATION OF T-CELL EPITOPES

The delineation of T-cell epitopes requires the identification of a minimal fragment of the relevant protein required to stimulate an effector population, and identification of the MHC allele involved in the presentation of that fragment/epitope. The general approach is to test antigen-specific effector T-cell populations for recognition of APC presenting various forms of the protein. APC expressing different MHC alleles can be used to define the MHC allele(s) involved in the presentation of a particular epitope. Truncated expression vectors, recombinant protein fragments, and synthetic peptides are used to define a minimal epitope within the protein necessary for activation of the clonal effector population. In general, the minimal epitope is defined as the smallest peptide that is recognized efficiently by the effector population. As discussed above, minimal class I-restricted epitopes are usually 8–10 aa in length. Defined minimal epitopes are usually active as synthetic peptides at concentrations much lower than those necessary for slightly longer or shorter peptides. It is more difficult to define minimal class II-restricted epitopes because peptides can extend out of the class II peptide binding site at either end.

The delineation of T-cell epitopes in the HIV-1 env protein has been accomplished using several types of *in vitro* assays for T-cell recognition. Interpretation of the published data requires understanding of the advantages and limitations of each approach. Therefore, a brief description of these assays is given below.

The most common assay for detecting antigen-specific CTL is the ^{51}Cr release assay. Effector CTL are mixed with appropriate target APC that have been previously labeled with $Na^{51}CrO_4$. If the effector population contains cells that are capable of lysing the target cells, ^{51}Cr is released into the supernatant, where it can be readily quantitated by γ counting. The amount of lysis attributable to cytolytic activity of the effector cells is typically calculated using the formula: % specific lysis = [(experimental counts − media control)/(detergent control − media control)] × 100. The CTL assay is extremely sensitive, and can detect lysis of target cells pulsed with picomolar concentrations of the appropriate antigenic peptides. Although the ^{51}Cr release assay is typically used to detect class I-restricted, $CD8^+$ CTL, $CD4^+$ CTL can also be detected in this assay. Therefore, for mixed populations of effector cells, additional steps must be taken to establish the phenotype of the cells causing the lysis in this assay. Phenotype can be determined by depletion of effector populations using anti-CD4 or anti-CD8 antibodies followed by complement-mediated lysis or physical separation techniques. A further potential complication in CTL assays using mixed populations of effector cells is that antibody-dependent, env-specific lysis by $CD16^+$ NK cells can be observed in freshly isolated effector cell populations taken from infected individuals. Precautions must therefore be taken to rule out such lysis in studies involving freshly isolated effector cell populations from infected individuals.

For $CD4^+$ T cells, different assays are often used, since many $CD4^+$ T cells do not have the ability to lyse APC. Activation of T_h is characterized by proliferation and secretion of cytokines, such as interleukin 2 (IL-2). Proliferation can be detected by determining the incorporation of [^{3}H]thymidine, and IL-2 production can be detected by appropriate bioassays or by ELISA methods. IL-2 production is frequently measured by determining the incorporation of [^{3}H]thymidine by an IL-2-dependent T-cell line.

For each type of assay, an effector T-cell population is mixed with APC expressing the relevant antigen. Several different types of T-cell and APC populations have been used. T-cell epitopes can be delineated using polyclonal populations of T cells or T-cell clones. The use of clonal effector populations allows detailed analysis of the epitope. HIV-1-specific T-cell clones have been isolated from HIV-1-seropositive humans, naive seronegative individuals, recipients of various experimental AIDS vaccines, and immunized mice. The tissue sources used have included mononuclear cells isolated from spleen, lymph nodes, cerebrospinal fluid, bronchoalveolar washes, and peripheral blood. Various restimulation strategies, either antigen-specific or nonspecific, have been used to induce T-cell activation and proliferation *in vitro*.

In the case of class I-restricted epitopes, the most frequently used target cells are autologous or MHC-mismatched Epstein–Barr virus-transformed B lymphoblastoid cell lines (B-LCL), which are typically infected with vaccinia virus vectors encoding the recombinant protein of interest, or exposed in culture to a peptide of interest prior to the assay. These B-LCL are easily grown in culture and are good targets for vaccinia virus infection. Recombinant vaccinia virus vectors have been useful in the elucidation of T-cell responses to the HIV-1 env protein. Because vaccinia replicates in the cytosol, the HIV-1 rev dependence of the export of env mRNA from the nucleus is not an issue, and the env protein can be readily expressed in cells infected with recombinant vaccinia vectors. Thus, B-LCL of known HLA type can also be used to determine the general MHC restriction of T-cell clones. Certain B-cell lines, such as the C1R line which does not express MHC I, can be coinfected with vaccinia vectors bearing known MHC I alleles in order to further dissect the

MHC I restriction of CTL clones. Other target cells have also been used, including fibroblasts and HIV-1-infected cells.

When target cells expressing an appropriate MHC allele are incubated in culture with a synthetic peptide encompassing a T-cell epitope, the target cells acquire the capacity to activate T cells specific for the epitope. It is uncertain whether presentation of these peptides occurs following binding to previously empty cell surface MHC molecules, displacement of natively processed self peptides from cell surface MHC molecules, or association with MHC molecules following cellular uptake. By incubating target cells bearing the appropriate MHC molecule with various synthetic peptides representing overlapping epitopes within the protein of interest, the minimum epitope necessary for T-cell activation can be defined.

7. T-CELL EPITOPES IN THE HIV-1 ENV PROTEIN

A summary of defined T-cell epitopes in the env protein is given in Figs. 2 and 3 and Table I. It is important to note that some of the epitopes have been defined in detailed studies using T-cell clones, with clear delineation of the boundaries of the epitope and the MHC restriction element utilized. In contrast, some of the epitopes have been identified only in studies using polyclonal T-cell populations from infected individuals or immunized experimental animals. In many of these studies, the epitope boundaries and presenting MHC molecules have not been defined. Many overlapping epitopes are shown. In general, these

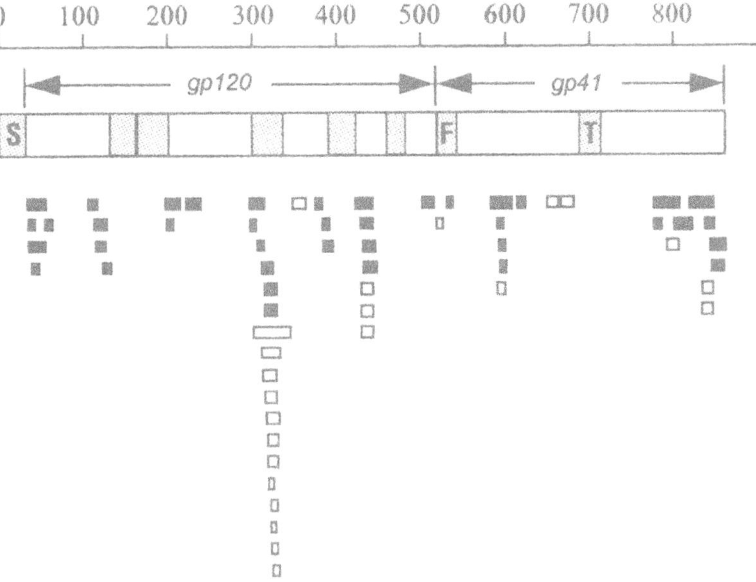

FIGURE 2. Class I-restricted epitopes in the HIV-1 env protein. The positions of published human (dark boxes) and murine (open boxes) T-cell epitopes are shown. Also shown are the hydrophobic signal (S), fusion (F), and transmembrane (T) domains to the env protein and the five hypervariable regions (V1–5) of gp120.

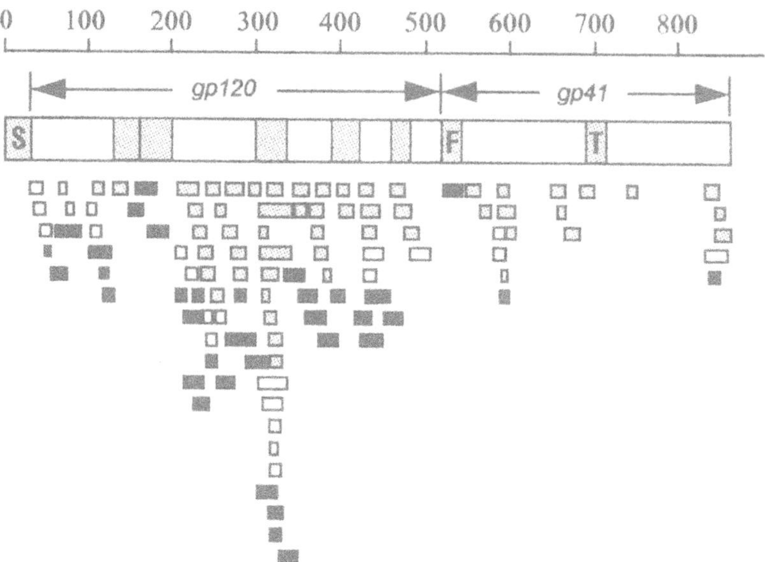

FIGURE 3. Class II-restricted epitopes in the HIV-1 env protein. The positions of published human (shaded boxes), murine (open boxes), and nonhuman primate (dark boxes) T-cell epitopes are shown. Also shown are the hydrophobic signal (S), fusion (F), and transmembrane (T) domains of the env protein and the five hypervariable regions (V1–5) of gp120.

were identified in different studies using the same or overlapping peptides and are not necessarily distinct, particularly in case where restriction elements have not been identified.

7.1. Class I-Restricted Epitopes

Several interesting conclusions may be drawn from the accumulated data on defined T-cell epitopes in the env protein. First, epitopes are located throughout the molecule. Distinct topological domains of the molecule including gp120, and the extracellular and cytoplasmic domains of gp41, all contain multiple epitopes. Given that many of the epitopes were identified in studies in which the effector cells were obtained from infected individuals, it appears that all parts of the protein are subject to processing for class I-restricted antigen presentation. This is interesting in the sense that the currently accepted paradigm for class I-restricted antigen processing does not provide a convenient explanation for the processing of epitopes in the extracellular domains of plasma membrane proteins (see below). It is important to remember that, in a given individual, only a small subset of the total env epitopes will be presented because each individual inherits at most two different alleles at each of the three class I loci (HLA A, B, and C in humans). For example, from a single seronegative individual immunized with a recombinant vaccinia vector carrying the HIV-1 *env* gene, env-specific clones restricted to HLA A3.1, B18, and B35 were isolated along with three different class II-restricted clones.

A second feature of interest is the location of epitopes in relationship to the distribution of variability within the protein. At first glance, there appears to be a paucity of defined epitopes within the V1, V2, V4, and V5 hypervariable regions of gp120. However, it is important to remember that virtually all assays of env-specific CTL have utilized env antigen derived from standard reference isolates of HIV-1 such as LAI. Therefore, in any given infected individual, the CTL generated *in vivo* in response to the infecting strain of the virus may not be detectable in *in vitro* assays using lab strain-based antigens, particularly if the epitopes recognized are in hypervariable regions of the molecules. Bollinger and colleagues have recently isolated from infected individuals env-specific CTL clones that recognize target cells expressing env protein from donor-derived HIV-1 isolate, but not targets expressing env protein from a reference laboratory strain of HIV-1 (R. C. Bollinger, unpublished results). It is thus likely that the use of antigen preparations derived from laboratory strains of HIV-1 significantly underestimates the total anti-env response in infected individuals, particularly with respect to epitopes in the hypervariable regions.

It is also important to point out that many of the epitopes listed were identified in studies in which synthetic peptides were used as immunogens. Because many investigators have focused on the delineation of epitopes in conserved regions of the env protein, we have much more information about epitopes in conserved regions. Thus, because some of the approaches used to define epitopes introduce a bias against epitopes in variable regions of the env protein, it is not yet possible to conclude that there is a true paucity of epitopes in these regions, a finding that might reflect selective pressure to eliminate these epitopes. Interestingly, epitopes have been defined in the V3 loop, reflecting the intense interest in this region of the molecule (see below). Thus, despite the ostensible paucity of epitopes in some of the hypervariable regions of the env protein, it is likely that epitopes are located throughout the molecule.

7.2. Class II-Restricted Epitopes in the Env Protein

As is the case with the class I-restricted epitopes described above, there are fewer defined epitopes within the most variable regions of the env protein. This likely reflects the same ascertainment biases described above. In studies using effector cell populations from infected individuals, *in vitro* assays using antigens based on laboratory strains such as LAI will fail to identify many T-cell clones specific for epitopes in the variable regions of env. Studies of the response of immunized seronegative humans or experimental animals to env protein do not suffer from this bias, and in these studies, epitopes have been detected in variable regions. In the same manner, studies of the *in vitro* responses of T cells isolated from HIV-1-seronegative individuals to env proteins or peptides have detected epitopes in variable regions of the protein (see Table I).

There does appear to be a paucity of defined epitopes in the cytoplasmic domain of gp41. This could reflect the fact that, in infected cells, the cytoplasmic domain of the protein may have less access to class II processing compartments than the ecto-domain.

8. ADDITIONAL ASPECTS OF ANTIGEN PROCESSING OF THE ENV PROTEIN: SOME EXCEPTIONS TO THE RULES

Recent work has revealed that the generalized antigen processing pathways detailed above are not the only ones that cells use to process the HIV-1 env protein for presentation to T cells. Alternative pathways have now been defined. Understanding these alternative

TABLE I. Env Epitopes Published through October 1995[a]

Position[b]	Sequence	MHC restriction	Minimal epitope defined?	Assay[c]	Clone?	Species[d]	Other strains[e]	Status/ vaccine[f]	Reference
31–55	TEKLWVTVYYGVPVWKEATTTLFCA	B18		C	yes	H		vac	Johnson *et al.* (1994a)
32–44	EQLWVTVYYGVPV			P		M		pep	Sastry and Arlinghaus (1991)
33–42	KLWVTVYYGV			C		H		sp	Dupuis *et al.* (1995)
34–55	LWVTVYYGVPVWKEATTTLFCA	A2		C		H		sn & sp	Dadaglio *et al.* (1991)
37–46	TVYYGVPVWK	A3.1	yes	C	yes	H	+	vac	Johnson *et al.* (1994a,b)
38–48	VYYGVPVWKEA			P		M		pep	Sastry and Arlinghaus (1991)
41–54	GVPVWKEATTLFC			P		M		pep	Sastry and Arlinghaus (1991)
45–55	WKEATTTLFCA			P		P		pep	Nehete *et al.* (1993)
52–61	LFCASDAKAY			C		H		sp	Lieberman *et al.* (1992)
54–74	CASDAKAYDTEVHNVWATHAC			P		P		pep	Eriksson *et al.* (1993)
65–75	AHKVWATHACV			P		M		pep	Sastry and Arlinghaus (1991)
65–89	VHNVWATHACVPTDPNPQEVVLVNV			P		P		pep	Eriksson *et al.* (1993)
74–85	CVPTNPVPQEVV			P		M		pep	Sastry and Arlinghaus (1991)
74–105	CVPTDPNPQEVVLVNVTENFNMWKN DMVEQMH			C, P		H		sp/vac	Ratto *et al.* (1995)
98–109	NNMVEQMHEDII			P		M		pep	Sastry and Arlinghaus (1991)
101–126	VEQMHEDIISLWDQSLKPCVKLTPLC			P		P		pep	Eriksson *et al.* (1993)
102–114	EQMHEDIISLWDQ			P		M		pep	Sastry and Arlinghaus (1991)
105–117	HEDIISLWDQSLK			2		H		sp	Clerici *et al.* (1989)
105–117	HEDIISLWDQSLK			P		H		vac	Berzofsky *et al.* (1988)
105–117	HEDIISLWDQSLK			P		M		pep	Cease *et al.* (1987)
105–117	HEDIISLWDQSLK			C, P, 2		H		snx	Pinto *et al.* (1995)
105–117	HEDIISLWDQSLK			2		H		snx	Clerici *et al.* (1992)
111–126	LWDQSLKPCVKLTPLC	Bw60 A2		C		H		pep & rec	Macatonia *et al.* (1991)
112–124	WDQSLKPCVKLTP			P		P		pep	Hosmalin *et al.* (1991)
112–123	WDQSLKPCVKLT	A2, A1 B8		C		H		sp	Clerici *et al.* (1991b)
118–130	PCVKLTPLCVSLK			P		P		pep	Nehete *et al.* (1993)
121–129	KLTPLCVTL			C		H		sp	Dupuis *et al.* (1995)

131–146	TDLGKATNTNSSNWKE		P		H		sn	Manca *et al.* (1991)
147–169	SSSGRMIMEKGEIKNCSFNISTS		P		P		pep	Eriksson *et al.* (1993)
157–181	GEIKNCSFNISTSIRGKVQKEYAFF		P		P		pep	Vahlne *et al.* (1991)
157–181	GEIKNCSFNISTSIRGKVQKEYAFF	class I class II	P		P		pep	Eriksson *et al.* (1993)
170–197	IRGKVQKEYAFFYKLDIIPIDNDTTSYS		P		P		pep	Eriksson *et al.* (1993)
193–212	TTSYTLTSCNTSVITQACPK	A2	C		H		sp & sn	Dadaglio *et al.* (1991)
197–205	KLTSCNTSV	A2.1	C		H		sp	Brander *et al.* (1995)
204–216	SVITQACSKVSFE		P		M		pep	Sastry and Arlinghaus (1991)
204–216	SVITQACPKVSFE		P		P		pep	Nehete *et al.* (1993)
206–230	ITQACPKVSFEPIPIHYCAPAGFAI	class II	C	yes	H		vac	Johnson *et al.* (1994a)
211–235	PKVSFEPIPIHYCAPAGFAILKCNN		P		P		pep	Eriksson *et al.* (1993)
215–228	FEPIPIHYCAFPGF		P		M		pep	Sastry and Arlinghaus (1991)
217–236	PIPIHYCAPAGFAILKCNNK		C		H		sp	Lieberman *et al.* (1992)
221–234	HYCAPAGFAILKCN		P		H		sn	Praud *et al.* (1994)
224–242	APAGFAILKCNNKTFNGTG		P		P		pep	Eriksson *et al.* (1993)
225–240	PAGFAILKCNNKTFNY	DQ1	P	yes	H	+/−	sn	Manca *et al.* (1993)
231–246	CNNKTFNGKGPCTNVS		P	yes	H		sn	Manca *et al.* (1991)
235–250	NKTFNGKGPCTNVSTY	DQ1	P	yes	H	+/−	sn	Manca *et al.* (1993)
236–246	KKFNGTGPCTN		P		M		pep	Sastry and Arlinghaus (1991)
240–252	GTGPCTNVSTVQC		P		M		pep	Sastry and Arlinghaus (1991)
240–252	GTGPCTNVSTVQC		P		P		pep	Nehete *et al.* (1993)
241–256	PCTNVSTVQCTHGIRP		P	yes	H		sn	Manca *et al.* (1991)
245–260	TNVSTVQCTHGIRPIY	DQ1	P	yes	H	+	sn	Manca *et al.* (1993)
250–263	VQCTHGIRPVVSTQ		P		M		pep	Sastry and Arlinghaus (1991)
251–266	THGIRPIVSTQLLLNG		P		H		sn	Manca *et al.* (1991)
253–274	THGIRPVVSTQLLLNGSLAEEE		P		P		pep	Vahlne *et al.* (1991)
253–274	THGIRPVVSTQLLLNGSLAEEE		P		P		pep	Eriksson *et al.* (1993)
254–263	VVSTQLLLNG		P		H		sp	Pugliese *et al.* (1992)
261–276	QLLLNGSLAEEEVVIR		P		H		sn	Manca *et al.* (1991)
262–284	TQLLLNGSLAEEEVVIRSANFTD		P		H		sp	Bell *et al.* (1992)
263–297	QLLLNGSLAEEEVVIRSVNFTDNAKTII VQLNTSV		P		P		pep	Eriksson *et al.* (1993)
269–283	EVVIRSANFTDNAKT		P		H		sp	Wahren *et al.* (1989)

(*continued*)

TABLE I. (*Continued*)

Position[b]	Sequence	MHC restriction	Minimal epitope defined?	Assay[c]	Clone?	Species[d]	Other strains[e]	Status/ vaccine[f]	Reference
271–286	EEVVIRSDNFTNNAKT			P		H		sn	Manca *et al.* (1991)
274–288	SANFTDNAKTIIVQL			P		H		sp	Wahren *et al.* (1989)
275–300	VVIRSVNFTDNAKTIIVQLNTSVEIN			P		P		pep	Eriksson *et al.* (1993)
288–311	TIIVQLNTSVEINCTRPNNNTRKR			P		P		pep	Eriksson *et al.* (1993)
294–303	NESVAINCVT	DR2 (w15)	yes	P	yes	H		rec	Botarelli *et al.* (1991)
296–312	SVEINCTRPNNNTRKSI	A2		C		H		sn & sp	Dadaglio *et al.* (1991)
297–303	VEINCTR?	class I	yes	C		H		sp	Moukrim and Achour (1995)
300–339	NCTRPNNNTRKRIRIQRGPGRAFVTIG KIGNMRQAHCNIS	H-2[d]		C		M	+/−	pep	Layton *et al.* (1993)
301–325	CTRPNNNTRKRIRIQRGPGRAFVTI			P		P		pep	Eriksson *et al.* (1993)
301–336	NNTRKRIRIQRGPGRAFVTIGKIGNMR QAHCNISRA	D[d]		P, C		M		pep	Kingsman *et al.* (1995)
301–337	CTRPNNNTRKSIRIQRGPGRAFVTIGK IGNMRQAHCN	DR3		P	yes	H	−	sn	Fernandez *et al.* (1995)
303–312	RPNNNTRKSI	B7	yes	C	yes	H	+/−	sp	Safrit *et al.* (1994a)
306–328	NNTRKSIRIQRGPGRAFVTIGKI			C, P		H		sp	Ratto *et al.* (1995)
306–329	NNTRKSIRIQRGPGRAFVTIGKIG			C		M		pep	Nehete *et al.* (1995a)
306–329	NNTrksihiQRGPGRafyttgkilG[h]			2, 3, P		M	+/−	pep	Estaquier *et al.* (1993)
307–315	NTRKSIRIQ	DRB1 *0101		P	yes	H	−	sn	Fernandez *et al.* (1995)
307–326	NTRKSIRIQRGPGRAFVTIG	DRB1 *0101		P	yes	H	+/−	sn	Fernandez *et al.* (1995)
309–323	IRQGPGRAFVTIGKI			P		H		sp	Wahren *et al.* (1989)
310–327	KSIRIQRGPGRAFVTIGK	Dd		C		M	+	pep	Nardelli and Tam (1993)
310–327	KRKRIHIGPGRAFYTTKN	D[d]		C		M	+	pep	Nardelli and Tam (1993)
312–327	IRIQRGPGRAFVTIGK			C		M		pep	Deprez *et al.* (1995)
312–327	IRIQRGPGRAFVTIGK	D[d]		C		M		pep	Choppin *et al.* (1990)
312–331	IRIQRGPGRAFVTIGKIGNM			P		P		pep	Eriksson *et al.* (1993)
312–335	IRIQRGPGRAFVTIGKIGNMRQAH			P		P		pep	Vahlne *et al.* (1991)
312–329	NNTRKSIRIQRGPGRAFVTIGKIG			P		H		vac	Gorse *et al.* (1992)

313–326	RIGPGRAFVTIG			C		M		pep	Wagner *et al.* (1992)
313–327	RIQRGPGRAFVTIGK			P		M		bac	Charbit *et al.* (1993)
313–327	RIQRGPGRAFVTIGK			C		M		pep	Wagner *et al.* (1992)
313–327	RIQRGPGRAFVTIGK			C		M		bac	Kameoka *et al.* (1994)
313–327	RIQRGPGRAFVTIGK	A2		C		H		sn & sp	Dadaglio *et al.* (1991)
313–325	RIQRGPGRAFVTI	I-A^d	yes	P		M		pep	Takeshita *et al.* (1995)
313–327	RIQRGPGRAFVTIGK	H-2^u		C		M		pep	Shirai *et al.* (1993)
		H-2^p							
		H-2^d							
313–327	RIQRGPGRAFVTIGK	D^d		C		M		pep	Takahashi *et al.* (1989a)
313–327	RIQRGPGRAFVTIGK	Ak, Ek		P		M		pep	Takahashi *et al.* (1994a)
313–327	RIQRGRPGRAFVTIGK	A11		C		H	–	vac	Achour *et al.* (1994)
313–327	RIQRGRGPGRAFVTIGK			P		P	+	sp	Nehete *et al.* (1995b)
313–327	RIQRGPGRAFVTIGK	D^d		P	yes	M		pep	Moore and Fox (1994)
313–327	RIQRGPGRAFVTIGK			C, P, 2		H	+	snx	Pinto *et al.* (1995)
313–327	RIQRGPGRAFVTIGK	D^d		C		M		pep	Shirai *et al.* (1994)
313–327	RIQRGPGRAFVTIGK			P		H		pep	Baier *et al.* (1995)
313–327	RIQRGPGRAFVTIGK			2		H		sp	Clerici *et al.* (1989)
313–327	RIQRPGRAFVTIGK	class I		C		M		rec	Takahashi *et al.* (1990b)
313–327	RIQRGPGRAFVTIGK	H-2^d		C		M		vac	Takahasi *et al.* (1988)
313–327	RIQRGPGRAFVTIGK	A2, A3		C		H		vac	Achour *et al.* (1993)
313–327	RIQRGPGRAFVTIGK	H-2^d		2, C		M		pep	Lasarte *et al.* (1995)
313–327	RIQRGPGRAFVTIGK	D^d		C		M	–	vac	Takahashi *et al.* (1989a)
313–327	SIHIGPGRAFYATGD	D^d		C		M	+	pep	Casement *et al.* (1995)
313–327	GIAIGPGRTLYAREK	D^d		C		M	+/–	pep	Casement *et al.* (1995)
313–327	RIQRGPGRAFVTIGK	D^d		C		M	–	pep	Casement *et al.* (1995)
313–327	RIHIGPGRAFYTTKN	D^d		C		M	+	pep	Casement *et al.* (1995)
313–327	RIQRGPGRAFVTIGK			P, C		M		dna	Okuda *et al.* (1995)
313–327	RIQRGPGRAFVTIGK	D^d		C		M		pep	Sastry *et al.* (1992)
313–327	RIQRGPGRAFVTIGK	D^d, A^d		P, C		M		pep	Takahashi *et al.* (1990a)
313–327	RIQRGPGRAFVTIGK	D^d		C		M	–	vac	Takahashi *et al.* (1989b)
313–327	RIQRGPGRAFVTIGK	D^d		C		M	–	vac	Takahashi *et al.* (1989a)

(*continued*)

TABLE I. (*Continued*)

Position[b]	Sequence	MHC restriction	Minimal epitope defined?	Assay[c]	Clone?	Species[d]	Other strains[e]	Status/ vaccine[f]	Reference
313–327	RIQRGPGRAFVTIGK	H-2^{d} H-2^{a} H-2^{p} H-2^{u} H-2^{q}		C		M	–	pep	Shirai *et al.* (1992)
313–328	RIQRGPGRAFYTTKN			2		H		snx	Clerici *et al.* (1992)
313–328	RIHIGPGRAFYTTKN			2		H		snx	Clerici *et al.* (1992)
313–329	RIQRGPGRAFVTIGKIG			C		M		pep	Nehete *et al.* (1995a)
314–328	GRAFVTIGKIGNMRQ			P		H		sp	Wahren *et al.* (1989)
315–323	IQRGPGRAFV	D^{d}	yes	C, IFNγ	yes	M		pep	Takeshita *et al.* (1995)
315–329	RAFVTIGKIGNMRQA	D^{d} I-A^{d}		P, C		M		pep	More and Fox (1993)
316–324	RGPGRAFVT	D^{d}		C		M		vac	Bergmann *et al.* (1994)
316–325	RGPGRAFVTI	D^{d}		C	Hy[g]	M		pep	Kozlowski *et al.* (1992)
316–325	RGPGRAFVTI	H-2^{d}		C	Hy[g]	M		pep	Kozlowski *et al.* (1993)
316–325	RGPGRAFVTI	D^{d}	yes	C		M		pep	Takahashi *et al.* (1993)
316–329	RGPGRAFVTIGKIG			C		M		pep	Nehete *et al.* (1995a)
317–325	GPGRAFVTI	D^{d}, L^{d}		C		M		vac	Bergmann *et al.* (1994)
318–326	PGRAFVTIG	D^{d}	yes	C		M		vac	Bergmann *et al.* (1994)
320–329	RAFVTIGKIG			C		M		pep	Nehete *et al.* (1995a)
326–348	GKIGNMRQAHCNISRAKWNNTLK			P		P		pep	Eriksson *et al.* (1993)
332–346	RQAHCNISRAKWNNT	I-A^{d}		P	yes	M		pep	Warren and Thomas (1992)
332–358	RQAHCNISRAKWNNTLKQIDSKLREQF			P		P		pep	Eriksson *et al.* (1993)
342–366	KWNNTLKQIDSKLREQFGNNKTIIF	class II		C	yes	H		vac	Johnson *et al.* (1994a)
346–359	QIVKKLREQFGNNK			P		H		sp	Krowka *et al.* (1990)
348–362	KQIDSKLREQFGNNK	H-2^{d}		C		M		vac	Takahashi *et al.* (1988)
349–370	QIDSKLREQFGNNKTIIFKQSS			P		P		pep	Eriksson *et al.* (1993)
359–382	GNNKTIIFKQSSGGDPEIVTHSFN			P		P		pep	Eriksson *et al.* (1993)
369–383	SSGGDPEIVTHSFNC			P		H		sp	Wahren *et al.* (1989)
367–377	KQSSGGDPEIV			P, 2		H		sp	Schrier *et al.* (1989)

369–383	PEIVTHSFNCGGEFF			P		H		sp	Wahren *et al.* (1989)
371–386	PEIVMHSFNCRGEFFY			P		H		sn	Manca *et al.* (1991)
372–394	GDPEIVTHSFNCGGEFFYCNSTQ			P		P		pep	Eriksson *et al.* (1993)
374–380	PEIVTHS	A2		C		H		sn & sp	Dadaglio *et al.* (1991)
381–388	FNCGGEFF	Cw4	yes	C	yes	H	+/−	sp	Johnson *et al.* (1993)
381–392	KNCGGEFFYCNS	A2		C		H		sn & sp	Dadaglio *et al.* (1991)
383–405	CGGEFFYCNSTQLFNSTWFNSTW			P		P		pep	Eriksson *et al.* (1993)
394–408	TWFNSTWSTKGSNNT			P		H		sp	Wahren *et al.* (1989)
399–413	TWSTKGSNNTEGSDT			P		H		sp	Wahren *et al.* (1989)
415–434	GSDTITLPCRIKQIINMWQK			P		P		pep	Eriksson *et al.* (1993)
415–434	GSDTITLPCRIKQFINMWQE	DR4 Dw10		P, C	yes	H		sn	Siliciano *et al.* (1988), Polydefkis *et al.* (1990)
415–431	GSDTITLPCRIKQFINM	DRab1 *0402	yes	P	yes	H		sn	Olsen *et al.* (1994)
421–440	LPCRIKQFINMWQEVGKAMY	A2		C		H		sn	Dadaglio *et al.* (1991)
421–434	LPCRIKQFINMWQE	DR4 Dw10	yes	P, C	yes	H	+/−	sn	Siliciano *et al.* (1988)
421–434	LPCRIKQFINMWQE	DR4	yes	P	yes	H	+/−	sn	Callahan *et al.* (1990)
423–449	CRIKQIINMWQKVGKAMYAPPISGQIR			P		P		pep	Eriksson *et al.* (1993)
424–438	INMWQEVGKAMYAPP			P		H		sp	Wahren *et al.* (1989)
426–441	KQIINMWQEVGKAMYA			2		H		snx	Clerici *et al.* (1992)
426–441	KQIINMWQEVGKAMYA			C, P, 2		H	+	snx	Pinto *et al.* (1995)
426–441	KQIINMWQEVGKAMYA	H-2[b] H-2[a]		C		M		pep	Shirai *et al.* (1992)
426–441	KQIINMWQEVGKAMYA	class II		P	Hy[g]	M		pep	Boehncke *et al.* (1993)
426–441	KQIINMWQEVGKAMYA			P		P		pep	Yasutomi *et al.* (1993a)
426–441	KQIINMWQEVGKAMYA			P		H		pep	Baier *et al.* (1995)
426–441	KQIINMWQEVGKAMYA			2		H		sp	Clerici *et al.* (1989)
426–441	KQIINMWQEVGKAMYA			P		H		sn	Berzofsky *et al.* (1988)
426–441	KQIINMWQEVGKAMYA			P		M		pep	Cease *et al.* (1987)
(426–441): (301–321)	KQIINMWQEVGKAMYA: CTRPNYNKRKRIHIGPGRA	D[d]		C		M		pep	Hart *et al.* (1991)
(426–441): (301–321)	KQIINMWQEVGKAMYA: CTRPNYNKRKRIHIGPGRA	class I		C		P		pep	Haynes *et al.* (1993)

(continued)

TABLE I. (*Continued*)

Position[b]	Sequence	MHC restriction	Minimal epitope defined?	Assay[c]	Clone?	Species[d]	Other strains[e]	Status/ vaccine[f]	Reference
(426–441):	KQIINMWQEVGKAMYA: EGCTPYDINQML	class I		C		P		pep	Haynes *et al.* (1993)
426–449	KQIINMWQEVGKAMYAPPISGQIR	class II		P		M		pep	Shirai *et al.* (1994)
426–450	KQFINMWQEVGKAMYAPPISGQIRC			P, 2R, 2		P		rec	Lusso *et al.* (1988)
428–443	FINMWQEVGKAMYAPP	A2, A1, B8		C		H		sp	Clerici *et al.* (1991a)
428–443	FINMWQEVGKAMYAPP			P		P		pep	Hosmalin *et al.* (1991)
445–458	SGQIRCSSNITGLL			P		P		pep	Eriksson *et al.* (1993)
450–471	CSSNITGLLLTRDGGNSNNESE			P		P		pep	Eriksson *et al.* (1993)
459–473	GNSNNESEIFRPGGG			P		H		sp	Wahren *et al.* (1989)
466–481	FRPGGGDMRDNWRSEL			P		H		sp	Krowka *et al.* (1990)
474–488	DMRDNWRSELYKYKV			P		H		sp	Wahren *et al.* (1989)
481–504	RDNWRSELYKYKVVKIEPLGVAPT	class II		P		M		pep	Shirai *et al.* (1994)
484–498	YKYKVVKIEPLGVAP			P		H		sp	Wahren *et al.* (1989)
494–513	VKIEPLGVAPTKAKRRVVQR	A2		C		H		sn & sp	Dadaglio *et al.* (1991)
504–517	TKAKRRVVEREKRA			C		H		sp	Clerici *et al.* (1993a)
(517–528): (426–441): (301–321)	AVGIGALFLGFL: KQIINMWQEVGKAMYA: CTRPNYNKRKRIHIGPGRA:FYTTK	D^d		C		M		pep	Hart *et al.* (1991)
519–543	GIGALFLGFLGAAGSTMGARSMTLT			P		P		pep	Nehete *et al.* (1993)
527–535	FLAAGSTM	A2.1		C		H		sp	Brander *et al.* (1995)
546–645	ARQLLSGIVQQQNNLLRAIEAQQHLLQ LTVWGIKQLQARILAVERYLKDQQLLG IWGCSGKLICTTAVPWNASWSNKSLE QIWNNMTWMEWDREINNYTS	class II		C	yes	H	+	rec	Orentas *et al.* (1990)
547–561	GIVQQQNNLLRAIEA			P		H		sp	Wahren *et al.* (1989)
562–576	QQKLLQLTVWFIKQL			P		H		sp	Wahren *et al.* (1989)
580–591	QLQARILAVERY	class II	yes	P		M		pep	Brown *et al.* (1995)
580–604	QLQARILAVERYLKDQQLLGIWGCS			C		H		sp	Jassoy *et al.* (1992)
584–595	RILAVERYDQ	DPw4.2	yes	C	yes	H	+/−	vac	Hammond *et al.* (1991)

584–593	RILAVERYLK	class II	yes	P		M		pep	Brown *et al.* (1995)
586–598	LAVERYLKDQQLL			P		P		pep	Nehete *et al.* (1993)
587–596	AVERYLKDQQ	D^d	yes	P	yes	M		pep	Brown *et al.* (1995)
589–597	ERYLKDQQL	B14	yes	C	yes	H		sp	Kalams *et al.* (1994)
589–597	ERYLKDQQL	B14	yes	C	yes	H	+/−	sp	Johnson *et al.* (1992)
589–599	ERYLKDQQLLG	B8		C	yes	H		sp	Johnson *et al.* (1992)
591–598	YLKDQQLL	B8	yes	C		H	+/−	sp	Johnson *et al.* (1992)
591–598	YLKDQQLL	A24	yes	C	yes	H	+/−	sp	Dai *et al.* (1992)
593–604	LGIWGCSGKLIC		yes	P		H		sp	Bell *et al.* (1992)
611–619	TAVPWNASW	B35	yes	C	yes	H		vac	Johnson *et al.* (1994a)
647–661	IHSLIEESQNQQEKN	H-2^d		C		M		vac	Takahashi *et al.* (1988)
652–666	EESQNQQEKNEQELL			P		H		sp	Wahren *et al.* (1989)
655–667	QNQQEKNEQELLE			P, 2		H		sp	Schrier *et al.* (1989)
667–681	ELDWASLWNWFNIT	H-2^d		C		M		vac	Takahashi *et al.* (1988)
672–686	ASLWNWFNITNWLWY			P		H		sp	Wahren *et al.* (1989)
682–696	IKLFIMIVGGLVGLR			P		H		sp	Wahren *et al.* (1989)
706–725	VLSIVNRVRQGYSPLSFQTH	A32		C	yes	H		sp	Safrit *et al.* (1994b)
737–749	GIEEEGGERDRDR			P, 2		H		sp	Schrier *et al.* (1989)
774–782	HRLRDLLLI		yes	C	yes	H	+/−	sp	Safrit *et al.* (1994b)
775–785	RLRDLLLIVTR	A31	yes	C	yes	H	+/−	sp	Safrit *et al.* (1994b)
776–785	LRDLLLIVTR	A3.1	yes	C	yes	H	+/−	sp	Takahashi *et al.* (1991)
786–807	IVELLGRRGWEALKYWWNLLQY	B27		C		H		sp	Lieberman *et al.* (1992)
790–804	LGRRGWEALKYWWNL	H-2^d		C		M		vac	Takahashi *et al.* (1988)
800–821	YWWNLLQYWSQELKNSAVNLLN			C		H		sp	Lieberman *et al.* (1992)
817–827	SLLNATDIAV	A2	yes	C	yes	H	+	sp	Dupuis *et al.* (1995)
818–827	LLNATDIAV	A2	yes	C	yes	H	+	sp	Dupuis *et al.* (1995)
818–827	LLNATDIAV			C		H		sp	Dupuis *et al.* (1995)
830–858	GTDRVIEVVQGAYRAIRHIPRRIRQGLER	class II		P		M		pep	Shirai *et al.* (1994)
832–858	DRVIEVVQGAYRAIR			C, P 2		H		snx	Pinto *et al.* (1995)
832–846	DRVIEVVQGAYRAIR	H-2^u H-2^p H-2^d		C		M		pep	Shirai *et al.* (1993)

(continued)

TABLE I. (*Continued*)

Position[b]	Sequence	MHC restriction	Minimal epitope defined?	Assay[c]	Clone?	Species[d]	Other strains[e]	Status/ vaccine[f]	Reference
832–846	DRVIEVVQGAYRAIR	$H\text{-}2^d$ H-2a $H\text{-}2^p$ $H\text{-}2^u$ $H\text{-}2^q$		C		M		pep	Shirai *et al.* (1992)
832–846	DRVIEVVQGAYRAIR			2		H		sp	Clerici *et al.* (1989)
832–846	DRVIEVVQGAYRAIR			2		H		snx	Clerici *et al.* (1992)
833–841	RVIEVLQRA			C		H		sp	Dupuis *et al.* (1995)
834–848	VIEVVQGACRAIRHI			P		P		pep	Hosmalin *et al.* (1991)
834–848	VIEVVQGACRAIRHI	A2, A1 B8		C		H		sp	Clerici *et al.* (1991b)
842–861	YRAIRHIPRRIRQGLERILL	A30 B8		C		H		sp	Lieberman *et al.* (1992)
847–861	KIPRRIRQFLERILL			P		H		sp	Wahren *et al.* (1989)

[a]In the absence of definitive data on the phenotype of the responding cells, epitopes eliciting proliferative responses have been listed as class II-restricted epitopes whereas epitopes detected in CTL assays have been listed as class I-restricted epitopes. The caveats discussed in the text apply to this classification.
[b]The corresponding position (amino acid number) of the epitope based on the reference HIV-1 LAI isolate.
[c]The assay used to detect T-cell activity. C, CTL assay; P, proliferation assay; numbers, assay detecting secretion of interleukin (IL) of that number.
[d]Species from which the effector cells were isolated. H, human; M, mouse; P, nonhuman primate.
[e]Ability of the effector population to recognize various strains of HIV-1. (+) indicates that the effector population was able to recognize the corresponding epitope sequence of more than one HIV-1 strain; (−) indicates that the effector population was unable to recognize one or more strains of HIV-1.
[f]The vaccination status or HIV-1 serological status of the individual from whom effector T cells were isolated. sp, HIV-1-seropositive human; sn, HIV-1-seronegative human; snx, HIV-1-seronegative human with suspected exposure to the virus; vac, live viral vaccine; dna, naked DNA vaccine; pep, peptide-based vaccine; rec, recombinant HIV-1 protein vaccine; bac, bacterial vaccine vector.
[g]T-cell hybridoma.
[h]Lowercase letters indicate positions at which peptide synthesis was partially degenerate.

antigen processing pathways may be important for the development of vaccines and immunotherapeutics and for understanding certain aspects of AIDS pathogenesis.

The processing of the HIV-1 env protein, and of viral env proteins in general, for recognition by $CD8^+$ T cells presents an interesting biological puzzle. The ecto-domain of gp160 is cotranslationally translocated into the ER lumen, and is biochemically undetectable in the cytoplasm. The theory that only cytosolic proteins can be presented in the context of class I MHC molecules would therefore predict that epitopes in the ecto-domain of gp160 should not be presented. However, as shown in Fig. 2, numerous $CD8^+$ T-cell epitopes have been defined in gp120 and in the extracellular domain of gp41. Two general pathways for presentation of ecto-domain epitopes can be envisioned. First, processing reactions may occur in the ER after translocation of the ecto-domain of gp160 into the lumen of the ER. This processing pathway should not be dependent on the TAP transporters. Second, a low level of mislocalization of gp160 to the cytosol may allow for cytosolic processing by the normal class I processing pathway. This pathway should be strictly dependent on the TAP transporters.

Recent studies have shown that certain HIV-1 env epitopes can be processed in the ER. This conclusion was reached based on the observation that some env epitopes can be presented by the cell lines T2 and .174, both of which have homozygous deletions encompassing the genes for TAP-1 and TAP-2. Using a panel of $CD8^+$ CTL clones, Hammond *et al.* (1995) have recently demonstrated efficient presentation of two gp120 epitopes (the A3.1-restricted epitope 37-46, and the B18-restricted epitope 31-55) in both cell lines. Successful TAP-1/2-independent processing of the epitopes was found to be dependent on the translocation of gp160 into the ER and independent of CD4/gp120 interactions. Presentation was not affected by retention of the protein in the ER/*cis*-Golgi, suggestive of processing within the ER. Several other HIV-1 env epitopes tested were not able to undergo this TAP-independent ER processing reaction.

In order to test the hypothesis that some class I-restricted epitopes in the gp160 ecto-domain are derived from gp160 molecules that were mislocalized to the cytoplasm, Ferris and colleagues (Ferris *et al.*, 1996) analyzed the presentation of a TAP-1/2-dependent gp41 epitope, 611-TAVPW*N*A*S*W-619, which contains an N-linked glycosylation signal. Functional and biochemical studies showed that a B35-restricted CTL clone specific for this epitope recognized a nonglycosylated form of this epitope, suggesting that the substrate for processing of the env protein for class I-restricted recognition is env protein that does not become glycosylated at the relevant Asn residue. Because glycosylation occurs immediately after translocation of NXS/T sequences into the ER, it is possible that some of the env protein that is processed is derived from a small fraction of the newly synthesized protein that fails to translocate into the ER. Another possible explanation for the TAP-dependent processing of epitopes containing N-linked glycosylation sites is that env protein in the ER either escapes glycosylation or becomes partially deglycosylated and then gains access to the cytosol where it enters the standard class I antigen processing pathway.

9. THE PROBLEM OF gp160 GLYCOSYLATION

As mentioned above, the env protein is heavily glycosylated. The presence of these bulky sugar side chains creates special problems for immune recognition of the virus. In addition to influencing epitope recognition by host antibodies (Skehel *et al.*, 1984), the glycosylation state of an epitope can alter its recognition by T cells. This phenomenon must be taken into account when designing immunotherapeutic or vaccination strategies.

Botarelli *et al.* (1991) describe a series of experiments involving human volunteers vaccinated with recombinant unglycosylated gp120 synthesized intracellularly in yeast. A fraction of the gp120-specific CD4$^+$ T cells cloned from the volunteers could recognize unglycosylated gp120, but were unable to recognize the native glycosylated protein expressed in CHO cells. The minimal epitope of one such clone, 292-*N*E*S*VAI*N*C*T*-300, contains two N residues which are glycosylated in native gp120.

This work has some important implications. First, it implies that vaccines involving unglycosylated recombinant protein or unglycosylated synthetic peptides might elicit some responding CD4$^+$ T cells that are not capable of recognizing glycosylated env protein synthesized in natural infection. The converse possibility must also be considered. In a more extensive series of experiments involving an ovalbumin epitope, Ishioka and colleagues report results similar to those of Botarelli, and also describe an epitope in which the presence of a carbohydrate moiety is, in fact, important for T-cell recognition (Ishioka *et al.*, 1992). If this is the case, then strategies utilizing synthetic peptides for detecting CD4$^+$ T-cell responses in experimental vaccinees and in infected individuals might underestimate the actual CD4$^+$ T-cell response to the native glycosylated protein.

These issues could be of less concern in the analysis of CD8$^+$ T-cell epitopes. As mentioned above, the majority of env epitopes are thought to be TAP-dependent and may be derived by processing of nonglycosylated env protein mislocalized to the cytosol.

10. SYNTHETIC PEPTIDES IN VACCINE STRATEGIES

Many studies of T-cell epitopes in the env protein have been motivated by interest in the concept of synthetic peptide vaccines. In mice, injection of epitopic peptides in Freund's adjuvant (Aichele *et al.*, 1990; Fayolle *et al.*, 1991; Gao *et al.*, 1991; Hart *et al.*, 1991; Schulz *et al.*, 1991; Nehete *et al.*, 1995a), iscoms (Takahashi *et al.*, 1990b), liposome capsules (Watari *et al.*, 1987), or in the absence of adjuvant (Carbone and Bevan, 1989; Ishioka *et al.*, 1989; Lasarte *et al.*, 1992, 1995; Nehete *et al.*, 1995a) can elicit CTL responses to the peptide. Several human trials of peptide vaccine strategies have also been undertaken (Kahn *et al.*, 1992; Schwander *et al.*, 1994; Rubinstein *et al.*, 1995). The mechanism by which class I-restricted responses to exogenous peptides are elicited is unknown. Since exogenous peptide added to cultured cells can apparently bind to vacant class I molecules on the cell surface, it is possible that the exogenous peptides are presented on the class I molecules of APCs *in vivo* by this route. It has also been suggested that, under special circumstances, macrophages can endocytose and process exogenous proteins for presentation on MHC I molecules (Rock *et al.*, 1993; Huang *et al.*, 1994; Reimann *et al.*, 1994). This pathway could conceivably play a role in the priming of T-cell responses following peptide vaccination.

One advantage of peptide-based vaccines is that they have less potential risk than strategies involving recombinant live viral vaccines. A second potential advantage of peptide-based vaccine strategies is that peptides representing many different HIV-1 strains could be injected. For example, Casement *et al.* (1995) recently used a cocktail of peptides from various HIV-1 strains to elicit a broad CD8$^+$ response in mice to a range of different strain epitopes from a region of the highly polymorphic V3 loop of gp120.

It has been suggested that because anti-HIV-1 antibody might facilitate infection of macrophages, it might be desirable to induce a CD8$^+$ CTL response in the absence of an antibody response in vaccinees (Takahashi *et al.*, 1993). Peptide vaccine strategies have been shown to elicit CD8$^+$ CTL responses in the apparent absence of CD4$^+$ T-cell or antibody responses (Lasarte *et al.*, 1995). One line of evidence suggesting that an antibody-less response could be protective comes from studies demonstrating "CTL only" responses to HIV-1 in persistently seronegative individuals known to have been exposed to the virus (Borkowsky *et al.*, 1990; Cheynier *et al.*, 1992; Kelker *et al.*, 1992; Clerici *et al.*, 1991, 1992, 1993b, 1994; Rowland *et al.*, 1993; DeMaria *et al.*, 1994; Langlade *et al.*, 1994; Pinto *et al.*, 1995). Recent evidence also indicates that certain specialized APCs, which can bind virions coated with otherwise neutralizing antibody, may facilitate HIV-1 infection of $CD4^+$ T cells (Heath *et al.*, 1995). This finding casts doubt on the potential value of neutralizing antibody responses. Thus, peptide vaccine strategies could conceivably be useful in eliciting only certain arms of the immune response.

11. THE P18 PEPTIDE

Perhaps the single most studied peptide shown to contain an HIV-1 env protein T-cell epitope is the "P18" peptide (313-RIQRGPGRAFVTIGK-327) representing a sequence from the HIV-1 IIIB strain V3 hypervariable loop, which is also a major target of strain-specific neutralizing antibody responses. Takahashi and colleagues first identified this epitope in the form of a peptide containing an immunodominant class I-restricted epitope recognized by T-cell lines isolated from mice immunized with a vaccinia vector carrying the HIV-1 env gene (Takahashi *et al.*, 1988). The peptide has been used in a gamut of studies, including a large number of peptide vaccine strategies (see Table I).

Research by Kozlowski and colleagues has since shown that proteases found in fetal calf serum, such as angiotensin-1 converting enzyme (ACE) and others, act on P18 to produce a ten-amino-acid peptide better able to stimulate a mouse T-cell hybridoma (Kozlowski *et al.*, 1992, 1993). Similar results have been reported in systems involving epitopes from influenza nucleoprotein (Sherman *et al.*, 1992) and ovalbumin (Falo *et al.*, 1992). The experiments also demonstrate that the sequence surrounding an epitope in a synthetic peptide can influence its antigenicity and that the action of extracellular proteases might be very important for the immunogenicity of synthetic peptide vaccines. These poorly understood extracellular peptide processing reactions should be considered in the interpretation of studies involving peptide antigens.

An obvious drawback to peptide-based vaccination approaches is that they depend on prior knowledge of the anchor residues necessary for peptide binding to each vaccinee's MHC molecules. Since MHC alleles are so highly polymorphic, it is difficult to design a mixture of peptides that will elicit T-cell responses in an entire population of humans. In addition, analysis of peptide vaccine systems has typically relied on restimulation of T cells in the presence of cognate peptide. Since this procedure enriches tremendously for peptide-specific T cells, it is hard to guess the magnitude of the original *in vivo* responses. The magnitude of immune response to synthetic peptides must be further assessed before their usefulness is established.

12. CONCLUSIONS

Class I- and class II-restricted epitopes are located throughout the HIV-1 env protein. The analysis of these epitopes has provided new insights into antigen processing pathways and vaccine design strategies. It is likely that the env protein of HIV-1 will become the best understood viral antigen and that knowledge gained from the study of epitopes in the env protein will be useful in the design of vaccines for other viral illnesses.

REFERENCES

Achour, A., Picard, O., M'Bika, J. P., Willer, A., Snart, R., Bizzini, B., Carelli, C., Burny, A., and Zagury, D., 1993, Envelope protein and p18(IIIB) peptide recognized by cytotoxic T lymphocytes from humans immunized with human immunodeficiency virus envelope, *Vaccine* **11**:609–701.

Achour, A., Lemhammedi, S., Picard, O., M'Bika, J. P., Zagury, J. F., Moukrim, Z., Willer, A., Beix, F., Burny, A., and Zagury, D., 1994, Cytotoxic T lymphocytes specific for HIV-1 gp160 antigen and synthetic P18IIIB peptide in an HLA-A11-immunized individual, *AIDS Res. Hum. Retrovir.* **10**:19–25.

Aichele, P., Hengartner, H., Zinkernagel, R. M., and Schulz, M., 1990, Antiviral cytotoxic T cell response induced by in vivo priming with a free synthetic peptide, *J. Exp. Med.* **171**:1815–1820.

Akiyama, K., Yokota, K., Kagawa, S., Shimbara, N., Tamura, T., Akioka, H., Nothwang, H. G., Noda, C., Tanaka, K., and Ichihara, A., 1994, cDNA cloning and interferon gamma down-regulation of proteasomal subunits X and Y, *Science* **265**:1231–1234.

Allan, J. S., Coligan, J. E., Barin, F., McLane, M. F., Sodroski, J. G., Rosen, C. A., Haseltine, W. A., Lee, T. H., and Essex, M., 1985, Major glycoprotein antigens that induce antibodies in AIDS patients are encoded by HTLV-III, *Science* **228**:1091–1094.

Amigorena, S., Drake, J. R., Webster, P., and Mellman, I., 1994, Transient accumulation of new class II MHC molecules in a novel endocytic compartment in B lymphocytes [see comments], *Nature* **369**:113–120.

Attaya, M., Jameson, S., Martinez, C. K., Hermel, E., Aldrich, C., Forman, J., Lindahl, K. F., Bevan, M. J., and Monaco, J. J., 1992, Ham-2 corrects the class I antigen-processing defect in RMA-S cells, *Nature* **355**: 647–649.

Baier, G., Baierbitterlich, G., Looney, D. J., and Altman, A., 1995, Immunogenic targeting of recombinant peptide vaccines to human antigen-presenting cells by chimeric anti-HLA-DR and anti-surface immunoglobulin D antibody Fab fragments in vitro, *J. Virol.* **69**:2357–2365.

Belich, M. P., Glynne, R. J., Senger, G., Sheer, D., and Trowsdale, J., 1994, Proteasome components with reciprocal expression to that of the MHC-encoded LMP proteins, *Curr. Biol.* **4**:769–776.

Bell, S. J., Cooper, D. A., Kemp, B. E., Doherty, R. R., and Penny, R., 1992, Definition of an immunodominant T cell epitope contained in the envelope gp41 sequence of HIV-1, *Clin. Exp. Immunol.* **87**:37–45.

Bergmann, C. C., Tong, L., Cua, R. V., Sensintaffar, J. L., and Stohlman, S. A., 1994, Cytotoxic T cell repertoire selection. A single amino acid determines alternative class I restriction, *J. Immunol.* **152**:5603–5612.

Berzofsky, J. A., Bensussan, A., Cease, K. B., Bourge, J. F., Cheynier, R., Lurhuma, Z., Salaun, J. J., Gallo, R. C., Shearer, G. M., and Zagury, D., 1988, Antigenic peptides recognized by T lymphocytes from AIDS viral envelope-immune humans, *Nature* **334**:706–708.

Bjorkman, P. J., Saper, M. A., Samraoui, B., Bennett, W. S., Strominger, J. L., and Wiley, D. C., 1987, The foreign antigen binding site and T cell recognition regions of class I histocompatibility antigens, *Nature* **329**:512–518.

Boehncke, W. H., Takeshita, T., Pendleton, C. D., Houghten, R. A., Sadegh, N. S., Racioppi, L., Berzofsky, J. A., and Germain, R. N., 1993, The importance of dominant negative effects of amino acid side chain substitution in peptide–MHC molecule interactions and T cell recognition, *J. Immunol.* **150**:331–341.

Bollinger, R. C., Quinn, T. C., Liu, A. Y., Stanhope, P. E., Hammond, S. A., Viveen, R., Clements, M. L., and Siliciano, R. F., 1993, Cytokines from vaccine-induced HIV-1 specific cytotoxic T lymphocytes: Effects on viral replication, *AIDS Res. Hum. Retrovir.* **9**:1067–1077.

Bollinger, R. C., Egan, M. A., Chun, T., Mathieson, B., and Siliciano, R. F., 1996, Cellular immune responses to HIV-1 in progressive and non-progressive infections [review], *AIDS* (in press).

Borkowsky, W., Krasinski, K., Moore, T., and Papaevangelou, V., 1990, Lymphocyte proliferative responses to HIV-1 envelope and core antigens by infected and uninfected adults and children, *AIDS Res. Hum. Retrovir.* **6**:673–678.

Botarelli, P., Houlden, B. A., Haigwood, N. L., Servis, C., Montagna, D., and Abrignani, S., 1991, N-glycosylation of HIV-gp120 may constrain recognition by T lymphocytes, *J. Immunol.* **147**:3128–3132.

Brander, C., Pichler, W. J., and Corradin, G., 1995, Identification of HIV protein-derived cytotoxic T lymphocyte (CTL) epitopes for their possible use as synthetic vaccine, *Clin. Exp. Immunol.* **101**:107–113.

Brown, J. H., Jardetzky, T. S., Gorga, J. C., Stern, L. J., Urban, R. G., Strominger, J. L., and Wiley, D. C., 1993,

Three-dimensional structure of the human class II histocompatibility antigen HLA-DR1 [see comments], *Nature* **364:**33–39.

Brown, L. E., White, D. O., Agius, C., Kemp, B. E., Yatzakis, N., Poumbourios, P., Mcphee, D. A., and Jackson, D. C., 1995, Synthetic peptides representing sequences within gp41 of HIV as immunogens for murine T- and B-cell responses, *Arch. Virol.* **140:**635–654.

Callahan, K. M., Fort, M. M., Obah, E. A., Reinherz, E. L., and Siliciano, R. F., 1990, Genetic variability in HIV-1 gp120 affects interactions with HLA molecules and T cell receptor, *J. Immunol.* **144:**3341–3346.

Carbone, F. R., and Bevan, M. J., 1989, Induction of ovalbumin-specific cytotoxic T cells by in vivo peptide immunization, *J. Exp. Med.* **169:**603–612.

Casement, K. S., Nehete, P. N., Arlinghaus, R. B., and Sastry, K. J., 1995, Cross-reactive cytotoxic T lymphocytes induced by V3 loop synthetic peptides from different strains of human immunodeficiency virus type 1, *Virology* **211:**261–267.

Cease, K. B., Margalit, H., Cornette, J. L., Putney, S. D., Robey, W. G., Ouyang, C., Streicher, H. Z., Fischinger, P. J., Gallo, R. C., DeLisi, C., and Berzofsky, J. A., 1987, Helper T-cell antigenic site identification in the acquired immunodeficiency syndrome virus gp120 envelope protein and induction of immunity in mice to the native protein using a 16-residue synthetic peptide [published erratum appears in *Proc. Natl. Acad. Sci. USA* 1988 **85:**8226], *Proc. Natl. Acad. Sci. USA* **84:**4249–4253.

Charbit, A., Martineau, P., Ronco, J., Leclerc, C., Lo, M. R., Michel, V., O'Callaghan, D., and Hofnung, M., 1993, Expression and immunogenicity of the V3 loop from the envelope of human immunodeficiency virus type 1 in an attenuated aroA strain of Salmonella typhimurium upon genetic coupling to two Escherichia coli carrier proteins, *Vaccine* **11:**1221–1228.

Chen, Z. W., Shen, L., Miller, M. D., Ghim, S. H., Hughes, A. L., and Letvin, N. L., 1992, Cytotoxic T lymphocytes do not appear to select for mutations in an immunodominant epitope of simian immunodeficiency virus gag. *J. Immunol.* **149:**4060–4066.

Cheynier, R., Langlade, D. P., Marescot, M. R., Blanche, S., Blondin, G., Wain, H. S., Griscelli, C., Vilmer, E., and Plata, F., 1992, Cytotoxic T lymphocyte responses in the peripheral blood of children born to human immunodeficiency virus-1-infected mothers, *Eur. J. Immunol.* **22:** 2211–2217.

Choppin, J., Martinon, F., Gomard, E., Bahraoui, E., Connan, F., Bouillot, M., and Levy, J. P., 1990, Analysis of physical interactions between peptides and HLA molecules and application to the detection of human immunodeficiency virus 1 antigenic peptides, *J. Exp. Med.* **172:**889–899.

Clerici, M., Stocks, N. I., Zajac, R. A., Boswell, R. N., Bernstein, D. C., Mann, D. L., Shearer, G. M., and Berzofsky, J. A., 1989, Interleukin-2 production used to detect antigenic peptide recognition by T-helper lymphocytes from asymptomatic HIV-seropositive individuals, *Nature* **339:**383–385.

Clerici, M., Berzofsky, J. A., Shearer, G. M., and Tacket, C. O., 1991a, Exposure to human immunodeficiency virus (HIV) type I indicated by HIV-specific T helper cell responses before detection of infection by polymerase chain reaction and serum antibodies [corrected] [published erratum appears in *J. Infect Dis.* 1991 **164:**832], *J. Infect. Dis.* **164:**178–182.

Clerici, M., Lucey, D. R., Zajac, R. A., Boswell, R. N., Gebel, H. M., Takahashi, H., Berzofsky, J. A., and Shearer, G. M., 1991b. Detection of cytotoxic T lymphocytes specific for synthetic peptides of gp160 in HIV-seropositive individuals, *J. Immunol.* **146:**2214–2219.

Clerici, M., Giorgi, J. V., Chou, C. C., Gudeman, V. K., Zack, J. A., Gupta, P., Ho, H. N., Nishanian, P. G., Berzofsky, J. A., and Shearer, G. M., 1992, Cell-mediated immune response to human immunodeficiency virus (HIV) type 1 in seronegative homosexual men with recent sexual exposure to HIV-1 [see comments], *J. Infect. Dis.* **165:**1012–1019.

Clerici, M., Shearer, G., Hounsell, E. F., Jameson, B., Habeshaw, J., and Dalgleish, A. G., 1993a, Alloactivated cytotoxic T cells recognize the carboxy-terminal domain of human immunodeficiency virus-1 gp120 envelope glycoprotein, *Eur. J. Immunol.* **23:**2022–2025.

Clerici, M., Sison, A. V., Berzofsky, J. A., Rakusan, T. A., Brandt, C. D., Ellauri, M., Villa, M., Colie, C., Venzon, D. J., Sever, J. L., and Shearer, J. M., 1993b, Cellular immune factors associated with mother-to-infant transmission of HIV, *AIDS* **7:**1427–1433.

Clerici, M., Levin, J. M., Kessler, H. A., Harris, A., Berzofsky, J. A., Landay, A. L., and Shearer, G. M., 1994, HIV-specific T-helper activity in seronegative health care workers exposed to contaminated blood, *J. Am. Med. Assoc.* **271:**42–46.

Collins, E. J., Garboczi, D. N., and Wiley, D. C., 1994, Three-dimensional structure of a peptide extending from one end of a class I MHC binding site, *Nature* **371:**626–629.

Cooney, E. L., Collier, A. C., Greenberg, P. D., Coombs, R. W., Zarling, J., Arditti, D. E., Hoffman, M. C., Hu, S. L., and Corey, L., 1991, Safety of and immunological response to a recombinant vaccinia virus vaccine expressing HIV envelope glycoprotein [see comments], *Lancet* **337**:567–572.

Cooney, E. L., McElrath, M. J., Corey, L., Hu, S. L., Collier, A. C., Arditti, D., Hoffman, M., Coombs, R. W., Smith, G. E., and Greenberg, P. D., 1993, Enhanced immunity to human immunodeficiency virus (HIV) envelope elicited by a combined vaccine regimen consisting of priming with a vaccinia recombinant expressing HIV envelope and boosting with gp160 protein, *Proc. Natl. Acad. Sci. USA* **90**:1882–1886.

Dadaglio, G., Leroux, A., Langlade, D. P., Bahraoui, E. M., Traincard, F., Fisher, R., and Plata, F., 1991, Epitope recognition of conserved HIV envelope sequences by human cytotoxic T lymphocytes, *J. Immunol.* **147:** 2302–2309.

Dai, L. C., West, K., Littaua, R., Takahashi, K., and Ennis, F. A., 1992, Mutation of human immunodeficiency virus type 1 at amino acid 5858 on gp41 results in loss of killing by CD8+ A24-restricted cytotoxic T lymphocytes, *J. Virol.* **66**:3151–3154.

DeMaria, A., Cirillo, C., and Moretta, L., 1994, Occurrence of human immunodeficiency virus type 1 (HIV-1)-specific cytolytic T cell activity in apparently uninfected children born to HIV-1-infected mothers, *J. Infect. Dis.* **170**:1296–1299.

Deprez, B., Gras, M. H., Martinon, F., Gomard, E., Levy, J. P., and Tartar, A., 1995, Pimelautide or trimexautide as built-in adjuvants associated with an HIV-1-derived peptide: Synthesis and in vivo induction of antibody and virus-specific cytotoxic T-lymphocyte-mediated response, *J. Med. Chem.* **38**:459–465.

DeVita, V. T., Jr., Hellman, S., Rosenberg, S. A., and Allen, J. R., eds., 1988, *AIDS: Etiology, Diagnosis, Treatment and Prevention*, second edition, Lippincott, Philadelphia.

Dolin, R., Graham, B. S., Greenberg, S. B., Tacket, C. O., Belshe, R. B., Midthun, K., Clements, M. L., Gorse, G. J., Horgan, B. W., Atmar, R. L., Karzon, D. T., Bonnez, W., Fernie, B. F., Montefiori, D. C., Stablein, D. M., Smith, G. E., and Koff, W. C., 1991, The safety and immunogenicity of a human immunodeficiency virus type 1 (HIV-1) recombinant gp160 candidate vaccine in humans. NIAID AIDS Vaccine Clinical Trials Network, *Ann. Intern. Med.* **114**:119–127.

Dupuis, M., Kundu, S. K., and Merigan, T. C., 1995, Characterization of HLA-A-*-0201-restricted cytotoxic T cell epitopes in conserved regions of the HIV type 1 gp160 protein, *J. Immunol.* **155**:2232–2239.

Earl, P. L., Doms, R. W., and Moss, B., 1990, Oligomeric structure of the human immunodeficiency virus type 1 envelope glycoprotein, *Proc. Natl. Acad. Sci. USA* **87**:648–652.

Earl, P. L., Koenig, S., and Moss, B., 1991, Biological and immunological properties of human immunodeficiency virus type 1 envelope glycoprotein: Analysis of proteins with truncations and deletions expressed by recombinant vaccinia viruses, *J. Virol.* **65**:31–41.

Egan, M. A., Pavlat, W. A., Tartaglia, J., Paoletti, E., Weinhold, K. J., Clements, M. L., and Siliciano, R. F., 1995, Induction of human immunodeficiency virus type 1 (HIV-1)-specific cytolytic T lymphocyte responses in seronegative adults by a nonreplicating, host-range-restricted canarypox vector (ALVAC) carrying the HIV-1MN env gene, *J. Infect. Dis.* **171**:1623–1627.

Eriksson, K., Horal, P., Svennerholm, B., Jeansson, S., Vahlne, A., Holmgen, J., and Czerkinsky, C., 1993, Systematic identification of T-cell activating epitopes on the human immunodeficiency virus type 1 envelope glycoprotein gp120 in primates immunized with synthetic peptides, *Vaccine* **11**:859–865.

Estaquier, J., Boutillon, C., Gras, M. H., Ameisen, J. C., Capron, A., Tartar, A., and Auriault, C., 1993, Comprehensive delineation of antigenic and immunogenic properties of peptides derived from the nef HIV-1 regulatory protein [review], *Vaccine* **11**:1083–1092.

Falo, L. J., Colarusso, L. J., Benacerraf, B., and Rock, K. L., 1992, Serum proteases alter the antigenicity of peptides presented by class I major histocompatibility complex molecules, *Proc. Natl. Acad. Sci. USA* **89**:8347–8350.

Fayolle, C., Deriaud, E., and Leclerc, C., 1991, In vivo induction of cytotoxic T cell response by a free synthetic peptide requires CD4+ T cell help, *J. Immunol.* **147**:4069–4073.

Fernandez, M. H., Faith, A., Higgins, J. A., Weber, J., and Rees, A., 1995, The effect of a single amino acid substitution within the V3 loop of HIV-1 gp120 on HLA-DR1-restricted CD4 T-cell recognition, *Immunology* **85**:176–183.

Ferris, R. L., Shen, X. F., Buck, C., Hammond, S. A., Woods, A. S., Cotter, R. J., Takiguchi, M., Igarashi, Y., Ichikawa, Y., and Siliciano, R. F., 1996, Class I-restricted presentation of an HIV-1 gp41 epitope containing an N-linked glycosylation site: Implications for the mechanism of processing of viral envelope proteins, *J. Immunol.* **156**:834–840.

Fisher, A. G., Ensoli, B., Looney, D., Rose, A., Gallo, R. C., Saag, M. S., Shaw, G. M., Hahn, B. H., and Wong, S. F., 1988, Biologically diverse molecular variants within a single HIV-1 isolate, *Nature* **334**:444–447.

Fruh, K., Gossen, M., Wang, K., Bujard, H., Peterson, P. A., and Yang, Y., 1994, Displacement of housekeeping proteasome subunits by MHC-encoded LMPs: A newly discovered mechanism for modulating the multicatalytic proteinase complex, *EMBO J.* **13**:3236–3244.

Gao, X. M., Zheng, B., Liew, F. Y., Brett, S., and Tite, J., 1991, Priming of influenza virus-specific cytotoxic T lymphocytes in vivo by short synthetic peptides, *J. Immunol.* **147**:3268–3273.

Gelderblom, H. R., Reupke, H., and Pauli, G., 1985, Loss of envelope antigens of HTLV-III/LAV, a factor in AIDS pathogenesis? [letter], *Lancet* **2**:1016–1017.

Gelderblom, H. R., Hausmann, E. H., Ozel, M., Pauli, G., and Koch, M. A., 1987, Fine structure of human immunodeficiency virus (HIV) and immunolocalization of structural proteins, *Virology* **156**:171–176.

Gorse, G. J., Belshe, R. B., Newman, F. K., and Frey, S. E., 1992, Lymphocyte proliferative responses following immunization with human immunodeficiency virus recombinant GP160. The NIAID AIDS Vaccine Clinical Trials Network, *Vaccine* **10**:383–388.

Guagliardi, L. E., Koppelman, B., Blum, J. S., Marks, M. S., Cresswell, P., and Brodsky, F. M., 1990, Colocalization of molecules involved in antigen processing and presentation in an early endocytic compartment [review], *Nature* **343**:133–139.

Hahn, B. H., Gonda, M. A., Shaw, G. M., Popovic, M., Hoxie, J. A., Gallo, R. C., and Wong, S. F., 1985, Genomic diversity of the acquired immune deficiency syndrome virus HTLV-III: Different viruses exhibit greatest divergence in their envelope genes, *Proc. Natl. Acad. Sci. USA* **82**:4813–4817.

Hahn, B. H., Shaw, G. M., Taylor, M. E., Redfield, R. R., Markham, P. D., Salahuddin, S. Z., Wong, S. F., Gallo, R. C., Parks, E. S., and Parks, W. P., 1986, Genetic variation in HTLV-III/LAV over time in patients with AIDS or at risk for AIDS, *Science* **232**:1548–1553.

Hammond, S. A., Obah, E., Stanhope, P., Monell, C. R., Strand, M., Robbins, F. M., Bias, W. B., Karr, R. W., Koenig, S., and Siliciano, R. F., 1991, Characterization of a conserved T cell epitope in HIV-1 gp41 recognized by vaccine-induced human cytolytic T cells, *J. Immunol.* **146**:1470–1477.

Hammond, S. A., Bollinger, R. C., Stanhope, P. E., Quinn, T. C., Schwartz, D., Clements, M. L., and Siliciano, R. F., 1992, Comparative clonal analysis of human immunodeficiency virus type 1 (HIV-1)-specific CD4+ and CD8+ cytolytic T lymphocytes isolated from seronegative humans immunized with candidate HIV-1 vaccines, *J. Exp. Med.* **176**:1531–1542.

Hammond, S. A., Johnson, R. P., Kalams, S. A., Walker, B. D., Takiguchi, M., Safrit, J. T., Koup, R. A., and Siliciano, R. F., 1995, An epitope-selective transporter associated with antigen presentation (TAP)-1/2-independent pathway and a more general TAP-1/2-dependent antigen-processing pathway allow recognition of the HIV-1 envelope glycoprotein by CD8+ CTL, *J. Immunol.* **154**:6140–6156.

Hart, M. K., Weinhold, K. J., Scearce, R. M., Washburn, E. M., Clark, C. A., Palker, T. J., and Haynes, B. F., 1991, Priming of anti-human immunodeficiency virus (HIV) CD8+ cytotoxic T cells in vivo by carrier-free HIV synthetic peptides, *Proc. Natl. Acad. Sci. USA* **88**:9448–9452.

Haynes, B. F., Yasutomi, Y., Torres, J. V., Gardner, M. B., Langlios, A. J., Bolognesi, D. P., Matthews, T. J., Scearce, R. M., Jones, D. M., Moody, M. A., McDanal, C., Heinly, C., Bergamo, B., Palker, T. J., and Letvin, N. L., 1993, Use of synthetic peptides in primates to induce high-titered neutralizing antibodies and MHC class I-restricted cytotoxic T cells against acquired immunodeficiency syndrome retroviruses: An HLA-based vaccine strategy, *Trans. Assoc. Am. Physicians* **106**:33–41.

Heath, S. L., Tew, J. G., Szakal, A. K., and Burton, G. F., 1995, Follicular dendritic cells and human immunodeficiency virus infectivity, *Nature* **377**:740–744.

Heemels, M. T., and Ploegh, H., 1995, Generation, translocation, and presentation of MHC class I-restricted peptides [review], *Annu. Rev. Biochem.* **64**:463–491.

Hosmalin, A., Nara, P. L., Zweig, M., Lerche, N. W., Cease, K. B., Gard, E. A., Markham, P. D., Putney, S. D., Daniel, M. D., Desrosiers, R. C., and Berzofsky, J. A., 1991, Priming with T helper cell epitope peptides enhances the antibody response to the envelope glycoprotein of HIV-1 in primates, *J. Immunol.* **146**:1667–1673.

Howard, J. C., 1995, Supply and transport of peptides presented by class I MHC molecules [review], *Curr. Opin. Immunol.* **7**:69–76.

Huang, A. Y., Golumbek, P., Ahmadzadeh, M., Jaffee, E., Pardoll, D., and Levitsky, H., 1994, Bone marrow-derived cells present MHC class I-restricted tumour antigens in priming of antitumour immune responses [review], *Ciba Found. Symp.* **187**:229–240.

Ishioka, G. Y., Colon, S., Miles, C., Grey, H. M., and Chesnut, R. W., 1989, Induction of class I MHC-restricted, peptide-specific cytolytic T lymphocytes by peptide priming in vivo, *J. Immunol.* **143**:1094–1100.

Ishioka, G. Y., Lamont, A. G., Thomson, D., Bulbow, N., Gaeta, F. C., Sette, A., and Grey, H. M., 1992, MHC interaction and T cell recognition of carbohydrates and glycopeptides, *J. Immunol.* **148**:2446–2451.

Jassoy, C., Johnson, R. P., Navia, B. A., Worth, J., and Walker, B. D., 1992, Detection of a vigorous HIV-1-specific cytotoxic T lymphocyte response in cerebrospinal fluid from infected persons with AIDS dementia complex, *J. Immunol.* **149:**3113–3119.

Jassoy, C., Harrer, T., Rosenthal, T., Navia, B. A., Worth, J., Johnson, R. P., and Walker, B. D., 1993, Human immunodeficiency virus type 1-specific cytotoxic T lymphocytes release gamma interferon, tumor necrosis factor alpha (TNF-alpha), and TNF-beta when they encounter their target antigens, *J. Virol.* **67:**2844–2852.

Johnson, R. P., Trocha, A. Buchanan, T. M., and Walker, B. D., 1992, Identification of overlapping HLA class I-restricted cytotoxic T cell epitopes in a conserved region of the human immunodeficiency virus type 1 envelope glycoprotein: Definition of minimum epitopes and analysis of the effects of sequence variation, *J. Exp. Med.* **175:**961–971.

Johnson, R. P., Trocha, A., Buchanan, T. M., and Walker, B. D., 1993, Recognition of a highly conserved region of human immunodeficiency virus type 1 gp120 by an HLA-Cw4-restricted cytotoxic T-lymphocyte clone, *J. Virol.* **67:**438–445.

Johnson, R. P., Hammond, S. A., Trocha, A., Siliciano, R. F., and Walker, B. D., 1994a, Induction of a major histocompatibility complex class I-restricted cytotoxic T-lymphocyte response to a highly conserved region of human immunodeficiency virus type 1 (HIV-1) gp120 in seronegative humans immunized with a candidate HIV-1 vaccine, *J. Virol.* **68:**3145–3153.

Johnson, R. P., Hammond, S. A., Trocha, A., Siliciano, R. F., and Walker, B. D., 1994b, Epitope specificity of MHC restricted cytotoxic T lymphocytes induced by candidate HIV-1 vaccine, *AIDS Res. Hum. Retrovir.* **10**(Suppl. 2)**:**573–575.

Kahn, J. O., Stites, D. P., Scillian, J., Murcar, N., Stryker, R., Volberding, P. A., Naylor, P. H., Goldstein, A. L., Sarin, P. S., Simmon, V. F., Warg, S. S., and Heseltine, P., 1992, A phase I study of HGP-30, a 30 amino acid subunit of the human immunodeficiency virus (HIV) p17 synthetic peptide analogue sub-unit vaccine in seronegative subjects, *AIDS Res. Hum. Retrovir.* **8:**1321–1325.

Kalams, S. A., and Walker, B. D., 1994, The cytotoxic T-lymphocyte response in HIV-1 infection [review], *Clin. Lab. Med.* **14:**271–299.

Kalams, S. A., Johnson, R. P., Trocha, A. K., Dynan, M. J., Ngo, H. S., D'Aquila, R. T., Kurnick, J. T., and Walker, B. D., 1994, Longitudinal analysis of T cell receptor (TCR) gene usage by human immunodeficiency virus 1 envelope-specific cytotoxic T lymphocyte clones reveals a limited TCR repertoire, *J. Exp. Med.* **179:**1261–1271.

Kameoka, M., Nishino, Y., Matsuo, K., Ohara, N., Kimura, T., Yamazaki, A., Yamada, T., and Ikuta, K., 1994, Cytotoxic T lymphocyte response in mice induced by a recombinant BCG vaccination which produces an extracellular alpha antigen that fused with the human immunodeficiency virus type 1 envelope immunodominant domain in the V3 loop, *Vaccine* **12:**153–158.

Kelker, H. C., Seidlin, M., Vogler, M., and Valentine, F. T., 1992, Lymphocytes from some long-term seronegative heterosexual partners of HIV-infected individuals proliferate in response to HIV antigens, *AIDS Res. Hum. Retrovir.* **8:**1355–1359.

Kelly, A., Powis, S. H., Kerr, L. A., Mockridge, I., Elliott, T., Bastin, J., Uchanska, Z. B., Ziegler, A., Trowsdale, J., and Townsend, A., 1992, Assembly and function of the two ABC transporter proteins encoded in the human major histocompatibility complex, *Nature* **355:**641–644.

Kingsman, A. J., Burns, N. R., Layton, G. T., and Adams, S. E., 1995, Yeast retrotransposon particles as antigen delivery systems, *Ann. N.Y. Acad. Sci.* **754:**202–213.

Kleijmeer, M. J., Kelly, A., Geuze, H. J., Slot, J. W., Townsend, A., and Trowsdale, J., 1992, Location of MHC-encoded transporters in the endoplasmic reticulum and cis-Golgi, *Nature* **357:**342–344.

Koenig, S., Earl, P., Powell, D., Pantaleo, G., Merli, S., Moss, B., and Fauci, A. S., 1988, Group-specific, major histocompatibility complex class I-restricted cytotoxic responses to human immunodeficiency virus 1 (HIV-1) envelope proteins by cloned peripheral blood T cells from an HIV-1-infected individual, *Proc. Natl. Acad. Sci. USA* **85:**8638–8642.

Koup, R. A., Safrit, J. T., Cao, Y., Andrews, C. A., McLeod, G., Borkowsky, W., Farthing, C., and Ho, D. D., 1994, Temporal association of cellular immune responses with the initial control of viremia in primary human immunodeficiency virus type 1 syndrome, *J. Virol.* **68:**4650–4655.

Kozlowski, S., Corr, M., Takeshita, T., Boyd, L. F., Pendleton, C. D., Germain, R. N., Berzofsky, J. A., and Margulies, D. H., 1992, Serum angiotensin-1 converting enzyme activity processes a human immunodeficiency virus 1 gp160 peptide for presentation by major histocompatibility complex class I molecules, *J. Exp. Med.* **175:**1417–1422.

Kozlowski, S., Corr, M., Shirai, M., Boyd, L. F., Pendleton, C. D., Berzofsky, J. A., and Margulies, D. H., 1993,

Multiple pathways are involved in the extracellular processing of MHC class I-restricted peptides, *J. Immunol.* **151:**4033–4044.

Krowka, J., Stites, D., Debs, R., Larsen, C., Fedor, J., Brunette, E., and Duzgunes, N., 1990, Lymphocyte proliferative responses to soluble and liposome-conjugated envelope peptides of HIV-1, *J. Immunol.* **144:** 2535–2540.

Langlade, D. P., Ngo, G., Huong, N., Ferchal, F., and Oksenhendler, E., 1994, Human immunodeficiency virus (HIV) nef-specific cytotoxic T lymphocytes in noninfected heterosexual contact of HIV-infected patients [see comments], *J. Clin. Invest.* **93:**1293–1297.

Lasarte, J. J., Sarobe, P., Gullon, A., Prieto, J., and Borras, C. F., 1992, Induction of cytotoxic T lymphocytes in mice against the principal neutralizing domain of HIV-1 by immunization with an engineered T-cytotoxic–T-helper synthetic peptide construct, *Cell. Immunol.* **141:**211–218.

Lasarte, J. J., Sarobe, P., Prieto, J., and Borrascuesta, F., 1995, In vivo cytotoxic T-lymphocyte induction may take place via CD8(+) T helper lymphocytes, *Res. Immunol.* **146:**35–44.

Lasky, L. A., Nakamura, G., Smith, D. H., Fennie, C., Shimasaki, C., Patzer, E., Berman, P., Gregory, T., and Capon, D. J., 1987, Delineation of a region of the human immunodeficiency virus type 1 gp120 glycoprotein critical for interaction with the CD4 receptor, *Cell* **50:**975–985.

Layton, G. T., Harris, S. J., Gearing, A. J., Hill, P. M., Cole, J. S., Griffiths, J. C., Burns, N. R., Kingsman, A. J., and Adams, S. E., 1993, Induction of HIV-specific cytotoxic T lymphocytes in vivo with hybrid HIV-1 V3:Ty-virus-like particles, *J. Immunol.* **151:**1097–1107.

Lieberman, J., Fabry, J. A., Kuo, M. C., Earl, P., Moss, B., and Skolnik, P. R., 1992, Cytotoxic T lymphocytes from HIV-1 seropositive individuals recognize immunodominant epitopes in Gp160 and reverse transcriptase, *J. Immunol.* **148:**2738–2747.

Lusso, P., Markham, P. D., Ranki, A., Earl, P., Moss, B., Dorner, F., Gallo, R. C., and Krohn, K. J., 1988, Cell-mediated immune response toward viral envelope and core antigens in gibbon apes (Hylobates lar) chronically infected with human immunodeficiency virus-1, *J. Immunol.* **141:**2467–2473.

Macatonia, S. E., Patterson, S., and Knight, S. C., 1991, Primary proliferative and cytotoxic T-cell responses to HIV induced in vitro by human dendritic cells, *Immunology* **74:**399–406.

Manca, F., Habeshaw, J., and Dalgleish, A., 1991, The naive repertoire of human T helper cells specific for gp120, the envelope glycoprotein of HIV, *J. Immunol.* **146:**1964–1971.

Manca, F., Habeshaw, J. A., Dalgleish, A. G., Fenoglio, D., Li, P. G., and Sercarz, E. E., 1993, Role of flanking variable sequences in antigenicity of consensus regions of HIV gp120 for recognition by specific human T helper clones, *Eur. J. Immunol.* **23:**269–274.

Miskovsky, E. P., Liu, A. Y., Pavlat, W., Viveen, R., Stanhope, P. E., Finzi, D., Fox, W., Hruban, R. H., Podack, E. R., and Siliciano, R. F., 1994, Studies of the mechanism of cytolysis by HIV-1-specific CD4+ human CTL clones induced by candidate AIDS vaccines, *J. Immunol.* **153:**2787–2799.

Modrow, S., Hahn, B. H., Shaw, G. M., Gallo, R. C., Wong, S. F., and Wolf, H., 1987, Computer-assisted analysis of envelope protein sequences of seven human immunodeficiency virus isolates: Prediction of antigenic epitopes in conserved and variable regions, *J. Virol.* **61:**570–578.

Monaco, J. J., Cho, S., and Attaya, M., 1990, Transport protein genes in the murine MHC: Possible implications for antigen processing, *Science* **250:**1723–1726.

Moore, J. P., McKeating, J. A., Weiss, R. A., and Sattentau, Q. J., 1990, Dissociation of gp120 from HIV-1 virions induced by soluble CD4 [see comments], *Science* **250:**1139–1142.

Moore, M. W., Carbone, F. R., and Bevan, M. J., 1988, Introduction of soluble protein into the class I pathway of antigen processing and presentation, *Cell* **54:**777–785.

Moore, R. L., and Fox, B. S., 1993, Immunization of mice with human immunodeficiency virus glycoprotein gp160 peptide 315–329 induces both class I- and class II-restricted T cells: Not all T cells can respond to whole molecule stimulation, *AIDS Res. Hum. Retrovir.* **9:**51–59.

Moore, R. L., and Fox, B. S., 1994, CD4+ class I-restricted T cells specific for HIV gp160 315–329, *Cell. Immunol.* **154:**43–53.

Morrison, L. A., Lukacher, A. E., Braciale, V. L., Fan, D. P., and Braciale, T. J., 1986, Differences in antigen presentation to MHC class I- and class II-restricted influenza virus-specific cytolytic T lymphocyte clones, *J. Exp. Med.* **163:**903–921.

Moukrim, Z., and Achour, A., 1995, Cytotoxic T lymphocytes specific for the synthetic VEINCTR peptide, a sequence found within the fas molecule and env gp120 in the blood of HIV-1 seropositive individuals, *Cell. Mol. Biol.* **41:**439–444.

Nardelli, B., and Tam, J. P., 1993, Cellular immune responses induced by in vivo priming with a lipid-conjugated multimeric antigen peptide, *Immunology* **79**:355–361.

Nehete, P. N., Satterfield, W. C., Matherne, C. M., Arlinghaus, R. B., and Sastry, K. J., 1993, Induction of human immunodeficiency virus-specific T cell responses in rhesus monkeys by synthetic peptides from gp160, *AIDS Res. Hum. Retrovir.* **9**:235–240.

Nehete, P. N., Casement, K. S., Arlinghaus, R. B., and Sastry, K. J., 1995a, Studies on in vivo induction of HIV-1 envelope-specific cytotoxic T lymphocytes by synthetic peptides from the V3 loop region of HIV-1 IIIB gp120, *Cell. Immunol.* **160**:217–223.

Nehete, P. M., Murthy, K. K., Satterfield, W. C., Arlinghaus, R. B., and Sastry, K. J., 1995b, Studies on V3-specific cross-reactive T-cell responses in chimpanzees chronically infected with HIV-1(IIIB), *AIDS* **9**:567–572.

Okuda, K., Bukawa, H., Hamajima, K., Kawamoto, S., Sekigawa, K. I., Yamada, Y., Tanaka, S. I., Ishii, N., Aoki, I., Nakamura, M., Yamamoto, H., Cullen, B. R., and Fukushima, J., 1995, Induction of potent humoral and cell-mediated immune responses following direct injection of DNA encoding the HIV type 1 env and rev gene products, *AIDS Res. Hum. Retrovir.* **11**:933–943.

Olson, R. R., Reuter, J. J., McNicholl, J., Alber, C., Klohe, E., Callahan, K., Siliciano, R. F., and Karr, R. W., 1994, Acidic residues in the DR beta chain third hypervariable region are required for stimulation of a DR(α, β 1*0402)-restricted T-cell clone, *Hum. Immunol.* **41**:193–200.

Orentas, R. J., Hildreth, J. E., Obah, E., Polydefkis, M., Smith, G. E., Clements, M. L., and Siliciano, R. F., 1990, Induction of CD4+ human cytolytic T cells specific for HIV-infected cells by a gp160 subunit vaccine, *Science* **248**:1234–1237.

Ortmann, B., Androlewicz, M. J., and Cresswell, P., 1994, MHC class I/beta 2-microglobulin complexes associate with TAP transporters before peptide binding, *Nature* **368**:864–867.

Phillips, R. E., Rowland, J. S., Nixon, D. F., Gotch, F. M., Edwards, J. P., Ogunlesi, A. O., Elvin, J. G., Rothbard, J. A., Bangham, C. R., Rizza, C. R., and McMichael, A. J., 1991, Human immunodeficiency virus genetic variation that can escape cytotoxic T cell recognition [see comments], *Nature* **354**:453–459.

Pinto, L. A., Sullivan, J., Berzofsky, J. A., Clerici, M., Kessler, H. A., Landay, A. L., and Shearer, G. M., 1995, Env-specific cytotoxic T lymphocyte responses in HIV seronegative health care workers occupationally exposed to HIV-contaminated body fluids, *J. Clin. Invest.* **96**:867–876.

Plata, F., Autran, B., Martins, L. P., Wain, H. S., Raphael, M., Mayaud, C., Denis, M., Guillon, J. M., and Debre, P., 1987, AIDS virus-specific cytotoxic T lymphocytes in lung disorders, *Nature* **328**:348–351.

Polydefkis, M., Koenig, S., Flexner, C., Obah, E., Gebo, K., Chakrabarti, S., Earl, P. L., Moss, B., and Siliciano, R. F., 1990, Anchor sequence-dependent endogenous processing of human immunodeficiency virus 1 envelope glycoprotein gp160 for CD4+ T cell recognition, *J. Exp. Med.* **171**:875–887.

Powis, S. J., Townsend, A. R., Deverson, E. V., Bastin, J., Butcher, G. W., and Howard, J. C., 1991, Restoration of antigen presentation to the mutant cell line RMA-S by an MHC-linked transporter, *Nature* **354**:528–531.

Praud, C., Jurcevic, S., L'Faqihi, F. E., Guiraud, M., dePreval, C., and Thomsen, M., 1994, Promiscuous and specific binding of HIV peptides to HLA-DR1 and DR103. Impact on T-cell repertoire of nonimmunized individuals, *Hum. Immunol.* **41**:56–60.

Pugliese, O., Viora, M., Camponeschi, B., Fei, P. C., Caprilli, F., Chersi, A., Evangelista, M., diMassimo, A. M., and Colizzi, V., 1992, A gp120 HIV peptide with high similarity to HLA class II beta chains enhances PPD-specific and autoreactive T cell activation. *Clin. Exp. Immunol.* **90**:170–174.

Rammensee, H. G., 1995, Chemistry of peptides associated with MHC class I and class II molecules [review], *Curr. Opin. Immunol.* **7**:85–96.

Ratto, S., Sitz, K. V., Scherer, A. M., Manca, F., Loomis, L. D., Cox, J. H., Redfield, R. R., and Birx, D. L., 1995, Establishment and characterization of human immunodeficiency virus type 1 (HIV-1) envelope-specific CD4(+) T lymphocyte lines from HIV-1-seropositive patients, *J. Infect. Dis.* **171**:1420–1430.

Redfield, R. R., Birx, D. L., Ketter, N., Tramont, E., Polonis, V., Davis, C., Brundage, J. F., Smith, G., Johnson, S., Fowler, A., Wierzba, T., Schafferman, A., Volvitz, F., Oster, C., and Burke, D. S., 1991, A phase I evaluation of the safety and immunogenicity of vaccination with recombinant gp160 in patients with early human immunodeficiency virus infection. Military Medical Consortium for Applied Retroviral Research [see comments], *N. Engl. J. Med.* **324**:1677–1684.

Reimann, J., Bohm, W., and Schirmbeck, R., 1994, Alternative processing pathways for MHC class I-restricted epitope presentation to CD8+ cytotoxic T lymphocytes [review], *Biol. Chem. Hoppe Seyler* **375**:731–736.

Robey, W. G., Safai, B., Oroszlan, S., Arthur, L. O., Gonda, M. A., Gallo, R. C., and Fischinger, P. J., 1985, Characterization of envelope and core structural gene products of HTLV-III with sera from AIDS patients, *Science* **228**:593–595.

Rock, K. L., Rothstein, L., Gamble, S., and Fleischacker, C., 1993, Characterization of antigen-presenting cells that present exogenous antigens in association with class I MHC molecules, *J. Immunol.* **150:**438–446.

Rowell, J. F., Ruff, A. L., Guarnieri, F. G., Staveleyocarroll, K., Lin, X. L., Tang, J., August, J. T., and Siliciano, R. F., 1995a, Lysosome-associated membrane protein-1-mediated targeting of the HIV-1 envelope protein to an endosomal/lysosomal compartment enhances its presentation to MHC class II-restricted T cells, *J. Immunol.* **155:**1818–1828.

Rowell, J. F., Stanhope, P. E., and Siliciano, R. F., 1995b, Endocytosis of endogenously synthesized HIV-1 envelope protein—Mechanism and role in processing for association with class II MHC, *J. Immunol.* **155:**473–488.

Rowland, J. S., Nixon, D. F., Aldhous, M. C., Gotch, F., Ariyoshi, K., Hallam, N., Kroll, J. S., Froebel, K., and McMichael, A., 1993, HIV-specific cytotoxic T-cell activity in an HIV-exposed but uninfected infant, *Lancet* **341:**860–861.

Rubinstein, A., Goldstein, H., Pettoello, M. M., Mizrachi, Y., Bloom, B. R., Furer, E., Althaus, B., Que, J. U., Hasler, T., and Cryz, S. J., 1995, Safety and immunogenicity of a V3 loop synthetic peptide conjugated to purified protein derivative in HIV-seronegative volunteers, *AIDS* **9:**243–251.

Saag, M. S., Hahn, B. H., Gibbons, J., Li, Y., Parks, E. S., Parks, W. P., and Shaw, G. M., 1988, Extensive variation of human immunodeficiency virus type-1 in vivo, *Nature* **334:**440–444.

Safrit, J. T., Lee, A. Y., Andrews, C. A., and Koup, R. A., 1994a, A region of the third variable loop of HIV-1 gp120 is recognized by HLA-B7-restricted CTLs from two acute seroconversion patients, *J. Immunol.* **153:**3822–3830.

Safrit, J. T., Andrews, C. A., Zhu, T., Ho, D. D., and Koup, R. A., 1994b, Characterization of human immunodeficiency virus type 1-specific cytotoxic T lymphocyte clones isolated during acute seroconversion: Recognition of autologous virus sequences within a conserved immunodominant epitope, *J. Exp. Med.* **179:**463–472.

Sastry, K. J., and Arlinghaus, R. B., 1991, Identification of T-cell epitopes without B-cell activity in the first and second conserved regions of the HIV Env protein, *AIDS* **5:**699–707.

Sastry, K. J., Nehete, P. N., Venkatnarayanan, S., Morkowski, J., Platsoucas, C. D., and Arlinghaus, R. B., 1992, Rapid in vivo induction of HIV-specific CD8+ cytotoxic T lymphocytes by a 15-amino acid unmodified free peptide from the immunodominant V3-loop of GP120, *Virology* **188:**502–509.

Schrier, R. D., Gnann, J. J., Landes, R., Lockshin, C. Richman, D., McCutchan, A., Kennedy, C., Oldstone, M. B., and Nelson, J. A., 1989, T cell recognition of HIV synthetic peptides in a natural infection, *J. Immunol.* **142:** 1166–1176.

Schulz, M., Zinkernagel, R. M., and Hengartner, H., 1991, Peptide-induced antiviral protection by cytotoxic T cells, *Proc. Natl. Acad. Sci. USA* **88:**991–993.

Schwander, S., Opravil, M., Luthy, R., Hanson, D. G., Schindler, J., Dawson, A., Letwin, B., and Dietrich, M., 1994, Phase I/II vaccination study of recombinant peptide F46 corresponding to the HIV-1 transmembrane protein coupled with 2.4 dinitrophenyl (DNP) Ficoll, *Infection* **22:**86–91.

Shepherd, J. C., Schumacher, T. N., Ashton, R. P., Imaeda, S., Ploegh, H. L., Janeway, C. J., and Tonegawa, S., 1993, TAP1-dependent peptide translocation in vitro is ATP dependent and peptide selective [published erratum appears in *Cell* 1993 **75:**613], *Cell* **74:**577–584.

Sherman, L. A., Burke, T. A., and Biggs, J. A., 1992, Extracellular processing of peptide antigens that bind class I major histocompatibility molecules, *J. Exp. Med.* **175:**1221–1226.

Shirai, M., Pendleton, C. D., and Berzofsky, J. A., 1992, Broad recognition of cytotoxic T cell epitopes from the HIV-1 envelope protein with multiple class I histocompatibility molecules, *J. Immunol.* **148:**1657–1667.

Shirai, M., Vacchio, M. S., Hodes, R. J., and Berzofsky, J. A., 1993, Preferential V beta usage by cytotoxic T cells cross-reactive between two epitopes of HIV-1 gp160 and degenerate in class I MHC restriction, *J. Immunol.* **151:**2283–2295.

Shirai, M., Pendleton, C. D., Ahlers, J., Takeshita, T., Newman, M., and Berzofsky, J. A., 1994, Helper-cytotoxic T lymphocyte (CTL) determinant linkage required for priming of anti-HIV CD8+ CTL in vivo with peptide vaccine constructs, *J. Immunol.* **152:**549–556.

Siliciano, R. F., Lawton, T., Knall, C., Karr, R. W., Berman, P., Gregory, T., and Reinherz, E. L., 1988, Analysis of host–virus interactions in AIDS with anti-gp120 T cell clones: Effect of HIV sequence variation and a mechanism for CD4+ cell depletion, *Cell* **54:**561–575.

Siliciano, R. F., Knall, C., Lawton, T., Berman, P., Gregory, T., and Reinherz, E. L., 1989, Recognition of HIV glycoprotein gp120 by T cells. Role of monocyte CD4 in the presentation of gp120, *J. Immunol.* **142:**1506–1511.

Skehel, J. J., Stevens, D. J., Daniels, R. S., Douglas, A. R., Knossow, M., Wilson, I. A., and Wiley, D. C., 1984, A carbohydrate side chain on hemagglutinins of Hong Kong influenza viruses inhibits recognition by a monoclonal antibody, *Proc. Natl. Acad. Sci. USA* **81:**1779–1783.

Spies, T., and DeMars, R., 1991, Restored expression of major histocompatibility class I molecules by gene transfer of a putative peptide transporter [see comments], *Nature* **351**:323–324.

Spies, T., Bresnahan, M., Bahram, S., Arnold, D., Blanck, G., Mellins, E., Pious, D., and DeMars, R., 1990, A gene in the human major histocompatibility complex class II region controlling the class I antigen presentation pathway [see comments], *Nature* **348**:744–747.

Stanhope, P. E., Clements, M. L., and Siliciano, R. F., 1993a, Human CD4+ cytolytic T lymphocyte responses to a human immunodeficiency virus type 1 gp160 subunit vaccine, *J. Infect. Dis.* **168**:92–100.

Stanhope, P. E., Liu, A. Y., Pavlat, W., Pitha, P. M., Clements, M. L., and Siliciano, R. F., 1993b, An HIV-1 envelope protein vaccine elicits a functionally complex human CD4+ T cell response that includes cytolytic T lymphocytes, *J. Immunol.* **150**:4672–4686.

Stein, B. S., and Engleman, E. G., 1990, Intracellular processing of the gp160 HIV-1 envelope precursor. Endoproteolytic cleavage occurs in a cis or medial compartment of the Golgi complex, *J. Biol. Chem.* **265**: 2640–2649.

Stern, L. J., Brown, J. H., Jardetzky, T. S., Gorga, J. C., Urban, R. G., Strominger, J. L., and Wiley, D. C., 1994, Crystal structure of the human class II MHC protein HLA-DR1 complexed with an influenza virus peptide, *Nature* **368**:215–221.

Suh, W. K., Cohen, D. M., Fruh, K., Wang, K., Peterson, P. A., and Williams, D. B., 1994, Interaction of MHC class I molecules with the transporter associated with antigen processing, *Science* **264**:1322–1326.

Takahashi, H., Cohen, J., Hosmalin, A., Cease, K. B., Houghten, R., Cornette, J. L., DeLisi, C., Moss, B., Germain, R. N., and Berzofsky, J. A., 1988, An immunodominant epitope of the human immunodeficiency virus envelope glycoprotein gp160 recognized by class I major histocompatibility complex molecule-restricted murine cytotoxic T lymphocytes, *Proc. Natl. Acad. Sci. USA* **85**:3105–3109.

Takahashi, H., Houghten, R., Putney, S. D., Margulies, D. H., Moss, B., Germain, R. N., and Berzofsky, J. A., 1989a, Structural requirements for class I MHC molecule-mediated antigen presentation and cytotoxic T cell recognition of an immunodominant determinant of the human immunodeficiency virus envelope protein, *J. Exp. Med.* **170**:2023–2035.

Takahashi, H., Merli, S., Putney, S. D., Houghten, R., Moss, B., Germain, R. N., and Berzofsky, J. A., 1989b, A single amino acid interchange yields reciprocal CTL specificities for HIV-1 gp160, *Science* **246**:118–121.

Takahashi, H., Germain, R. N., Moss, B., and Berzofsky, J. A., 1990a, An immunodominant class I-restricted cytotoxic T lymphocyte determinant of human immunodeficiency virus type 1 induces CD4 class II-restricted help for itself, *J. Exp. Med.* **171**:571–576.

Takahashi, H., Takeshita, T., Morein, B., Putney, S., Germain, R. N., and Berzofsky, J. A., 1990b, Induction of CD8+ cytotoxic T cells by immunization with purified HIV-1 envelope protein in ISCOMs [see comments], *Nature* **344**:873–875.

Takahashi, H., Dai, L. C., Fuerst, T. R., Biddison, W. E., Earl, P. L., Moss, B., and Ennis, F. A., 1991, Specific lysis of human immunodeficiency virus type 1-infected cells by a HLA-A3.1-restricted CD8+ cytotoxic T-lymphocyte clone that recognizes a conserved peptide sequence within the gp41 subunit of the envelope protein, *Proc. Natl. Acad. Sci. USA* **88**:10277–10281.

Takahashi, H., Nakagawa, Y., Yokomuro, K., and Berzofsky, J. A., 1993, Induction of CD8+ cytotoxic T lymphocytes by immunization with syngeneic irradiated HIV-1 envelope derived peptide-pulsed dendritic cells, *Int. Immunol.* **5**:849–857.

Takeshita, T., Takahashi, H., Kozlowski, S., Ahlers, J. D., Pendleton, C. D., Moore, R. L., Nakagawa, Y., Yokomuro, K., Fox, B. S., Margulies, D. H., and Berzofsky, J. A., 1995, Molecular analysis of the same HIV peptide functionally binding to both a class I and a class II MHC molecule, *J. Immunol.* **154**:1973–1986.

Townsend, A. R., Rothbard, J., Gotch, F. M., Bahadur, G., Wraith, D., and McMichael, A. J., 1986, The epitopes of influenza nucleoprotein recognized by cytotoxic T lymphocytes can be defined with short synthetic peptides, *Cell* **44**:959–968.

Trowsdale, J., Hanson, I., Mockridge, I., Beck, S., Townsend, A., and Kelly, A., 1990, Sequences encoded in the class II region of the MHC related to the 'ABC' superfamily of transporters [see comments], *Nature* **348**: 741–744.

Tulp, A., Verwoerd, D., Dobberstein, B., Ploegh, H. L., and Pieters, J., 1994, Isolation and characterization of the intracellular MHC class II compartment [see comments], *Nature* **369**:120–126.

Vahlne, A., Horal, P., Eriksson, K., Jeansson, S., Rymo, L., Hedstrom, K. G., Czerkinsky, C., Holmgren, J., and Svennerholm, B., 1991, Immunizations of monkeys with synthetic peptides disclose conserved areas on gp120 of human immunodeficiency virus type 1 associated with cross-neutralizing antibodies and T-cell recognition, *Proc. Natl. Acad. Sci. USA* **88**:10744–10748.

Van, K. L., Ashton, R. P., Ploegh, H. L., and Tonegawa, S., 1992, TAP1 mutant mice are deficient in antigen presentation, surface class I molecules, and CD4-8+ T cells, *Cell* **71**:1205–1214.

Wagner, R., Modrow, S., Boltz, T., Fliessbach, H., Niedrig, M., Von Brunn, A., and Wolf, H., 1992, Immunological reactivity of a human immunodeficiency virus type I derived peptide representing a consensus sequence of the GP120 major neutralizing region V3, *Arch. Virol.* **127**:139–152.

Wahren, B., Rosen, J., Sandstrom, E., Mathiesen, T., Modrow, S., and Wigzell, H., 1989, HIV-1 peptides induce a proliferative response in lymphocytes from infected persons, *J. Acq. Immune Defic. Syndr.* **2**:448–456.

Walker, B. D., Chakrabarti, S., Moss, B., Paradis, T. J., Flynn, T., Durno, A. G., Blumberg, R. S., Kaplan, J. C., Hirsch, M. S., and Schooley, R. T., 1987, HIV-specific cytotoxic T lymphocytes in seropositive individuals, *Nature* **328**:345–348.

Wang, B., Boyer, J., Srikantan, V., Ugen, K., Gilbert, L., Phan, C., Dang, K., Merva, M., Agadjanyan, M. G., Newman, M., Carrano, R., Mccallus, D., Coney, L., Williams, W. V., and Weiner, D. B., 1995, Induction of humoral and cellular immune responses to the human immunodeficiency type 1 virus in nonhuman primates by in vivo DNA inoculation, *Virology* **211**:102–112.

Warren, A. P., and Thomas, D. B., 1992, Class II (I-Ad) restricted T-cell recognition of the V3 loop region of HIV-1 gp120, *AIDS Res. Hum. Retrovir.* **8**:559–564.

Watari, E., Dietzschold, B., Szokan, G., and Heber, K. E., 1987, A synthetic peptide induces long-term protection from lethal infection with herpes simplex virus 2, *J. Exp. Med.* **165**:459–470.

Willey, R. L., Rutledge, R. A., Dias, S., Folks, T., Theodore, T., Buckler, C. E., and Martin, M. A., 1986, Identification of conserved and divergent domains within the envelope gene of the acquired immunodeficiency syndrome retrovirus, *Proc. Natl. Acad. Sci. USA* **83**:5038–5042.

Willey, R. L., Smith, D. H., Lasky, L. A., Theodore, T. S., Earl, P. L., Moss, B., Capon, D. J., and Martin, M. A., 1988, In vitro mutagenesis identifies a region within the envelope gene of the human immunodeficiency virus that is critical for infectivity, *J. Virol.* **62**:139–147.

Yasutomi, Y., Palker, T. J., Gardner, M. B., Haynes, B. F., and Letvin, N. L., 1993a, Synthetic peptide in mineral oil adjuvant elicits simian immunodeficiency virus-specific CD8+ cytotoxic T lymphocytes in rhesus monkeys, *J. Immunol.* **151**:5096–5105.

Yasutomi, Y., Reimann, K. A., Lord, C. I., Miller, M. D., and Letvin, N. L., 1993b, Simian immunodeficiency virus-specific CD8+ lymphocyte response in acutely infected rhesus monkeys, *J. Virol.* **67**:1707–1711.

Yewdell, J. W., Bennink, J. R., and Hosaka, Y., 1988, Cells process exogenous proteins for recognition by cytotoxic T lymphocytes, *Science* **239**:637–640.

CHAPTER 3

B-CELL SITES IN THE HIV GLYCOPROTEINS

EWA BJÖRLING and ERLING NORRBY

1. B-CELL IMMUNE RESPONSES AGAINST HIV

HIV, like other lentiviruses, has the capacity to direct the synthesis of a large number of different proteins. Some of these proteins participate in the formation of virus particles, whereas other proteins of a nonstructural nature appear in infected cells and may be released by secretion or in connection with a possible death of such cells. Each of these different proteins has a varying number of immunogenic sites, which may elicit humoral as well as cell-mediated responses. An acute infection with HIV as a consequence can lead to the mobilization of a large spectrum of immune responses. It is a daunting task to define the dynamics and specificities of these reactions. A considerable amount of information has already accumulated in this field, but more knowledge is needed to provide a comprehensive understanding of the complete relationship. There are three major contexts in which knowledge of HIV immunobiology is applicable.

1. Serodiagnosis and seroepidemiology. Qualified serodiagnosis may aid not only in demonstrating occurrence or absence of infection but also in defining risks for transmission, including the special situation of child·exposure during pregnancy and delivery, in evaluating possibilities for long-term survival, and in understanding mechanisms of pathogenesis. Potentially cell tropism characteristics depend on particular structural features in immunogenic sites of the virus.
2. Development of tools for active and passive immune intervention.
3. Evaluation of protein function and interaction. Site-specific immunological reagents allow studies of the maturation and chemical modification of proteins, as well as their aggregation into oligomers or other functional interactions and changes in folding reflecting functional alterations or denaturation phenomena.

EWA BJÖRLING and ERLING NORRBY • Microbiology and Tumorbiology Center, Karolinska Institute, S-171 77 Stockholm, Sweden.

Immunology of HIV Infection, edited by Sudhir Gupta. Plenum Press, New York, 1996.

In this chapter we will summarize the current knowledge on the regions of the envelope glycoproteins of subtypes HIV-1 and HIV-2 that have been identified as antigenic and immunogenic sites recognized by antibodies. Many techniques are used for identification of these sites. We refer to other reviews (Neurath, 1993) for discussion of available techniques and for evaluation of possibilities and limitations in their application.

Throughout the presentation the term *antigenic* or *immunogenic site(s)* will be used. Both linear sites defined by peptide reagents and discontinuous sites will be discussed. A single site may contain one or many epitopes and we employ the latter term only when it has been identified with a clonal immune reagent.

2. BASIC PROPERTIES OF THE TWO SURFACE GLYCOPROTEINS

Both HIV-1 and HIV-2 have been discovered as causative agents of AIDS (Barré-Sinoussi *et al.*, 1983; Popovic *et al.*, 1984; Clavel *et al.*, 1986), and much knowledge about their molecular characteristics, mechanisms of gene expression, and genomic complexity has been unraveled since then. Many isolates of both HIV-1 and HIV-2 have been characterized by nucleotide sequencing (Myers *et al.*, 1993) and from these studies we have learned that genetic variation is a hallmark of this kind of virus, and that a consequence of this is alteration of structure, function, and immunogenicity within a single individual throughout the lifelong infection with HIV.

Two proteins derive from cleavage of the HIV-1 envelope (env) precursor product, the large glycosylated outer protein gp120 and the transmembranous protein gp41. The corresponding cleavage products for HIV-2 are gp125 and gp36, respectively. The envelope proteins play an important role in interactions with cellular receptor membrane, in membrane fusion effects, and in initiation of signal transduction into cells.

There is approximately only 40% sequence homology among gp120 from distinct HIV-1 isolates (Myers *et al.*, 1992), and there are only ten short completely conserved stretches in gp120. The cysteine residues involved in the formation of disulfide bridges are conserved in both gp120 and gp41, which suggests that the basic structure of these two envelope proteins is conserved among different HIV isolates (Myers *et al.*, 1994). The two glycoproteins are known to be highly antigenic and immunogenic. The large glycoprotein shows a diversity in the number and relative positions of the glycosylation sites in different HIV strains. These variations may influence the specific immunogenicity of the protein (Alexander and Elder, 1984). Extensive base changes in the hypervariable regions which contain half of the potential N-linked glycosylation sites of the highly glycosylated gp120 protein are one source of variation in glycosylation. There are 24 *N*-glycosylation sites in gp120 from HIV-1 IIIB (Leonard *et al.*, 1990). Elimination of *N*-glycosylation sites around the CD4 binding site has resulted in reduction of virus infectivity (Dirckx *et al.*, 1990).

The variability in gp120 between HIV-1 strains is unevenly distributed along the molecule. Modrow *et al.* (1987) compared the predicted amino acid sequences of different HIV-1 envelope proteins based on nucleotide sequences and found five hypervariable regions (V1–V5) and five conserved regions (C1–C5) (Fig. 1). The hypervariable regions consist of up to 80 aa, which are surrounded by cysteines, suggesting that they form loops. These loops most likely are exposed at the surface of gp120. Mapping of structures on the HIV gp120 indicates that by way of contrast many conserved regions may be inaccessible for antibodies in the natural configuration. Antibodies to sites hidden in native gp120 may

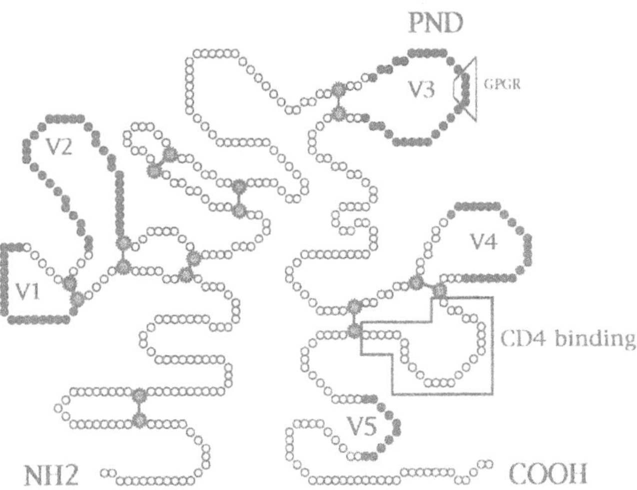

FIGURE 1. Schematic diagram of gp120 of HIV-1 adapted from Leonard *et al.* (1990). The variable amino acid residues in the five hypervariable regions of Modrow *et al.* (1987), V1–V5, are indicated as solid circles. Cysteine residues are indicated as large dark circles connected to each other with disulfide bonds. Open circles represents amino acid residues in the constant regions. The relatively conserved amino acids (GPGR) located at the tip of the V3 loop, the principal neutralizing domain (PND), and the CD4 binding site are enclosed in polygons.

be induced by vaccination with partially denatured proteins (De Santis *et al.*, 1993), but not by natural HIV infection.

Because of this sequence variability both intrasubtypically and between the different subtypes, the results of B-cell site mapping with one HIV isolate may not be applicable to other isolates.

Variability in Amino Acid Sequence of HIV Envelope Glycoproteins

The two HIV serotypes show an amino acid homology of about 60% in both *gag* and *pol* gene products whereas the envelope proteins are only distantly related, with about 40% identity (Guyader *et al.*, 1987). The sequence variability is higher for the large glycoprotein than for the transmembranous glycoprotein (Fig. 2). HIV-2 is closely related to simian immunodeficiency virus (SIV), and shows a 70–80% overall amino acid sequence homology with SIV isolated from macaques (SIVmac) (Murphey-Corb *et al.*, 1986). No corresponding nonhuman primate lentivirus relative of HIV-1 has as yet been identified. The primate lentiviruses are classified according to their phylogenetic relationships, which have been determined by comparing their nucleotide sequence. The most common approach is to assess how often particular clusters of sequences are found when the data are randomly resampled (Felsenstein, 1985). The classification of a phylogenetic tree of primate lentiviruses leads to a first level of five different lineages, and the second level of classification is to identify subgroups within each of these five clusters (Myers *et al.*, 1993, 1994; Louwagie *et al.*, 1993; Jin *et al.*, 1994; Breuer *et al.*, 1995).

Classification of different HIV-1 shows that at present one main group (group M) and one outliner group (group O) exist (Myers *et al.*, 1993). The main group is further divided into eight genetic subtypes A–H (Sharp *et al.*, 1994). In the commencement of the HIV

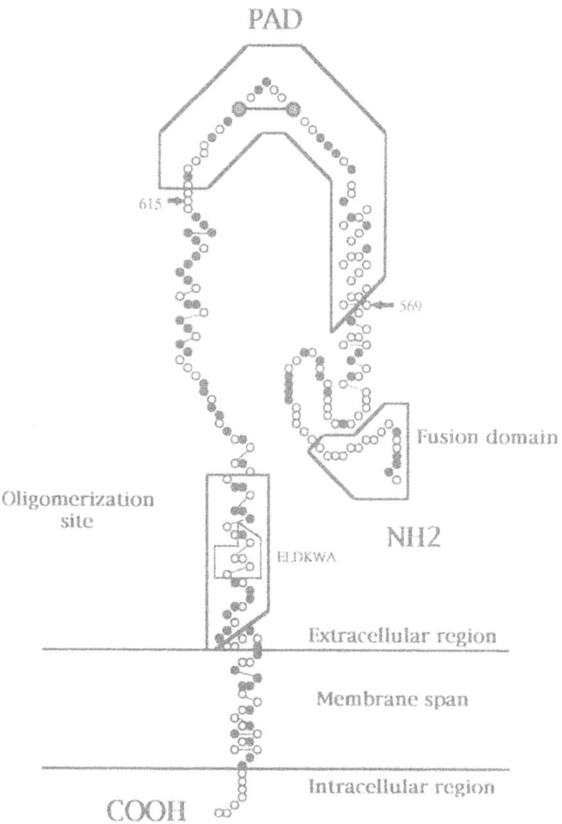

FIGURE 2. Schematic diagram of gp41 of HIV-1 adapted from Gallaher *et al.* (1989). Variable and constant amino acid residues according to the published HIV-1 sequence HXB2 (Myers *et al.*, 1990) are shown as solid and open circles, respectively. The principal antigenic domain, PAD (aa 570–613), the fusion domain important for mediating fusion between HIV-1 virions and cells (aa 512–527), and the gp41 oligomerization site are shown in polygons. The amino acid sequence ELDKWA in the external domain of gp41 recognized by a human neutralizing antibody is also indicated.

research efforts, primary HIV isolates were classified as African or North American, but with the availability of sequences from several isolates this terminology has become obsolete. The prototypic "North American" cluster which now include isolates from all continents has been named subtype B (Myers *et al.*, 1992). Cluster D contains the viruses initially classified as "African isolates." Viruses of subtype A are from Central Africa, subtype C contains isolates from South Africa and India, and subtype E is the dominant subtype in Thailand. The more recently identified cluster subtypes F–H include viruses from different parts of the world (Zaire, Gabon, Brazil, India, and Romania). Subtypes B and D seem to be more closely related to each other, and this finding supports the theory that the viruses in North America (cluster B) originate from Central African viruses (cluster D).

The studies of genetic subtypes are helpful for comparison of immunobiological characteristics and for interpretation of the diversity found in different geographical regions. Understanding the molecular epidemiology of HIV infection may have a possible relevance in vaccine design. Today there are few data on correlation between immunobiological properties such as cross neutralization and subtype-specific serological reactivity, and characteristics. In a recent study HIV-1 primary isolates from different geographical regions, representing genetic subtypes A–E, have been characterized in autologous and heterologous neutralization with a broad panel of human HIV-positive sera. No clear pattern of genetic subtype-specific neutralization could be seen (E.-M. Fenyö, personal communication).

HIV-2, the second type of lentivirus discovered to cause immunodeficiency in humans, was first isolated from a West African patient (Clavel *et al.*, 1986; Kanki *et al.*, 1987; Albert *et al.*, 1987). HIV-2 infection has today been documented in Africa, Europe, the Americas, and Asia, but is still mostly confined to West Africa and Portugal. HIV-2 has been divided into five different subtypes, A to E, and nearly all of them have been identified in West Africa. More recently epidemic spreading of HIV-2 subtype A isolates was demonstrated to occur in India. The most common subtypes today are A and B, which both are prevalent throughout West Africa, while subtypes C–E are represented by only a few isolates.

3. POSTINFECTION AND POSTIMMUNIZATION IMMUNE RESPONSES

The first reports characterizing the antibody response to HIV-1 infection were presented in the mid-1980s (Allan *et al.*, 1985; Robey *et al.*, 1985), and soon thereafter virus neutralizing activity in sera from HIV-infected individuals was detected (Robert-Guroff *et al.*, 1985; Weiss *et al.*, 1985). gp120 seems to be the most important target for the neutralizing antibodies (Robey *et al.*, 1986; Javaherian *et al.*, 1989; Steimer *et al.*, 1991). Antibody responses to the surface glycoproteins are either neutralizing or nonneutralizing, and can be subdivided into strain, group, type, or intertype specific reactions. Several studies with native and denatured gp120 have shown that the majority of antibodies in sera from HIV-positive individuals are directed against conformational antigenic sites. These sites contain amino acids that are discontiguous in the linear sequence but have a physical proximity in the properly folded protein (Ho *et al.*, 1991a; Steimer *et al.*, 1991; Moore and Ho, 1993).

The primary neutralizing anti-HIV-1 antibody response is strain specific and directed against the V3 loop (Weiss *et al.*, 1986; Nara *et al.*, 1987; Profy *et al.*, 1990; Steimer *et al.*, 1991; Kang *et al.*, 1991). However, HIV-1 frequently escapes neutralization, as evidenced by absence of autologous neutralizing antibodies to later isolates (Albert *et al.*, 1990; Nara *et al.*, 1990; Tremblay and Weinberg, 1990; von Gegerfelt *et al.*, 1991; Arendrup *et al.*, 1992). Sequential isolates from a laboratory worker accidentally infected with HIV-1 were shown to contain an amino acid substitution that resulted in resistance against neutralization by an anti-V3 monoclonal antibody (di Marzo Veronese *et al.*, 1993). This finding gives strong support to the concept that the initial antibody response is functional, since these antibodies appear to impose a specific selection pressure on the virus. The mechanism behind the development of neutralization resistance is not fully understood, but most likely involves mutations within and outside the V3 region in the envelope glycoproteins. Infected individuals eventually appear to be unable to produce neutralizing antibodies to the new antigenic variants and this inability together with a possible selection for viruses with an altered host cell tropism is likely to contribute to disease progression. Several explanations for this inability have been suggested including genetic diversification overwhelming of the immune system (Nowak *et al.*, 1991), selective B-cell anergy (Lane *et al.*, 1983), and "the original antigenic sin" (Hoskins *et al.*, 1979).

At a later phase a more broadly reactive virus neutralizing activity in the sera of HIV-1-infected individuals can be found. Antibodies responsible for neutralizing activity have been characterized to predominantly identify discontinuous sites and of particular importance in this context may be discontinuous structures of this kind responsible for the CD4 binding in the native gp120 (Steimer *et al.*, 1991; Kang *et al.*, 1991; McKeating *et al.*, 1992a; Nakamura *et al.*, 1992; Thali *et al.*, 1992; Posner *et al.*, 1993). Anti-CD4 antibodies seem to be associated with long-term controlled infection and are lost in individuals with disease progression (Cavacini *et al.*, 1993).

HIV-1 and HIV-2 share morphological and genomic structures, and consequently also biological properties. In spite of the low degree of homology found in the envelope glycoproteins, HIV-1 and HIV-2 use the same receptor, the CD4 molecule, present on the surface of helper T lymphocytes and cells of the macrophage/monocyte lineage (Sattentau *et al.*, 1988), and the replicative capacity of the virus strain correlates with the clinical severity of the infection in individuals (Åsjö *et al.*, 1986). HIV-2 has also been reported to have a lower physiopathological potential than HIV-1 (Gody *et al.*, 1988; De Cock *et al.*, 1990). A high degree of genetic variability in the *env* gene of HIV-1 has been demonstrated in studies of sequential isolates from the same patient (Hahn *et al.*, 1986; Simmonds *et al.*, 1991; Holmes *et al.*, 1992) and within a single patient isolate (Saag *et al.*, 1988; Meyerhans *et al.*, 1989). Sequential isolation of HIV-2 from experimentally infected macaques showed that in contrast to HIV-1, the V1 and V2 regions of HIV-2 seem to be highly conserved during the course of infection in macaques (Tolle *et al.*, 1994).

We have shown that individuals with HIV-2 infection, in contrast to HIV-1 (Albert *et al.*, 1990), retain the capability to neutralize autologous virus throughout the course of disease, and this may in part explain why HIV-2 appears to be less pathogenic than HIV-1 (Björling *et al.*, 1993). These findings have been supported by a large epidemiological study by Kanki *et al.* (1994), in which it was demonstrated that the heterosexual spread of HIV-2 is significantly slower than that of HIV-1, and that the disease development was reduced in HIV-2 infection (Marlink *et al.*, 1994), which suggests that HIV-2 has a lower virulence compared to HIV-1. It appears also that HIV-2-infected individuals are often protected against subsequent HIV-1 infection, and this may be a result of cross-reactive immunity to epitopes conserved between HIV-1 and HIV-2 (Travers *et al.*, 1995).

HIV-2 infections, like HIV-1 infections, result in the production of neutralizing antibodies predominantly directed against regions in the envelope glycoprotein (Weiss *et al.*, 1985; Ranki *et al.*, 1987), and there is also *in vitro* evidence of cross-neutralizing antibodies (Weiss *et al.*, 1988; Böttiger *et al.*, 1989, 1990).

Understanding the specificity and effect of sites that are accessible to neutralizing antibodies is the most important knowledge for construction of a non-replicating immunogen based on envelope proteins. Matters like immunodominance, immunoprotection, and immune potentiating effects need to be considered in this context.

By use of synthetic peptides many groups have mapped linear sites for both monoclonal reagents and polyclonal sera. This is an efficient method to mimic selected moieties of large protein molecules. This type of site mapping data primarily yields information about antigenic linear sites. One potential advantage is that the peptide often only partly mimics the correct folding of a conformational site on the native protein and the internal structure of the epitope could then be modified to make it more potent to induce a more broadly reactive immune response than the natural pathogen sequence (Berzofsky, 1993). In the effort to design a synthetic peptide vaccine against HIV, Palker *et al.* (1989) constructed T1-SP10 which included peptides corresponding to the V3 loop of gp120 and the T1 epitope in the CD4 binding region. This construct induced high titers of neutralizing antibodies in several animal species. By construction of chimeric *gag*–V3 viruslike particles, Luo *et al.* (1992) showed that the gag protein is highly immunogenic and could be an approach for HIV synthetic vaccine development.

4. DISCONTINUOUS EPITOPES AND LINEAR SITES IN HIV GLYCOPROTEINS

Extensive mapping of immunoreactive sites in the envelope glycoproteins has shown that there are only a few linear sites that are both neutralizing and immunodominant. By comparison of serum antibody neutralizing activity against common HIV-1 strains with serum antibody binding activity against different peptides corresponding to overlapping regions of the entire envelope, two immunodominant linear neutralizing regions in gp120 have been defined: the V3 region and the carboxy-terminal region of gp120. Using the same approach, two regions in gp41, corresponding to aa 647–671 and 732–746, were also found. The following is a summary of the most important findings of antigenic and immunogenic sites in a sequential presentation from the amino-terminal C1 region of the large glycoprotein to the carboxy-terminus of the transmembranous protein of HIV-1 and HIV-2, respectively.

4.1. The C1 Region in gp120

Serological data indicate that the immunogenicity is low for this region (Moore *et al.*, 1993a). In another study, van Tijn *et al.* (1989) showed that the C1 region (aa 55–65) harbors an antigenic site for human anti-HIV-1 sera. Several murine mAbs have been developed against this region, and aa 30–53, 61–70, and 91–110 have been mapped for antibody binding (Åkerblom *et al.*, 1990; di Marzo Veronese *et al.*, 1992; Kusk *et al.*, 1992; Nakamura *et al.*, 1992; Niedrig *et al.*, 1992). One mouse mAb directed against aa 64–78 decreased cell-to-cell spread of HIV-1 (Niedrig *et al.*, 1992). Nakamura *et al.* (1992) showed that a mAb directed against the C1 region could block monomeric gp120 binding to CD4.

In the C1 region of HIV-2 a linear antigenic site (aa 44–56) for human HIV-2 antibody-positive sera has been indicated (Norrby *et al.*, 1991; Mannervik *et al.*, 1992).

4.2. The V1 and V2 Regions in gp120

The V2 region is contained in a loop stabilized by a disulfide bond and is closely linked to a loop including the first variable (V1) domain (Leonard *et al.*, 1990; Fig. 1). These two sequential disulfide-linked loops have been demonstrated to represent an antigenic site in tests with human HIV-1-positive sera (van Tijn *et al.*, 1989; Moore *et al.*, 1993b) and also to be capable of mediating neutralization. Pincus *et al.* (1994) showed that affinity-purified human anti-V1 antibodies could neutralize HIV-1 IIIB. A weak reactivity with human sera containing HIV-1 antibodies could also be seen with a peptide (aa 135–152) corresponding to the V1 region of HIV-1_{BRU} (Norrby *et al.*, 1991). One linear site mediating neutralization was identified in the V1 region (aa 119–137) of HIV-2 by peptide immunization of guinea pigs (Björling *et al.*, 1991).

The V2 region is important in HIV-1 gp120 function, since it was found that the amino acid sequence in this region influences the replication capacity of the virus (Sullivan *et al.*, 1993) as well as in tropism (Westervelt *et al.*, 1992; Koito *et al.*, 1994). A hypervariable locus in the HIV-1 V2 region has been suggested to be predictive for conversion from non-synctium-inducing (NSI) to syncytium-inducing (SI) phenotype (Groenink *et al.*, 1993).

The V2 loop harbors both linear and conformation-dependent epitopes. Kayman (1994) have shown that 50% of HIV-1 antibody-positive human sera reacted with a fusion protein containing the V1/V2 domain, indicating that this region is important for antibody recognition. Studies with peptides representing linear sites of the V2 region showed that one immunodominant region for human HIV-1 antibody-positive sera is located in the central part of the V1/V2 region (Moore *et al.*, 1993a). Peptide immunization of rats could elicit strain-restricted neutralizing antibodies directed to the V2 region (Davis *et al.*, 1993).

Accumulated evidence shows that the V2 region is an important target for neutralizing antibodies, most of which, however, are strain specific and recognize conformationally sensitive structures located at the central portion of V2. A number of recent reports (Ho *et al.*, 1991a; Fung *et al.*, 1992; McKeating *et al.*, 1993; Moore *et al.*, 1993a; Sullivan *et al.*, 1993; Warrier *et al.*, 1994; Shotton *et al.*, 1995) have described neutralizing monoclonal antibodies directed against epitopes in the V1 and V2 region, many of which are dependent on protein glycosylation and/or conformation. Gorny *et al.* (1994) have derived a human monoclonal antibody directed against the V2 region (697/30D) that was shown to have neutralizing activity against some primary isolates but not against laboratory strains of HIV-1.

Also in the case of HIV-2 there are data indicating that the V2 region is important as a target for antibody binding. Recent results from our laboratory show that the majority of a panel of human HIV-2 sera recognize overlapping peptides corresponding to the central and C-terminal part of the HIV-2 V2 region (aa 160–189, 189–205) (Öhman *et al.*, unpublished data). Babas *et al.* (1994) have immunized rabbits with peptides corresponding to the V2 region of HIV-2, but these sera were unable to inhibit syncytium formation induced by HIV-2 *in vitro*.

4.3. The C2 Region in gp120

Four of the eight conserved potential glycosylation sites are located within the C2 region (Willey *et al.*, 1986). Removal of any one of these sites by site-directed mutagenesis markedly reduced virus infectivity (Willey *et al.*, 1988). In another study Ho *et al.* (1988) could show neutralization of different HIV-1 isolates by antisera raised against synthetic peptides corresponding to the C2 domain. In the C2 region of HIV-2 a linear antigenic site reacting with antibodies in human HIV-2 antibody-positive sera has been demonstrated (Mannervik *et al.*, 1992).

4.4. The V3 Region, the Principal Neutralizing Domain

Already in early studies the V3 loop was identified as the principal neutralizing determinant (Javaherian *et al.*, 1989). Since then much attention has been focused on this region. In the original studies it was demonstrated that peptides corresponding to the V3 region could elicit neutralizing antibodies and that most of the neutralizing activity from experimentally infected or gp120-vaccinated animals was directed against the V3 domain (Matthews *et al.*, 1986; Putney *et al.*, 1986; Robey *et al.*, 1986; Goudsmit *et al.*, 1988; Rusche *et al.*, 1988; Javaherian *et al.*, 1989, 1990; LaRosa *et al.*, 1990). This region, the principal neutralizing domain (PND: Fig. 1), is associated with aa 296–343, depending on the HIV-1 isolate, and forms a loop as a result of disulfide bonding between the cysteines at each end. The amino acids at the tip of the loop are relatively conserved (Fig. 1), and display only limited variation among virus isolates from different parts of the world. Substitutions within the V3 region, particularly at the tip of the loop, lead to pronounced changes of virus infectivity, syncytium formation, and the cellular tropism (Levy, 1993). Also, changes outside the V3 loop can influence the structure and function of the PND (Stamatatos and Cheng-Mayer, 1993). Different studies of blocking of neutralization by peptides have shown that the major part of neutralizing capacity of the HIV-1 isolate MN and IIIB of anti-HIV-1 human sera could be adsorbed with HIV-1 V3 loop peptides (aa 304–318) (Broliden *et al.*, 1992; Vogel *et al.*, 1994).

Several studies have characterized the HIV-1 V3 region using human monoclonal antibodies derived from infected individuals (Scott *et al.*, 1990; Gorny *et al.*, 1991). Many human anti-V3 mAbs have been isolated that have neutralizing capacity, and most of them are directed against the tip of the V3 loop (Scott *et al.*, 1990; Gorny *et al.*, 1991; Tilley *et al.*, 1991; Karwowska *et al.*, 1992a). Even though it must be concluded that the V3 region is important in human neutralizing antibody responses, it should be kept in mind that most of the relevant studies were performed with T-cell-line-adapted viruses. Neutralization of primary HIV-1 isolates appears to be a strikingly different matter.

In neutralization of HIV-1-derived primary isolates from all six genome clusters by human mAbs directed against the V3 loop—447/52-D and 19b (Moore *et al.*, 1994)—T-cell-adapted HIV-1 isolates were shown to be sensitive to neutralization, but primary isolates were much less reactive with these mAbs. Although mAb 19b showed a broad reactivity including strains outside subtype B, it neutralized primary isolates only with a limited efficiency. In contrast to the restricted reactivity of the V3 mAbs, the mAbs interfering with CD4 binding used in the same study showed a much broader reactivity against the different subtypes and some of them could neutralize primary isolates from all subtypes represented, A to F.

Using peptides representing regions of the glycoprotein gp125 of HIV-2 to screen HIV-2 human antibody-positive sera, several groups have defined the HIV-2 V3 region as a linear antibody binding site (de Wolf *et al.*, 1991; Norrby *et al.*, 1991; Jones *et al.*, 1992; Mannervik *et al.*, 1992).

Characterization of the potential neutralization activity of antibodies reacting with HIV-2 gp125 has produced conflicting results. There are a few reports which describe failure to induce neutralizing antibodies to the HIV-2 V3 region by peptide immunization (Robert-Guroff *et al.*, 1992; Babas *et al.*, 1994). In our laboratory we have identified the homologue of the HIV-1 V3 loop as a target for neutralization of HIV-2, by raising or neutralizing animal sera with peptide immunization, by blocking of neutralizing capacity of anti-HIV-2 human sera by peptides corresponding to the V3 loop (aa 311–330, 318–337), and by development of neutralizing murine mAbs directed against the V3 loop of HIV-2 (Björling *et al.*, 1991, 1994). Fine mapping of important individual amino acids for antibody binding in this region, showed two antigenic sites with conserved motif within V3: Phe-His-Ser (aa 315–317) and Trp-Cys-Arg (aa 329–331). Potentially these two sites can interact to represent a single discontinuous antigenic site.

Matsushita *et al.* (1995) recently presented findings supporting these results in studies of a neutralizing murine mAb directed against the HIV-2 V3 region. This mAb was mapped to a six-amino-acid segment with the core sequence His-Tyr-Gln (aa 316–318), and partly overlaps with the neutralizing site earlier described by us (Björling *et al.*, 1994). Traincard *et al.* (1994) have developed still another mAb against the V3 region of HIV-2, but this antibody does not neutralize the virus. Broad cross-neutralizing activity including many primary HIV-2 isolates from Guinea Bissau was demonstrated with guinea pig hyperimmune sera against V3 loop peptides (Björling *et al.*, 1994). It should be emphasized in this context that the V3 amino acid sequences of HIV-2 isolates show a more stable picture with only 7% variation as compared to 16% found in different HIV-1 strains (LaRosa *et al.*, 1990).

4.5. The C3 Region in gp120

This region is predicted to be very poorly accessible from the surface of gp120 and there are few reports concerning immunogenicity of this part of the envelope glycoprotein. Michel *et al.* (1988) immunized rabbits with a recombinant HIV-hepatitis B surface antigen and could induce anti-HIV neutralizing antibodies directed against the C3 and V4 regions. One murine mAb reacting with a linear C3 HIV-2 site has been described (Matsushita *et al.*, 1995), but this mAb only showed a weak neutralizing activity. Kusk *et al.* (1992) have defined aa 355–365 as important for antibody binding of antibodies in human anti-HIV-1 sera.

4.6. The Fourth Domain, Including the "CD4 Binding Region"

The C4 region was shown early on to be important for CD4 binding (Fig. 1), since deletion of a stretch of 12 amino acids could abolish the ligand activity (Lasky *et al.*, 1987), and mAbs directed to this region can block CD4 binding (Dowbenko *et al.*, 1988; Sun *et al.*, 1989; Cordell *et al.*, 1991; McKeating *et al.*, 1992a; Nakamura *et al.*, 1992). These early findings led to the conclusion that a short linear site in C4 is important in CD4 binding. Since then, other studies have shown that amino acid substitutions also outside the C4 domain could abolish the CD4 binding to gp120, and hence that CD4 binding must be dependent on structures including stretches of amino acids from different regions of gp120 which fold to physical proximity in the native protein (Olshevsky *et al.*, 1990). A single amino acid in C4 of HIV-1, Trp-427, appears to play a particularly critical role in CD4 binding (Cordonnier *et al.*, 1989; Olshevsky *et al.*, 1990). HIV-2 shows a similar picture with Trp-428 playing a corresponding role (Keller *et al.*, 1993).

The C4 domain has been shown to be an antigenic region since HIV-1-positive human sera react with C4 peptides (Norrby *et al.*, 1991; Moore *et al.*, 1993b). For HIV-2 there is only a weak reactivity of human sera against peptides representing this region (Norrby *et al.*, 1991).

mAbs directed against the C4 region have been used for probing the structure of the C4 and V4 domains and their interactions with the V3 loop. mAbs that recognized conformation-sensitive C4 structures failed to bind to gp120 when the sequence of the V3 loop was changed (Moore *et al.*, 1993b). One mAb binding a linear site in the V4 region has been developed. This mAb was derived from an animal immunized with denatured gp160

(Abacioglu *et al.*, 1994) and binds to aa 392–402, a region that does not seem to be exposed on the surface of native gp120, or possibly may be sterically sheltered by heavy glycosylation of the V4 loop. Sera from mice immunized with baculovirus-expressed envelope glycoproteins showed a limited reactivity to peptides representing the V4 region of HIV-1 (Bristow *et al.*, 1994). In HIV-2 there is a linear site in the V4 region that appears to be antigenic in human HIV-2 antibody-positive sera (Mannervik *et al.*, 1992; Öhman *et al.*, unpublished data).

4.7. The Carboxy-Terminal Part of gp120, the Fifth Region

The carboxy-terminal part of C5 harbors an immunodominant site that reacts with the majority of HIV-1- and HIV-2-positive sera (Palker *et al.*, 1987; Norrby *et al.*, 1991, Broliden *et al.*, 1992). The amino-terminal part of C5 in native gp120 is predicted to contain a long stretch that is inaccessible for antibody binding (Moore *et al.*, 1994). Broliden *et al.* (1992) have shown that seroreactivity against a C5 peptide (aa 489–508) correlates with neutralization of IIIB, and furthermore that this peptide blocks neutralizing activity of human anti-HIV-1 sera. In another study rabbit sera raised against a recombinant C5 fragment were shown to neutralize HIV-1 (Charbit *et al.*, 1990).

This region is unique in that it shows homology to HLA. A monoclonal antibody, M38, displayed the capacity to react with both gp120 and HLA class I heavy chain. Its target site has been mapped to the carboxy-terminal part of the C5 region, and within the $\alpha 1$ domain of HLA heavy chain (Grassi *et al.*, 1991; Lopalco *et al.*, 1993).

In HIV-2 we have defined two overlapping peptides (aa 472–493, 489–509) that could induce neutralizing antibodies in animals and also mediate a certain blocking of neutralization of human anti-HIV-2 sera (Björling *et al.*, 1991, 1994). One reactive region in V5 of HIV-2 has also been identified with human anti-HIV-2 sera (Mannervik *et al.*, 1992).

4.8. The Transmembranous Protein, gp41

The transmembranous protein gp41 of HIV-1 is responsible for viral fusion to the target cell and for syncytium formation (Sodroski *et al.*, 1986; Kowalski *et al.*, 1987). In analogy the same properties reside in the gp36 protein of HIV-2. A highly immunodominant region, the principal antigenic domain (PAD; Fig. 2)—in HIV-1 gp41 and in HIV-2 gp36—has been mapped to aa 570–613 and 595–614, respectively, by demonstration of strongly reactive peptides (Chiodi *et al.*, 1987; Gnann *et al.*, 1987; Norrby *et al.*, 1987, 1991; Klasse *et al.*, 1988; Schrier *et al.*, 1988; Horal *et al.*, 1991; Oldstone *et al.*, 1991). Using peptide-specific mAbs the PAD in HIV-1 has been demonstrated to harbor two different sites in the central part of the region (Norrby *et al.*, 1989). This site harbors the only intramolecular loop of gp41 (Fig. 2) and this loop structure has been reported to include sites mediating neutralization (conflicting data), enhancement of HIV infection, and antibody-dependent cell-mediated cytotoxicity (Schrier *et al.*, 1988; Tyler *et al.*, 1990; Robinson *et al.*, 1991). This region and a second immunodominant region in gp41 corresponding to aa 644–663 have been identified also in studies with human mAbs (Teeuwsen *et al.*, 1990; Xu *et al.*, 1991).

Vanini *et al.* (1993) have used purified gp41 directed human antibodies for mapping of sites critical for membrane fusion and four sites (aa 583–591, 595–599, 603–609, and 664–673) were found to possibly be involved in the fusion process. Reduction in the antibody titers of antibodies directed against three of these sites correlated with disease progression.

Several targets for neutralization in the gp41 have been identified. One site is located in the amino-terminal part of gp41 (aa 503–532) by Chanh *et al.* (1986) and Ho *et al.* (1987). The corresponding neutralization domain has recently been identified in the HIV-2 gp36 by peptide immunization of guinea pigs (Öhman *et al.*, unpublished data).

The only epitope in a protein other than gp120 recognized by a potent neutralizing human mAb, designated 2F5 (Muster *et al.*, 1994), corresponds to the specific sequence ELDKWA in the external domain of gp41 (Conley *et al.*, 1994; Fig. 2). This epitope on gp41 is represented among HIV-1 envelope sequences from different geographic locations, and in concordance with this, mAb 2F5 was capable of neutralizing both lymphoid cell culture-adapted HIV-1 variants and several HIV-1 primary isolates. The sequence ELDKWA has also been inserted into an immunogenic site of influenza virus hemagglutinin and used for immunization of mice. These hyperimmune sera neutralized HIV-1 (Muster *et al.*, 1994).

Broad neutralization of HIV-1 has also been correlated with seroreactivity of human anti-HIV-1 sera to peptides mimicking two conserved regions in gp41: aa 652–666 (which include the sequence ELDKWA recognized by mAb 2F5) and aa 732–746 (Broliden *et al.*, 1992). These peptides displayed a capacity to block the neutralizing activity in the human sera. Sites in the intracytoplasmic domain somewhat unexpectedly also have been reported to be an antigenic region for anti-HIV-1 human antibodies (Kennedy *et al.*, 1986) and induce *in vitro* neutralizing HIV-1 and HIV-2 antibodies in rabbits and guinea pigs, respectively (Chanh *et al.*, 1986; Ho *et al.*, 1987; Dalgleish *et al.*, 1988; Björling *et al.*, 1991). This HIV-1 region was also found to be a potent immunogen when inserted in the VP1 domain of poliovirus (Evans *et al.*, 1989). This epitope most probably is not exposed at the surface of mature virions; speculatively, it may be recognizable by antibodies after the CD4 binding when the virus and cell membrane are in close apposition and thus block the fusion process. More work is needed to clarify the *in vivo* relevance of the reported results, since most of the studies on anti-gp41-neutralizing antibodies have been performed in animals.

4.9. Discontinuous Epitopes in gp120 and gp41

Later during the course of the HIV infection, broadly neutralizing antibodies appear, and these are believed to be directed predominantly against non-V3 epitope(s) of gp120 (Ho *et al.*, 1991b). Several broadly cross-reactive human mAbs that block gp120–CD4 binding have been described (Ho *et al.*, 1991b; Karwowska *et al.*, 1992a) and in some cases the epitopes recognized have been characterized (Ho *et al.*, 1991b; Posner *et al.*, 1991; Tilley *et al.*, 1991; Thali *et al.*, 1991, 1992; Karwowska *et al.*, 1992b; McKeating *et al.*, 1992b). One of these antibodies (F105) showed a reduced capacity to react with gp120 after introduction of changes in four different regions: aa 256–257 (C2), 368–370 (C3), 421 (C4), and 470–484 (C5) (Thali *et al.*, 1991). This finding supports the hypothesis that the CD4 binding site is discontinuous and includes amino acid stretches from more than one of these regions (Ardman *et al.*, 1990; Olshevsky *et al.*, 1990). Ho *et al.* (1991b) have reported another human monoclonal neutralizing antibody 15e that has the capacity to block gp120–CD4 interaction. mAb 15e does not react with nonglycosylated gp120 made by *Escherichia coli*, suggesting that carbohydrate residues may be essential for the recognition.

By using recombinant DNA technology to express Fab antibody molecules by the phage-display library method, a potent neutralizing antibody reacting with a discontinuous site has been isolated (Barbas *et al.*, 1992). This antibody IgG1b12 was reconstructed from Fab 12, a human antigen binding antibody fragment. The Fab 12 fragment was obtained from a seropositive HIV-1 individual by panning with soluble gp120 from HIV-1_{LAI}. The IgG1b12 antibody has been shown to effectively neutralize many HIV-1 primary isolates as well as HIV-1 laboratory strains (Burton *et al.*, 1994). With the same technique, Roben *et al.* (1994) and Ditzel *et al.* (1995) have developed neutralizing recombinant human antibodies to conformational epitopes that are dependent on the V3 region, the V2 region, and the region important for CD4 binding, respectively.

Several other human mAbs directed against discontinuous epitopes in gp41 have been produced (Grunow *et al.*, 1988; Sugano *et al.*, 1988; Tyler *et al.*, 1990), but none of these mAbs could neutralize HIV.

5. EPILOGUE

During the past decade a remarkable wealth of information on the immunochemistry and immunobiology of the glycoproteins of HIV-1 and HIV-2 has been accumulated. Many techniques have been employed to identify antigenic and immunogenic sites in the different virus proteins. A relatively large number of linear highly antigenic sites in the heavily glycosylated surface protein were identified by use of the synthetic peptide technique.

A range of discontinuous sites were also identified in tests with clonal immune reagents. Parts of the protein that were critically involved were identified using site-directed mutagenesis and tests with antigenic protein fragments. In spite of the knowledge gained, many central questions remain unanswered. What is the extent of variations in immunogenic properties of the virus in the infected individual and in virus strains of different epidemic origins? How do such variations influence pathogenesis and possibilities for immune interventions? What is the influence of host cell adaptation in viral immunogenic properties? What are the critical features in virus-load relationships and what causes the immune system to break down rapidly in some individuals and not in others? What effect will suppression of virus load at the time of the primary infection have on long-term events? Will it be acceptable to tolerate a vaccine-induced infection permissive immunity safeguarding against development of disease? The questions are many and some answers are difficult to reach and hence slow in coming.

Attempts to develop vaccines, which are in urgent demand, have met with frustrations. There still is a long way to go before a nonreplicating component vaccine and in particular a synthetic vaccine preventing AIDS can be developed. Attainment of the goal of sterilizing immunity may be exceedingly difficult. The need to develop a cross-protective immunity also including primary isolate of virus deserves further studies. On the positive side, however, it should be mentioned that HIV-1 infection in chimpanzees has been blocked by immune intervention and preexposure immunity in monkeys has been proven to block or markedly suppress the extent of primary virus replication. A consequence of the reduced virus load in the latter situation can be a delayed or complete blocking of the development of AIDS in experimental animals.

The relatively high stability of the PND of HIV-2 as compared to the corresponding site in HIV-1 is of interest in selection of a target system for development and explorative testing of a vaccine. In this context, it has been suggested that an HIV-2 postinfection immunity may block or delay the development of AIDS following a subsequent HIV-1 infection.

Future breakthroughs in our understanding of HIV immunobiology may provide tools for immune protective interventions with the ultimate goal of preventing the deadly disease

AIDS. Even though stumbling blocks have been encountered, there are reasons to maintain a reserved optimism in these endeavors. The advance of knowledge will continue and this advance will create new possibilities.

REFERENCES

Abacioglu, Y. H., Fouts, T. R., Laman, J. D., Claassen, E., Pincus, S. H., Moore, J. P., Roby, C. A., and Kamin-Lewis, R., 1994, Epitope mapping and topology of baculovirus-expressed HIV-1 gp160 determined with panel of murine monoclonal antibodies, *AIDS Res. Hum. Retrovir.* **10(4)**:371–381.

Åkerblom, L., Hinkula, J., Broliden, P.-A., Makitalo, B., Fridbreger T., and Rosen, J., 1990, Neutralizing cross-reactive and non-neutralizing monoclonal antibodies to HIV-1 gp120, *AIDS* **4**:953–960.

Albert, J., Bredberg, U., Chiodi, F., Böttiger, B., Fenyö, E.-M., Norrby, E., and Biberfeld, G., 1987, A new human retrovirus isolate of West African origin and its relationship to HTLV-IV, LAV-II and HTLV-IIIB, *AIDS Res. Hum. Retrovir.* **3**:3–10.

Albert, J., Abrahamsson, B., Nagy, K., Aurelius, E., Gaines, H., Nyström, G., and Fenyö, E. M., 1990, Rapid development of isolate-specific neutralizing antibodies after primary HIV-1 infection and consequent emergence of virus variants which resist neutralization by autologous sera, *AIDS* **4**:107–112.

Alexander, S., and Elder, J. H., 1984, Carbohydrate dramatically influences immune reactivity of antisera to viral glycoprotein antigens, *Science* **226**:1328–1330.

Allan, J. S., Coligan, J. E., Barin, F., McLane, M. F., Sodroski, J. F., Rosen, C. A., Haseltine, W. A., Lee, T. H., and Essex, M., 1985, Major glycoprotein antigens that induce antibodies in AIDS patients are encoded by HTLV-III, *Science* **228**:1091–1094.

Ardman, B., Kowalski, M., Bristol, J., Haseltine, W., and Sodroski, J., 1990, Effects of CD4 binding of anti-peptide sera to the fourth and fifth conserved domains of HIV-1 gp120, *J. Acq. Immune Defic. Syndr.* **3**:206–214.

Arendrup, M., Nielsen, C., Hansen, J. E., Pedersen, C., Mathiesen, L., and Nielsen, J. O., 1992, Autologous HIV-1 neutralizing antibodies: Emergence of neutralization-resistant escape virus and subsequent development of virus neutralizing antibodies, *J. Acq. Immune Defic. Syndr.* **5**:303–307.

Åsjö, B., Morfeldt-Månsson, L., Albert, J., Biberfeld, G., Karlsson, A., Lidman, K., and Fenyö, E.-M., 1986, Replicative capacity of human immunodeficiency virus from patients with varying severity of HIV infection, *Lancet* **2**:660–662.

Babas, T., Benichou, S., Guetard, D., Montagnier, L., and Bahraoui, E., 1994, Specificity of antipeptide antibodies produced against V2 and V3 regions of the external envelope of human immunodeficiency virus type 2, *Mol. Immunol.* **31**:361–369.

Barbas, C. F., III, Björling, E., Chiodi, F., Dunlop, N., Cababa, D., Jones, T. M., Zebedee, S. L., Persson, M. A., Nara, P. L., Norrby, E., and Burton, D. R., 1992, Recombinant human Fab fragments neutralize human type 1 immunodeficiency virus in vitro, *Proc. Natl. Acad. Sci. USA* **89**:9339–9343.

Barré-Sinoussi, F., Cherman, F. C., Rey, F., Nugeyre, M., Chamaret, S., Gruest, J., Dauguet, C., Axler-Blin, C., Brun-Vezinet, F., Rouzioux, C., Rozenbaum, W., and Montagnier, L., 1983, Isolation of a T-lymphotropic retrovirus from a patient at risk for acquired immune deficiency syndrome (AIDS), *Science* **220**:868–870.

Berzofsky, J. A., 1993, Epitope selection and design of synthetic vaccines. Molecular approaches to enhancing immunogenicity and cross-reactivity of engineered vaccines, *Ann. N.Y. Acad. Sci.* **690**:256–264.

Björling, E., Broliden, K., Bernardi, D., Utter, G., Thorstensson, R., Chiodi, F., and Norrby, E., 1991, Hyperimmune antisera against synthetic peptides representing the glycoprotein of human immunodeficiency virus type 2 can mediate neutralization and antibody-dependent cytotoxic activity, *Proc. Natl. Acad. Sci. USA* **88**:6082–6086.

Björling, E., Scarlatti, G., von Gegerfelt, A., Albert, J., Biberfeld, G., Chiodi, F., Norrby, E., and Fenyö, E.-M., 1993, Autologous neutralizing antibodies prevail in HIV-2 but not in HIV-1 infection, *Virology* **193**:528–530.

Björling, E., Chiodi, F., Utter, G., and Norrby, E., 1994, Two V3 associated important neutralizing domains in the envelope glycoprotein gp125 of human immunodeficiency virus type 2, *J. Immunol.* **152**:1952–1959.

Böttiger, B., Karlsson, A., Naucler, A., Andreasson, P. Å., Mendes Costa, C., and Biberfeld, G., 1989, Cross-neutralizing antibodies against HIV-1 (HTLV-IIIB and HTLV-III RF) and HIV-2 (SBL-6669 and a new isolate SBL-K135), *AIDS Res. Hum. Retrovir.* **5**:511–519.

Böttiger, B., Karlsson, A., Andreasson, P. Å., Naucler, A., Mendes Costa, C., Norrby, E., and Biberfeld, G., 1990, Envelope cross reactivity between human immunodeficiency virus type 1 and 2 detected by different serological methods: Correlation between cross neutralization and reactivity against the main neutralizing site, *J. Virol.* **64**:3492–3499.

Breuer, J., Douglas, N. W., Goldman, N., and Daniels, R. S., 1995, Human immunodeficiency virus type 2 (HIV-2) *env* gene analysis: Prediction of glycoprotein epitopes important for heterotypic neutralization and evidence for three genotype clusters within the HIV-2a subtype, *J. Gen. Virol.* **76**:333–345.

Bristow, R. G., Douglas, A. R., Skehel, J. J., and Daniels, R. S., 1994, Analysis of murine antibody responses to baculovirus-expressed human immunodeficiency virus type 1 envelope glycoproteins, *J. Gen. Virol.* **75**: 2089–2095.

Broliden, P.-A., von Gegerfelt, A., Clapham, P., Rosen, J., Fenyö, E.-M., Wahren, B., and Broliden, K., 1992, Identification of human neutralization-inducing regions of the human immunodeficiency virus type 1 envelope glycoproteins, *Proc. Natl. Acad. Sci. USA* **89**:461–465.

Burton, D. R., Pyati, J., Koduri, R., Sharp, S. J., Thornton, G. B., Parren, P. W., Sawyer, L. S., Hendry, R. M., Dunlop, N., Nara, P. L., Lamacchia, M., Garratty, E., Stiehm, E. R., Bryson, Y. J., Cao, Y., Moore, J. P., Ho, D. D., and Barbas, C. F., III, 1994, Efficient neutralization of primary isolates of HIV-1 by a recombinant human monoclonal antibody, *Science* **266**:1024–1027.

Cavacini, L. A., Emes, C. L., Power, J., Underdahl, J., Goldstein, R., Mayer, K., and Posner, M. R., 1993, Loss of serum antibodies to a conformational epitope of HIV-1/gp120 identified by a human monoclonal antibody is associated with disease progression, *J. Acq. Immune Defic. Syndr.* **6**:1093–1102.

Chanh, T., Dreesman, G., Kanda, P., Linette, G., Sparrow, J., Ho, D., and Kennedy, R., 1986, Induction of anti-HIV neutralizing antibodies by synthetic peptides, *EMBO J.* **11**:3065–3071.

Charbit, A., Molla, A., Ronco, J., Clement, J. M., Favier, V., Bahraoui, E. M., Montagnier, L., Leguern, A., and Hofnung, M., 1990, Immunogenicity and antigenicity of conserved peptides from the envelope of HIV-1 expressed at the surface of recombinant bacteria, *AIDS* **4**:545–551.

Chiodi, F., von Gegerfelt, A., Albert, J., Fenyö, E.-M., Gaines, H., von Sydow, M., Biberfeld, G., Parks, E., and Norrby, E., 1987, Site directed ELISA with synthetic peptides representing the HIV transmembrane glycoprotein, *J. Med. Virol.* **23**:1–9.

Clavel, F., Guetard, D., Brun-Vezinet, F., Chamaret, S., Rey, M. A., Santos-Ferreria, M. O., Laurent, A. G., Dauguet, C., Katlama, C., Rouzioux, C., Klatzmann, D., Champalimaud, J. L., and Montagnier, L., 1986, Isolation of a new human retrovirus from West African patients with AIDS, *Science* **233**:343–346.

Conley, A. J., Kessler, J. A., II, Boots, L. J., Tung, J.-S., Arnold, B., Keller, P. M., Shaw, A., and Emini, E., 1994, Neutralization of divergent human immunodeficiency virus type 1 variants and primary isolates by IAM-41-2F5, an anti-gp41 human monoclonal antibody, *Proc. Natl. Acad. Sci. USA* **91**:3348–3352.

Cordell, J., Moore, J. P., Dean, C. J., Klasse, P. J., Weiss, R. A., and McKeating, J. A., 1991, Rat monoclonal antibodies to non-overlapping epitopes of HIV-1 gp120 block CD4 binding *in vitro*, *Virology* **185**:72–79.

Cordonnier, A., Montagnier, L., and Emerman, M., 1989, Single amino acid changes in HIV envelope affect viral tropism and receptor binding, *Nature* **340**:571–574.

Dalgleish, A. G., Chanh, T. C., Kennedy, R. C., Kanda, P., Clapham, P. R., and Weiss, R. A., 1988, Neutralization of diverse HIV-1 strains by monoclonal antibodies raised against a gp41 synthetic peptide, *Virology* **165**: 209–215.

Davis, D., Stephens, D.M., Carne, C. A., and Lachmann, P. J., 1993, Antisera raised against the second variable region of the external envelope glycoprotein of human immunodeficiency virus type 1 cross-neutralize and show an increased neutralization index when they act together with antisera to the V3 neutralization epitope, *J. Gen. Virol.* **74**:2609–2617.

De Cock, K. M., Odehouri, K., Colebunders, R. L., Adjorlolo, G., Lafontaine, M. F., Porter, A., Gnaore, E., Diaby, L., Moreau, J., Heyward, W. L., Kadio, A., Heroin, P., Kanga, J.-M., Beda, B., Niamkey, E., Achi, Y., Coulibaly, N., Attia, Y., Giordano, C., Rayfield, M., and Schochetman, G., 1990, A comparison of HIV-1 and HIV-2 infections in hospitalized patients in Abidjan, Cote d'Ivoire, *AIDS* **4**:443–448.

De Santis, C., Robbioni, P., Langhi, R., Lopalco, L., Siccardi, A. G., Beretta, A., and Roberts, N. J., Jr., 1993, Cross-reactive response to human immunodeficiency virus type 1 (HIV-1) gp120 and HLA class I heavy chains induced by receipt of HIV-1-derived envelope vaccines, *J. Infect. Dis.* **168**:1396–1403.

de Wolf, F., Meloen, R. H., Bakker, M., Barin, F., and Goudsmit, J., 1991, Characterization of human antibody-binding sites on the external envelope of human immunodeficiency virus type 2, *J. Gen. Virol.* **72**:1261–1267.

di Marzo Veronese, F., Rahman, R., Pal, R., Boyer, C., Romano, J., Kalyasaraman, U. S., Nair, B. C., Gallo, R. C., and Sarngadharan, M. G., 1992, Delineation of immunoreactive, conserved regions in the external envelope glycoprotein of the HIV-1, *AIDS Res. Hum. Retrovir.* **8**:1125–1132.

di Marzo Veronese, F., Reitz, M. S., Jr., Gupta, G., Robert-Guroff, M., Boyer-Thompson, C., Louie, A., Gallo,

R. C., and Lusso, P., 1993, Loss of a neutralizing epitope by a spontaneous point mutation in the V3 loop of HIV-1 isolated from an infected laboratory worker, *J. Biol. Chem.* **268:**25894–25901.

Dirckx, L., Lindemann, D., Ette, R., Manzoni, C., Moritz, D., and Mous, J., 1990, Mutation of conserved N-glycosylation sites around the CD4-binding site of human immunodeficiency virus type 1 gp120 affects viral infectivity, *Virus Res.* **18:**9–20.

Ditzel, H. J., Binley, J. M., Moore, J. P., Sodroski, J., Sullivan, N., Sawyer, L. S., Hendry, R. M., Yang, W. P., Barbas, C. F., III, and Burton, D. R., 1995, Neutralizing recombinant human antibodies to a conformational V2 and CD4-binding site-sensitive epitope of HIV-1 gp120 isolated by using an epitope-masking procedure, *J. Immunol.* **154:**893–906.

Dowbenko, D., Nakamura, G., Fennie, C., Shimasaki, C., Riddle, L., Harris, R., Gregory, T., and Lasky, L., 1988, Epitope mapping of the human immunodeficiency virus type 1 gp120 with monoclonal antibodies, *J. Virol.* **62:**4703–4711.

Evans, L. A., Thomson-Honnebier, G., Steimer, K., Paoletti, E., Perkus, M. E., Hollander, H., and Levy, J. A., 1989, Antibody-dependent cellular cytotoxicity is directed against both the gp120 and gp41 envelope proteins of HIV, *AIDS* **3:**273–276.

Felsenstein, J., 1985, Confidence limits on phylogenies: An approach using the bootstrap, *Evolution* **39:**783–791.

Fung, M. S. C., Sun, C. R. Y., Gordon, W. L., Liou, R. S., Chang, T. W., Sun, W. N. C., Daar, E. S., and Ho, D. D., 1992, Identification and characterization of a neutralization site within the second variable region of human immunodeficiency virus type 1 gp120, *J. Virol.* **66:**848–856.

Gallaher, W. R., Ball, J. M., Garry, R. F., Griffin, M. C., and Montelaro, R. C., 1989, A general model for the transmembrane proteins of HIV and other retroviruses, *AIDS Res. Hum. Retrovir.* **5:**431–440.

Gnann, J. W., Nelson, J. A., and Oldstone, M. B., 1987, Fine mapping of an immunodominant domain in the transmembrane glycoprotein of HIV, *J. Virol.* **61:**2639–2641.

Gody, M., Quattara, S. A., and de The, G., 1988, Clinical experience of AIDS in relation to HIV-1 and HIV-2 infection in a rural hospital in Ivory Coast, West Africa, *AIDS* **2:**433–436.

Gorny, M. K., Xu, J. Y., Gianakakos, V., Karwowska, S., Williams, C., Sheppard, H. W., Hanson, C. V., and Zolla-Pazner, S., 1991, Production of site directed neutralizing human monoclonal antibodies against the third variable domain of the HIV-1 envelope glycoprotein, *Proc. Natl. Acad. Sci. USA* **88:**3238–3241.

Gorny, M. K., Moore, J. P., Karwowska, S., Sodroski, J., Williams, C., Burda, S., Boots, L. J., and Zolla-Pazner, S., 1994, Human anti-V2 monoclonal antibody that neutralizes primary but not laboratory isolates of HIV-1, *J. Virol.* **68:**8312–8320.

Goudsmit, J., Boucher, C. A. B., Meloen, R. H., Epstein, L. G., Smit, L., van der Hoek, L., and Bakker, M., 1988, Human antibody response to a strain-specific HIV-1 gp120 epitope associated with cell fusion inhibition, *AIDS* **2:**157–164.

Grassi, F., Meneveri, R., Gullberg, M., Lopalco, L., Rossi, G. B., Lanza, P., De Santis, C., Brattsand, G., Butto, S., Ginelli, E., Beraetta, A., and Siccardi, A. G., 1991, Human immunodeficiency virus type 1 gp120 mimics a hidden monomorphic epitope borne by class I major histocompatibility complex heavy chains, *J. Exp. Med.* **174:**53–62.

Groenink, M., Fouchier, R. A., Broersen, S., Baker, C. H., Koot, M., van't Wout, A. B., Huisman, H. G., Miedema, F., Tersmette, M., and Schuitemaker, H., 1993, Relation of phenotype evolution of HIV-1 to envelope V2 configuration, *Science* **260:**1513–1516.

Grunow, R., Jahn, S., Porstmann, T., Kiessig, S. S., Steinkellner, S. H., Steindl, F., Mattanovich, D., Gurtler, L., Deinhardt, F., Katinger, H., and von Baehr, R., 1988, The high efficiency, human B cell immortalizing heteromyeloma CB-F7. Production of human monoclonal antibodies to human immunodeficiency virus, *J. Immunol. Methods* **106:**257–265.

Guyader, M., Emerman, M., Sonigo, P., Clavel, F., Montagnier, L., and Alizon, M., 1987, Genome organization and transactivation of the human immunodeficiency virus type 2, *Nature* **326:**662–669.

Hahn, B. H., Shaw, G. M., Taylor, M. E., Redfield, R. R., Markham, P. D., Salahuddin, S. Z., Wong-Staal, F., Gallo, R. C., Parks, E. S., and Parks, W. P., 1986, Genetic variation in HTLV-III/LAV over time in patients with AIDS, *Science* **232:**1548–1553.

Ho, D. D., Sarngadharan, M. G., Hirsch, M. S., Schooley, R. T., Rota, T. R., Kennedy, R. C., Chanh, T. C., and Sato, V. L., 1987, Human immunodeficiency virus neutralizing antibodies recognize several conserved domains on the envelope glycoproteins, *J. Virol.* **61:**2024–2028.

Ho, D. D., Kaplan, I. E., Rackauskas, I. E., and Gurney, M. E., 1988, Second conserved domain of gp120 is important for viral infectivity and antibody neutralization, *Science* **239:**1021–1023.

Ho, D. D., Fung, M. S., Cao, Y., Li, X. L., Sun, C., Chang, T. W., and Sun, N. C., 1991a, Another discontinuous epitope on glycoprotein gp120 that is important in HIV-1 neutralization is identified by a monoclonal antibody, *Proc. Natl. Acad. Sci. USA* **88:**8849–8852.

Ho, D. D., McKeating, J. A., Li, X. L, Moudgil, T., Daar, E. S., Sun, N. C., and Robinson, J. E., 1991b, A conformational epitope on gp120 important in CD4 binding and HIV-1 neutralization identified by a human monoclonal antibody, *J. Virol.* **65:**489–493.

Holmes, E. C., Zhang, L. Q., Simmonds, P., Ludlam, C. A., and Leigh Brown, A. J., 1992, Convergent and divergent sequence evolution in the surface envelope glycoprotein of human immunodeficiency virus type 1 within a single infected patient, *Proc. Natl. Acad. Sci. USA* **89:**4835–4839.

Horal, P., Svennerholm, B., Jeansson, S., Rymo, L., Hall, W. W., and Vahlne, A., 1991, Continuous epitopes of the HIV-1 transmembrane glycoprotein and reactivity of human sera to synthetic peptides representing various HIV-1 isolates, *J. Virol.* **65:**2718–2723.

Hoskins, T. W., Davies, J. R., Smith, A. J., Miller, C. L., and Allchin, A., 1979, Assessment of inactivated influenza-A vaccine after three outbreaks of influenza A at Christ's Hospital, *Lancet* **1:**33–35.

Javaherian, K., Langlois, A. J., McDanal, C., Ross, K. L., Eckler, L. I., Jellis, C. L., Profy, A. T., Rusche, J. R., Bolognesi, D. P., Putney, S. D., and Matthews, T. J., 1989, Principal neutralizing domain of the human immunodeficiency virus type 1 envelope protein, *Proc. Natl. Acad. Sci. USA* **86:**6768–6772.

Javaherian, K., Langlois, A. J., LaRosa, G. J., Profy, A. T., Bolognesi, D. P., Herlihy, W. C., Putney, S. D., and Matthews, T. J., 1990, Broadly neutralizing antibodies elicited by the hypervariable neutralizing determinant of HIV-1, *Science* **250:**1590–1593.

Jim, M. J., Hui, H., Robertson, D. L., Muller, M. C., Barré-Sinoussi, F., Hirsch, V. M., Allan, J. S., Shaw, P. M., and Hahn, B. H., 1994, Mosaic genome structure of simian immunodeficiency virus from West African green monkeys, *EMBO J.* **13:**2935–2947.

Jones, I. M., Morikawa, Y., Fenouillet, E., and Moore, J. P., 1992, Antigenicity of the HIV-2 V3 loop, *AIDS* **6:** 888–889.

Kang, C. Y., Nara, P., Chamat, S., Caralli, V., Ryskamp, T., Haigwood, N., Newman, R., and Kohler, H., 1991, Evidence for non V3 specific neutralizing antibodies that interfere with gp120/CD4 binding in human immunodeficiency infected humans, *Proc. Natl. Acad. Sci. USA* **88:**6171–6175.

Kanki, P. J., M'Boup, S., Ricard, D., Barin, F., Denis, F., Boye, C., Sangare, L., Travers, K., Albaum, M., Marlink, R., Romet-Lemonne, J.-L., and Essex, M., 1987, Human T-lymphotropic virus type 4 and the human immunodeficiency virus in West Africa, *Science* **236:**827–831.

Kanki, P., Travers, K., M'Boup, S., Hsieh, C.-C., Marlink, R. G., Guéye-Ndiaye, A., Siby, T., Thior, I., Herandez-Avila, M., Sankalé, J.-L., Ndoye, I., and Essex, M. E., 1994, Slower heterosexual spread of HIV-2 than HIV-1. *Lancet* **343:**943–946.

Karwowska, S., Gorny, M. K., Buchbinder, A., and Zolla-Pazner, S., 1992a, Type-specific human monoclonal antibodies cross-react with the V3 loop of various HIV-1 isolates, in: *Vaccines 92* (F. Brown, R. M. Chanock, H. S. Ginsberg, and R. A. Lerner, eds.), Cold Spring Harbor Laboratory Press, Cold Spring Harbor, NY, p. 171.

Karwowska, S., Gorny, M. K., Buchbinder, A., Gianakakos, V., Williams, C., Fuerst, T., and Zolla-Pazner, S., 1992b, Production of human monoclonal antibodies specific for conformational and linear non-V3 epitopes of gp120, *AIDS Res. Hum. Retrovir.* **8:**1099–1106.

Kayman, S. C., Revesz, K., Chen, H., Kopelman, R., and Pinter, A., 1994, Presentation of native epitopes in the V1/V2 and V3 regions of human immunodeficiency virus type 1 gp120 by fusion glycoproteins containing isolated gp120 domains, *J. Virol.* **68:**400–410.

Keller, R., Peden, K., Paulous, S., Montagnier, L., and Cordonnier, A., 1993, Amino acid changes in the fourth conserved region of human immunodeficiency virus type 2 strain HIV-2_{ROD} envelope glycoprotein modulate fusion, *J. Virol.* **67:**6253–6258.

Kennedy, R. C., Henkel, R. D., Pauletti, D., Allan, J. S., Lee, T. H., Essex, M., and Dreesman, G. R., 1986, Antiserum to a synthetic peptide recognizes the HTLV-III envelope glycoprotein, *Science* **231:**1556–1559.

Klasse, P. J., Pipkorm, R., and Blomberg, J., 1988, Presence of antibodies to a putatively immunosuppressive part of HIV envelope glycoprotein gp41 is strongly associated with health among HIV-positive subjects, *Proc. Natl. Acad. Sci. USA* **85:**5225–5229.

Koito, A., Harrowe, G., Levy, J. A., and Cheng-Mayer, C., 1994, Functional role of the V1/V2 region of human immunodeficiency virus type 1 envelope glycoprotein gp120 in infection of primary macrophages and soluble CD4 neutralization, *J. Virol.* **68:**2253–2259.

Kowalski, M., Potz, J., Basiripour, L., Dorfman, T., Goh, W. C., Terwilliger, E., Dayton, A., Rosen, C., Haseltine, W., and Sodroski, J., 1987, Functional regions of the envelope glycoprotein of human immunodeficiency virus type 1, *Science* **237:**1351–1355.

Kusk, P., Holmback, K., Lindhardt, B. O., Hulgaard, E. F., and Bugge, T. H., 1992, Mapping of two new human B-cell epitopes on HIV-1 gp120, *AIDS* **6**:1451–1456.

Lane, H. C., Masur, H., Edgar, L. C., Whalen, G., Rook, A. H., and Fauci, A. S., 1983, Abnormalities of B-cell activation and immunoregulation in patients with acquired immunodeficiency syndrome, *N. Engl. J. Med.* **309**:453–458.

LaRosa, G. J., Davide, J. P., Weinhold, K., Waterbury, J., Profy, A., Lewis, J., Langlois, A., Dreesman, G., Boswell, R., Shadduck, P., Holley, L., Karplus, M., Bolognesi, D., Matthews, T., Emini, E., and Putney, S., 1990, Conserved sequence and structural elements in the HIV-1 principal neutralizing determinant, *Science* **249**:932–935.

Lasky, L. A., Nakamura, G., Smith, D. H., Fennie, C., Shimasaki, C., Patzer, E., Berman, P., Gregory, T., and Capon, D. J., 1987, Delineation of a region of the human immunodeficiency virus type 1 gp120 glycoprotein critical for interaction with the CD4 receptor, *Cell* **50**:975–985.

Leonard, C. K., Spellman, M. W., Riddle, L., Harris, R. J., Thomas, J. N., and Gregory, T. J., 1990, Assignment of intrachain disulfide bonds and characterization of potential glycosylation sites of the type 1 recombinant human immunodeficiency virus envelope glycoprotein (gp120) expressed in Chinese hamster ovary cells, *J. Biol. Chem.* **265**:10373–10382.

Levy, J., 1993, Pathogenesis of human immunodeficiency virus infection, *Microbiol. Rev.* **57**:183–289.

Lopalco, L., De Santis, C., Meneveri, R., Longhi, R., Ginelli, E., Grassi, F., Siccardi, A. G., and Beretta, A., 1993, Human immunodeficiency virus type 1 gp120 C5 region mimics the HLA class alpha-1 peptide-binding domain, *Eur. J. Immunol.* **23**:2016–2021.

Louwagie, J., McCutchan, F. E., Peeters, M., Brennan, T. P., Sanders-Buell, E., Eddy, G. A., van der Groen, G., Fransen, K., Gershy-Damet, G.-M., Deleys, R., and Burke, D. S., 1993, Phylogenetic analysis of *gag* genes from 70 international HIV-1 isolates provides evidence for multiple genotypes, *AIDS* **7**:769–780.

Luo, L., Li, Y., Cannon, P. M., Kim, S., and Yong Kang, C., 1992, Chimeric gag-V3 virus-like particles of human immunodeficiency virus induce virus neutralizing antibodies, *Proc. Natl. Acad. Sci. USA* **89**:10527–10531.

McKeating, J., Thali, M., Furman, C., Karwowska, S., Gorny, M. K., and Cordell, J., 1992a, Amino acid residues of the HIV-1 gp120 critical for binding of rat and human neutralizing antibodies that block the gp120–sCD4 interaction, *Virology* **190**:134–142.

McKeating, J., Moore, J., Ferguson, M., Marsden, H. S., Graham, S., Almond, J. W., Evans, D. J., and Weiss, R. A., 1992b, Monoclonal antibodies to the C4 region of HIV-1 gp120: Use in topological analysis of a CD4 binding site. *AIDS Res. Hum. Retrovir.* **8**:451–459.

McKeating, J. A., Shotton, C., Cordell, J., Graham, S., Balfe, P., Sullivan, N., Charles, M., Page, M., Blomstedt, A., Olofsson, S., Kayman, S. C., Wu, Z., Pinter, A., Dean, C., Sodroski, J., and Weiss, R. A., 1993, Characterization of neutralizing monoclonal antibodies to linear and conformation-dependent epitopes within the first and second variable domains of human immunodeficiency virus type 1 gp120, *J. Virol.* **67**:4932–4944.

Mannervik, M., Putkonen, P., Ruden, U., Kent, K. A., Norrby, E., Wahren, B., and Broliden, P.-A., 1992, Identification of B-cell antigenic sites on HIV-2 gp125, *J. Acq. Immune Defic. Syndr.* **5**:177–187.

Marlink, R., Kanki, P., Thior, I., Travers, K., Eisen, G., Siby, T., Traore, I., Hsieh, C.-C., Dia, M. C., Gueye, E. H., Hellinger, J., Gueyé-Ndiaye, A., Sankalé, J.-L., Ndoye, I., Mboup, S., and Essex, M., 1994, Reduced rate of disease development after HIV-2 infection as compared to HIV-1 *Science* **265**:1587–1590.

Matsushita, S., Matsumi, S., Yoshimura, K., Morikita, T., Murakami, T., and Takatsuki, K., 1995, Neutralizing monoclonal antibodies against human immunodeficiency virus type 2 gp120, *J. Virol.* **69**:3333–3340.

Matthews, T. J., Langlois, A. J., Robey, W. G., Chang, N. T., Gallo, R. C., Fischinger, P. J., and Bolognesi, D. P., 1986, Restricted neutralization of divergent human T-lymphotropic virus type III isolates by antibodies to the major envelope glycoprotein, *Proc. Natl. Acad. Sci. USA* **83**:9709–9713.

Meyerhans, A., Cheynier, R., Albert, J., Seth, M., Kwok, S., Sninsky, J., Morfeldt-Månson, L., Åsjö, B., and Wain-Hobson, S., 1989, Temporal fluctuations in HIV quasispecies *in vivo* are not reflected by sequential HIV isolations, *Cell* **58**:901–910.

Michel, M. L., Mancini, M., Sobczak, E., Favier, V., Guetard, D., Bahraoui, E. M., and Tollais, P., 1988, Induction of anti human immunodeficiency virus (HIV) neutralizing antibodies in rabbits immunized with recombinant HIV-hepatitis B surface antigen particle, *Proc. Natl. Acad. Sci. USA* **85**:7957–7960.

Modrow, S., Hahn, B. H., Shaw, G. M., Gallo, R. C., Wong-Staal, F., and Wolf, H., 1987, Computer assisted analysis of envelope protein sequences of seven human immunodeficiency virus isolates: Prediction of antigenic epitopes in conserved and variable regions, *J. Virol.* **61**:570–578.

Moore, J. P., and Ho, D. D., 1993, Antibodies to discontinuous or conformationally sensitive epitopes on the gp120 glycoprotein of HIV type 1 are highly prevalent in sera of infected humans, *J. Virol.* **67**:863–867.

Moore, J., Sattentau, Q., Yoshiyama, H., Thali, M., Charles, M., Sullivan, N., Poon, S.-W., Fung, M. S., Traincard, F., Pincus, M., Robey, G., Robinson, J. E., Ho, D. D., and Sodroski, J., 1993a, Probing the structure of the V2 domain of HIV type 1 surface glycoprotein gp120 with a panel of eight monoclonal antibodies: Human immune response to the V1 and V2 domains, *J. Virol.* **67:**6136–6151.

Moore, J. P., Thali, M., Jameson, B. A., Vignaux, F., Lewis, G. K., Poon, S. W., Charles, M. A., Fung, M. S., Sun, B., Durda, P. M., Åkerblom, L., Wahren, B., Ho, D. D., Sattentau, Q., and Sodroski, J., 1993b, Immunochemical analysis of the gp120 surface glycoprotein of human immunodeficiency virus type 1: Probing the structure of the C4 and V4 domains and the interaction of the C4 domain with the V3 loop, *J. Virol.* **67:**4785–4796.

Moore, J. P., McCutchan, F. E., Poon, S. W., Mascola, J., Liu, J., Cao, Y., and Ho, D. D., 1994, Exploration of antigenic variation in gp120 from clades A through F of human immunodeficiency virus type 1 by using monoclonal antibodies, *J. Virol.* **68:**8350–8364.

Murphey-Corb, M., Martin, L. N., Rangan, S. R., Baskin, G. B., Gormus, B. J., Wolf, R. H., Andes, W. A., West, M., and Montelaro, R. C., 1986, Isolation of an HTLV-III related retrovirus from macaques with simian AIDS and its possible origin in asymptomatic mangabeys, *Nature* **321:**435–437.

Muster, T., Guinea, R., Trkola, A., Purtscher, M., Klima, A., Steindl, F., Palese, P., and Katinger, H., 1994, Cross-neutralizing activity against divergent human immunodeficiency virus type 1 isolates induced by the gp41 sequence ELDKWAS, *J. Virol.* **68:**4031–4034.

Myers, G., Korber, B., Smith, R. F., Berzofsky, J. A., and Pavlakis, G. N., 1992, *Human Retroviruses and AIDS 1992*, Los Alamos National Laboratory, Los Alamos, NM.

Myers, G., Korber, B., Smith, R. F., Berzofsky, J. A., and Pavlakis, G. N., 1993, *Human Retroviruses and AIDS 1993*, Los Alamos National Laboratory, Los Alamos, NM.

Myers, G., Korber, B., Jeang, K. T., Henderson, L., Wain-Hobson, S., and Pavlakis, G. N., 1994, *Human Retroviruses and AIDS 1994*, Los Alamos National Laboratory, Los Alamos, NM.

Myers, G., Rabson, A. B., Berzofsky, J. A., Smith, T. F., and Wong-Staal, F., 1990, *Human Retroviruses and AIDS 1990*, Los Alamos National Laboratory, Los Alamos, NM.

Nakamura, G. R., Byrn, R., Rosenthal, K., Porter, J. P., Hobbs, M. R., Riddle, L., Eastman, D. J., Dowbenko, D., Gregory, T., Fendly, B. M., and Berman, P. W., 1992, Monoclonal antibodies to the extracellular domain of HIV-1 IIIB gp160 that neutralize infectivity, block binding to CD4 and react with diverse isolates, *AIDS Res. Hum. Retrovir.* **8:**1875–1885.

Nara, P. L., Robey, W. G., Arthur, L. O., Asher, D. M., Wolff, A. V., Gibbs, C. J., Jr., Gajdusek, D. C., and Fischinger, P. J., 1987, Persistent infection of chimpanzees with HIV: Serological responses and properties in re-isolated viruses, *J. Virol.* **61:**3173–3180.

Nara, P. L., Smith, L., Dunlop, N., Hatch, W., Merges, M., Waters, D., Kelliher, J., Gallo, R. C., Fischinger, P. J., and Goudsmit, J., 1990, Emergence of viruses resistant to neutralization by V3 specific antibodies in experimental human immunodeficiency virus type 1 IIIB infection of chimpanzees, *J. Virol.* **64:**3779–3791.

Neurath, A. R., 1993, B cell antigenic site mapping of HIV-1 glycoproteins, in: *Chemical Immunology*, Volume 56 (L. Aldorini, B. Arai, F. W. Fitch, K. Ishizaka, P. J. Lachmann, and B. H. Waksman, eds.), Karger, Basel, pp. 34–60.

Niedrig, M., Harthus, H. P., Hinkula, J., Broker, M., Bickhard, H., Pauli, G., Gelderblom, H. R., and Wahren, B., 1992, Inhibition of viral replication by monoclonal antibodies directed against HIV gp120, *J. Gen. Virol.* **73:**2451–2455.

Norrby, E., Biberfeld, G., Chiodi, F., von Gegerfelt, A., Naucler, A., Parks, E., and Lerner, R., 1987, Discrimination between antibodies to HIV and to related retroviruses using site-directed serology, *Nature* **329:**248–250.

Norrby, E., Parks, D. E., Utter, G., Houghten, R. A., and Lerner, R. A., 1989, Immunochemistry of the dominating antigenic region Ala582 to Cys604 in the transmembranous protein of simian and human immunodeficiency virus, *J. Immunol.* **143:**3602–3608.

Norrby, E., Putkonen, P., Böttiger, B., Utter, G., and Biberfeld, G., 1991, Comparison of linear antigenic sites in the envelope proteins of human immunodeficiency virus (HIV) type 2 and type 1, *AIDS Res. Hum. Retrovir.* **7:**279–285.

Nowak, M. A., Anderson, R. A., McLean, A. R., Wolfs, T. F. W., Goudsmit, J., and May, R. M., 1991, Antigenic diversity thresholds and the development of AIDS, *Science* **254:**963–969.

Oldstone, M. B., Tishon, A., Lewicki, H., Dyson, H. J., Feher, V. A., Assa-Munt, N., and Wright, P. E., 1991, Mapping the anatomy of the immunodominant domain of the HIV gp41 transmembrane protein: Peptide conformation analysis using monoclonal antibodies and proton nuclear magnetic resonance spectroscopy, *J. Virol.* **65:**1727–1734.

Olshevsky, U., Helseth, E., Furman, C., Li, J., Haseltine, W., and Sodroski, J., 1990, Identification of individual human immunodeficiency virus type 1 gp120 amino acids important for CD4 receptor binding, *J. Virol.* **64:**5701–5707.

Palker, T. J., Matthews, T. J., Clark, M. E., Ciancole, G. J., Randall, R. R., Langlois, A. J., White, G. C., Safai, B., Snyderman, R., Bolognesi, D. P., and Haynes, B. F., 1987, A conserved region at the COOH terminus of human immunodeficiency virus gp120 envelope protein contains an immunodominant epitope, *Proc. Natl. Acad. Sci. USA* **84:**2479–2483.

Palker, T. J., Matthews, T. J., Langlois, A., Tanner, M. E., Martin, M. E., Scearce, R. M., Kim, J. E., Berzofsky, J. A., Bolognesi, D. P., and Haynes, B. F., 1989, Polyvalent human immunodeficiency virus synthetic immunogen comprised of envelope gp120 T helper cell sites and B cell neutralization epitopes, *J. Immunol.* **142:**3612–3619.

Pincus, S. H., Messer, K. G., Nara, P. L., Blattner, W. A., Colclough, G., and Reitz, M., 1994, Temporal analysis of the antibody response to HIV envelope protein in HIV-1 infected laboratory workers, *J. Clin. Invest.* **93:** 2505–2513.

Popovic, M., Sarngadharan, M. G., Read, E., and Gallo, R. C., 1984, Detection, isolation, and continuous production of cytopathic retroviruses (HTLV-III) from patients with AIDS and pre-AIDS, *Science* **224:** 497–500.

Posner, M., Hideshima, T., Cannon, T., Mukherjee, M., Mayer, K. H., and Byrn, R. A., 1991, An IgG human monoclonal antibody which reacts with HIV-1 gp120 inhibits virus binding to cells, and neutralizes infection, *J. Immunol.* **146:**4325–4332.

Posner, M. R., Cavacini, L. A., Emes, C., Power, J., and Byrn, R., 1993, Neutralization of HIV-1 by F105, a human monoclonal antibody to the CD4 binding site of gp120, *J. Acq. Immune Defic. Syndr.* **6:**7–14.

Profy, A., Salinas, P., Eckler, L., Dunlop, N., Nara, P., and Putney, S., 1990, Epitopes recognized by the neutralizing antibodies of an HIV-1-infected individual, *J. Immunol.* **144:**4641–4647.

Putney, S. D., Matthews, T. J., Robey, W. G., Lynn, D. L., Robert-Guroff, M., Mueller, W. T., Langlois, A., Ghrayeb, J., Petteway, S. R., Weinhold, K. J., Fischinger, P. J., Wong-Staal, F., Gallo, R. C., and Bolognesi, D. P., 1986, HTLV-III/LAV-neutralizing antibodies to an E. coli-produced fragment of the virus envelope, *Science* **234:**1392–1395.

Ranki, A., Weiss, S. H., Valle, S. L., Antonen, J., and Krohn, K. J. E., 1987, Neutralizing antibodies in HIV (HTLV-III) infection: Correlation with clinical outcome and antibody response against different viral proteins, *Clin. Exp. Immunol.* **69:**231–239.

Roben, P., Moore, J. P., Thali, M., Sodroski, J., Barbas, C. F., III, and Burton, D. R., 1994, Recognition properties of a panel of human recombinant Fab fragments to the CD4 binding site of gp120 that show differing abilities to neutralize human immunodeficiency virus type 1, *J. Virol.* **68:**4821–4828.

Robert-Guroff, M., Brown, M., and Gallo, R. C., 1985, HTLV-III neutralizing antibodies in patients with AIDS and AIDS related complex, *Nature* **316:**72–74.

Robert-Guroff, M., Aldrich, K., Muldoon, R., Stern, T. L., Bansal, G. P., Matthews, T. J., Markham, P. D., Gallo, R. C., and Franchini, G., 1992, Cross-neutralization of human immunodeficiency virus type 1 and 2 and simian immunodeficiency virus isolates, *J. Virol.* **66:**3602–3608.

Robey, W. G., Safai, B., Oroszlan, S., Arthur, L. O., Gonda, M. A., Gallo, R. C., and Fischinger, P. J., 1985, Characterization of envelope and core structural gene products of HTLV-III with sera from AIDS patients, *Science* **228:**593–595.

Robey, W. G., Arthur, L. O., Matthews, T. J., Langlois, A., Copeland, T. D., Lerche, N. W., Oroszlan, S., Bolognesi, D. P., Gilden, A. V., and Fischinger, P. J., 1986, Prospect for prevention of human immunodeficiency virus infection: Purified 120kDa envelope glycoprotein induces neutralizing antibody, *Proc. Natl. Acad. Sci. USA* **83:**7023–7027.

Robinson, W. E., Jr., Gorny, M. K., Xu, J. Y., Mitchell, W. M., and Zolla-Pazner, S., 1991, Two immunodominant domains of gp41 bind antibodies which enhance HIV-1 infection *in vitro*, *J. Virol.* **65:**4169–4176.

Rusche, J. R., Javaherian, K., McDanal, C., Petro, J., Lynn, D. L., Grimalia, R., Langlois, A., Gallo, R. C., Arthur, L. O., Fischinger, P. J., Bolognesi, D. P., Putney, S., and Matthews, T. J., 1988, Antibodies that inhibit fusion of HIV-1 infected cells bind to 24 amino acid sequence of the viral envelope, gp120, *Proc. Natl. Acad. Sci. USA* **85:**3198–3202.

Saag, M. S., Hahn, B. H., Gibbons, J., Li, Y., Parks, E. S., Parks, W. P., and Shaw, G. M., 1988, Extensive variation of human immunodeficiency virus type 1 *in vivo*, *Nature* **334:**440–444.

Sattentau, Q. J., Clapham, P., Weiss, R. A., Beverly, P., Montagnier, L., Alhalabi, M. F., Gluckmann, J. C., and Klatzmann, D., 1988, The human and simian immunodeficiency viruses HIV-1, HIV-2 and SIV interact with similar epitopes in their cellular receptor, the CD4 molecule, *AIDS* **2:**101–105.

Schrier, R. D., Gnann, J. W., Jr., Langlois, A. J., Shriver, K., Nelson, J. A., and Oldstone, M. B., 1988, B and T-lymphocyte responses to an immunodominant epitope of human immunodeficiency virus, *J. Virol.* **62:** 2531–2536.

Scott, C. F., Jr., Silver, S., Profy, A. T., Putney, S. D., Langlois, A., Weinhold, K., and Robinson, J. E., 1990, Human monoclonal antibody that recognizes the V3 region of HIV gp120 and neutralizes the human T-lymphotropic virus type III-MN strain, *Proc. Natl. Acad. Sci. USA* **87:**8597–8600.

Sharp, P. M., Robertson, D. L., Gao, F., and Hahn, B. H., 1994, Origins and diversity of human immunodeficiency viruses, *AIDS* **8(Suppl. 1):**S27–S42.

Shotton, C., Arnold, C., Sattentau, Q., Sodroski, J., and McKeating, J. A., 1995, Identification and characterization of monoclonal antibodies specific for polymorphic antigenic determinants within the V2 region of the human immunodeficiency virus type 1 envelope glycoprotein, *J. Virol.* **69:**222–230.

Simmonds, P., Zhang, L. Q., McOmish, F., Balfe, P., Ludlam, C. A., and Leigh Brown, A. J., 1991, Discontinuous sequence change of human immunodeficiency virus (HIV) type 1 *env* sequences in plasma viral and lymphocyte-associated proviral populations *in vivo*: Implications for models of HIV pathogenesis, *J. Virol.* **65:**6266–6275.

Sodroski, J., Goh, W. C., Rosen, K., Campbell, K., and Haseltine, W. A., 1986. Role of the HTLV-III/LAV envelope in syncytium formation and cytopathicity, *Nature* **322:**470–474.

Stamatatos, L., and Cheng-Mayer, C., 1993, Evidence that the structural conformation of envelope gp120 affects human immunodeficiency virus type 1 infectivity, host range and syncytium forming ability, *J. Virol.* **67:**5635–5639.

Steimer, K. S., Scandella, C. J., Stiles, P. V., and Haigwood, N. L., 1991, Neutralization of divergent HIV-1 isolates by conformation dependent human antibodies to gp 120, *Science* **254:**105–108.

Sugano, T., Musuho, Y., Matsumoto, Y., Lake, D., Gschwind, C., Petersen, E. A., and Hersh, E. M., 1988, Human monoclonal antibody against glycoproteins of human immunodeficiency virus, *Biochem. Biophys. Res. Commun.* **155:**1105–1112.

Sullivan, N., Thali, M., Furman, C., Ho, D. D., and Sodroski, J., 1993, Effect of amino acid changes in the V1/V2 region of the human immunodeficiency virus type 1 gp120 glycoprotein on subunit association, syncytium formation, and recognition by a neutralizing antibody, *J. Virol.* **67:**3674–3679.

Sun, N. C., Ho, D. D., Sun, C. R., Liou, R. S., Gordon, W., Fung, M. S., Li, X. L., Ting, R. C., Lee, T. H., Chang, N. T., and Chang, T.-W., 1989, Generation and characterization of monoclonal antibodies to the putative CD-4-binding domain of HIV-1 gp120, *J. Virol.* **63:**3579–3585.

Teeuwsen, V. J. P., Sieblink, K. H. J., Crush-Stanton, S., Swerdlow, B., Schalken, J. J., Goudsmir, J., van de Akker, R., Stukart, M. J., Vytdehaag, F. G., and Osterhaus, A. D., 1990, Production and characterization of a human monoclonal antibody, reactive with a conserved epitope on gp41 of human immunodeficiency virus type 1, *AIDS Res. Hum. Retrovir.* **6:**381–392.

Thali, M., Olshevsky, U., Furman, C., Gabuzda, D., Posner, M., and Sodroski, J., 1991, Characterization of a discontinuous HIV-1 gp120 epitope recognized by a broadly reactive neutralizing human monoclonal antibody, *J. Virol.* **65:**6188–6193.

Thali, M., Furman, C., Ho, D. D., Robinson, J., Tilley, S., Pinter, A., and Sodroski, J., 1992, Discontinuous conserved neutralization epitopes overlapping the CD4 binding region of the HIV-1 gp120 envelope glycoprotein, *J. Virol.* **66:**5635–5641.

Tilley, S. A., Honnen, W. J., Racho, M., Hilgartner, M., and Pinter, A., 1991, A human monoclonal antibody against CD4 binding site of HIV-1 gp120 exhibits potent, broadly neutralizing activity, *Res. Virol.* **142:**247–259.

Tolle, T., Petry, H., Bachmann, B., Hunsmann, G., and Luke, W., 1994, Variability of the env gene in cynomolgus macaques persistently infected with human immunodeficiency virus type 2 strain ben, *J. Virol.* **68:**2765–2771.

Traincard, R., Rey-Cuille, M. A., Huon, I., Dartevelle, S., Mazie, J. C., and Benichou, S., 1994, Characterization of monoclonal antibodies to human immunodeficiency virus type 2 envelope glycoproteins, *AIDS Res. Hum. Retrovir.* **10:**1659–1667.

Travers, K., Mboup, S., Marlink, R., Guéye-Ndiaye, A., Siby, T., Thior, I., Traore, I., Dieng-Sarr, A., Sankalé, J.-L., Mullins, C. Ndoye, I., Hsieh, C.-C., Essex, M., and Kanki, P., 1995, Natural protection against HIV-1 infection provided by HIV-2, *Science* **268:**1612–1615.

Tremblay, M., and Weinberg, M. A., 1990, Neutralization of multiple HIV-1 isolates from a single subject by autologous sequential sera, *J. Infect. Dis.* **162:**735–737.

Tyler, D. S., Stanley, S. D., Zolla-Pazner, S., Gorny, M. K., Shadduck, P., Langlois, A. J., Matthews, T. J., Bolognesi, D. P., Palker, T. J., and Weinhold, K. J., 1990, Identification of sites within gp41 that serve as targets for antibody-dependent cellular cytotoxicity by using human monoclonal antibodies, *J. Immunol.* **145**:3276–3282.

Vanini, S., Longhi, R., Lazzarin, A., Vigo, E., Siccardi, A. G., and Viale, G., 1993, Discrete regions of HIV-1 gp41 defined by syncytia-inhibiting affinity-purified human antibodies, *AIDS* **7**:167–174.

van Tijn, D. A., Boucher, C. A., Bakker, M., and Goudsmit, J., 1989, Antigenicity of linear B cell epitopes in the C1, V1 and V3 region of HIV-1 gp120, *J. Acq. Immune Defic. Syndr.* **2**:303–306.

Vogel, T., Kurth, R., and Norley, S., 1994, The majority of neutralizing Abs in HIV-1 infected patients recognize linear V3-loop sequences. Studies using HIV-1_{MN} multiple antigenic peptides, *J. Immunol.* **153**:1895–1904.

von Gegerfelt, A., Albert, J., Morfeldt-Månson, L., Broliden, K., and Fenyö, E.-M., 1991, Isolate-specific neutralizing antibodies in patients with progressive HIV-1-related disease, *Virology* **185**:162–168.

Warrier, S. V., Pinter, A., Honnen, W. J., Girard, M., Muchmore, E., and Tilley, S. A., 1994, A novel, glycan-dependent epitope in the V2 domain of human immunodeficiency virus type 1 gp120 is recognized by a highly potent, neutralizing chimpanzee monoclonal antibody, *J. Virol.* **68**:4636–4642.

Weiss, R. A., Clapham, P. R., Weber, J., Cheingsong-Popov, R., Dalgleish, A., Carne, A., Weller, I., and Tedder, R. S., 1985, Neutralisation of human T-lymphotropic virus type III by sera of AIDS and AIDS-risk patients, *Nature* **316**:69–72.

Weiss, R. A., Clapham, P. R., Weber, J. N. N., Dalgleish, A. G., Lasky, L. A., and Berman, P. W., 1986, Variable and conserved neutralization antigens of HIV, *Nature* **324**:572–575.

Weiss, R. A., Clapham, P., Weber, J. N., Whitby, D., Tedder, R. S., O'Connor, T., Chamaret, S., and Montagnier, L., 1988, HIV-2 antisera cross-neutralise HIV-1, *AIDS* **2**:95–100.

Westervelt, P., Trowbridge, D. B., Epstein, L. G., Blumberg, B. M., Li, Y., Hahn, B. H., Shaw, G. M., Price, R. W., and Ratner, L., 1992, Macrophage tropism determinants of human immunodeficiency virus type 1 in vivo, *J. Virol.* **66**:2577–2582.

Willey, R. L., Rutledge, R. A., Dias, S., Folks, T., Theodore, T., Buckler, C. E., and Martin, M. A., 1986, Identification of conserved and divergent domains within the envelope gene of the acquired immunodeficiency syndrome retrovirus, *Proc. Natl. Acad. Sci. USA* **83**:5038–5042.

Willey, R. L., Smith, L. A., Lasky, L. A., Theodore, T. S., Earl, P. L., Moss, B., Capon, D. J., and Martin, M. A., 1988, In vitro mutagenesis identifies a region within the envelope gene of the human immunodeficiency virus that is critical for infectivity, *J. Virol.* **62**:139–147.

Xu, J. Y., Gorny, M. K., Palker, T., Karwowska, S., and Zolla-Pazner, S., 1991, Epitope mapping of two immunodominant domains of gp41, the transmembrane protein of HIV-1, using 10 human monoclonal antibodies, *J. Virol.* **65**:4832–4838.

CHAPTER 4

LYMPHOCYTE ADHESION CORECEPTORS AND THEIR ROLES IN HIV-1 REPLICATION

JEFFREY A. LEDBETTER

1. INTRODUCTION

T cells recognize and respond to antigen during contact with B cells and other antigen-presenting cells (APC) (for review see Clark and Ledbetter, 1994). The specificity of the T-cell response is determined when the T-cell receptor (TCR) recognizes peptide antigens bound to MHC class I or class II molecules on the APC. However, engagement of the TCR alone is not sufficient for induction of a T-cell response (Bretscher and Cohn, 1970; Mueller *et al.*, 1989; Tan *et al.*, 1993). The affinity of the TCR for peptide/MHC complexes is low (Matsui *et al.*, 1991), and APCs may express only small numbers of each immunogenic peptide. Although the low affinity and high off rate of TCR binding may allow multiple interactions with a restricted number of antigens (Valitutti *et al.*, 1995), additional adhesion interactions are required to stabilize the T cell/APC cellular conjugates (Clark and Ledbetter, 1994). These accessory adhesion events also supplement and modify the intracellular signals that are transmitted to both the T cell and the APC. Altered signals to T cells that may lead to inactivation or anergy can occur either by specific blocking of adhesion receptors (Ledbetter *et al.*, 1995) or via presentation of modified peptide antigens (Madrenas *et al.*, 1995; Sloan-Lancaster *et al.*, 1994). Our understanding of these accessory receptor interactions that make critical contributions to the T cell and APC activation response continues to grow rapidly. Here I will review some of the better-characterized adhesion and signaling molecules of T cells and APC, including CD4, CD8, CD2, CD28, CD40, and β2 integrins. These molecules and their counterreceptors are important for replication of HIV-1, since the signals they provide have dramatic effects on the amounts of virus released from stimulated T cells (Diegel *et al.*, 1993; Smithgall *et al.*, 1995; Pinchuk *et al.*, 1994; Moran *et al.*, 1993).

JEFFREY A. LEDBETTER • Bristol-Myers Squibb Pharmaceutical Research Institute, Seattle, Washington 98121.

Immunology of HIV Infection, edited by Sudhir Gupta. Plenum Press, New York, 1996.

2. STRUCTURE OF THE T-CELL ANTIGEN RECEPTOR

The antigen receptor complex of T cells is composed of the α,β or γ,δ dimers that contact peptide/MHC complexes, and the CD3 signal-transducing chains γ, δ, ε, and ζ. Although the TCR/CD3 complex does not contain intrinsic tyrosine kinase activity, the CD3 chains become phosphorylated on tyrosine residues very rapidly during T-cell activation (for review see Weiss and Littman, 1994). Two Src family kinases, $p59^{fyn}$ (Fyn) and $p56^{lck}$ (Lck), have been demonstrated to play critical and nonoverlapping roles in this activation response. Fyn interacts directly with the CD3 complex (Timson Gauen *et al.*, 1992), whereas Lck binds to the cytoplasmic tails of the CD8, CD4, and CD2 coreceptors (Rudd *et al.*, 1988; Veillette *et al.*, 1988). CD3 cross-linking activates Fyn (Tsygankov *et al.*, 1992), whereas CD2, CD4, or CD8 cross-linking activates Lck (Veillette *et al.*, 1989; Danielian *et al.*, 1991). The interaction of TCR/CD3 with CD2, CD4, or CD8 that occurs during T-cell binding to APC results in strong amplification of tyrosine phosphorylation in T cells through increased Lck-mediated phosphorylation of CD3 signaling chains. This means that the T-cell antigen receptor that is formed during T-cell/APC interactions is composed of TCR/CD3 and other coreceptors including CD4 or CD8, CD2, CD28, and CD18. Additional molecules such as CD45 and CD5 are also components of the activated T-cell receptor. The stoichiometries of TCR/CD3 associations with these coreceptors has a strong influence on the T-cell response.

In addition to binding to T-cell coreceptors, Lck also can associate with the IL-2 receptor (Kobayashi *et al.*, 1993) and has been found to contribute to T-cell activation and cytokine gene expression through a mechanism that is independent of its association with CD4 or CD8 (Weiss and Littman, 1994). Another cytoplasmic tyrosine kinase, ZAP70, is also critical for T-cell activation and functions downstream of the Src family kinases (Chan *et al.*, 1991; Iwashima *et al.*, 1994; Wange *et al.*, 1993; Timson Gauen *et al.*, 1994). The sequential activation of Src family kinases followed by cytosolic kinases of the ZAP70 family such as $p72^{syk}$, is common to other lymphocyte receptors that lack intrinsic tyrosine kinase activity, including the Fc receptors on monocytes and mast cells, and the B-cell antigen receptor (Weiss and Littman, 1994).

3. SIGNALS FROM THE T-CELL ANTIGEN RECEPTOR

The sites of tyrosine phosphorylation on the CD3 signaling chains are contained within an approximately 26-residue motif termed AHR1 or TAM sequences (Wange *et al.*, 1993; Timson Gauen *et al.*, 1994). This motif allows the formation of a signaling complex at the membrane that includes ZAP70 kinase (Hatada *et al.*, 1995) and additional effector molecules, including phospholipase C γ1 (PLCγ1), PI-3 kinase, and linker proteins including growth factor receptor-bound protein 2 (Grb2), human Son of Sevenless (hSos) (Bowtell *et al.*, 1992), and pp35/36 (Nel *et al.*, 1995; Gilliland *et al.*, 1992). The signaling complexes form primarily through interactions of the SH2 and SH3 domains contained in the proteins. The SH2 domains bind to phosphotyrosyl peptide motifs formed after tyrosine kinase activation (Songyang *et al.*, 1994; Pawson and Gish, 1992), whereas the SH3 domains bind to proline-rich motifs that are independent of tyrosine phosphorylation (Ren *et al.*, 1993; Lim *et al.*, 1994). The complexes form to propagate the signal originating at the TCR/CD3 receptor to key enzymes that redistribute to the membrane during T-cell activation. Several signaling pathways originate from these complexes, including activation of both PLCγ1 and ras (Pastor *et al.*, 1995), indicating that they may be coordinately regulated.

One early signaling pathway that was recognized in T cells activated by TCR/CD3 cross-linking was an increase in cytoplasmic calcium concentration (Weiss and Littman, 1994). The calcium increase is the result of inositol 1,4,5-trisphosphate (IP_3-mediated release of intracellular calcium, followed by the opening of plasma membrane calcium channels. The signal originates with the tyrosine phosphorylation and activation of PLCγ1 (Weiss and Littman, 1994), an enzyme that generates IP_3 and DG, second messengers for both calcium mobilization and protein kinase C activation. PLCβ is also expressed in T cells and responds to stimulation of chemokine receptors but not the TCR/CD3 or coreceptor cross-linking.

Both Src family and ZAP70 kinases are important for PLCγ1 phosphorylation, since calcium signaling defects in kinase-negative patients (Arpaia *et al.*, 1994; Chan *et al.*, 1994) or cell lines have been found. After TCR/CD3 cross-linking, PLCγ1 associates with a T-cell-specific linker protein pp35/36 through SH2 interactions (Gilliland *et al.*, 1992), and with the CD3 ζ chain. PLCγ1 translocates to the membrane and requires an association with the cytoskeletal protein profilin for regulation by tyrosine phosphorylation (Todderud *et al.*, 1990). The signal from PLCγ1 activation is essential for T-cell activation, since the immunosuppressants cyclosporin and FK506 inhibit the calcium-dependent phosphatase calcineurin. Calcineurin activation is required for the translocation to the nucleus by the nuclear factor of activated T cells (NF-AT) during activation of the IL-2 gene (Sigal and Dumont, 1992).

The activation of PLCγ1 in T cells by tyrosine phosphorylation is regulated both by the TCR/CD3 complex and by T-cell coreceptors, including CD2, CD18 (LFA-1), CD4, and CD8. For example, cross-linking of CD3 together with CD2, CD18, CD4, or CD8 with antibodies increases the calcium signal by enhancing the tyrosine phosphorylation of PLCγ1 (Ledbetter *et al.*, 1988; Kanner *et al.*, 1992, 1993). Under natural conditions, these coreceptors interact with the TCR/CD3 complex during APC binding to T cells. When expression levels of TCR/CD3 are low, as in immature T cells in the thymus, antibody cross-linking studies have shown that the activation of PLCγ1 is even more dependent on coreceptor interaction with the TCR/CD3 complex (Turka *et al.*, 1991; Gilliland *et al.*, 1991). The mechanism for this synergy is likely to be the recruitment of additional coreceptor-associated Lck to the TCR/CD3 to enhance the phosphorylation of tyrosines within the AHRI motifs of the CD3 chains, resulting in more ZAP70 recruitment and PLCγ1 activation in the signaling complexes (Sancho *et al.*, 1992).

Another signal that is required for T-cell responses is the activation of the guanine nucleotide binding (G) protein $p21^{ras}$ (see Pastor *et al.*, 1995, for review). Constitutively active $p21^{ras}$ synergizes with calcium signals in the activation of the IL-2 gene, and a dominant negative $p21^{ras}$ inhibits IL-2 gene expression (Baldari *et al.*, 1995; Owaki *et al.*, 1993). Activation of $p21^{ras}$ initiates a cascade of kinase interactions first by activating the Raf-1 kinase through a GTP-dependent association of ras with Raf-1 (Koide *et al.*, 1993; Nassar *et al.*, 1995). Raf-1 activates mitogen-activated kinase kinase (MKK) that in turn activates extracellular signal-regulated kinases (ERKs) (Izquierdo *et al.*, 1993; Howe *et al.*, 1992). The signal converges on the regulation of the transcription factor NF-AT, a complex of AP1 and a member of the c-rel family of transcription factors (NF-ATp) (Rao, 1994). AP-1 is composed of c-jun and c-fos, and regulation by ERKs may occur via activation of transcription factors necessary for the induction of the c-fos gene (Marais *et al.*, 1993).

Activation of $p21^{ras}$ after stimulation of the TCR/CD3 complex is primarily mediated by the guanine nucleotide exchange factor, hSos. hSos is a component of the signaling complex that assembles at the membrane through protein–protein interactions with the linker molecules pp35/36 and Grb2 (Buday *et al.*, 1994; Nel *et al.*, 1995). GTPase-activation proteins for ras (ras-GAP) act as negative regulators of $p21^{ras}$, and stimulation of the TCR/CD3 complex has been reported to inhibit the activity of ras-GAP (Graves *et al.*, 1991). Therefore, the overall activation of $p21^{ras}$ is likely to be regulated by a combination of hSos and ras-GAP activities after antigen recognition.

Another putative guanine nucleotide exchange factor, Vav, is phosphorylated on tyrosine residues after antigen receptor stimulation in lymphocytes. Gene knock-out experiments have shown that vav-deficient mice have severely impaired T-cell development, and T cells that are present are hyporesponsive to antigen (Tarakhovsky *et al.*, 1995; Zhang *et al.*, 1995; Fischer *et al.*, 1995). Although vav could function in guanine nucleotide exchange for $p21^{ras}$ *in vitro* (Gulbins *et al.*, 1993), expression of active vav in fibroblasts did not cause activation of $p21^{ras}$ (Bustelo *et al.*, 1994). Therefore, the function of vav in lymphocyte activation is still uncertain.

The CD2, CD4, and CD8 coreceptors provide signals to T cells that depend primarily on physical interactions with the TCR/CD3 complex to increase tyrosine phosphorylation of the CD3 AHRI motifs. These molecules constitutively associate with TCR/CD3, probably at a low stoichiometry. Increased CD4 association with TCR/CD3 was shown to occur during T cell–APC binding (Kupfer *et al.*, 1987). It is likely that during cellular interactions, the stoichiometry of CD2, CD4, and β2 integrins associated with TCR/CD3 increases via redistribution of ligand/adhesion coreceptors to sites of cell/cell contact. If CD2, CD4, CD8, or β2 integrins are coclustered with TCR/CD3 using mAbs, there is a powerful synergy in activation signals (Kanner *et al.*, 1992; Ledbetter *et al.*, 1989). In contrast, many studies have shown that cross-linking of CD4, CD8, or CD2 independently of TCR/CD3 delivers signals to T cells that are inhibitory for T-cell activation (Miller *et al.*, 1993; Ohno *et al.*, 1991; Ledbetter *et al.*, 1988), even though the associated Lck kinase is activated under these conditions (Danielian *et al.*, 1991; Veillette *et al.*, 1989; Ledbetter *et al.*, 1995). This means that "remote" signals through these coreceptors given by a mAb or by a cell other than the APC would be expected to inhibit rather than augment an antigen-specific response. One response of T cells to CD4 cross-linking that may contribute to inhibition is the expression of the FAS receptor. The FAS receptor transmits signals that lead to apoptosis in T cells and other lymphoid and nonlymphoid cells (Nagata and Suda, 1995). There is evidence that T cells from HIV-1-positive individuals are sensitive to apoptosis from FAS triggering, possibly as a consequence of CD4 signals delivered by HIV-1 gp120 envelope glycoprotein binding to CD4 (Terai *et al.*, 1991; Banda *et al.*, 1992; Westendorp *et al.*, 1995; Wang *et al.*, 1994). Therefore, the signals delivered by coreceptors when they are bound without coordinated engagement of the TCR are not sufficient for T-cell proliferation but in the case of CD4 can sensitize T cells to subsequent apoptotic signals.

The CD28 receptor is a critical T-cell coreceptor (Linsley and Ledbetter, 1993) that differs from CD2, CD4, or CD8 in that CD28 can function at least partially independently of TCR/CD3. Soluble antibody binding to CD28 can deliver "remote" stimulatory signals needed for T-cell activation without depending on cross-linking of CD28 with TCR/CD3 (Moretta *et al.*, 1985; Martin *et al.*, 1986; Ledbetter *et al.*, 1985). CD28 also differs from other T-cell coreceptors since only CD28 has been found to contribute to IL-2 gene activation through a mechanism that is calcium independent and partially resistant to inhibition by cyclosporine (June *et al.*, 1987). CD28 is known to signal through a protein tyrosine kinase-dependent mechanism that involves the activation of the Src family kinases Lck and Fyn, and the Tec family kinase itk/emt (August and Dupont, 1994; Hutchcroft and Bierer, 1994; August *et al.*, 1994). Following CD28 cross-linking, CD28 is phosphorylated on a tyrosine residue to form a high-affinity binding site for the SH2 domain of the p85 subunit of phosphatidylinositol-3 kinase (PI-3K) (Prasad *et al.*, 1994; Stein *et al.*, 1994; Truitt *et al.*, 1994). PI-3K binds tightly to CD28 after activation, and is thought to transmit some of the critical signals, since mutation of the PI-3K SH2 binding site on CD28 prevented CD28 function in transfected cells (Pages *et al.*, 1994; Stein *et al.*, 1994). However, in T cells, there is evidence that PI-3K also associates with CD4 and TCR/CD3 after T-cell activation (Thompson *et al.*, 1992), so it is unlikely that activation of PI-3K fully explains the signaling of the CD28 receptor. CD28 cross-linking also contributes to the activation of PLCγ1 through tyrosine phosphorylation of this enzyme (Lu *et al.*, 1992; Ledbetter and Linsley, 1992), and mediates a calcium-dependent and cyclosporine-sensitive arm of the CD28 signal. Another protein strongly phosphorylated after CD28 activation is the vav proto-oncogene (Nunes *et al.*, 1995). CD28 cross-linking with mAbs but not with natural ligand could activate ERK2, suggesting the possibility of CD28 contributions to $p21^{ras}$ activation (August and Dupont, 1995; Nunes *et al.*, 1995). However, none of the linker proteins Grb2, Shc, or pp35/36, or the guanine nucleotide exchange factor hSos have been found to be associated with CD28 after activation (Pastor *et al.*, 1995). The CD28 receptor has been reported to play an important role in the activation of a kinase related to ERK2, called Jun N-terminal kinase (JNK) (Su *et al.*, 1994). JNK activation is important for activation of c-jun, and could synergize with ERK activation of c-fos gene expression to form active AP1 heterodimers. JNK is also required for the activation of the ATF2 transcription factor that binds to the promoters of many genes (Gupta *et al.*, 1995). Evidence has also been presented that CD28 cross-linking induces 5-lipoxygenase activation and production of reactive oxygen intermediates (Los *et al.*, 1995), and can stimulate sphingomyelin-ceramide turnover (Chan and Ochi, 1995).

4. SIGNALS FROM THE IL-2 RECEPTOR

Although expression of cytokines by T cells depends on signals from TCR/CD3 and coreceptors, cell cycle progression requires signals through the IL-2 receptor (IL-2R). The IL-2R is composed of three subunits, α, β, and γ. The α chain is not expressed on resting T cells, and its expression early after T-cell activation confers high-affinity IL-2 binding. The β and γ chains are responsible for signal transduction through the activation of tyrosine kinases, including Lck and Janus kinases (JAK1 and JAK3) (Beadling *et al.*, 1994). Lck and JAK kinases bind to distinct regions of the β chain (Kobayashi *et al.*, 1993; Ihle *et al.*, 1994), and β-chain knock-out mice exhibit dysregulated T-cell activation and autoimmunity (Suzuki *et al.*, 1995). JAK kinases phosphorylate on tyrosine residues and activate transcription factors termed STATS (Signal transducers and activators of transcription) that migrate to the nucleus after cytokine stimulation (Ihle *et al.*, 1994). The IL-2R γ chain is a common component of the receptor for other cytokines in addition to IL-2, including IL-4, IL-7, IL-9, and IL-15. The JAK–STAT pathway is constitutively activated in T cells transformed by HTLV-1, a human lymphotropic virus that leads to T-cell leukemia (Migone *et al.*, 1995).

The IL-2R transmits some signals in common with the TCR/CD3 complex, including activation of $p21^{ras}$ (Ravichandran and Burakoff, 1994; Graves *et al.*, 1992). However, unlike TCR/CD3 stimulation, there is no activation of PLCγ1 after IL-2 stimulation, and no downstream calcium mobilization or activation of PKC (Mills *et al.*, 1986). The IL-2R also differs from the TCR/CD3 complex in that the tyrosine kinases activated by IL-2 are not directed toward vav or PI-3K. Although a functional IL-2R is needed for T-cell replication, the IL-2 signals do not seem to be involved in stimulation of HIV-1 replication (Moran *et al.*, 1993; Poli and Fauci, 1992). Therefore, there is not a straightforward correlation between T-cell growth and HIV-1 replication in infected T cells.

The genes responsible for several inherited immunodeficiency diseases in humans have been found to involve lymphocyte receptors or their signal transduction pathways. For example, lymphocyte adhesion deficiency (LAD) results from defects in the β2 integrins and leads to increased susceptibility to bacterial infections (Kishimoto *et al.*, 1987; Bowen *et al.*, 1982). The CD40 receptor is also critical for B-cell differentiation, since mutations in the X-linked gene encoding the CD40 ligand gp39 cause hyper IgM syndrome (Aruffo *et al.*, 1993; Allen *et al.*, 1993; DiSanto *et al.*, 1993; Graf *et al.*, 1992). The inability to activate the CD40 receptor in these patients results in failure to produce antibodies of the IgG isotypes. Defects in the IL-2 receptor γ chain itself (Noguchi *et al.*, 1993) or in the STAT transcription factors that transduce the IL-2 signal to the nucleus cause severe combined immune deficiency (SCID) (Macchi *et al.*, 1995). Mutations in lymphocyte tyrosine kinases including ZAP70 in T cells (Arpaia *et al.*, 1994; Chan *et al.*, 1994) and Btk in pre-B cells (Tsukada *et al.*, 1995; Vetrie *et al.*, 1995) also result in immunodeficiency diseases that have been understood at the molecular level only in the past several years. The variety of genetic defects that can result in immunodeficiency disease underscores the delicate balance of receptors and signals maintained by a competent immune system.

During acquired immunodeficiency disease there is a disruption of normal receptor and activation functions involving the CD4 receptor and signals through the T-cell receptor. The depletion of glutathione and resulting oxidative stress, possibly related to high levels of TNF-α, is also likely to be important in the disruption of activation signals in lymphocytes and resulting immunosuppression in AIDS patients (for review, see Roederer *et al.*, 1993). The potent effects of oxidative stress on lymphocytes seem to be caused both by direct polyclonal tyrosine kinase activation (Schieven *et al.*, 1993; Schieven and Ledbetter, 1995) and by uncoupling of TCR/CD3 signal transduction (Flescher *et al.*, 1994; Schieven *et al.*, 1994; Kavahagh *et al.*, 1993). The combination of signals from CD4 and oxidative stress may work together to cause high sensitivity of CD4 cells to apoptosis from the FAS death receptor.

5. RECEPTOR SIGNALS THAT REGULATE HIV-1 REPLICATION IN INFECTED CELLS

Although IL-2R signals do not increase HIV-1 replication in T cells (Moran *et al.*, 1993; Poli and Fauci, 1992), there is evidence that signals through the TCR/CD3 complex and through the costimulatory receptors engaged during contact with APC have potent effects on HIV-1 replication. Stimulation of $CD4^+$ T cells from peripheral blood of HIV-1 seropositive donors resulted in high levels of HIV-1 production *in vitro* when the activation signal caused T-cell interactions with APC. For example, the ability of soluble anti-CD3 mAbs to induce T-cell proliferation is known to depend on binding of the mAb to T cells via CD3 and to APC via Fc receptors. Immobilized anti-CD3 mAbs can induce T-cell proliferation without a requirement for APC Fc receptor binding. Surprisingly, soluble anti-CD3 induced large amounts of HIV-1 replication with very little T-cell proliferation, whereas immobilized anti-CD3 induced much less virus but more T-cell proliferation (Moran *et al.*, 1993). By separation of blood monocytes and CD4 T cells from seropositive donors, it was found that either of these populations could serve as the source of virus when added together with the complementary population from virus-negative donors during *in vitro* stimulation. This means that the signals provided by the APC/T-cell interaction create the right environment for high levels of HIV-1 replication and spread.

Other pathways of mitogenic T-cell activation that depend on APC/T-cell interactions, including staphylococcal enterotoxin superantigens, also induced very high levels of HIV-1 replication (Moran *et al.*, 1993). Normal blood dendritic cells that can induce T-cell proliferation in the absence of exogenous antigen also stimulated HIV-1 replication in T cells (Pinchuk *et al.*, 1994). Both the CD28 and CD40 receptors have been identified as critical components of the dendritic cell/T-cell interaction that promotes HIV-1 replication (Pinchuk *et al.*, 1994; Weissman *et al.*, 1995). These results suggest the possibility that coreceptor signals may be critical for driving HIV-1 replication in lymphoid organs where cell contact and adhesion is favored. In addition, dendritic cell support of HIV-1 replication in T cells is associated with resistance to neutralization by anti-HIV-1 antibodies (Heath *et al.*, 1995).

An important role of T-cell coreceptor signals in HIV-1 replication was directly demonstrated by the effects of specific inhibitors of lymphocyte adhesion/coreceptor molecules during virus replication *in vitro* (Table I). Inhibition of the CD28 receptor using soluble CTLA4-Ig prevented HIV-1 replication in T cells stimulated with either soluble anti-CD3 or staphylococcal enterotoxin superantigens (Diegel *et al.*, 1993; Smithgall *et al.*, 1995). The inhibition of virus by CTLA4-Ig occurred even at low concentrations of the inhibitor that were not effective in blocking T-cell proliferation (Smithgall *et al.*, 1995). Higher concentrations of CTLA4-Ig blocked both virus replication and T-cell proliferation. Similarly, inhibition of the CD2 coreceptor pathway with anti-CD2 mAbs or anti-LFA-3 (CD58) mAbs also blocked virus replication by over 90% without preventing T-cell proliferation (Diegel *et al.*, 1993). The β2 integrins also play an important role, since

TABLE I. Inhibition of HIV-1 Replication by Blocking T-Cell Adhesion/Coreceptor Binding[a]

Adhesion/ coreceptor	Inhibitor	% inhibition of HIV replication	References
CD28	CTLA4-Ig	72–98	Diegel *et al.* (1993), Smithgall *et al.* (1995), Pinchuk *et al.* (1994)
	Anti-CD80		
CD2	Anti-CD2 Fab	82–95	Diegel *et al.* (1993)
	Anti-CD2 sFv		
CD58 (LFA-3)	Anti-LFA-3	96	Diegel *et al.* (1993)
CD18	Anti-CD18 $F(ab')_2$	84–95	Diegel *et al.* (1993)
	Anti-ICAM-1	98	

[a]HIV-1 replication in peripheral blood mononuclear cells (depleted of $CD8^+$, B cells, and NK cells) from seropositive donors was induced by accessory-cell-dependent T-cell activation (soluble anti-CD3 mAb, staphylococcal enterotoxin superantigens, or blood dendritic cells).

the CD18 mAb 60.3 that inhibits adhesion through this pathway also blocked HIV-1 replication when T cells were stimulated by mechanisms that depend on T-cell/APC engagement (Diegel *et al.*, 1993). CD18 also mediates syncytium formation during HIV-1 replication (Valentin *et al.*, 1990). Stimulation of CD40 enhanced the ability of dendritic cells to support HIV-1 replication in T cells, and the response to CD40 stimulation was the result of increased expression of CD28 ligands (CD80 and CD86) on the dendritic cells (Pinchuk *et al.*, 1994). These results suggest that inhibition of specific coreceptors on T cells or APC may selectively inhibit HIV-1 replication without completely blocking T-cell function. Coreceptor inhibitors may be useful for reducing virus load *in vivo*, perhaps in combination with antiviral drug therapy. The reduction in virus replication would likely slow the rate of selection of drug-resistant viral mutants. Such a strategy of dual inhibition could also alter the course of the virus-specific immune response, both by reducing antigen levels and by directly altering signaling pathways from the lymphocyte coreceptors.

REFERENCES

Allen, R. C., Armitage, R. J., Conley, M. E., Rosenblatt, H., Jenkins, N. A., Copeland, N. G., Bedell, M. A., Edelhoff, S., Disteche, C. M., Simoneaux, D. K., Fanslow, W. C., Belmont, J., and Spriggs, M. K., 1993, CD40 ligand gene defects responsible for X-linked hyper-IgM syndrome, *Science* **259**:990–993.

Arpaia, E., Shahar, M., Dadi, H., Cohen, A., and Roifman, C. M., 1994, Defective T cell receptor signaling and CD8+ thymic selection in humans lacking zap-70 kinase, *Cell* **76**:947–958.

Aruffo, A., Farrington, M., Hollenbaugh, D., Li, X., Milatovich, A., Nonoyama, S., Bajorath, J., Grosmaire, L. S., Stenkamp, R., Neubauer, M., Roberts, R. L., Noelle, R. J., Ledbetter, J. A., Francke, U., and Ochs, H. D., 1993, The CD40 ligand, gp39, is defective in activated T cells from patients with X-linked hyper-Igm syndrome, *Cell* **72**:291–300.

August, A., and Dupont, B., 1994, Activation of src family kinase lck following CD28 crosslinking in the Jurkat leukemic cell line, *Biochem. Biophys. Res. Commun.* **199**:1466–1473.

August, A., and Dupont, B., 1995, Activation of extracellular signal-regulated protein kinase (ERK/MAP kinase) following CD28 cross-linking: Activation in cells lacking p56lck, *Tissue Antigens* **46**:155–162.

August, A., Gibson, S., Kawakamis, Y., Kawakamis, T., Mills, G. B., and Dupont, B., 1994, CD28 is associated with and induces the immediate tyrosine phosphorylation and activation of the tec family kinase itk/tsk/emt in the Jurkat leukemic T-cell line, *Proc. Natl. Acad. Sci. USA* **91**:9347–9351.

Baldari, C. T., Macchia, G., and Telford, J. L., 1995, Interleukin-2 promoter activation in T-cells expressing activated Ha-ras, *J. Biol. Chem.* **267**:4289–4291.

Banda, N. K., Bernier, J., Kurahara, D. K., Kurrle, R., Haigwood, N., Sekaly, R. P., and Finkel, T. H., 1992, Crosslinking CD4 by human immunodeficiency virus gp120 prime cells for activation-induced apoptosis, *J. Exp. Med.* **176**:1099–1106.

Beadling, C., Guschin, D., Witthuhn, B. A., Ziemiecki, A., Ihle, J. N., Kerr, I. M., and Cantrell, D. A., 1994, Activation of JAK kinases and STAT proteins by interleukin-2 and interferon alpha, but not the T cell antigen receptor, in human T lymphocytes, *EMBO J.* **13**:5605–5615.

Bowen, T. J., Ochs, H. D., Altman, L. C., Price, T. H., Van Epps, D. E., Brautigan, D. L., Rosin, R. E., Perkins, W. D., Babior, B. M., Klebanoff, S. J., and Wedgwood, R. J., 1982, Severe recurrent bacterial infections associated with defective adherence and chemotaxis in two patients with neutrophils deficient in a cell-associated glycoprotein, *J. Pediatr.* **101**:932–940.

Bowtell, D., Fu, P., Simon, M., and Senior, P., 1992, Identification of murine homologues of the Drosophila son of sevenless gene: Potential activators of ras, *Proc. Natl. Acad. Sci. USA* **89**:6511–6515.

Bretscher, P., and Cohn, M., 1970, A theory of self–nonself discrimination, *Science* **169**:1042–1049.

Buday, L., Egan, S. E., Rodriquez, V. P., Cantrell, D. A., and Downward, J., 1994, A complex of Grb2 adaptor protein, Sos exchange factor, and a 36-kDa membrane-bound tyrosine phosphoprotein is implicated in ras activation in T cells, *J. Biol. Chem.* **269**:9019–9023.

Bustelo, X. R., Suen, K. L., Leftheris, K., Meyers, C. A., and Barbacid, M., 1994, Vav cooperates with Ras to transform rodent fibroblasts but is not a Ras GDP/GTP exchange factor, *Oncogene* **9**:2405–2413.

Chan, A. C., Irving, B. A., Fraser, J. D., and Weiss, A., 1991, The zeta chain is associated with a tyrosine kinase and upon T-cell antigen receptor stimulation associates with ZAP-70, a 70-kDa tyrosine phosphoprotein, *Proc. Natl. Acad. Sci. USA* **88**:9166–9170.

Chan, A. C., Kadlecek, T. A., Elder, M. E., Filipovich, A. H., Kuo, W. L., Iwashima, M., Parslow, T. G., and Weiss, A., 1994, ZAP-70 deficiency in an autosomal recessive form of severe combined immunodeficiency. *Science* **264**:1599–1601.

Chan, G., and Ochi, A., 1995, Sphingomyelin-ceramide turnover in CD28 costimulatory signaling, *Eur. J. Immunol.* **25**:1999–2004.

Clark, E. A., and Ledbetter, J. A., 1994, How B and T cells talk to each other, *Nature* **367**:425–429.

Danielian, S., Fagard, R., Alcover, A., Acuto, O., and Fischer, S., 1991, The tyrosine kinase activity of p56lck is increased in human T cells activated va CD2, *Eur. J. Immunol.* **21**:1967–1970.

Diegel, M. L., Moran, P. A., Gilliland, L. K., Damle, N. K., Hayden, M. S., Zarling, J. M., and Ledbetter, J. A., 1993, Regulation of HIV production by blood mononuclear cells from HIV-infected donors: II. HIV-1 production depends on T cell–monocyte interaction, *AIDS Res. Hum. Retrovir.* **9**:465–473.

DiSanto, J. P., Bonnefoy, J. Y., Gauchat, J. F., Fischer, A., and de Saint-Basile, G., 1993, CD40 ligand mutations in X-linked immunodeficiency with hyper-IgM, *Nature* **361**:541–543.

Fischer, K.-D., Zmuidzinas, A., Gardner, S., Barbacid, M., Bernstein, A., and Guidos, C., 1995, Defective T-cell receptor signalling and positive selection of Vav-deficient CD4+ CD8+ thymocytes, *Nature* **374**:474–476.

Flescher, E., Ledbetter, J. A., Schieven, G. L., Vela-Roch, N., Fossum, D., Dang, H., Ogawa, N., and Tralal, N., 1994, Longitudinal exposure of human T lymphocytes to weak oxidative stress suppresses transmembrane and nuclear signal transduction, *J. Immunol.* **153**:4880–4889.

Gilliland, L. K., Teh, H. S., Uckun, F. M., Norris, N. A., Schieven, G. L., and Ledbetter, J. A., 1991, CD4 and CD8 are positive regulators of T cell receptor signal transduction in early T cell differentiation, *J. Immunol.* **146**:1759–1765.

Gilliland, L. K, Schieven, G. L., Norris, N. A., Kanner, S. B., Aruffo, A., and Ledbetter, J. A., 1992, Lymphocyte lineage-restricted tyrosine-phosphorylated proteins that bind PLC-gamma-1 SH2 domains, *J. Biol. Chem.* **267**:13610–13616.

Graf, D., Korthauer, U., Mages, H. W., Senger, G., and Kroczek, R. A., 1992, Cloning of TRAP, a ligand for CD40 on human T cells, *Eur. J. Immunol.* **22**:3193.

Graves, J. D., Downward, J., Rayter, S., Warne, P., Tutt, A. L., Glennie, M., and Cantrell, D. A., 1991, CD2 antigen mediated activation of the guanine nucleotide binding proteins p21ras in human T lymphocytes, *J. Immunol.* **146**:3709–3712.

Graves, J. D., Downward, J., Izquierdo-Pastor, M., Rayter, S., Warne, P. H., and Cantrell, D. A., 1992, The growth factor IL-2 activates p21ras proteins in normal human T lymphocytes, *J. Immunol.* **148**:2417–2422.

Gulbins, E., Coggeshall, K. M., Gottfried, B., Katzav, S., Burn, P., and Altman, A., 1993, Tyrosine kinase-stimulated guanine nucleotide exchange activity of vav in T cell activation, *Science* **260**:822–825.

Gupta, S., Campbell, D., Derijard, B., and Davis, R. J., 1995, Transcription factor ATF2 regulation by the JNK signal transduction pathway, *Science* **267**:389–393.

Hatada, M. H., Lu, X., Laird, E. R., Green, J., Morgenstern, J. P., Lou, M., Marr, C. S., Phillips, T. B., Ram, M. K., Theriault, K., Zoller, M. J., and Karas, J. L., 1995, Molecular basis for interaction of the protein tyrosine kinase ZAP-70 with the T-cell receptor, *Nature* **377**:32–38.

Heath, S. L., Tew, J. G., Szakal, A. K., and Burton, G. F., 1995, Follicular dendritic cells and human immunodeficiency virus infectivity, *Nature* **377**:740–744.

Howe, L. R., Leevers, S. J., Gomez, N., Nakielny, S., Cohen, P., and Marshall, C. J., 1992, Activation of the MAP kinase pathway by the protein kinase raf, *Cell* **71**:335–342.

Hutchcroft, J. E., and Bierer, B. E., 1994, Activation-dependent phosphorylation of the T-lymphocyte surface receptor CD28 and associated proteins, *Proc. Natl. Acad. Sci. USA* **91**:3260–3264.

Ihle, J. N., Witthuhn, B. A., Quelle, F. W., Yamamoto, K., Thierfelder, W. E., Kreider, B., and Silvennoinen, O., 1994, Signaling by the cytokine receptor superfamily: JAKs and STATs, *Trends Biochem. Sci.* **19**:222–227.

Iwashima, M., Irving, B. A., van Oers, N. S., Chan, A. C., and Weiss, A., 1994, Sequential interactions of the TCR with two distinct cytoplasmic tyrosine kinases, *Science* **263**:1136–1139.

Izquierdo, M., Leevers, S. J., Marshall, C. J., and Cantrell, D., 1993, p21ras couples the T cell antigen receptor to extracellular signal-regulated kinase 2 in T lymphocytes, *J. Exp. Med.* **178**:1199–1208.

June, C. H., Ledbetter, J. A., Gillespie, M. M., Lindsten, T., and Thompson, C. B., 1987, T-cell proliferation involving the CD28 pathway is associated with cyclosporine-resistant interleukin 2 gene expression, *Mol. Cell. Biol.* **7**:4472–4481.

Kanner, S. B., Damle, N. K., Blake, J., Aruffo, A., and Ledbetter, J. A., 1992, CD2/LFA-3 ligation induces phospholipase-C gamma-1-tyrosine phosphorylation and regulates CD3 signaling, *J. Immunol.* **148:**2023–2029.

Kanner, S. B., Grosmaire, L. S., Ledbetter, J. A., and Damle, N. K., 1993, Beta2-integrin LFA-1 signaling through phospholipase C-gammal activation, *Proc. Natl. Acad. Sci. USA* **90:**7099–7103.

Kavahagh, T. J., Grossmann, A., Jinneman, J. C., Kanner, S. B., White, C. C., Eaton, D. L., Ledbetter, J. A., and Rabinovitch, P. S., 1993, The effect of 1-chloro-2,4-dinitrobenzene exposure on antigen receptor (CD3)-stimulated transmembrane signal transduction in purified subsets of human peripheral blood lymphocytes, *Toxicol. Appl. Pharmacol.* **119:**91–99.

Kishimoto, T. K., Hollander, N., Roberts, T. M., Anderson, D. C., and Springer, T. A., 1987, Heterogeneous mutations in the beta subunit common to the LFA-1, Mac-1, and p150,95 glycoproteins cause leukocyte adhesion deficiency, *Cell* **50:**193–202.

Kobayashi, N., Kono, T., Hatakeyama, M., Minami, Y., Miyazaki, T., Perlmutter, R. M., and Taniguchi, T., 1993, Functional coupling of the src-family protein tyrosine kinases p59fyn and p53/56lyn with the interleukin 2 receptor: Implications for redundancy and pleiotropism in cytokine signal transduction, *Proc. Natl. Acad. Sci. USA* **90:**4201–4205.

Koide, H., Satoh, T., Nakafuku, M., and Kaziro, Y., 1993, GTP-dependent association of Raf-1 with Ha-Ras: Identification of Raf as a target downstream of Ras in mammalian cells, *Proc. Natl. Acad. Sci. USA* **90:**8683–8686.

Kupfer, A., Singer, S. J., Janeway, C. A. J., and Swain, S. L., 1987, Coclustering of CD4 (L3T4) molecule with the T-cell receptor is induced by specific direct interaction of helper T cells and antigen-presenting cells, *Proc. Natl. Acad. Sci. USA* **84:**5888–5892.

Ledbetter, J. A., and Linsley, P. S., 1992, CD28 receptor crosslinking induces tyrosine phosphorylation of PLCy-1, *Adv. Exp. Med. Biol.* **323:**23–27.

Ledbetter, J. A., Martin, P. J., Spooner, C. E., Wofsy, D., Tsu, T. T., Beatty, P. G., and Gladstone, P., 1985, Antibodies to Tp67 and Tp44 augment and sustain proliferative responses of activated T cells, *J. Immunol.* **135:**2331–2336.

Ledbetter, J. A., June, C. H., Rabinovitch, P. S., Grossmann, A., Tsu, T. T., and Imboden, J. B., 1988, Signal transduction through CD4 receptors: Stimulatory vs. inhibitory activity is regulated by CD4 proximity to the CD3/T cell receptor, *Eur. J. Immunol.* **18:**525–532.

Ledbetter, J. A., Norris, N. A., Grossmann, A., Grosmaire, L. S., June, C. H., Uckun, F. M., Cosand, W. L., and Rabinovitch, P. S., 1989, Enhanced transmembrane signalling activity of monoclonal antibody heteroconjugates suggests molecular interactions between receptors on the T cell surface, *Mol. Immunol.* **26:**137–145.

Ledbetter, J. A., Schieven, G. L., and Linsley, P. S., 1995, Biological inhibitors of lymphocyte co-receptors for antigen-specific immunosuppression, in: *Graft-versus-Host Disease*, 2nd ed. (J. Ferrara and J. Deeg, eds.), Dekker, New York, in press.

Lim, W. A., Richards, F. M., and Fox, R. O., 1994, Structural determinants of peptide-binding orientation and of sequence specificity in SH3 domains, *Nature* **372:**375–379.

Linsley, P. S., and Ledbetter, J. A., 1993, The role of the CD28 receptor during T cell responses to antigen, *Annu. Rev. Immunol.* **11:**191–212.

Los, M., Schenk, H., Hexel, K., Baeuerle, P. A., Droge, W., and Schulze-Osthoff, K., 1995, IL-2 gene expression and NF-kappaB activation through CD28 requires reactive oxygen production by 5-lipoxygenase, *EMBO J.* **14:**3731–3740.

Lu, Y., Granelli-Piperno, A., Bjorndahl, J. M., Phillips, C. A., and Trevillyan, J. M., 1992, CD28-induced T cell activation. Evidence for a protein-tyrosine kinase signal transduction pathway, *J. Immunol.* **149:**24–29.

Macchi, P., Villa, A., Giliani, S., Sacco, M. G., Frattini, A., Porta, F., Ugazio, A. G., Johnston, J. A., Candotti, F., O'Shea, J. J., Vezzoni, P., and Notarangelo, L. D., 1995, Mutations of Jak-3 gene in patients with autosomal severe combined immune deficiency (SCID), *Nature* **377:**65–68.

Madrenas, J., Wange, R. L., Wang, J. L., Isakov, N., Samelson, L. E., and Germain, R. N., 1995, Zeta phosphorylation without ZAP-70 activation induced by TCR antagonists or partial agonists, *Science* **267:**515–518.

Marais, R., Wynne, J., and Treisman, R., 1993, The SRF accessory protein Elk-1 contains a growth factor-regulated transcriptional activation domain, *Cell* **73:**381–393.

Martin, P. J., Ledbetter, J. A., Morishita, Y., June, C. H., Beatty, P. J., and Hansen, J. A., 1986, A 44 kDa cell surface homodimer regulates interleukin 2 production by activated human T lymphocytes, *J. Immunol.* **136:**3282–3287.

Matsui, K., Boniface, J. J., Reay, P. A., Schild, H., Fazekas de St Groth, B., and Davis, M. M., 1991, Low affinity interaction of peptide–MHC complexes with T cell receptors, *Science* **254:**1788–1791.

Migone, T.-S., Lin, J.-X., Cereseto, A., Mulloy, J. C., O'Shea, J. J., Franchini, G., and Leonard, W. J., 1995, Constitutively activated Jak-STAT pathway in T cells transformed with HTLV-1, *Science* **269:**79–85.

Miller, G., Hochman, P. S., Meier, W., Tizard, R., Bixler, S., Rosa, M., and Wallner, B. P., 1993, Specific interaction of LFA-3 with CD2 can inhibit T cell responses, *J. Exp. Med.* **178:**211–222.

Mills, G. B., Stewart, D. J., Mellors, A., and Gelfand, E. W., 1986, Interleukin 2 does not induce phosphatidylinositol hydrolysis in activated T cells, *J. Immunol.* **136:**3019–3024.

Moran, P. A., Diegel, M. L., Sias, J. C., Ledbetter, J. A., and Zarling, J. M., 1993, Regulation of HIV production by blood mononuclear cells from HIV-infected donors: I. Lack of correlation between HIV-1 production and T cell activation, *AIDS Res. Hum. Retrovir.* **9:**455–464.

Moretta, A., Pantaleo, G., Lopez-Botet, M., and Moretta, L., 1985, Involvement of T44 molecules in an antigen-independent pathway of T cell activation, *J. Exp. Med.* **162:**823–838.

Mueller, D. L., Jenkins, M. K., and Schwartz, R. H., 1989, Clonal expansion vs functional clonal inactivation: A costimulatory pathway determines the outcome of T cell receptor occupancy, *Annu. Rev. Immunol.* **7:** 445–489.

Nagata, S., and Suda, T., 1995, Fas and Fas ligand: lpr and gld mutations, *Immunol. Today* **16:**39–43.

Nassar, N., Horn, G., Herrmann, C., Scherer, A., McCormick, F., and Wittinghofer, A., 1995, The 2.2 A crystal structure of the Ras-binding domain of the serine/threonine kinase c-Rafl in complex with RaplA and a GTP analogue, *Nature* **375:**554–560.

Nel, A. E., Gupta, S., Lee, L., Ledbetter, J. A., and Kanner, S. B., 1995, Ligation of the T-cell antigen receptor (TCR) induces association of hSosl, AZP-70, PLC-gammal and other phosphoproteins with Grb2 and the zeta-chain of the TCR, *J. Biol. Chem.* **270:**18428–18436.

Noguchi, M., Yi, H., Rosenblatt, H. M., Filipovich, A. H., Adelstein, S., Modi, W. S., McBride, O. W., and Leonard, W. J., 1993, Interleukin-2 receptor gamma chain mutation results in X-linked severe combined immunodeficiency in humans, *Cell* **73:**147–157.

Nunes, J. A., Collette, Y., Truneh, A., Olive, D., and Cantrell, D. A., 1995, The role of p21ras in CD28 signal transduction: Triggering of CD28 with antibodies, but not the ligand B7-1, activates p21ras, *J. Exp. Med.* **180:**1067–1076.

Ohno, H., Nakamura, T., Yagita, H., Okumura, K., Taniguchi, M., and Saito, T., 1991, Induction of negative signal through CD2 during antigen-specific T cell activation, *J. Immunol.* **147:**2100–2106.

Owaki, H., Varma, R., Gillis, B., Bruder, J. T., Rapp, U. R., Davis, L. S., and Geppert, T. D., 1993, Raf-1 is required for T cell IL2 production, *EMBO J.* **12:**4367–4373.

Pages, F., Ragueneau, M., Rottapel, R., Truneh, A., Nunes, J., Imbert, J., and Olive, D., 1994, Binding of phosphatidylinositol-3-OH kinase to CD28 is required for T-cell signalling, *Nature* **369:**327–329.

Pastor, M. I., Reif, K., and Cantrell, D., 1995, The regulation and function of p21ras during T-cell activation and growth, *Immunol. Today* **16:**159–164.

Pawson, T., and Gish, G. D., 1992, SH2 and SH3 domains: From structure to function, *Cell* **71:**359–362.

Pinchuk, L. M., Polacino, P. S., Agy, M. B., Klaus, S. J., and Clark, E. A., 1994, The role of CD40 and CD80 accessory cell molecules in dendritic cell-dependent HIV-1 infection, *Immunity* **1:**317–325.

Poli, G., and Fauci, A. S., 1992, The effect of cytokines and pharmacologic agents on chronic HIV infection, *AIDS Res. Hum. Retrovir.* **8:**191–197.

Prasad, K. V., Cai, Y. C., Raab, M., Duckworth, B., Cantley, L., Shoelson, S. E., and Rudd, C. E., 1994, T-cell antigen CD28 interacts with the lipid kinase phosphatidylinositol 3-kinase by a cytoplasmic Tyr(P)-Met-Xaa-Met motif, *Proc. Natl. Acad. Sci. USA* **91:**2834–2838.

Rao, A., 1994, NF-ATp: A transcription factor required for the co-ordinate induction of several cytokine genes, *Immunol. Today* **15:**274–281.

Ravichandran, K. S., and Burakoff, S. J., 1994, The adapter protein Shc interacts with the interleukin-2 (IL-2) receptor upon IL-2 stimulation, *J. Biol. Chem.* **269:**1599–1602.

Ren, R., Mayer, B. J., Cicchetti, P., and Baltimore, D., 1993, Identification of a ten-amino acid proline-rich SH3 binding site, *Science* **259:**1157–1161.

Roederer, M., Staal, F. J. T., Anderson, M., Rabin, R., Raju, P. A., and Herzenberg, L. A., 1993, Disregulation of leukocyte glutathione in AIDS, *Ann. N.Y. Acad. Sci.* **677:**113–125.

Rudd, C. E., Trevillyan, J. M., Dasgupta, J. D., Wong, L. L., and Schlossman, S. F., 1988, The CD4 receptor is complexed in detergent lysates to a protein-tyrosine kinase (pp58) from human T lymphocytes, *Proc. Natl. Acad. Sci. USA* **85:**5190–5194.

Sancho, J., Ledbetter, J. A., Choi, M. S., Kanner, S. B., Deans, J. P., and Terhorst, C., 1992, CD3-zeta surface expression is required for CD4-p56lck-mediated upregulation of T cell antigen receptor-CD3 signaling in T cells, *J. Biol. Chem.* **267:**7871–7879.

Schieven, G. L., and Ledbetter, J. A., 1995, Activation of tyrosine kinase signal pathways by radiation and oxidative stress, *Trends Endocrinol. Metab.* **5**:383–388.

Schieven, G. L., Kirihara, J. M., Burg, D. L., Geahlen, R. L., and Ledbetter, J. A., 1993, p72syk tyrosine kinase is activated by oxidizing conditions which induce lymphocyte tyrosine phosphorylation and Ca^{2+} signals, *J. Biol. Chem.* **268**:16688–16692.

Schieven, G. L., Mittler, R. S., Nadler, S. G., Kirihara, J. M., Bolen, J. B., Kanner, S. B., and Ledbetter, J. A., 1994, ZAP-70 tyrosine kinase, CD45 and T cell receptor involvement in UV and H_2O_2 induced T cell signal transduction, *J. Biol. Chem.* **269**:20718–20726.

Sigal, N. H., and Dumont, F. J., 1992, Cyclosporin A, FK506, and rapamycin: Pharmacologic probes of lymphocyte signal transduction, *Annu. Rev. Immunol.* **10**:519–560.

Sloan-Lancaster, J., Shaw, A. S., Rothbard, J. B., and Allen, P. M., 1994, Partial T cell signaling: Altered phospho-zeta and lack of ZAP70 recruitment in APL-induced T cell anergy, *Cell* **79**:913–922.

Smithgall, M. D., Wong, J. G. P., Linsley, P. S., and Haffar, O. K., 1995, Costimulation of CD4+ T cells via CD28 modulates human immunodeficiency virus type 1 infection and replication in vitro, *AIDS Res. Hum. Retrovir.* **11**:885–892.

Songyang, Z., Shoelson, S. E., Chaudhuri, M., Gish, G., Pawson, T., Haser, W. G., King, F., Roberts, T., Ratnofsky, S., Lechleider, R. J., Neel, B. G., Birge, R. B., Fajardo, J. E., Chou, M. M., Hanafusa, H., Schaffhausen, B., and Cantley, L. C., 1994, SH2 domains recognize specific phosphopeptide sequences, *Cell* **72**:767–778.

Stein, P. H., Fraser, J. D., and Weiss, A., 1994, The cytoplasmic domain of CD28 is both necessary and sufficient for costimulation of interleukin-2 secretion and association with phosphatidylinositol 3′-kinase, *Mol. Cell. Biol.* **14**:3392–3402.

Su, B., Jacinto, E., Hibi, M., Kallunki, T., Karin, M., and Ben-Neriah, Y., 1994, JNK is involved in signal integration during costimulation of T lymphocytes, *Cell* **77**:727–736.

Suzuki, H., Kundig, T. M., Furlonger, C., Wakeham, A., Timms, E., Matsuyama, T., Schmits, R., Simard, J. J. L., Ohashi, P. S., Griesser, H., Taniguchi, T., Paige, C. J., and Mak, T. W., 1995, Deregulated T cell activation and autoimmunity in mice lacking interleukin-2 receptor beta, *Science* **268**:1472–1480.

Tan, P., Anasetti, C., Hansen, J. A., Melrose, J., Brunvand, M., Bradshaw, J., Ledbetter, J. A., and Linsley, P. S., 1993, Induction of alloantigen-specific hyporesponsiveness in human T lymphocytes by blocking interaction of CD28 with its natural ligand B7/BB1, *J. Exp. Med.* **177**:165–173.

Tarakhovsky, A., Turner, M., Schaal, S., Mee, P. J., Duddy, L. P., Rajewsky, K., and Tybulewicz, V. L. J., 1995, Defective antigen receptor-mediated proliferation of B and T cells in the absence of Vav, *Nature* **374:** 467–470.

Terai, C., Kornbluth, R. S., Pauza, C. D., Richman, D. D., and Carson, D. A., 1991, Apoptosis as a mechanism of cell death in cultured T lymphoblasts acutely infected with HIV-1, *J. Clin. Invest.* **87**:1710–1715.

Thompson, P. A., Gutkind, J. S., Robbins, K. C., Ledbetter, J. A., and Bolen, J. B., 1992, Identification of distinct populations of PI-3 kinase activity following T cell activation, *Oncogene* **7**:719–725.

Timson Gauen, L. K., Kong, A. N., Samelson, L. E., and Shaw, A. S., 1992, p59fyn tyrosine kinase associates with multiple T-cell receptor subunits through its unique amino-terminal domain, *Mol. Cell. Biol.* **12**:5438–5446.

Timson Gauen, L. K., Zhu, Y., Letourneur, F., Hu, Q., Bolen, J. B., Matis, L. A., Klausner, R. D., and Shaw, A. S., 1994, Interactions of p59fyn and ZAP-70 with T-cell receptor activation motifs: Defining the nature of a signalling motif, *Mol. Cell. Biol.* **14**:3729–3741.

Todderud, G., Wahl, M. I., Rhee, S. G., and Carpenter, G., 1990, Stimulation of phospholipase C-gamma 1 membrane association by epidermal growth factor, *Science* **249**:296–298.

Truitt, K. E., Hicks, C. M., and Imboden, J. B., 1994, Stimulation of CD28 triggers an association between CD28 and phosphatidylinositol 3-kinase in Jurkat T cells, *J. Exp. Med.* **179**:1071–1076.

Tsukada, S., Saffran, D. C., Rawlings, D. J., Parolini, O., Allen, R. C., Klisak, I., Sparkes, R. S., Kubagawa, H., Mohandas, T., Quan, S., Belmont, J. W., Cooper, M. D., Conley, M. E., and Witte, O. N., 1995, Deficient expression of a B cell cytoplasmic tyrosine kinase in human X-linked agammaglobulinemia, *Cell* **72:** 279–290.

Tsygankov, A. Y., Broker, B. M., Fargnoli, J., Ledbetter, J. A., and Bolen, J. B., 1992, Activation of tyrosine kinase p60fyn following T cell antigen receptor crosslinking, *J. Biol. Chem.* **267**:18259–18262.

Turka, L. A., Linsley, P. S., Paine, R., Schieven, G. L., Thompson, C. B., and Ledbetter, J. A., 1991, Signal transduction via CD4, CD8, and CD28 in mature and immature thymocytes: Implications for thymic selection, *J. Immunol.* **146**:1428–1436.

Valentin, A., Lundin, K., Patarroyo, M., and Asjoe, B., 1990, The leukocyte adhesion glycoprotein CD18 participates in HIV-1 induced syncytia formation in monocytoid and T-cells, *J. Immunol.* **144**:934–937.

Valitutti, S., Muller, S., Cella, M., Padovan, E., and Lanzavecchia, A., 1995, Serial triggering of many T-cell receptors by a few peptide–MHC complexes, *Nature* **375**:148–151.

Veillette, A., Bookman, M. A., Horak, E. M., and Bolen, J. B., 1988, The CD4 and CD8 T cell surface antigens are associated with the internal membrane tyrosine-protein kinase p56lck, *Cell* **55**:301–308.

Veillette, A., Bookman, M. A., Horak, E. M., Samelson, L. E., and Bolen, J. B., 1989, Signal transduction through the CD4 receptor involves the activation of the internal membrane tyrosine-protein kinase p56lck, *Nature* **338**:257–259.

Vetrie, D., Vorechovsky, I., Sideras, P., Holland, J., Davies, A., Flinter, F., Hammarstrom, L., Kinnon, K., Levinsky, R., Bobrow, M., Smith, C. I. E., and Bentley, D. R., 1995, The gene involved in X-linked agammaglobulinaemia (XLA) is a member of the src family of protein-tyrosine kinases, *Nature* **361**:226–233.

Wang, Z.-Q., Dudhane, A., Orlikowsky, T., Clarke, K., Li, X., Darzynkiewicz, Z., and Hoffmann, M. K., 1994, CD4 engagement induces Fas antigen-dependent apoptosis of T cells in vivo, *Eur. J. Immunol.* **24**:1549–1552.

Wange, R. L., Malek, S. N., Desiderio, S., and Samelson, L. E., 1993, Tandem SH2 domains of ZAP-70 bind to T cell antigen receptor zeta and CD3 epsilon from activated Jurkat T cells, *J. Biol. Chem.* **268**:19797–19801.

Weiss, A., and Littman, D. R., 1994, Signal transduction by lymphocyte antigen receptors, *Cell* **76**:263–274.

Weissman, D., Li, Y., Orenstein, J. M., and Fauci, A. S., 1995, Both a precursor and a mature population of dendritic cells can bind HIV, *J. Immunol.* **155**:4111–4117.

Westendorp, M. O., Frank, R., Ochsenbauer, C., Stricker, K., Dheln, J., Walczak, H., Debatin, K.-M., and Krammer, P. H., 1995, Sensitization of T cells to CD95-mediated apoptosis by HIV-1 Tat and gp120, *Nature* **375**:497–503.

Zhang, R., Alt, F. W., Davidson, L., Orkin, S. H., and Swat, W., 1995, Defective signalling through the T- and B-cell antigen receptors in lymphoid cells lacking the vav proto-oncogene, *Nature* **374**:470–473.

SECTION II

IMMUNOPATHOGENESIS

CHAPTER 5

HIV IN LYMPH NODE AND THYMUS

DHAVALKUMAR D. PATEL, LAURA P. HALE,
and BARTON F. HAYNES

1. INTRODUCTION

CD4, the receptor for HIV-1 on host immune cells, is expressed at varying levels on a wide variety of immune cell types. Many of the stromal and lymphoid cell types of the thymus and lymph nodes express CD4 and are infected by HIV during the course of systemic HIV infection. However, a variety of cell types in lymph node and thymus are damaged in HIV infection either as a direct consequence of HIV infection, or as a consequence of being targeted for damage by anti-HIV immune responses.

In the end stages of AIDS, both the thymus and lymph nodes are progressively depleted of $CD4^+$ lymphoid cells, and their respective microenvironments are damaged. In this chapter, we summarize the effects of progressive HIV infection on lymph nodes and thymus, and discuss the ramifications of HIV effects on lymph nodes and thymus on the possibility of reconstituting immune function in AIDS.

2. LYMPH NODE

2.1. Normal Lymph Node Architecture

Lymph nodes are encapsulated lymphoid organs that receive and filter lymph from specific anatomic sites. Afferent lymphatics drain into the subcapsular sinus located directly below the capsule, while efferent lymphatics exist at the lymph node hilum (Fig. 1). Lymph nodes are also connected to the venous circulation via specialized venules with plump endothelial cells termed *high endothelial venules*.

Lymph nodes are divided into four main anatomic compartments, each of which is the

DHAVALKUMAR D. PATEL and BARTON F. HAYNES • Departments of Medicine and Immunology, and Center for AIDS Research, Duke University Medical Center, Durham, North Carolina 27710. LAURA P. HALE • Department of Pathology, Duke University Medical Center, Durham, North Carolina, 27710.
Immunology of HIV Infection, edited by Sudhir Gupta. Plenum Press, New York, 1996.

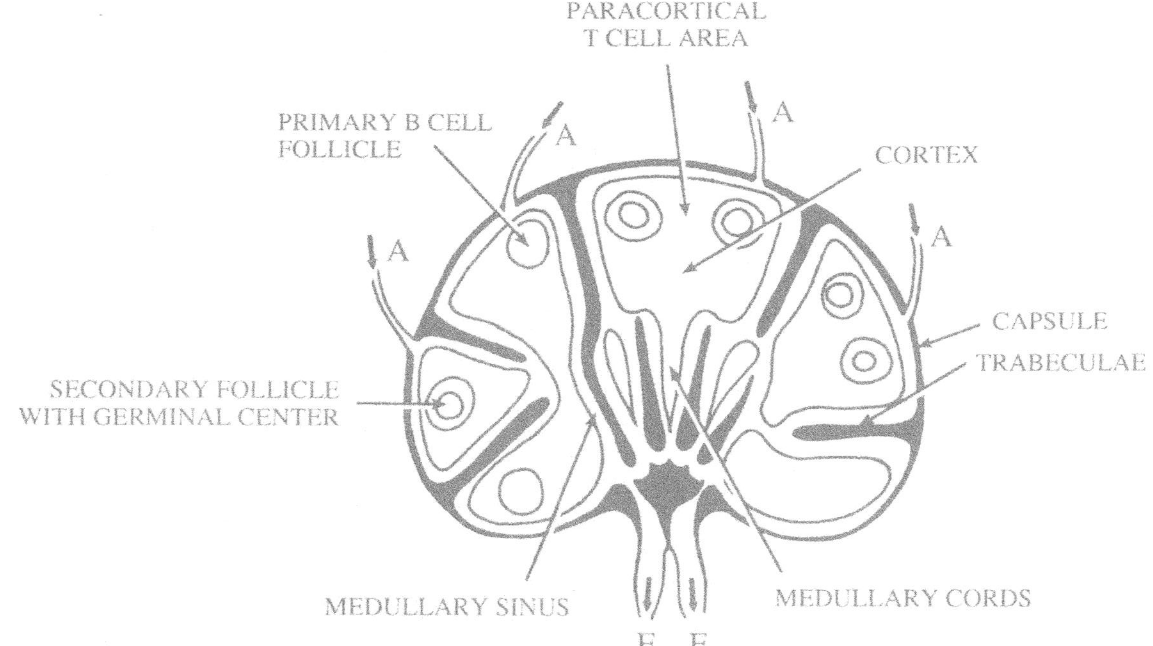

FIGURE 1. Schematic representation of lymph node architecture. Lymph flows into nodes via afferent lymphatics (A) and leaves nodes via efferent lymphatics (E). B-cell areas are primary and secondary follicles in lymph node cortex, while T cells are concentrated in paracortical areas. (Reproduced with permission from Haynes, in *Harrison's Principles of Internal Medicine*, 12th ed., McGraw–Hill.)

primary location for specific immunologic reactions: the follicles (generation of B-cell precursors of plasma cells), the paracortex (expansion and activation of T lymphocytes involved in cellular immune responses), the medullary cords (formation of antibody-secreting plasma cells), and the sinuses (removal and processing by macrophages of antigens from incoming lymph) (van der Valk and Meijer, 1992) (Fig. 1).

Follicles are round collections of cells usually present near the lymph node capsule. Primary follicles are composed predominantly of B cells expressing IgM and IgD. A secondary follicle occurs when a germinal center develops in a primary follicle in response to antigenic stimulation, leading to the formation of antibody-secreting cells as well as memory B cells. The germinal center appears pale with standard histochemical stains, with a darker-staining rim (Fig. 2A). The outer rim of the germinal center (mantle zone) is comprised of small B lymphocytes that express surface (s) IgM and IgD, similar to those B lymphocytes present in a primary follicle. This rim of B cells is less distinct than the analogous marginal zone of B cells seen around germinal centers in the spleen (van den Oord *et al.*, 1986).

Lymph node germinal centers contain B cells in multiple stages of activation and differentiation (Hsu and Jaffe, 1984). Plasma cells, immunoblasts, and small numbers of $CD4^+$ helper T cells are also occasionally present. The composition of a germinal center varies as the immune response progresses, beginning with large noncleaved cells, followed by macrophages, follicular dendritic cells, and centrocytes. Macrophages present within

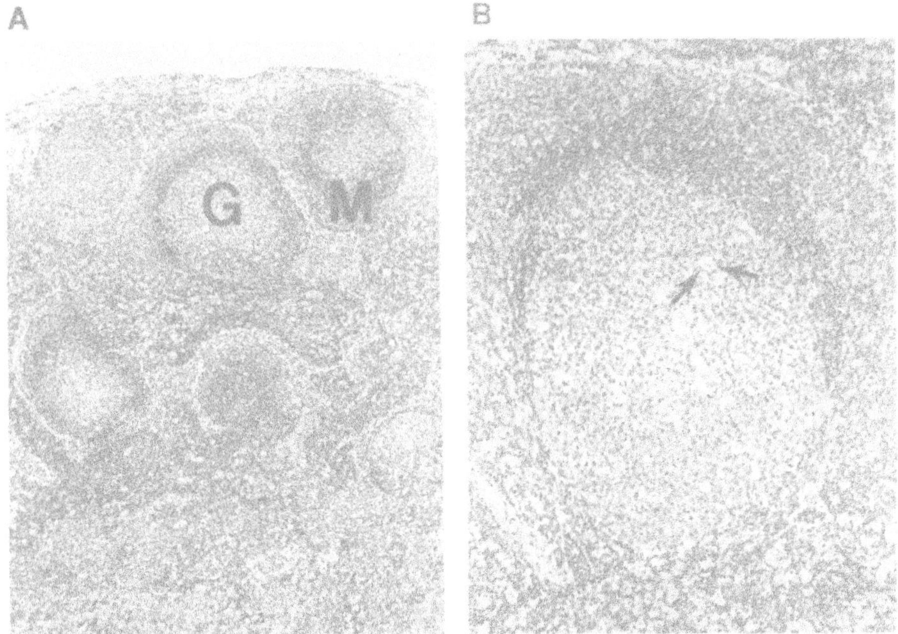

FIGURE 2. Reactive lymph node. (A) Reactive normal lymph node characterized by multiple small round follicles with well-developed germinal centers (G) and defined mantle zones (M), low-power view. (B) Magnification view of a reactive secondary follicle, demonstrating a germinal center. Note the "starry sky" appearance within the germinal center and para cortex indicating prominence of tingible body macrophages (arrows).

germinal centers are called tingible body macrophages because their cytoplasm contains phagocytosed debris from cells that have undergone apoptosis (Fig. 2B).

Follicular dendritic cells (FDCs) have medium to large nuclei that may be binucleate, with a fine chromatin pattern and inconspicuous nucleoli. The cytoplasm of dendritic cells is difficult to visualize on standard histologic sections, but may be seen with immunohistochemical reagents such as anti-CD35 (C3b receptor) mAb (van der Valk *et al.*, 1984) and anti-CD83 (HB15) mAb (Engel and Tedder, 1994). Because lymph node FDCs are adherent to other adjacent FDCs via desmosomes and form a complex reticular supporting meshwork, FDCs are also referred to as dendritic reticular cells. FDCs are derived from bone marrow, express major histocompatibility complex (MHC) class II antigens, and serve as efficient antigen-presenting cells for B and T lymphocytes (Tew *et al.*, 1990; Steinman *et al.*, 1993). Because FDCs are long-lived and retain antigen for long periods of time, they likely function in induction and maintenance of memory B- and T-cell immune responses (Donaldson *et al.*, 1986; Steinman, 1991; Steinman *et al.*, 1993). MHC class II-positive, bone marrow-derived Langerhans cells are also present in the lymph node cortex and function in antigen presentation to T and B cells (Steinman, 1991).

The lymph node paracortex is the region adjacent to and between B-cell follicles, and extends into the deeper layers of the lymph node. The majority of the cells in the paracortex are $CD3^+$ T lymphocytes (Stein *et al.*, 1980). The paracortex is an important site of T-cell immune responses, with formation of antigen-specific effector and memory T cells (Stevens *et al.*, 1982). T lymphocytes recruited from the blood enter the lymph node via high endothelial venules located primarily within the paracortex. The CD4:CD8 ratio of T cells in lymph node paracortical areas is normally 3–4:1 (Hsu *et al.*, 1983; Poppeman *et al.*, 1981).

Located in the deeper regions of the lymph node, the medullary cords are dark-staining because of their high cellular content. They are adjacent to and separated by the lighter-staining, less cellular sinuses. The predominant cell types within the medullary cords are plasma cells, plasmacytoid B lymphocytes, T lymphocytes that regulate antibody formation, and macrophage antigen-presenting cells (van der Valk and Meijer, 1992).

Lymph node sinuses are channels for the flow of lymph through the lymph node. Endothelium partially lines the largest sinus which is the subcapsular sinus present beneath the capsule. As sinuses travel toward the hilum, endothelial cells become sparse and the sinuses become lined with macrophages. The sinus macrophages are thus the first hematopoietic cells to encounter antigen in the incoming lymph and remove antigens for processing and presentation to B and T lymphocytes.

2.2. HIV Infection of Lymph Nodes

One of the earliest clinical signs of HIV infection is the development of generalized lymphadenopathy. Our understanding of HIV infection of lymph nodes is based on histologic studies from the early 1980s when lymph node biopsies were routinely performed for diagnosis (Armstrong *et al.*, 1985; Tenner-Racz *et al.*, 1985, 1986; Le Tourneau *et al.*, 1986; Biberfeld *et al.*, 1987). From those and later histopathologic studies, at least three distinct histologic patterns in lymph nodes from HIV patients have emerged: (1) follicular hyperplasia and lysis, (2) follicular involution, and (3) lymphocyte depletion patterns (Jaffe, 1994; Ioachim, 1994). Sequential HIV-infected lymph node biopsies have demonstrated progression from follicular hyperplasia to follicular involution to lymphocyte depletion patterns with time, which correlates with decrease in $CD4^+$ cells (Krueger *et al.*, 1991), development of opportunistic infections, and mortality (Chadburn *et al.*, 1989). It must be noted, however, that the patterns of lymph node changes seen in early to mid stages of HIV infection are not specific (Ioachim *et al.*, 1983; Ewing *et al.*, 1985; Stanley and Frizzera, 1986). Similar changes can be seen in other conditions including lymph node draining sites of bacterial infections, and in lymph nodes in rheumatoid arthritis (Nosanchuk and Schnitzer, 1969), syphilis (Jaffe, 1994), and Castleman's disease (Keller *et al.*, 1972).

2.2.1. Follicular Hyperplasia

The generalized lymph node enlargement associated with early HIV infection ($CD4^+$ T lymphocyte count > 500/mm^3) is manifested histologically by florid or explosive follicular hyperplasia (Fig. 3A). Follicles are increased in number and markedly enlarged, with development of large irregularly shaped germinal centers that may have serpentine, dumbbell, or serrated configurations (Fig. 4A). Mantle zones are frequently decreased in size as a result of the high proliferative rate of the germinal center cells (Jaffe, 1994) and may be disrupted or absent. Follicles may contain large numbers of tingible body macrophages, with a prominent "starry sky" pattern. Plasma cells and infiltrates of small lymphocytes, including $CD8^+$ T cells, may also be seen within follicles. Small hemorrhages may be present adjacent to germinal centers (Fig. 3A) (Chadburn *et al.*, 1989). Follicular

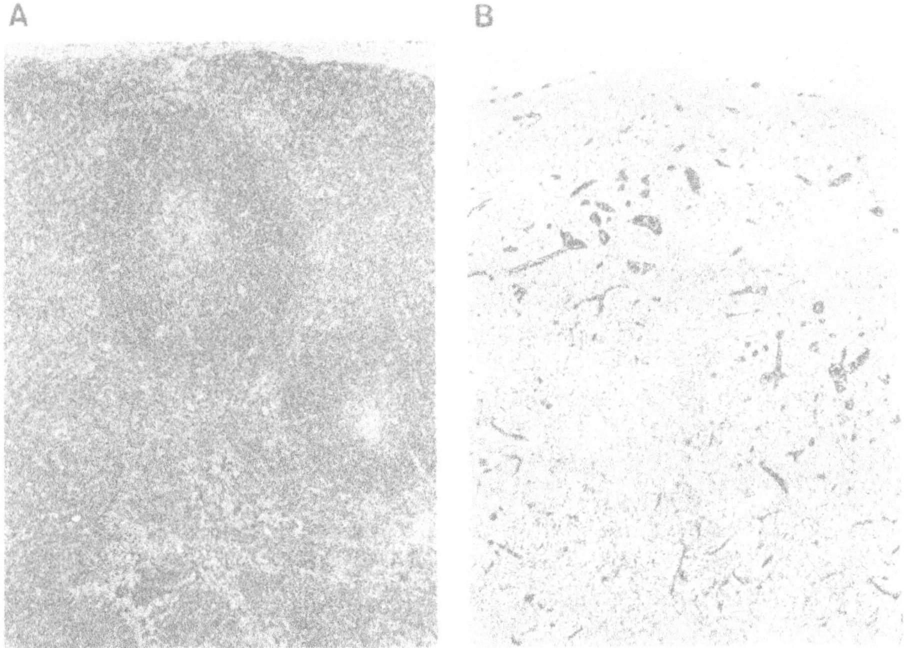

FIGURE 3. Lymph node in early and late HIV infection. (A) Photomicrograph of follicular hyperplasia in a patient with early HIV infection, with a large germinal center, focally attenuated mantle zone, and focal hemorrhage. (B) Lymph node in the late stages of AIDS. This lymph node obtained at autopsy from a patient with AIDS demonstrates loss of follicular architecture, marked lymphodepletion, and vascular proliferation, accentuated here by vascular congestion.

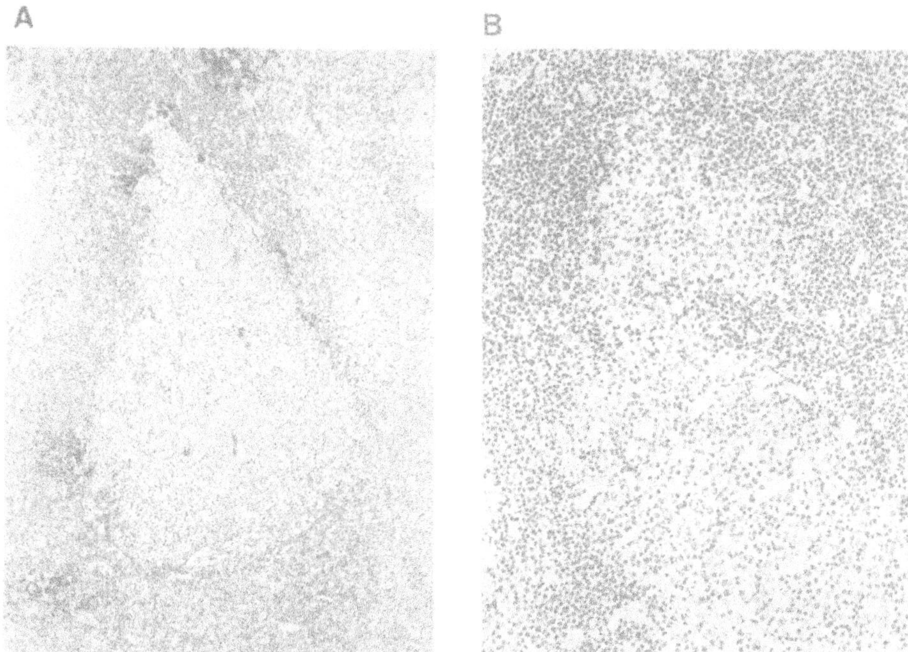

FIGURE 4. Follicular lysis. In the intermediate stages of HIV infection, after follicular hyperplasia, germinal centers may become large and irregularly shaped as shown in panel A, with follicular lysis which is characterized by infiltration of small lymphocytes. (B) Higher-power magnification of an irregularly shaped germinal center in a patient with AIDS showing disruption of the follicular dendritic cell network and infiltration of the germinal center with small lymphocytes.

hyperplasia is thought to occur as a result of expansion of the FDC network and normal immune activation in response to antigenic challenge (Pantaleo *et al.*, 1994). However, follicular hyperplasia may not only be related to direct infection of lymphocytes by HIV, but may result from HIV-derived products such as Tat because mice transgenic for the tat gene product develop lymphoid hyperplasia in spleen, lymph node, and lung (Vellutini *et al.*, 1995).

Warthin–Finkeldey-like giant cells, comprised of mulberrylike clusters of lymphocytes, have also been described in HIV-infected lymph nodes (Chadburn *et al.*, 1989; Ioachim, 1994; Jaffe, 1994; Burke *et al.*, 1994). These giant cells are not specific for HIV infection, but are also seen in viral infections such as measles; they likely represent the syncytium-inducing properties of these viruses. Warthin–Finkeldey giant cells have also been described in reactive and neoplastic lymphoid disorders, with no evidence of viral infection (Kjeldsberg and Kim, 1981).

2.2.2. Follicular Lysis

"Follicular lysis" or follicular fragmentation also occurs in the early stages of HIV infection and is characterized by the infiltration of cytotoxic T lymphocytes from the mantle zone into the germinal center (Fig. 4B), and has been reported to be relatively specific for

HIV infection (Devergne *et al.*, 1991). In normal lymph nodes, serine esterase B (a cytotoxic granule constituent that is transcribed by activated cytotoxic T lymphocytes and natural killer cells) mRNA expression is limited to cells present in interfollicular (paracortical) areas. In HIV-infected lymph nodes, however, Devergne *et al.* (1991) showed that cells expressing serine esterase B mRNA were also present within follicles, and serine esterase B mRNA expression was associated with local presence of HIV antigens and RNA. Thus, activated cytotoxic T cells present within follicles in HIV-infected lymph nodes likely contribute to anti-HIV cellular immune responses, resulting in the characteristic histologic picture of follicular lysis. B cells may fill the sinuses in HIV-infected lymph nodes, and they may also be prominent in paracortical areas of HIV-infected lymph nodes (Sohn *et al.*, 1985).

2.2.3. Follicular Involution

As HIV infection progresses, lymph nodes are progressively destroyed and demonstrate involution with small, hypocellular, often hyalinized germinal centers, relative paracortical hyperplasia, and vascular proliferation (Fig. 3B). This stage histologically resembles the hyaline vascular type of Castleman's disease and mantle zone lymphoma but can be distinguished from the latter by the lack of the interfollicular vascular network seen in Castleman's disease and by the presence of polyclonal B-cell surface markers in HIV infection (Chadburn *et al.*, 1989; Knowles, 1992). While follicular involution is associated with intermediate-stage disease, it may be seen in a limited fashion in combination with follicular hyperplasia in early stage disease (Jaffe, 1994).

2.2.4. Lymphocyte Depletion

Lymph nodes in late HIV infection ($CD4^+$ T lymphocyte count $< 200/mm^3$) exhibit marked lymphodepletion, with absence of follicular architecture and depletion of FDCs. The majority of cells present are histiocytes and plasma cells. Vascular proliferation may be prominent (Fig. 3B). This pattern is most often seen at autopsy, as these lymph nodes are small and infrequently biopsied. Follicular involution and lymphocyte depletion histologic patterns are correlated with progression to AIDS and death caused by opportunistic infections (Chadburn *et al.*, 1989). The disappearance of germinal centers from lymph nodes in late stages of HIV disease suggests that $CD4^+$ cells are necessary for the functional integrity of the germinal centers (Fox *et al.*, 1991).

2.2.5. HIV Replication in Lymph Node: Role of Follicular Dendritic Cells

The follicular hyperplasia stage of HIV infection of lymph nodes is associated with replication of HIV in $CD4^+$ T lymphocytes and trapping of virions in immune complexes on FDCs. While HIV particles were clearly shown to be present in lymph node germinal centers by electron microscopy and immunohistology (Armstrong *et al.*, 1985; Tenner-Racz *et al.*, 1985, 1986; Le Tourneau *et al.*, 1986; Biberfeld *et al.*, 1987), early studies utilizing Southern blotting led some investigators to conclude that little or no HIV replication occurred in lymph nodes (Baroni *et al.*, 1988; Uccini *et al.*, 1989). More sensitive techniques such as in situ hybridization, quantitative PCR, and in situ PCR, however, have demonstrated that the lymph node is actually a reservoir of HIV (Emilie *et al.*, 1990; Fox *et al.*,

1991; Pantaleo *et al.*, 1991, 1993c; Embretson *et al.*, 1993). In fact, the levels of viral burden and viral replication at this early stage of HIV infection are far greater in lymph node compared to the peripheral blood (Pantaleo *et al.*, 1991, 1993c). Embretson *et al.* (1993) using in situ PCR showed that about 25% of CD4+ T lymphocytes within germinal centers were infected with HIV. These cells may be the primary target of CTLs infiltrating germinal centers during follicular lysis.

In the early asymptomatic stages of HIV infection, the frequency of circulating HIV-infected CD4+ T lymphocytes is low, with low levels or absence of virions in the plasma (Ho *et al.*, 1989; Coombs *et al.*, 1989). These observations led to the hypothesis of "clinical latency" after HIV infection. However, studies comparing HIV viral burden in peripheral blood and in lymphoid organs including lymph node, tonsils, and adenoids from the same individual indicate that frequencies of HIV-infected CD4+ cells from lymphoid organs are 0.5 to 1.0 log higher than from peripheral blood (Pantaleo *et al.*, 1993a,b). In some cases, HIV RNA was detectable in mononuclear cells from lymph node but not from peripheral blood from the same individual (Pantaleo *et al.*, 1993a,b). These results indicate that the lymphoid organs function as major reservoirs for HIV during early, clinically latent stages of infection.

During the early (latent) stages of HIV infection, viral particles in the lymph node are restricted to the germinal centers associated with FDCs (Fig. 5B) (Tenner-Racz *et al.*, 1986; Biberfeld *et al.*, 1987). HIV accumulates in germinal centers complexed with immunoglobulin and complement (immune complexes) trapped on the villus processes of FDCs, consistent with their role in antigen clearance and presentation (Tew *et al.*, 1990; Fox *et al.*, 1991; Spiegel *et al.*, 1992). Viral replication at this stage is low (Fig. 5A,C). Contrary to their role in immune activation, however, HIV–immune complexes trapped on FDCs serve as a source of infection for susceptible cells (Heath *et al.*, 1995) leading to increased viral replication in the intermediate stages of clinical latency (Fig. 5D,F). As antigen-activated lymphocytes migrate into and throughout the lymph node during antigen-stimulated immune responses, they may encounter HIV–immune complexes on the surface of FDCs and become infected, thus contributing to the slow decline in CD4+ cells observed clinically. As disease progresses within a given lymph node, virus is trapped in some germinal centers and not others because of follicular involution (Fig. 5E).

In the late stages of HIV infection of the lymph node, the germinal centers are involuted and lymph node architecture destroyed, with loss of virus-trapping capabilities of the node (Fig. 5G–I). The efficiency of viral trapping corresponds to the integrity of the FDC network (Pantaleo *et al.*, 1993a,b). The effect of FDC loss on immune function may be twofold: loss of FDCs may allow development of viremia and increased numbers of infected cells as a result of lack of viral trapping, and/or loss of the FDC network may inhibit normal antigen-specific responses via ineffective antigen presentation and inadequate maintenance of T and B memory responses (Pantaleo *et al.*, 1993c).

CD4+ T cells, macrophages, and FDCs may be damaged or destroyed in HIV infection as a result of cytopathic effects from direct HIV infection, or from indirect effects of HIV infection. Indirect effects of HIV infection include the killing of both HIV-infected and -uninfected lymph node cells by anti-HIV CD8+ cytotoxic T lymphocytes (CTLs), and by HIV protein products by mechanisms including apoptosis or programmed cell death in immune and stromal cells (Ameisen and Capron, 1991).

Involvement of the lymph node in the earliest stages of HIV infection immediately following exposure to the virus but before follicular hyperplasia has not been well charac-

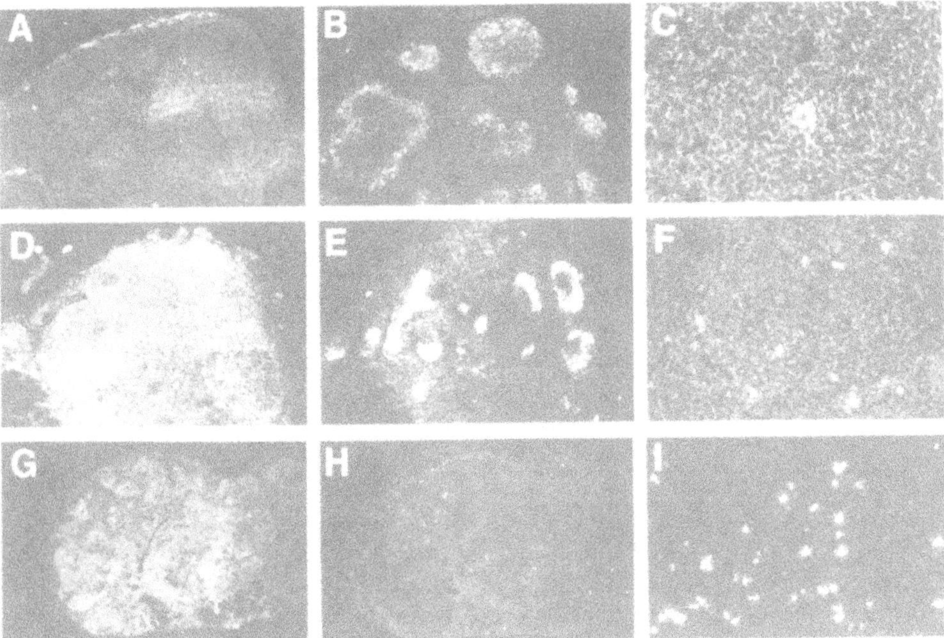

FIGURE 5. *In situ* hybridization of HIV RNA in different stages of lymph node infection with HIV. (A–C) Early stage of HIV infection. (A) Darkfield image of lymph node not digested with protease showing little HIV replication. (B) After protease digestion, HIV RNA in extracellular virus particles is localized to the area of germinal centers. Note the large irregularly shaped germinal center on the left. (C) High-power darkfield image without protease digestion of a single cell in the paracortical area with active HIV replication. (D–F) Intermediate stage of HIV infection. (D) The darkfield image without protease digestion shows diffuse reactivity in the paracortical areas. (E) After protease digestion, high levels of extracellular virus particles trapped on follicular dendritic cells are seen in some, but not all, follicles. (F) A high-power darkfield view without protease digestion shows HIV replication in a number of cells in the paracortical area. (G–I) Late stage of HIV infection. (G) A darkfield image without protease digestion reveals disruption of the lymph node architecture with absent germinal centers. (H) Only a modest increase in HIV RNA signal is noted with protease digestion consistent with the loss of virus-trapping ability of the lymph node as a result of the degeneration and death of follicular dendritic cells. (I) High-magnification view without protease digestion showing numerous cells with large amounts of HIV replication. (Reproduced with permission from Pantaleo *et al.*, 1993, *Nature* **362:**355–358.)

terized. However, many similarities exist between HIV and simian immunodeficiency virus (SIV), and the kinetics of SIV infection of the lymph node have been better characterized (Wyand *et al.*, 1989; Reimann *et al.*, 1994; Chakrabarti *et al.*, 1994a,b; Baskin *et al.*, 1995). In SIVmac251 infection, active viral replication was noted 7–14 days after infection, particularly in $CD4^+$ lymphocytes and macrophages in the subcapsular sinuses indicating an entry of infected cells via the afferent lymphatics (Reimann *et al.*, 1994; Chakrabarti *et al.*, 1994a,b). At day 14, neutralizing antibodies to SIVmac251 appeared and peripheral blood as well as lymph node $CD8^+$ T lymphocytes increased concomitant with clearance of p27 antigenemia (Reimann *et al.*, 1994). HIV-specific CTLs first appeared at day 7 postinoculation (Reimann *et al.*, 1994). This was also associated with a change in lymph node virus localization to FDCs and decrease in viral replication (Reimann *et al.*, 1994; Chakrabarti *et al.*, 1994a,b; Baskin *et al.*, 1995) similar to the follicular hyperplasia stage of HIV infection.

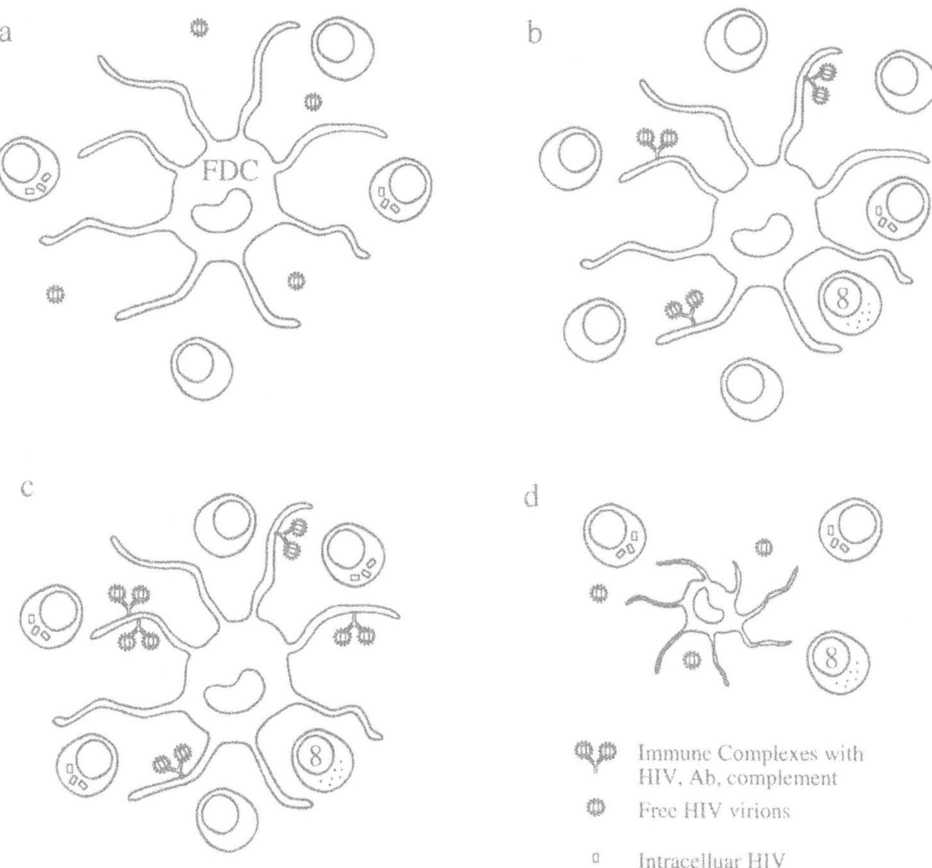

FIGURE 6. Schematic representation of the different stages of HIV infection of the lymph node. (a) Virus dissemination; (b) Early stage follicular hyperplasia; (c) Intermediate stage follicular involution; (d) End stage lymphocyte depletion. Follicular dendritic cells (FDCs) and cytotoxic T lymphocytes (8) are labeled. $CD4^+$ T lymphocytes infected with HIV (intracytoplasmic rectangles), HIV-infected macrophages (not shown), and free virions are present at the earliest stages of virus dissemination after inoculation with HIV. Once an immune response has been generated, HIV virions are trapped in immune complexes by FDCs at the follicular hyperplasia stage seen in the early stages of clinical latency. CTL infiltration of follicles (follicular lysis) also occurs at this stage. Because of infection of $CD4^+$ T lymphocytes by HIV–immune complexes trapped on FDC, virus replication slowly increases with degeneration and involution of follicles. During the stage of clinical AIDS, the lymph node microenvironment is destroyed and FDCs no longer trap HIV–immune complexes.

Extrapolation of data from SIV studies combined with the current knowledge about HIV suggests that HIV infection of the lymph node proceeds as follows (Fig. 6). After inoculation, HIV travels as free virions or in the form of infected $CD4^+$ T lymphocytes to lymph node and infects $CD4^+$ macrophages lining the lymph node sinusoids and $CD4^+$ T lymphocytes within the cortex (Fig. 6A). After a period of about 2 weeks, viral replication is markedly reduced by the host immune response in the form of neutralizing antibodies and HIV-specific CTLs. Anti-HIV antibodies (either neutralizing or not) form immune complexes with free HIV particles and the immune complexes are trapped by FDCs (Fig. 6B) at the follicular hyperplasia (early clinical latency) stage. In addition to serving a role in immune activation, the HIV–immune complexes trapped on FDCs infect resident and trafficking $CD4^+$ T lymphocytes and increase viral load (intermediate follicular involution stage) (Fig. 6C). With progressive infection and depletion of circulating $CD4^+$ T lymphocytes, marked lymphoid depletion and destruction of the lymph node microenvironment occurs with progression to clinical AIDS (Fig. 6D).

2.2.6. Cytokine Effects

Constitutive cytokine expression in HIV-infected lymph nodes includes large amounts of IFN-γ and IL-10 produced by $CD8^+$ cells, with low to undetectable IL-2 and IL-4 regardless of the stage of disease. $CD4^+$ cells account for very little of the cytokine mRNA in lymph nodes (Graziosi *et al.*, 1994). IFN-γ induces retention of lymphocytes in the lymph node, which may contribute to the observed lymphadenopathy (Westermann *et al.*, 1993).

The role of apoptosis in immune development and normal cellular functions has only recently been understood. Apoptosis is readily observed in normal lymph nodes, where it is primarily limited to the germinal centers. However, comparative studies of HIV-infected lymph nodes demonstrate a three- to fourfold increase in apoptosis in cortex, paracortex, and sinuses, involving CD8+ T and B cells as well as $CD4^+$ T cells. This increased apoptosis is histologically manifested by "mottling" or a starry sky pattern resulting from increased tingible body macrophages which ingest apoptotic debris. The intensity of apoptosis is apparently related to the general state of immune activation and does not correlate with the clinical stage of HIV disease or with viral burden (Muro-Cacho *et al.*, 1995). Activated or resting $CD4^+$ and $CD8^+$ T cells and thymocytes from healthy HIV-negative donors undergo apoptosis in response to stimulation through the T-cell receptor complex in the absence of accessory cells, which is associated with IFN-γ expression in the absence of IL-2 expression. Thus, the cytokine profile in HIV lymph nodes may lead to increased apoptosis in cells receiving aberrant activation signals during HIV infection (Groux *et al.*, 1993).

3. THYMUS

The thymus is essential for the normal initial development of T cells, and infection of the thymus and postthymic regenerating T cells with HIV results in a deficiency in the regenerative capability of the T-cell arm of the immune system. In this section, we will briefly review the normal intrathymic development of T cells and the effect of HIV infection on thymic structure and function.

3.1. Normal Thymic Architecture and Ontogeny

The thymus is a complex encapsulated lymphoid organ consisting of T lymphocytes at all stages of maturation and the nonlymphoid stroma of thymic epithelial cells, fibroblasts, endothelial cells, macrophages, and dendritic cells. The postnatal thymus is a multilobulated structure with three distinct zones (the subcapsular cortical, inner cortical, and medullary zones) within each lobule (Haynes, 1984) (Fig. 7). The cortex is characterized by its high content of lymphocytes (predominantly immature T cells), and the medulla is characterized by collections of terminally differentiated thymic epithelial cells and cell debris termed *Hassall's bodies*. Mature lymphocytes reside in the medulla. The

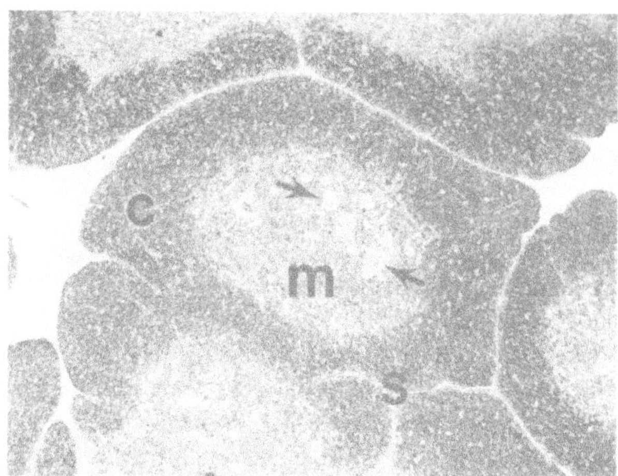

FIGURE 7. Normal thymus architecture. Photomicrograph of a hematoxylin and eosin-stained section of human thymus. Shown is a section through one lobule of a postnatal human thymus. The cortical (c) and medullary (m) zones are indicated. Lobules are separated by fibrous septa (s) which are contiguous with the fibrous capsule. Also shown are Hassall's bodies (arrows) which are characteristic of the medullary zone of human thymus. (Reproduced with permission from Patel and Haynes, in *Encyclopedia of Human Biology*, 2nd ed., Academic Press.)

human subcapsular cortex and inner cortex both contain immature T lymphocytes but differ in that the subcapsular cortical epithelium is Thy-1 $(CDw90)^{+}$ and ectodermally derived and the inner cortical epithelium is $CDw90^{-}$ and of endodermal origin (Ritter *et al.*, 1981; Haynes *et al.*, 1984).

The human thymus begins to develop as early as 4 weeks after fertilization at which time the primitive thymic rudiment is formed from ectoderm of the third pharyngeal cleft and endoderm of the third pharyngeal pouch (Haynes, 1984). With colonization of the human thymic rudiment at 8 weeks of gestation by T-lymphocyte precursors, there is an explosive expansion of all cell types within the thymus, and the thymus becomes lobulated (Haynes and Heinly, 1995). The thymus reaches its maximum absolute weight at puberty (Suster and Rosai, 1992), then begins a long slow process of involution. The connective tissue septa become replaced by adipose tissue; however, adipose tissue does not infiltrate into the thymic parenchyma (Fig. 8). The number of cortical thymocytes decreases, and the medulla decreases in size, with blurring of the corticomedullary distinction. Hassall's bodies may become cystic, and in thymocyte-depleted thymus from many causes, epithelial remnants may become spindled or form epithelial rosette-like structures, similar to those seen in the thymic dysplasia of congenital immunodeficiencies (Rosai and Levine, 1976). However, despite the involuted appearance, terminal deoxynucleotidyl transferase (TdT)-positive immature thymocytes can be documented even in thymus from elderly persons (Steinmann, 1986; Hirokawa *et al.*, 1982), indicative of ongoing thymopoiesis.

3.2. Intrathymic T-Lymphocyte Development

Beginning with their migration to the thymus, $CD34^{+}CD7^{+ or -}$ T-lymphocyte precursors undergo proliferation, positive selection, and negative selection to develop into mature

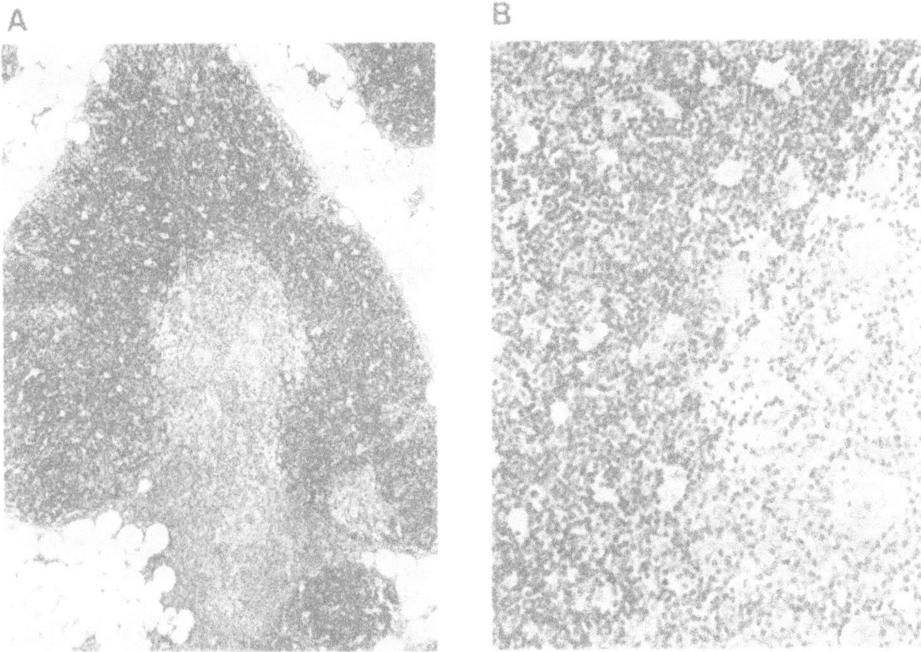

FIGURE 8. Age-related changes in the thymus. (A) Low-power photomicrograph of a section of normal thymus from a 38-year-old woman. Note the fatty infiltration of the thymus, but maintenance of the corticomedullary junction. (B) In this higher-power view, the cortex is highly lymphoid while the medulla has Hassall's bodies but fewer numbers of lymphocytes.

immunocompetent T lymphocytes capable of specific interactions with self-major histocompatibility complex (MHC) antigens in the recognition of foreign antigens (MHC restriction). The most immature subset of thymocytes express surface CD34, but do not have CD3/T-cell receptor (TCR) complex, CD4, or CD8 molecules on their surface and are referred to as triple-negative (TN) cells (Fig. 9). TN immature T lymphocytes proliferate, expand to become $CD4^{+}CD8^{+}$ double-positive (DP) cortical thymocytes and also begin to express low levels of the CD3/TCR complex. During the DP stage, thymocytes are selected to either die by apoptosis or proliferate based on the specificity of their TCR (von Boehmer *et al.*, 1989; Marrack *et al.*, 1993). Thymocytes are programmed to die in situ unless they express TCR capable of recognizing foreign peptides in the context of self-MHC molecules and are positively selected to survive and proliferate. Proliferation of immature TN thymocytes and positive selection of DP thymocytes occurs through interactions with thymic fibroblasts and thymic epithelial cells and is triggered by thymic epithelial cell-derived cytokines (Denning *et al.*, 1988). Thymocytes that express TCRs with a nonspecific, high affinity for self-MHC molecules are eliminated by negative selection when their TCRs engage MHC molecules on thymic macrophages and dendritic cells. Thymocytes that express self-reactive TCRs are also deleted via negative selection.

The final stage of intrathymic T-cell development involves the selective loss of either CD4 or CD8 on DP thymocytes yielding positively selected single-positive (SP) $CD4^{+}$ or $CD8^{+}$ thymocytes in the thymic medulla. At this stage, mature medullary thymocytes

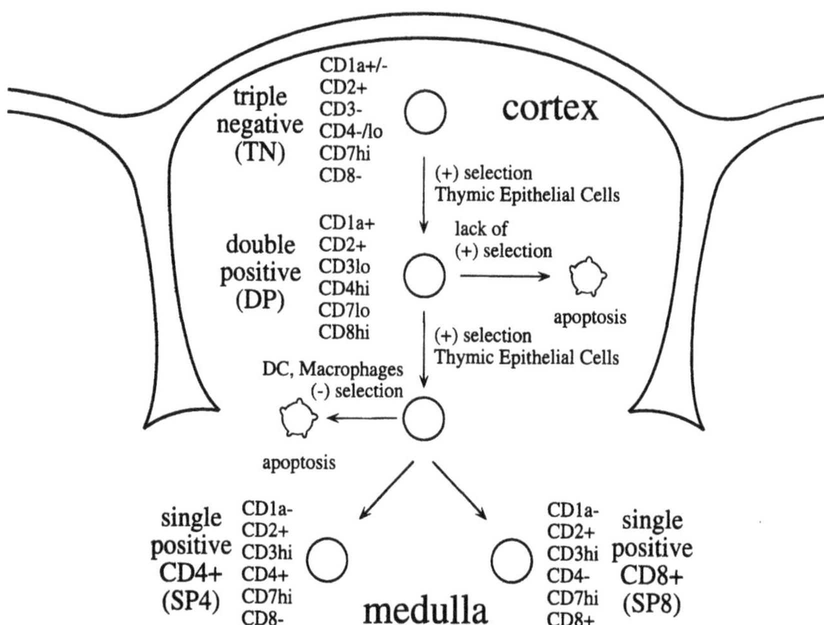

FIGURE 9. Schematic of the intrathymic development of T cells. Intrathymic development of T cells occurs in three general stages: the triple-negative (TN), double-positive (DP), and single-positive (SP) stages. T-lymphocyte precursors (TN) initially migrate to the thymus and reside in the subcapsular cortical and inner cortical regions. By direct contact with thymic stromal cells and by cytokines liberated from thymic stromal cells, TN cells are induced to proliferate and differentiate into double-positive thymocytes. DP thymocytes that are CD3/TCR lo+ and that are able to interact with self-MHC molecules of cortical epithelium are induced to proliferate (positive selection) and those thymocytes with TCR that cannot interact with self-MHC die by programmed cell death (apoptosis). DP cells also undergo negative selection by macrophages and dendritic cells primarily at the corticomedullary junction to delete thymocytes with TCR that react nonspecifically with self-MHC and with TCR that recognize self-antigens. The selected single-positive thymocytes reside in the medulla and likely undergo further maturation steps before their export to the periphery.

express either CD4 or CD8 in association with high levels of the CD3/TCR complex. Despite a mature surface phenotype, medullary thymocytes are not yet totally immunocompetent in that they will not proliferate in response to stimulation with either phytohemagglutinin or concanavalin A without exogenous IL-2. The specific molecules and mechanisms that mediate the export of mature single-positive T lymphocytes from the thymus are not known.

3.3. HIV Infection of Thymus

Early work by Joshi and Oleske (1985, 1990) describing the histopathology of thymic biopsies in children with AIDS, and autopsy studies of AIDS patients (Reichert *et al.*, 1983; Elie *et al.*, 1983; Seemayer *et al.*, 1984; Joshi *et al.*, 1984; Guarda *et al.*, 1984; Welch *et al.*, 1984; Grody *et al.*, 1985) has formed the initial basis of our understanding of the pathophysiology of HIV infection of the thymus. Joshi and Oleske (1985) identified three different histopathologic patterns in thymic biopsies from children with AIDS: thymitis, severe stress-related changes termed *precocious involution*, and thymic dysplasia. By comparison with autopsy studies and studies in the SCID-hu mouse model (see below), thymitis likely represents an early stage in the HIV infection of the thymus and thymic involution, including dysplasia, represents the late stages of HIV infection.

3.3.1. HIV-Induced Thymitis

HIV-induced thymitis is characterized by the presence of germinal centers in the thymic medulla and, in some cases, the presence of plasma cells and lymphocytes obscuring the thymic corticomedullary junction. In HIV-associated thymitis, the anatomic location and weight of the thymus are normal (Joshi and Oleske, 1985). This stage of HIV infection appears to be similar to the follicular hyperplasia with irregularly shaped follicles, $CD8^+$ T-cell infiltration of the follicles, and fragmentation of the FDC network seen in lymph nodes associated with early HIV infection (Joshi and Oleske, 1985; Prevot *et al.*, 1992). The amount of follicular hyperplasia seen in the thymus in early HIV infection is variable but can be of such magnitude that the thymus is abnormally enlarged (Prevot *et al.*, 1992).

3.3.2. HIV-Induced Thymic Involution

In the later stages of HIV infection, there is marked involution of the thymus with severe thymocyte depletion, loss of corticomedullary distinction, and depletion of cortical thymic epithelial cells (Fig. 10). There may also be a variable amount of infiltration of plasma cells (Seemayer *et al.*, 1984) and $CD68^+$ tissue macrophages (Papiernik *et al.*, 1992) in the fat adjacent to cords of involuted thymus. The blood vessels may be hyalinized to show an onion-skin pattern. The amount of thymic involution is much greater than that expected from the patient's age and the chronic nature of the patient's illness.

Thymic dysplasia with epithelial rosette formation (Seemayer *et al.*, 1984) and calcification or loss of Hassall's bodies (Elie *et al.*, 1983; Seemayer *et al.*, 1984; Grody *et al.*, 1985; Schuurman *et al.*, 1989) has frequently been associated with thymic involution in AIDS, and may represent the latest stages of HIV infection of the thymus (Fig. 10B). These changes are similar to those observed in congenital immunodeficiency diseases such as severe combined immunodeficiency (SCID) in which lymphoid development does not occur. In fact, Schuurman *et al.* (1988) found no major difference between the histopathologic appearance of the thymus in patients with AIDS and patients with congenital immunodeficiencies. In many cases, the loss of Hassall's bodies may not be complete (Savino *et al.*, 1986) and they may become calcified (Reichert *et al.*, 1983). Hassall's bodies are swirls of terminally differentiated medullary thymic epithelium that are analogous to the stratum spinosum and stratum corneum of skin (Haynes, 1984; Lobach *et al.*, 1985; Patel *et al.*, 1995). Thus, Hassall's bodies disappear from thymus when there is disruption of thymic epithelial growth and maturation. In HIV-induced thymic atrophy, thymic epithelial growth arrest may occur via loss of the thymic lymphoid component, immune-mediated damage to thymic epithelial cells (Savino *et al.*, 1986), or direct HIV-induced effects on thymic epithelium (Schnittman *et al.*, 1991; Stanley *et al.*, 1993). All of these mechanisms may play a role in HIV-mediated thymus damage. It has been demonstrated that normal development of the thymic microenvironment is dependent on the lymphoid component of the thymus (van Ewijk *et al.*, 1994). For example, Hassall's bodies do not develop in human thymic ontogeny until several weeks after colonization and expansion of the lymphoid component (Haynes *et al.*, 1984; Haynes and Heinly, 1995), and in cases where the lymphoid component never develops

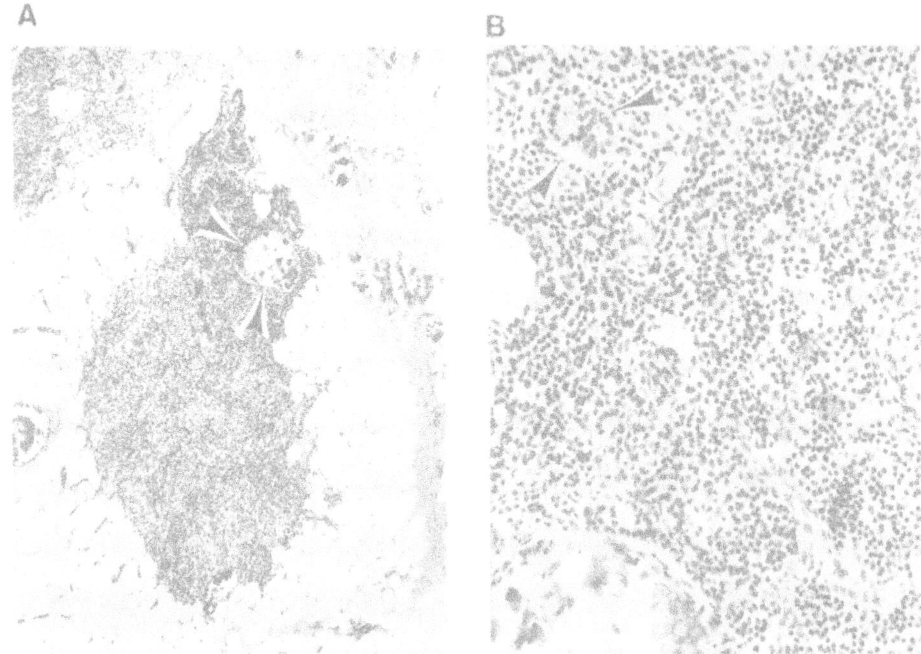

FIGURE 10. Thymus in the late stages of AIDS. (A) Low-power photomicrograph of thymus obtained at autopsy from a 42-year-old male with AIDS. The thymus is markedly atrophic, with loss of corticomedullary distinction, thymocyte depletion, and rare, generally calcified Hassall's bodies (arrowheads). (B) Higher-magnification view demonstrating pseudoglandular epithelial "rosettes" (arrowheads) and condensation of epithelial islands.

(X-linked SCID, adenosine deaminase deficiency, purine nucleoside phosphorylase deficiency), Hassall's bodies do not form. Thus, development of both the lymphoid and stromal components of the thymus are closely linked.

3.3.3. Thymocytes in HIV Infection

While it had been hypothesized that the severe lymphodepletion seen in the thymus from patients with end-stage AIDS was related to infection and destruction of lymphocytes by HIV (Reichert *et al.*, 1983; Seemayer *et al.*, 1984), this point was not clear because HIV was not as easily identified in the thymus as it was in the blood or lymph nodes of patients with AIDS. Several groups showed that unfractionated human thymocytes in vitro were susceptible to HIV infection (Schnittman *et al.*, 1990; Tremblay *et al.*, 1990; Tanaka *et al.*, 1992), and Schnittman *et al.* (1990) went on to fractionate subsets of thymocytes to show that not only were the $CD4^+$ mature medullary thymocytes infectable by HIV, but that HIV infects the immature $CD3^{lo}CD4^+CD8^+$ double-positive thymocytes, double-positive thymocyte clones, and $CD3^-CD4^-CD8^-$ triple-negative thymocytes in vitro. Further, they showed that the triple-negative thymocytes expressed low levels of surface CD4 and that infection of $CD7^+$ triple-negative thymocytes was blocked by anti-CD4 mAb OKT4a. Later, Valentin *et al.* (1994) subfractionated the triple-negative thymocytes based on CD1a expression where the $CD1a^-$ triple-negative cells (presumably the most immature thymocytes) were not infectable by HIV, but the CD1a$^+$ triple-negative cells that were also CD2$^+$ and CD7$^+$ were infectable by HIV. In this case, infection of CD1a$^+$CD2+CD7+ triple-negative cells with HIV was blocked by anti-CD4 mAb OKT4a but not by mAb to CD8. Taken together, these data suggest that one of the major mechanisms by which HIV-mediated lymphodepletion occurs in vivo in the thymus is via HIV infection of thymocytes at all stages of maturation.

While the data on infectivity of HIV in thymocyte subsets in vitro provided compelling evidence that thymocytes were permissive for HIV infection, many questions remained about the pathophysiology of HIV infection of the thymus in vivo. One of the important steps toward a better understanding of the pathophysiology of HIV was provided by McCune *et al.* (1988) who established an animal model, the SCID-hu mouse, whereby human thymus development could be recapitulated in an animal model by transplantation of human fetal liver and thymus under the renal capsule of immunodeficient SCID mice. Using the SCID-hu mouse model, Nakimawa *et al.* (1988) were able to document HIV infection of the human thymus. HIV infection with the SM, TY, and EW isolates of HIV peaked at 3–4 weeks in the cortex of SCID-hu thymus, and by 5 weeks, double-positive cells were eliminated or significantly decreased with an inversion of the CD4:CD8 ratio (Bonyhadi *et al.*, 1993; Aldrovandi *et al.*, 1993). Infection of triple-negative, double-positive, and CD4$^+$ single-positive thymocytes by HIV as shown by the in vitro studies was certainly plausible because all of these cell types express surface CD4. However, using the SCID-hu mouse, Stanley *et al.* (1993) showed by RT-PCR that CD8$^+$ single-positive thymocytes were clearly infected in vivo by the JR-CSF isolate of HIV. Stanley *et al.* (1993) hypothesized that HIV infection of this subset of thymocytes could result from either infection of more immature CD8$^+$ single-positive thymocytes when they still expressed low levels of CD4, downregulation of CD4 on infected double-positive cells, preferential maturation of infected immature thymocytes along the CD8$^+$ single-positive pathway, or that CD8$^+$ single-positive thymocytes could become infected by a non-CD4-dependent cell–cell contact mechanism.

Another important finding from the SCID-hu mouse work was that the different isolates of HIV had varying effects on the thymus. While the SM, TY, and EW isolates of HIV were clearly thymocytotropic resulting in marked lymphodepletion and inversion of the thymocyte CD4:CD8 ratio, the JR-CSF isolate was less thymocytotropic than other HIV strains and showed delayed kinetics of thymus infection with no inversion of the thymocyte CD4:CD8 ratio (Bonyhadi *et al.*, 1993; Aldrovandi *et al.*, 1993; Stanley *et al.*, 1993). Similar findings have been noted in the SIV model where SIV(ΔB670) infection resulted in profound thymocyte depletion (Baskin *et al.*, 1991) while SIVmac251 was not thymocytotropic (Muller *et al.*, 1993). Infection with SIVmac251 did, however, result in moderate thymic lymphodepletion that was associated with the loss of cortical thymic epithelial cells and dendritic cells. Similarly, human thymic epithelial cells are destroyed in infection with JR-CSF, but not in infection with SM (Stanley *et al.*, 1993). These studies have led us to hypothesize that, for some strains of HIV, infection/destruction of the thymic stroma can occur and that this can result in altered thymopoiesis.

3.3.4. Thymic Epithelial Cells

Thymic epithelial cells are essential for normal thymopoiesis, and are required for proliferation and positive selection and proliferation of immature thymocytes. In evaluating thymic tissue from autopsies of AIDS patients, Seemayer *et al.* (1984) originally proposed that thymic epithelial cell injury likely occurs as a primary pathogenic event because of the loss of Hassall's bodies. Savino *et al.* (1986) noted thymic epithelial cell damage in HIV infection with loss of the fine reticular pattern of epithelium and emergence of round or spindle-shaped cells that formed large epithelial keratin-positive clusters within areas of thymic epithelial cell damage. Because of the deposition of IgA, IgG, IgM, C3, C4, and C1q on thymic epithelial cells in HIV-infected thymus, Savino *et al.* (1986) hypothesized that thymic epithelial cells could be destroyed by an autoimmune mechanism, but they were not able to find thymic epithelial cell-specific antibodies in the serum. With the cross-reactivity of anti-gp41 mAbs with thymic epithelial cells (K. Casey and B. Haynes, unpublished data), autoimmune mechanisms of thymic epithelial cell destruction in HIV infection are plausible. Similar cross-reactivity of anti-HTLV-I core antibodies with human thymic epithelium has been reported as well (Haynes *et al.*, 1983), and it is probable that similar immunopathologic processes occur in both HIV-1 and HTLV-I that result in thymic epithelial cell damage and ineffective thymopoiesis. Clearly, immunosuppression occurs in both types of retroviral infections.

Whether thymic epithelial cells are actually infected by HIV is controversial. Numazaki *et al.* (1989) suggested that cultured thymic epithelial cells were able to be infected with $HIV_{IIIB/LAI}$ in vitro with cytopathic effects including epithelial giant cell formation and a more differentiated surface phenotype, but neither they nor Schnittman *et al.* (1991) could document a productive infection of TE cells in vitro. In the SCID-hu model, Stanley *et al.* (1993) showed by electron microscopy that thymic epithelial cells of $HIV_{JR\text{-}CSF}$-infected thymus could endocytose $HIV_{JR\text{-}CSF}$ but not HIV_{SM} with large amounts of $HIV_{JR\text{-}CSF}$ RNA documented in thymic epithelial cell cytoplasm by in situ hybridization. Thymic epithelial cell destruction was readily apparent after 2 weeks of $HIV_{JR\text{-}CSF}$ infection of thymus in SCID-hu mice, well before the onset of lymphodepletion. In SIV(ΔB670) infection of rhesus monkeys, thymic epithelial cells were not affected (Baskin *et al.*, 1991). However, with SIVmac251 infection, cortical thymic epithelial cells selectively became necrotic and died (Muller *et al.*, 1993). A productive infection of thymic epithelial cells could not be documented with either JR-CSF infection of SCID-hu thymus or SIVmac251 infection of rhesus monkey thymus. Moreover, no free virus particles could be found in the thymus of SIVmac251-infected monkeys, suggesting that the lymphodepletion observed in SIVmac251 infection may be related either to a defect in thymopoiesis or to autoimmune mechanisms. Thymic epithelial cells do not need to be productively infected by HIV to be damaged by HIV. Ameisen and Capron (1991) hypothesized that programmed cell death in HIV-uninfected cells could be induced by HIV products without direct infection of cells by HIV. For example, in rodent neurons, CD4-independent binding of HIV gp120 has been shown to induce a calcium flux in neurons leading to cell death (Dreyer *et al.*, 1990). Taken together, these data suggest that defective T-cell development resulting from destruction of the cortical thymic epithelial cell component of the thymic microenvironment is a plausible mechanism for the lymphodepletion seen in the thymus during HIV infection.

3.3.5. Dendritic Cells

Dendritic cells play a major role in the pathogenesis of HIV infection in lymph nodes, but their role in thymic dysfunction in HIV infection of the thymus is less clear. Naparsteck *et al.* (1982) demonstrated recirculation back to the thymus of antigen-primed, postthymic T cells, suggesting that the thymic medulla of postpubertal thymuses can function like lymph node as a site of antigen activation of memory T cells, an event that requires dendritic cells.

Clearly when germinal centers are present in thymus, normal dendritic cell function including filtering of antigens such as whole virus particles is inferred to occur. Few studies have critically analyzed the role of dendritic cells in HIV pathophysiology in the thymus. Muller *et al.* (1993) noted in thymuses of SIVmac251-infected monkeys that interdigitating dendritic cells were destroyed by cytolysis, while Baskin *et al.* (1991) believed that macrophages in the cortex of SIV(ΔB670)-infected thymus were SIV-infected. Valentin *et al.* (1994) demonstrated that purified $CD1a^+CD2^-CD3^-CD4^-CD7^-CD8^-CD14^-$ thymic cells (presumably dendritic cells, see Table I) were infectable in vitro by HIV. Thus, it is likely that dendritic cells may play a similar key role in the thymus as they do in lymph node regarding antigen-presenting cell functions, and their destruction in the thymus in HIV infection is likely an important pathologic event. HIV-infected dendritic cells, monocytes, or $CD4^+$ thymocytes may serve as a reservoir to infect either $CD8^+$ single-positive thymocytes or thymic epithelial cells by a mechanism similar to that seen by Bourinbain and Phillips (1991) where HIV-infected monocyte contact with intestinal epithelial cells resulted in HIV uptake by epithelial cells in phagocytic endosomes.

3.3.6. Natural Killer Cells

Natural killer (NK) cell activity during HIV infection is functionally defective (Poli *et al.*, 1985; Sirianni *et al.*, 1990; Scott-Algara *et al.*, 1992). NK cells clearly develop extrathymically, but can also arise from NK precursors within the thymus (Denning *et al.*, 1991). Whether this is related to a selective depletion of NK cells (Vuillier *et al.*, 1988) and/or NK suppressor factors liberated during HIV infection (Goicoa *et al.*, 1995) is controversial. NK cells do not express high levels of either surface CD4 molecules (Table I) or CD4 mRNA, but have been reported to be infectable in vitro by $HIV_{IIIB/LAI}$ (Schnittman *et al.*, 1990; Chehimi *et al.*, 1991).

3.4. Assessing Thymic Function in HIV Infection and the Role of Thymic Transplantation and Thymus-Derived Hormones in the Treatment of AIDS

The thymus is not necessary for normal T-lymphocyte function in the adult, because a subset of mature postthymic peripheral T lymphocytes are self-renewing (Fig. 11) (Stutman, 1978; Brearley *et al.*, 1987). However, when the normal T-lymphocyte pool of cells is destroyed by infection with HIV or chemotherapy for cancer, the thymus may be necessary

TABLE I. Surface Phenotype of Leukocytes in the Thymus

Cell type	CD1a	CD2	CD3	CD4	CD7	CD8	CD14	CD16	CD34
TN thymocyte	−/+	+	−	−/lo	−/lo/hi	−	−	−	+
DP thymocyte	+	+	lo	+	lo	+	−	−	−
SP4 thymocyte	−	+	hi	+	hi	−	−	−	−
SP8 thymocyte	−	+	hi	−/lo	hi	+	−	−	−
NK cell precursor	−	+	−	−/lo	hi	−	−	−	−
NK cell	−	+	−	−/lo	hi	+	−	+	−
Macrophage	−	−	−	lo	−	−	+	−	−
Dendritic cell	+	−	−	lo	−	−	−	−	−

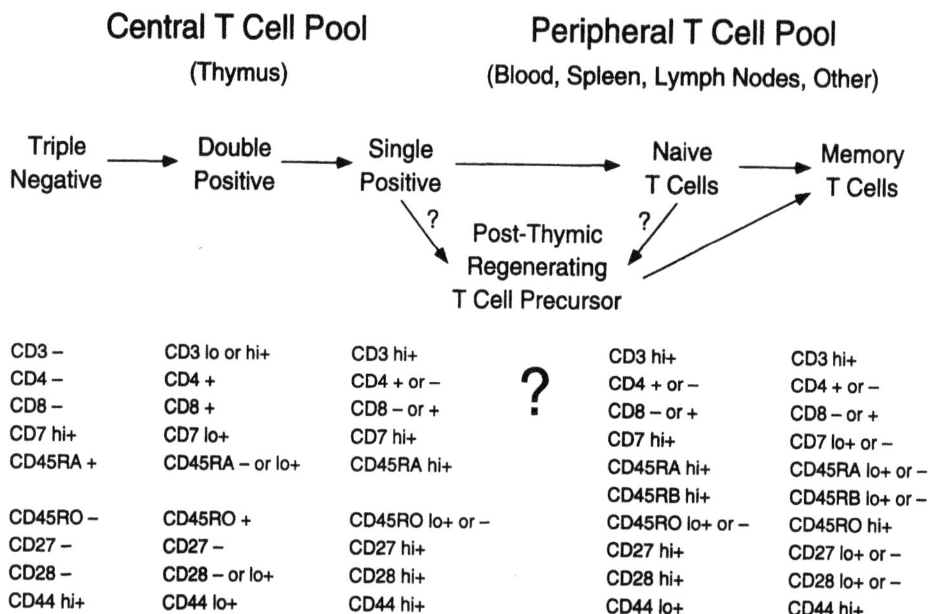

FIGURE 11. Relationship of pre- and postthymic T-cell precursors to naive and memory T cells.

in the adult for complete regeneration of T lymphocytes. Studies with patients undergoing intensive chemotherapy for cancer have shown that T-cell regeneration is dependent on a functional thymus, and that the capacity of the thymus to support T-cell regeneration is inversely correlated with age and size of the thymus (Mackall *et al.*, 1995).

Because of the pronounced lymphodepletion and destruction of the thymus, intrathymic T-cell development does not likely occur in the late stages of HIV infection (Schnittman *et al.*, 1990; Haynes and Denning, 1992). The lack of effective thymopoiesis in late-stage HIV infection has been inferred primarily from studies evaluating thymic morphology in AIDS and from studies of thymic component infectability in vitro. Recent work evaluating CD45 isoform expression by T-cell subsets has provided evidence that thymopoiesis in AIDS is indeed defective. In the periphery, naive T lymphocytes that have yet to be exposed to a specific antigen express the CD45RA and RB isoforms of CD45; and, after antigen exposure, memory T lymphocytes express the CD45RO isoform and lose CD45RA and RB (Trowbridge and Thomas, 1994). Recently it has been shown that reappearance of peripheral blood CD4$^+$ T cells following antiretroviral chemotherapy in AIDS is likely to be the result of regeneration of peripheral postthymic CD45RO$^+$ memory T lymphocytes, not the appearance of newly developed CD45RA$^+$ naive T lymphocytes produced in the thymus (Ho *et al.*, 1995; Roederer, 1995).

Thus, HIV infection of the thymus results in a thymic microenvironment that shares many characteristics with certain congenital immunodeficiencies. Because of success in treating congenitally immunodeficient patients with thymic transplantation (Hong *et al.*, 1976; Hong, 1986), several groups have attempted to reconstitute the T-cell arm of the immune system in AIDS with thymic transplantation. While engraftment of the thymus did occur in some cases (Hong, 1986), immune system reconstitution did not occur (Ciobanu *et al.*, 1985; Hong, 1986; Danner *et al.*, 1986; Phair, 1986; Dwyer *et al.*, 1987; Dupuy *et al.*,

1991). Based on decreased thymus-derived hormones thymopoietin, thymosin, and thymulin in patients with HIV infection (Dardenne *et al.*, 1983; Naylor *et al.*, 1986; Savino *et al.*, 1986), several investigators have attempted immunologic reconstitution by administration of thymus-derived hormones to patients with AIDS. While some investigators noted a transient improvement in CD4 counts, overall survival was not affected by thymic hormone treatment (Aiuti *et al.*, 1983; Clumeck *et al.*, 1985; Schulof *et al.*, 1986; Valesini *et al.*, 1987; Chachoua *et al.*, 1989; Silvestris *et al.*, 1989; Hermans and Clumeck, 1989).

It is not surprising that thymic transplantation alone did not lead to immune system reconstitution in AIDS. For immune reconstitution in AIDS to have a lasting salutory effect: (1) both the thymic microenvironment and progeny of differentiating stem cells will need to be resistant to HIV infection, (2) the patient's bone marrow and immune compartments will need to be prepared by chemotherapy to receive stem cell (bone marrow) allografts, and (3) it is likely that it will be advantageous to decrease viral load to the lowest possible level prior to and during immune reconstitution.

Thus, thymic transplantation in AIDS will likely have the greatest chance of boosting T-cell immune function if: (1) the thymic graft is partially HLA-matched to the patient's HLA type, (2) thymic transplantation is combined with bone marrow transplantation, and (3) bone marrow transplantation is undertaken with prior ablative chemotherapy and involves use of a strategy to protect developing immune cells from new HIV infection (i.e., gene therapy).

Finally, recent data suggest that host HLA or HLA-linked genes determine the quality of the host immune response to HIV, i.e., certain HLA antigens are associated with long-term survival states while others are associated with rapid progression to AIDS (reviewed in Haynes *et al.*, 1996). Thus, if bone marrow and thymic allografting could be achieved using partially HLA-matched tissues that also express HLA antigens associated with long-term survival with HIV infection, one might be able to reconstruct a more effective immune system regarding HIV infection, and possibly negate the need for gene therapy to protect the new immune system. Successful immune cell reconstitution will depend on conducting appropriate clinical trials, simultaneous with incisive basic research into molecular mechanisms of regulation of hematopoiesis.

4. SUMMARY

It is clear that the effects of HIV infection of both thymus and lymph nodes profoundly limit the ability of immune cell regeneration to compensate for HIV-induced T-cell destruction. The T-cell arm of the immune system in AIDS is most likely depleted both because of destruction of the central T cell regenerative microenvironment in the thymus and because of destruction of the peripheral postthymic regenerating T-cell pool present in lymph nodes, gut-associated lymphoid tissue, and spleen. Given that the pathobiology of HIV effects on the immune system is now becoming clear, investigators are guardedly optimistic regarding finding ways to successfully reconstitute the immune system in AIDS.

REFERENCES

Aiuti, F., Buscino, L., Fiorilli, M., Galli, E., Quinti, I., Rossi, P., Seminara, R., and Goldstein, G., 1983, Thymopoietin pentapeptide treatment of primary immunodeficiencies, *Lancet* **1**:551–554.

Aldrovandi, G. M., Feuer, G., Gao, L., Jamieson, B., Kristeva, M., Chen, I. S. Y., and Zack, J. A., 1993, The SCID-hu mouse as a model for HIV-1 infection, *Nature* **363**:732–736.

Ameisen, J.-C., and Capron, A., 1991, Cell dysfunction and depletion in AIDS: The programmed cell death hypothesis, *Immunol. Today* **12**:102–105.

Armstrong, J. A,. Dawkins, R. L., and Horne, R., 1985, Retroviral infection of accessory cells and the immunological paradox in AIDS, *Immunol. Today* **6**:121–122.

Baroni, C. D., Pezzella, F., Pezzella, M., Macchi, B., Vitolo, D., Uccini, S., and Ruco, L. P., 1988, Expression of HIV in lymph node cells of LAS patients. Immunohistology, in situ hybridization and identification of target cells, *Am. J. Pathol.* **133**:498–506.

Baskin, G. B., Murphey-Corb, M., Martin, L. N., Davison-Fairburn, B., and Kuebler, D., 1991, Thymus in simian immunodeficiency virus-infected rhesus monkeys, *Lab. Invest.* **65**:400–407.

Baskin, G. B., Martin, L. N., Murphey-Corb, M., Hu, F. S., Kuebler, D., and Davison, B., 1995, Distribution of SIV in lymph nodes of serially sacrificed rhesus monkeys, *AIDS Res. Hum. Retrovir.* **11**:273–285.

Biberfeld, P., Ost, A., Portwit, A., Sandsted, B., Pallesen, G., Bottiger, B., Morfelt-Mansson, L., and Biberfeld, G., 1987, Histopathology and immunohistology of HTLV-III/LAV related lymphadenopathy and AIDS, *Acta Pathol. Microbiol. Immunol. Scand.* **95**:47–65.

Bonyhadi, M. L., Rabin, L., Salimi, S., Brown, D. A., Kosek, J., McCune, J. M., and Kaneshima, H., 1993, HIV induces thymus depletion *in vivo*, *Nature* **363**:728–736.

Bourinbain, A. S., and Phillips, D. M., 1991, Transmission of human immunodeficiency virus from monocytes to epithelia, *J. Acq. Immune Defic. Syndr.* **4**:56–63.

Brearley, S., Gentle, T. A., Baynham, M. I., Roberts, K. D., Abrams, L. D., and Thompson, R. A., 1987, Immunodeficiency following neonatal thymectomy in Man, *Clin. Exp. Immunol.* **70**:322–327.

Burke, A. P., Anderson, D., Mannan, P., Ribas, J. L., Liang, Y.-H., Smialek, J., and Virmani, R., 1994, Systemic lymphadenopathic histology in human immunodeficiency virus-1-seropositive drug addicts without apparent acquired immunodeficiency syndrome, *Hum. Pathol.* **25**:248–256.

Chachoua, A., Green, M. D., Valentine, F., and Muggia, F. M., 1989, Phase I/II trial of thymostimulin in opportunistic infections of the acquired immune deficiency syndrome, *Cancer Invest.* **7**:225–229.

Chadburn, A., Metroka, C., and Mouradian, J., 1989, Progressive lymph node histology and its prognostic value in patients with acquired immunodeficiency syndrome and AIDS-related complex, *Hum. Pathol.* **20**:579–587.

Chakrabarti, L., Cumont, M. C., Montagnier, L., and Hutrel, B., 1994a, Variable course of primary simian immunodeficiency virus infection in lymph nodes: Relation to disease progression, *J. Virol.* **68**:6634–6643.

Chakrabarti, L., Isola, P., Cumont, M. C., Claessens-Maire, M. A., Hutrel, M., Montagnier, L., and Hutrel, B., 1994b, Early stages of simian immunodeficiency virus infection in lymph nodes. Evidence for high viral load and successive populations of target cells, *Am. J. Pathol.* **144**:1226–1237.

Chehimi, J., Bandyopadhyay, S., Prakash, K., Perussia, B., Hassan, N. F., Kawashima, H., Campbell, D., Kornbluth, J., and Starr, S. E., 1991, In vitro infection of natural killer cells with different human immunodeficiency virus type 1 isolates, *J. Virol.* **65**:1812–1822.

Ciobanu, N., Paietta, E., Karten, M., Ramos, S., Wiernik, P. H., and Naylor, P., 1985, Thymus fragment transplantation in the acquired immunodeficiency syndrome, *Ann. Intern. Med.* **103**:479.

Clumeck, N., Cran, S., Van de Perre, P., Lemone-Mascart, F., Duchateau, J., and Bolla, K., 1985, Thymopentin treatment in AIDS and pre-AIDS patients, *Surv. Immunol. Res.* **4**:58S–62S.

Coombs, R. W., Collier, A. C., Allain, J. P., Nikora, B., Leuter, M., Gjerset, G. F., and Corey, L., 1989, Plasma viremia in human immunodeficiency virus infection, *N. Engl. J. Med.* **321**:1626–1631.

Danner, S. A., Schuurman, H.-J., Lange, J. M. A., Meyling, F. H. J. G., Schellekens, P. T., Huber, J., and Kater, L., 1986, Implantation of cultured thymic fragments in patients with acquired immunodeficiency syndrome, *Arch. Intern. Med.* **146**:1133–1136.

Dardenne, M., Bach, J.-F., and Safai, B., 1983, Low serum thymic hormone levels in patients with acquired immunodeficiency syndrome, *N. Engl. J. Med.* **309**:48–49.

Denning, S. M., Kurtzberg, J., Le, P. T., Tuck, D. T., Singer, K. H., and Haynes, B. F., 1988, Human thymic epithelial cells directly induce autologous immature thymocyte activation, *Proc. Natl. Acad. Sci. USA* **85**: 3125–3129.

Denning, S. M., Jones, D. M., Ware, R. E., Weinhold, K. J., Brenner, M. B., and Haynes, B. F., 1991, Analysis of clones derived from human CD7+, CD4−, CD8−, CD3− thymocytes, *Int. Immunol.* **3**:1015–1024.

Devergne, O., Peuchmaur, M., Crevon, M. C., Trapani, J. A., Maillot, M. C., Galanaud, P., and Emilie, D., 1991, Activation of cytotoxic cells in hyperplastic lymph nodes from HIV-infected patients, *AIDS* **5**:1071–1079.

Donaldson, S. L., Kosco, M. H., Szakal, A. K., and Tew, J. G., 1986, Localization of antibody-forming cells in draining lymphoid organs during long term maintenance of the antibody response, *J. Leukocyte Biol.* **40:** 147–157.

Dreyer, E. B., Kaiser, P. K., Offermann, J. T., and Lipton, S. A., 1990, HIV-1 coat protein neurotoxicity prevented by calcium channel antagonists, *Science* **248:**364–367.

Dupuy, J.-M., Gilmore, N., Goldman, H., Tsoukas, C., Pekovic, D., Chausseau, J.-P., Duperval, R., Joly, M., Pelletier, L., and Thibaudeau, Y., 1991, Thymic epithelial cell transplantation in patients with acquired immunodeficiency syndrome: Evidence for infection by HIV-1 of newly differentiated T cells at the site of transplantation, *Thymus* **17:**205–218.

Dwyer, J. M., Wood, C. C., McNamara, J., and Kinder, B., 1987, Transplantation of thymic tissue into patients with AIDS: An attempt to reconstitute the immune system, *Arch. Intern. Med.* **147:**513–517.

Elie, R., Larouche, A. C., Arnoux, E., Guerin, J.-M., Pierre, G., Malebranche, R., Seemayer, T. A., Dupuy, J.-M., Russo, P., and Lapp, W. S., 1983, Thymic dysplasia in acquired immunodeficiency syndrome, *N. Engl. J. Med.* **308:**841–842.

Embretson, J., Zupancic, M., Ribas, J. L., Burke, A., Tenner-Racz, K., Racz, P., and Haase, A. T., 1993, Massive covert infection of helper T lymphocytes and macrophages by HIV during the incubation period of AIDS, *Nature* **362:**359–362.

Emilie, D., Peuchmaur, M., Maillot, M. C., Crevon, M. C., Brousse, N., Delfraissy, J. F., Dormont, J., and Galanaud, P., 1990, Production of interleukins in human immunodeficiency virus-1-replicating lymph nodes, *J. Clin. Invest.* **86:**148–159.

Engel, P., and Tedder, T. F., 1994, New CD from the B cell section of the Fifth International Workshop on Human Leukocyte Differentiation Antigens, *Leuk. Lymphoma* **13S:**61–64.

Ewing, E. P., Chandler, R. W., Spira, T. J., Byrnes, R. K., and Chan, W. C., 1985, Primary lymph node pathology in AIDS and AIDS-related lymphadenopathy, *Arch. Pathol. Lab. Med.* **109:**977–981.

Fox, C. H., Tenner-Racz, K., Racz, P., Firpo, A., Pizzo, P. A., and Fauci, A. S., 1991, Lymphoid germinal centers are reservoirs of human immunodeficiency virus type 1 RNA, *J. Infect. Dis.* **164:**1051–1057.

Goicoa, M. A., Sen, L., Iannitelli, P. S., Diez, R. A., and Estevez, M. E., 1995, Natural killer suppressor factors in sera from HIV-infected subjects, *Scand. J. Immunol.* **41:**523–528.

Graziosi, C., Pantaleo, G., Gantt, K. R., Fortin, J.-P., Demarest, J. F., Cohen, O. J., Sekaly, R. P., and Fauci, A. S., 1994, Lack of evidence for the dichotomy of TH1 and TH2 predominance in HIV-infected individuals, *Science* **265:**248–252.

Grody, W. W., Fligiel, S., and Naeim, F., 1985, Thymus involution in the acquired immunodeficiency syndrome, *Am. J. Clin. Pathol.* **84:**85–95.

Groux, H., Monte, D., Plouvier, B., Capron, A., and Ameisen, J.-C., 1993, CD3-mediated apoptosis of human medullary thymocytes and activated peripheral T cells: Respective roles of interleukin-1, interleukin-2, interferon-gamma and accessory cells, *Eur. J. Immunol.* **23:**1623–1629.

Guarda, L. A., Luna, M. A., Smith, J. L., Jr., Mansell, P. W. A., Gyorkey, F., and Roca, A. N., 1984, Acquired immune deficiency syndrome: Postmortem findings, *Am. J. Clin. Pathol.* **81:**549–557.

Haynes, B. F., 1984, The human thymic microenvironment, *Adv. Immunol.* **36:**87–142.

Haynes, B. F., and Denning, S. M., 1992, Lymphopoiesis, in: *The Molecular Basis of Blood Diseases*, 2nd ed. (G. Stamatoyannopoulos, A. Nienhuis, P. Majerus, and H. Varmus, eds.), Saunders, Philadelphia, pp. 425–462.

Haynes, B. F., and Heinly, C. S., 1995, Early human T cell development: Analysis of the human thymus at the time of initial entry of hematopoietic stem cells into the fetal thymic microenvironment, *J. Exp. Med.* **181:** 1445–1458.

Haynes, B. F., Robert-Guroff, M., Metzgar, R. S., Franchini, G., Kalyanaraman, V. S., Palker, T. J., and Gallo, R. C., 1983, Monoclonal antibody against human T cell leukemia virus p19 defines a human thymic epithelial antigen acquired during ontogeny, *J. Exp. Med.* **157:**907–920.

Haynes, B. F., Scearce, R. M., Lobach, D. F., and Hensley, L. L., 1984, Phenotypic characterization and ontogeny of mesodermal-derived and endocrine epithelial components of the human thymic microenvironment, *J. Exp. Med.* **159:**1149–1168.

Haynes, B. F., Panataleo, G., and Fauci, A. S., 1996, Towards an understanding of the correlates of protective immunity to HIV infection, *Science* **271:**324–328.

Heath, S. L., Tew, J. G., Tew, J. G., Szakal, A. K., and Burton, G. F., 1995, Follicular dendritic cells and human immunodeficiency virus infectivity, *Nature* **377:**740–744.

Hermans, P., and Clumeck, N., 1989, Preliminary results on clinical and immunological effects of thymus hormone preparations in AIDS, *Med. Oncol. Tumor Pharmacother.* **6:**55–58.

Hirokawa, K., McClure, J. E., and Goldstein, A. L., 1982, Age-related changes in localization of thymosin in the human thymus, *Thymus* **4:**19–29.

Ho, D. D., Moudgil, T., and Alam, M., 1989, Quantitation of human immunodeficiency virus type 1 in the blood of infected persons, *N. Engl. J. Med.* **321:**1621–1625.

Ho, D. D., Perelson, A. S., and Shaw, G. M., 1995, Cyclosporin A, a reply, *Nature* **375:**198.

Hong, R., 1986, Reconstitution of T-cell deficiency by thymic hormone or thymus transplantation therapy, *Clin. Immunol. Immunopathol.* **40:**136–141.

Hong, R., Santosham, M., Schulte-Wisserman, H., Horowitz, S., Hsu, S. H., and Winkelstein, J. A., 1976, Reconstitution of B and T lymphocyte function in severe combined immunodeficiency disease after transplantation with thymic epithelium, *Lancet* **2:**1270–1272.

Hsu, S. M., and Jaffe, E. S., 1984, Phenotypic expression of B lymphocytes. 2. Immunoglobulin expression of germinal center cells, *Am. J. Pathol.* **114:**396–402.

Hsu, S. M., Cossman, J., and Jaffe, E. S., 1983, Lymphocyte subsets in normal human lymphoid tissue, *Am. J. Clin. Pathol.* **80:**21–30.

Ioachim, H. L., 1994, Human immunodeficiency virus lymphadenitis, in: *Lymph Node Pathology*, 2nd ed., Lippincott, Philadelphia, pp. 73–82.

Ioachim, H. L., Lerner, C. W., and Tapper, M. L., 1983, The lymphoid lesions associated with the acquired immunodeficiency syndrome, *Am. J. Surg. Pathol.* **7:**543–553.

Jaffe, E. S., 1994, Reactive lymph node hyperplasias, in: *Surgical Pathology of the Lymph Nodes and Related Organs*, Saunders, Philadelphia, pp. 102–106.

Joshi, V. V., and Oleske, J. M., 1985, Pathologic appraisal of the thymus gland in acquired immunodeficiency syndrome in children: A study of four cases and a review of the literature, *Arch. Pathol. Lab. Med.* **109:** 142–146.

Joshi, V. V., and Oleske, J. M., 1990, Morphological findings in children with acquired immunodeficiency syndrome: Pathogenesis and clinical implications, *Pediatr. Pathol.* **10:**155–165.

Joshi, V. V., Oleske, J. M., Minnefor, A. B., Singh, R., Bokhari, T., and Rapkin, R. H., 1984, Pathology of suspected acquired immunodeficiency syndrome in children: A study of eight cases, *Pediatr. Pathol.* **2:**71–87.

Keller, A. R., Hochholzer, L., and Castleman, B., 1972, Hyaline-vascular and plasma cell types of giant lymph node hyperplasia of the mediastinum and other location, *Cancer* **29:**670–683.

Knowles, D., 1992, *Neoplastic Hematopathology*, Williams & Wilkins, Baltimore, pp. 431–436.

Krueger, G. R., Ablashi, D. V., Lusso, P., and Josephs, S. F., 1991, Immunological dysregulation of lymph nodes in AIDS patients, *Curr. Top. Pathol.* **84:**157–188.

Le Tourneau, A., Audouin, J., Diebold, J., Marche, C., Tircottet, V., and Reynes, M., 1986, LAV-like viral particles in lymph node germinal centers in patients with persistent lymphadenopathy syndrome and the acquired immunodeficiency syndrome-related complex. An ultrastructural study of 30 cases, *Hum. Pathol.* **17:**1047–1053.

Lobach, D. F., Scearce, R. M., and Haynes, B. F., 1985, The human thymic microenvironment: Phenotypic characterization of Hassall's bodies with the use of monoclonal antibodies, *J. Immunol.* **134:**250–257.

McCune, J. M., Nakimawa, R., Kaneshima, H., Schultz, L. D., Lieberman, M., and Weissman, I. L., 1988, The SCID-hu mouse: Murine model for the analysis of human hemolymphoid differentiation and function, *Science* **241:**1632–1639.

Mackall, C. L., Fleisher, T. A., Brown, M. R., Andrich, M. P., Chen, C. C., Feuerstein, I. M., Horowitz, M. E., Magrath, I. T., Shad, A. T., Steinberg, S. M., Wexler, L. H., and Gress, R. E., 1995, Age, thymopoiesis, and CD4+ T-lymphocyte regeneration after intensive chemotherapy, *N. Engl. J. Med.* **332:**143–149.

Marrack, P., Hugo, P., McCormack, J., and Kappler, J., 1993, Death and T cells, *Immunol. Rev.* **133:**119–129.

Muller, J. G., Krenn, V., Schindler, C., Czub, S., Stahl-Hennig, C., Coulibaly, C., Hunsmann, G., Kneitz, C., Kerkau, T., Rethwilm, A., terMeulen, V., and Muller-Hermelink, H. K., 1993, Alterations of thymus cortical epithelium and interdigitating dendritic cells but no increase of thymocyte cell death in the early course of simian immunodeficiency virus infection, *Am. J. Pathol.* **143:**699–713.

Muro-Cacho, C. A., Pantaleo, G., and Fauci, A. S., 1995, Analysis of apoptosis in lymph nodes of HIV-infected persons. Intensity of apoptosis correlates with the general state of activation of the lymphoid tissue and not with stage of disease or viral burden, *J. Immunol.* **154:**5555–5566.

Nakimawa, R., Kaneshima, H., Lieberman, M., Weissman, I. L., and McCune, J. M., 1988, Infection of the SCID-hu mouse by HIV-1, *Science* **242:**1684–1686.

Naparstek, Y., Holoshitz, J., Eisentein, S., Reshef, T., Rappaport, S., Chemke, J., Ben-Nun, A., and Cohen, I. R., 1982, Effector T lymphocyte line cells migrate to the thymus and persist there, *Nature* **300:**262–264.

Naylor, P. H., Friedman-Klein, A., Hersch, E., Erdos, M., and Goldstein, A. L., 1986, Thymosin beta-1 and thymosin beta-4 in serum: Comparison of normal, cord, homosexual, and AIDS serum, *Int. J. Immunopharmacol.* **8:**667–676.

Nosanchuk, J. S., and Schnitzer, B., 1969, Follicular hyperplasia in lymph nodes from patients with rheumatoid arthritis, *Cancer* **24:**334–354.

Numazaki, K., Goldman, H., Bai, X.-Q., Wong, I., and Wainberg, M. A., 1989, Effects of infection by HIV-1, cytomegalovirus, and human measles virus on cultured human thymic epithelial cells, *Microbiol. Immunol.* **33:**733–745.

Pantaleo, G., Graziosi, C., Butini, L., Pizzo, P. A., Schnittman, S. M., Kotler, D. P., and Fauci, A. S., 1991, Lymphoid organs function as major reservoirs for human immunodeficiency virus, *Proc. Natl. Acad. Sci. USA* **88:**9838–9842.

Pantaleo, G., Graziosi, C., and Fauci, A. S., 1993a, The pathogenesis of human immunodeficiency virus infection, *N. Engl. J. Med.* **328:**327–335.

Pantaleo, G., Graziosi, C., and Fauci, A. S., 1993b, The role of lymphoid organs in the pathogenesis of HIV infection, *Semin. Immunol.* **5:**157–163.

Pantaleo, G., Graziosi, C., Demarest, J. F., Butini, L., Montroni, M., Fox, C. H., Orenstein, J. M., Kotler, D. P., and Fauci, A. S., 1993c, HIV infection is active and progressive in lymphoid tissue during the clinically latent stage of disease, *Nature* **362:**355–358.

Pantaleo, G., Graziosi, C., Demarest, J. F., Cohen, O. J., Vaccarezza, M., Gantt, K., Muro-Cacho, C., and Fauci, A. S., 1994, Role of lymphoid organs in the pathogenesis of human immunodeficiency virus (HIV) infection, *Immunol. Rev.* **140:**105–130.

Papiernik, M., Brossard, Y., Mulliez, N., Roume, J., Brechot, C., Barin, F., Goudeau, A., Bach, J.-F., Griscelli, C., Henrion, R., and Vazeux, R., 1992, Thymic abnormalities in fetuses aborted from human immunodeficiency virus type 1 seropositive women, *Pediatrics* **89:**297–301.

Patel, D. D., Whichard, L. P., Radcliff, G., Denning, S. M., and Haynes, B. F., 1995, Characterization of human thymic epithelial cell surface antigens: Phenotypic similarity of thymic epithelial cells to epidermal keratinocytes, *J. Clin. Immunol.* **15:**80–91.

Phair, J., 1986, Therapy for acquired immunodeficiency syndrome: Implantation of cultured thymic fragments, *Arch. Intern. Med.* **146:**1074–1075.

Poli, G., Introna, M., Zanaboni, F., Peri, G., Carbonari, M., Aiuti, F., Lazzarin, A., Moroni, M., and Mantovani, A., 1985, Natural killer cells in intravenous drug abusers with lymphadenopathy syndrome, *Clin. Exp. Immunol.* **62:**128–135.

Poppeman, S., Bhen, A. K., Reinherz, E. L., McCluskey, R. T., and Schlossman, S. F., 1981, Distribution of T cell subsets in human lymph nodes, *J. Exp. Med.* **153:**30–41.

Prevot, S., Audouin, J., Andre-Bougaran, J., Griffais, R., Le Tourneau, A., Fournier, J. G., and Diebold, J., 1992, Thymic pseudotumorous enlargement due to follicular hyperplasia in human immunodeficiency virus seropositive patient, *Am. J. Clin. Pathol.* **97:**420–425.

Reichert, C. M., O'Leary, T. J., Levens, D. L., Simrell, C. R., and Macher, A. M., 1983, Autopsy pathology in the acquired immunodeficiency syndrome, *Am. J. Pathol.* **112:**357–382.

Reimann, K. A., Tenner-Racz, K., Racz, P., Montefiori, D. C., Yasutomi, Y., Lin, W., Ransil, B. J., and Letvin, N. L., 1994, Immunopathogenic events in acute infection of rhesus monkeys with simian immunodeficiency virus of macaques, *J. Virol.* **68:**2362–2370.

Ritter, M. A., Sauvage, C. A., and Cotmore, S. F., 1981, The human thymus microenvironment: *In vivo* identification of thymic nurse cells and other antigenically distinct subpopulations of epithelial cells, *Immunology* **44:**439–446.

Roederer, M., 1995, T-cell dynamics of immunodeficiency, *Nature Med.* **1:**621–622.

Rosai, J., and Levine, G. D., 1976, *Tumors of the Thymus: Atlas of Tumor Pathology*, 2nd series, fascicle 13, Armed Forces Institute of Pathology, Washington, DC.

Savino, W., Dardenne, M., Marche, C., Trophilme, D., Dupuy, J.-M., Pekovic, D., Lapointe, N., and Bache, J.-F., 1986, Thymic epithelium in AIDS: An immunohistologic study, *Am. J. Pathol.* **122:**302–307.

Schnittman, S. M., Denning, S. M., Greenhouse, J. J., Justement, J. S., Baseler, M., Kurtzberg, J., Haynes, B. F., and Fauci, A. S., 1990, Evidence for susceptibility of intrathymic T cell precursors and their progeny carrying T cell antigen receptor phenotypes $TCR\alpha\beta^+$ and $TCR\gamma\delta^+$ to human immunodeficiency virus infection: A mechanism for CD4+ (T4) lymphocyte depletion, *Proc. Natl. Acad. Sci. USA* **87:**7727–7731.

Schnittman, S. M., Singer, K. H., Greenhouse, J. J., Stanley, S. K., Whichard, L. P., Le, P. T., Haynes, B. F., and Fauci, A. S., 1991, Thymic microenvironment induces HIV expression. Physiologic secretion of IL-6 by thymic epithelial cells up-regulates virus expression in chronically infected cells, *J. Immunol.* **147:**2553–2558.

Schulof, R. S., Simon, G. L., Sztein, M. B., Parenti, D. M., DiGioia, R. A., Courtless, J. W., Orenstein, J. M., Kessler, C. M., Kind, P. D., Schlesselman, S., Paxton, H. M., Robert-Guroff, M., Naylor, P. H., and Goldstein, A. L., 1986, Phase I/II trial of thymosin fraction 5 and thymosin alpha one in HTLV-III seropositive subjects, *J. Biol. Response Modif.* **5:**429–443.

Schuurman, H. J., van Barlen, J., Krone, W. J. A., and Huber, J., 1988, The thymus in the acquired immune deficiency syndrome, in: *Thymus Update 1: The Microenvironment of the Human Thymus* (M. D. Kendall and M. A. Ritter, eds.), Harwood Academic Publishers, Chur, Switzerland, pp. 171–189.

Scott-Algara, D., Vuillier, F., Cayota A., and Dighiero, G., 1992, Natural killer (NK) cell activity during HIV infection: A decrease in NK activity is observed at the clonal level and is not restored after in vitro long-term culture of NK cells, *Clin. Exp. Immunol.* **90:**181–187.

Seemayer, T. A., Laroche, A. C., Russo, P., Malebranche, R., Arnoux, E., Guerin, J.-M., Pierre, G., Dupuy, J. M., Gartner, J. G., Lapp, W. S., Spira, T. J., and Elie, R., 1984, Precocious thymic involution manifest by epithelial injury in the acquired immunodeficiency syndrome, *Hum. Pathol.* **15:**469–474.

Silvestris, F., Gernone, A., Frassanito, M. A., and Dammacco, F., 1989, Immunologic effects of long-term thymopentin treatment in patients with HIV-induced lymphadenopathy syndrome, *J. Lab. Clin. Med.* **113:** 139–144.

Sirianni, M. C., Tagliaferri, F., and Aiuti, F., 1990, Pathogenesis of the natural killer cell deficiency in AIDS, *Immunol. Today* **11:**81–82.

Sohn, C. C., Sheibani, K., Winberg, C. D., and Rappaport, H., 1985, Monocytoid B lymphocytes: Their relation to the patterns of the acquired immunodeficiency syndrome (AIDS) and AIDS-related lymphadenopathy, *Hum. Pathol.* **16:**979–985.

Spiegel, H., Herbst, H., Niedobitek, G., Foss, H. D., and Stein, H., 1992, Follicular dendritic cells are a major reservoir for human immunodeficiency virus type 1 in lymphoid tissues facilitating infection of CD4+ T helper cells, *Am. J. Pathol.* **140:**15–22.

Stanley, M. W., and Frizzera, G., 1986, Diagnostic specificity of histologic features in lymph node biopsy specimens from patients at risk for the acquired immunodeficiency syndrome, *Hum. Pathol.* **17:**1231–1239.

Stanley, S. K., McCune, J. M., Kaneshima, H., Justement, J. S., Sullivan, M., Boone, E., Baseler, M., Adelsberger, J., Bonyhadi, M., Orenstein, J., Fox, C. H., and Fauci, A. S., 1993, Human immunodeficiency virus infection of the human thymus and disruption of the thymic microenvironment in the SCID-hu mouse, *J. Exp. Med.* **178:**1151–1163.

Stein, H., Bork, A., Tolksdorf, G., Lennert, K., Rodt, H., and Gerdes, J., 1980, Immunohistologic analysis of the organization of normal lymphoid tissue and non-Hodgkin's lymphomas, *J. Histochem. Cytochem.* **28:**746–760.

Steinman, R. M., 1991, The dendritic cell system and its role in immunogenicity, *Annu. Rev. Immunol.* **9:**271–296.

Steinman, R. M., Witmer-Pack, M., and Inaba, K., 1993, Dendritic cells: Antigen presentation, accessory function and clinical relevance, *Adv. Exp. Med. Biol.* **329:**1–9.

Steinmann, G. G., 1986, Changes in human thymus during aging, *Curr. Top. Pathol.* **75:**43–88.

Stevens, S. K., Weismann, I. L., and Butcher, E. C., 1982, Differences in the migration of T and B lymphocytes: Organ-selective localization in vivo and the role of lymphocyte–endothelial cell recognition, *J. Immunol.* **128:**844–851.

Stutman, O., 1978, Intrathymic and extrathymic T cell maturation, *Immunol. Rev.* **42:**138–184.

Suster, S., and Rosai, J., 1992, Thymus, in: *Histology for Pathologists* (S. S. Sternberg, ed.), Raven Press, New York, pp. 261–277.

Tanaka, K. E., Hatch, W. C., Kress, Y., Soeiro, R., Calvelli, T., Rashbaum, W., Rubinstein, A., and Lyman, W. D., 1992, HIV-1 infection of human fetal thymocytes, *J. Acq. Immune Defic. Syndr.* **5:**94–101.

Tenner-Racz, K., Racz, P., Dietrich, M., and Karin, P., 1985, Altered dendritic follicular cells and virus-like particles in AIDS and AIDS related lymphadenopathy, *Lancet* **1:**105–106.

Tenner-Racz, K., Racz, P., Bofill, M., Sculz-Meyer, A., Dietrich, M., Kern, P., Weber, J., Pinching, A. J., Veronese-Dimarzo, F., Popovic, M., Klatzmann, D., Gluckman, J. C., and Janossy, G., 1986, HTLV-III/LAV viral antigens in lymph nodes of homosexual men with persistent generalized lymphadenopathy and AIDS, *Am. J. Pathol.* **123:**9–15.

Tew, J. G., Kosco, M. H., Burton, G. F., and Szakal, A. K., 1990, Follicular dendritic cells as accessory cells, *Immunol. Rev.* **117:**185–211.

Tremblay, M., Numazaki, K., Goldman, H., and Wainberg, M. A., 1990, Infection of human thymic lymphocytes by HIV-1, *J. Acq. Immune Defic. Syndr.* **3:**356–360.

Trowbridge, I. S., and Thomas, M. L., 1994, CD45: An emerging role as a protein tyrosine phosphatase required for lymphocyte activation and development, *Annu. Rev. Immunol.* **12:**85–116.

Uccini, S., Monardo, F., Vitolo, D., Faggioni, A., Gradilone, A., Agliano, A. M., Manzari, V., Ruco, L. P., and Baroni, C. D., 1989, Human immunodeficiency virus (HIV) and Epstein–Barr virus (EBV) antigens and genome in lymph nodes of HIV-positive patients affected by persistent generalized lymphadenopathy, *Am. J. Clin. Pathol.* **92:**729–735.

Valentin, H., Nugeyre, M.-T., Vuillier, F., Boumsell, L., Schmid, M., Barre-Sinoussi, F., and Pereira, R., 1994, Two subpopulations of human triple-negative thymic cells are susceptible to infection by human immunodeficiency virus type 1 in vitro, *J. Virol.* **68:**3041–3050.

Valesini, G., Barnaba, V., Benvenuto, R., Balsano, F., Mazzanti, P., and Cazzola, P., 1987, A calf thymus acid lysate improves clinical symptoms and T-cell defects in the early stages of HIV infection: Second report, *Eur. J. Cancer Clin. Oncol.* **23:**1915–1919.

van der Oord, J. J., de Wolf-Peeters, C., and Desmet, V. J., 1986, The marginal zone of the human reactive lymph node, *Am. J. Clin. Pathol.* **86:**475–479.

van der Valk, P., and Meijer, C. J. L. M., 1992, Reactive lymph nodes, in: *Histology for Pathologists* (S. S. Sternberg, ed.), Raven Press, New York, pp. 233–251.

van der Valk, P., van der Loo, E. M., Jansen, J., Daha, M. R., and Meijer, C. J. L. M., 1984, Analysis of lymphoid and dendritic cells in human lymph node, tonsil, and spleen. A study using monoclonal and heterologous antibodies, *Virchow Arch. B* **45:**169–185.

van Ewijk, W., Shores, E. W., and Singer, A., 1994, Crosstalk in the mouse thymus, *Immunol. Today* **15:**214–217.

Vellutini, C., Horschowski, N., Philippon, V., Gambarelli, D., Nave, K. A., and Filippi, P., 1995, Development of lymphoid hyperplasia in transgenic mice expressing the HIV tat gene, *AIDS Res. Hum. Retrovir.* **11:**21–29.

von Boehmer, H., Teh, H. S., and Kisielow, P., 1989, The thymus selects the useful, neglects the useless and destroys the harmful, *Immunol. Today* **10:**57–61.

Vuillier, F., Bianco, N. E., Montagnier, L., and Dighiero, G., 1988, Selective depletion of low-density $CD8^+$, $CD16^+$ lymphocytes during HIV infection, *AIDS Res. Hum. Retrovir.* **4:**121–129.

Welch, K., Finkbeiner, W., Alpers, C. E., Blumenfield, W., Davis, R. L., Smuckler, E. A., and Beckstead, J. H., 1984, Autopsy findings in the acquired immune deficiency syndrome, *J. Am. Med. Assoc.* **252:**1152–1159.

Westermann, J., Persin, S., Matyas, J., van der Meide, P., and Pabst, R., 1993, IFN-gamma influences the migration of thoracic duct B and T lymphocyte subsets in vivo, *J. Immunol.* **150:**3843–3852.

Wyand, M. S., Ringler, D. J., Naidu, Y. M., Mattmuller, M., Chalifoux, L. V., Sehgal, P. K., Daniel, M. D., Desrosiers, R. C., and King, N. W., 1989, Cellular localization of simian immunodeficiency virus in lymphoid tissues. II. In situ hybridization, *Am. J. Pathol.* **134:**385–393.

CHAPTER 6

EFFECTS OF HIV-1 AND HIV-1 ENVELOPE GLYCOPROTEINS ON SIGNALING PATHWAYS IN HUMAN T LYMPHOCYTES

SUDHIR GUPTA

1. INTRODUCTION

HIV-1 infection is unique with regard to immune responses, in which there is evidence for immune paradox, i.e., both immune activation and immune suppression. Immune stimulation is evident by elevated levels of various cytokines and hyperimmunoglobulinemia, whereas immune suppression is associated with quantitative and qualitative deficiency of T cells, especially of CD4+ T cells (reviewed in Fauci, 1988). It appears that HIV-1 or its envelope glycoproteins (gp160, gp120) can induce these paradoxical changes by various mechanisms, including blocking CD4–major histocompatibility complex (MHC) class II interaction and by altering signal transduction pathway. In this chapter, I will review the role of HIV-1 and its glycoproteins in activation and downregulation of signaling pathways in human T cells.

2. SIGNALING PATHWAYS IN T CELLS

Antigen is presented to T cells in the context of the MHC and elicits a response that involves an interaction between T-cell receptor (TCR) and the accessory structures CD4/CD8. However, current evidence suggests that the TCR recognition of antigen bound to MHC is insufficient to induce T-cell clonal expansion or generate effector functions. In order for CD4+ helper T cells to produce significant levels of interleukin 2 (IL-2) to initiate an autocrine-driven T-cell clonal expansion, there is a requirement for "costimulatory" signals provided by an interaction between CD28 on T cells and B7 on antigen-presenting

---

SUDHIR GUPTA • Division of Basic and Clinical Immunology, University of California, Irvine, California 92697.

Immunology of HIV Infection, edited by Sudhir Gupta. Plenum Press, New York, 1996.

cells. The subject of signaling pathways in lymphocytes has been reviewed recently (Rudd *et al.*, 1994; June *et al.*, 1994; Weiss and Littman, 1994; Ledbetter, this volume). I will briefly review the subject as a prelude to changes in signaling pathways following infection with HIV or binding with HIV envelope glycoproteins.

T cells express several src-related protein tyrosine kinases (PTKs), including $p56^{lck}$ and $p59^{fynT}$. The CD4 molecule is associated with $p56^{lck}$, whereas $p59^{fynT}$ interacts with TCRζ chain and CD3 γ, δ, and ε chains through its N-terminus. $p56^{lck}$ appears to play a role in a variety of T-cell functions, including thymocyte differentiation, cytolytic function, CD4 endocytotic trafficking, cytokine production, T-cell apoptosis, and T-cell signaling. $p59^{fynT}$ kinase, in a nonobligatory fashion, is associated with certain T-cell functions, including Ca^{2+} release and T-cell proliferation. T-cell signaling *per se* appears to be only minimally affected by $p59^{fynT}$. Both $p56^{lck}$ and $p59^{fynT}$ kinases are activated by receptor cross-linking resulting in the phosphorylation of various targets. CD4 $p56^{lck}$ phosphorylates the TCRζ chain. TCRζ chain phosphorylation can be induced by cross-linking of TCR and CD4 coreceptor stimulation. The phosphorylation of TCRζ chain creates binding sites for the PTK-Zap70, which then phosphorylates downstream substrates such as phospholipase Cγ (PLCγ) and possibly mitogen-activated kinases (MAP-2 kinase). Phosphorylated TCRζ also binds to the intracellular SH2 domain containing (SHC) adaptor protein. SHC protein activates $p21^{ras}$ by means of intermediate Grb-2 and a guanine nucleotide releasing protein (mSos). PLCγ catalyzes the hydrolysis of phosphoinositide 4,5-diphosphate (PIP_2) to generate inositol 1,4,5-trisphosphate (IP_3) and diacylglycerol (DAG), thereby mobilizing intracellular Ca^{2+} and stimulation of protein kinase C (PKC). These events lead to a cascade of events resulting in the activation of nuclear transcription factors necessary for initiating transcription of cytokine genes (especially the IL-2 gene).

Recently it has been shown that other intracellular proteins may also be recruited to the TCR/CD3–CD4 complex in a tyrosine phosphorylation-independent fashion providing a potentially distinct signaling pathway from the TCR/CD3–$p59^{fynT}$ and CD4 $p56^{lck}$ complexes. The SH3 domain of $p56^{lck}$ and $p59^{fynT}$ binds the lipid kinase PI 3 kinase. PI 3 kinase can act on PI, PIP and PIP_2 phosphate to generate PI_3. CD4 $p56^{lck}$ also associates with PI 4 kinase which also takes part in PI turnover. The proximity of PI 4 kinase with PLCγ could facilitate the generation of PI_3 and DAG.

The stimulation of resting T cells with CD28 alone does not result in significant T-cell activation; however, CD28 stimulation in conjunction with TCR stimulation produces dramatic augmentation of T-cell responses, including cytokine production. Therefore, it is clear that the B7–CD28 interactions provide secondary "costimulatory" signal to T cells. B7.1 was recently designated as CD80. The cytoplasmic domain of B7 isoform (7.2) contains three potential sites for phosphorylation by PKC. It is also possible that the cytoplasmic domain of B7.2 has a function in signal transduction. The hallmark of CD28-mediated signal transduction is the production of cytokines, including IL-2, that are resistant to cyclosporin A (CSA). Two signal pathways are coupled to CD28, one that is dominant in activated T cells and is CSA sensitive, and another that occurs in naive T cells and is CSA resistant. In activated T cells, interaction between high-affinity B7 family ligands and CD28 receptor results in phosphorylation of residues in the CD28 motif by a PTK. PI 3 kinase binds to the site and initiates signal via tyrosine phosphorylation of PLCγ1. In naive T cells, possible interaction between low-affinity B7 ligands and CD28 results in signaling that is CSA resistant. In summary, the effects of ligation of CD28 receptor on early signaling events (either by cross-linking or ligation with B7) include: (1) increased tyrosine phosphorylation of cellular substrates in activated T cells, (2) PLCγ phosphorylation in activated T cells, (3) increased intracellular Ca^{2+} in T-cell lines but not in resting T cells, (4) lack of synergy with TCR in increasing intracellular Ca^{2+}, (5) association of CD28 with p85α subunit of PI 3 kinases and appearance of IP_3 metabolites in T-cell lines, (6) activation of raf-1 kinase activity (along with TCR and CD4 cross-linking) in resting T cells, and (7) increased intracellular cGMP.

3. INTERACTION BETWEEN HIV-1 AND CD4

CD4 serves as a major receptor for HIV-1. Interaction of HIV-1 (or gp160/120) with the CD4 molecule results in immune activation, immune suppression, syncytium formation, and priming for apoptosis (Shalaby *et al.*, 1987; Mann *et al.*, 1987; Chirmule *et al.*, 1988, 1990; Diamond *et al.*, 1988; Weinhold *et al.*, 1989; Yoshida *et al.*, 1992; Banda *et al.*, 1992). A number of experimental strategies, including random and site-directed mutagenesis studies performed on membrane or soluble CD4 molecules, have led to mapping of the HIV-1 gp120 high-affinity primary binding site to a region encompassing amino acid residues 39–59 within the first NH_2-terminal domain D1 of CD4. The crystal structure of the first two domains (D1, D2) on recombinant CD4 molecules has shown that these residues belong to a protruding region constituted by strands C′, C″, D, and corresponding loops (Ryu *et al.*, 1990; Wang *et al.*, 1990). Recently, it has been demonstrated that CD4 appears to interact with MHC class II molecules primarily through the HIV gp120 binding site and possibly through a second minor interaction site mapped on the same face of the molecule (Houlgatte *et al.*, 1994). The carbohydrate residues of gp120 contribute significantly to the affinity of the gp120–CD4 interaction.

4. PHOSPHORYLATION OF CD4

There are conflicting reports on the role of CD4 phosphorylation in HIV infection. Fields *et al.* (1988) demonstrated that binding of HIV-1 to CD4 induces PKC-dependent phosphorylation of the CD4 molecule in peripheral blood T cells and $CD4^+$ T-cell line. In contrast, Hoxie *et al.* (1988) were unable to demonstrate phosphorylation of CD4 in peripheral blood T cells and T-cell line, using purified gp120. A possible explanation for this discrepancy may be that an additional interaction between intact virus (in addition to gp120) and CD4 molecule is necessary for phosphorylation of CD4. Gaulton *et al.* (1992), using uninfected and chronically infected cell lines, showed that (1) at the basal level, there was no detectable phosphorylation of CD4 in uninfected or HIV-1-infected cell lines and (2) no or minimal phosphorylation of CD4 was induced by anti-CD3 monoclonal antibody, although normal CD4 phosphorylation was observed with the PKC activator PDBu (phorbol 12,13-dibutyrate). This would suggest that TCR/CD3-mediated CD4 phosphorylation is via non-PKC kinase, or else different PKC isozymes may be involved in TCR/CD3 activation as compared to those in phorbol ester activation (perhaps most of the isoforms are activated). Phorbol diester directs PKC-dependent phosphorylation of all three cytoplasmic serine residues on the CD4 molecule (Shin *et al.*, 1990). The sites for anti-CD3-induced serine phosphorylation on CD4 have not been mapped. Therefore, it is also possible that alterations in the availability of specific serine residues within CD4 to CD3-induced phosphorylation of HIV-infected cells may be involved.

In the following discussion the effect of interactions between HIV-1 or gp160/120 and CD4 on T lymphocytes will be discussed on upstream signal pathway (e.g., protein tyrosine kinase, inositol phosphate metabolism, and intracellular calcium) and downstream signaling pathway (PKC, nuclear transcription factors, and cytokine genes).

5. EFFECTS OF HIV-1/gp160/gp120 ON PROTEIN TYROSINE KINASES

CD4 is physically associated with protein tyrosine kinase (PTK), the $p56^{lck}$. Protein $p56^{lck}$ is encoded by the *lck* proto-oncogene. $p56^{lck}$ is highly phosphorylated *in vivo* on a tyrosine residue (Tyr-505). However, phosphorylation of Tyr-505 is not mediated by $p56^{lck}$ by itself; autophosphorylation of $p56^{lck}$ occurs on Tyr-384. It has been observed that the cross-linking of CD4 increases the activity of $p56^{lck}$ and the activators of PKC cause dissociation of CD4 and $p56^{lck}$. This would suggest that the $p56^{lck}$ can be affected by modulation of the CD4 molecule. Since HIV-1/gp160/120 binds to CD4 and downregulates CD4 expression, a number of investigators have examined the effect of gp160/gp120 or peptides derived from gp120 sequences on $p56^{lck}$. There are conflicting reports on the ability of HIV-1/gp160/gp120 to activate CD4-associated $p56^{lck}$. Horak *et al.* (1990) showed that neither HIV-1 nor gp120 activated $p56^{lck}$ in an alloreactive IL-2-dependent T-cell clone, and both failed to alter the composition of cellular phosphotyrosine-containing proteins. Kaufmann *et al.* (1992) also failed to demonstrate activation of $p56^{lck}$ by gp120. In contrast, Juszczac *et al.* (1991) observed that gp120 induced a rapid increase in CD4-associated $p56^{lck}$ tyrosine kinase activity and autophosphorylation of $p56^{lck}$ in the CEM T-cell line. This effect was greater when gp120–CD4 was cross-linked by anti-gp120. Furthermore, they showed that long-term exposure of cells to gp120 resulted in almost complete dissociation of $p56^{lck}$ from CD4 and downregulation of surface CD4. The $p56^{lck}$ dissociation preceded the downregulation of CD4. Soula *et al.* (1992) also observed a rapid activation of $p56^{lck}$ kinase activity and autophosphorylation following binding of HIV-1 gp160 with CD4 on Jurkat T cells. Cefai *et al.* (1992) observed that the prolonged exposure of P28D $CD4^+$ T-cell clones to HIV-1 gp120 resulted in cointernalization of gp120 and CD4 with a concomitant loss of surface CD4, alteration in the steady-state levels of CD4 mRNA, and loss of CD4-associated $p56^{lck}$. These events were associated with depressed response of T-cell clone to antigen and anti-CD3 monoclonal antibody. Furthermore, the removal of exogenous gp120 resulted in the release of internalized gp120 in degraded form and restoration of CD4 and $p56^{lck}$. These changes were associated with restoration of CD3/TCR-mediated responses. These data suggest that downregulation of CD4 and CD4-associated $p56^{lck}$ is involved in gp120- or HIV-1-mediated inhibition of CD3/TCR-mediated activation of T cells. Cohen *et al.* (1992) have reported induction of tyrosine phosphorylation of several proteins (135-, 95-, 50- to 60-, and 30-kDa substrates) in Jurkat T cells cocultured with a cell line expressing gp120 and gp41. Hivroz *et al.* (1993) studied PTK activity of $p56^{lck}$ in the HUT78 T-cell line and resting T cells following CD4 binding of gp160/120 and derived peptides mimicking CD4 binding sites, amino acid residues 418 to 459. They showed that gp160/120 induces a rapid rise in the catalytic activity of $p56^{lck}$ as evidenced by both enhanced autophosphorylation of $p56^{lck}$ and phosphorylation of an exogenous substrate. They demonstrated phosphorylation of tyrosine residues on 35-, 60-, 70-, and 120-kDa proteins. These changes were amplified by cross-linking of gp120. The enhanced activity preceded CD4/$p56^{lck}$ dissociation. Activation was dependent on CD4 association with $p56^{lck}$, since gp120 failed to induce $p56^{lck}$ activation in $CD8^+$ T cells and HUT78 T cells expressing mutated or truncated form of CD4 unable to associate with $p56^{lck}$. Furthermore, they showed that synthetic peptides derived from gp120 sequences (encompassing residues 418 to 459 found to be involved in binding to CD4) also increased $p56^{lck}$ activity. Their findings suggested that $p56^{lck}$ activation by gp120 probably does not require CD4 cross-linking and the resulting pattern of cell protein phosphorylation on tyrosine residues is distinct from that induced by CD4 cross-linking. Goldman *et al.* (1994) have demonstrated that gp120 ligation of CD4 in HPB cells activates the CD4-associated tyrosine kinase $p56^{lck}$ and inactivates TCR function by uncoupling the receptor from early signaling events, i.e., protein tyrosine phosphorylation and intracellular calcium mobilization. They observed that the degree of tyrosine phosphorylation was more pronounced with gp120 and anti-gp120 as compared to cross-linking of CD4 with anti-CD4 antibody. They also showed that TCRζ chain phosphorylation was not a necessary step in gp120-induced TCR desensitization in the T-cell line tested. It appears that the TCR signaling defect induced by CD4 ligation with gp120 and anti-gp120 involves uncoupling from PTK activation and negative signal is not related to downregulation of CD3. According to these investigators, the possible mechanisms involve either $p56^{lck}$ sequestration or inactivation of the $p56^{lck}$ required for TCR function. The protein tyrosine phosphorylation following stimulation with anti-CD3 and anti-CD28 has also been studied in purified $CD4^+$ T cells from 25 asymptomatic patients with HIV-1 infection (Cayota *et al.*, 1994). A defective tyrosine phosphorylation was observed following stimulation with immobilized anti-CD3 monoclonal antibody. This defect was observed primarily in patients who demonstrated poor proliferative response to anti-CD3, and was associated with increased levels of $p59^{fyn}$ and decreased cellular levels of $p56^{lck}$. These investigators also studied the role of CD28 as a "costimulatory" signal. Anti-CD28 augmented the proliferative response of anti-CD3 in CD4 cells from patients; however, it failed to correct the tyrosine phosphorylation defect in HIV-infected patients. These data would suggest a role of $p59^{fyn}$ and $p56^{lck}$ in hyporesponsiveness of T cells in early stages of HIV infection.

6. EFFECTS OF HIV-1/gp160/gp120 ON PI KINASES, INTRACELLULAR CALCIUM, AND INOSITOL PHOSPHATE METABOLISM

Prasad *et al.* (1993) examined the effect of HIV on PI 4 kinase activity. As with the PI 3 kinases, the cross-linking of CD4 receptor, either by antibody or by HIVgp120, induces an increase in CD4 precipitable PI 4 kinase activity.

Several investigators have examined the effects of HIV-1, gp160, or gp120 on intracellular calcium and inositol phosphate metabolism. Gupta and Vayuvegula (1987) were the first to demonstrate that chronic infection of the $CD4^+$ T-cell line H9 with HIV-1 was associated with increased levels of intracellular calcium and depolarization of plasma membrane, suggesting a state of activation. Furthermore, they demonstrated that these HIV-1-infected cells were no longer responsive to signaling by anti-CD3 monoclonal antibody or phytohemagglutinin (PHA) as determined by rise in intracellular calcium, whereas uninfected cells responded to these stimuli normally. Nye and Pinching (1990) also reported that chronically HIV-1-infected H9 cells show increased levels of intracellular calcium, IP_3 and IP_4. *In vitro* activation of these cells with PHA resulted in reduction in previously elevated IP3, whereas an attenuated intracellular calcium rise was observed with PHA and anti-CD3 monoclonal antibodies. Kornfeld *et al.* (1988) also showed that binding of gp120 to the CD4 surface protein of resting uninfected T cells activates the IP_3 and calcium signal pathway. In addition, they observed an associated increase in the expression of IL-2 receptor (IL-2R). Neudorf *et al.* (1990) also observed that the binding of gp120 with CD4 resulted in increased intracellular calcium mobilization. In contrast, Mittler and Hoffman (1989) and Horak *et al.* (1990) failed to observe any changes in intracellular calcium or expression of IL-2R and transferrin receptor following binding or cross-linking of gp120 to CD4. Kaufmann *et al.* (1992), using purified gp120 from HIV-1-infected cells and recombinant gp120, did not observe any significant changes in inositol phosphate metabolism, intracellular calcium, or PKC translocation. Orloff *et al.* (1991) also reported that the binding of HIV-1 to $CD4^+$ T cells does not induce calcium influx or lead to activation of PKC.

In contrast to direct activation of T cells by HIV-1 and its envelope glycoproteins, interaction and binding of HIV-1 or gp120/gp160 to CD4 leads to inhibition of signaling of CD4 T cells via TCR/CD3 complex or CD4. Goldman *et al.* (1994) have shown that pretreatment of $CD4^+$ T cells with gp120 leads to decreased rise of intracellular calcium following stimulation with anti-CD4 antibody. This inhibitory effect was not related to downregulation of cell surface CD3 expression. Linette *et al.* (1988) showed that normal T cells infected *in vitro* with HIV-1 failed to demonstrate intracellular calcium mobilization and lymphocyte proliferation following activation with anti-CD3 antibody. However, HIV-1-infected T cells responded to anti-CD2 stimulation by increased intracellular calcium mobilization. Cefai *et al.* (1990) reported similar results. They demonstrated that both HIV-1 gp160 and gp120 specifically inhibited phosphoinositide transduction pathway, intracellular calcium mobilization, changes in intracellular pH, and lymphocyte proliferation, when stimulated with anti-CD3 or anti-TCR α/β monoclonal antibody. In contrast, no inhibitory effect was observed on any of these parameters when cells were stimulated with anti-CD2 antibody. These investigators did not observe any downregulation of CD3/TCR or CD2 expression. Nye *et al.* (1992) demonstrated that lymphocytes from HIV-1-infected individuals with progressive disease failed to convert IP_4 to IP_3, the inositol 1,3,4,5-tetrakisphosphate 5 phosphomonoesterase (PME) activity being the first affected, while activity of 3-phosphomonoesterase remains until the advanced stage of disease. Accumulation of IP_4 interferes with calcium homeostasis. Gupta (1993) also reported that lymphocytes from patients with progressive HIV disease failed to normalize T-cell responses (proliferation and IL-2R expression) on activation with PMA and calcium ionophore, suggesting a defect in downstream signaling pathway. Jabado *et al.* (1994) also demonstrated that gp120 inhibits T-cell proliferation induced by PMA. Therefore, it appears that the inhibition by gp120 cross-linking of CD4 is at least in part related to a negative signal downregulation. These results are consistent with earlier observations of Oyaizu *et al.* (1990) who reported inhibition of IL-2 mRNA by HIV-1 gp120. Corado *et al.* (1991) demonstrated that HIV-1 gp160 and synthetic peptides derived from gp160 sequence and analogous to the putative binding site of gp160 to CD4 (residues 418–460) inhibited adhesion between $CD4^+$ T and B cells. The authors proposed several mechanisms; however, they suggested that this inhibitory effect is mediated by negative signaling through CD4.

7. EFFECTS OF HIV-1/gp160/gp120 ON PROTEIN KINASE C

Gupta *et al.* (1994) have shown that recombinant gp120 induces activation of both calcium-dependent (PKCα,β) and calcium-independent PKC isoforms (PKCδ,ε,ζ). Zorn *et al.* (1990) demonstrated that HIV-1 gp120 activates nuclear PKC from splenic lymphocytes and rat hippocampus. Vasoactive intestinal peptide (VIP), which has considerable sequence homology with gp120, was also found to activate PKC in similar systems. Zauli *et al.* (1994) reported increased PKC activity in hematopoietic progenitor-like cells (TF-1) following engagement of CD4 by HIV-1. In contrast, Kaufmann *et al.* (1992), using purified gp120, and Orloff *et al.* (1991), using HIV-1, did not observe any translocation or activation of PKC in T cells. The reasons for these discrepancies are not apparent. However, the data on HIV-1- or gp160/120-induced PKC-dependent phosphorylation of CD4 would support the observations that the binding of CD4 to HIV-1 or its envelope protein apparently leads to PKC activation.

8. EFFECTS OF HIV-1/gp160/gp120 ON NUCLEAR TRANSCRIPTION FACTORS

Chirmule *et al.* (1994) demonstrated that HIV-1 gp160–CD4 interaction in T cells and T-cell lines resulted in the activation of NF-κB complex consisting of p^{56}, p^{50}, and *c-rel* proteins. Furthermore, gp160-induced activation of NF-κB (transcription factor for cytokines, including IL-2) was abrogated by PKC inhibitors, suggesting a role of PKC in gp160-induced activation of NK-κB. These investigators (Chirmule *et al.*, 1995) also showed that gp160 induces an activation of AP-1 (activated protein-1, another transcription factor for IL-2) that was dependent on tyrosine phosphorylation. The stimulatory effects of gp160 were mediated through the CD4 molecule. Furthermore, they showed that AP-1 complex was comprised of Fos and Jun proteins. The treatment of T cells with gp160 resulted in inhibition of anti-CD3-induced IL-2 secretion. Jabado *et al.* (1994) examined the effect of gp120 on binding activity of nuclear transcriptional factors (NF-κB, AP-1, and NF-AT) involved in IL-2 gene transcription. They observed that ligation of peripheral blood $CD4^{+}$ T cells with gp120 specifically inhibited the binding activity of all three nuclear factors induced by T-cell activation with anti-CD3 + PKC activator and calcium ionophore + PKC activator. Since $p21^{ras}$-mediated cascade of events may form a common pathway for the regulation of these transcription factors, an inhibitory effect of CD4 ligation with HIV on $p21^{ras}$ could explain this inhibitory effect on the binding activity of nuclear transcription factors. Consistent with these findings are the observations of Oyaizu *et al.* (1990) who showed that HIV-1 gp120 inhibits the IL-2 gene but has no effect on IL-2 gene transcription.

9. CONCLUSION

In summary, it appears that the interaction of HIV-1 or its envelope glycoproteins (gp120 and gp160) leads to initial activation of both up- and downstream signaling pathways, followed by changes that lead to defective response to stimulation by mitogens or antigens via TCR. There is much controversy with regard to the stimulatory effect of HIV/gp160/120 on signal transduction, whereas its negative effect on signal transduction is better established. Some of these events are observed *in vivo* as well. The inhibitory effects of HIV-1/HIV-1gp160/120 are not related to downregulation of cell surface CD3 or phosphorylation of TCRζ chain, and appear to involve uncoupling of CD4 from protein tyrosine kinase activation. The precise mechanisms for some of these paradoxical effects of HIV-1 gp160/120 interactions remain to be elucidated. The role of loss of calcium homeostasis in HIV infection should be further explored with regard to its inhibitory effect on signal transduction. The influence of HIV-1/gp160/gp120 on other downstream signaling components (i.e., $p21^{ras}$, MAP-2 kinases) remains to be studied. Several other proteins (in addition to gp160/120) may also be involved in abnormalities of signal transduction pathways in HIV. These include Nef and Tat regulatory proteins. The role of these proteins in signal transduction (positive or negative) in T lymphocytes remains to be explored. Furthermore, HIV-1 gp41 appears to play a regulatory role in the function of T cells (Schwartz *et al.*, this volume). The effects of gp41 on signal transduction remain to be investigated. B lymphocytes from patients with HIV display poor proliferative response and specific antibody responses. However, signaling pathways have not been explored in humans. Recently, Selvey *et al.* (1995), studying mice with a retrovirus-induced AIDS (MAIDS), have observed defects in calcium influx, tyrosine phosphorylation of Ig-α, Ig-β, and undefined protein of 80 kDa, following cross-linking of surface IgM with anti-IgM. Furthermore, they failed to detect a number of other tyrosine phosphorylation events (PI 3 kinase, *syk* kinase, phosphorylation of GTPase-activating protein) in MAIDS B cells. The effects of HIV-1 and gp160/gp120 on signaling pathways in human macrophages and B lymphocytes need to be explored.

REFERENCES

Banda, N. K., Bernier, J., Kurahara, D. K., Kurrle, R., Haigwood, N., Sekaly, R.-P., and Finkel, T. H., 1992, Crosslinking CD4 by human immunodeficiency virus gp120 primes T cells for activation-induced apoptosis, *J. Exp. Med.* **176:**1099–1106.

Cayota, A. F., Vuiller, F., Siliciano, J., and Dighiero, G., 1994, Defective protein tyrosine phosphorylation and altered levels of $p59^{fyn}$ and $p56^{lck}$ in CD4 T cells from HIV-1-infected patients, *Int. Immunol.* **6:**611–621.

Cefai, D., Debre, P., Kaczorek, M., Idziorek, T., Autran, B., and Bismuth, G., 1990, Human immunodeficiency virus 1 glycoprotein gp120 and gp160 specifically inhibit the CD3/T cell antigen receptor phosphoinositol pathway, *J. Clin. Invest.* **86:**2117–2124.

Cefai, D., Ferrer, M., Serpente, N., Idziorek, T., Dautry-Varsat, A., Debre, P., and Bismuth, G., 1992, Internalization of HIV glycoprotein gp120 is associated with down-modulation of membrane CD4 $p56^{lck}$, *J. Immunol.* **149:**285–294.

Chirmule, N., Kalyanaraman, V., Oyaizu, N., and Pahwa, S., 1988, Inhibitory influences of envelope glycoproteins of HIV-1 on normal immune responses, *J. AIDS* **1:**425–430.

Chirmule, N., Kalyanaraman, V. S., Oyaizu, N., Slade, H. B., and Pahwa, S., 1990, Inhibition of functional properties of tetanus antigen-specific T-cell clones by envelope glycoprotein 120 of human immunodeficiency virus, *Blood* **75:**152–159.

Chirmule, N., Kalyanaraman, V. S., and Pahwa, S., 1994, Signal transduced through the CD4 molecule on T lymphocytes activate NF-kB, *Biochem. Biophys. Res. Commun.* **203:**498–505.

Chirmule, N., Goonewardena, H., Pahwa, S., Pasieka, R., Kalyanaraman, V. S., and Pahwa, S., 1995, HIV-1 envelope glycoproteins induce activation of activated protein-1 in CD4+ T cells, *J. Biol. Chem.* **270:**19364–19369.

Cohen, D. I., Tani, Y., Tian, H., Boone, E., Samelson, L. E., and Lane, H. C., 1992, Participation of tyrosine phosphorylation in the cytopathic effect of human immunodeficiency virus-1, *Science* **256:**542–545.

Corado, J., Mazerolles, F., LeDeist, F., Barbat, C., Kaczorek, M., and Fischer, A., 1991, Inhibition of CD4+ T cell activation and adhesion by peptides derived from the gp160, *J. Immunol.* **147:**475–482.

Diamond, D. C., Sleckman, B. P., Gregory, T., Lasky, L. A., Greenstein, J. L., and Burakoff, S. J., 1988, Inhibition of CD(+) T cell function by the HIV envelope protein gp120, *J. Immunol.* **141:**3715–3717.

Fauci, A. S., 1988, The human immunodeficiency virus: Infectivity and mechanisms of pathogenesis, *Science* **239:**617–623.

Fields, A. P., Bednarik, D. P., Hess, A., and May, W. S., 1988, Human immunodeficiency virus induces phosphorylation of its cell surface receptor, *Nature* **333:**278–280.

Gaulton, G. N., Brass, L. F., Kozbor, D., Pletcher, C. H., and Hoxie, J. A., 1992, Inhibition of T cell antigen receptor-dependent phosphorylation of CD4 in human immunodeficiency virus type 1 infected cells, *J. Biol. Chem.* **267:**4102–4109.

Goldman, F., Jensen, W. A., Johnson, G. L., Heasley, L., and Cambier, J. C., 1994, gp120 ligation of CD4 induces $p56^{lck}$ activation and TCR desensitization independent of TCR tyrosine phosphorylation, *J. Immunol.* **153:**2905–2917.

Gupta, S., 1993, Signal transduction defect in the acquired immunodeficiency syndrome and AIDS-related complex, *Thymus* **22:**83–90.

Gupta, S., and Vayuvegula, B., 1987, Human immunodeficiency virus-associated changes in signal transduction, *J. Clin. Immunol.* **7:**486–489.

Gupta, S., Aggarwal, S., Kim, C., and Gollapudi, S., 1994, Human immunodeficiency virus-1 gp120 induces changes in protein kinase C isozymes—A preliminary report, *Int. J. Immunopharmacol.* **16:**197–204.

Hivroz, C., Mazerolles, F., Soula, M., Fagard, R., Graton, S., Meloche, S., Sekaly, R.-P., and Fischer, A., 1993, Human immunodeficiency virus gp120 and derived peptides activate protein tyrosine kinase $p56^{lck}$ in human CD4 T lymphocytes, *Eur. J. Immunol.* **23:**600–607.

Horak, I. D., Popovic, M., Horak, E. M., Lucas, P. J., Gress, R. E., June, C. H., and Bolen, J. B., 1990, No T-cell tyrosine protein kinase signalling or calcium mobilization after CD4 association with HIV-1 or HIV-1 gp120, *Nature* **348:**557–560.

Houlgatte, R., Scarmato, P., Marhomy, S. E., Martin, M., Ostankovitch, M., Lafosse, S., Vervisch, A., Auffray, C., and Tonneau, D. P., 1994, MHC class II antigens and the HIV envelope glycoprotein gp120 bind to the same face of CD4, *J. Immunol.* **152:**4475–4488.

Hoxie, J. A., Rackowski, J. L., Haggarty, B. S., and Gaulton, G. N., 1988, T4 endocytosis and phosphorylation induced by phorbol esters but not not by mitogen or HIV infection, *J. Immunol.* **140:**786–795.

Jabado, N., LeDeist, F., Fischer, A., and Hivroz, C., 1994, Interaction of HIV gp120 and anti-CD4 antibodies with CD4 molecule on human CD4+ T cells inhibits the binding activity of NFAT, NF-kB and AP-1, three nuclear factors regulating interleukin-2 gene enhancer activity, *Eur. J. Immunol.* **24:**2646–2652.

June, C. H., Bluestone, J. A., Nadler, L. M., and Thompson, C. B., 1994, The B7 and CD28 receptor families, *Immunol. Today* **15:**321–331.

Juszczak, R. J., Turchin, J., Truneh, A., Culp, J., and Kassis, S., 1991, Effect of human immunodeficiency virus gp120 glycoprotein on the association of the protein tyrosine kinase $p56^{lck}$ with the CD4 on human T lymphocytes, *J. Biol. Chem.* **266:**11176–11183.

Kaufmann, R., Laroche, D., Buchner, K., Hucho, F., Rudd, C., Lindschau, P., Ludwig, A., Hoer, E., Oberdisse, E., Kopp, J., Korner, I. J., and Repke, H., 1992, The HIV-1 surface protein gp120 has no effect on transmembrane signal transduction, *J. AIDS* **15:**760–770.

Kornfeld, H., Cruickshank, W. W., Pyle, S., Berman, J. S., and Center, D. M., 1988, Lymphocyte activation by HIV-1 envelope glycoprotein, *Nature* **335:**445–454.

Linette, G. P., Hartzman, R. J., Ledbetter, J. A., and June, C. H., 1988, HIV-1 infected T cells show a selective signaling defect after perturbation of CD3/antigen receptor, *Science* **241:**573–576.

Weiss, A., and Littman, D. R., 1994, Signal transduction by lymphocyte antigen receptors, *Cell* **76:**263–274.

Mann, D., Lasane, F., Popovic, M., Arthur, L. O., Robe, G. W., Blattner, W. A., and Newman, M. J., 1987, HTLV III large envelope glycoprotein (gp120) suppresses PHA-induced lymphocyte blastogenesis, *J. Immunol.* **138:**2640–2644.

Mittler, R. S., and Hoffman, M. K., 1988, Synergism between HIV gp120 and gp120-specific antibody in blocking human T cell activation, *Science* **245:**1380–1382.

Neudorf, S. M. L., Jones, M. M., McCarthy, B. M., Harmony, J. A. K., and Choi, E. M., 1990, The CD4 molecule transmits biochemical information important in the regulation of T lymphocyte activity. *Cell Immunol.* **125:**301–314.

Nye, K. E., and Pinching, A. J., 1990, HIV infection of H9 lymphoblastoid cells chronically activates the inositol polyphosphate pathway, *AIDS* **4:**41–45.

Nye, K. E., Riley, G. A., and Pinching, A. J., 1992, The defect seen in the PI hydrolysis pathway in HIV infected lymphocytes and lymphoblastoid cells is due to inhibition of the 1,4,5 triphosphate, 1,3,4,5 tetrakisphosphate and 5-phosphomonoesterase, *Clin. Exp. Immunol.* **89:**89–93.

Orloff, G. M., Kennedy, M. S., Dawson, C., and McDougal, J. S., 1991, HIV-1 binding to CD4 T cells does not induce a Ca^{++} influx or lead to activation of protein kinases, *AIDS Res. Hum. Retrovir.* **7:**587–593.

Oyaizu, N., Chirmule, N., Kalyanaraman, V. S., Hall, W. W., Good, R. A., and Pahwa, S., 1990, Human immunodeficiency virus type 1 envelope glycoprotein gp120 produces immune defects in CD4+ T lymphocytes by inhibiting interleukin 2 mRNA, *Proc. Natl. Acad. Sci. USA* **87:**2379–2383.

Prasad, K. V. S., Kapeller, R., Janssen, O., Duke-Cohan, J. S., Cantley, L. C., and Rudd, C. E., 1993, Phosphatidylinositol (PI) 3-kinase binding to the CD4–$p56^{lck}$ complex: The $p56^{lck}$ SH3 domain binds to PI 3-kinase but not PI 4-kinase, *Mol. Cell. Biol.* **13:**7708–7717.

Rudd, C. E., Janssen, O., Cai, Y.-C., de Silva, A. J., Raab, M., and Prasad, K. V. S., 1994, Two step TCRζ/CD3-CD4 and CD28 signaling in T cells: SH2/SH3 domains, protein-tyrosine and lipid kinases, *Immunol. Today* **15:** 225–234.

Ryu, S. E., Kwong, P. D., Truneh, A., Porter, T. G., Arthos, J., Rosenberg, M., Dai, X., Xuong, N. H., Axel, R., Sweet, R. W., and Hendrickson, W. A., 1990, Crystal structure of an HIV-binding recombinant fragment of human CD4, *Nature* **348:**419–426.

Selvey, L. A., Morse, H. C., III, June, C. H., and Hodes, R. J., 1995, Analysis of antigen receptor signaling in B cells from mice with retrovirus-induced acquired immunodeficiency syndrome, *J. Immunol.* **154:**171–179.

Shalaby, M. R., Krowka, J. F., Gregory, T. J., Hirabayashi, S. E., McCabe, S. M., Kaufman, D. S., Stites, D. P., and Ammann, A. J., 1987, The effects of human immunodeficiency virus recombinant envelope glycoprotein on immune cell functions in vitro, *Cell Immunol.* **110:**140–148.

Shin, J., Doyle, C., Yang, Z., Kappes, D., Strominger, J. L., 1990, Structural features of the cytoplasmic region of CD4 required for internalization, *EMBO J.* **9:**425–434.

Soula, M., Fagard, R., and Fischer, S., 1992, Interaction of human immunodeficiency virus glycoprotein 160 with CD4 in Jurkat cells increases $p56^{lck}$ autophosphorylation and kinase activity, *Int. Immunol.* **4:**295–299.

Wang, J., Yan, Y., Garrett, T. P. J., Liu, J., Rogers, D. W., Garlick, R. L., Tarr, G. E., Husain, Y., Reinherz, E. L., and Harrison, S. C., 1990, Atomic structure of a fragment of human CD4 containing two immunoglobulin-like-domains, *Nature* **348:**411–418.

Weinhold, K. J., Lyerly, H. K., Stanley, H. D., Austin, A. A., Matthews, T. J., and Bolognesi, D. P., 1989, HIV-1 gp120-mediated immune suppression and lymphocyte destruction in the absence of viral infection, *J. Immunol.* **142:**3091–3097.

Yoshida, H., Kaga, K., Moroi, Y., Kimura, G., and Momoto, K., 1992, The effect of $p56^{lck}$, a lymphocyte-specific protein tyrosine kinase on syncytium formation by HIV envelope glycoprotein, *Int. Immunol.* **4:**233–242.

Zauli, G., Furlini, G., Vitale, M., Re, M. C., Gibellini, D., Zamai, L., and Visani, G., 1994, CD4 engagement by HIV-1 in TF-1 hematopoietic progenitor cells increases protein kinase C activity and reduces intracellular Ca^{++} levels, *Microbiologica* **17:**85–92.

Zorn, N. E., Weill, C. L., and Russell, D. H., 1990, The HIV protein GP120 activates nuclear protein kinase C in nuclei from lymphocytes and brain. *Biochem. Biophys. Res. Commun.* **166:**1133–1139.

CHAPTER 7

LYMPHOCYTE APOPTOSIS IN HIV INFECTION

NAOKI OYAIZU and SAVITA PAHWA

1. INTRODUCTION

Human immunodeficiency virus (HIV-1) is the etiologic agent of acquired immunodeficiency syndrome (AIDS). Our understanding of the complexities of pathogenic mechanisms of HIV disease is still evolving; however, the mechanism whereby HIV-1 infection leads to profound depletion of CD4 T cells remains one of the central unsolved problems in AIDS research. In the past several years, there has been a dichotomy between virological and immunological viewpoints in understanding HIV-mediated cytopathicity, the former emphasizing killing of infected CD4 cells by HIV and the latter emphasizing indirect mechanisms wherein HIV or its soluble component(s) alter CD4 T-cell function and induce susceptibility to apoptosis.

Apoptosis is a morphologically defined process, characterized by the condensation of the nucleus and cytoplasm and a distinctive pattern of chromosomal DNA fragmentation. The designation and concept of apoptosis was introduced in 1972 and it has reemerged, after more than 15 years of dormancy, as one of the most vigorously investigated areas in biology. Demonstration of apoptosis in the immune system, shown at first for immature thymocytes, has subsequently been demonstrated in mature peripheral T lymphocytes as well. With the demonstration that accelerated apoptosis does exist in HIV infection, HIV cytopathicity as well has been reevaluated in the light of apoptosis induction. Two recent provocative studies conducted in HIV-infected patients treated with antiretroviral agents have highlighted the dynamic inverse relationship between plasma virus burden and CD4 T cells (Wei *et al.*, 1995; Ho *et al.*, 1995). Using mathematical models, the authors estimated that 10^9 virions were produced and that 5% of the pool of CD4 T cells was destroyed and replenished daily. Although these studies have been largely interpreted to implicate destruction of productively infected cells *in vivo*, direct evidence of death of infected cells was not provided in

NAOKI OYAIZU and SAVITA PAHWA • Department of Pediatrics, North Shore University Hospital–Cornell University Medical College, Manhasset, New York 11030.

Immunology of HIV Infection, edited by Sudhir Gupta. Plenum Press, New York, 1996.

either study. On the other hand, compelling evidence has recently emerged indicating that uninfected cells, not productively infected cells, preferentially undergo apoptosis (Su *et al.*, 1995a; Finkel *et al.*, 1995). In a recent study of lymph nodes from HIV-infected individuals and from SIV-infected macaques, DNA fragmentation was rarely detected in productively infected cells, whereas HIV RNA was rarely detected in apoptotic cells (Finkel *et al.*, 1995), thereby implicating occurrence of apoptosis predominantly in bystander (uninfected) cells rather than in the productively infected cells themselves.

Thus, even after one and a half decades of intensive studies, the exact mechanisms underlying HIV-mediated cytopathicity are still enigmatic and need closer scrutiny. The immunological and virological viewpoints should eventually reconcile with each other. The purpose of this chapter is to summarize current information about the regulatory mechanisms of T-cell apoptosis and the role of apoptosis in HIV pathogenesis with the goal of providing an integrated view of HIV cytopathicity.

2. HIV-MEDIATED CYTOPATHICITY—VIROLOGIC VIEWPOINT

Earlier studies have suggested that the cytopathic effects of HIV-1 consist of syncytium formation and single-cell lysis. The tropism of HIV-1 for CD4-bearing lymphocytes is related to the high-affinity binding of the viral envelope protein gp120 to its receptor, the CD4 molecule. Following receptor binding, gp120 and gp41 mediate the fusion of viral and host cell membranes and allow virus entry into the target cells. A similar process mediated by the HIV-1 envelope proteins expressed on the surface of productively infected cells leads to fusion of these cells with surrounding $CD4^+$ cells. The resulting syncytia exhibit membrane fragility and eventually die (Lifson *et al.*, 1986; Sodroski *et al.*, 1986). Single-cell lysis, in addition to syncytium formation, has been shown to contribute to the cytopathic effects associated with HIV-1 infection and accounts for the destruction of most HIV-1-infected cells in tissue culture (Somasundaran and Robinson, 1987; Kowalski *et al.*, 1991; Bergeron and Sodroski, 1992). Major mechanisms that have been suggested to explain single-cell lysis include the following: (1) single-cell killing occurs as a consequence of alterations in the lipid composition of host membrane after HIV infection which results in increased membrane permeability (Cloyd and Lynn, 1991); (2) massive viral budding results in cell death by injuring the external cell membrane (Stevenson *et al.*, 1988); and (3) toxic effects of env expression lead to cell death (Koga *et al.*, 1992). However, the precise molecular basis of single-cell lysis has not been elucidated. In addition, cytopathicity has mainly been measured by means of vital dye exclusion tests in these studies and thus involvement of the apoptotic process has not been evaluated. Importantly, single-cell lysis appears to be dependent on target cell CD4 expression (DeRossi *et al.*, 1986). This requirement is supported by the observation that cells expressing very low levels of CD4 emerge following HIV-1 infection and exhibit little or no cytopathic effects despite the production of large amounts of HIV (Kowalski *et al.*, 1991). This observation suggests that budding of the virus does not necessarily cause cell death in the productively infected cells, and HIV cytopathicity may mainly be operative at the time of virus entry. In 1991, several groups demonstrated that acute HIV infection *in vitro* led to lymphocyte death via a mechanism of apoptosis (Terai *et al.*, 1991; Laurent-Crawford *et al.*, 1991) and this was blocked by anti-gp120 antibodies. Later, env gene expression alone was shown to be able to trigger target-cell apoptosis (Laurent-Crawford *et al.*, 1993; Lu *et al.*, 1994). These studies strongly suggested that toxic effects of env could, at least in part, be ascribed to its apoptosis-inducing ability. However, the degree of contribution of env-mediated cytotoxicity via a membrane fusion event and subsequent direct damage of cell membrane versus that of an indirect mechanism via apoptosis induction should be defined more precisely. Whether the cytopathic effect of HIV is initiated on virus entry or is operative during productive infection remains to be defined as well. It should be noted that most of the virological studies have been conducted utilizing transformed lymphoblastoid or monocytoid cell lines. Recent studies have revealed that these cell lines differ from their normal counterparts with respect to their sensitivity for undergoing apoptosis. Some cell lines are extremely sensitive for apoptosis whereas others are fairly resistant (X. Su *et al.*, 1995). Thus, care should be taken in interpreting the data to avoid an over- or underestimation of the role of apoptosis. Finally, all of these studies have been conducted *in vitro* and there is still little evidence of how HIV exerts it cytopathic effect *in vivo.*

3. HIV-MEDIATED CYTOPATHICITY—IMMUNOLOGIC VIEWPOINT

From the immunologic viewpoint, mechanisms postulated to be involved in HIV-mediated cytopathicity include cytotoxic T-lymphocyte (CTL) response, antibody-dependent complement-mediated cytotoxicity (ADCC), HIV-induced autoimmune attack on host immune cells, and T-cell apoptosis. In this chapter, we will focus on the T-cell apoptosis associated with HIV infection.

4. ACTIVATION-INDUCED T-CELL DEATH (AICD) VIA APOPTOSIS

The physiologic cell death during embryogenesis, metamorphosis, endocrine-dependent tissue atrophy, and normal tissue turnover is called *programmed cell death* (PCD) (Kerr *et al.*, 1972; Wyllie *et al.*, 1980). Most of PCD is manifested by apoptosis, a process of cell death characterized by condensation and segmentation of nuclei with extensive fragmentation of chromosomal DNA into nucleosome units. The concept of apoptosis was first introduced in the field of immunology as a mechanism of thymic negative selection, enabling the host to eliminate autoreactive thymocytes (central tolerance). Subsequently, it has been shown that the apoptotic process is operative in the periphery, thereby contributing to the maintenance of constant numbers of lymphocytes and elimination of autoreactive T cells having specificities for antigens that were not presented in the thymus (peripheral tolerance). Homeostasis of multicellular organisms including the immune system is controlled not only by the proliferation and differentiation of cells but also by cell death.

The number of T cells specific for any given antigen is initially small. Activation of T cells on recognition of foreign antigen leads to clonal expansion in order to mount an efficient host immune response against the offending pathogen. Cells that have been repeatedly stimulated with specific antigen undergo apoptosis, probably as a shut-off mechanism to terminate immune response. This process is termed *activation-induced cell death* (Ucker *et al.*, 1989).

5. MOLECULAR REGULATION OF T-CELL APOPTOSIS

As outlined in Fig. 1, two components broadly regulate mammalian cell apoptosis: multiple upstream cell-lineage-specific apoptosis-priming processes, which eventually funnel into a downstream death-specific pathway. Recent evidence indicates that this death-specific process utilizes a functionally common pathway, which is regulated by evolutionarily conserved molecules such as the Bcl-2 family of proteins and proteases of the interleukin-1β converting enzyme (ICE) family. In this section, we will focus our discussion on Fas and its ligand system as a major mechanism to explain AICD in T cells with special reference to cytokine involvement and will refer to current knowledge of death signaling since all of these components are intimately related to HIV pathogenesis.

5.1. Fas Antigen and Its Ligand as Major Components of AICD

Activation-induced cell death was first described in T-cell hybridomas (Ashwell *et al.*, 1987). These cells undergo apoptosis on stimulation with antigens, mitogens, or antibodies for TCR/CD3. Many recent studies point toward the importance of Fas antigen and its interaction with Fas ligand (Fas-L) in the induction of peripheral T-cell apoptosis (Nagata

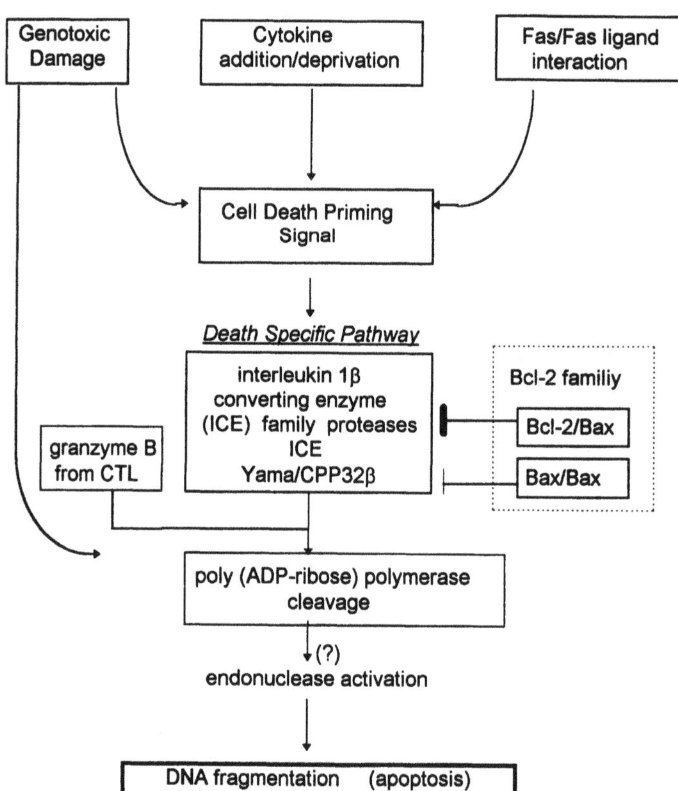

FIGURE 1. Regulation of apoptosis in T lymphocytes. Apoptosis-inducing signals funnel into a death-specific process. Bcl-2 family of proteins operates as an apoptosis-repressor system in this death-specific pathway.

and Goldstein, 1995). Human Fas antigen, designated as CD95, is a 36-kDa type I transmembrane glycoprotein identical to APO-1 and Fas-L is a 40-kDa type II membrane protein. They belong to the nerve growth factor (NGF)/tumor necrosis factor receptor (TNF-R) and TNF family of surface molecules, respectively (Yonehara *et al.*, 1989; Suda *et al.*, 1993). Addition of anti-Fas antibody (which mimics natural Fas-L) results in apoptosis induction in sensitive cells expressing this antigen. While Fas antigen can be expressed in a variety of tissues/cells including activated lymphocytes, the expression of Fas-L appears to be restricted to the T lineage of cells (Suda *et al.*, 1995). Major breakthroughs elucidating the pivotal role of the Fas/Fas-L system in regulating physiologic T-cell apoptosis have come from studies in autoimmune-prone mice. Mice homozygous for *lpr* mutation (*lpr*) and for *gld* mutation (*gld*) both develop massive lymphadenopathy composed of T cells and lupuslike autoimmune syndrome with aging (Cohen and Eisenberg, 1991). The *lpr* mutation affects the structural gene for mouse Fas antigen (Watanabe-Fukunaga *et al.*, 1992a,b) and the *gld* mutation is a point mutation of mouse Fas-L (Takahashi *et al.*, 1994; Lynch *et al.*, 1994). Although the role of Fas/Fas-L interaction in the thymus has not been elucidated completely, negative selection in the thymus is largely normal in these animals; rather, their peripheral T cells have been shown to be resistant to activation-induced apoptosis (Herron *et al.*, 1993; Russell *et al.*, 1993; Singer and Abbas, 1994). Recently, the presence of *lpr*-type Fas gene mutation has been identified in humans (Fisher *et al.*, 1995). Affected individuals show a T-lymphocyte proliferative disorder with various degrees of autoimmune symptoms. These studies implicate the pivotal role of Fas/Fas-L interaction in maintaining consistency of T-cell numbers and self tolerance.

Consistent with this notion is a growing body of evidence suggesting that Fas/Fas-L interaction is a major molecular mechanism regulating physiologic T-cell death. Several groups have recently provided compelling evidence that Fas/Fas-L interaction is critical for activation-induced T-cell death (Cheng *et al.*, 1994; Alderson *et al.*, 1995; Brunner *et al.*, 1995; Dhein *et al.*, 1995; Ju *et al.*, 1995). These studies revealed that autocrine Fas/Fas-L interaction is essential for TCR activation-induced death of alloreactive T-cell clones, T hybridoma cells, transformed Jurkat cells, and nontransformed preactivated T cells. All of these studies show that TCR stimulation induces the expression of Fas and its ligand on these cells and that killing can be inhibited by blocking Fas/Fas-L interaction by the addition of reagents such as soluble Fas decoy molecules. Thus, Fas/Fas-L interaction appears to be critical for activation-induced T-cell death and the maintenance of peripheral tolerance. Fas/Fas-L interaction is involved not only in AICD but also in cytotoxic T-cell-mediated killing (Ju *et al.*, 1994). It has been demonstrated that perforin and granzyme A from $CD8^+$ CTL can induce lysis/apoptosis in target cells as a classical mechanism of CTL activity (Heusel *et al.*, 1994). Some cytotoxic T cells obtained from perforin-deficient mice still retain the capacity to kill target cells and this was shown to be mediated through Fas/Fas-L interaction (Käji *et al.*, 1994; Kojima *et al.*, 1994).

5.2. Bcl-2 Family as Repressor for Apoptosis

It is becoming increasingly apparent that the susceptibility of target T cells to undergo apoptosis is largely regulated by the Bcl-2 family of proteins (Fig. 2). The bcl-2 gene is a proto-oncogene initially found at the breakpoint of the t(14;18) chromosomal translocation of human follicular lymphomas (Bakhshi *et al.*, 1985). Bcl-2 is an intracellular membrane protein and has been shown to block apoptosis in many experimental systems. Conversely,

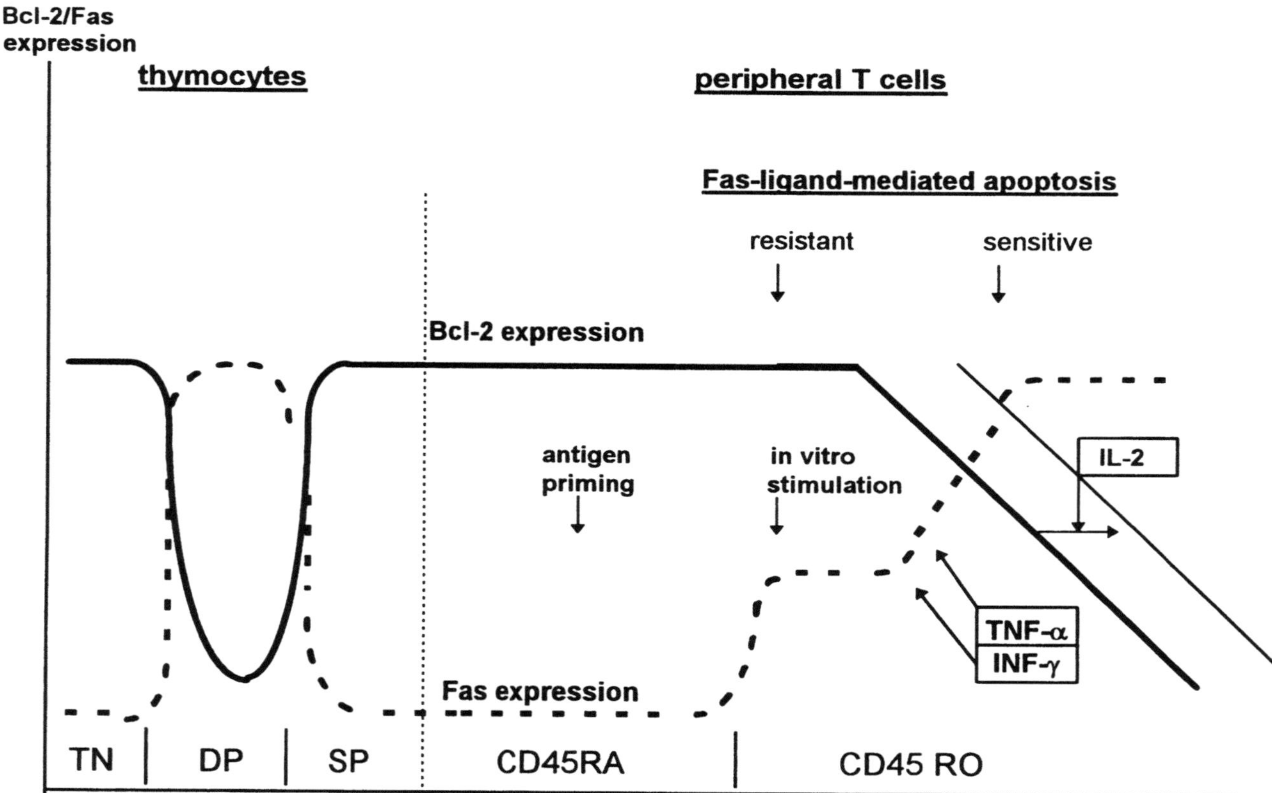

FIGURE 2. Thymocyte development and differentiation of peripheral T cells is intimately associated with reciprocal expression of Bcl-2 and Fas antigen. Gradual transition of high Bcl-2/low Fas expression of CD45RA$^+$ naive T cells to low Bcl-2/high Fas expression in CD45RO$^+$ memory T cell defines the susceptibility for Fas-ligand-mediated apoptosis. Cytokines TNF-α and IFN-γ are able to upregulate Fas while IL-2 upregulates Bcl-2 expression. TN, CD3/4/8 triple-negative; DP, CD4/CD8 double-positive; SP, CD4 or CD8 single-positive thymocytes.

lymphocytes from bcl-2 knock-out mice exhibit a markedly shortened life span and the number of mature T and B cells decrease with time, and almost completely disappear 2 months after birth (Nakayama *et al.*, 1994). Reciprocal expression of bcl-2 and Fas is a common feature of developmental/activational stages of T cells that are intimately associated with apoptosis induction (Fig. 2). In the periphery, naive T cells express abundant bcl-2 with little Fas expression, whereas memory CD45R0^{+} T cells express significantly decreased bcl-2 with increased expression of Fas (Miyawaki *et al.*, 1992; Gratiot-Deans *et al.*, 1994). After repeated activation of T cells *in vitro*, bcl-2 levels are diminished and this is associated with increased Fas expression (Yoshino *et al.*, 1994; Salmon *et al.*, 1994). This inverse relationship between bcl-2 and Fas is also demonstrated during the course of acute viral infection *in vivo* (Uehara *et al.*, 1992). In brief, for peripheral mature T cells, the gradual loss of Bcl-2 and gain of Fas expression are two features that are associated with an increased susceptibility to apoptosis.

The Bcl-2 proteins themselves comprise a family in which new members are being recognized with increasing frequency. An expanding family of Bcl-2-related proteins share two conserved regions referred to as Bcl-2 homology 1 and 2 (BH1 and BH2) domains. One member is Bax which heterodimerizes with Bcl-2 and a recent study indicates that this heterodimer formation is essential in order for bcl-2 to exert its antiapoptotic action (Oltvai *et al.*, 1993; Yin *et al.*, 1994) (Fig. 2). Three new members of Bcl-2 family proteins, Bcl-X (Boise *et al.*, 1993), Bad (Yang *et al.*, 1995), and Bak (Chittenden *et al.*, 1995), and a novel Bcl-2-binding protein, BAG-1, have been reported recently (Takayama *et al.*, 1995). Thus, the Bcl-2 family is composed of a complex machinery in which competing dimerizations eventually define its cell death-repressing activity.

5.3. Cell Death Signal

5.3.1. Fas Signaling

Although T cells upregulate Fas/Fas-L expression within 24 h of TCR stimulation, they only became sensitive to anti-Fas-mediated apoptosis several days later (Owen-Schaub *et al.*, 1992) (Fig. 3). Freshly isolated peripheral T cells are fairly resistant to Fas-based apoptosis although they express substantial amounts of Fas antigen. In contrast, T cells obtained from HIV-infected patients express augmented Fas and are extremely sensitive to anti-Fas-mediated apoptosis (Katsikis *et al.*, 1995). This observation suggests that Fas-mediated apoptosis is regulated not only by its ligand expression, but also by a permissive signaling pathway downstream to Fas receptor. In this regard, at least two mechanisms have been shown to explain this activity; one is the functional regulation of the Fas receptor itself and the other is regulation of the bcl-2 family's counterdeath activity. Deletion mapping analysis has identified a negative regulatory domain mapped to the C-terminal 15 amino acids of Fas that suppresses Fas-generated signals leading to cell death (Itoh *et al.*, 1993). A novel protein tyrosine phosphatase FAP-1 (*F*as-*a*ssociated *p*hosphatase) has recently been identified which was found to preferentially interact with the C-terminal negative regulatory domain of Fas (Sato *et al.*, 1995). FAP-1 thus appears to be a negative regulator of Fas-mediated death signal. Fas-sensitive T-cell lines were found to lack this protein and the induction of FAP-1 expression in these cell lines resulted in their gaining resistance to Fas-mediated apoptosis. The involvement of tyrosine kinase activities in mediating Fas-based death signaling is evidenced in human T-cell lines (Eischen *et al.*, 1994). Several studies

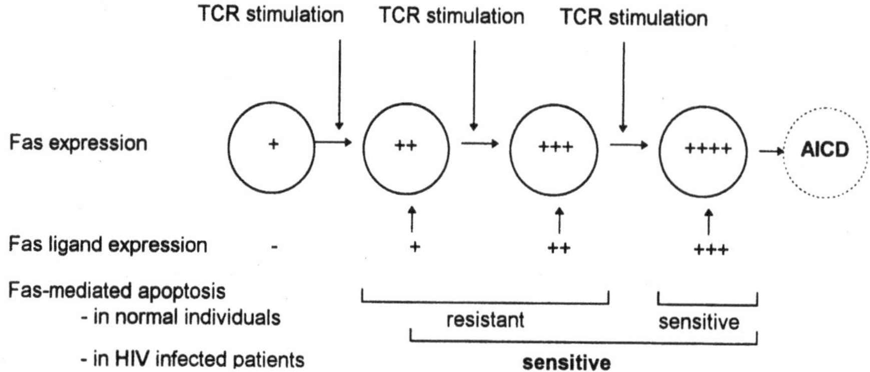

FIGURE 3. Fas/Fas ligand expression in activation-induced cell death. TCR stimulation leads to both Fas and its ligand expression within 24 hr. However, Fas/Fas-L expression *per se* is not sufficient to trigger apoptosis in freshly isolated peripheral T cells. In contrast, T cells from HIV-infected individuals are extremely sensitive to apoptosis induction in response to anti-Fas treatment.

indicate that the bcl-2 family death repressor system is operative downstream to the Fas signal. It has previously been shown that overexpression of bcl-2 partially blocks Fas- and p55 TNF-R-mediated death signal (Itoh *et al.*, 1993). Further, coexpression of BAG-1 and Bcl-2 were shown to provide markedly increased protection from cell death induced by anti-Fas antibody (Takayama *et al.*, 1995). These studies indicate that the levels of expression of these molecules constitute the regulatory mechanisms which define the Fas-mediated death signal. With respect to the nature of Fas signaling, in addition to protein tyrosine kinase pathway, ligation of Fas has been shown to result in the stimulation of the sphingomyelin signaling pathway to produce ceramides, which, in turn, induce Ras activation and apoptosis (Gulbins *et al.*, 1995). Addition of ceramide has previously been shown to induce apoptosis in the HL-60 leukemic cell line (Obeid *et al.*, 1993) and TNF-α has been shown to induce sphingomyelin hydrolysis as well (Weigmann *et al.*, 1994). This observation is intriguing since increased levels of ceramide have been reported in lymphocytes obtained from HIV-infected individuals (Van Veldhoven *et al.*, 1992) and in HIV-infected HL-60 cells (Rivas *et al.*, 1994).

5.3.2. Role of Proteases in Mediating the Death Signal

It has previously been shown that apoptosis induced by TCR activation, like other routes to physiologic cell death, depends on the activity of a serine or cysteine protease (Sarin *et al.*, 1993; Sarin *et al.*, 1994). Several lines of evidence now support the notion that interleukin-1β converting enzyme (ICE), which is a cysteine protease and a homologue of the product of the nematode *Caenorhabditis elegans* cell-death gene, ced-3, which is essential for apoptosis, is also involved in the mammalian cell-death signal including Fas signaling (Kuida *et al.*, 1995; Enari *et al.*, 1995; Los *et al.*, 1995). However, although ICE knock-out mice display resistance to anti-Fas-induced apoptosis in thymocytes, these mice developed normally, with no obvious defects in physiologic cell death. This observation implies that there may be another protease that plays a key role in mammalian apoptosis. In fact, another ICE-like cysteine protease designated as Yama or CPP32β has recently been identified (Fernandes-Alnermri *et al.*, 1994; Tewari *et al.*, 1995; Nicholson *et al.*, 1995). Yama/CPP32β, when activated, cleaves poly(ADP-ribose) polymerase to a specific 85-kDa form. Since poly(ADP-ribose) polymerase cleavage is a biochemical event observed in virtually every form of apoptosis examined including Fas- and TNF-mediated apoptosis (Kaufman *et al.*, 1993; Tewari *et al.*, 1995), Yama/CPP32β might play a central, universal role in mammalian apoptosis (see Fig. 1).

As described above, our understanding of the mechanisms of physiologic T-cell death has been advancing at an extraordinary pace. Based on this updated information, we will rereview HIV-mediated apoptosis induction in the following sections.

6. ACCELERATED LYMPHOCYTE APOPTOSIS ASSOCIATED WITH HIV INFECTION

Since 1991, a number of laboratories have demonstrated that *in vitro* infection of mononuclear cells with HIV (Terai *et al.*, 1991; Laurent-Crawford *et al.*, 1991) led to apoptotic cell death and that lymphocytes obtained from HIV-infected individuals manifested accelerated apoptosis (Meyaard *et al.*, 1992; Lewis *et al.*, 1994). The percentage of cells undergoing apoptosis in the acute phase of primary HIV infection has been shown to be higher than in asymptomatic individuals (Meyaard *et al.*, 1994), but even in the asymptomatic patient, 15–40% of cultured peripheral T cells (degree varies with culture period and the method employed) spontaneously undergo apoptosis, a level that is much higher than in uninfected controls (Oyaizu *et al.*, 1993; Carbonari *et al.*, 1994; Meyaard *et al.*, 1994). A discrepancy exists between the number of HIV-infected cells and the percentage of cells undergoing apoptosis in peripheral circulation. Considering the fact that productively infected cells are barely detectable in peripheral circulation in the asymptomatic stage (Schnittman *et al.*, 1992; Saksela *et al.*, 1994), direct cytopathic effect of HIV (or requirement for productive infection) cannot account for the observed substantial degree of apoptosis in peripheral circulation. In addition, analysis of the phenotype of cells undergoing apoptosis has revealed that not only $CD4^+$ T cells but also $CD8^+$ T cells undergo accelerated apoptosis in HIV infection (Meyaard *et al.*, 1992, 1994; Lewis *et al.*, 1994). Apoptotic death of cells has been shown not to be quantitatively correlated with the presence of syncytium-inducing (SI) and non-syncytium-inducing (NSI) HIV variants, suggesting that *in vitro* HIV cytopathicity does not correlate with *in vivo* apoptotic cell death (Meyaard *et al.*, 1994). However, a significantly lesser degree of apoptotic cell death has been reported in patients with HIV-2 infection, whose clinical course is much milder, as compared to those with HIV-1 infection (Jaleco *et al.*, 1994). In addition to these *in vitro* studies, experimental infection in animal models of the human immune system utilizing mice with severe combined immunodeficiency (SCID) reconstituted with human fetal liver and thymus (SCID-hu mice) showed rapid induction of apoptosis in thymocytes, far in excess of the numbers of productively infected cells, which resulted in marked reduction of single $CD4^+$ T cells (Su *et al.*, 1995a; Bonyhadi *et al.*, 1993). The relevance of these findings has been further extended by the observation of accelerated levels of peripheral blood T-cell apoptosis in primate and feline models of pathogenic lentiviral infections that cause AIDS-like diseases (Del Llano *et al.*, 1993; Bishop *et al.*, 1993). Based on these findings, it was proposed that apoptosis might be a major contributor to the depletion of $CD4^+$ T cells in

HIV infection and immune-based mechanisms (described below) for elimination of non-infected cells have been implicated.

7. MECHANISM(S) TO EXPLAIN HIV-ASSOCIATED APOPTOSIS

Studies described in the preceding section clearly indicate that in addition to direct HIV-mediated cytopathicity, immune mechanisms play a dominant role in the global deterioration of the immune system including destruction of $CD4^+$ T cells. Several mechanisms have been proposed to account for the observed accelerated T-cell apoptosis which can basically be categorized as (1) HIV envelope protein-mediated clustering of CD4 molecules (CD4 cross-linking) and subsequent aberrant signaling to T cells; (2) involvement of cytokine/cytokine receptors including Fas/Fas-L system; (3) involvement of accessory cells as inducers of apoptosis acting directly and indirectly; (4) possible superantigen activity encoded by HIV products or cofactors; and (5) structural components of HIV (other than env) playing a role in T-cell apoptosis. All of these proposed mechanisms are not mutually exclusive, but rather may be interrelated.

7.1. HIV gp120-Mediated CD4 Cross-Linking and Its Role in Apoptosis

7.1.1. Soluble gp120 as a Functional Inhibitor for CD4 T Cells

Earlier studies conducted by others and ourselves have revealed that many of the immunological abnormalities observed in HIV infection such as suppression of T helper function and B-cell hyperactivation did not require productive HIV infection, and that structural components of HIV could mediate these activities since addition of whole virus extracts also induced these phenomena *in vitro* (Pahwa *et al.*, 1985). Subsequently, together with the advance in our understanding of the mechanism of T-cell activation, the inhibitory effect of gp120 on T-cell activation is now firmly established. Exogenously provided soluble gp120 has been shown to inhibit antigen-specific T-cell activation (see Fig. 4) as demonstrated by (1) defective TCR-mediated signaling as manifested by failure of triggering of phosphatidylinositol turnover and (2) reduced T-cell proliferative response and IL-2 mRNA induction and secretion (Diamond *et al.*, 1988; Chirmule *et al.*, 1990; Oyaizu *et al.*, 1990). These inhibitory effects of gp120 could be ascribed to its high-affinity binding to the CD4 molecule, thereby interfering with the interaction of CD4 with its natural ligand, class II MHC, which is critical for mediating optimal TCR signaling (Oyaizu *et al.*, 1992). Thus, HIV envelope protein clearly comprises one of the HIV-specific detrimental components by selectively inhibiting antigen-specific T-helper-cell activation (or conversely as an inducer of T-cell unresponsiveness).

7.1.2. CD4XL as a Mechanism for Physical Elimination of T Cells

The original study conducted by Newell and colleagues, demonstrating that *in vitro* CD4XL of purified murine $CD4^+$ T cells with anti-CD4 antibody followed by subsequent TCR stimulation led to T-cell apoptosis (Newell *et al.*, 1990), suggested that gp120 may contribute to physical elimination of CD4 T cells as well. In fact, these findings were reproduced in humans by CD4XL using HIV gp120 and anti-gp120 antibody (Banda *et al.*,

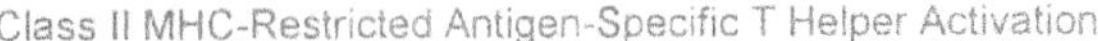

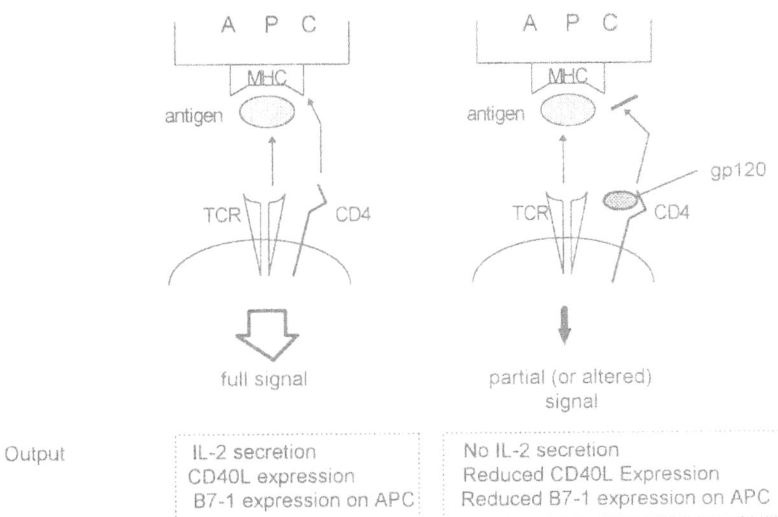

FIGURE 4. HIV gp120-mediated functional inhibition of T-helper-cell activation. gp 120 binds to CD4, thereby blocking physiological CD4–MHC class II interaction. This interference leads to partial (impaired) activation of T cells in the context of antigen-specific MHC class II-restricted T-cell activation.

1992). What is the *in vivo* relevance of this observation? In the setting of HIV infection, the likelihood of CD4XL occurring *in vivo* is extremely high. Ligation of CD4 molecules could result either from circulating HIV envelope protein [patients with HIV infection have circulating and cell-associated gp120, both free and complexed with anti-gp 120 antibodies (Oh *et al.*, 1992; Amadori *et al.*, 1992)] or from autoantibodies to CD4 cells, cell-free virus, or infected cells expressing gp120. A probable site where CD4 ligation may occur is in the lymph nodes where T lymphocytes traffic into the germinal centers and are exposed to abundant HIV virions trapped in the processes of follicular dendritic cells. However, this phenomenon by itself would not explain the loss of $CD8^+$ T cells which also undergo accelerated apoptosis in HIV infection. TCR-activation equivalent events *in vivo* also should be defined, although persistent and chronic HIV infection by itself is a likely candidate for continuous T-cell activation. We have shown that cross-linking of CD4 molecules, if performed in unfractionated peripheral blood mononuclear cells (PBMC) instead of purified CD4 T cells, induces apoptosis in T cells without the need for secondary TCR activation (Oyaizu *et al.*, 1993), and upregulates Fas antigen in both CD4 and CD8 T cells (Oyaizu *et al.*, 1994). Depletion of accessory cells results in failure of induction of T-cell apoptosis. Other lines of evidence for the role of gp120 in T-cell apoptosis induction have been derived from the observations that (1) HIV-mediated apoptosis induction is blocked by the addition of anti-gp120 antibodies (Terai *et al.*, 1991) and (2) env gene expression by itself has been shown to be sufficient to induce apoptosis in T-cell lines (Laurent-Crawford *et al.*, 1993; Lu *et al.*, 1994). Further, it has recently been shown that preactivated T cells undergo apoptosis following gp120 treatment (Foster *et al.*, 1995). These *in vitro* experimental systems demonstrating that CD4XL leads to T-cell apoptosis are

TABLE I. *In Vitro* Models of HIV gp120/CD4 Cross-Linking-Induced T-Cell Apoptosis

Cell culture system	Mode of CD4XL/env gene expression	Post-CD4XL TCR stimulation	References
Utilizing normal cells			
Murine CD4 T cells	anti-CD4 mAb-mediated	Yes	Newell *et al.* (1990)
Human CD4 T cells	gp120 + anti-gp120	Yes	Banda *et al.* (1992)
PBMC	anti-CD4 mAb-mediated	No	Oyaizu *et al.* (1993)
TSST-1-activated PBMC	gp120 + anti-gp120	No	Foster *et al.* (1995)
Utilizing transformed cells			
CD4 T-cell line (CEM)	env gene expression	No	Laurent-Crawford *et al.* (1993)
Monocytoid cell line (U937)	env gene expression	No	Lu *et al.* (1994)

summarized in Table I. Collectively, these studies strongly suggest that HIV gp120, in addition to functioning as an inhibitor for CD4 T-cell activation, further compromises the immune system by promoting physical elimination of T cells by gp120-mediated CD4XL (see Fig. 5). In this context, elucidation of the molecular mechanisms of gp120-mediated apoptosis induction is of extreme importance.

7.2. Role of Cytokines in HIV-Associated Apoptosis

7.2.1. Cytokine Dysregulation in HIV Infection

Based on the cytokine produced, a response can be classified as being of type 1 or type 2 with IL-2, IFN-γ, and IL-12 representing type 1 cytokines, regulating cell-mediated immunity; IL-4, IL-5, and IL-10 are type 2 cytokines linked to humoral immunity (Salgame *et al.*, 1991). Cytokines TNF-α, GM-CSF, and IL-6 are not specifically categorized. A major source of these latter cytokines is the macrophage which also secretes IL-10 and IL-12. Cytokine secretion pattern in T cells is intimately regulated by their differentiation stages. Naive T cells can only secrete their own autocrine growth factor IL-2 after initial antigen stimulation, and following differentiation into effector cells, they undergo polarization to secrete either type 1 or type 2 or both (type 0) cytokines, and finally, terminally differentiated memory T cells gradually lose the capacity to produce IL-2 while retaining the capacity to secrete IFN-γ and IL-4 (Salmon *et al.*, 1994). As described earlier, this gradual maturation of T cells is also intimately associated with reciprocal expression of Bcl-2 and Fas antigen expression, namely, high Bcl-2/low Fas to low Bcl-2/high Fas transition defines the susceptibility for apoptosis. In accordance with this view, recent studies have revealed that exogenously supplemented IL-2 resulted in increase of Bcl-2 (Miyazaki *et al.*, 1995) which is associated with increased cell survival in memory T cells (Akbar *et al.*, 1993) (Fig. 2).

One of the characteristic immunologic disorders associated with HIV infection is increased production of a number of cytokines. Although some researchers have proposed that HIV disease progression is associated with a shift in cytokine pattern from type 1 to type 2, based on the cytokine secretion profile in response to *in vitro* stimulation (Clerici and Shearer, 1993; Clerici *et al.*, 1993), the dominant *in vivo* response in HIV infection appears to be increased TNF-α, IFN-γ, IL-10, and IL-6 with constantly reduced IL-2 as determined by studying plasma levels and constitutive lymphocyte cytokine mRNA expression pattern

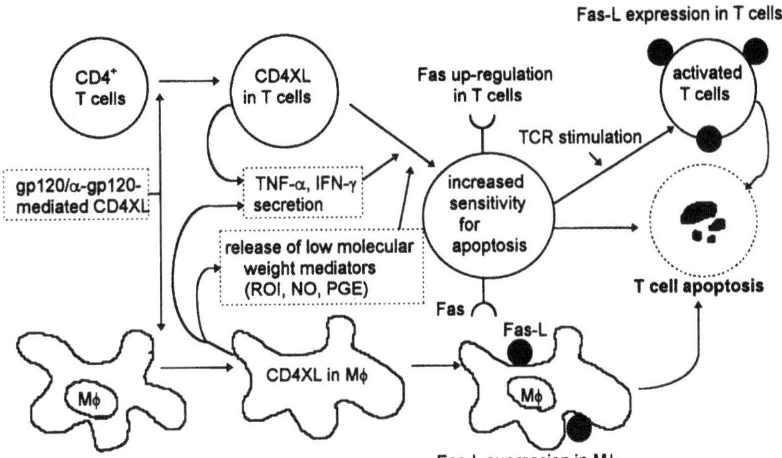

FIGURE 5. CD4 cross-linking-induced T-cell apoptosis. A hypothetical model of CD4 cross-linking (XL)-mediated apoptosis induction. $CD4^+$ T cells and/or macrophages are subject to CD4XL through interaction with HIV virions or with envelope proteins gp120/anti-gp120 antibodies. These CD4XL reagents lead to cytokine secretion including TNF-α and IFN-γ which in turn upregulate Fas antigen expression on T cells. CD4XL may lead to Fas-L expression on macrophages. Interaction of macrophage-derived Fas-L with Fas-expressing T cells would trigger apoptosis. Induced cytokines and macrophage-derived low-molecular-weight chemical mediators (such as ROI, NO, PGE) play a promotive role for increasing sensitivity to target cells for Fas-mediated death signaling.

(Lahdevirta *et al.*, 1988; Graziosi *et al.*, 1994). Of interest is the finding that IL-2 and IFN-γ, hitherto considered to be coordinately controlled, are affected differently in HIV infection (Fan *et al.*, 1993).

7.2.2. Role of gp120/CD4XL in Cytokine Dysregulation

One possible mechanism for the selective upregulation of cytokines in patients can be explained by the cytokine-inducible abilities of gp120. CD4–gp120 interaction not only provides a critical step for HIV infection but also elicits a CD4-mediated signal into the target cells. HIV-1 gp120 has been shown to induce a variety of cytokines including TNF-α, IL-6, IL-1, GM-CSF, IFN-β from T cells or macrophages through its interaction with CD4 molecules (Wahl *et al.*, 1989; Clouse *et al.*, 1991; Oyaizu *et al.*, 1991; Rieckmann *et al.*, 1991; Than *et al.*, 1994; Gessani *et al.*, 1994). Further, we have demonstrated that a similar cytokine pattern can be induced *in vitro* by performing CD4XL in PBMC of HIV-seronegative donors, which contributed to apoptosis induction (see below). As described earlier, recent studies have clearly elucidated the pivotal role of Fas/Fas-L interaction in T-cell apoptosis induction. We have examined whether CD4XL affects Fas expression and found that CD4XL results in increased expression of Fas in T cells (Oyaizu *et al.*, 1994). Unexpectedly, not only CD4 T cells but also CD8 T cells showed increased Fas expression on CD4XL and this was achieved in the absence of accessory cells. Further, CD4XL was found to result in induction of cytokines TNF-α and IFN-γ in the absence of IL-2 and IL-4 and both of the induced cytokines contributed to Fas upregulation. Neutralizing antibodies to TNF-α and to IFN-γ both blocked CD4XL-induced Fas upregulation and apoptosis induction (Oyaizu *et al.*, 1994). As described in the preceding section, in the context of antigen-induced T-cell activation, gp120 has been shown to selectively suppress antigen-driven IL-2 secretion in CD4 T cells (Oyaizu *et al.*, 1990). Recent studies have revealed that exogenously supplemented IL-2 results in increase of Bcl-2 (Miyazaki *et al.*, 1995) and IL-2 has been reported to provide a protective effect on T-cell apoptosis after antigen stimulation (Leonardo, 1991). These results may explain the increase in CD4 cell counts observed in HIV-infected patients during the clinical trial with IL-2 in HIV-infected patients (Kovacs *et al.*, 1995).

Collectively, these findings suggest that the interaction between HIV-1 envelope protein and CD4 molecules, operating at an interface of HIV virion and host immune system, and the subsequent CD4XL mechanism could explain the observed constitutive and discordant cytokine expression in HIV-infected patients. Endogenous cytokine imbalance, with high proinflammatory cytokines such as TNF-α and deficient IL-2 appear to serve as conditions that facilitate apoptosis induction.

7.2.3. Cytokine Dysregulation and Apoptosis

Several lines of evidence support the notion that CD4XL-mediated aberrant cytokine secretion and subsequent Fas upregulation may contribute to the observed accelerated T-cell apoptosis in HIV infection. First, under a variety of cell culture conditions including studies with normal peripheral T cells, both TNF-α and IFN-γ play a promotive role for T-cell apoptosis (Grell *et al.*, 1994; Liu and Janeway, 1990; Groux *et al.*, 1993; Novelli *et al.*, 1994; Tartaglia *et al.*, 1993). Moreover, TNF-α and IFN-γ may independently mediate signals for apoptosis; Fas expression and Fas-mediated cytotoxicity have been found to be greatly increased on target cells by treatment with these cytokines (Yonehara *et al.*, 1989; Itoh *et al.*, 1991; Oyaizu *et al.*, 1994). The fact that ligation of Fas leads to stimulation of sphingomyelin hydrolysis to produce ceramide (Gulbins *et al.*, 1995) and the abilities of TNF-α and IFN-γ to induce sphingomyelin hydrolysis (Obeid *et al.*, 1993) may explain the synergistic effects of these cytokines in increasing the sensitivity of target cells for Fas-based cytotoxicities.

With respect to the interrelationship between CD4XL-mediated T-cell apoptosis and the requirement for Fas antigen in this process, strong evidence has been derived from the study showing that administration of anti-CD4 mAb *in vivo* resulted in CD4 T-cell depletion through apoptosis in normal mice but this was not observed in Fas-defective *lpr* mice (Wang *et al.*, 1994a). In the setting of HIV infection and the involvement of Fas-based cytotoxicity, the following is known: (1) selective anti-Fas antibody-mediated killing occurs in chronically HIV-infected, but not uninfected, cells (Kobayashi *et al.*, 1990), (2) we and others have observed that Fas expression is significantly increased in both $CD4^+$ and $CD8^+$ T cells of HIV-infected individuals (Debatin *et al.*, 1994; McCloskey *et al.*, 1995; Krowka *et al.*, 1994), and (3) unlike cells of uninfected individuals, $CD4^+$ and $CD8^+$ T cells from HIV-infected individuals have recently been shown to undergo marked apoptosis *in vitro* in response to anti-Fas antibody (Katsikis *et al.*, 1994). Collectively, these findings strongly suggest that CD4XL-mediated aberrant cytokine secretion and subsequent Fas upregulation may largely contribute to the observed accelerated T-cell apoptosis in HIV disease (Fig. 5).

Recent findings indicate that two cytokines secreted by accessory cells may participate in the regulation of T-cell apoptosis in HIV infection: IL-10 promotes T-cell apoptosis and IL-12 prevents it (Clerici *et al.*, 1995). However, because of the complex nature of cytokine cross talk and because of the pleiotropic nature of cytokine function, it is difficult to conclusively establish which cytokine is protective or promotive for apoptosis induction in the setting of HIV infection and this subject requires further studies.

7.3. Role of Accessory Cells in HIV-Associated Apoptosis

In the setting of T-cell apoptosis induction in HIV infection, several studies implicate the regulatory role of accessory cells: (1) Monocytes/macrophages and dendritic cells have been shown to act as reservoirs of HIV thereby providing HIV virions and the HIV-1 external envelope protein gp120 to target T cells (Pope *et al.*, 1994). (2) Antigen-presenting cell (APC) dysfunction as a result of HIV infection may cause defective T-cell activation and subsequent apoptosis. In this regard, it has previously been reported that anti-CD28 antibody provided a rescue signal to block patients' T-cell apoptosis *in vitro* (Groux *et al.*, 1992) and treatment with anti-CTLA4 antibodies *in vitro* has recently been shown to promote apoptosis (Gribben *et al.*, 1995). Thus, interaction of costimulatory molecules between APCs and T cells, particularly the interaction of B7 family of proteins and CD28/CTLA4, is currently under intensive investigation. In fact, we have shown that pretreatment of gp120 resulted in inhibition of anti-CD3-induced CD40L expression in T cells which in turn led to reduced B7-1 expression on APCs (Chirmule *et al.*, 1995). However, whether interactions of these molecules are directly regulating T-cell apoptosis or indirectly regulating it via induction of cytokines is not known. (3) Monocytes/macrophages are the most likely source of pro-apoptosis-inducing cytokines as well as pro-apoptosis-inducing low-molecular-weight molecules such as reactive oxygen intermediates (ROI), prostaglandins (PGs), and nitric oxide (NO) (Buttke and Sandstrom, 1994). In addition to these possibilities, as described earlier, CD4XL performed in purified T cells is not sufficient for apoptosis induction. Preactivation of T cells (Foster *et al.*, 1995), a second stimulus via the TCR (Newell *et al.*, 1990; Banda *et al.*, 1992), or the presence of accessory cells (Oyaizu *et al.*, 1993) are necessary for CD4XL-induced T-cell apoptosis (Table I). Addition of cytokines TNF-α and/or IFN-γ to peripheral T cells by themselves is insufficient to induce apoptosis even though these cytokines can upregulate Fas (Oyaizu *et al.*, 1994). These results point to the important role of accessory cells (and TCR stimulation) and the necessity of other factor(s) in inducing T-cell apoptosis. Apparently, the most likely candidate for such a factor is Fas-L. It is unclear whether death of activated T cells is suicidal, or whether Fas-L is provided by neighboring cells including activated T cells or even APCs, although exclusive expression of Fas-L in T-lineage cells has recently been reported (Suda *et al.*, 1995). Nonetheless, CD4XL alone appears to be sufficient to induce T-cell apoptosis in the presence of accessory cells. This view is consistent with a recent study demonstrating that administration of gp120 and anti-gp120 antibodies into human $CD4^+$-expressing transgenic mice was sufficient to induce depletion of human $CD4^+$-expressing murine T lymphocytes *in vivo* without TCR stimulation (Wang *et al.*, 1994b). Several other studies point to the regulatory role of accessory cells (particularly of macrophages) in inducing HIV-mediated T-cell depletion. The dominant role of noncytopathic macrophage-tropic HIV strains in CD4 T-cell depletion has been observed in SCID mice reconstituted with human PBL (Mosier *et al.*, 1993). A regulatory role of macrophages in T-cell apoptosis can be deduced from the nonhuman primate model as well. HIV-1 is able to establish persistent infection in both humans and chimpanzees; while human infection leads to AIDS, in the chimpanzee, HIV infection does not cause AIDS-like disease (Watanabe *et al.*, 1991; Johnson *et al.*, 1993). HIV fails to infect monocytes in chimpanzees (Gendelman *et al.*, 1991) and accelerated apoptosis does not occur in T cells from HIV-infected chimpanzees (Schuitemaker *et al.*, 1993).

7.4. Possible Role of Superantigen Encoded by HIV or by Cofactor

Because some animal retroviruses such as mouse mammary tumor virus (MMTV) or defective murine leukemia virus encode superantigen activity (Hügin *et al.*, 1991), and the latter has been shown to cause AIDS-like disease (Aziz *et al.*, 1989), it has been proposed that HIV may encode a superantigen and thereby play a role in disease pathogenesis. Although this is a very intriguing hypothesis, there is no convincing evidence in its favor. Similarly, it has been proposed that dual infection with other microorganisms such as mycoplasma which may encode superantigen activity may thereby act as an important cofactor for disease progression. However, evidence for this possibility is also inconclusive.

7.5. Other HIV Components Involved in T-Cell Apoptosis

In addition to envelope protein, other viral factor(s) such as Tat protein have been proposed to play a role in T-cell apoptosis induction in HIV infection. Two recent reports indicate that HIV Tat may play a role in promoting T-cell apoptosis (Li *et al.*, 1995; Westendorp *et al.*, 1995). However, this issue is currently controversial since other investigators have provided evidence implicating Tat as playing a protective role for apoptosis in T cells (Zauli *et al.*, 1993; Gibellini *et al.*, 1995). The bases for contradictory data, which may arise from differences in experimental systems or materials used, are currently unknown. However, given the observation that productively infected cells barely undergo apoptosis *in vivo*, it is intriguing to speculate that HIV may encode a protective factor for apoptosis as this would explain the remarkable persistence of the disease.

8. WHAT IS GOING ON *IN VIVO*?

As referred to in the Introduction, Wei *et al.* and Ho *et al.* showed that treatment of patients with various anti-HIV drugs, which were designed to affect only new rounds of infection, resulted in a rapid reduction of free viruses in plasma and this reduction was accompanied by an increase in the number of circulating $CD4^+$ T cells (Wei *et al.*, 1995; Ho *et al.*, 1995). These studies reaffirmed that the long clinical latent phase is not a period of viral inactivity but underscored an extraordinarily active replication of virus and dynamic compensation of CD4 T cells from peripheral lymphoid pool occurring in this phase. Another important finding in these studies is that, in contrast to the genomic RNA pattern which showed rapid emergence of drug-resistant mutants, analysis of proviral DNA in peripheral lymphocytes revealed a high proportion of wild-type provirus. This finding suggests that dynamic viral replication is occurring in peripheral lymphoid organs rather than in peripheral circulation. The background of these studies lies in the rediscovery of sequestration and heavy viral burden in the lymphoid organs where 98% of lymphocytes reside. Recent studies of Finkel *et al.* indicate that viral RNA and apoptotic cells are predominantly colocalized in the secondary follicle of infected lymph node but that apoptosis predominantly occurs in uninfected cells and not in productively infected cells. These findings led the authors to conclude that HIV-infected cells do not die by apoptosis, but rather that HIV induces apoptosis in bystander cells. Because of the lack of noninfected control preparations, interpretation of their data is still open to question; the observation by itself is important and intriguing because these approaches finally and directly shed light on the fundamental question of how HIV kills cells *in vivo*. The observation that increased lymphocyte apoptosis occurs in the HIV-infected lymph node has been confirmed in a more recent study (Muro-Cacho *et al.*, 1995). Clearly, an *in vivo* framework is needed to understand how different cells and their microenvironment might be involved in the induction of HIV replication and how the virus exerts its cytopathic effects. In the final section, we will discuss histopathological considerations regarding the possible events occurring in the lymph node in HIV infection.

9. HISTOPATHOLOGICAL CONSIDERATION OF HIV PATHOGENESIS

T cells are densely populated in paracortical regions where they may be activated by recognizing antigen presented on APCs, such as dendritic cells or macrophages. Once activated, T cells and antigen-bearing B cells migrate (or form) into primary follicle where B cells interact with follicular dendritic cells (FDCs). FDCs have unique properties and are capable of trapping immune complexes (IC) and retaining them on their surface for a long period of time (van den Eterwegh *et al.*, 1992; Joling *et al.*, 1993). This interaction leads to the formation of a finely structured germinal center (GC) where B cells undergo terminal differentiation (Clark and Ledbetter, 1994).

Studies of the lymph nodes from SIV-infected macaques have revealed that in the first week postinoculation, SIV RNA-positive cells were found in a high number in macrophages scattered in the subcapsular sinuses and in T cells scattered in the paracortical areas. A shift in the pattern of viral infection was observed 2 weeks after inoculation, with a concentration of viral RNA in the GC of the developing follicle. As the secondary follicle developed, FDCs constituted a reticular network in the GC and retained large amounts of SIV virions (Chakrabarti *et al.*, 1994a,b). This pattern, namely scattered distribution of productively infected cells in paracortical areas and intense extracellular association of FDCs, persists for at least several months and is consistent with observations of Pantaleo *et al.* (1993b) and Embretson *et al.* (1993) who have conducted studies in HIV-infected lymph nodes. Histopathology of HIV-infected lymph nodes shows features consistent with *in situ* hybridization studies of viral distribution. The follicle includes significantly hyperplastic GC with extensive cytolysis and phagocytosis of nuclear debris by tangible body macrophages (O'Hara, 1989). These histopathological observations point to a major battlefield between HIV and the host immune system in secondary lymphoid follicles. Although few T cells and macrophages (tangible body macrophages) are present in the GC, many $CD4^+$ T cells reside in apical zones of secondary follicles; infiltration of GC with $CD8^+$ T cells is reported to be a specific feature of HIV infection (O'Hara, 1989) and a recent study implicates HIV-specific $CD8^+$ CTL infiltration of splenic white pulps, the anatomically equivalent site of lymph node follicles (Cheynier *et al.*, 1994). Several lines of data implicate a distinctive feature of GC T cells: (1) most GC T cells have the phenotype of activated memory-type CD4 T cells (Bowen *et al.*, 1991); (2) on antigenic stimulation *in vivo*, many GC T cells, but not T cells in paracortical areas, have been shown to actively proliferate as determined by incorporation of bromodeoxyuridine (Fuller *et al.*, 1993); (3) studies utilizing adoptive transfer of antigen-specific transgenic T cells to syngeneic mice have revealed that only specific antigen-activated T cells can gain access to the GC (Kearney *et al.*, 1994); (4) by employing *in situ* hybridization for detecting cytokine mRNA, selective enrichment of lymphokine-producing T cells occurs in GC as compared to T cells in paracortical areas (Emille *et al.*, 1990). As mentioned above, ultrastructural and immunohistochemical studies reveal a tremendous amount of extracellular association of HIV virions with FDCs in the form of immune complexes (Pantaleo *et al.*, 1993b; Embretson *et al.*, 1993; Joling *et al.*, 1993). Therefore, GC might provide a special milieu for T cells to undergo CD4XL. CD4XL could lead to TNF-α and IFN-γ secretion (Oyaizu *et al.*, 1991). An important aspect of the CD4XL-induced cytokine secretion in HIV pathogenesis is the capacity of these cytokines to induce HIV replication. Among them, TNF-α is particularly important since it has been shown that TNF-α alone is able to upregulate HIV replication and synergizes with IL-6, GM-CSF, and IFN-γ (Duh *et al.*, 1989; Poli *et al.*, 1990; Biswas *et al.*, 1992; Biswas *et al.*, 1994). It is thus possible that HIV production is amplified via a CD4XL mechanism in GC and this may explain why GC harbor a heavy viral burden and CD4XL may be the primary

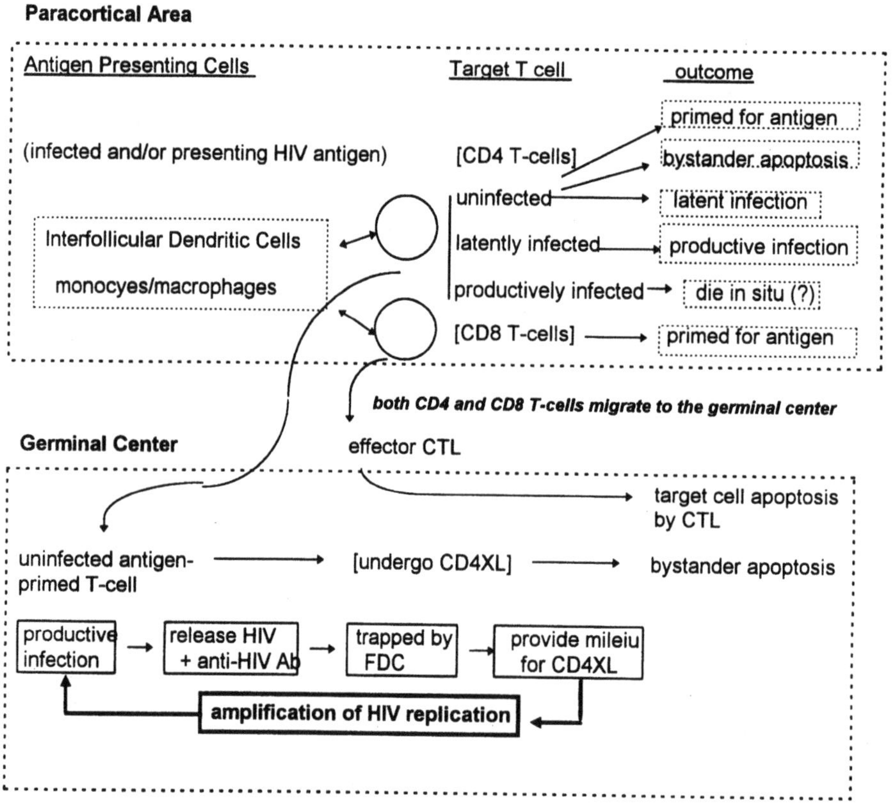

Paracortical Area
Antigen Presenting Cells
Target T cell
outcome
primed for antigen
(infected and/or presenting HIV antigen)
[CD4 T-cells]
bystander apoptosis
uninfected
latent infection
Interfollicular Dendritic Cells
latently infected
productive infection
monocyes/macrophages
productively infected
die in situ (?)
[CD8 T-cells]
primed for antigen
both CD4 and CD8 T-cells migrate to the germinal center
Germinal Center
effector CTL
target cell apoptosis by CTL
uninfected antigen-primed T-cell
[undergo CD4XL]
bystander apoptosis
productive infection
release HIV + anti-HIV Ab
trapped by FDC
provide mileiu for CD4XL
amplification of HIV replication

FIGURE 6. Immunohistopathological events occurring in the lymph node in HIV infection. HIV-infected macrophages and/or HIV antigen-bearing dendritic cells act as antigen-presenting cells for T cells in the paracortical areas. These interactions lead to antigen-specific activation as well as to the establishment of infection in target T cells. Activated T cells migrate to the germinal center where they undergo further activation and promote HIV replication.

mechanism that maintains high levels of HIV replication. Collectively, secondary follicles (including GC) may be the major site where CD4 (and CD8) T-cell destruction and dynamic HIV replication occurs through a complex series of immune cell interactions (Fig. 6).

10. CONCLUSIONS

Certainly, AIDS is a primary consequence of continuous, high-level replication of HIV, leading to virus- and immune-mediated killing of CD4 lymphocytes. Whether or not apoptosis is the primary mechanism of death of productively infected cells, apoptosis comprises a major mechanism of cell death in HIV-infected individuals including cell types not necessarily permissive to infection with HIV. It should be emphasized that HIV-mediated cell death mechanisms should be evaluated separately in uninfected cell systems and in productively infected cell systems to dissect possible opposing mechanisms, which may be operative. Nonetheless, it becomes clear that the critical interface is the interaction between viral envelope protein and target cell CD4 molecules under a specific immuno-anatomical milieu. This interface might also bridge immunological and virological mechanisms operative in HIV pathogenesis. Intensive analysis of this interaction reflecting *in vivo* circumstances may eventually solve the central question in AIDS pathogenesis of how HIV kills lymphocytes.

ACKNOWLEDGMENTS. This work has been supported by National Institutes of Health Grants AI28281, HD26606 and DA05061.

REFERENCES

Akbar, A. N., Borthwick, N., Salmon, M., Gombert, W., Bofill, M., Shamsadeen, N., Pilling, D., Pett, S., Grundy, J. E., and Janossy, G., 1993, The significance of low bcl-2 expression by CD45R0 T cells in normal individuals and patients with acute viral infections: The role of apoptosis in T cell memory, *J. Exp. Med.* **178**:427–438.

Alderson, M. R., Tough, T. W., Davis-Smith, T., Braddy, S., Falk, B., Schooley, K. A., Goodwin, R. G., Smith, C. A., Ramsdell, F., and Lynch, D. H., 1995, Fas ligand mediates activation-induced cell death in human T lymphocytes, *J. Exp. Med.* **181**:71–77.

Amadori, A., Silvestro, G. D., Zamarchi, R., Veronese, M. L., Mazza, M. R., Schiavo, G., Panozzo, M., DeRossi, A., Ometto, L., Mous, J., Barelli, A., Borri, A., Salmaso, L., and Chieco-Bianchi, L., 1992, CD4 epitope masking by gp120/anti-gp120 antibody complexes: A potential mechanism for CD4+ cell function down-regulation in AIDS patients, *J. Immunol.* **148**:2709–2716.

Ashwell, J. D., Cunningham, R. E., Noguchi, P. D., and Hernandez, D., 1987, Cell growth cycle block of T cell hybridomas upon activation with antigen, *J. Exp. Med.* **165**:173–194.

Aziz, D. C., Hanna, Z., and Jolicoeur, P., 1989, Severe immunodeficiency disease induced by a defective murine leukemia virus, *Nature* **338**:505–508.

Bakhshi, A., Jensen, J. P., Goldman, P., Wright, J. J., McBride, O. W., Epstein, A. L., and Korsmeyer, S. J., 1985, Cloning the chomosomal breakpoint of t(14;18) human lymphomas: Clustering around JH on chromosome 14 and near a transcriptional unit on 18, *Cell* **41**:889–906.

Banda, N. K., Bernier, J., Kurahara, D. K., Kurrle, R., Haigwood, N., Sekaly, R.-P., and Finkel, T. H., 1992, Crosslinking CD4 by human immunodeficiency virus gp120 primes t cells for activation-induced apoptosis, *J. Exp. Med.* **176**:1099–1106.

Bergeron, L., and Sodroski, J., 1992, Dissociation of unintegrated viral DNA accumulation from single-cell lysis induced by human immunodeficiency virus type 1, *J. Virol.* **66**:5777–5787.

Bishop, S. A., Gruffydd-Jones, T. J., Harbour, D. A., and Stokes, C. R., 1993, PCD (apoptosis) as a mechanism of cell death in PBMC from cats infected with feline immunodeficiency virus (FIV), *Clin. Exp. Immunol.* **93:** 65–71.

Biswas, P., Poli, G., Kinter, A. L., Justment, J. S., Stanley, S. K., Maury, W. J., Bressler, P., Orenstein, J. M., and Fauci, A. S., 1992, Interferon-gamma induces the expression of human immunodeficiency virus in persistently infected promonocytic cells (U1) and redirects the production of virions to intracytoplasmic vacuoles in phorbol myristate acetate-differentiated U1 cells, *J. Exp. Med.* **176:**739–750.

Biswas, P., Poli, G., Orenstein, J. M., and Fauci, A. S., 1994, Cytokine-mediated induction of human immunodeficiency virus (HIV) expression and cell death in chronically infected U1 cells: Do tumor necrosis factor alpha and gamma interferon selectively kill HIV-infected cells? *J. Virol.* **68:**2598–2604.

Boise, L. H., Gonzalez-Garcia, M., Postema, C. E., Ding, L., Lindsten, T., Turka, L. A., Mao, X., Nunez, G., and Thompson, C. B., 1993, bcl-x, bcl-2-related gene that functions as a dominant regulator of apoptotic cell death, *Cell* **74:**597–608.

Bonyhadi, M. L., Rabin, L., Salimi, S., Brown, D. A., Kosek, J., McCune, J. M., and Kaneshima, H., 1993, HIV induces thymus depletion in vivo, *Nature* **363:**728–732.

Bossu, P., Singer, G. G., Andres, P., Ettinger, R., Marshak-Rothstein, A., and Abbas, A., K., 1994, Mature CD4+ T lymphocytes from MRL/lpr mice are resistant to receptor-mediated tolerance and apoptosis, *J. Immunol.* **151:**7233–7239.

Bowen, M. B., Butch, A. W., Parvin, C. A., Levine, A., and Nahm, M. H., 1991, Germinal center T cells are distinct helper-inducer T cells, *Hum. Immunol.* **31:**67–76.

Brunner, T., Mogill, R., LaFace, D., Yoo, N. J., Mahboul, A., Echeverri, F., Martin, S. J., Force, W. R., Lynch, D. H., Ware, C. F., and Green, D. R., 1995, Cell-autonomous Fas (CD95)/Fas-ligand interaction mediates activation-induced apoptosis in T-cell hybridoma, *Nature* **373:**441–444.

Buttke, T. M., and Sandstrom, P. A., 1994, Oxidative stress as a mediator of apoptosis, *Immunol. Today* **15:**209–213.

Carbonari, M., Cibati, M., Cherchi, M., Sbarigia, D., Pesce, A. M., Dell'Anna, L., Modica, A., and Fiorilli, M., 1994, Detection and characterization of apoptotic peripheral blood lymphocytes in human immunodeficiency virus infection and cancer chemotherapy by a novel flow immunocytometric method, *Blood* **83:**1268–1277.

Chakrabarti, L., Cumont, M.-C., Montagnier, L., and Hurtrel, B., 1994a, Variable course of primary simian immunodeficiency virus infection in lymph nodes: Relation to disease progression, *J. Virol.* **68:**6634–6642.

Chakrabarti, L., Isola, P., Cumont, M.-C., Claessens-Maire, M.-A., Hurtrel, M., Montagnier, L., and Hurtrel, B., 1994b, Early stages of simian immunodeficiency virus infection in lymph nodes, *Am. J. Pathol.* **144:**1226–1237.

Cheng, J., Zhou, T., Liu, C., Shapiro, J. P., Brauer, M. J., Kiefer, M. C., Barr, P. J., and Mounz, J. D., 1994, Protection from Fas-mediated apoptosis by a soluble form of the Fas molecule, *Science* **263:**1759–1762.

Cheynier, R., Henrichwark, S., Hadida, F., Pelletier, E., Oksenhendler, E., Autran, B., and Wain-Hobson, S., 1994, HIV and T cell expansion in splenic white pulps is accompanied by infiltration of HIV-specific cytotoxic T lymphocytes, *Cell* **78:**373–387.

Chirmule, N., Karyanaraman, V. S., Oyaizu, N., Slade, H., and Pahwa, S., 1990, Inhibition of functional properties of tetanus antigen-specific T cell clones by envelope glycoproteins of HIV-1, *Blood* **75:**152–159.

Chirmule, N., McCloskey, T. W., Hu, R., Kalyanaraman, V. S., and Pahwa, S., 1995, HIV gp120 inhibits T cell activation by interfering with expression of costimulatory molecules CD40 ligand and CD80 (B71), *J. Immunol.* **155:**917–924.

Chittenden, T., Harrington, E. A., O'Conner, R., Flemington, C., Lutz, R. J., Evan, G. I., and Guild, B. C., 1995, Induction of apoptosis by the Bcl-2 homologue Bak, *Nature* **374:**733–739.

Clark, E. A., and Ledbetter, J. A., 1994, How B and T cells talk to each other, *Nature* **367:**425–428.

Clerici, M., and Shearer, G. M., 1993, A Th1-Th2 switch is a critical step in the etiology of HIV infection, *Immunol. Today* **14:**107–110.

Clerici, M., Hakim, F. T., Venzon, D. J., Blatt, S., Hendrix, C. W., Wynn, T. A., and Shearer, G. M., 1993, Changes in interleukin-2 and interleukin-4 production in asymptomatic, human immunodeficiency virus-seropositive individuals, *J. Clin. Invest.* **91:**759–765.

Clerici, M., Sarin, A., Coffman, R. L., Wynn, T. A., Blatt, S., Hendrix, C. W., Wolf, S. F., Shearer, G. M., and Henkart, P. A., 1995, Type 1/type 2 cytokine modulation of T-cell programmed cell death as a model for human immunodeficiency virus pathogenesis, *Proc. Natl. Acad. Sci. USA* **91:**11811–11815.

Clouse, K. A., Cosentino, L. M., Weih, K. A., Pyle, S. W., Robbins, P. B., Hochstein, H. D., Natarajan, V., and Farrar, W. L., 1991, The HIV-1 gp120 envelope protein has the intrinsic capacity to stimulate monokine secretion, *J. Immunol.* **147:**2892–2901.

Cloyd, M. W., and Lynn, W. S., 1991, Perturbation of host-cell membrane is a primary mechanism of HIV cytopathicity, *Virology* **181:**307–309.

Cohen, P. L., and Eisenberg, R. A., 1991, Lpr and gld: Single gene models of systemic autoimmunity and lymphoproliferative disease, *Annu. Rev. Immunol.* **9:**243–262.

Debatin, K.-M., Fahrig-Faissner, A., Enenkel-Stoodt, S., Kreuz, W., Benner, A., and Krammer, P. H., 1994, High expression of Apo-1 (CD95) on T lymphocytes from human immunodeficiency virus-1-infected children, *Blood* **83:**3101–3103.

Del Llano, A. M., Amerio-Puig, J. P., Kraiselburd, E. N., Kessler, M. J., Malaga, C. A., and Lavergne, J. A., 1993, The combined assessment of cellular apoptosis, mitochondrial function and proliferative response to pokeweed mitogen has prognostic value in SIV infection, *J. Med. Primatol.* **22:**194–200.

DeRossi, A., Franchini, G., Aldovini, A., DelMistro, A., Chieco-Bianchi, L., Gallo, R., and Wong-Staal, F., 1986, Differential response to the cytopathic effects of human T-cell lymphotropic virus III (HTLV-III) superinfection in T4+ (helper) and T8+ (suppressor) T-cell clones transformed by HTLV-1, *Proc. Natl. Acad. Sci. USA* **83:**4297–4301.

Dhein, J., Walczac, H., Baumler, C., Debatin, K.-M., and Krammer, P. H., 1995, Autocrine T-cell suicide mediated by APO-1/(Fas/CD95), *Nature* **373:**438–441.

Diamond, D. C., Sleckman, B. P., Gregory, T., Lasky, L. A., Greenstein, J. L., and Burakoff, S. J., 1988, Inhibition of CD4+ T cell function by the HIV envelope protein gp120, *J. Immunol.* **141:**3715–3717.

Duh, E. J., Maury, W. J., Folks, T. M., Fauci, A. S., and Rabson, A., 1989, Tumor necrosis factor-alpha activates human immunodeficiency virus type 1 through induction of nuclear factor binding to the NF-kB sites in the long terminal repeat, *Proc. Natl. Acad. Sci. USA* **86:**5974–5978.

Eischen, C. M., Dick, C. J., and Leibson, P. J., 1994, Tyrosine kinase activation provides an early and requisite signal for Fas-induced apoptosis, *J. Immunol.* **153:**1947–1954.

Embretson, J., Zupancic, M., Ribas, J. L., Burke, A., Racz, P., Tenner-Racz, K., and Haase, A. T., 1993, Massive covert infection of helper T lymphocytes and macrophages by HIV during the incubation period of AIDS, *Nature* **362:**359–362.

Emille, D., Permutter, M., Malliot, M. C., Brousse, N., Delfraissy, J. F., Dormont, J., and Galanaud, P., 1990, Production of interleukins in human immunodeficiency virus-1-replicating lymph nodes, *J. Clin. Invest.* **86:** 148–159.

Enari, M., Hug, H., and Nagata, S., 1995, Involvement of an ICE-like protease in Fas-mediated apoptosis, *Nature* **375:**78–81.

Fan, J., Bass, H. Z., and Fahey, J. L., 1993, Elevated INF-γ and decreased IL-2 gene expression are associated with HIV infection, *J. Immunol.* **151:**5031–5040.

Fernandes-Alnemri, T., Litwack, G., and Alnemri, E. S., 1994, CPP32, a novel human apoptotic protein with homology to *Caenorhabdtis elegans* cell death protein Ced-3 and mammalian interleukin-1β-converting enzyme, *J. Biol. Chem.* **269:**30761–30764.

Finkel, T. H., Tudor-Williams, G., Banda, N. K., Cotton, M. F., Curiel, T., Monks, C., Baba, T. W., Ruorecht, R. M., and Kupfer, A., 1995, Apoptosis occurs predominantly in bystander cells and not in productively infected cells of HIV- and SIV-infected lymph nodes, *Nature Med.* **1:**129–134.

Fisher, G. H., Rosenberg, F. J., Straus, S. E., Dale, J. K., Middleton, L. A., Lin, A. Y., Strober, W., Lenardo, M. J., and Puck, J. M., 1995, Dominant interfering Fas gene mutations impair apoptosis in a human autoimmune lymphoproliferative syndrome, *Cell* **81:**935–946.

Foster, S., Beverley, P., and Aspinall, R., 1995, gp120-induced programmed cell death in recently activated T cells without subsequent ligation of the T cell receptor, *Eur. J. Immunol.* **25:**1778–1782.

Fuller, K. A., Kanagawa, O., and Nahm, M. H., 1993, T cells within germinal centers are specific for the immunizing antigen, *J. Immunol.* **151:**4505–4512.

Gendelman, H. E., Ehrlich, G. D., Baca, L. M., Conley, S., Ribas, J., Kalter, D. C., Melzer, M. S., Poiez, B. J., and Nara, P., 1991, The inability of human immunodeficiency virus to infect chimpanzee monocytes can be overcome by serial passage in vivo, *J. Virol.* **65:**3853–3863.

Gessani, S., Puddu, P., Varano, B., Borghi, P., Conti, L., Fantuzzi, L., and Belardelli, F., 1994, Induction of beta interferon by human immunodeficiency virus type 1 and its gp120 protein in human monocyte macrophage, *J. Virol.* **68:**1983–1986.

Gibellini, D., Caputo, A., Celeghini, C., Bassini, A., La Placa, M., Capitani, S., and Zauli, G., 1995, Tat-expressing Jurkat cells show an increased resistance to different apoptotic stimuli, including acute human immunodeficiency virus-type 1 (HIV-1) infection, *Br. J. Haematol.* **89:**24–33.

Gratiot-Deans, J., Merino, R., Nunez, G., and Turka, L. A., 1994, Bcl-2 expression during T cell development:

Early loss and late return occur at specific stages of commitment to differentiation and survival, *Proc. Natl. Acad. Sci. USA* **91**:10685–10689.

Graziosi, C., Pantaleo, G., Gantt, K. R., Fortin, J.-P., Demarrest, J. F., Cohen, O. J., Sèkaly, R. P., and Fauci, A. S., 1994, Lack of evidence for the dichotomy of Th1 and Th2 predominance in HIV-infected individuals, *Science* **265**:248–252.

Grell, M., Zimmermann, G., Hülser, D., Pfizenmaier, K., and Scheurich, P., 1994, TNF receptors TR60 and TR80 can mediate apoptosis via induction of distinct signal pathways, *J. Immunol.* **153**:1963–1972.

Gribben, J. G., Freeman, G. J., Boussiotis, V. A., Rennert, P., Jellis, C., Greenfield, E., Barber, M., Restivo, V. A., Jr., Ke, X., Gray, G., and Nadler, L. K., 1995, CTLA4 mediates antigen-specific apoptosis of human T-cells, *Proc. Natl. Acad. Sci. USA* **92**:811–815.

Groux, H., Torpier, G., Montè, D., Mounton, Y., Capon, A., and Ameisen, J.-C., 1992, Activation-induced death by apoptosis in CD4+ T cells from human immunodeficiency-infected asymptomatic individuals, *J. Exp. Med.* **175**:331–340.

Groux, H., Monte, D., Plouvier, B., Capon, A., and Ameisen, J.-C., 1993, CD3-mediated apoptosis of human medullary thymocytes and activated T cells: Respective roles of interleukin-1, interleukin-2, interferon-γ and accessory cells, *Eur. J. Immunol.* **23**:1623–1629.

Gulbins, E., Bissonnette, R., Mahboubi, A., Martin, S., Nishioka, W., Brunner, T., Baier, G., Baier-Bitterlich, G., Byrd, C., Lang, F., Kolesnick, R., Altman, A., and Green, D., 1995, Fas-induced apoptosis is mediated via a ceramide-initiated Ras signaling pathway, *Immunity* **2**:341–351.

Herron, L. R., Eisenberg, R. A., Roper, E., Kakkanaiah, V. N., Cohen, P. P. L., and Kotzin, B. L., 1993, Selection of the T cell receptor repertoire in lpr mice, *J. Immunol.* **151**:3450–3459.

Heusel, J., Wesselschmidt, R. L., Shresta, S., Russel, J. H., and Ley, T. J., 1994, Cytotoxic lymphocytes require granzyme B for the rapid induction of DNA fragmentation and apoptosis in allogeneic target cells, *Cell* **76**:977–987.

Ho, D. D., Neumann, A. U., Perelson, A. S., Chen, W., Leonard, J. M., and Markowitz, M., 1995, Rapid turnover of plasma virions and CD4 lymphocytes in HIV-1 infection, *Nature* **373**:123–126.

Hügin, A. W., Vacchio, M. S., and Morse, H. C., III, 1991, A virus-encoded "superantigen" in a retrovirus-induced immunodeficiency syndrome of mice, *Science* **252**:424–427.

Itoh, N., and Nagata, S., 1993, A novel protein domain required for apoptosis. Mutational analysis of human Fas antigen, *J. Biol. Chem.* **268**:10932–10937.

Itoh, N., Yonehara, S., Ishii, A., Yonehara, M., Mizushima, S., Sameshima, M., Hase, A., Seto, Y., and Nagata, N., 1991, The polypeptide encoded by the cDNA for human cell surface antigen Fas can mediate apoptosis, *Cell* **66**:233–243.

Itoh, N., Tsujimoto, Y., and Nagata, S., 1993, Effect of bcl-2 on Fas antigen-mediated cell death, *J. Immunol.* **151**:621–627.

Jaleco, A. C., Covas, M. J., and Victorino, R. M. M., 1994, Analysis of lymphocyte cell death and apoptosis in HIV-2-infected patients, *Clin. Exp. Immunol.* **98**:185–189.

Johnson, B. K., Stone, G. A., Godec, M. S., Asher, D. M., Gajdusek, D. C., and Gibbs, C. J., Jr., 1993, Long-term observations of human immunodeficiency virus-infected chimpanzees, *AIDS Res. Hum. Retrovir.* **9**:375–378.

Joling, P., Bakker, L. J., Strijp, J. A. G., Meerloo, T., de Graaf, L., Dekker, M. E. M., Goudsmit, J., Verhoef, J., and Schuurman, H.-J., 1993, Binding of human immunodeficiency virus type-1 to follicular dendritic cells in vitro is complement dependent, *J. Immunol.* **150**:1065–1073.

Ju, S. T., Cui, H., Panka, D., Ettinger, R., and Marshak-Rothstein, A., 1994, Participation of target Fas protein in apoptosis pathway induced by CD4+ Th1 and CD8+ cytotoxic T cells, *Proc. Natl. Acad. Sci. USA* **91**:4185–4189.

Ju, S. T., Panka, D. J., Cui, H., Ettinger, R., El-Khatib, M., Sherr, D. H., Stanger, B. Z., and Marshak-Rothstein, A., 1995, Fas (CD95)/FasL interactions required for programmed cell death after T cell activation, *Nature* **373**:444–448.

Käji, D., Vignaux, F., Lederman, B., Bürki, K., Depraetere, V., Nagata, S., Hengartner, H., and Golstein, P., 1994, Fas and perforin pathways as major mechanisms of T cell-mediated cytotoxicity, *Science* **265**:528–530.

Katsikis, P. D., Wunderlich, E. S., Smith, C. A., Herzenberg, L. A., and Herzenberg, L. A., 1995, Fas antigen stimulation induces marked apoptosis of T Lymphocytes in human immunodeficiency virus-infected individuals, *J. Exp. Med.* **181**:2029–2036.

Kaufman, S. H., Desnoyers, S., Ottaviano, Y., Davidson, N. E., and Poirier, G. G., 1993, Specific proteolytic cleavage of poly(ADP-ribose) polymerase: An early marker of chemotherapy-induced apoptosis, *Cancer Res.* **53**:3976–3985.

Kearney, E. R., Pape, K. A., Loh, D. Y., and Jenkins, M. K., 1994, Visualization of peptide-specific T cell immunity and peripheral tolerance induction in vivo, *Immunity* **1**:327–339.

Kerr, J. F. R., Wyllie, A. H., and Currie, A. R., 1972, Apoptosis: A basic biological phenomenon with wide ranging implication in tissue kinetics, *Br. J. Cancer* **26**:239–257.

Kobayashi, N., Hamamoto, Y., Yamamoto, N., Ishii, A., Yonehara, M., and Yonehara, S., 1990, Anti-Fas monoclonal antibody is cytocidal to human immunodeficiency virus-infected cells without augmenting viral replication, *Proc. Natl. Acad. Sci. USA* **87**:9620–9624.

Koga, Y., Nakamura, K., Sasaki, M., Kimura, G., and Nomoto, K., 1992, The difference in gp160 and gp120 of HIV type 1 in the induction of CD4 downregulation preceding single-cell killing, *Virology* **201**:137–141.

Kojima, H., Someya-Shinohara, Y., Takagaki, Y., Ohno, H., Saito, T., Katayama, T., Yagita, H., Okumura, K., Shinkai, Y., Alt, F. W., Matsuzaki, A., Yonehara, S., and Takayama, H., 1994, Two distinct pathways of specific killing revealed by perforin mutant cytotoxic T lymphocytes, *Immunity* **1**:357–364.

Kovacs, J. A., Baseler, M., Dewar, R. J., Vogel, S., Davey, R. T., Jr., Falloon, J., Polis, M. A., Walker, R. E., Stevens, R., Salzman, N. P., Metcalf, J. A., Masur, H., and Lane, H. C., 1995, Increases in CD4 T lymphocytes with intermittent courses of interleukin-2 in patients with human immunodeficiency virus infection, *N. Engl. J. Med.* **332**:567–575.

Kowalski, M., Bergerson, L., Dorfman, T., Haseltine, W., and Sodorski, J., 1991, Attenuation of human immunodeficiency virus type 1 cytopathic effect by a mutation affecting the transmembrane envelope protein, *J. Virol.* **65**:281–291.

Krowka, J. F., Sheppard, H. W., Acher, M. S., Fitzpatrick, P., Kiefer, M. C., Pavioff, N., and Barr, P. J., 1994, Soluble CD95 inhibits HIV-related apoptosis, *Xth Int. Conf. AIDS, Yokohama* (Abstr. #PA0105).

Kuida, K., Lippke, J. A., Ku, G., Harding, M. W., Livingston, D. J., Su, M. S., and Flavell, R. A., 1995, Altered cytokine export and apoptosis in mice deficient in interleukin-1β converting enzyme, *Science* **267**:2000–2003.

Lahdevirta, J., Maury, C. P. J., Teppo, A.-M., and Repo, H., 1988, Elevated levels of circulating cachectin/tumor necrosis factor in patients with acquired immunodeficiency syndrome, *Am. J. Med.* **85**:289–291.

Laurent-Crawford, A. G., Krust, B., Muller, S., Riviere, Y., Rey-Culle, M.-A., Bechet, J. M., Montagnier, L., and Hovanessian, A. G., 1991, The cytopathic effect of HIV is associated with apoptosis, *Virology* **185**:829–839.

Laurent-Crawford, A. G., Krust, B., Muller, S., Riviere, Y., Desgranges, C., Muller, S., Kieny, M. P., Daugust, C., and Hovanessian, A. G., 1993, Membrane expression of HIV envelope glycoprotein triggers apoptosis in CD4 cells, *AIDS Res. Hum. Retrovir.* **9**:761–773.

Leonardo, M. J., 1991, Interleukin-2 programs mouse αβ T lymphocytes for apoptosis, *Nature* **363**:858–861.

Lewis, D. E., Ng Tang, D. S., Adu-Oppong, A., Schober, W., and Rodgers, J. R., 1994, Anergy and apoptosis in CD8+ T cells from HIV-infected persons, *J. Immunol.* **153**:412–420.

Li, C., Friedman, D. J., Wang, C., Metelev, V., and Pardee, A. B., 1995, Induction of apoptosis in uninfected lymphocytes by HIV-1 tat protein, *Science* **268**:429–431.

Lifson, J. D., Feinberg, M. B., Reyes, G. R., Rabin, L., Banapour, B., Chakrabarti, S., Moss, B., Wong-Staal, F., Steimer, K. S., and Engleman, E. B., 1986, Induction of CD4-dependent cell fusion by the HTLVIII/LAV envelope protein, *Nature* **323**:725–728.

Liu, Y., and Janeway, C. A., Jr., 1990, Interferon γ plays a critical role in induced cell death of effector T cell: A possible third mechanism of self-tolerance, *J. Exp. Med.* **172**:1735–1739.

Los, M., de Craen, M. V., Penning, L. C., Schenk, H., Westendorp, M., Baeuerie, P. A., Dröge, W., Krammer, P. H., Fiers, W., and Schulze-Osthoff, K., 1995, Requirement of an ICE/CED-3 protease for Fas/Apo-1-mediated apoptosis, *Nature* **375**:81–83.

Lu, Y.-Y., Koga, Y., Tanaka, K., Sasaki, M., Kimura, G., and Nomotom, K., 1994, Apoptosis induced in CD4+ cells expressing gp160 of human immunodeficiency virus type 1, *J. Virol.* **68**:390–399.

Lynch, D. H., Watson, M. L., Alderson, M. R., Baum, P. R., Miller, R. E., Tough, T., Gibson, M., Davis-Smith, T., Smith, C. A., Hunter, K., Bhat, D., Din, W., Goodwin, R. G., and Seldin, M. F., 1994, The mouse Fas-ligand gene is mutated in gld mice and is part of TNF family gene cluster, *Immunity* **1**:131–136.

McCloskey, T. W., Oyaizu, N., Kaplan, M., and Pahwa, S., 1995, Expression of the Fas antigen in patients infected with human immunodeficiency virus, *Cytometry* **22**:111–114.

Meyaard, L., Otto, S. A., Jonker, R. R., Mijnster, M. J., Keet, R. P. M., and Miedema, F., 1992, Programmed death of T cells in HIV-1 infection, *Science* **257**:217–219.

Meyaard, L., Otto, S. A., Keet, R. P. M., Roos, M. T. L., and Miedema, F., 1994, Programmed death of T cells in human immunodeficiency virus infection, *J. Clin. Invest.* **93**:982–988.

Miyawaki, T., Uehara, T., Nibu, R., Tsuji, T., Yachie, A., Yonehara, S., and Taniguchi, N., 1992, Differential expression of apoptosis-related Fas antigen on lymphocyte subpopulation in human peripheral blood, *J. Immunol.* **149**:3753–3758.

Miyazaki, T., Liu, Z.-J., Kawahara, A., Minami, Y., Yamada, K., Tsujimoto, Y., Barsoumian, E. L., Perimutter, R. M., and Taniguchi, T., 1995, Three distinct IL-2 signaling pathways mediated by bcl-2, c-myc, and lck cooperate in hematopoietic cell proliferation, *Cell* **81**:223–231.

Mosier, D. E., Gulizia, R. J., MacIsaac, P. D., Torbett, B. E., and Levy, J. A., 1993, Rapid loss of CD4+ T cells in human-PBL-SCID mice by noncytopathic HIV isolates, *Science* **260**:689–692.

Muro-Cacho, C. A., Pantaleo, G., and Fauci, A. S., 1995, Analysis of apoptosis in lymph nodes of HIV-infected persons, *J. Immunol.* **154**:5555–5566.

Nagata, S., and Goldstein, P., 1995, The Fas death factor, *Science* **267**:1449–1456.

Nakayama, K., Nakayama, K.-I., Negishi, I., Kuida, K., Sawa, H., and Loh, D. Y., 1994, Target disruption of Bcl-2αβ in mice: Occurrence of gray hair, polycystic kidney disease, and lymphocytopenia, *Proc. Natl. Acad. Sci. USA* **91**:3700–3704.

Newell, M. K., Haughn, L. J., Maroun, C. R., and Julius, M. H., 1990, Death of mature T cells by separate ligation of CD4 and the T-cell receptor for antigen, *Nature* **347**:286–289.

Nicholson, D. W., Ali, A., Thornberry, N. A., Vaillancourt, J. P., Ding, C. K., Gallant, M., Gareau, Y., Griffin, P. R., Labelle, M., Lazebnik, Y. A., Munday, N. A., Raju, S. M., Smulson, M. E., Yamin, T.-T., Yu, V. L., and Miller, D. K., 1995, Identification and inhibition of the ICE/CED-3 protease necessary for mammalian apoptosis, *Nature* **376**:37–43.

Novelli, F., Pierro, F., diCelle, P. F., Bertini, S., Affaticati, P., Garotta, G., and Forni, G., 1994, Environmental signals influence expression of the IFN-γ receptor on human T cells control whether IFN-γ promotes proliferation or apoptosis, *J. Immunol.* **152**:496–504.

Obeid, L. M., Linardic, C. M., Karolak, L. A., and Hannun, Y. A., 1993, Programmed cell death induced by ceramide, *Science* **259**:1769–1771.

Oh, S.-K., Cruikshank, W. W., Raina, J., Blanchard, G. C., Adler, W. H., Walker, J., and Kornfeld, H., 1992, Identification of HIV-1 envelope glycoprotein in the serum of AIDS and ARC patients, *J. Acq. Immune Defic. Syndr.* **5**:251–256.

O'Hara, C. J., 1989, Lymphoid system, in: *Pathology and Pathophysiology of AIDS and HIV-Related Diseases* (S. J. Harawi and C. J. O'Hara, eds.) Chapman & Hall, London, pp. 136–183.

Oltvai, Z., Milliman, C. L., and Korsmeyer, S. J., 1993, Bcl-2 heterodimerizes in vivo with a conserved homolog, Bax, that accelerates programmed cell death, *Cell* **74**:609–619.

Owen-Schaub, L. B., Yonehara, S., Crump, W. L., III, and Grimm, E. A., 1992, DNA fragmentation and cell death is selectively triggered in activated human lymphocytes by Fas antigen engagement, *Cell. Immunol.* **140**: 197–295.

Oyaizu, N., Chirmule, N., Ohnishi, Y., Kalyanaraman, V. S., and Pahwa, S., 1991, Human immunodeficiency virus type 1 envelope glycoprotein gp120 and gp160 induce interleukin-6 production in CD4+ T-cell clones, *J. Virol.* **65**:6277–6282.

Oyaizu, N., Chirmule, N., Kalyanaraman, V. S., Hall, W. W., Good, R. A., and Pahwa, S., 1990, Human immunodeficiency virus type 1 envelope protein gp120 produces immune defects in CD4+ T lymphocytes by inhibiting interleukin 2 mRNA, *Proc. Natl. Acad. Sci. USA* **87**:2379–2383.

Oyaizu, N., Chirmule, N., and Pahwa, S., 1992, Role of CD4 molecule in the induction of interleukin 2 and interleukin 2 receptor in class II major histocompatibility complex-restricted antigen specific T helper clones, *J. Clin. Invest.* **89**:1807–1816.

Oyaizu, N., McCloskey, T. W., Coronesi, M., Chirmule, N., Kalyanaraman, V. S., and Pahwa, S., 1993, Accelerated apoptosis in peripheral blood mononuclear cells (PBMC) from human immunodeficiency virus type-1 infected patients and in CD4 cross-linked PBMCs from normal individuals, *Blood* **82**:3392–3400.

Oyaizu, N., McCloskey, T. W., Soe Than, Hu, R., Kalyanaraman, V. S., and Pahwa, S., 1994, Crosslinking of CD4 molecules up-regulates Fas antigen expression in lymphocytes by inducing interferon γ and tumor necrosis factor-α secretion, *Blood* **84**:2622–2631.

Pahwa, S., Pahwa, R., Saxinger, C., Gallo, R. C., and Good, R. A., 1985, Influence of the human T-lymphotropic virus/lymphadenopathy-associated virus on functions of human lymphocytes: Evidence for immunosuppressive effects and polyclonal B-cell activation by banded viral preparations, *Proc. Natl. Acad. Sci. USA* **82**:8198–8202.

Pantaleo, G., Graziosi, C., and Fauci, A. S., 1993a, The immuno-pathogenesis of human immunodeficiency virus infection, *N. Engl. J. Med.* **328**:327–335.

Pantaleo, G., Graziosi, C., Demarest, J. F., Butini, L., Montroni, M., Fox, C. H., Orenstein, J. M., Kotler, D. P., and Fauci, A. S., 1993b, HIV infection is active and progressive in lymphoid tissue during the clinically latent stage of disease, *Nature* **362**:355–358.

Poli, G., Bressler, P., Kinter, A., Duh, E., Timmer, W. C., Rabson, A., Justement, J. S., Stanley, S., and Fauci, A. S., 1990, Interleukin 6 induces human immunodeficiency virus expression in infected monocytic cells alone and in synergy with tumor necrosis factor α by transcriptional and post-transcriptional mechanisms, *J. Exp. Med.* **172**:151–158.

Pope, M., Betjes, M. G. H., Romani, N., Hirmand, H., Cameron, P. U., Hoffman, L., Gezelter, S., Schuler, G., and Steinman, R. M., 1994, Conjugate of dendritic cells and memory T lymphocytes from skin facilitate productive infection of HIV-1, *Cell* **78**:389–398.

Rieckmann, P., Poli, G., Fox, C. H., Kehrl, J. H., and Fauci, A. S., 1991, Recombinant gp120 specifically enhances tumor necrosis factor-α production and Ig secretion in B lymphocytes from HIV-infected individuals but not from seronegative donors, *J. Immunol.* **147**:2922–2927.,

Rivas, C. I., Golde, D. W., Vera, J. C., and Kolesnick, R. N., 1994, Involvement of the sphingomyelin pathway in autocrine tumor necrosis factor signaling for human immunodeficiency virus production in chronically infected HL-60 cells, *Blood* **83**:2191–2197.

Russell, J., Rush, B., Weaver, C., and Wang, R., 1993, Mature T cells of autoimmune lpr/lpr mice have a defect in antigen-stimulated suicide, *Proc. Natl. Acad. Sci. USA* **90**:4409–4413.

Saksela, K., Stevens, C., Rubinstein, P., and Baltimore, D., 1994, Human immunodeficiency virus type 1 mRNA expression in peripheral blood cells predicts disease progression independently of the numbers of CD4+ lymphocytes, *Proc. Natl. Acad. Sci. USA* **91**:1104–1108.

Salgame, P., Abrams, J. S., Clayberger, C., Goldstein, H., Convit, J., Modlin, R. T., and Bloom, B. R., 1991, Differential lymphokine profile of functional subsets of human CD4 and CD8 T cell clone, *Science* **254**: 279–282.

Salmon, M., Pilling, D., Borthwick, N. J., Viner, N., Janossy, G., Bacon, P. A., and Akbar, A. N., 1994, The progressive differentiation of primed T cells is associated with an increased susceptibility to apoptosis, *Eur. J. Immunol.* **24**:892–899.

Sarin, A., Adams, D. H., and Henkart, P. A., 1993, Protease inhibitors selectively block T-cell receptor-triggered programmed cell death in a murine T cell hybridoma and activated peripheral T-cells, *J. Exp. Med.* **178**:1693–1700.

Sarin, A., Clerici, M., Blatt, S. P., Hendrix, C. W., Shearer, G. M., and Henkart, P. A., 1994, Inhibition of activation-induced programmed cell death and restoration of defective immune responses of HIV+ donors by cysteine protease inhibitors, *J. Immunol.* **153**:862–872.

Sato, T., Irie, S., Kitada, S., and Reed, J. C., 1995, FAP-1: A protein tyrosine phosphatase that associates with Fas, *Science* **268**: 411–415.

Schnittman, S. M., Psallidopoulos, M., Lane, H. C., Thompson, L., Baseler, M., Massari, F., Fox, C. H., Salzmann, N. P., and Fauci, A. S., 1992, The reservoir for HIV-1 in human peripheral blood is a T cell that maintains expression of CD4, *Science* **245**:305–308.

Schuitemaker, H., Meyaard, L., Kootstra, N. A., Dubbes, R., Otto, S. A., Termette, M., Heeney, J. L., and Miedema, F., 1993, Lack of T cell dysfunction and programmed cell death in human immunodeficiency virus type 1-infected chimpanzees correlates with absence of monocytotropic variants, *J. Infect. Dis.* **168**:1140–1147.

Singer, G. G., and Abbas, A. K., 1994, The Fas antigen is involved in peripheral but not thymic deletion of T lymphocytes in T cell receptor transgenic mice, *Immunity* **1**:365–371.

Sodroski, J., Goh, W. C., Rosen, C. A., Campbell, K., and Haseltine, W., 1986, Role of the HTLV-III/LAV envelope in syncytium formation and cytopathicity, *Nature* **322**:470–474.

Somasundaran, M., and Robinson, H. L., 1987, A major mechanism of human immunodeficiency virus-induced cell killing does not involve cell fusion, *J. Virol.* **61**:3114–3119.

Stevenson, M., Meier, C., Mann, A. M., Chapman, N., and Wasiak, W., 1988, Envelope glycoprotein of HIV induces interference and cytolysis resistance in CD4+ cells: Mechanism for persistence in AIDS, *Cell* **53**:483–496.

Su, L., Kanesima, H., Bonyhadi, M., Salimi, S., Kraft, D., Rabin, L., and McCune, J. M., 1995a, HIV-1-induced thymocyte depletion is associated with indirect cytopathicity and infection of progenitor cells in vivo, *Immunity* **2**:25–36.

Su, X., Zhou, T., Wang, Z., Yang, P., Jope, R. S., and Mountz, J. D., 1995b, Defective expression of hematopoietic cell protein phosphatase (HCP) in lymphoid cells blocks Fas-mediated apoptosis, *Immunity* **2**:353–362.

Suda, T., Takahashi, T., Golstein, P., and Nagata, S., 1993, Molecular cloning and expression of the Fas ligand, a novel member of the tumor necrosis factor family, *Cell* **75**:1169–1178.

Suda, T., Okazaki, T., Naito, Y., Yokota, T., Arai, N., Ozaki, S., Nakao, K., and Nagata, S., 1995, Expression of Fas ligand in cells of T cell lineage, *J. Immunol.* **154:**3806–3813.

Takahashi, T., Tanaka, M., Brannan, C. I., Jenkins, N. A., Copeland, N. G., Suda, T., and Nagata, S., 1994, Generalized lymphoproliferative disease in mice, caused by a point mutation in the Fas ligand, *Cell* **76:** 969–976.

Takayama, S., Sato, T., Krajewski, S., Kochel, K., Irie, S., Millan, J., and Reed, J. C., 1995, Cloning and functional analysis of BAG-1: A novel Bcl-2 binding protein with anti-cell death activity, *Cell* **80:**279–284.

Tartaglia, L. A., Ayres, T. M., Wong, G. H. W., and Goeddel, D. V., 1993, A novel domain within the 55 kd TNF receptor signals cell death, *Cell* **74:**845–853.

Terai, C., Kornbluth, R. S., Pavia, D., Richman, D. D., and Carson, D. A., 1991, Apoptosis as a mechanism of cell death in cultured T lymphoblasts acutely infected with HIV-1, *J. Clin. Invest.* **87:**1710–1715.

Tewari, M., Quan, L. T., O'Rourke, K., Desnoyers, S., Zeng, Z., Beidler, D. R., Poirier, G. G., Salvesen, G. S., and Dixit, V. M., 1995, Yama/CPP32β, a mammalian homolog of CED-3, is a CrmA-inhibitable protease that cleaves the death substrate poly(ADP-ribose) polymerase, *Cell* **81:**801–809.

Than, S., Oyaizu, N., Kalyanaraman, V. S., and Pahwa, S., 1994, Effect of HIV-1 envelope protein gp160 on cytokine production from cord blood T cells, *Blood* **84:**184–188.

Ucker, D. S., Aswell, J. D., and Nickas, G., 1989, Activation-driven T cell death I. Requirements for de novo transcription and translation and association of genome fragmentation, *J. Immunol.* **143:**3461.

Uehara, T., Miyawaki, T., Ohta, K., Tamaru, Y., Yokoi, T., Nakamura, S., and Taniguchi, A., 1992, Apoptotic cell death of primed CD45R0+ T lymphocytes in Epstein–Barr virus-induced infectious mononucleosis, *Blood* **80:**452–458.

van den Eterwegh, A. J. M., Laman, V. D., Schellekens, M. M., Boersma, W. J. A., and Claassen, E., 1992, Complement-mediated follicular localization of T-independent type-2 antigens: The role of marginal zone macrophage, *Eur. J. Immunol.* **22:**719–726.

Van Veldhoven, P. P., Matthews, T. J., Bolognasi, D. P., and Bell, R. M., 1992, Change in bioactive lipids, alkyacylglycerol and ceramide, occur in HIV-infected cells, *Biochem. Biophys. Res. Commun.* **187:**209–216.

Wahl, L. M., Corcoran, M. L., Pyle, S. W., Arthur, L. O., Harel-Bellan, A., and Farrar, W., 1989, Human immunodeficiency virus glycoprotein (gp120) induction of monocyte arachidonic acid metabolites and interleukin 1, *Proc. Natl. Acad. Sci. USA* **86:**621–625.

Wang, J., Stolman, S. A., and Dennert, G., 1994, TCR cross-linking induces CTL death via internal action of TNF, *J. Immunol.* **152:**3824–3832.

Wang, Z., Dudhane, A., Orlikowsky, T., Clarke, K., Li, X., Darzynkeiwicz, Z., and Hoffmann, M. K., 1994a, CD4 engagement induces Fas antigen-dependent apoptosis in vivo, *Eur. J. Immunol.* **24:**1549–1552.

Wang, Z., Orlikowsky, T., Dudhane, A., Clarke, K., Li, X., Darzynkeiwicz, Z., and Hoffmann, M. K., 1994b, Deletion of T lymphocytes in human CD4 transgenic mice induced by HIV-gp120 and gp120-specific antibodies from AIDS patients, *Eur. J. Immunol.* **24:**1553–1557.

Watanabe, M., Ringler, D. J., Fultz, P. N., MacKey, J. J., Boyson, J. E., Levine, C. G., and Letvin, N. L., 1991, A chimpanzee-passaged human immunodeficiency virus isolate is cytopathic for chimpanzee cells but does not induce disease, *J. Virol.* **65:**3344–3348.

Watanabe-Fukunaga, R., Brannan, C. I., Copeland, N. G., Jenkins, N. A., and Nagata, S., 1992a, Lymphoproliferation disorder in mice explained by defects in Fas antigen that mediates apoptosis, *Nature* **356:**314–317.

Watanabe-Fukunaga, R., Brannan, C. I., Ito, N., Yonehara, S., Copeland, N. G., Jenkins, N. A., and Nagata, S., 1992b, The cDNA structure, expression, and chromosomal assignment of the mouse Fas antigen, *J. Immunol.* **148:**1274–1279.

Wei, X., Ghosh, S. K., Taylor, M. E., Johnson, V. A., Emini, E. A., Deutsch, P., Lifson, J. D., Bonhoeffer, S., Nowak, M. A., Hahn, B. H., Saag, M. S., and Shaw, G. M., 1995, Viral dynamics in human immunodeficiency virus type 1 infection, *Nature* **373:**117–122.

Weigmann, K., Schütze, S., Machleidt, T., Witte, D., and Krönke, M., 1994, Functional dichotomy of neutral and acid sphingomyelinases in tumor necrosis factor signaling, *Cell* **78:**1005–1015.

Westendorp, M. O., Frank, R., Ochsenbauer, C., Stricker, K., Dhein, J., Walczak, H., Debatin, K.-M., and Krammer, P. H., 1995, Sensitization of T cells to CD95-mediated apoptosis by HIV-1 and gp120, *Nature* **375:**495–500.

Wyllie, A. H., Kerr, J. F. R., and Currie, A. R., 1980, Cell death: The significance of apoptosis, *Int. Rev. Cytol.* **68:**251–306.

Yang, E., Zha, J., Jockel, J., Boise, L. H., Thompson, C. B., and Korsmeyer, S. J., 1995, Bad, a heterodimeric partner for Bcl-xL and Bcl-2, displaces Bax and promote cell death, *Cell* **80:**285–291.

Yin, X.-M., Oltvai, Z. N., and Korsmeyer, S. J., 1994, BH1 and BH2 domains of Bcl-2 are required for inhibition of apoptosis and heterodimerization with Bax, *Nature* **369:**321–323.

Yonehara, S., Ishii, A., and Yonehara, M., 1989, A cell-killing monoclonal antibody (anti-Fas) to a cell surface antigen co-downregulated with the receptor of tumor necrosis factor, *J. Exp. Med.* **169:**1747–1756.

Yoshino, T., Kondo, E., Cao, L., Takahashi, K., Hayashi, K., Nomura, S., and Akagi, T., 1994, Inverse expression of bcl-2 protein and Fas antigen in lymphoblasts in peripheral lymph nodes and activated peripheral blood T and B lymphocytes, *Blood* **83:**1856–1861.

Zauli, G., Gibellini, D., Milani, D., Mazzoni, M., Borgatti, P., La Placa, M., and Capitani, S., 1993, Human immunodeficiency virus type 1 tat protein protects lymphoid, epithelial, and neuronal cell lines from death by apoptosis, *Cancer Res.* **53:**4481–4485.

CHAPTER 8

BIOLOGICAL ACTIVITIES OF HIV-SPECIFIC PEPTIDES

STANLEY A. SCHWARTZ, MADHAVAN P. N. NAIR, and LINDA B. LUDWIG

1. INTRODUCTION

Infection with different viruses may produce immunologic dysfunctions in the host ranging from immunodeficiency states to autoimmune disorders. Generally it was assumed that these actions were related to the direct effects, including infection, of whole virions on target cells. These concepts became more sharply focused with the identification of the human immunodeficiency virus type 1 (HIV-1) and the recognition that it can infect a critical cell involved in the regulation of the immune response of humans, namely, the $CD4^+$ T lymphocyte. Earlier studies focused on the direct infection of $CD4^+$ cells by HIV-1 as the primary mechanism underlying the pathogenesis of the acquired immunodeficiency syndrome (AIDS). With the isolation and purification of HIV-1, it was shown that whole virions and crude extracts therefrom could induce *in vitro* some of the immunologic phenomena that were observed in clinical disease. It has been well documented that AIDS patients manifest a variety of immune dysfunctions including decreased lymphocyte proliferative responses to mitogens and antigens, decreased cellular cytotoxic activities and polyclonal B-lymphocyte activation (for a review see de Martini and Parker, 1989). However, the earlier observation that there was a poor correlation of peripheral virus load with extent of disease suggested that other, extrainfectious mechanisms may be contributing to disease progression. This led to our hypothesis that soluble factors such as proteins encoded by the HIV genome and shed by infected cells may also be involved in the pathogenesis of AIDS. Through the important observations of Fauci and his colleagues, we now know that the major repository of HIV in the infected host is the lymph nodes (Pantaleo *et al.*, 1991, 1993). Thus, while there may be a paucity of $CD4^+$ infected cells in the peripheral circulation of the infected host, significant viral proliferation and accumulation occurs in the lymph nodes.

STANLEY A. SCHWARTZ, MADHAVAN P. N. NAIR, and LINDA B. LUDWIG • Department of Medicine, State University of New York at Buffalo, Buffalo General Hospital, Buffalo, New York 14203.
Immunology of HIV Infection, edited by Sudhir Gupta. Plenum Press, New York, 1996.

Although these more recent studies now explain the earlier apparent paradox of relatively low numbers of infected cells in the peripheral blood even in patients with advanced disease, they do not negate the hypothesis that extrainfectious mechanisms (e.g., immunoregulatory, HIV-specific, soluble products) may also contribute to the pathogenesis of AIDS.

Our research group proposed the concept of the potential role of immunoregulatory HIV gene products in the pathogenesis of AIDS in 1988 when we examined several recombinant and synthetic HIV peptides as candidates for an HIV vaccine (Nair *et al.*, 1988). Initially we screened these peptides for biological activities prior to their use in clinical trials. We were impressed to observe that they were not inert in various *in vitro* assays, suggesting caution in considering their use as possible vaccine candidates. With this observation we hypothesized that various HIV peptides had potent biological activities which could contribute to the pathogenesis and progression of AIDS in addition to the direct infection of target cells. This chapter will review current evidence supporting this hypothesis.

2. ENVELOPE GLYCOPROTEINS

HIV-1 envelope and core proteins have been the subject of considerable investigation as vaccine candidates. Hence, we have substantial information regarding their biological activities. Earlier studies demonstrated that crude preparations of HIV-1 could induce lymphocyte proliferative responses, polyclonal B-cell activation, and suppression of B-cell proliferation to exogenous activators *in vitro* (Schnittman *et al.*, 1986; Pahwa *et al.*, 1985, 1986). However, since HIV-1 is a membrane-budding virus and whole virions also contain host cell membrane antigens, it remained to be determined which specific molecular components of the virus were responsible for the observed biological activities. As demonstrated in our initial investigations, a panel of pure, recombinant, and synthetic HIV-1 envelope peptides expressed significant immunoregulatory activities *in vitro* (Nair *et al.*, 1988). These peptides have been previously described (Crowl *et al.*, 1985; Certa *et al.*, 1986; Shoeman *et al.*, 1987). Furthermore, they were considered as potential candidates for an HIV-1 vaccine. Our original studies focused on gp41 and included the following peptide constructs, all of which include sequences from gp41: (1) a recombinant fusion product, env–gag, consisting of an 80-amino-acid sequence from the surface glycoprotein, gp41, and a 190-amino-acid sequence from the internal core protein, P24; (2) env-80 dihydrofolate reductase (DHFR), a synthetic oligonucleotide-based recombinant envelope peptide corresponding to a superconserved region of gp41; and (3) the synthetic peptides, env 487–511 and env 578–608. We demonstrated that the env–gag peptide could stimulate significant proliferation of peripheral blood lymphocytes (PBL) from normal donors *in vitro*. Moreover, env–gag is a potent polyclonal B-lymphocyte activator, capable of inducing substantial production of IgG from PBL from healthy donors *in vitro*. Paradoxically, however, env–gag could suppress pokeweed mitogen-induced immunoglobulin synthesis by normal PBL. In addition, we showed that the other HIV peptides, env-80 DHFR, env 487–511, and env 578–608, also could induce proliferation of PBL *in vitro*. Lastly, env–gag was capable of activating mitosis in both $CD3^+$ and $CD3^-$ PBL. Since all of these effects were mediated by peptides bearing sequences from gp41, it is evident that they were independent of binding to the CD4 receptor. Moreover, our data also demonstrated that specific domains of the entire gp41 molecule are biologically active. The mechanisms underlying these effects and the pathway(s) of signal transduction remain to be determined. Thus, these were the initial studies demonstrating that pure, HIV-1 peptides had significant immunoregulatory activities.

Earlier we reported that natural killer (NK) cell activity was depressed in intravenous drug abusers at high risk of HIV-1 infections (Nair *et al.*, 1986). Subsequently, others have demonstrated that NK cell dysfunction is a frequent finding among patients infected with HIV-1 as reviewed by Siranni *et al.* (1990) and Brenner *et al.* (1989). NK cells do not manifest the CD4 receptor for HIV-1 but may be infected by HIV-1 (Ruscetti *et al.*, 1986; Robinson *et al.*, 1988). Thus, we recently studied the effects of the above-mentioned HIV-1 gp41 peptides on the NK functions of lymphocytes from healthy donors. Data presented in Fig. 1 demonstrate the dose response effects of several peptides on the NK activities of normal lymphocytes. Cells were incubated for 72 hr with different peptides and assayed for NK cytotoxicity against the erythroleukemia cell line, K562, a standard NK cell target. The results are reported as percent inhibition of NK activity related to treatment with HIV-1 peptides calculated by comparison with the cytotoxicity produced by untreated, control lymphocytes. The fusion peptide, env–gag, at 10 and 50 ng/ml produced 30.5% ($p < 0.025$) and 20.8% ($p < 0.05$) suppression of cytotoxicity, respectively. However, env–gag at both lower (5 ng/ml) and higher (100 ng/ml) concentrations produced negligible suppression, 5 and 10%, respectively. A recombinant HIV peptide, env-DHFR, and a synthetic HIV peptide, env 578–608, produced negligible suppression of the NK activities of normal lymphocytes after culture for 72 hr. The effects of these latter peptides were also examined earlier after 24 and 48 hr of incubation with NK effector cells and no significant effects on cytotoxicity were observed (data not presented). Another synthetic peptide, env 487–511,

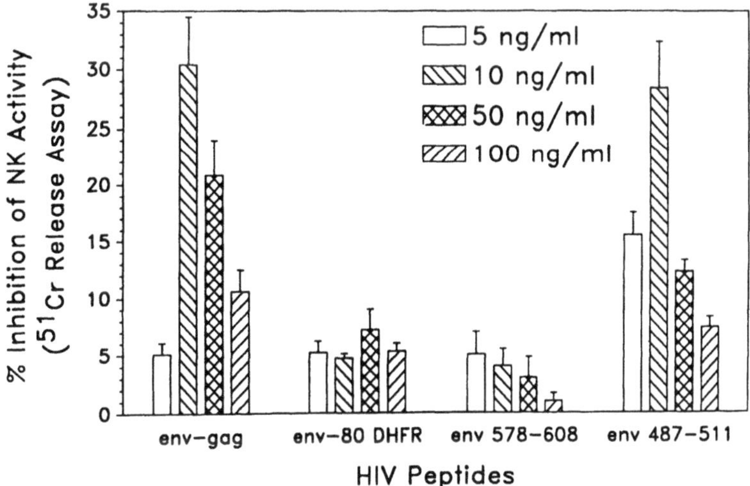

FIGURE 1. Effect of HIV peptides on the NK activity of normal lymphocytes. PBL (1×10^6) were cultured with varying concentrations of HIV peptides for 72 hr, washed, and tested for NK activity against K562 target cells at a 50:1 effector-to-target (E:T) cell ratio. Results are expressed as percent inhibition of NK activity calculated on the basis of the cytotoxicity obtained with untreated cultures. Cytotoxic activities of untreated lymphocytes varied from 30 to 40% at the 50:1 E:T cell ratio. Values are the mean ± S.D. of three experiments performed in triplicate. A description of the various HIV-1 peptides used can be found in the text.

manifested significant suppression (28.6%, $p < 0.02$) of the NK activities of normal PBL at a concentration of 10 ng/ml; however, other concentrations, 5, 50, and 100 ng/ml, did not produce any significant suppression.

Studies were also undertaken to examine the effects of direct addition of env–gag peptides without preincubation on the NK activity of lymphocytes from both normal donors and patients with AIDS. The number of $CD4^+$ cells were 50, 730, 120, 190, 60, 142, and 127 per mm^3 for patients 1, 2, 3, 4, 5, 7, and 8, respectively. When PBL from healthy donors as well as AIDS patients were mixed with the env–gag peptide and washed immediately and tested for NK activity (0 hr), no significant effect was observed (data not presented). However, when env–gag was added to the reaction mixture of effector and target cells and allowed to remain during the 4-hr assay period, significant suppression of NK activity occurred with lymphocytes from AIDS patients but no significant suppression was observed with normal lymphocytes (Table I). For example, direct addition of env–gag peptide significantly suppressed the NK activities of lymphocytes from AIDS patients #3 (36% suppression, $p < 0.0002$), #4 (45% suppression, $p < 0.0032$), #6 (25% suppression, $p < 0.0249$), #7 (45% suppression, $p < 0.0007$), and #8 (63% suppression, $p < 0.0200$). Moderate but not statistically significant suppression (20%) of the NK activity of lympho-

TABLE I. Direct Addition of HIV env–gag Peptide on the NK Activity of Lymphocytes from Normal Donors and AIDS Patients[a]

Source of lymphocytes	Treatment of lymphocytes	% Cytotoxicity[b]	
Normals	Medium	41.2 ± 5.0	$p < 0.31$[c]
	+ Env–gag	36.7 ± 4.7	
AIDS patients[d]			
# 1	Medium	28.3 ± 3.4	$p < 0.2844$
	+ Env–gag	23.7 ± 3.6	
# 2	Medium	32.8 ± 4.8	$p < 0.2098$
	+ Env–gag	26.0 ± 3.6	
# 3	Medium	60.1 ± 3.0	$p < 0.0002$
	+ Env–gag	38.3 ± 4.8	
# 4	Medium	16.8 ± 2.4	$p < 0.0032$
	+ Env–gag	9.2 ± 2.2	
# 5	Medium	28.7 ± 3.6	$p < 0.2017$
	+ Env–gag	24.1 ± 4.1	
# 6	Medium	22.7 ± 2.0	$p < 0.0249$
	+ Env–gag	17.0 ± 2.0	
# 7	Medium	26.3 ± 3.6	$p < 0.0007$
	+ Env–gag	14.5 ± 2.4	
# 8	Medium	25.7 ± 5.3	$p < 0.0200$
	+ Env–gag	9.4 ± 2.4	

[a]Env–gag peptide was added directly to the mixture of effector and target cells to obtain a final concentration of 50 ng/ml and NK activity against K562 targets was measured at a 50:1 E:T cell ratio in a 4-hr ^{51}Cr release assay (no preincubation of effector cells with env–gag peptides was performed).
[b]Values represent mean percent cytotoxicity ± S.D. of five separate experiments performed in triplicate using lymphocytes from healthy donors.
[c]Statistical significance of the difference was determined by two sample "t" test analyses between treated and untreated cultures.
[d]Lymphocytes from eight different AIDS patients were tested for their NK activity in five separate experiments; one normal lymphocyte sample was included in each experiment as a control for the AIDS sample.

cytes from patient #2 occurred with the addition of env–gag peptide. Lymphocytes from patients #1 and #5 treated with the env–gag peptide showed negligible suppression (16% each, $p < 0.2$) which was comparable to control lymphocytes (11% suppression, $p < 0.31$).

In summary, our observations on the effect of HIV peptides on NK functions are complex but consistent. Thus when lymphocytes from healthy donors were precultured with peptides containing domains from either gp120 or gp41, suppression of NK activity occurred following a unimodal dose response curve. However, when the fusion peptide, env-gag, consisting of sequences from the envelope glycoprotein, gp41, and the core protein, p24, was added directly without preculture to peripheral blood lymphocytes from healthy donors and patients with AIDS, the NK activities of only the AIDS patients were selectively suppressed. Furthermore, this effect can be mediated by selected domains of gp41 as demonstrated by the use of specific synthetic peptides from gp41. It has been reported that gp120 appears to inhibit $CD4^+$ T-lymphocyte functions by suppressing the expression of IL-2 and its subsequent synthesis (Oyaizu *et al.*, 1990; Liegler and Stites, 1994). However, it has not been determined if this also is the mechanism underlying the suppression of NK activity by peptides of gp41. We are currently attempting to resolve this question. In the experiments above it was observed that env–gag had a very restricted concentration range for inducing biological effects and concentrations above and below this range were not active. This is consistent with a similar narrow concentration range of env–gag on other lymphocyte functions described in our previous report (Nair *et al.*, 1988). Furthermore, the direct addition of env–gag peptide to a mixture of effector and target cells in a 4-hr ^{51}Cr release assay for NK activity, selectively inhibited the NK activity of PBL only from AIDS patients. This suppression did not correlate with the number of $CD4^+$ cells present and supports our hypothesis that HIV-1 peptides may be noninfectious mediators of disease progression in HIV-1 infections. We are currently trying to determine if the selective suppression of the NK activity of PBL from AIDS patients in these direct addition experiments is caused either by blocking binding of effectors to target cells or by inhibition of their lytic functions.

Pahwa and her colleagues have made significant progress in defining the biological effects of HIV envelope peptides. In their earlier investigations they utilized unfractionated protein extracts from purified, disrupted, whole virus preparations (Pahwa *et al.*, 1985, 1986). However, subsequent experiments employed pure envelope glycoproteins. Specifically they showed that native gp120 from HIV-1 could inhibit proliferation of lymphocytes from normal donors in response to treatment with anti-CD3 monoclonal antibodies and specific antigens such as tetanus toxoid (Chirmule *et al.*, 1988). The mechanism underlying these effects appears to be inhibition of IL-2 gene expression with a secondary inhibition of the expression of the α chain of the IL-2 receptor (Oyaizu *et al.*, 1990). However, all of these effects could be abrogated by the addition of IL-2 to the cultures.

3. REGULATORY PROTEINS

3.1. General Discussion

The complex retrovirus HIV-1 also encodes a set of proteins that play a critical role in regulating viral gene expression. One of the features distinguishing the replication cycle of a complex retrovirus, such as HIV-1, from the simple retroviruses is the presence and requirement for the multiply spliced viral transcripts encoding the nuclear regulatory proteins (Cullen, 1992). Whereas the simple retroviruses, once in proviral form, are able to utilize host cell transcription factors to produce a high level of proviral transcripts, the complex retroviruses require the viral regulatory factors tat and rev, in addition to the host cell transcriptional machinery, for efficient viral gene expression (Cullen, 1992; Varmus and Brown, 1989; Sodroski *et al.*, 1984, 1985). The HIV-1 proteins, tat, rev, and nef, are synthesized early following establishment of the proviral form of the virus. The initial population of HIV-1 transcripts reaching the cell cytoplasm appear to be exclusively in the form of small, multiply spliced mRNAs encoding these viral regulatory proteins (Cullen, 1992; Sodroski *et al.*, 1984, 1985, 1986; Arya *et al.*, 1985; Feinberg *et al.*, 1986). The regulatory proteins tat and rev act *in trans* to directly regulate HIV-1 gene expression (Cullen, 1992). The nef gene product, unlike tat and rev, is not required for HIV-1 replication in culture, although some have found that it can enhance the replication of certain HIV-1 isolates in culture (Terwilliger *et al.*, 1991). That nef plays an important role, however, in the viral life cycle is suggested by the conservation of the nef open reading frame in all primate lentiviruses (Myers and Pavlakis, 1991). Each of these HIV-1 regulatory proteins will be discussed with respect to potential mechanisms of activity during the HIV-1 life cycle within the cell, as compared and contrasted with observed, external, extrainfectious effects on surrounding immune cells that may be contributing to the pathogenesis of AIDS.

3.2. Tat

Of the various regulatory gene products of HIV-1, the transactivator of transcription (tat) protein is considered important for viral replication since replication cannot proceed in its absence. This protein is concentrated in the nucleus and nucleolus of HIV-1-infected cells (Ruben *et al.*, 1989; Rappaport *et al.*, 1989). The tat protein binds to a pyrimidine bulge in the stem loop of the transactivation response (TAR) RNA structure found at the 5′ end of all HIV-1 mRNAs. Although several cellular proteins are known to bind to the TAR RNA (Gatignol *et al.*, 1989; Marciniak *et al.*, 1990a,b), their precise roles have not been clearly elucidated.

The apparent molecular size of tat is 15.5 kDa, with the full-length protein consisting of 86 amino acids. The tat protein is encoded by two exons. The first encodes amino acid residues 1 through 72, while the second encodes 14 C-terminal residues containing an arginine–glycine–aspartic acid (RGD) sequence near the C-terminal region. Mutational studies and the use of synthetic proteins have helped to identify the functional domains on the tat protein. In addition to the basic domain consisting of an arginine-rich motif common to other sequence-specific RNA-binding proteins, tat contains two other distinct functional domains (Lazinski *et al.*, 1989). One domain (amino acids 22–37) includes a clustering of seven cysteine residues in a highly conserved motif. This domain binds Zn^{2+} and assists in dimerization. A group of acidic residues forming part of an amphipathic, α-helical structure at the N-terminus is proposed as the activation domain of tat (Frankel *et al.*, 1988; Rappaport *et al.*, 1989). The polypeptide product of the first exon exhibits two important domains while a basic domain consisting of an arginine-rich sequence (amino acids 38–58) is responsible for targeting tat to the nucleus (Endo *et al.*, 1989) and for its transactivation properties (Mann and Frankel, 1991; Endo *et al.*, 1989). The amino acid sequence 73–86, encoded by the second exon, also contains transactivation activity similar to amino acid sequence 38–58. This led to the conclusion that residues 73–86 are unnecessary for transactivation activity (Cullen, 1986; Muesing *et al.*, 1987; Frankel and Pabo, 1988). The second exon encodes amino acids 73–86 which contain an RGD sequence (amino acids 78–80) (Brake *et al.*, 1990). The biological function(s) of this domain is unknown although studies have shown that it possesses potential binding properties to integrin receptors on cells and also may contribute to the stabilization of the tat–TAR complex.

In most cellular contexts, the basal transcriptional activity of the HIV-1 long terminal repeat (LTR) is quite low (Garcia *et al.*, 1987; Nabel and Baltimore, 1987). Of the early gene products, tat is one of the first to exert its effect on the HIV-1 LTR, and functionally results in a large (100-fold) increase in HIV-1 LTR-dependent gene expression (Sodroski *et al.*, 1985; Arya *et al.*, 1985). This enhanced proviral transcription leads to further accumulation of tat and a second regulatory protein, rev, as well as nef. Rev inhibits the further synthesis of multiply spliced mRNAs, and facilitates the appearance of the unspliced and singly spliced mRNAs that encode the HIV-1 structural proteins in the cytoplasm, where translation can occur (Felber *et al.*, 1989; Feinberg *et al.*, 1986; Hanly *et al.*, 1989; Malim *et al.*, 1989). Both a functional tat gene product, and a *cis*-acting target sequence for tat called the transactivation response element (TAR) are required for HIV-1 replication (Rosen *et al.*, 1985; Fisher *et al.*, 1986; Dayton *et al.*, 1986).

TAR is an RNA sequence containing a 59-nucleotide stem loop structure and is present at the 5′ end of all HIV-1 transcripts (Rosen *et al.*, 1985; Muesing *et al.*, 1987; Jacobovits *et al.*, 1988; Hauber and Cullen, 1988). While the *in vitro* interaction between tat and TAR occurs at the site of a small, pyrimidine-rich bulge, mutations of the 6-nucleotide terminal loop sequence of TAR are equally deleterious *in vivo*, suggesting that other factors or cellular proteins capable of interacting with either TAR or tat are important for tat function *in vivo* (Feng and Holland, 1988; Berkhout and Jeang, 1989; Dingwall *et al.*, 1990; Selby *et al.*, 1989; Roy *et al.*, 1990a,b; Weeks and Crothers, 1991; Sumner-Smith *et al.*, 1991).

While many studies demonstrate that tat increases the steady-state level of transcripts, there has been controversy regarding the mechanism. It is probable that tat functions at several interrelated levels to manipulate HIV-1 gene expression, with recent evidence suggesting a major role in promoting transcription elongation (Rittner *et al.*, 1995; Selby *et al.*, 1989; Laspia *et al.*, 1989; Southgate and Green, 1991; Sharp and Marciniak, 1989; Kao *et al.*, 1987; Cullen, 1990; Ratnasabapathy *et al.*, 1990; Feinberg *et al.*, 1991; Kessler and Mathews, 1991; Marciniak *et al.*, 1990a,b). In addition, in a *Xenopus* oocyte system, tat was shown to exert a posttranscriptional effect (Braddock *et al.*, 1989). It has been proposed that tat functions as a sequence-specific, RNA-binding, antitermination protein (Selby *et al.*, 1989; Greenblatt *et al.*, 1993). Mutants of tat produce viral transcripts that hybridize to proximal HIV DNA (promoter) sequences, but not to sequences farther away from the promoter region. In the presence of tat, however, long HIV-1 viral transcripts are produced that hybridize to sequences spanning the length of the HIV transcription unit. Thus, the presence of tat interacting with TAR near the 5′ end of all HIV-1 transcripts enables RNA polymerase II, presumably in conjunction with cellular protein(s), to synthesize through a transcriptional block (Greenblatt *et al.*, 1993). The C-terminal basic domain of the tat protein is responsible for TAR binding, and is required for nuclear and nucleolar localization (Hauber *et al.*, 1989; Ruben *et al.*, 1989; Siomi *et al.*, 1990).

The powerful transactivation capabilities of tat, and the potential of tat interaction with other cellular proteins have led to recent proposals of tat activation occurring independently of the TAR element (Harrich *et al.*, 1990; Taylor *et al.*, 1992b, 1995; Buonaguro *et al.*, 1992;

Howcroft *et al.*, 1993). These models propose that tat engages in protein–protein interaction (directly or indirectly via an "adaptor protein") with yet other transcriptional factors that then exhibit enhanced binding to their target sequences, such as the NF-κB element. This transactivation capability may play a role in the observed mitogenic effects of extracellular HIV-1 tat that promotes the G1–S transition of endothelial cells and is believed to be involved, along with inflammatory cytokines, in the induction of Kaposi's sarcoma (Fiorelli *et al.*, 1995).

Although tat is essential for viral replication, it has been observed that its actions may not be restricted to HIV replication, and also involve pleiotropic effects on the immune, vascular, and central nervous systems of the host. Earlier studies showed that tat may be concentrated *in vivo* in lymphoid tissues at sites where HIV-1 replication is most active during the clinically latent period of infection (Embretson *et al.*, 1993; Pantaleo *et al.*, 1993).

In vitro studies demonstrated that tat is secreted by HIV-infected or tat-transfected cells into extracellular medium, is taken up by cells (Frankel and Pabo, 1988), reaches the nucleus (Mann and Frankel, 1991), and manifests either stimulatory or inhibitory effects (Ensoli *et al.*, 1993; Viscidi *et al.*, 1989). Earlier studies have shown that tat stimulates cell adhesion and growth by interaction of its RGD sequences with the integrins $\alpha5\beta1$ and $\alpha_v\beta3$, the receptors for extracellular matrix fibronectin and vitronectin, respectively (Barillari *et al.*, 1992, 1993). The basic region of tat has been shown to bind with the target through interaction with the integrin $\alpha_v\beta5$ (Vogel *et al.*, 1993). Zauli *et al.* (1993) showed that constitutively expressed tat protected lymphoid, epithelial, and neuronal cells from apoptosis induced by serum starvation.

In transfection experiments, tat demonstrated the capacity to induce dysregulation of various growth factors and inflammatory cytokine genes. Sastry *et al.* (1990) demonstrated the induction of TNF β gene expression in Raji cells transfected with the HIV-1 tat gene. They suggested that tat may be associated with the induction of TNF β genes which in turn may stimulate growth in a variety of cell types. The possibility that tat could affect the transcription of the IL-6 gene, which contains NF-κB and NF-IL-6 enhancer elements, was examined by Scala *et al.* (1994). They demonstrated that by cotransfecting the P IL 6Pr-CAT and tat-expressing pSVT8 plasmid in MC3-lymphoblastoid or in HeLa epithelial cells, tat transactivates the human IL-6 promoter. Buonaguro *et al.*(1992, 1994) have shown that HIV-1 tat protein transactivates the expression of TNF α and β genes, but not IL-1 and IL-6 genes in monocytic (U937), T-lymphocytic (H-9 and Jurkat), and epithelial (COS-1) cell lines transiently or permanently expressing tat gene. Tat-transfected H-9 cells also secreted higher levels of IL-10, a Th-2-derived cytokine, whereas rIL-10 inhibited HIV-1 replication in infected monocytes and PBMCs suggesting a role of IL-10 in the long latency between HIV-1 infection and development of AIDS (Masood *et al.*, 1994). Further, the tat-transfected H-9 cell line when stimulated with mitogen, showed a significant decrease in IL-2 mRNA and protein as well as expression of IL-2 receptor α and β chains, whereas IL-4R expression was unchanged (Puri *et al.*, 1995). These observations suggest that the immunosuppressive effects of tat, at least in part, may be mediated through the dysfunction of the expression of various cytokines. However, Westendorp *et al.* (1994) using IL-2 promoter chloramphenicol acetyltransferase (CAT) constructs, and IL-2-secreting Jurkat T cells showed that endogenous and exogenous tat enhances IL-2 expression in activated T cells.

Viscidi *et al.* (1989) showed that both recombinant and synthetic tat protein significantly inhibited soluble tetanus toxoid and Candida antigen induced lymphoproliferative response of PBMCs, while tat did not modulate mitogen (PHA or Con A)-induced lymphocyte proliferative responses. Since tat had no effect on mitogenesis, it was suggested that tat may interfere with signal transduction via the T-cell antigen receptor or with the production of cytokines that mediate inhibition. Further, treatment of vascular cells with tat also was shown to increase expression of the receptor for tat. Recombinant tat peptides increased immunoglobulin G and IL-6 production *in vitro* by normal uninfected PBMCs suggesting that tat can function in the absence of any other viral proteins (Rautonen *et al.*, 1984). Recently, Chirmule *et al.* (1995) reported that synthetic tat peptide inhibited the proliferative responses of $CD4^+$ lymphocytes stimulated by specific antigens and both $CD4^+$ and $CD8^+$ T cells treated with anti-$CD3^+$ monoclonal antibodies. These effects appear to be mediated by inhibition of IL-2 mRNA expression, independent of IL-2 receptor expression.

Increased levels of transforming growth factor (TGF) β1 have been observed in AIDS patients (Allen *et al.*, 1991) and spontaneous *in vitro* production of TGF β1 by PBMCs from AIDS patients also was reported (Kekow *et al.*, 1990). Therefore, TGF β1 seems to play a significant role in the pathogenesis of HIV infections (Allen *et al.*, 1991). TGF β1 also has been shown to mediate the spread of HIV-1 to uninfected macrophages (Lazdins *et al.*, 1991a,b). However, the role of HIV-1 tat proteins on TGF β1 production and activity has not been clearly elucidated. Earlier studies also have shown the transactivation of TGF β1 promoter by HIV-1 tat (Lotz *et al.*, 1990). Zauli *et al.* (1992) showed that HIV-1 tat protein significantly induced the production of TGF β1 by bone marrow cells from normal subjects, suggesting that HIV tat protein could contribute to the derangement of hematopoiesis in HIV-infected subjects.

Other studies also demonstrated a significant role of tat protein in the development of Kaposi's sarcoma (KS) by acting at both extracellular and nuclear levels presumably mediated through transactivation of cellular genes for cytokines such as TNF, TGF β, basic fibroblast growth factor (bFGF), and IL-6 (Ensoli *et al.*, 1990, 1991, 1994; Albini *et al.*, 1994, 1995a). Previously it was shown that transgenic mice bearing the tat gene developed KS-like lesions suggesting that tat itself or tat-induced factors may promote KS (Ensoli *et al.*, 1991). Further, recombinant tat protein induced the proliferation of AIDS-KS cells, and the proliferation could be blocked by specific anti-tat antibodies (Ensoli *et al.*, 1991) and tissue inhibitor of metalloproteinase-2 (Albini *et al.*, 1994). Barillari *et al.* (1992 and 1993) recently showed that tat promotes adhesion of AIDS-KS and normal vascular cells and this was associated with the RGD sequence, probably through interaction with integrin receptors ($\alpha5\beta1$ and $\alpha_v\beta3$), the expression of which could be upregulated by the same cytokine (conditioned medium from activated T cells) that promotes the cell adhesion. In AIDS-KS the developmental cytokine bFGF plays a prominent role in the growth of KS cells in an autocrine fashion, stimulating the endothelial migration, invasion, and proliferation, events that are required for angiogenesis (Folkman and Klagsbrun, 1987). It has been shown that bFGF and tat synergize in inducing an angiogenic KS lesion in mice, presumably by upregulating matrix proteins (Ensoli *et al.*, 1994), and tat mimics heparin binding angiogenic growth factors (Albini *et al.*, 1995b). HIV-1 tat is also known to modulate major histocompatibility complex class I genes (Howcroff *et al.*, 1993) and the manganese superoxide dismutase gene (Flores *et al.*, 1993). In summary, these *in vitro* and *in vivo* studies clearly demonstrate that tat modulates a number of immunological events that directly or indirectly lead to transactivation of HIV-1 provirus. This, in turn, leads to the emergence of HIV-1 from the latent state to clinically active disease.

3.3. Rev

Rev is believed to mediate or enable the export of the larger unspliced or singly spliced HIV-1 mRNA from the nucleus to the cytoplasm. In the absence of functional rev protein ("regulator of virion protein expression"), only the multiply spliced, approximately 2-kb mRNAs encoding tat, rev, and nef are found in the cytoplasm of the cell (Sodroski *et al.*, 1986; Feinberg *et al.*, 1986). As the level of HIV-1 gene expression increases secondary to tat, a switch to the presence of 4- and 9-kb viral mRNA transcripts is observed in the cytoplasm concomitantly with a reduction in the amount of the multiply spliced mRNA encoding the regulatory proteins (Sodroski *et al.*, 1986; Feinberg *et al.*, 1986; Kim *et al.*, 1989a; Malim *et al.*, 1988). While rev protein is required for stimulation of the transport of singly spliced and unspliced HIV-1 RNA species to the cytoplasm, it does not alter the pattern of HIV-1 RNA expression in the cell nucleus, where unspliced viral transcripts can be detected even prior to rev production (Felber *et al.*, 1989; Hammarskjold *et al.*, 1989; Malim *et al.*, 1990). The switch to the late, structural phase with expression of the virion gag, pol, and env and vif, vpr, and vpu proteins appears to require a critical level of rev (Emerman *et al.*, 1989; Cochrane *et al.*, 1990a). The rev protein, thereby, acts as a negative regulator of its own synthesis, while inducing the appearance of the structural gene transcripts in the cell cytoplasm (Malim *et al.*, 1988).

The action of the rev transactivator is mediated by its specific interaction with a highly structured RNA target sequence, the rev response element (RRE) (Malim *et al.*, 1990; Cochrane *et al.*, 1990a,b; Emerman *et al.*, 1989; Daly *et al.*, 1989; Zapp and Green, 1989; Rosen *et al.*, 1988). The initial rev binding appears to engage a structured 13-nucleotide sequence element within the full-length, 234-nucleotide RRE, although the remainder of the RRE structure may be important for stabilizing or presenting this small sequence (Heaphy *et al.*, 1990; Huang *et al.*, 1991; Tiley *et al.*, 1992). The rev RNA-binding domain contains a basic, arginine-rich motif which is responsible for sequence-specific interaction of rev with RRE and for nuclear/nucleolar localization (NL) (Berger *et al.*, 1991; Cochrane *et al.*, 1990a,b; Malim *et al.*, 1989a). Rev function also depends on areas adjacent to the NL domain that enable multimerization of rev on the RRE (Malim and Cullen, 1991; Olsen *et al.*, 1990). In addition, rev contains a leucine-rich domain that may be involved in interaction with a component of the nuclear RNA transport or splicing machinery (Malim *et al.*, 1991).

Experiments with genes mutated at 5′ or 3′ splice sites have given further insight into how the interaction of rev protein and the RRE might stimulate the transport of unspliced or singly spliced HIV-1 mRNAs. Typically, mRNAs with a single 5′ or 3′ splice site mutation are not transported to the cytoplasm because of the formation and lack of release of assembled spliceosome(s). The interaction of rev protein with the RRE releases this prohibition, perhaps by enabling transport through the nuclear pore despite the presence of spliceosome or by triggering release of the spliceosome. Experiments with engineered mRNAs containing both an RRE and a mutated 5′ or 3′ splice site have shown that the presence of rev, despite incomplete splicing, enables the transport of these mRNAs into the cell cytoplasm (Malim *et al.*, 1990; Chang and Sharp, 1989). Possibly, rev protein functions by selectively channeling mRNA across the nuclear-envelope pore complex (Felber *et al.*, 1989; Malim *et al.*, 1990). Thus, while the actual mechanism by which rev accomplishes this has not been fully elucidated, this represents an area of intense investigation. The role of rev in the correct localization and subsequent efficient translation of viral mRNA is fundamental to the survival of HIV-1, inasmuch as the absence of rev inhibits viral expression. Mechanisms for the correct localization of mRNA analogous to rev-mediated functions also might be expected to be important for host cellular survival and potentially shared by cellular regulatory processes. Hence, it is not surprising that human nucleic acid sequences exist that are shared with the HIV-1 rev gene (Horwitz *et al.*, 1992). Even more intriguing and pertinent to the extrainfectious contributions of HIV-1 proteins or gene products to the pathogenesis of AIDS is the recent description of an antisense oligomer complementary to the rev gene of HIV-1 inducing massive splenomegaly and polyclonal hypergammaglobulinemia in mice (Branda *et al.*, 1993). This response to a rev antisense DNA is particularly interesting in view of the polyclonal B-cell activation described in patients with AIDS.

3.4. Nef

The third early gene product, nef, is an HIV-1 regulatory protein whose biological function is poorly understood. The nef gene product is a myristylated phosphoprotein that is found associated with cell cytoplasmic membrane structures (Hammes *et al.*, 1989). Some have ascribed properties typical of the G-protein family of signal transduction proteins to nef, but confirmation of this has not been reported (Guy *et al.*, 1987; Nebreda *et al.*, 1991). Inhibition of HIV-1 LTR-specific gene expression, no effect, or even enhanced replication of certain HIV-1 isolates by nef in culture have all been described (Terwilliger *et al.*, 1986, 1991; Kim *et al.*, 1989b). Thus, continuing controversy surrounds the cellular effects of the nef protein and the role of nef in the HIV-1 replication cycle. However, nef appears to have some major effects on T-cell function by downregulating CD4 expression or interfering with TCR-mediated signal transduction (Garcia and Miller, 1991). Recently, when two protein isoforms of nef were compared for effects on $CD4^+$ cells, the 27-kDa (nef 27), but not the 25-kDa (nef 25) form of the protein electroporated into T cells was able to reduce the surface expression of CD4 and IL-2R (Greenway *et al.*, 1994). Thus, production of nef 27 during HIV-1 infection may contribute to the immunodeficiency observed with AIDS by impairing expression of two critical T-cell surface molecules important for cellular proliferation (Garcia and Miller, 1991; Greenway *et al.*, 1994). Regulation of B-lymphocyte activity has recently been attributed to HIV-1 nef protein (Chirmule *et al.*, 1994). They showed that a recombinant nef protein could induce polyclonal B-cell differentiation *in vitro* through a proposed mechanism that involves the induction of IL-6 by monocytes and the direct interaction of T and B lymphocytes through upregulation of adhesion molecules.

4. NEUROMODULATION BY HIV-1 PROTEINS

AIDS encephalopathy is a serious complication of infections with HIV-1. In perinatal HIV-1 infections, the neurologic manifestations usually present early in the course of disease and tend to be reversible on institution of antiviral therapy. However, AIDS dementia, which occurs as a later manifestation of HIV-1 infections in adults, often is irreversible. Furthermore, while it is known that HIV-1 can infect brain macrophages and microglia, considerable controversy surrounds the issue of whether neurons of the CNS can be infected with HIV-1. There are studies that support both positions. Nevertheless, current evidence demonstrates that soluble HIV-1 gene products may be neurotoxic. Early in the course of HIV-1 infections the encephalopathy may be reversible, but after prolonged neurotoxic activity the neuropathology becomes irreversible. Previous investigations demonstrated that gp120 could suppress the growth of neuronal cells *in vitro*, supporting the hypothesis that certain HIV-1 soluble gene products are neurotoxic (Kaiser *et al.*, 1990). The role of gp120 as a mediator of AIDS-associated neurotoxicity has been extensively reviewed recently (Brenneman *et al.*, 1994; Dawson and Dawson, 1994).

Studies by Bernton *et al.* (1992) demonstrated that supernates from HIV-infected human monocyte cultures were toxic *in vitro* to neuronal cell growth using fetal rat brain cortical explant cultures. This neurotoxic activity was mediated by the excitatory amino acid (EAA) agonist, *N*-methyl-D-aspartic acid (NMDA). Neurotoxicity induced by gp120 could be inhibited by different NMDA antagonists (Sindou *et al.*, 1994; Lipton, 1992a,b). Also it has been proposed that both gp120 and NMDA may exert their neurotoxic effects through the induction of protein kinase C translocation from the cytosol to the cell membrane by two different pathways (Ushijima *et al.*, 1994). Other potential mechanisms of gp120-mediated neurotoxicity have been described including inhibition of myelination (Kimura-Kuroda *et al.*, 1994) and complement-dependent cytotoxicity of neurons (Apostolski *et al.*, 1994). Indirect mechanisms of gp120-induced neurotoxicity also have been proposed. Pulliam *et al.* (1993) demonstrated in a human brain tissue system that HIV-1 gp120 did not directly cause neuronal cell death. Rather, it caused specific dysfunctions and/or death of astrocytes and they proposed that this could indirectly in turn affect the neurons. Others have demonstrated that binding of gp120 to the CD4 receptor of monocytoid cells may induce the production of neurotoxins by the latter (Giulian *et al.*, 1993).

We subsequently reported that the HIV-1 recombinant fusion protein, env–gag, can augment the neurotoxicity mediated by NMDA *in vivo* (Barks *et al.*, 1993). Using 7-day-old rat pups, HIV peptides ± NMDA were injected stereotactically into the dorsal hippocampus. Doses of either env–gag (100 ng) or NMDA (5 nmole) which did not cause any neuropathology when injected alone, produced significant loss of pyramidal cells and gross lesions of the hippocampus when injected together. While these results demonstrate that peptides from HIV-1 can potentiate EAA-mediated neurotoxicity, the specific mechanisms underlying this effect remain to be determined. We are actively engaged in elucidating these mechanisms.

5. SUMMARY

In this chapter we provide substantial evidence that soluble HIV-1 gene products have potent biological effects on host cells. Many of these actions parallel dysfunctions manifested by patients with AIDS. These include pathogenic effects on both the immune and central nervous systems. Consequently, the observations described herein support a model that proposes that in addition to the direct effects of HIV-1 infections on the host, progression of disease can also be mediated by indirect, extrainfectious mechanisms such as biologically active, HIV-1-specific proteins and peptides. Such observations augur for caution in the use of HIV-1-specific peptides as vaccine candidates, particularly in individuals who are already infected. Nevertheless, we must be vigilant for the lessons to be learned from such investigations. They also may yield unique, new immunotherapeutic agents derived from HIV peptides which may be useful in the therapy of other diseases associated with dysregulation of the immune system.

ACKNOWLEDGMENTS. Some of our research described herein was supported by grant R01 MH47225 from the National Institute of Mental Health and by a grant from the Margaret Duffy and Robert Cameron Troup Fund of the Buffalo General Hospital. The authors express their sincere appreciation to Carol Sperry and Gerry Sobkowiak for their excellent secretarial assistance.

REFERENCES

Albini, A., Fontanini, G., Masiello, L., Tacchetti, C., Bigini, D., Luzzi, P., Noonan, D. M., and Stetler-Stevenson, W. G., 1994, Angiogenic potential in vivo by Kaposi's sarcoma cell-free supernatants and HIV-1 tat product: Inhibition of KS-like lesions by tissue inhibitor of metalloproteinase, *AIDS* **8:**1237–1244.

Albini, A., Barillari, G., Benelli, R., Gallo, R. C., and Ensoli, B., 1995a, Angiogenic properties of human immunodeficiency virus type 1 Tat protein, *Proc. Natl. Acad. Sci. USA* **92:**4838–4842.

Albini, A., Benelli, R., Masiello, L., Rusnati, M., Giunciuglio, D., Rubartelli, A., Ziche, M., Soldi, R., Bussolino, F., Presta, M., and Noonan, D., 1995b, HIV-1 Tat mimics heparin-binding angiogenic growth factors, *AIDS Res. Hum. Retrovir.* **11:**S115.

Allen, J. B., Wong, H. L., Guyre, P. M., Simon, G. L., and Wahl, S. M., 1991, Association of circulating receptor FcγRIII-positive monocytes in AIDS patients with elevated levels of transforming growth factor-β, *J. Clin. Invest.* **87:**1773–1779.

Apostolski, S., McAlarney, T., Hays, A. P., and Latov, N., 1994, complement dependent cytotoxicity of sensory ganglion neurons mediated by gp120 glycoprotein of HIV-1, *Immunol. Invest.* **23:**47–52.

Arya, S. D., Guo, C., Josephs, S. F., and Wong-Staal, F., 1985, Trans-activator gene of human T-lymphotrophic virus type III (HTLV-III), *Science* **229:**69–73.

Barillari, G., Buonaguro, L., Fiorelli, V., Hoffman, J., Michaels, F., Gallo, R. C., and Ensoli, B., 1992, Effects of cytokines from activated immune cells on vascular cell growth and HIV-1 gene expression; implications for AIDS-Kaposi's sarcoma pathogenesis, *J. Immunol.* **149:**3727–3734.

Barillari, G., Gendelman, R., Gallo, R. C., and Ensoli, B., 1993, The Tat protein of human immunodeficiency virus type 1, a growth factor for AIDS Kaposi sarcoma and cytokine-activated vascular cells, induces adhesion of the same cell types by using integrin receptors recognizing the RGD amino acid sequence, *Proc. Natl. Acad. Sci. USA* **90:**7941–7945.

Barks, J. D., Nair, M. P. N., Schwartz, S. A., and Silverstein, F. S., 1993, Potentiation of N-methyl-D-aspartate mediated brain injury by a human immunodeficiency virus-1-derived peptide in perinatal rodents, *Pediatr. Res.* **34:**192–198.

Berger, J., Aepinus, C., Dobrovnik, M., Fleckenstein, B., Hauber, J., and Bohnlein, E., 1991, Mutational analysis of functional domains in the HIV-1 Rev trans-regulatory protein, *Virology* **183:**630–635.

Berkhout, B., and Jeang, K. T., 1989, Trans-activation of human immunodeficiency virus type 1 is sequence specific for both the single-stranded bulge and loop of the trans-acting-responsive hairpin: A quantitative analysis, *J. Virol.* **63:**5501–5504.

Bernton, E. W., Bryant, H. U., Decoster, M. A., Orenstein, J. M., Ribas, J. L., Meltzer, M. S., and Gendeman, H. E., 1992, No direct neuronotoxicity by HIV-1 virions or culture fluids from HIV-1-infected T cells or monocytes, *AIDS Res. Hum. Retrovir.* **8:**495–503.

Braddock, M., Chambers, A., Wilson, W., Esnouf, M. P., Adam, S. E., Kingsman, A. J., and Kingsman, S. M., 1989, HIV-1 TAT "activates" presynthesized RNA in the nucleus, *Cell* **58:**269–279.

Brake, D. A., Debouch, C., and Biesecke, C., 1990, Identification of an Arg-Gly-Asp (RGD) cell adhesion site in human immunodeficiency virus type 1 transactivation protein, tat, *J. Cell Biol.* **111:**1275–1281.

Branda, R. F., Moore, A. L., Mathews, L., McCormack, J. J., and Zon, G., 1993, Immune stimulation by an antisense oligomer complementary to the *rev* gene of HIV-1, *Biochem. Pharmacol.* **45:**2037–2043.

Brenneman, D. E., McCune, S. K., Mervis, R. F., and Hill, J. M., 1994, gp120 as an etiologic agent for neuroAIDS: Neurotoxicity and model systems, *Adv. Neuroimmunol.* **4:**157–165.

Brenner, B. G., Dascal, A., Margolese, R. G., and Wainberg, M. A., 1989, Natural killer cell function in patients with acquired immunodeficiency syndrome and related diseases, *J. Leuk. Biol.* **46:**75–83.

Buonaguro, L., Barillari, G., Chang, H. K., Bohan, C. A., Kao, V., Morgan, R., Gallo, R. C., and Ensoli, B., 1992,

Effects of the human immunodeficiency virus type 1 Tat protein on the expression of inflammatory cytokines, *J. Virol.* **66:**7159–7167.

Buonaguro, L., Buonaguro, F. M., Giraldo, G., and Ensoli, B., 1994, The human immunodeficiency virus type 1 tat protein transactivates tumor necrosis factor β gene expression through a TAR-like structure, *J. Virol.* **68:** 2667–2682.

Certa, U., Bannwarth, W., Stuber, D., Gentz, B., Lanzer, M., LeGrice, B., Guillot, F., Wendler, I., Hunsmann, G., Bujard, H., and Mous, J., 1986, Subregions of a conserved part of the HIV gp41 transmembrane protein are differentially recognized by antibodies of infected individuals, *EMBO J.* **5:**3051–3056.

Chang, D. D., and Sharp, P. A., 1989, Regulation by HIV Rev depends upon recognition of splice sites, *Cell* **59:**789–795.

Chirmule, N., Kalyanaraman, V., Oyaizu, N., and Pahwa, S., 1988, Inhibitory influences of envelope glycoproteins of HIV-1 on normal immune responses, *J. Acq. Immune Defic. Syndr.* **1:**425–430.

Chirmule, N., Oyaizu, N., Saxinger, C., and Pahwa, S., 1994, Nef protein of HIV-1 has B-cell stimulatory activity, *AIDS* **8:**733–734.

Chirmule, N., Than, S., Khan, S. A., and Pahwa, S., 1995, Human immunodeficiency virus Tat induces functional unresponsiveness in T cells, *J. Virol.* **69:**492–498.

Cochrane, A. W., Chen, C. H., and Rosen, C., 1990a, Specific interaction of the HIV Rev transactivator protein with a structured region in the env mRNA, *Proc. Natl. Acad. Sci. USA* **87:**1198–1201.

Cochrane, A. W., Perkins, A., and Rosen, C. A., 1990b, Identification of sequences important in the nucleolar localization of human immunodeficiency virus Rev: Relevance of nucleolar localization to function, *J. Virol.* **64:**881–885.

Crowl, R., Ganguly, K., Gordon, M., Conroy, R., Schaber, R., Corney, R., Schaber, M., Kramer, R., Shaw, G., Wong-Staal, F., and Reddy, R. P., 1985, HTLV-III env gene products synthesized in E. coli are recognized by antibodies present in the drts of AIDS patients, *Cell* **41:**979–986.

Cullen, B. R., 1986, Trans-activation of human immunodeficiency virus occurs via a bimodal mechanism, *Cell* **46:**973–982.

Cullen, B. R., 1990, The HIV-1 Tat protein: An RNA sequence-specific processivity factor, *Cell* **63:**655–657.

Cullen, B. R., 1992, Mechanism of action of regulatory proteins encoded by complex retroviruses, *Microbiol. Rev.* **56:**375–394.

Daly, T., Cook, K., Gray, G., Maione, T., and Rusche, J., 1989, Specific binding of HIV-1 recombinant Rev protein to the Rev-responsive element in vitro, *Nature* **342:**816–819.

Dawson, T. M., and Dawson, V. L., 1994, gp120 neurotoxicity in primary cortical cultures, *Adv. Neuroimmunol.* **4:**167–173.

Dayton, A. I., Sodroski, J. G., Rosen, C. A., Goh, W. C., and Haseltine, W. A., 1986, The trans-activator gene of the human T cell lymphotropic virus type III is required for replication, *Cell* **44:**941–947.

de Martini, R. M., and Parker, J. W., 1989, Immunologic alterations in human immunodeficiency virus infection: A review, *J. Clin. Lab. Anal.* **3:**56–70.

Dingwall, C., Ernberg, I., Gait, M. J., Green, S. M., Heaphy, S., Karn, J., Lowe, A. D., Singh, M., and Skinner, M. A., 1990, HIV-1 Tat protein stimulates transcription by binding to a U-rich bulge in the stem of the TAR RNA structure, *EMBO J.* **9:**4145–4153.

Embretson, J., Zupancic, M., Ribas, J. L., Burke, A., Tenner-Racz, J., and Haase, A. T., 1993, Massive covert infection of helper T lymphocytes and macrophages by HIV during the incubation period of AIDS, *Nature* **362:**359–362.

Emerman, M., Vazeux, R., and Peden, K., 1989, The rev gene product of the human immunodeficiency virus affects envelope-specific RNA localization, *Cell* **57:**1155–1165.

Endo, S., Kubota, S., Siomi, H., Adachi, A., Oroszlan, S., Maki, M., and Hatanaka, M., 1989, A region of basic amino-acid cluster in HIV-1 Tat protein is essential for transacting activity and nuclear localization, *Virus Genes* **3:**99–110.

Ensoli, B., Barillari, G., Zaki Salahuddin, S. Z., Gallo, R. C., and Wong-Staal, F., 1990, Tat protein of HIV-1 stimulates growth of cells derived from Kaposi's sarcoma lesions of AIDS patients, *Nature* **345:**84–86.

Ensoli, B., Barillari, G., and Gallo, R. C., 1991, Pathogenesis of AIDS associated Kaposi's sarcoma, *Hematol. Oncol. Clin. North Am.* **5:**281–295.

Ensoli, B., Buonaguro, L., Barillari, G., Fiorelli, V., Gendelman, R., Morgan, R. A., Wingfield, P., and Gallo, R. C., 1993, Release, uptake, and effects of extracellular human immunodeficiency virus type 1 Tat protein on cell growth and viral transactivation, *J. Virol.* **67:**277–287.

Ensoli, B., Gendelman, R., Markham, P., Fiorelli, V., Colombini, S., Raffeld, M., Cafaro, A., Chang, H.-K., Brady,

J. N., and Gallo, R. C., 1994, Synergy between basic fibroblast growth factor and HIV-1 Tat protein in induction of Kaposi's sarcoma, *Nature* **371:**674–680.

Feinberg, M. B., Jarrett, R. F., Aldovini, A., Gallo, R. C., and Wong-Staal, F., 1986, HTLV-III expression and production involve complex regulation at the levels of splicing and translation of viral RNA, *Cell* **46:** 807–817.

Feinberg, M. B., Baltimore, D., and Frankel, A. D., 1991, The role of Tat in the human immunodeficiency virus life cycle indicates a primary effect on transcriptional elongation, *Proc. Natl. Acad. Sci. USA* **88:**4045–4049.

Felber, B. K., Hadzopoulou-Cladaras, M., Cladaras, C., Copeland, T., and Pavlakis, G. N., 1989, Rev protein of human immunodeficiency virus type 1 affects the stability and transport of the viral mRNA, *Proc. Natl. Acad. Sci. USA* **86:**1495–1499.

Feng, S., and Holland, E. C., 1988, HIV-1 tat trans-activation requires the loop sequence within tar, *Nature* **334:**165–167.

Fiorelli, V., Gendelman, R., Samaniego, F., Markham, P. D., and Ensoli, B., 1995, Cytokines from activated T cells induce normal endothelial cells to acquire the phenotypic and functional features of AIDS-Kaposi's sarcoma spindle cells, *J. Clin. Invest.* **95:**1723–1734.

Fisher, A. G., Feinberg, M. B., Josephs, S. F., Harper, M. E., Marselle, L. M., Reyes, G., Gonda, M. A., Aldovini, A., Debouk, C., Gallo, R. C., and Wong-Staal, F., 1986, The trans-activator gene of HTLV-III is essential for virus replication, *Nature* **320:**367–371.

Flores, S. C., Marecki, J. C., Harper, K. P., Bose, S. K., Nelson, S. K., and McCord, J. M., 1993, Tat protein of human immunodeficiency virus type 1 represses expression of magnanese superoxide dismutase in HeLa cells, *Proc. Natl. Acad. Sci. USA* **90:**7632–7636.

Folkman, J., and Klagsbrun, M., 1987, Angiogenic factors, *Science* **235:**442–447.

Frankel, A. D., and Pabo, C. O., 1988, Cellular uptake of the Tat protein from human immunodeficiency virus, *Cell* **55:**1189–1193.

Frankel, A. D., Bredt, D. S., and Pabo, C. O., 1988, Tat protein from human immunodeficiency virus forms a metal-linked dimer, *Science* **240:**70–73.

Garcia, J. V., and Miller, A. D., 1991, Serine phosphorylation-independent downregulation of cell-surface CD4 by nef, *Nature* **350:**508–511.

Garcia, J. A., Wu, F. K., Mitsuyasu, R., and Gaynor, R. B., 1987, Interactions of cellular proteins involved in the transcriptional regulation of the human immunodeficiency virus, *EMBO J.* **6:**3761–3770.

Gatignol, K. A., Kumar, A., Rabson, A., and Jeang, K. T., 1989, Identification of cellular proteins that bind to the human immunodeficiency virus type 1 trans-activation-response TAR element RNA, *Proc. Natl. Acad. Sci. USA* **86:**7828–7832.

Giulian, D., Wendt, E., Vaea, K., and Noonan, C. A., 1993, The envelope glycoprotein of human immunodeficiency virus type 1 stimulates release of neurotropins from monocytes, *Proc. Natl. Acad. Sci. USA* **90:**2769–2773.

Greenblatt, J., Nodwell, J. R., and Mason, S. W., 1993, Transcriptional antitermination, *Nature* **364:**401.

Greenway, A. L., McPhee, D. A., Grgacic, E., Hewish, D., Lucantoni, A., Macreadie, I., and Azad, A., 1994, Nef 27, but not the Nef 25 isoform of human immunodeficiency virus-type 1 pNL4.3 down-regulates surface CD4 and IL-2R expression in peripheral blood mononuclear cells and transformed T cells, *Virology* **198:** 245–256.

Guy, B., Kieny, M. P., Riviere, Y., Peuch, C. L., Dott, K., Girard, M., Montagnier, L., and Lecocq, J. P., 1987, HIV F/3′orf encodes a phosphorylated GTP-binding protein resembling an oncogene product, *Nature* **330:**266–269.

Hammarskjold, J. L., Heimer, J., Hammarskjold, B., Sangwan, I., Albert, L., and Rekosh, D., 1989, Regulation of human immunodeficiency virus env expression by the rev gene product, *J. Virol.* **63:**1959–1966.

Hammes, S. R., Dixon, E. P., Malim, M. H., Cullen, B. R., and Greene, W. C., 1989, Nef protein in human immunodeficiency virus type 1: Evidence against its role as a transcriptional inhibitor, *Proc. Natl. Acad. Sci. USA* **86:**9549–9553.

Hanly, S. M., Rimsky, L. T., Malim, M. H., Kim, J. H., Hauber, J., Dodon, M. D., Lee, S. Y., Maizel, J. V., Cullen, B. R., and Greene, W. C., 1989, Comparative analysis of the HTLV-1 Rex and HIV-1 Rev trans-regulatory proteins and their RNA response elements, *Genes Dev.* **3:**1534–1544.

Harrich, D., Garcia, J., Mitsuyasu, R., and Gaynor, R. B., 1990, TAR independent activation of the human immunodeficiency virus in phorbol ester stimulated T lymphocytes, *EMBO J.* **9:**4417–4423.

Hauber, J., and Cullen, B., 1988, Mutational analysis of the transactivation-responsive region of the human immunodeficiency virus type 1 long terminal repeat, *J. Virol.* **62:**673–679.

Hauber, J., Malim, M. H., and Cullen, B. R., 1989, Mutational analysis of the conserved basic domain of the human immunodeficiency virus tat protein, *J. Virol.* **63:**1181–1187.

Heaphy, S., Dingwall, C., Ernberg, I., Gait, M. J., Green, S. M., Karn, J., Lowe, A. D., Singh, M., and Skinner, M. A., 1990, HIV-1 regulator of virion expression (Rev) protein binds to an RNA stem-loop structure located within the Rev response element region, *Cell* **60**:685–693.

Horwitz, M. S., Boyce-Jacino, M. T., and Faras, A. J., 1992, Novel human endogenous sequences related to human immunodeficiency virus type I, *J. Virol.* **66**:2170–2179.

Howcroft, T., Strebel, K. K., Martin, M. A., and Singer, D. S., 1993, Repression of MHC class I gene promoter by two exon Tat of HIV, *Science* **260**:1320–1322.

Huang, X., Hope, T. J., Bond, B. L., McDonald, D., Grahl, K., and Parslow, T. G., 1991, Minimal Rev-response element for type 1 human immunodeficiency virus, *J. Virol.* **65**:2131–2134.

Jakobovits, A., Smith, D. H., Jakobovits, E. B., and Capon, D. J., 1988, A discrete element 3′ of human immunodeficiency virus 1 (HIV-1) and HIV-2 mRNA initiation sites mediates transcriptional activation by an HIV trans-activator, *Mol. Cell. Biol.* **8**:2555–2561.

Kaiser, P. T., Offermann, J. T., and Lipton, S. A., 1990, Neuronal injury due to HIV-1 envelope protein is blocked by anti-gp120 antibodies but not by anti-CD43 antibodies, *Neurology* **40**:1757–1761.

Kao, S. Y., Calman, A. F., Luciw, P. A., and Peterlin, B. M., 1987, Anti-termination of transcription within the long terminal repeat of HIV-1 by tat gene product, *Nature* **330**:489–493.

Kekow, J., Wachsman, W., McCutchan, J. A., Cronin, M., Carson, D. A., and Lotz, M., 1990, Transforming growth factor b1 and non-cytopathic mechanisms of immunodeficiency in human immunodeficiency virus infection, *Proc. Natl. Acad. Sci. USA* **87**:8321–8325.

Kessler, M., and Mathews, M. B., 1991, Tat transactivation of the human immunodeficiency virus type 1 promoter is influenced by basal promoter activity and the simian virus 40 origin of DNA replication, *Proc. Natl. Acad. Sci. USA* **88**:10018–10022.

Kim, S., Byrn, R., Groopman, J., and Baltimore, D., 1989a, Temporal aspects of DNA and RNA synthesis during human immunodeficiency virus infection: Evidence for differential gene expression, *J. Virol* **63**:3708–3713.

Kim, S., Ikeuchi, K., Byrn, R., Groopman, J., and Baltimore, D., 1989b, Lack of a negative influence on viral growth by the nef gene of human immuno-deficiency virus type 1, *Proc. Natl. Acad. Sci. USA* **86**:9544–9548.

Kimura-Kuroda, J., Nagashima, K., and Yasui, K., 1994, Inhibition of myelin formation by HIV-1 gp120 in rat cerebral cortex, *J. Virol.* **137**:81–99.

Laspia, K. M. F., Rice, A. P., and Mathews, M. B., 1989, HIV-1 Tat protein increases transcriptional initiation and stabilized elongation, *Cell* **59**:283–292.

Lazdins, J. K., Klimkait, T., Alteri, E., Walker, M., Woods-Kook, K., Cox, D., Bilbe, G., Shipman, R., Cerletti, N., and McMaster, G., 1991a, TGF-β up regulator of HIV replication in macrophages, *Res. Virol.* **142**:239–242.

Lazdins, J. K., Klimkait, T., Woods-Kook, K., Walker, M., Altern, E., Cox, D., Cerletti, N., Shipman, R., Bilbe, G., and McMaster, G., 1991b, In vitro effect of transforming growth factor-β on progression of HIV-1 infection in primary mononuclear phagocytes, *J. Immunol.* **147**:120–127.

Lazinski, D., Grzadzielska, E., and Das, A., 1989, Sequence-specific recognition of RNA hairpins by bacteriophage antiterminators requires a conserved arginine-rich motif, *Cell* **59**:207–218.

Liegler, T. J. and Stites, D. P., 1994, HIV-1 gp120 and anti-gp120 induce reversible unresponsiveness in peripheral CD4 T lymphocytes, *J. Acq. Immune Defic. Syndr.* **7**:340–348.

Lipton, S. A., 1992a, Requirement for macrophages in neuronal injury induced by HIV envelope protein gp120, *Neuroreport* **3**:913–915.

Lipton, S. A., 1992b, Memantine prevents HIV coat protein-induced neuronal injury in vitro, *Neurology* **42**:1403–1405.

Lotz, M., Keckow, J., Cronin, M. T., McCutchan, J. A., Clark-Lewis, I., Carson, D. A., and Wachsman, W., 1990, Induction of transforming growth factor b (TGFb) by HIV-1 Tat: A noncytopathic pathway of immunodeficiency in HIV infection, *FASEB J.* **4**:A1861.

Malim, M. H., and Cullen, B. R., 1991, HIV-1 structural gene expression requires the binding of multiple Rev monomers to the viral RRE: Implications for HIV-1 latency, *Cell* **65**:241–248.

Malim, M. H., Hauber, J., Fenrick, R., and Cullen, B. R., 1988, Immuno-deficiency virus rev trans-activator modulates the expression of the viral regulatory genes, *Nature* **335**:181–183.

Malim, M. H., Hauber, J., Le, S.-Y., Maizel, J. V., and Cullen, B. R., 1989a, The HIV-1 rev trans-activator acts through a structured target sequence to activate nuclear export of unspliced viral mRNA, *Nature* **338**: 254–257.

Malim, M. H., Bohnlein, S., Hauber, J., and Cullen, B. R., 1989b, Functional dissection of the HIV-1 Rev trans-activator-derivation of a trans-dominant repressor of Rev function, Cell **58**:205–214.

Malim, M. H., Tiley, L. S., McCarn, D. F., Rusche, J. R., Hauber, J., and Cullen, B. R., 1990, HIV-1 structural gene expression requires binding of the Rev trans-activator to its RNA target sequence, *Cell* **60**:675–683.

Malim, M. H., McCarn, D. F., Tiley, L. S., and Cullen, B. R., 1991, Mutational definition of the human immunodeficiency type 1 Rev activation domain, *J. Virol.* **65**:4248–4254.

Mann, D. A., and Frankel, A. D., 1991, Endocytosis and targeting of exogenous HIV-1 Tat protein, *EMBO J.* **10**:1733–1739.

Marciniak, R. A., Calnan, B. J., Frankel, A. D., and Sharp, P. A., 1990a, HIV-1 Tat protein trans-activates transcription in vitro, *Cell* **63**:791–802.

Marciniak, R. A., Garcia-Blanco, M. A., and Sharp, P. A., 1990b, Identification and characterization of a HeLa nuclear protein that specifically binds to the trans-activation-response (TAR) element of human immunodeficiency virus, *Proc. Natl. Acad. Sci. USA* **87**:3624–3628.

Masood, R., Lunardi-Iskandar, Y., Zhang, M. T., Law, R. E., Huang, C. L., Puri, R. K., Levine, A. M., and Gill, P. S., 1994, IL-10 inhibits HIV-1 replication and is induced by tat, *Biochem. Biophys. Res. Commun.* **202**:374–383.

Muesing, M. A., Smith, D. H., and Capon, D. J., 1987, Regulation of mRNA accumulation by a human immunodeficiency virus trans-activator protein, *Cell* **48**:691–701.

Myers, G., and Pavlakis, G. N., 1991, Evolutionary potential of complex retroviruses, in: *Viruses: The Retroviridae*, Volume 1 (R. R. Wagner, H. Fraenkel-Conrat, and J. Levy, eds.), Plenum Press, New York, pp 1–37.

Nabel, G., and Baltimore, D., 1987, An inducible transcription factor activates expression of human immunodeficiency virus in T cells, *Nature* **326**:711–713.

Nair. M. P. N., Laign, T. J., and Schwartz, S. A., 1986, Decreased natural and antibody-dependent cellular cytotoxic activities in intravenous drug abusers, *Clin. Immunol. Immunopathol.* **38**:68–78.

Nair, M. P. N., Pottathil, R., Heimer, E. P., and Schwartz, S. A., 1988, Immunoregulatory activities of human immunodeficiency virus (HIV) proteins: Effect of HIV recombinant and synthetic peptides on immunoglobulin synthesis and proliferative responses by normal lymphocytes, *Proc. Natl. Acad. Sci. USA* **85**:6498–6502.

Nebreda, A. R., Bryan, T., Segade, F., Wingfield, P., Venkatesan, S., and Santos, E., 1991, Biochemical and biological comparison of HIV-1 NEF and ras gene product, *Virology* **183**:151–159.

Olsen, H. S., Cochrane, A. W., Dillon, P. J., Nalin, C. M., and Rosen, C. A., 1990, Interaction of the human immunodeficiency virus type 1 Rev protein with a structured region in env mRNA is dependent on multimer formation mediated through a basic stretch of amino acids, *Genes Dev.* **4**:1357–1364.

Oyaizu, N., Chirmule, N., Kalyanaraman, V. S., Hall, W. W., Pahwa, R., Shuster, M., and Pahwa, S., 1990, Human immunodeficiency virus type 1 envelope glycoprotein gp120 produces immune defects in CD4+ T lymphocytes by inhibiting interleukin 2 mRNA, *Proc. Natl. Acad. Sci. USA* **87**:2379–2387.

Pahwa, S., Pahwa, R., Saxinger, C., Gallo, R. C., and Good, R. A., 1985, Influence of the human T-lymphotropic virus/lymphadenopathy-associated virus on functions of human lymphocytes: Evidence for immunosuppressive effects and polyclonal B-cell activation by banded viral preparations, *Proc. Natl. Acad. Sci. USA* **82:** 8198–8202.

Pahwa, S., Pahwa, R., Good, R. A., Gallo, R. C., and Saxinger, C., 1986, Stimulatory and inhibitory influences of human immunodeficiency virus on normal B lymphocytes, *Proc. Natl. Acad. Sci. USA* **83**:9124–9128.

Pantaleo, G., Graziosi, C., Butini, L., Pizzo, P. A., Schnittman, S. M., Kotler, D. P., and Fauci, A. S., 1991, Lymphoid organs function as major reservoirs for human immunodeficiency virus, *Proc. Natl. Acad. Sci. USA* **88**:9838–9842.

Pantaleo, G., Graziosi, C., Demarest, H. F., Butini, L., Montroli, M., Fox, C. H., Orenstein, J. M., Kotler, D., and Fauci, A. S., 1993, HIV infection is active and progressive in lymphoid tissue during the clinically latent stage of the disease, *Nature* **362**:355–358.

Pulliam, L., West, D., Haigwood, N., and Swanson, R. A., 1993, HIV-1 envelope gp120 alters astrocytes in human brain cultures, *AIDS Res. Hum. Retrovir.* **9**:439–444.

Puri, R. K., Leland, P., and Aggarwal, B. B., 1995, Constitutive expression of human immunodeficiency virus type 1 tat gene inhibits interleukin 2 and interleukin 2-receptor expression in a human CD4+ T lymphoid (H9) cell line, *AIDS Res. Hum. Retrovir.* **11**:31–40.

Rappaport, J., Lee, S. J., Khalili, K., and Wong-Staal, F., 1989, The acidic amino-terminal region of the HIV-1 TAT protein constitutes an essential activating domain, *New Biol.* **1**:101–110.

Ratnasabapathy, R., Sheldon, M., Johal, L., and Hernandez, N., 1990, The HIV-1 long terminal repeat contains an unusual element that induces the synthesis of short RNAs from various mRNA and snRNA promoters, *Genes Dev.* **64**:2061–2074.

Rautonen, J., Rautonen, N., Martin, N. L., and Wara, D. W., 1994, HIV type 1 Tat protein induces immunoglobulin and interleukin 6 synthesis by uninfected peripheral blood mononuclear cells, *AIDS Res. Hum. Retrovir.* **10:**781–785.

Rittner, K., Churcher, M. J., Gait, M. J., and Karn, J., 1995, The human immunodeficiency virus long terminal repeat includes a specialized initiator element which is required for tat-responsive transcription, *J. Mol. Biol.* **248:**562–580.

Robinson, W. E., Jr., Mitchell, W. M., Chambers, W. H., Schuffman, S. J., Montefiori, D. C., and Oeltmann, T. N., 1988, Natural killer cell infection and inactivation in vitro by the human immunodeficiency virus, *Pathology* **19:**535–540.

Rosen, C. A., Sodroski, J. G., and Haseltine, W. A., 1985, The location of cis-acting regulatory sequences in the human T cell lymphotropic virus type III (HTLV-III/LAV) long terminal repeat, *Cell* **41:**813–823.

Rosen, C. A., Terwilliger, E., Dayton, A., Sodroski, J. G., and Haseltine, W. A., 1988, Intragenic cis-acting gene-responsive sequences of the human immunodeficiency virus, *Proc. Natl. Acad. Sci. USA* **85:**2071–2075.

Roy, S., Delling, U., Chen, C. H., Rosen, C. A., and Sonenberg, N., 1990a, A bulge structure in HIV-1 TAR RNA is required for Tat binding and Tat-mediated trans-activation, *Genes Dev.* **4:**1365–1373.

Roy, S., Parkin, N. T., Rosen, C. A., Itovitch, J., and Sonenberg, N., 1990b, Structural requirements for trans-activation of human immunodeficiency virus type 1 long terminal repeat-directed gene expression by tat: Importance of base pairing, loop sequence, and bulges in the tat-responsive sequence, *J. Virol.* **64:**1402–1406.

Ruben, S., Perkins, A., Purcell, R., Joung, K., Sia, R., Burghoff, R., Haseltine, W. A., and Rosen, C. A., 1989, Structural and functional characterization of human immunodeficiency virus tat protein, *J. Virol.* **63:**1–8.

Ruscetti, F. W., Mikovits, J. A., Kalyanaraman, V. S., Overton, R., Stevenson, H., Stromberg, K., Herberman, R. B., Farrar, W. L., and Ortaldo, J. R., 1986, Analysis of effector mechanisms against HTLV-I- and HTLV-III/LAV-infected lymphoid cells, *Immunology* **136**:3619–3624.

Sastry, K. J., Reddy, H. R., Pandita, R., Totpal, K., and Aggarwal, B. B., 1990, HIV-1 tat gene induces tumor necrosis factor-b (lymphotoxin) in a human b-lymphoblastoid cell line, *J. Biol. Chem.* **265:**20091–20093.

Scala, G., Ruocco, M. R., Ambrosino, C., Mallardo, M., Giordano, V., Baldassarre, F., Dragonetti, E., Quinto, I., and Venuta, S., 1994, The expression of the interleukin 6 gene induced by the human immunodeficiency virus type 1 Tat protein, *J. Exp. Med.* **179:**961–971.

Schnittman, S. M., Lane, H. C., Higgins, S., Folks, T., and Fauci, A. S., 1986, Direct polyclonal activation of human B lymphocytes by acquired immunodeficiency virus, *Science* **233:**1084–1086.

Selby, M. J., Bain, E. S., Luciw, P. A., and Peterlin, B. M., 1989, Structure, sequence, and position of the stem-loop in tar determine transcriptional elongation by tat through the HIV-1 long terminal repeat, *Genes Dev.* **3:** 547–558.

Sharp, P. A., and Marciniak, R. A., 1989, HIV TAR: An RNA enhancer, *Cell* **59:**229–230.

Shoeman, R. L., Young, D., Pottathil, R., Victor, J., Conroy, R. R., Crowl, R. M., Coleman, T., Heimer, E., Lai, C. Y., and Ganguly, L., 1987, Comparison of recombinant human immunodeficiency virus gag precursor and gag/env fusion proteins and a synthetic env pepetide as diagnostic reagents, *Anal. Biochem.* **161:**370–379.

Sindou, P., Couratier, P., Esclaire, F., Yardin, C., Bousseau, A., and Hugon, J., 1994, Prevention of HIV coat protein (gp120) toxicity in cortical cell cultures by riluzole, *J. Neurol. Sci.* **126:**133–137.

Siomi, H., Shida, H., Maki, M., and Hatanaka, M., 1990, Effects of a highly basic region of human immunodeficiency virus Tat protein on nucleolar localization, *J. Virol.* **64:**1803–1807.

Siranni, M. C., Tagliaferri, F., and Aiuti, F., 1990, Pathogenesis of natural killer cell deficiency in AIDS, *Immunol. Today* **11:**81–82.

Sodroski, J. G., Rosen, C. A., and Haseltine, W. A., 1984, Trans-acting transcriptional activation of the long terminal repeat of human T lymphotropic viruses in infected cells, *Science* **225:**381–421.

Sodroski, J. R., Patarca, C., Rosen, C., Wong-Staal, F., and Haseltine, W., 1985, Location of the trans-activating region on the genome of human T-cell lymphotropic virus type III, *Science* **229:**74–77.

Sodroski, J., Goh, W. C., Rosen, C., Dayton, A., Terwilliger, E., and Haseltine, W. A., 1986, A second post-transcriptional transactivator gene required for the HTLV-III replication, *Nature* **321:**412–417.

Southgate, C. D., and Green, M. R., 1991, The HIV-1 Tat protein activates transcription from an upstream DNA-binding site: Implications for Tat function, *Genes Dev.* **5:**2496–2507.

Sumner-Smith, M., Roy, S., Barnett, R., Reid, L. S., Kuperman, R., Delling, U., and Sonenberg, N., 1991, Critical chemical features in trans-acting-responsive RNA are required for interaction with human immunodeficiency virus type 1 TAT protein, *J. Virol.* **65:**5196–5202.

Taylor, J. P., Cupp, C., Diaz, A., Chowdhury, M., Khalili, K., Jimenez, S. A., and Amini, S., 1992a, Activation of expression of genes coding for extra-cellular matrix proteins in Tat-producing glioblastoma cells, *Proc. Natl. Acad. Sci. USA* **89:**9617–9621.

Taylor, J. P., Pomerantz, R., Bagasra, O., Chowdhury, M., Rappaport, J., Khalili, K., and Amini, S., 1992b, TAR-independent transactivation by Tat in cells derived from the CNS: A novel mechanism of HIV-1 gene regulation, *EMBO J.* **11**:395–403.

Taylor, J. P., Pomerantz, R. J., Oakes, J. W., Khalili, K., and Amini, S., 1995, A CNS-enriched factor that binds to NF-kappa B and is required for interaction with HIV-1 tat, *Oncogene* **10**:395–400.

Terwilliger, E., Sodroski, J. G., Rosen, C. A., and Haseltine, W. A., 1986, Effects of mutations with the 3′ orf open reading frame region of human T-cell lymphotrophic virus type III (HTLV-III/LAV) on replication and cytopathogenicity, *J. Virol.* **60**:754–760.

Terwilliger, E. F., Langhoff, E., Gabuzda, D., Zazopoulos, E., and Haseltine, W. A., 1991, Allelic variation in the effects of the nef gene on replication of human immunodeficiency virus type 1, *Proc. Natl. Acad. Sci. USA* **88**:10971–10975.

Tiley, L. S., Malim, M. H., Tewary, H. K., Stockley, P. G., and Cullen, B. R., 1992, Identification of a high-affinity RNA-binding site for the human immunodeficiency virus type 1 Rev protein, *Proc. Natl. Acad. Sci. USA* **89**:758–762.

Ushijima, H., Ando, S., Kunisada, T., Schroder, H. C., Klocking, H. P., Kijjoa, A., and Muller, W. E., 1993, HIV-1 gp120 and MNDA induce protein kinase C translocation differentially in rat primary neuronal cultures, *J. Acq. Immune Defic. Syndr.* **6**:339–343.

Varmus, H., and Brown, P., 1989, Retroviruses, in: *Mobile DNA* (D. E. Berg and M. M. Howe, eds.), American Society for Microbiology, Washington, DC, pp. 53–108.

Viscidi, R. P., Mayur, K., Lederman, H. M., and Frankel, A. D., 1989, Inhibition of antigen-induced lymphocyte proliferation by Tat protein from HIV-1, *Science* **246**:1606–1608.

Vogel, B. F., Lee, S. S., Hildebrand, A., Craig, W., Pierschbacher, M. D., Wong-Staal, F., and Ruoslahti, E., 1993, A novel integrin specificity exemplified by binding of the a_vb_5 integrin to the basic domain of the HIV tat protein and vitronectin, *J. Cell Biol.* **121**:461–468.

Weeks, K. M., and Crothers, D. M., 1991, RNA recognition by Tat-derived peptides: Interaction in the major groove, *Cell* **66**:577–588.

Westendorp, M. O., Li-Weber, M., Frank, R. W., and Krammer, P. H., 1994, Human immunodeficiency virus type 1 tat upregulates interleukin-2 secretion in activated T cells, *J. Virol.* **68**:4177–4185.

Zapp, M., and Green, M., 1989, Sequence-specific RNA binding by the HIV-1 Rev protein, *Nature* **342**:714–716.

Zauli, G., Re, M. C., Furlini, G., Giovannini, M., and La Placa, M., 1991, Evidence for an HIV-1 mediated suppression of in vitro growth of enriched (CD-34+) hematopoietic progenitors, *J. AIDS* **4**:1251–1253.

Zauli, G., Davis, B. R., Re, B. R., Visani, M. C., Furlini, G., and La Placa, M., 1992, Tat protein stimulates production of transforming growth factor-β by marrow macrophages: A potential mechanism for HIV-1 induced hematopoietic suppression, *Blood* **80**:3036–3043.

Zauli, G., Gibellini, D., Milani, D., Mazzoni, M., Borgatti, P., La Placa, M., and Capitani, S., 1993, Human immunodeficiency virus type 1 Tat protein protects lymphoid, epithelial and neuronal cell lines from death by apoptosis, *Cancer Res.* **53**:4481–4485.

CHAPTER 9

PHENOTYPE AND FUNCTION OF T CELLS IN HIV DISEASE

JANIS V. GIORGI

1. OVERVIEW

Phenotype refers to the unique collection of antigens expressed on the surface of a cell. For clinical and research purposes, phenotypic analyses on lymphocytes are typically done using flow cytometry on peripheral blood and can be done on lymphoid tissue. Flow cytometric measurements utilize monoclonal antibodies (mAb) against cell surface differentiation antigens to enumerate lymphocyte subsets that have distinct functional activities, lineages, and maturational states (Giorgi, 1992b; Giorgi *et al.*, 1992). Major lymphocyte subtypes ($CD4^+$ T, $CD8^+$ T, natural killer, and B cells) as well as subsets of these populations can be discriminated.

Cell surface molecules recognized by mAb include those that react with maturation or activation antigens or receptors for cytokines. The close correlation of lymphocyte phenotype with function and differentiation state results from the fact that many cell surface molecules play a role in specific lymphocyte functions such as antigen recognition, lysis of virus-infected cells, and immune regulation. Lymphocyte function can be measured *in vitro* in assays designed to detect these activities.

Each lymphocyte subset has distinct functions that are reflected in its phenotype. In the past, most of our knowledge about which immune functions were mediated by phenotypically identified lymphocyte subsets came from studies on healthy control donors. Investigations of HIV infection have provided a unique opportunity to identify which cells produce cytokines or mediate effector functions *in vivo* during antigen stimulation. Consequently, insight into the association between lymphocyte function and cell surface marker expression has been extended significantly.

JANIS V. GIORGI • Department of Medicine, Jonsson Comprehensive Cancer Center, UCLA AIDS Institute and the Multicenter AIDS Cohort Study, UCLA Schools of Medicine and Public Health, Los Angeles, California 90095.

Immunology of HIV Infection, edited by Sudhir Gupta. Plenum Press, New York, 1996.

2. IMMUNOPHENOTYPES: ALTERATIONS IN NUMBERS OF T-LYMPHOCYTE SUBSETS

2.1. $CD4^+$ Cell Phenotypes

2.1.1. Stages of Total $CD4^+$ Cell Numerical Decline

Phenotypic alterations in $CD4^+$ cells of HIV-infected subjects are summarized in Table I. Decreases in $CD4^+$ cell absolute numbers and percentages and decreased CD4:CD8 ratios (the number of $CD4^+$ cells/mm^3 divided by the number of $CD8^+$ cells/mm^3) occur from approximately the time of HIV infection onward. These decreases are associated with the length of time individuals have been HIV-infected and are predictors of disease progression. The Centers for Disease Control and Prevention 1993 surveillance case definition of AIDS includes persons with a circulating $CD4^+$ cell count of $\leqslant 200/\text{mm}^3$ regardless of whether or not clinical AIDS symptoms are present (Centers for Disease Control and Prevention, 1992). In contrast, in adult controls (a population of uninfected homosexual men), the $CD4^+$ cell absolute number, percentage, and CD4:CD8 ratio (mean $\pm$ S.D.) were $898 \pm 318/\text{mm}^3$, $44.5 \pm 8.2\%$, and 1.58 ± 0.66, respectively (Taylor *et al.*, 1989). As compared with adults, healthy uninfected newborns have roughly similar $CD4^+$ cell percentages and CD4:CD8 ratios but have about three times as many $CD4^+$ T lymphocytes/mm^3 as a result of relative lymphocytosis that gradually resolves by age 6 or 7 (Hannet *et al.*, 1992).

Decreases in circulating $CD4^+$ cell levels in adults and children occur in four stages (Giorgi, 1992a). In stage 1 there is a rapid drop in $CD4^+$ cell levels that occurs over the first 12–18 months of infection (Zaunders *et al.*, 1995; Giorgi, 1992a). For example, Los Angeles participants in the Multicenter AIDS Cohort Study (MACS) who had a known date of seroconversion during the study dropped from a mean $CD4^+$ cell number of 945/mm^3 at their last seronegative visit to 740/mm^3, 697/mm^3, and 634/mm^3 at 6, 12, and 18 months later, respectively (decreases relative to baseline of 22, 26, and 33%, respectively). A transient more profound drop and rapid partial rebound in $CD4^+$ cell levels may occur during the first few weeks of the acute infection syndrome but it occurs so rapidly that, if it is a frequent event, it is not observed in most donors. Stage 2, which is characterized by a period of stable or slowly declining $CD4^+$ cell counts that average around 500/mm^3, is highly variable in length. This plateau of $CD4^+$ cell levels is not observed in the most rapidly progressing infected individuals, but has now been shown to last for up to 15–20 years in long-term nonprogressors. Stage 3, which begins an average of 2 years prior to development of clinical AIDS and whose end is marked by the development of the first clinical AIDS diagnosis, is characterized by an accelerated rate of $CD4^+$ cell decline (Giorgi, 1992a). The median $CD4^+$ cell count at the time of AIDS diagnosis was 67/mm^3 with a 95% confidence interval of 58–84 (Taylor *et al.*, 1995). Stage 4, observed during the

TABLE I. Abnormal Phenotypes of $CD4^+$ T Cells

Asymptomatic	$\downarrow$ Total $CD4^+$ numbers and percentages compared with normal subjects $\uparrow$ Fas^+ cells
AIDS	Further $\downarrow$ total $CD4^+$ numbers and percentages Further $\uparrow$ Fas^+ cells $\uparrow$ $CD45RO^+CD38^+HLA\text{-}DR^+$ cells

last few years of life, is characterized by a variable but sometimes slower rate of $CD4^+$ cell loss. Circulating levels can be very low. In fact, a handful of people can live for months to years with almost no detectable circulating $CD4^+$ cells.

Throughout stages 1 and 2 of $CD4^+$ cell decline, the total T-cell number remains relatively constant. This has been hypothesized to result from a homeostatic mechanism that holds the circulating T-cell levels constant without regard to $CD4^+$ or $CD8^+$ phenotype (Margolick *et al.*, 1993, 1995; Adleman and Wofsy, 1993). Thus, as $CD4^+$ cells are depleted as a result of the pathogenic effects of HIV (or alternatively caused by immune clearance), both $CD4^+$ and $CD8^+$ cells are produced to replace them in a ratio of about 2:1 (the CD4:CD8 ratio of uninfected donors). Failure of T-cell homeostasis, a critical event during HIV disease, is evident in many individuals by a precipitous drop in total circulating T-cell (and total lymphocyte) numbers. This occurs coincident with stage 3 of $CD4^+$ cell decline. In MACS donors, this decline occurred on average 2 years before the onset of AIDS (Margolick *et al.*, 1995).

2.1.2. Selective Alterations in $CD4^+$ Cell Functional Subsets

As described later (Section 3.1.1), $CD4^+$ cells show defective responses on a per cell basis to recall antigens (such as tetanus toxoid, *Candida albicans*, or influenza) even in asymptomatic HIV-infected people. The *in vitro* response to recall antigens is an exclusive function of $CD4^+$ lymphocytes (i.e., $CD8^+$ T cells, NK cells, and B cells do not participate). Further, the $CD4^+$ cells that make this response must already have been sensitized to the specific antigen *in vivo* and hence are called "memory" cells. Memory $CD4^+$ cells are distinguished by their cell surface phenotype, i.e., $CD45RO^+/CD29^+/CD45RA^-$ (Merkenschlager *et al.*, 1988; Morimoto *et al.*, 1985; Tedder *et al.*, 1985). (CD45RO and CD45RA are the low- and high-molecular-weight isoforms, respectively, of the leukocyte common antigen; CD29 is the integrin β_1 subunit.) $CD4^+$ cells with the memory phenotype harbor more HIV provirus and hence are candidates for depletion by HIV cytopathic effects following activation and subsequent stimulation of viral replication (Schnittman *et al.*, 1990). Although it was initially believed that phenotypically defined memory cells were selectively decreased in HIV-infected people (Van Noesel *et al.*, 1990), other data (Chou *et al.*, 1994; Giorgi *et al.*, 1987a; Gupta, 1987) as well as the results of the Vth International Human Leukocyte Differentiation Antigen Workshop (Giorgi *et al.*, 1995) indicate that selective depletion of phenotypically defined memory $CD4^+$ cells does not occur even though loss of function can be easily documented. In fact, as $CD4^+$ cell levels drop near zero, there is actually a significant *increase* in the fraction of $CD4^+$ cells that express CD45RO (Giorgi *et al.*, 1995; Chou *et al.*, 1994). Thus, functional deficiency cannot be easily explained by phenotypic depletion. Meanwhile, as compared with uninfected controls, $CD4^+$ cells from HIV-infected people have a decreased fraction that expresses the CD28 costimulatory molecule (Caruso *et al.*, 1994; Borthwick *et al.*, 1994; Brinchmann *et al.*, 1994). This could contribute at least in part to the functional deficiency observed in their $CD4^+$ cells.

2.1.3. Activation Marker Expression on $CD4^+$ Cells

In very late HIV disease, most of the few remaining $CD4^+$ cells are $CD45RO^+$. This appears to reflect activation rather than memory because the cells respond poorly to recall antigen but express increased levels of several cell surface antigens that are associated with activation including HLA-DR (an MHC class II molecule), CD38 (an ectoenzyme described in Section 2.2.2), and Fas (a differentiation antigen that may mediate apoptotic cell death) (McCloskey *et al.*, 1995; Chou *et al.*, 1994; Kestens *et al.*, 1994). All of these activation antigens are expressed at high levels on $CD4^+$ cells after AIDS has developed but not during earlier stages of HIV disease. The elevation in HIV infection of the $CD4^+CD7^-CD57^+$ subset, a $CD4^+$ cell population that is rare in normal healthy subjects (Legac *et al.*, 1992), further implicates $CD4^+$ cell activation in AIDS pathogenesis. [The CD57 mAb is reactive with a carbohydrate moiety expressed on subsets of NK and T cells (McGarry *et al.*, 1983). The CD7 antigen, a T-cell-associated glycoprotein essential for T-cell function (Jung *et al.*, 1986), is expressed on immature and mature but not late-stage T cells.] The increased viral load observed in some HIV-infected people given the flu vaccine (O'Brien *et al.*, 1995) supports the conclusion that $CD4^+$ cell activation contributes to enhanced HIV replication (Zack *et al.*, 1990; Margolick *et al.*, 1987). Activated $CD4^+$ cells may also contribute to immunodeficiency because such cells cannot respond to new stimuli (Lees *et al.*, 1993).

2.1.4. Prognostic Value of $CD4^+$ Cell Decreases

$CD4^+$ cell counts have consistently been found to be strongly associated with the risk of progression to AIDS and death in HIV-infected individuals in all risk groups and across all stages of HIV disease (Centers for Disease Control and Prevention, 1994; Phillips *et al.*, 1991; Taylor *et al.*, 1989; Eyster *et al.*, 1987). For example, among homosexual men in the MACS who had been infected for at least 8 years, those with <200 $CD4^+$ cells/mm^3 had about a 70% chance of developing AIDS within the subsequent 3-year period while those with >500 $CD4^+$ cells/mm^3 had an incidence of new clinical AIDS diagnoses of 11%. In the same cohort, plasma RNA viral load had a similar prognostic value. $CD4^+$ cell number and viral load together provided more prognostic power than either alone but each was partially explained by the other.

$CD4^+$ cell percentage and CD4:CD8 ratio measurements are slightly more prognostic than $CD4^+$ cell absolute number (Taylor *et al.*, 1989). This would be expected to be especially useful in neonates and children under 7 years old in whom age-adjusted reference ranges must be used because of the relative lymphocytosis of childhood (Hannet *et al.*, 1992). In adults, CD4:CD8 ratio and $CD4^+$ cell percentage measurements are often used by physicians to verify whether decreases in $CD4^+$ cell absolute values are simply caused by fluctuations in absolute lymphocyte levels or likely reflect clinically significant events. None of the numerical alterations in phenotypically defined functional subpopulations of $CD4^+$ cells have proved to be strong independent predictors of outcome if the analyses take the predictive power of the absolute $CD4^+$ cell levels into account. The prognostic power of activation antigen expression on $CD4^+$ cells remains largely unexplored.

2.1.5. Immunophenotypes of $CD4^+$ Cells in Lymph Nodes

Studies in SIV-infected macaques indicate that $CD4^+$ cell loss in the blood is not reflected in the lymph nodes until the CD4:CD8 ratio drops to about 0.5 (Rosenberg *et al.*, 1993). Similar studies have not been done in humans. However, one recent study (Ramzaoui *et al.*, 1995) examined CD38 and HLA-DR antigen expression on $CD4^+$ cells in the lymph nodes of HIV-infected people and concluded that the distribution of activated cells was slightly different in the peripheral blood as compared with the nodes. Lymph nodes had fewer resting $CD4^+$ cells ($CD38^-$HLA-DR^-). In addition, the distribution of activated cells defined by HLA-DR and CD38 was different. The lymph nodes had more of the $CD4^+$ cells that might be considered the most activated ($CD38^+$HLA-DR^+) and no cells that expressed HLA-DR but not CD38 ($CD38^-$HLA-DR^+). These findings underscore the compartmentalization of the immune system between tissue and blood.

2.2. $CD8^+$ Cell Phenotypes

2.2.1. Alterations in Total $CD8^+$ Cell Numbers

Some of the numerous phenotypic alterations in $CD8^+$ cells of HIV-infected people are summarized in Table II. The average number of total circulating $CD8^+$ cells in uninfected people is around 500/mm^3. The $CD8^+$ cell count increases in most people at the time of HIV infection presumably related at least in part to the specific immune response of the host to the viral infection. $CD8^+$ cell levels may rise as high as 1000–2000/mm^3, i.e., several times the level in uninfected people. At a point about 2 years prior to AIDS development, presumably because of the loss of homeostatic control of lymphocyte levels mentioned earlier (Section 2.1.1), the $CD8^+$ cell levels drop to values similar to those observed in uninfected hosts (Margolick *et al.*, 1995).

2.2.2. Phenotypic Alterations in $CD8^+$ Cells that Reflect Activation

Results of the Vth International Human Leukocyte Differentiation Antigen Workshop (Giorgi *et al.*, 1995) confirmed that many of the previously reported phenotypic alterations in $CD8^+$ cells of HIV-infected people (reviewed in Autran and Giorgi, 1992) reflect $CD8^+$ T-cell activation. Many of the increased subsets are associated with cells that have cytotoxic T-lymphocyte (CTL) effector function. These include $CD8^+$ cells that express S6F1, a novel epitope of LFA-1 (Morimoto *et al.*, 1987), those that are $CD11b^-$, i.e., do not express CD11b, an integrin molecule (Reddy and Grieco, 1991), and those that are $CD45RO^+$ (Janossy *et al.*, 1993; Prince and Jensen, 1991a). Two of the first reports of lymphocyte subset changes in HIV disease found an increase in the $CD62L^-$ fraction of $CD8^+$ cells (Giorgi *et al.*, 1987b; Nicholson *et al.*, 1984). The CD62L molecule is the lymphocyte homing receptor required for lymphocyte adhesion to the high endothelial venules of peripheral lymphoid tissue (Camerini *et al.*, 1989). Again, the $CD62L^-$ fraction of $CD8^+$ T cells contains the cells with

TABLE II. Abnormal Phenotypes of $CD8^+$ T Cells

Asymptomatic	↑ CD38 and HLA-DR expression on $CD8^+$ cells
	↑ $CD28^-$ $CD8^+$ cell proportions
	↑ $CD45RO^+/RA^-$ $CD8^+$ cells
	Total $CD8^+$ cells elevated compared with normal controls
AIDS	Further ↑ of CD38 but not HLA-DR expression on $CD8^+$ cells
	↓ In number of resting HLA-DR^-CD38^- $CD8^+$ cells
	↓ In number of naive $CD45RA^+CD62L^+$ $CD8^+$ cells
	Total lymphocyte level and $CD8^+$ cell numbers ↓ as compared with asymptomatic subjects

CTL effector activity. $CD8^+$ T-cell activation, with the accompanying increase in the representation of $CD8^+$ cells that are $S6F1^+CD11b^-CD45RO^+Fas^+CD62L^-$, may in part reflect chronic HIV replication (Ferbas *et al.*, 1995). This conclusion is supported by the selective oligoclonal expansion of $CD8^+$ T cells with preferential donor-specific Vβ usage during both primary (Pantaleo *et al.*, 1994) and chronic (Kalams *et al.*, 1994) HIV disease.

Activation of the $CD8^+$ cells in HIV-infected people is also manifest by increased expression of HLA-DR and CD38 which is associated with stage of disease as illustrated in Fig. 1. CD38 is a multifunctional enzyme with activities that include NAD glycohydrolase, ADP-ribosyl cyclase, and cADPR hydrolase activity (Malavasi *et al.*, 1994). It may alter adenosine compounds outside the cell possibly producing second messengers that can be transported into the cell to support T-cell activation. Triggering CD38 in mature B cells prevents apoptosis (Zupo *et al.*, 1994) while its ligation on immature B cells suppresses lymphopoiesis (Kumagai *et al.*, 1995). HLA-DR is an MHC class II molecule whose upregulation by interferon-γ on antigen-presenting cells may enhance their activity

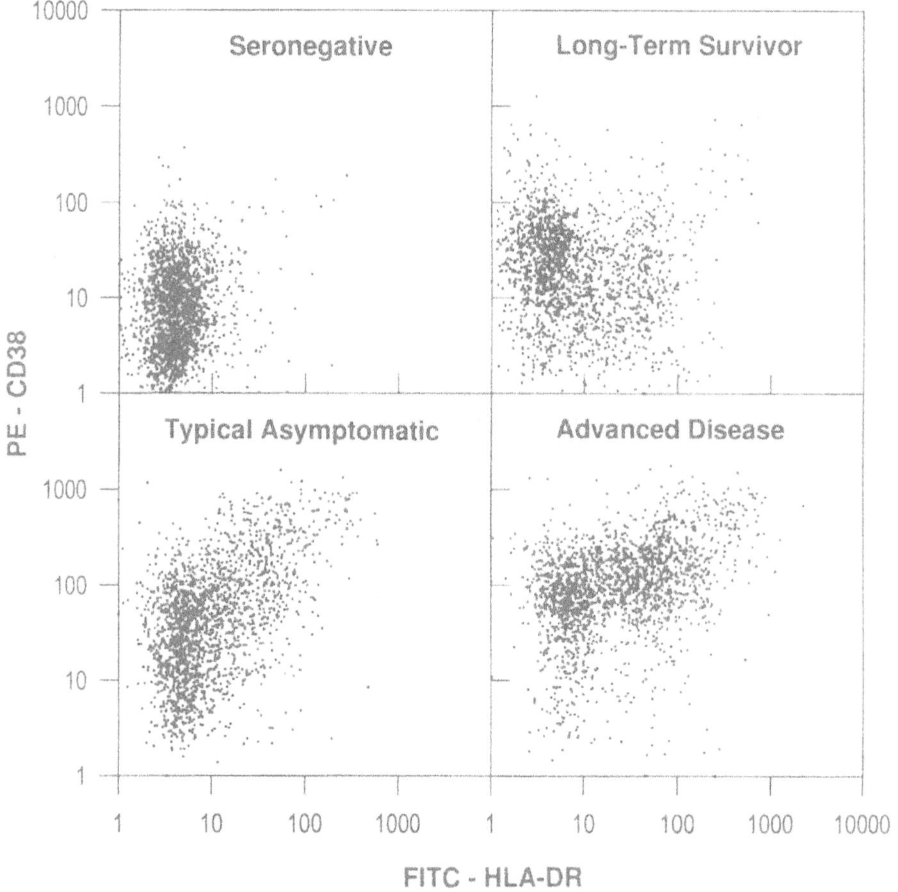

FIGURE 1. $CD8^+$ cell expression of the activation antigens CD38 and HLA-DR are elevated in HIV-infected people and reflect disease stage and prognosis (Giorgi *et al.*, 1993, 1994; Ho *et al.*, 1993).

(Martinez-Maza *et al.*, 1989). Although the function of these molecules on T cells is unknown, they are upregulated on T cells that are activated *in vivo* and *in vitro* (Mittler *et al.*, 1983; Hercend *et al.*, 1981) including anti-HIV-directed CTL effectors (Ho *et al.*, 1993).

Seronegative controls express very little CD38 or HLA-DR antigens on their $CD8^+$ cells (Fig. 1, Seronegative). A surge of $CD8^+$ cells that express elevated levels of HLA-DR and $CD38^+$ is observed around the time of seroconversion (Giorgi *et al.*, 1994). These activated cells probably include the CTL that develop at the time of acute HIV infection (Koup *et al.*, 1994). During the phase of HIV disease when $CD4^+$ levels are moderately stable in typical asymptomatic individuals whose disease progresses to AIDS over several years, there is usually an intermediate amount of both CD38 and HLA-DR expressed (Fig. 1, Typical Asymptomatic). A pattern of very high CD38 expression and only slightly elevated HLA-DR expression on $CD8^+$ cells is characteristic of AIDS (Fig. 1, Advanced Disease). In contrast, in long-term nonprogressors, HLA-DR expression remains slightly elevated but CD38 antigen expression is similar to levels in uninfected controls (Fig. 1, Long-Term Survivor). This and several other features of T-cell immunophenotype and function in long-term nonprogressors are summarized in Table III.

2.2.3. Selective Decreases in $CD8^+$ Cell Functional Subsets

One of the most striking phenotypic alterations in $CD8^+$ cells in HIV disease is an expansion of the $CD8^+CD28^-$ subset (Borthwick *et al.*, 1994; Brinchmann *et al.*, 1994; Lewis *et al.*, 1994; Saukkonen *et al.*, 1993; Landay *et al.*, 1993). CD28 is a costimulatory T-cell molecule whose triggering, which enhances IL-2 production (Fraser *et al.*, 1991), is essential to maximally support T-cell proliferative responses to antigen. The increase in the $CD8^+CD28^-$ subset in HIV disease explains, at least in part, the *in vitro* proliferative defect of T cells of HIV-infected people. The extent to which it is responsible *in vivo* for the immune deficiency that progressively overwhelms the immune defenses of the infected host remains to be resolved but is likely to be substantial.

While age-matched healthy heterosexual controls are usually an appropriate comparison group for studies of immune subset changes, this can be misleading when examining CD28 or CD57 expression in HIV-infected homosexual men. Uninfected homosexual men have an expansion of the $CD28^-CD8^+$ cell population as compared with age-matched heterosexual male controls (mean percent $CD28^-$ ~30, ~50, and ~65% in uninfected heterosexual men, uninfected homosexual men, and HIV-infected men, respectively). A similar situation exists for CD57 such that uninfected homosexual men have a fraction of $CD57^+$ cells that is elevated as compared with heterosexual male controls (Giorgi and Detels, 1989). These elevations in $CD57^+$ and $CD28^-$ subsets of $CD8^+$ cells, which are the

TABLE III. Features of T Cells of Long-Term Nonprogressors Who Have Undetectable Plasma HIV RNA (< ~300 copies/ml)[a]

CD4: CD8 ratio may be >1.0
$CD8^+$ cells show little activation and low CD38 antigen expression but have slightly elevated HLA-DR expression
Direct circulating anti-HIV CTL may not be detectable but other CTL responses remain intact
$CD8^+$ cells can be induced to make a soluble factor that suppresses HIV replication

[a]From Ferbas *et al.* (1995).

cause of the lower CD4:CD8 ratio in uninfected homosexual men versus heterosexual controls (Fahey *et al.*, 1984), are to our knowledge the only marked phenotypic differences that distinguish the lymphocyte subset distribution in homosexual versus heterosexual controls.

The finding in advanced HIV disease that there is a decrease in the naive $CD8^+$ cell subset, defined as $CD45RA^+CD62L^+$, sheds additional light on the cellular basis of the immune defects observed in HIV-infected people (Roederer *et al.*, 1995). This naive subset is the most immature of the circulating $CD8^+$ cells. While this population represents a major component of the $CD8^+$ cell compartment in uninfected people, these cells may be entirely absent in advanced HIV disease in adults (Roederer *et al.*, 1995) and children (Rabin *et al.*, 1995). This result suggests that the failure of the thymus to generate $CD8^+$ T cells may be as important to the ultimate collapse of the immune system in AIDS as thymic failure to generate $CD4^+$ cells. This failure may be caused by damage to the thymus as a result of HIV infection itself or host-mediated damage. Alternatively, it may be related to the exhaustion of $CD8^+$ T cells (Rocha *et al.*, 1995).

2.2.4. Prognostic Value of $CD8^+$ Cell Perturbations

Persistent $CD8^+$ T-cell activation, especially manifest by cell surface HLA-DR and CD38 antigen expression, is a hallmark of HIV infection. While increased levels of expression of CD38 on $CD8^+$ cells are strongly predictive of development of AIDS even after controlling for $CD4^+$ cell levels (Giorgi *et al.*, 1993; Levacher *et al.*, 1992), expression of HLA-DR in the absence of CD38 expression appears to be a marker of a successful protective immune response to chronic viral infection (Giorgi *et al.*, 1994). There are three possible reasons for the association of poor prognosis with high CD38 antigen expression on $CD8^+$ cells. First, it has been suggested that activities of $CD8^+$ cells including anti-HIV CTL (Ho *et al.*, 1993) and/or "promiscuous" killer T-cell activity (Vanham *et al.*, 1991) contribute to immune pathogenesis by lysing infected or uninfected $CD4^+$ cells in infected hosts. Second, high CD38 antigen expression may reflect immunologic immaturity of the $CD8^+$ cells (Salazar-Gonzalez *et al.*, 1985). Finally, CD38 antigen expression may simply reflect a cytokine-driven, normal biologic response to high viral load (Prince *et al.*, 1990). The association of HLA-DR expression with successful control of viral replication may be a reflection of an immune system that is still able to respond normally to antigenic stimulation.

As illustrated in Fig. 1, fluorescence staining of $CD8^+$ cells with CD38 and anti-HLA-DR mAb shows a broad range of reactivities. Conversion of these staining intensities into estimates of numbers of molecules indicates that $CD8^+$ T cells of control subjects express an average of approximately 500 molecules of each antigen while $CD8^+$ T cells of HIV-infected individuals express up to 15,000 of each (Liu *et al.*, 1996). Until recently, we and other investigators have used percentages of $CD8^+$ cells with reactivity of these mAb above the threshold of detection of the flow cytometer as the usual measure for these markers (Giorgi *et al.*, 1993; Autran and Giorgi, 1992; Yagi *et al.*, 1992; Kestens *et al.*, 1992; Prince and Jensen, 1991; Bogner *et al.*, 1990; Giorgi and Detels, 1989; Ziegler-Heitbrock *et al.*, 1988; Salazar-Gonzalez *et al.*, 1985). Widely different percentage readings from various investigators resulted because individual flow cytometers have different sensitivities (~300–3000 molecules). To overcome this difference, we have recently applied existing approaches to estimate the median relative fluorescence intensity (RFI) of CD38 and HLA-

DR antigen expression on CD8$^+$ T cells (Schwartz and Fernández-Repollet, 1993; Schmid *et al.*, 1988). RFI measurements reflect the continuum of expression of the increased CD38 and HLA-DR antigens on the CD8$^+$ T cells and appear to be amenable to standardization across flow cytometers and laboratories. CD38 RFI measurements are highly predictive of AIDS development.

Early work suggested that HLA-DR expression on CD8$^+$ cells might also be a marker of poor prognosis (Stites *et al.*, 1989). However, after controlling for CD4$^+$ cell levels, HLA-DR expression provides no additional prognostic power (Giorgi *et al.*, 1993). Using three-color analysis and combining HLA-DR with CD38 as shown in Fig. 1, increased HLA-DR but low CD38 expression is characteristic of the CD8$^+$ cells of stable long-term nonprogressors (Ferbas *et al.*, 1995). Likewise, development within a year of seroconversion of this population of CD8$^+$ cells is associated with stable disease and better outcome (Giorgi *et al.*, 1994).

2.2.5. Immunophenotypes of CD8$^+$ Cells in Lymph Nodes

The recent study cited above with regard to CD4$^+$ cells (Ramzaoui *et al.*, 1995) also examined CD8$^+$ cell expression of CD38 and HLA-DR antigens in the lymph nodes and blood of HIV-infected people. Distributions for resting versus activated CD8$^+$ cells were surprisingly similar to those for CD4$^+$ cells suggesting that the same mechanisms regulate differential distribution of T cells in the tissues versus the blood for the two major T-lymphocyte subsets. Lymph nodes had fewer resting CD8$^+$ cells (CD38$^-$HLA-DR$^-$) as compared with the peripheral blood. Also, the lymph nodes had more of the most activated CD8$^+$ cells (CD38$^+$HLA-DR$^+$) as compared with the blood, but unlike the blood had no cells that expressed only HLA-DR but not CD38 (CD38$^-$HLA-DR$^+$).

CD8$^+$ T cells in both the paracortical and germinal center areas of the lymph nodes of HIV-infected individuals demonstrate a number of unusual features (Bofill *et al.*, 1995). There is an increased frequency of CD45RO$^+$ cells and these have low levels of Bcl-2. As a result these cells are prone to apoptosis. Although these cells have the cell surface phenotype of CTL in that they are CD45RO$^+$ and express the cytotoxic granule-associated protein TIA-1, they do not have detectable perforin. Peripheral blood CD8$^+$ cells from the same donors also were CD45RO$^+$ and expressed TIA-1 as well as perforin. The lack of perforin in the CD8$^+$ lymph node cells suggests that these cells are not CTL effector cells but rather CTL precursors or end-stage CTL that are no longer functional.

3. ALTERATIONS IN FUNCTIONS OF T-LYMPHOCYTE SUBSETS

3.1. CD4$^+$ Cell Functions

3.1.1. Loss of Responses to Recall Antigens, Alloantigens, and Mitogens

CD4$^+$ cells respond to stimulation *in vitro* and *in vivo* by proliferating and producing cytokines. The classical marker for poor lymphocyte functional capacity is poor proliferation and cytokine production to various types of stimulation. Some stimuli, such as the T-cell mitogens PHA and Con A, induce responses in practically all CD4$^+$ cells. In contrast only about 1–3% of CD4$^+$ cells respond to each alloantigen. Only 0.1–0.3% respond to a given recall antigen (e.g., tetanus toxoid, *Candida albicans*, and influenza) which selectively stimulate "memory" cells, i.e., T cells that respond *in vivo* and *in vitro* to antigens to which the host has previously been sensitized. Recall antigens are often used in studies of HIV-induced dysfunction.

Some of the numerous features of $CD4^+$ cell dysfunction in HIV disease are listed in Table IV. The first report of a functional defect in purified $CD4^+$ T cells showed poor response in the autologous mixed leukocyte reaction (Gupta and Safai, 1983). Subsequently, a hierarchy of loss of proliferative responses to different kinds of stimuli was observed (Clerici *et al.*, 1989b; Lane *et al.*, 1985). Proliferative responses to soluble antigen are lost first, followed by loss of proliferative responses to alloantigen, and finally loss of proliferative responses to mitogens. Not surprisingly, production of IL-2 to these three classes of stimuli are also lost in a hierarchical fashion, since T-cell proliferation is dependent on production of this cytokine (Fan *et al.*, 1993; Clerici *et al.*, 1989a). Reduced IL-2 production and expression of IL-2R and transferrin receptor on $CD4^+$ cells of HIV-infected people as compared to levels induced when control $CD4^+$ cells are stimulated also contributes to the functional impairment (Gupta, 1986, 1993; Lees *et al.*, 1993; Fan *et al.*, 1993; Gruters *et al.*, 1990).

Selective loss of IL-2 production has also been implicated as the mechanism for early loss of CD3 mAb-induced T-cell proliferation in infected hosts (Gruters *et al.*, 1990). This assay has consistently been shown to be reliable in its ability to detect decreased T-cell function throughout the course of HIV disease (Miedema *et al.*, 1988). Duration of infection plays a role in the extent of functional immune deficiency (Gruters *et al.*, 1990; Giorgi *et al.*, 1987a). The qualitative $CD4^+$ T-cell dysfunction in HIV-infected people that is manifest as an inadequate *in vitro* response to recall antigen is one of the major immune defects that leads to AIDS. The *in vivo* response that is the clinical correlate of this *in vitro* measurement, i.e., the ability to control opportunistic infections via T-cell-mediated immunity, is central to HIV disease progression.

A number of mechanisms have been proposed to explain qualitative $CD4^+$ T-cell dysfunction. As noted above, a selective decrease in the phenotypically defined memory $CD4^+$ cells ($CD45RO^+CD29^+CD45RA^-$) does not seem to be the cause since a selective defect is not observed in HIV-infected subjects (Chou *et al.*, 1994; Giorgi *et al.*, 1987a; Gupta, 1987). Rather, the remaining cells do not function normally. This could reflect clonal deletion (Sabbaj *et al.*, 1992), glutathione deficiency (Staal *et al.*, 1992; Roederer *et al.*, 1991), defective protein tyrosine phosphorylation (Cayota *et al.*, 1994), or decreased protein kinase C activation as a result of HIV inhibition of inositol phospholipid turnover (Hofmann

TABLE IV. Abnormal Functions of $CD4^+$ T Cells

Asymptomatic	↓ Memory response to soluble antigens
	↓ Autologous mixed leukocyte reaction (reconstituted with IL-2)
	↓ Production of IL-2, IL-2R, and transferrin receptor
	↑ Apoptosis
AIDS	Further ↓ memory response to soluble antigens
	↓ Autologous mixed leukocyte reaction (not reconstituted with IL-2)
	Further ↓ production of IL-2, IL-2R, and transferrin receptor
	Further ↑ apoptosis
	↓ Response to mitogens

et al., 1990). In addition, the decreased expression of CD25 (IL-2 receptor α, p55) on $CD4^+$ cells in HIV infection may contribute to the decreased response to stimulation (Zola *et al.*, 1991; Hofmann *et al.*, 1991). Finally, shifts in the populations of cells secreting Th1- and Th2-like cytokines also contribute to immune dysfunction (Shearer and Clerici, 1992). Newly available methods to identify cytokines by intracellular staining allow identification of the relationship between phenotypic alterations in lymphocyte subsets and perturbations in cytokine profiles (Litton *et al.*, 1994; Jung *et al.*, 1993).

3.1.2. Apoptosis, Anergy, and Clonal Deletion of $CD4^+$ Cell Subsets

A number of additional basic immune mechanisms, discussed elsewhere throughout this book, contribute to the T-cell immune dysfunction observed *in vitro* and presumably *in vivo*. Apoptosis occurs in $CD4^+$ cells from HIV-infected people when the cells are cultured alone or with stimuli that activate through the CD3 molecule and the T-cell receptor (TCR) for antigen (Gougeon *et al.*, 1993; Meyaard *et al.*, 1992; Groux *et al.*, 1992). Cross-linking of HIV gp120 and the CD4 molecule primes $CD4^+$ cells from uninfected donors for this event (Banda *et al.*, 1992). Although the extent to which apoptosis contributes to $CD4^+$ cell dysfunction *in vivo* remains controversial, there is no doubt that apoptosis of cultured $CD4^+$ cells during *in vitro* assays could account for a major part of the immune dysfunction observed in most of the assays listed in Table IV. If cells do not even survive culture, they cannot contribute to the responses measured in most of these assays.

Another obvious contributor to immune dysfunction measured *in vitro* is the increased fraction of $CD28^-CD4^+$ cells in HIV disease (Caruso *et al.*, 1994; Borthwick *et al.*, 1994; Brinchmann *et al.*, 1994). The decreased fraction of this population would decrease the effective response of the total $CD4^+$ cell fraction even in the absence of other defects. Finally, whether clonal deletion of $CD4^+$ populations directed at certain antigens occurs selectively throughout the course of HIV disease remains unresolved (Schulick *et al.*, 1993; Sabbaj *et al.*, 1992). This is an important issue because if clones directed at certain antigens are selectively deleted through HIV cytopathic mechanisms, other proposed functional defects would likely play a less critical role. Obviously, selective clonal deletion of HIV-directed $CD4^+$ T cells could play an instrumental role in the failure of immune clearance in infected hosts.

3.1.3. Prognostic Value of $CD4^+$ Cell Functional Tests

The role of $CD4^+$ cells in providing immunologic help in the form of cytokines that are essential to support the cellular immune response implicates their functional activity as central to immune dysfunction in HIV disease and AIDS. Functional immune responses of $CD4^+$ cells measured as IL-2 production (Clerici *et al.*, 1989a) or proliferation to recall antigens (Clerici *et al.*, 1989b) or proliferation of $CD3^+$ cells to CD3 mAb stimulation (Miedema *et al.*, 1988) indicate that function is impaired even when $CD4^+$ cell counts are in the normal range. Prospective studies have shown prognostic value for impairment of $CD4^+$ cell function (Dolan *et al.*, 1995). Similarly, impairment of response of T cells to CD3 mAb stimulation has prognostic value in predicting the development of AIDS (Schellekens *et al.*, 1990). Impaired response to CD3 mAb stimulation most likely simultaneously reflects not only impaired $CD4^+$ cell response to recall antigens but also the increased proportions of $CD28^-CD8^+$ cells in HIV-infected people and induction of apoptosis in $CD4^+$ and $CD8^+$ cells as a result of CD3 stimulation (Gougeon *et al.*, 1993; Meyaard *et al.*, 1992; Groux *et al.*, 1992).

3.2. $CD8^+$ Cell Functions

3.2.1. Anti-HIV-Directed Responses

Abnormalities of $CD8^+$ cell function in HIV-infected people are summarized in Table V. Two types of anti-HIV-directed activities mediated by $CD8^+$ T cells are present in infected hosts, i.e., MHC class I-restricted CTL and suppression by a soluble factor (Walker and Plata, 1990; Walker and Levy, 1989). Both of these activities are present at higher levels during the asymptomatic period early after infection than later in disease and both have been implicated in protecting the infected host against disease progression (McMichael and Walker, 1994; Mackewicz *et al.*, 1991). Loss of HIV-directed CTL precursors occurs before loss of CTL precursors to other antigens (Carmichael *et al.*, 1993).

Fluorescence-activated cell sorting (FACS), used to isolate cells on the basis of cell surface phenotype, has been used to document that $CD8^+$ cells with effector CTL activity (also known as direct CTL activity) reside in the population of circulating activated $CD8^+$ cells that express elevated levels of HLA-DR (Ho *et al.*, 1993; Pantaleo *et al.*, 1990a) and CD38 (Ho *et al.*, 1993). Magnetic bead separation has been used to demonstrate that cells with anti-HIV suppressor activity are $CD28^+$ (Landay *et al.*, 1993). Meanwhile, $CD57^+CD8^+$ cells produce a soluble substance that inhibits T- and NK-cell cytotoxicity (Sadat-Sowti *et al.*, 1991). Production of this factor may contribute to the inability of anti-HIV CTL to clear HIV in the infected host.

3.2.2. "Promiscuous" Cytotoxic Activity

While specific CTL activity directed against HIV declines as HIV disease progresses, cytotoxic activity mediated against targets to which the effector cells are bound through CD3 mAb increases (Pantaleo *et al.*, 1990a). This non-MHC-restricted $CD8^+$ cell-mediated activity, also called *redirected killing* or *"promiscuous" cytotoxic activity*, appears to also be mediated by $CD38^+$ cells (Vanham *et al.*, 1991). It is a candidate mechanism of HIV-induced immunopathogenesis (Zarling *et al.*, 1990). The $CD8^+$ population that mediates this activity reacts with the unique unclustered mAb BY55 (Bensussan *et al.*, 1993). This mAb is reactive with only a few $CD8^+$ cells in seronegative controls and about 15–20% of $CD8^+$ cells in HIV-infected persons (Giorgi *et al.*, 1995; Bensussan *et al.*, 1993).

TABLE V. Abnormal Function of $CD8^+$ T Cells

Abnormality observed throughout disease	↑ Apoptosis
	↑ Promiscuous killing
	↓ Response to mitogens
	↓ Clonal frequency in growth assays
	↓ CTL precursor frequencies
Asymptomatic	Anti-HIV-specific CTL and viral suppressive activity present
AIDS	Anti-HIV-specific CTL and viral suppressive activity absent

3.2.3. Low Proliferative Potential in $CD8^+$ Cell Subpopulations

$CD8^+CD28^-$ cells from uninfected and HIV-infected people show almost no proliferation when incubated with T-cell stimuli including PHA and staphylococcal superantigens (Lewis *et al.*, 1994; Borthwick *et al.*, 1994; Brinchmann *et al.*, 1994). The lack of proliferative potential has been attributed to anergy, although in classical anergy, ligand interaction with the CD28 molecule must occur before the TCR engages peptide–MHC complex (Linsley and Ledbetter, 1993). This suggests that some other mechanism of nonresponsiveness could be responsible. Whatever the mechanism, the remarkable increase in the number of $CD28^-CD8^+$ cells that occurs in HIV disease (see Section 2.2.3) clearly contributes significantly to the poor proliferative response of PBMC from HIV-infected subjects. $CD28^-CD8^+$ cells, which undergo almost no cell division on stimulation, represent up to 90% of the T cells in cultures of PBMC from HIV-infected people. Separate studies extend this interpretation by showing that the expansion in HIV-infected people of activated $CD8^+$ cells with increased levels of HLA-DR expression is responsible for the poor *in vitro* responses to stimulation of their T cells (Bettens *et al.*, 1991).

3.2.4. Apoptosis and Decreased $CD8^+$ Cell Survival *in Vitro*

An additional factor that contributes to the functional defects of $CD8^+$ cells in HIV disease is their poor survival *in vitro* (Prince and Jensen, 1991b). Particularly activated $CD62L^-$ $CD45RO^+HLA\text{-}DR^+$ $CD8^+$ T cells do not survive well in culture either with or without stimulation (Prince and Czaplicki, 1989). Apoptosis of these cells has been implicated (Gougeon *et al.*, 1993; Meyaard *et al.*, 1992); levels of Fas antigen are elevated (McCloskey *et al.*, 1995) and Bcl-2 levels are decreased in a subpopulation of the $CD8^+$ cells (Bofill *et al.*, 1995). Addition of IL-2 to the cultures permitted survival of some of the $CD8^+$ cell populations (Prince and Czaplicki, 1989). Notably, the $HLA\text{-}DR^+$ $CD8^+$ cells have poor clonogenic frequency (Pantaleo *et al.*, 1990b). Poor cell survival may contribute to the proliferative defects even early in HIV disease (Bettens *et al.*, 1991). The proportion of $CD45RO^+$ $CD8^+$ cells increases progressively throughout the course of HIV disease and these cells have also been shown to die on activation, whereas $CD45RA^+$ $CD8^+$ cells do not (Janossy *et al.*, 1993).

4. SUMMARY

HIV-induced immunopathogenesis reflects both deterioration and activation of the immune system caused by HIV infection. Viral replication occurs unremittingly in the tissues and blood of the infected host. Decreasing $CD4^+$ cell levels are the primary marker of immune deficiency, but other aspects include the increase of $CD28^-CD8^+$ cells and decreases of $CD38^-HLA\text{-}DR^-$ (resting) and $CD45RA^+CD62L^+$ (naive) subsets of $CD8^+$ cells. Elevated expression of HLA-DR and CD38 antigens together with increased proportions of $CD8^+$ cells that have the cell surface phenotype of CTL provide evidence of $CD8^+$ cell activation throughout all stages of HIV disease. Numerical alterations in lymphocyte subsets may be the basis of many features of HIV-associated immune dysfunction. Increased proportions of cell subsets that undergo spontaneous or activation-induced apoptosis as well as increases in the representation of functionally inert populations of T cells also contribute to the functional defects.

REFERENCES

Adleman, L. M., and Wofsy, D., 1993, T-cell homeostasis: Implications in HIV infection, *J. AIDS* **6**:144–152.

Autran, B., and Giorgi, J. V., 1992, Activated CD8$^+$ cells in HIV-related diseases, in: *Immunodeficiency in HIV Infection and AIDS* (G. Janossy, B. Autran, and F. Miedema, eds.), Karger, Basel, pp. 171–184.

Banda, N. K., Bernier, J., Kurahara, D. K., Kurrle, R., Haigwood, N., Sekaly, R.-P., and Finkel, T. H., 1992, Crosslinking CD4 by human immunodeficiency virus gp120 primes T cells for activation-induced apoptosis, *J. Exp. Med.* **176**:1099–1106.

Bensussan, A., Rabian, C., Schiavon, V., Bengoufa, D., Leca, G., and Boumsell, L., 1993, Significant enlargement of a specific subset of CD3$^+$CD8$^+$ peripheral blood leukocytes mediating cytotoxic T-lymphocyte activity during human immunodeficiency virus infection, *Proc. Natl. Acad. Sci. USA* **90**:9427–9430.

Bettens, F., Pichler, C. E., Herrmann, B., De Weck, A. L., and Pichler, W. J., 1991, Selective stimulation of CD4$^+$ versus CD8$^+$ T-cell subsets in symptomatic and asymptomatic HIV-1-infected individuals, *AIDS Res. Hum. Retrovir.* **7**:773–780.

Bofill, M., Gombert, W., Borthwick, N. J., Akbar, A. N., McLaughlin, J. E., Lee, C. A., Johnson, M. A., Pinching, A. J., and Janossy, G., 1995, Presence of CD3$^+$CD8$^+$Bcl-2^{low} lymphocytes undergoing apoptosis and activated macrophages in lymph nodes of HIV-1$^+$ patients, *Am. J. Pathol.* **146**:1542–1555.

Bogner, J. R., Matuschke, A., Heinrich, B., Schreiber, M. A., Nerl, C., and Goebel, F., 1990, Expansion of activated T lymphocytes (CD3$^+$HLA/DR$^+$) detectable in early stages of HIV-1 infection, *Klin. Wochenschr.* **68**:393–396.

Borthwick, N. J., Bofill, M., Gombert, W. M., Akbar, A. N., Medina, E., Sagawa, K., Lipman, M. C., Johnson, M. A., and Janossy, G., 1994, Lymphocyte activation in HIV-1 infection. II. Functional defects of CD28$^-$ T cells, *AIDS* **8**:431–441.

Brinchmann, J. E., Dobloug, J. H., Heger, B. H., Haaheim, L. L., Sannes, M., and Egeland, T., 1994, Expression of costimulatory molecule CD28 on T cells in human immunodeficiency virus type 1 infection: Functional and clinical correlations, *J. Infect. Dis.* **169**:730–738.

Camerini, D., James, S. P., Stamenkovic, I., and Seed, B., 1989, Leu-8/TQ1 is the human equivalent of the Mel-14 lymph node homing receptor, *Nature* **342**:78–82.

Carmichael, A., Jin, X., Sissons, P., and Borysiewicz, L., 1993, Quantitative analysis of the human immunodeficiency virus type 1 (HIV-1)-specific cytotoxic T lymphocyte (CTL) response at different stages of HIV-1 infection: Differential CTL responses to HIV-1 and Epstein–Barr virus in late disease, *J. Exp. Med.* **177**: 249–256.

Caruso, A., Cantalamessa, A., Licenziati, S., Peroni, L., Prati, E., Martinelli, F., Canaris, A. D., Folghera, S., Gorla, R., Balsari, A., Cattaneo, R., and Turano, A., 1994, Expression of CD28 on CD8$^+$ and CD4$^+$ lymphocytes during HIV infection. *Scand. J. Immunol.* **40**:485–490.

Cayota, A., Vuillier, F., Siciliano, J., and Dighiero, G., 1994, Defective protein tyrosine phosphorylation and altered levels of p59^{fyn} and p56^{lck} in CD4 T cells from HIV-1 infected patients, *Int. Immunol.* **6**:611–621.

Centers for Disease Control and Prevention, 1992, 1993 Revised classification system for HIV infection and expanded surveillance case definition for AIDS among adolescents and adults, *MMWR* **41(No. RR-17)**:1–19.

Centers for Disease Control and Prevention, 1994, 1994 Revised guidelines for the performance of CD4$^+$ T-cell determinations in persons with human immunodeficiency virus (HIV) infections, *MMWR* **43(No. RR-3)**: 1–21.

Chou, C.-C., Gudeman, V., O'Rourke, S., Isacescu, V., Detels, R., Williams, G. J., Mitsuyasu, R. T., and Giorgi, J. V., 1994, Phenotypically defined memory CD4$^+$ cells are not selectively decreased in chronic HIV disease, *J. AIDS* **7**:665–675.

Clerici, M., Stocks, N. I., Zajac, R. A., Boswell, R. N., Bernstein, D. C., Mann, D. L., Shearer, G. M., and Berzofsky, J. A., 1989a, Interleukin-2 production used to detect antigenic peptide recognition by T-helper lymphocytes from asymptomatic HIV-seropositive individuals, *Nature* **339**:383–385.

Clerici, M., Stocks, N. E., Zajac, R. A., Boswell, R. N., Lucey, D. R., Via, C. S., and Shearer, G. M., 1989b, Detection of three distinct patterns of T helper cell dysfunction in asymptomatic, human immunodeficiency virus-seropositive patients: Independence of CD4$^+$ cell numbers and clinical staging, *J. Clin. Invest.* **84**: 1892–1899.

Dolan, M. J., Clerici, M., Blatt, S. P., Hendrix, C. W., Melcher, G. P., Boswell, R. N., Freeman, T. M., Ward, W., Hensley, R., and Shearer, G. M., 1995, *In vitro* T cell function, delayed-type hypersensitivity skin testing, and CD4$^+$ T cell subset phenotyping independently predict survival time in patients infected with human immunodeficiency virus, *J. Infect. Dis.* **172**:79–87.

Eyster, M. E., Gail, M. H., Ballard, J. O., Al-Mondhiry, H., and Goedert, J. J., 1987, Natural history of human immunodeficiency virus infections in hemophiliacs: Effects of T-cell subsets, platelet counts, and age, *Ann. Intern. Med.* **107**:1–6.

Fahey, J. L., Prince, H., Weaver, M., Groopman, J., Visscher, B., Schwartz, K., and Detels, R., 1984, Quantitative changes in T helper or T suppressor/cytotoxic lymphocyte subsets that distinguish acquired immune deficiency syndrome from other immune subset disorders, *Am. J. Med.* **76**:95–100.

Fan, J., Bass, H. Z., and Fahey, J. L., 1993, Elevated IFN-gamma and decreased IL-2 gene expression are associated with HIV infection, *J. Immunol.* **151**:5031–5040.

Ferbas, J., Kaplan, A. H., Hausner, M. A., Hultin, L. E., Matud, J. L., Liu, Z., Panicali, D. L., Ho, H.-N., Detels, R., and Giorgi, J. V., 1995, Viral burden in HIV-infected long-term survivors is a determinant of anti-HIV $CD8^+$ lymphocyte activity, *J. Infect. Dis.* **172**:329–339.

Fraser, J. D., Irving, B. A., Crabtree, G. R., and Weiss, A., 1991, Regulation of interleukin-2 gene enhancer activity by the T cell accessory molecule CD28, *Science* **251**:313–316.

Giorgi, J. V., 1992a, CD4 counts in relation to markers of immune activation, in: *Immunodeficiency in HIV Infection and AIDS* (G. Janossy, B. Autran, and F. Miedema, eds.), Karger, Basel, pp. 1–17.

Giorgi, J. V., 1992b, Introduction to Section on Immune Cell Phenotyping by Flow Cytometry, in: *Manual of Clinical Laboratory Immunology* (N. R. Rose, E. C. deMacario, J. L. Fahey, H. Friedman, and G. M. Penn, eds.), American Society of Microbiology, Washington, DC, pp. 156.

Giorgi, J. V., and Detels, R., 1989, T-cell subset alterations in HIV-infected homosexual men: NIAID Multicenter AIDS Cohort Study, *Clin. Immunol. Immunopathol.* **52**:10–18.

Giorgi, J. V., and Janossy, G., 1994, Flow cytometry studies in HIV disease: Relevance to AIDS vaccine development, *AIDS* **8**:s183–s193.

Giorgi, J. V., Fahey, J. L., Smith, D. C., Hultin, L. E., Cheng, H.-L., Mitsuyasu, R. T., and Detels, R., 1987a, Early effects of HIV on CD4 lymphocytes in vivo, *J. Immunol.* **138**:3725–3730.

Giorgi, J. V., Nishanian, P. G., Schmid, I., Hultin, L. E., Cheng, H.-L., and Detels, R., 1987b, Selective alterations in immunoregulatory lymphocyte subsets in early HIV (human T-lymphotropic virus type III/lymphadenopathy-associated virus) infection, *J. Clin. Immunol.* **7**:140–150.

Giorgi, J. V., Kesson, A. M., and Chou, C. C., 1992, Immunodeficiency and infectious diseases, in: *Manual of Clinical Laboratory Immunology* (N. R. Rose, E. C. deMacario, J. L. Fahey, H. Friedman, and G. M. Penn, eds.), American Society of Microbiology, Washington, DC, pp. 174–181.

Giorgi, J. V., Liu, Z., Hultin, L. E., Cumberland, W. G., Hennessey, K., and Detels, R., 1993, Elevated levels of $CD38^+CD8^+$ T cells in HIV infection add to the prognostic value of low $CD4^+$ T cell levels: Results of 6 years of follow-up, *J. AIDS* **6**:904–912.

Giorgi, J. V., Ho, H.-N., Hirji, K., Chou, C.-C., Hultin, L. E., O'Rourke, S., Park, L., Margolick, J. B., Ferbas, J., Phair, J. P., and the Multicenter AIDS Cohort Study, 1994, $CD8^+$ lymphocyte activation at HIV-1 seroconversion: Development of $HLA\text{-}DR^+CD38^-CD8^+$ cells is associated with subsequent stable $CD4^+$ cell levels, *J. Infect. Dis.* **170**:775–781.

Giorgi, J. V., Boumsell, L., and Autran, B., 1995, Reactivity of workshop T-cell section mAb with circulating $CD4^+$ and $CD8^+$ T cells in HIV disease and following *in vitro* activation, in: *Leucocyte Typing V: White Cell Differentiation Antigens* (S. F. Schlossman, L. Boumsell, W. Gilks, J. M. Harlan, T. Kishimoto, C. Morimoto, J. Ritz, S. Shaw, R. Silverstein, T. Springer, T. F. Tedder, and R. F. Todd, eds.), Oxford University Press, London, pp. 446–461.

Gougeon, M. L., Garcia, S., Heeney, J., Tschopp, R., Lecoeur, H., Guetard, D., Rame, V., Dauguet, C., and Montagnier, L., 1993, Programmed cell death in AIDS-related HIV and SIV infections, *AIDS Res. Hum. Retrovir.* **9**:553–563.

Groux, H., Torpier, G., Monté, D., Mouton, Y., Capron, A., and Ameisen, J. C., 1992, Activation-induced death by apoptosis in $CD4^+$ T cells from human immunodeficiency virus-infected asymptomatic individuals, *J. Exp. Med.* **175**:331–340.

Gruters, R. A., Terpstra, F. G., De Jong, R., Van Noesel, C. J. M., Van Lier, R. A. W., and Miedema, F., 1990, Selective loss of T cell functions in different stages of HIV infection: Early loss of anti-CD3-induced T cell proliferation followed by decreased anti-CD3-induced cytotoxic T lymphocyte generation in AIDS-related complex and AIDS, *Eur. J. Immunol.* **20**:1039–1044.

Gupta, S., 1986, Study of activated T cells in man. II. Interleukin 2 receptor and transferrin receptor expression on T cells and production of interleukin 2 in patients with acquired immune deficiency syndrome (AIDS) and AIDS-related complex, *Clin. Immunol. Immunopathol.* **38**:93–100.

Gupta, S., 1987, Subpopulations of $CD4^+$ ($T4^+$) cells in homosexual/bisexual men with persistent generalized lymphadenopathy, *Clin. Exp. Immunol.* **68**:1–4.

Gupta, S., 1993, Signal transduction defect in the acquired immunodeficiency syndrome and AIDS related complex, *Thymus* **22**:83–90.

Gupta, S., and Safai, B., 1983, Deficient autologous mixed lymphocyte reaction in Kaposi's sarcoma associated with deficiency of Leu-3$^+$ responder T cells, *J. Clin. Invest.* **71**:296–300.

Hannet, I., Erkeller-Yuksel, F., Lydyard, P., Deneys, V., and DeBruyére, M., 1992, Developmental and maturational changes in human blood lymphocyte subpopulations, *Immunol. Today* **13**:215–218.

Hercend, T., Ritz, J., Schlossman, S. F., and Reinherz, E. L., 1981, Comparative expression of T9, T10, and Ia antigens on activated human T cell subsets, *Hum. Immunol.* **3**:247–259.

Ho, H.-N., Hultin, L. E., Mitsuyasu, R. T., Matud, J. L., Hausner, M. A., Bockstoce, D., Chou, C.-C., O'Rourke, S., Taylor, J. M. G., and Giorgi, J. V., 1993, Circulating HIV-specific CD8$^+$ cytotoxic T cells express CD38 and HLA-DR antigens, *J. Immunol.* **150**:3070–3079.

Hofmann, B., Nishanian, P., Baldwin, R. L., Insixiengmay, P., Nel, A., and Fahey, J. L., 1990, HIV inhibits the early steps of lymphocyte activation, including initiation of inositol phospholipid metabolism, *J. Immunol.* **145**: 3699–3705.

Hofmann, B., Nishanian, P., Fahey, J. L., Esmail, I., Jackson, A. L., Detels, R., and Cumberland, W., 1991, Serum increases and lymphoid cell surface losses of IL-2 receptor CD25 in HIV infection: Distinctive parameters of HIV-induced change, *Clin. Immunol. Immunopathol.* **61**:212–224.

Janossy, G., Borthwick, N., Lomnitzer, R., Medina, E., Squire, S. B., Phillips, A. N., Lipman, M., Johnson, M. A., Lee, C., and Bofill, M., 1993, Lymphocyte activation in HIV-1 infection. I. Predominant proliferative defects among CD45RO$^+$ cells of the CD4 and CD8 lineages, *AIDS* **7**:613–624.

Jung, L. K. L., Fu, S. M., Hara, T., Kapoor, N., and Good, R. A., 1986, Defective expression of T cell-associated glycoprotein in severe combined immunodeficiency, *J. Clin. Invest.* **77**:940–946.

Jung, T., Schauer, U., Heusser, C., Neumann, C., and Rieger, C., 1993, Detection of intracellular cytokines by flow cytometry, *J. Immunol. Methods* **159**:197–207.

Kalams, S. A., Johnson, R. P., Trocha, A. K., Dynan, M. J., Ngo, H. S., D'Aquila, R. T., Kurnick, J. T., and Walker, B. D., 1994, Longitudinal analysis of T cell receptor (TCR) gene usage by human immunodeficiency virus 1 envelope-specific cytotoxic T lymphocyte clones reveals a limited TCR repertoire, *J. Exp. Med.* **179**:1261–1271.

Kestens, L., Vanham, G., Gigase, P., Young, G., Hannet, I., Vanlangendonck, F., Hulstaert, F., and Bach, B. A., 1992, Expression of activation antigens, HLA-DR and CD38, on CD8 lymphocytes during HIV-1 infections, *AIDS* **6**:793–797.

Kestens, L., Vanham, G., Vereecken, C., Vandenbruaene, M., Vercauteren, G., Colebunders, R. L., and Gigase, P. L., 1994, Selective increase of activation antigens HLA-DR and CD38 on CD4$^+$CD45RO$^+$ T lymphocytes during HIV-1 infection, *Clin. Exp. Immunol.* **95**:436–441.

Koup, R. A., Safrit, J. T., Cao, Y., Andrews, C. A., McLeod, G., Borkowsky, W., Farthing, C., and Ho, D. D., 1994, Temporal association of cellular immune responses with the initial control of viremia in primary human immunodeficiency virus type 1 syndrome, *J. Virol.* **68**:4650–4655.

Kumagai, M.-A., Coustan-Smith, E., Murray, D. J., Silvennoinen, O., Murti, K. G., Evans, W. E., Malavasi, F., and Campana, D., 1995, Ligation of CD38 suppresses human B lymphopoiesis, *J. Exp. Med.* **181**:1101–1110.

Landay, A. L., Mackewicz, C. E., and Levy, J. A., 1993, An activated CD4$^+$ T cell phenotype correlates with anti-HIV activity and asymptomatic clinical status, *Clin. Immunol. Immunopathol.* **69**:106–116.

Lane, H. C., Depper, J. M., Greene, W. C., Whalen, G., Waldmann, T. A., and Fauci, A. S., 1985, Qualitative analysis of immune function in patients with the acquired immunodeficiency syndrome: Evidence for a selective defect in soluble antigen recognition, *N. Engl. J. Med.* **313**:79–84.

Lees, O., Ramzaoui, S., Gilbert, D., Borsa, F., Humbert, G., Leblanc, D., Lagarde, M., and Tron, F., 1993, The impaired *in vitro* production of interleukin-2 in HIV infection is negatively correlated to the number of circulating CD4$^+$DR$^+$ T cells and is reversed by allowing T cells to rest in culture: Arguments for *in vivo* CD4$^+$ T cell activation, *Clin. Immunol. Immunopathol.* **67**:185–191.

Legac, E., Autran, B., Merle-Beral, H., Katlama, C., and Debré, P., 1992, CD4$^+$CD7$^-$CD57$^+$ T cells: A new T-lymphocyte subset expanded during human immunodeficiency virus infection, *Blood* **79**:1746–1753.

Levacher, M., Hulstaert, F., Tallet, S., Ullery, S., Pocidalo, J. J., and Bach, B. A., 1992, The significance of activation markers on CD8 lymphocytes in human immunodeficiency syndrome: Staging and prognostic value, *Clin. Exp. Immunol.* **90**:376–382.

Lewis, D. E., Tang, D. S. N., Adu-Oppong, A., Schober, W., and Rodgers, J. R., 1994, Anergy and apoptosis in CD8$^+$ T cells from HIV-infected person, *J. Immunol.* **153**:412–420.

Linsley, P. S., and Ledbetter, J. A., 1993, The role of the CD28 receptor during T cell responses to antigen, *Annu. Rev. Immunol.* **11**:191–212.

Litton, M. J., Sander, B., Murphy, E., O'Garra, A. O., and Abrams, J. S., 1994, Early expression of cytokines in lymph nodes after treatment in vivo with *Staphylococcus* enterotoxin B, *J. Immunol. Methods* **175**:47–58.

Liu, Z., Hultin, L. E., Cumberland, W. G., Hultin, P., Schmid, I., Matud, J. L., Detels, R., and Giorgi, J. V., 1996, Elevated relative fluorescence intensity of CD38 antigen expression on $CD8^+$ T cells is a marker of poor prognosis in HIV infection: Results of 6 years of follow-up, *Cytometry (Commun. Clin. Cytometry)* **26**:1–7.

McCloskey, T. W., Oyaizu, N., Kaplan, M., and Pahwa, S., 1995, Expression of the Fas antigen in patients infected with human immunodeficiency virus, *Cytometry* **22**:111–114.

McGarry, R. C., Helfand, S. L., Quarles, R. H., and Roder, J. C., 1983, Recognition of myelin-associated glycoprotein by the monoclonal antibody HNK-1, *Nature* **306**:376–378.

Mackewicz, C. E., Ortega, H. W., and Levy, J. A., 1991, $CD8^+$ cell anti-HIV activity correlates with the clinical state of the infected individual, *J. Clin. Invest.* **87**:1462–1466.

McMichael, A. J., and Walker, B. D., 1994, Cytotoxic T lymphocyte epitopes: Implications for HIV vaccines, *AIDS* **8**:S155–S173.

Malavasi, F., Funaro, A., Roggero, S., Horenstein, A., Calosso, L., and Mehta, K., 1994, Human CD38: A glycoprotein in search of a function, *Immunol. Today* **15**:95–97.

Margolick, J. B., Volkman, D. J., Folks, T. M., and Fauci, A. S., 1987, Amplification of HTLV-III/LAV infection by antigen-induced activation of T cells and direct suppression by virus of lymphocyte blastogenic responses, *J. Immunol.* **138**:1719–1723.

Margolick, J. B., Donnenberg, A. D., Muñoz, A., Park, L. P., Bauer, K. D., Giorgi, J. V., Ferbas, J., Saah, A. J., and the Multicenter AIDS Cohort Study, 1993, Changes in T and non-T lymphocyte subsets following seroconversion to HIV-1: Stable $CD3^+$ and declining CD3-populations suggest regulatory responses linked to loss of CD4 lymphocytes, *J. AIDS* **6**:153–161.

Margolick, J. B., Muñoz, A., Donnenberg, A. D., Park, L. P., Galai, N., Giorgi, J. V., O'Gorman, M. R. G., Ferbas, J., and the Multicenter AIDS Cohort Study, 1995, Failure of T-cell homeostasis preceeding AIDS in HIV-1 infection, *Nature Med.* **1**:674–680.

Martinez-Maza, O., Mitsuyasu, R. T., Miles, S. A., Giorgi, J. V., Heitjan, D. F., Sherwin, S. A., and Fahey, J. L., 1989, γ-interferon-induced monocyte major histocompatibility complex class II antigen expression in individuals with acquired immune deficiency syndrome, *Cell. Immunol.* **123**:316–324.

Merkenschlager, M., Terry, L., Edwards, R., and Beverley, P. C. L., 1988, Limiting dilution analysis of proliferative responses in human lymphocyte populations defined by the monoclonal antibody UCHL1: Implications for differential CD45 expression in T cell memory formation, *Eur. J. Immunol.* **18**:1653–1661.

Meyaard, L., Otto, S. A., Jonker, R. R., Mijnster, M. J., Keet, R. P. M., and Miedema, F., 1992, Programmed death of T cells in HIV-1 infection, *Science* **257**:217–219.

Miedema, F., Petit, A. J. C., Terpstra, F. G., Schattenkerk, J. K. M. E., De Wolf, F., Al, B. J. M., Roos, M., Lange, J. M. A., Danner, S. A., Goudsmit, J., and Schellekens, P. T. A., 1988, Immunological abnormalities in human immunodeficiency virus (HIV)-infected asymptomatic homosexual men: HIV affects the immune system before $CD4^+$ T helper cell depletion occurs, *J. Clin. Invest.* **82**:1908–1914.

Mittler, R. S., Rao, P. E., Talle, M. A., Look, R., and Goldstein, G., 1983, Cell membrane perturbation of resting T cells and thymocytes causes display of activation antigens, *J. Exp. Med.* **158**:99–111.

Morimoto, C., Letvin, N. L., Boyd, A. W., Hagan, M., Brown, H. M., Kornacki, M. M., and Schlossman, S. F., 1985, The isolation and characterization of the human helper inducer T cell subset, *J. Immunol.* **134**:3762–3769.

Morimoto, C., Rudd, C. E., Letvin, N. L., and Schlossman, S. F., 1987, A novel epitope of the LFA-1 antigen which can distinguish killer effector and suppressor effector cells in human CD8 cells, *Nature* **330**:479–480.

Nicholson, J. K. A., McDougal, J. S., Spira, T. J., Cross, G. D., Jones, B. M., and Reinherz, E. L., 1984, Immunoregulatory subsets of the T helper and T suppressor cell populations in homosexual men with chronic unexplained lymphadenopathy, *J. Clin. Invest.* **73**:191–201.

O'Brien, W. A., Grovit-Ferbas, K., Namazi, A., Ovcak-Derzic, S., Wang, H. J., Park, J., Yeramian, C., Mao, S. H., and Zack, J. A., 1995, Human immunodeficiency virus-type 1 replication can be increased in peripheral blood of seropositive patients after influenza vaccination, *Blood* **86**:1082–1089.

Pantaleo, G., De Maria, A., Koenig, S., Butini, L., Moss, B., Baseler, M., Lane, H. C., and Fauci, A. S., 1990a, $CD8^+$ T lymphocytes of patients with AIDS maintain normal broad cytolytic function despite the loss of human immunodeficiency virus-specific cytotoxicity, *Proc. Natl. Acad. Sci. USA* **87**:4818–4822.

Pantaleo, G., Koenig, S., Baseler, M., Lane, H. C., and Fauci, A. S., 1990b, Defective clonogenic potential of $CD8^+$

T lymphocytes in patients with AIDS: Expansion in vivo of a nonclonogenic CD3+CD8+DR+CD25− T cell population, **144**:1696–1704.

Pantaleo, G., Demarest, J. F., Soudeyns, H., Graziosi, C., Denis, F., Adelsberger, J. W., Borrow, P., Saag, M. S., Shaw, G. M., Sekaly, R. P., and Fauci, A. S., 1994, Major expansion of CD8+ T cells with a predominant Vβ usage during the primary immune response to HIV, *Nature* **370**:463–467.

Phillips, A. N., Lee, C. A., Elford, J., Janossy, G., Timms, A., Bofill, M., and Kernoff, P. B. A., 1991, Serial CD4 lymphocyte counts and development of AIDS, *Lancet* **337**:389–392.

Prince, H. E., and Czaplicki, C. D., 1989, Preferential loss of Leu 8−, CD45R−, HLA-DR+ CD8 cell subsets during *in vitro* culture of mononuclear cells from human immunodeficiency virus type I (HIV)-seropositive former blood donors, *J. Clin. Immunol.* **9**:421–428.

Prince, H. E., and Jensen, E. R., 1991a, Three-color cytofluorometric analysis of CD8 cell subsets in HIV-1 infection, *J. AIDS* **4**:1227–1232.

Prince, H. E., and Jensen, E. R., 1991b, HIV-related alterations in CD8 cell subsets defined by in vitro survival characteristics, *Cell. Immunol.* **134**:276–286.

Prince, H. E., Kleinman, S., Czaplicki, C., John, J., and Williams, A. E., 1990, Interrelationships between serologic markers of immune activation and T lymphocyte subsets in HIV infection, *J. AIDS* **3**:525–530.

Rabin, R. L., Roederer, M., Maldonado, Y., Petru, A., Herzenberg, L. A., and Herzenberg, L. A., 1995, Altered representation of naive and memory CD8 T cell subsets in HIV-infected children, *J. Clin. Invest.* **95**:2054–2060.

Ramzaoui, S., Jouen-Beades, F., Michot, F., Borsa-Lebas, F., Humbert, G., and Tron, F., 1995, Comparison of activation marker and TCR Vβ gene product expression by CD4+ and CD8+ T cells in peripheral blood and lymph nodes from HIV-infected patients, *Clin. Exp. Immunol.* **99**:182–188.

Reddy, M. M., and Grieco, M. H., 1991, Quantitative changes in T helper inducer (CD4+ CD45RA−), T suppressor inducer (CD4+ CD45RA+), T suppressor (CD8+ CD11b+), and T cytotoxic (CD8+ CD11b−) subsets in human immunodeficiency virus infection, *J. Clin. Lab. Anal.* **5**: 96–100.

Rocha, B., Grandien, A., and Freitas, A. A., 1995, Anergy and exhaustion are independent mechanisms of peripheral T cell tolerance, *J. Exp. Med.* **181**:993–1003.

Roederer, M., Staal, F. J. T., Osada, H., Herzenberg, L. A., and Herzenberg, L. A., 1991, CD4 and CD8 T cells with high intracellular glutathione levels are selectively lost as the HIV infection progresses, *Int. Immunol.* **3**: 933–937.

Roederer, M., Dubs, J. G., Anderson, M. T., Raju, P. A., and Herzenberg, L. A., 1995, CD8 naive T cell counts decrease progressively in HIV-infected adults, *J. Clin. Invest.* **95**:2061–2066.

Rosenberg, Y. J., Zack, P. M., White, B. D., Papermaster, S. F., and Lewis, M. G., 1993, Decline in the CD4+ lymphocyte population in the blood of SIV-infected macaques is not reflected in lymph nodes, *AIDS Res. Hum. Retrovir.* **9**:639–646.

Sabbaj, S., Para, M. F., Fass, R. J., Adams, P. W., Orosz, C. G., and Whitacre, C. C., 1992, Quantitation of antigen-specific immune responses in human immunodeficiency virus (HIV)-infected individuals by limiting dilution analysis, *J. Clin. Immunol.* **12**:216–224.

Sadat-Sowti, B., Debré, P., Idziorek, T., Guillon, J.-M., Hadida, F., Okzenhendler, E., Katlama, C., Mayaud, C., and Autran, B., 1991, A lectin-binding soluble factor released by CD8+CD57+ lymphocytes from AIDS patients inhibits T cell cytotoxicity, *Eur. J. Immunol.* **21**:737–741.

Salazar-Gonzalez, J. F., Moody, D. J., Giorgi, J. V., Martinez-Maza, O., Mitsuyasu, R. T., and Fahey, J. L., 1985, Reduced ecto-5′-nucleotidase activity and enhanced OKT10 and HLA-DR expression on CD8 (T-suppressor/cytotoxic) lymphocytes in the acquired immune deficiency syndrome: Evidence of CD8 cell immaturity, *J. Immunol.* **135**:1778–1785.

Saukkonen, J. J., Kornfeld, H., and Berman, J. S., 1993, Expansion of a CD8+CD28− cell population in the blood and lung of HIV-positive patients, *J. AIDS* **6**:1194–1204.

Schellekens, P. T. A., Roos, M. T. L., De Wolf, F., Lange, J. M. A., and Miedema, F., 1990, Low T-cell responsiveness to activation via CD3/TCR is a prognostic marker for acquired immunodeficiency syndrome (AIDS) in human immunodeficiency virus-1 (HIV-1)-infected men, *J. Clin. Immunol.* **10**:121–127.

Schmid, I., Schmid, P., and Giorgi, J. V., 1988, Conversion of logarithmic channel numbers into relative linear fluorescence intensity, *Cytometry* **9**:533–538.

Schnittman, S. M., Lane, H. C., Greenhouse, J., Justement, J. S., Baseler, M., and Fauci, A. S., 1990, Preferential infection of CD4+ memory T cells by human immunodeficiency virus type 1: Evidence for a role in the selective T-cell functional defects observed in infected individuals, *Proc. Natl. Acad. Sci. USA* **87**:6058–6062.

Schulick, R. D., Clerici, M., Dolan, M. J., and Shearer, G. M., 1993, Limiting dilution analysis of interleukin-2-producing T cells responsive to recall and alloantigens in human immunodeficiency virus-infected and uninfected individuals, *Eur. J. Immunol.* **23(2):**412–417.

Schwartz, A., and Fernández-Repollet, E., 1993, Development of clinical standards for flow cytometry, in: *Clinical Flow Cytometry* (A. L. Landay, K. A. Ault, K. D. Bauer, and P. S. Rabinovitch, eds.), The New York Academy of Sciences, New York, pp. 28–39.

Shearer, G. M., and Clerici, M., 1992, T helper cell immune dysfunction in asymptomatic, HIV-1-seropositive individuals: The role of TH1–TH2 cross regulation, in: *Regulation and Functional Significance of T-Cell Subsets* (R. L. Coffman, ed.), Karger, Basel, pp. 21–43.

Staal, F. J., Roederer, M., Israelski, D. M., Bubp, J., Mole, L. A., McShane, D., Deresinski, S. C., Ross, W., Sussman, H., Raju, P. A., Anderson, M. T., Moore, W., Ela, S. W., Herzenberg, L. A., and Herzenberg, L. A., 1992, Intracellular glutathione levels in T cell subsets decrease in HIV-infected individuals, *AIDS Res. Hum. Retrovir.* **8:**305–311.

Stites, D. P., Moss, A. R., Bacchetti, P., Osmond, D., McHugh, T. M., Wang, Y. J., Hebert, S., and Colfer, B., 1989, Lymphocyte subset analysis to predict progression to AIDS in a cohort of homosexual men in San Francisco, *Clin. Immunol. Immunopathol.* **52:**96–103.

Taylor, J. M. G., Fahey, J. L., Detels, R., and Giorgi, J. V., 1989, CD4 percentage, CD4 number, and CD4:CD8 ratio in HIV infection: Which to choose and how to use, *J. AIDS* **2:**114–124.

Taylor, J. M. G., Visscher, S. B., and Giorgi, J. V., 1995, $CD4^+$ T-cell number at the time of acquired immunodeficiency syndrome, *Am. J. Epidemiol.* **141:**645–651.

Tedder, T. F., Cooper, M. D., and Clement, L. T., 1985, Human lymphocyte differentiation antigens HB-10 and HB-11. II. Differential production of B cell growth and differentiation factors by distinct helper T cell subpopulations, *J. Immunol.* **134:**2989–2994.

Vanham, G., Kestens, L., Penne, G., Goilav, C., Gigase, P., Colebunders, R., Vandenbruaene, M., Goeman, J., Van Der Groen, G., and Ceuppens, J. L., 1991, Subset markers of $CD8^+$ cells and their relation to enhanced cytotoxic T-cell activity during human immunodeficiency virus infection, *J. Clin. Immunol.* **11:**345–355.

Van Noesel, C. J. M., Gruters, R. A., Terpstra, F. G., Schellekens, P. T. A., Van Lier, R. A. W., and Miedema, F., 1990, Functional and phenotypic evidence for a selective loss of memory T cells in asymptomatic human immunodeficiency virus-infected men, *J. Clin. Invest.* **86:**293–299.

Walker, B. D., and Plata, F., 1990, Cytotoxic T lymphocytes against HIV, *AIDS* **4:**177–184.

Walker, C. M., and Levy, J. A., 1989, A diffusible lymphokine produced by $CD8^+$ T lymphocytes suppresses HIV replication, *J. Immunol.* **66:**628–630.

Yagi, M. J., Chu, F.-N., Jiang, J. D., Wallace, J., Mason, P., Liu, Y., Carafa, J., and Bekesi, J. G., 1992, Increases in soluble CD8 antigen in plasma, and $CD8^+$ and $CD8^+CD38^+$ cells in human immunodeficiency virus type-1 infection, *Clin. Immunol. Immunopathol.* **63:**126–134.

Zack, J. A., Arrigo, S. J., Weitsman, S. R., Go, A. S., Haislip, A., and Chen, I. S. Y., 1990, HIV-1 entry into quiescent primary lymphocytes: Molecular analysis reveals a labile, latent viral structure, *Cell* **61:**213–222.

Zarling, J. M., Ledbetter, J. A., Sias, J., Fultz, P., Eichberg, J., Gjerset, G., and Moran, P. A., 1990, HIV-infected humans, but not chimpanzees, have circulating cytotoxic T lymphocytes that lyse uninfected $CD4^+$ cells, *J. Immunol.* **144:**2992–2998.

Zaunders, J., Carr, A., McNally, L., Penny, R., and Cooper, D. A., 1995, Effects of primary HIV-1 infection on subsets of $CD4^+$ and $CD8^+$ T lymphocytes, *AIDS* **9:**561–566.

Ziegler-Heitbrock, H. W. L., Stachel, D., Schlunk, T., Gürtler, L., Schramm, W., Fröschl, M., Bogner, J. R., and Riethmüller, G., 1988, Class II (DR) antigen expression on $CD8^+$ lymphocyte subsets in acquired immune deficiency syndrome (AIDS), *J. Clin. Immunol.* **8:**1–6.

Zola, H., Koh, L. Y., Mantzioris, B. X., and Rhodes, D., 1991, Patients with HIV infection have a reduced proportion of lymphocytes expressing the IL2 receptor p55 chain (TAC, CD25), *Clin. Immunol. Immunopathol.* **59:**16–25.

Zupo, S., Rugari, E., Dono, M., Taborelli, G., Malavasi, F., and Ferrarini, M., 1994, CD38 signaling by agonistic monoclonal antibody prevents apoptosis of human germinal center B cells, *Eur. J. Immunol.* **24:**1218–1222.

CHAPTER 10

CYTOTOXIC T-LYMPHOCYTE RESPONSES TO HIV

From Primary Infection to AIDS

BRIGITTE AUTRAN

The best candidates among host immune defenses for the control of HIV replication and spread in an infected individual are generally believed to be virus-specific cytotoxic T lymphocytes (CTLs), the natural function of which is to clear virus-infected cells (Cannon *et al.*, 1988; Plata, 1985; Plata *et al.*, 1987a; Engers *et al.*, 1984; Greenberg *et al.*, 1981; Buchmeier *et al.*, 1980; Leclerc and Cantor, 1980). Since the first characterizations of HIV-specific CTLs by our group and others (Plata *et al.*, 1987; Walker *et al.*, 1987), these CTL responses have been extensively studied and are characterized by an unusual intensity and polyclonality, as compared to CTL responses in other viral infections (Walker *et al.*, 1994a,b; Nixon and McMichael, 1991; Autran *et al.*, 1991; Letvin, 1991; Rivière *et al.*, 1989). The polyclonal HIV-specific CTLs are simultaneously directed against a large array of epitopes, most of which have been described in conserved areas from the complete set of the HIV-1 proteins. Multiple epitopes are also recognized in the context of the various MHC class I molecules in an individual's haplotype. The persistence of an HIV replication in the face of such vigorous immune responses indicates that CTLs are not efficient enough at controlling virus replication and spread. Despite these major advances in our knowledge of CTL responses in infected individuals, two major sets of questions remain incompletely elucidated.

The first question concerns the capacity of CTLs to confer protection against HIV-1 infection or disease and the mechanisms underlying the loss of CTL efficiency with disease progression. The HIV-specific CTLs are thought to be instrumental in the relative control of HIV after primary infection (Safrit *et al.*, 1994; Koup *et al.*, 1994) and correlate roughly with the maintenance of the clinically silent stage afterwards. However, an active HIV replication persists whatever the stage of the disease. CTLs ultimately fail to prevent the reascen-

BRIGITTE AUTRAN • Laboratoire d'Immunologie Cellulaire, URA CNRS 625–Hôpital Pitie-Salpêtrière, 75013 Paris, France.

Immunology of HIV Infection, edited by Sudhir Gupta. Plenum Press, New York, 1996.

sion of viral load with AIDS progression, while a decline of CTL activities directed against HIV is usually detected during AIDS (Hoffenbach *et al.*, 1989; Joly *et al.*, 1989). A viral escape to CTL control was proposed to explain such a phenomenon (Klenerman *et al.*, 1994, 1995; Couillin *et al.*, 1994; Phillips *et al.*, 1991), but remains highly debated and several lines of evidence rule out the hypothesis that a massive overgrowth of mutants might escape the highly polyclonal CTL responses developed by the host (Haas *et al.*, 1995a; Koup, 1994; Chen *et al.*, 1992; Meyerhans *et al.*, 1991).

The second question concerns the duality of CTL activities *in vivo*: protection or pathogenesis (Paul, 1995; Zinkernagel *et al.*, 1994)? The high levels of strongly activated HIV-specific CTLs that are directed against HIV-infected cells indeed probably limit the HIV infection but may also participate in the pathogenesis of the disease. Indeed the HIV-specific CTLs probably play a role in the destruction of the infected $CD4^+$ lymphocytes and in the disorganization of lymphoid organs, both representing major immune alterations characteristics of AIDS (Koenig *et al.*, 1995; Cheynier *et al.*, 1994; Jassoy *et al.*, 1992; Autran *et al.*, 1988; Meignan *et al.*, 1989; Sethi *et al.*, 1988; Plata *et al.*, 1987b). While the enigma of HIV infection persists (Baltimore, 1995), there is no doubt that the HIV-specific CTLs represent major goals for vaccination and immune therapies (Lieberman *et al.*, 1995; Koenig *et al.*, 1995; Walker *et al.*, 1994; Plata *et al.*, 1989). After description of the HIV-specific CTLs observed in infected individuals from seroconversion to AIDS, the remainder of the chapter focuses on these key questions.

1. CHARACTERIZATION OF CYTOTOXIC T LYMPHOCYTES SPECIFIC FOR HIV ANTIGENS: STRUCTURAL ANALYSIS

1.1. Detection of HIV-Specific CTL

After the onset of the AIDS epidemic in 1981, the first reports of HIV-specific CTLs to appear were by Walker and colleagues and our group in mid-1987 (Walker *et al.*, 1987; Plata *et al.*, 1987b). Since then a number of groups have contributed to the characterization of CTLs directed against HIV. These HIV-specific CTLs have been mainly detected in the peripheral blood of infected individuals because of the relative accessibility of blood leukocytes, but are also detectable in infected organs, such as the lungs (Autran *et al.*, 1988; Plata *et al.*, 1987b), lymph nodes (Cheynier *et al.*, 1994; Hadida *et al.*, 1992), and the central nervous system (CNS) (Jassoy *et al.*, 1992; Sethi *et al.*, 1987) (Table I).

1.1.1. Antigen Processing and Recognition by Virus-Specific CTL

The virus-immune CTLs recognize epitopes from structural proteins, such as external envelope and internal core proteins, as well as from nonstructural regulatory proteins. These epitopes are presented in the groove of MHC molecules on the infected cell surface (Bevan, 1995; Townsend *et al.*, 1985; Zinkernagel *et al.*, 1976). An antigen-specific but non-MHC-restricted cytolysis is usually attributed to ADCC and mediated by $CD16^+$ (FcRIII) non-T cells. The vast majority of virus-specific CTLs are $CD8^+$ T lymphocytes restricted by MHC class I molecules; they recognize 8- to 10-amino-acid-long antigenic peptides which are synthesized in the cytoplasm of the target cell, are processed through the ubiquitin–proteasome pathway, transported in the endoplasmic reticulum, and associated with MHC

TABLE I. Cytotoxic T Lymphocytes Specific for HIV Proteins in Infected Individuals

Compartments	HIV targets	References[a]
Infected tissues		
Lung	Env	Plata *et al.* (1987)
	Gag, Pol, Nef	Autran *et al.* (1988)
		Langlade-Demoyen *et al.* (1989)
		Hadida *et al.* (1992)
SNC	Env, Gag, Pol	Sethi *et al.* (1987)
		Jassoy *et al.* (1992)
Lymphoid organs	Env, Gag, Pol, Nef	Hoffenbach *et al.* (1989)
		Koup *et al.* (1991)
		Hadida *et al.* (1992)
		Cheynier *et al.* (1994)
Peripheral blood	Env, Gag, Pol, Nef, Vif, Rev	Walker *et al.* (1987)
		Koenig *et al.* (1988)
		Nixon *et al.* (1988)
		Rivière *et al.* (1989)
		Culmann *et al.* (1991)

[a]References mention only first descriptions and are not exhaustive.

class I molecules before being presented on the cell surface (Bevan, 1995; Rammensee *et al.*, 1993; Driscoll and Finley, 1992; Cox *et al.*, 1990). In contrast, MHC class II-restricted $CD4^+$ CTLs recognize 15-mers from exogenous antigens that are processed in the target cells (Long and Jacobson, 1989; Morrison *et al.*, 1986).

1.1.2. Effector CTLs and Precursors of CTLs Specific for HIV Antigen

Antiviral cytotoxic T cells are usually hardly detectable *in vitro* if they are not restimulated by cells bearing the appropriate combination of HLA molecules and viral antigens. In contrast, CTL responses directed against HIV antigens are readily detectable without any *in vitro* restimulation (Hong-Nerng *et al.*, 1993; Hadida *et al.*, 1992; Rivière *et al.*, 1989; Nixon *et al.*, 1988; Koenig *et al.*, 1988; Walker *et al.*, 1987; Plata *et al.*, 1987b). HIV-specific $CD8^+$ T cells are indeed detectable in fresh unstimulated cells and specific lysis is directed against antigens that are synthesized and processed in the target cell and is restricted by HLA molecules (McChesney *et al.*, 1990; Plata *et al.*, 1987b; Walker *et al.*, 1987). This unusual feature is related to the massive *in vivo* differentiation of effector CTLs directed at HIV antigens which infiltrate the infected organs and recirculate. This can be evidenced by demonstration of cytolytic granules and enzymes such as perforin and serine esterase in the cytoplasm of the tissue $CD8^+$ T cells (Tenner-Racz *et al.*, 1993; B. Autran, unpublished observations). Primary cytolysis can also be mediated by ADCC directed against native, nonprocessed gp120 on the target cell surface. In that case, the specific lysis is directed by gp120-specific antibodies and is not restricted by MHC molecules (McChesney *et al.*, 1990; Weinhold *et al.*, 1988).

The CTLs can also be amplified *in vitro* by restimulation with HIV-antigen-bearing cells, according to various protocols using stimulating cells that are infected with HIV (Nixon *et al.*, 1988) or rVV (Hosmalin *et al.*, 1990) or that are coated with appropriate peptides. This approach provides the opportunity to amplify and to detect memory CTLs of lower frequency or to induce *in vitro* differentiation of CTL precursors and of memory.

1.1.3. Construction of Target Cells for HIV-Specific CTL Analysis

Target cells expressing HIV proteins of endogenous origin are obtained either by HIV infection or by genetic engineering (Plata *et al.*, 1987b; Walker *et al.*, 1987). The latter approach is widely used; it can be achieved by transfecting both an HIV gene and a human MHC gene, as shown by our group who used murine mastocytoma cells doubly transfected with the HLA-A2 or -A3 gene and the HIV-1-LAI *env*, *gag*, or *nef* genes (Joly *et al.*, 1989; Hoffenbach *et al.*, 1989; Chenciner *et al.*, 1989; Langlade-Demoyen *et al.*, 1988; Plata *et al.*, 1987b). Most laboratories including ours also use autologous or HLA-matched Epstein–Barr virus (EBV)-transformed lymphoblasts that are infected by recombinant vaccinia viruses (rVV) encoding HIV-1 genes (Hadida *et al.*, 1992; Culmann *et al.*, 1991; Walker *et al.*, 1987, 1989; Rivière *et al.*, 1989; Koenig *et al.*, 1988; Nixon *et al.*, 1988; Moss and Flexner, 1987). Such strategy provides the opportunity to look for presentation of distinct HIV antigens by any of the HLA molecules. The HIV genes used in most studies originate from reference strains, frequently HIV-1-LAI or MN. Similar approaches can also be used for SIV genes (Bourgault *et al.*, 1994; Letvin, 1990). Recombinant vaccinia viruses can also incorporate truncated HIV genes, a procedure that allows the mapping of immunodominant regions in the various HIV genes (Lieberman *et al.*, 1992; Hosmalin *et al.*, 1990; Walker *et al.*, 1989). Target cells coated with exogenous HIV antigens were also used: $CD4^+$ target cells adsorbed with gp120 modeled mainly to an ADCC reactivity in the absence of antigen processing and/or presentation by MHC molecules (Weinhold *et al.*, 1988). Nevertheless, the use of $CD4^+$ activated helper T lymphocytes as presenting cells permitted the detection of $CD4^+$ restricted MHC class II CTLs specific for the envelope glycoprotein (Lanzavecchia *et al.*, 1988; Siliciano *et al.*, 1988). Finally, target cells can be coated with 8- to 15-amino-acid-long antigenic peptides that are efficiently presented in the groove of MHC antigens, provided they contain the appropriate anchor motif (Bevan, 1995; Falk *et al.*, 1991). This strategy allowed the mapping of the various CTL epitopes that are present on HIV proteins (Nixon *et al.*, 1988) and the analysis of the binding affinities (Couillin *et al.*, 1995; Choppin *et al.*, 1991), or the competition events that can occur as a consequence of sequence variations (Tussey *et al.*, 1995; Klenerman *et al.*, 1994; Gairin and Oldstone, 1992). HIV-infected cells can also be used as target cells, whether they are naturally infected (Plata *et al.*, 1987b) or infected *in vitro*.

1.1.4. Limiting Dilution Analysis for Estimation of HIV-Specific CTL Frequencies

Limiting dilution analysis (LDA) of CTLs allows estimating the relative frequencies of CTLs that are present in the various cell suspensions, according to the Poisson law. These frequencies are analyzed either without *in vitro* restimulation, thus measuring effector CTLs that are already differentiated *in vivo* (Hadida *et al.*, 1992; Hoffenbach *et al.*, 1989; Joly *et al.*, 1989), or after *in vitro* amplification, thus measuring the precursor and memory CTL frequencies (Klein *et al.*, 1995; Carmichael *et al.*, 1993; Gotch *et al.*, 1990; Hoffenbach *et al.*, 1989). In the latter case, however, several causes of errors are inherent in the method. First, the memory cells present in the tested suspension can be amplified *in vitro* together with precursor CTLs. Second, an inevitable bias of selection occurs among the precursor CTLs during the culture time period, since the clonogenic potential of precursor CTLs may decrease with disease progression (Pantaleo *et al.*, 1990). Recent discrepancies have also been found between LDA estimations and quantitative analysis of T-cell receptor usage that might reflect bias in both types of assays (Moss *et al.*, 1995).

1.2. HIV-1 Antigenic Specificities Recognized by CTLs

Highly polyclonal MHC-restricted CTLs are directed against the structural proteins, the Gag, Pol, Env protein products, and the accessory proteins, Nef, Vif, Rev, and Tat. Interestingly, Vif, Rev, and, mostly, Tat are poorly recognized by CTLs from HIV-infected individuals (Rivière *et al.*, 1989). The low frequency of CTLs directed against Tat contrasts to the major immunogenicity of the Tax protein from HTLV-1 in HTLV-1-positive patients (Koenig *et al.*, 1990), and might reflect the low production of these proteins in infected cells or an altered Tat presentation. The HIV-specific CTL responses are characterized by their intensity, their polyclonality, and their specificities for conserved regions of the proteins. They also use the complete set of the host HLA restricting elements to ensure the simultaneous recognition of high numbers of epitopes. These epitopes, however, are dependent on the processing constraints defined by viral sequences (Nietfeld *et al.*, 1995; Del Val *et al.*, 1991) or by host transporter genes (Hammond *et al.*, 1995), although the influence of TAP polymorphism on transport peptide variants is contested (Obst *et al.*, 1995). Several of these epitopes partially overlap each other and can be recognized in the context of several MHC class I or class II molecules, behaving as promiscuous epitopes as defined by Berzofsky *et al.* (1995), but only a few of them were defined as nonamers (Shirai *et al.*, 1992; Takeshita *et al.*, 1995; Johnson *et al.*, 1992; Takahashi *et al.*, 1992). Several regions or epitopes appear to be immunodominant for CTL recognition. Some shifts in immunodominant regions can be observed with progression of the disease (Nowak *et al.*, 1995; Haas *et al.*, 1995b; G. Haas, unpublished observations).

1.2.1. CTLs Specific for the Envelope Glycoprotein

The envelope gene products were the first CTL target to be determined (Plata *et al.*, 1987b; Walker *et al.*, 1987). The CTLs that recognize the envelop glycoproteins of HIV comprise both MHC-restricted CTLs and unrestricted ADCC cells. The Env proteins serve as target antigens for $CD8^+$ CTLs in association with a variety of MHC class I gene products, including HLA-A2, -A3, -A30, -B8, -B14, -B27 as shown in Table II (Shirai *et al.*, 1992; Rivière *et al.*, 1989; Plata *et al.*, 1987b; Walker *et al.*, 1987); gp 120-specific $CD4^+$ CTL clones restricted by HLA-DR2 and -DR4 molecules were also derived from peripheral blood lymphocytes (PBL) of HIV-infected or noninfected individuals (Lanzavecchia *et al.*, 1988; Siliciano *et al.*, 1988).

Several immunodominant CTL epitopes were identified both in gp120 and in gp41 (Table II). In spite of gp120 diversity among HIV isolates, many of these epitopes appear to be relatively well conserved and spread out along the entire sequence of the protein. This is evidenced by the high frequency of recognition of reference strain envelope gene products such as HIV-1-LAI or HIV-1-MN envelope which are recognized by 60% of a French cohort of 150 individuals (Rivière, 1989; Autran *et al.*, 1994). Moreover, several CTL Env epitopes (amino acids 112–124, 315–329, 428–443, and 834–848) defined in infected individuals, immunized mice, and seronegative human donors are also recognized by T-helper (Th)

TABLE II. HLA Class I-Restricted CTL Epitopes in the HIV-1 Envelope Glycoproteins

Amino acid numbering[a]	Sequences	HLA restricting elements	References
25–46	LWVTVYYGVPVWKEATTTLFCA	A2	Dadaglio *et al.* (1991)
37–46	TVYYGVPVWK	A3	Johnson *et al.* (1994)
112–124	WDQSLKPCVKLTP (T2)	A2	Clerici *et al.* (1992)
121–129	KLTPLCVTL	A2	Dupuis *et al.* (1995)
193–212	TTSYTLTSCNTSVITQACPK	A2	Dadaglio *et al.* (1991)
295–311	SVEINCTRPNNNTRKSI	A2	Dadaglio *et al.* (1991)
315–329	RIQRGPGRAFVTIGK (P18)	A2	Clerici *et al.* (1992)
374–381	PVEIVTHS	A2	Dadaglio *et al.* (1991)
380–388	SFNCGGEFF	Cw4	Johnson *et al.* (1994)
384–395	GGEFFYCNSTQL	A2	Plata *et al.* (1989)
421–440	LPCRIKQFINMWQEVGKAMY	A2	Dadaglio *et al.* (1991)
428–443	QKVGKAMYAPPISGQI (T1)	A2	Clerici *et al.* (1992)
494–513	VKIEPLGVAPTKAKRRVVQR	A2	Dadaglio *et al.* (1991)
584–591	ERYLKDQQ	A24	Dai *et al.* (1992)
584–592	ERYLKDQQL	B14	Johnson *et al.* (1992)
586–595	YRYLKDQQLL	B8	Johnson *et al.* (1992)
765–778	LRSLCLFSYHRLRD	A3.1	Takahashi *et al.* (1991)
788–809	IVELLGRRGWEALKYWWNLLQY	B27	Lieberman *et al.* (1992)
818–827	SLLNATVDIAV	A2	Dupuis *et al.* (1994)
834–848	QGACRAIRHIPRRIR (Th4)	A2	Clerici *et al.* (1992)
844–863	YRAIRHIPRRTRQGLERILL	A30, B8	Lieberman *et al.* (1992)

[a]According to the HIV-1-LAI sequence.

cells, suggesting that they can be bound by a diverse array of MHC molecules (Clerici *et al.*, 1992; Dadaglio *et al.*, 1991; Takahashi *et al.*, 1988). Finally, some of these T-cell epitopes overlap regions of Env recognized by neutralizing antibody or ADCC cells; for example, the 315–329 CTL epitope overlaps the 304–323 ADCC target and the 296–331 major neutralizing domain; the 428–433 CTL epitope overlaps the 423–437 neutralizing epitope. Others (amino acids 587–598 and 765–778) are in the immediate vicinity of B or Th epitopes, indicating their potential value in vaccine formulation (Dai *et al.*, 1992; Johnson *et al.*, 1992; Takahashi *et al.*, 1988). As mentioned above, Env-specific precursors can be primed *in vitro* in naive, seronegative, nonexposed individuals according to several stimulation protocols and induce both class I-restricted and class II-restricted (Berzofsky *et al.*, 1995; Stanhope *et al.*, 1993; Hoffenbach *et al.*, 1989; Lanzavecchia *et al.*, 1988; Siliciano *et al.*, 1988). Interestingly, the frequency of the precursors specific for Env appears to be extremely high in seronegative individuals (Hoffenbach *et al.*, 1989).

Therefore, several immunodominant and conserved regions have been described in the HIV-1 Env glycoprotein that might prove useful for eliciting cellular immunity in a genetically heterogeneous population (Egan *et al.*, 1995; Johnson *et al.*, 1994; Kundu *et al.*, 1992; Hammond *et al.*, 1991, 1992).

1.2.2. CTL Epitopes in the Core Protein

CTLs specific for the Gag gene products have been extensively studied in HIV-infected individuals (Buseyne *et al.*, 1993a; Gotch *et al.*, 1988; Nixon *et al.*, 1988). In contrast to the effector CTL responses to gP 120, the spontaneous Gag-specific lysis which can be detected *ex vivo* always appears to be MHC class I-restricted (Rivière *et al.*, 1989; Nixon *et al.*, 1988). As mentioned for the Env epitopes, several MHC class I gene products have been shown to present Gag antigens, including HLA-A2, -A33, -Bw6,-B8, -B12, -B14, -B27, -Bw52 (Table III). The CTL epitopes, rather than clustering in certain domains, are found along the entire Gag protein (Buseyne *et al.*, 1993a, 1994) as shown in Table III. An immunodominant Gag epitope, restricted by the HLA-B27 molecule, is located in a highly conserved region of p25, between amino acids 265 and 279 (Nixon *et al.*, 1988). Interestingly, this sequence is also recognized by Gag-specific antibodies in HIV-infected individuals (Nixon and McMichael, 1991). Other epitopes located in p14 (amino acids 418–443 and 446–460), or in p25 (amino acids 193–203 and 219–233), are recognized in association with the HLA-A2 molecule (Johnson *et al.*, 1991; Claverie *et al.*, 1988). A shift in the immunodominance of the various CTL epitopes has been proposed to be deleterious for CTL efficiency by Howak *et al.* (1995), as discussed below. The Gag protein also appears as a major target for CTL responses against SIV in infected monkeys, while a limited number of epitopes have been described (Letvin, 1990). Some studies showed a relationship between the Gag-specific precursor CTL frequencies and progression of the viral load,

TABLE III. HLA Class I-Restricted CTL Epitopes in the HIV-1 Gag Proteins

Amino acid numbering[a]	Sequences	HLA restricting elements	References
18–42	KIRLRPGGKKKYKLKHIVWASRELE	Bw62	Johnson *et al.* (1991)
20–28	RLRPGGKKK	A3	Johnson *et al.* (1991)
21–35	LRPGGKKKYKLKHIV	B8	Nixon and Mcmichael (1991)
77–85	SLYNTVATL	A2	Tsomides *et al.* (1991)
88–114	VHGAIGILILALAGLTAGGGALSLLLA (HGP30)	A2	Achour *et al.* (1990)
140–152	GQMVHQAISPRTL	Cw3	Littaua *et al.* (1991)
143–164	VHQAISPRTLNAWVKVVEEKAF	Bw57	Johnson *et al.* (1991)
153–173	NAWKVVEEKAFSPEVIPMFSA	Bw57	Johnson *et al.* (1991)
169–184	IPMFSALSEGATPQDL	B12(44)	Buseyne *et al.* (1993a)
173–194	SALSEGATPQDLNTMLNTVGGH	B14	Johnson *et al.* (1991)
183–197	DLNTMLNTVGGHQAA	B14	Nixon and Mcmichael (1991)
193–202	GHQAAQMLKE	A2	Claverie *et al.* (1988)
193–213	GHQAAQMLKETINEEAAEWDR	Bw52	Johnson *et al.* (1991)
219–232	AGPIAPGQMREPRG	A2	Claverie *et al.* (1988)
253–267	NPPIPVGEIYKRWII	B8	Gotch *et al.* (1990)
253–274	NPPIPVGEIYKRWIILGLNKIV	B8	Johnson *et al.* (1991)
254–262	PPIPVGEIY	B35	Rowland-Jones *et al.* (1995)
256–270	IPVGEIYKRWIILGL	B8	Buseyne *et al.* (1993a)
263–272	KRWIILGLNK	B27	Nixon *et al.* (1988)
263–277	KRWIILGLNKIVRMY	A33, B27	Nixon *et al.* (1988)
263–284	KRWIILGLNKIVRMYSPTSILD	Bw6	Johnson *et al.* (1991)
268–277	LGLNKIVRMY	Bw62	VanBaleen *et al.* (1991)
305–314	RAEQASQEVK	B14	Johnson *et al.* (1991)
323–337	VQNANPDCKYILKAL	B8	Nixon and Mcmichael (1991)
418–433	KEGHOMKDCTERQANF	A2	Claverie *et al.* (1988)
446–460	GNFLQSRPEPTAPPF	A2	Claverie *et al.* (1988)

[a]According to the HIV-1-LAI sequence.

suggesting that Gag-specific CTLs might be associated with protection against disease progression (Klein *et al.*, 1995). Therefore, the conserved Gag proteins are quite immunogenic and may prove valuable to include in an HIV vaccine.

1.2.3. CTL Epitopes in HIV-1 Reverse Transcriptase

The highly conserved Pol protein products are also detected by HIV-specific CTLs, as originally shown by Walker *et al.* (1989). CTLs are mostly directed against conserved epitopes as suggested by the high frequency of CTLs recognizing the HIV-1-LAI Pol-encoded antigens in 80% of cases in the French IMMUNOCO cohort (Autran *et al.*, 1994). However, the various epitopes recognized by CTLs in this protein have been less extensively studied to date (Table IV). The reverse transcriptase (RT) is the major CTL target but polymerase and integrase also function as targets for CTL recognition (Gomard *et al.*, personal communication). A limited number of CTL epitopes have been delineated in RT, in the context of HLA-A2, -A11, -B8, -B14, -Bw60. When focusing on RT: the NH_2-half of the RT is highly immunogenic in patients with more than 400 $CD4^+$ counts (N-terminal: 90%, versus C-terminal: 40% of patients), while at more advanced stages of disease CTLs were rather elicited to the COOH-moiety of RT (N-terminal: 20%, versus C-terminal: 100% of patients) (Haas *et al.*, 1995b; G. Haas, unpublished observations). A major epitope of the NH_2-half (amino acids 203–219) is recognized by both human and murine CTLs suggesting that it might bind to and be presented by a diverse array of MHC class I molecules (Hosmalin *et al.*, 1990). In the COOH-region, two immunogenic domains were found, containing epitopes located between pol (421–596) as well as (681–716) (Haas *et al.*, 1995b; G. Haas, unpublished observations). The persistence of an HIV-1 RT CTL recognition with disease progression, despite shifting of the immunodominant regions, appears therefore possible through an adaptation of the CTL repertoire, thus demonstrating the importance of a major polyclonality of the host HIV-specific CTL-mediated defenses. Such a shift in immunodominance might also allow the infected host to maintain CTL recognition of the highly conserved RT protein when subjected to the mutation pressure of anti-RT drugs.

TABLE IV. HLA Class I-Restricted CTL Epitopes in the HIV-1 RT

Amino acid numbering[a]	Sequences	HLA restricting elements	References
172–196	IETVPVKLKPGMDGPKVKQWPLTEE	B8	Walker *et al.* (1989)
203–219	EICTEMEKEGKISKIGP	A2	Hosmalin *et al.* (1990)
267–277	VLDVGDAYFSV	A2	Van der Burg *et al.* (1995)
325–334	AIFQSSMNTK	A11	Walker *et al.* (1989)
342–350	NPDIVIYQY	B35	Rowland-Jones *et al.* (1995)
342–366	NPDIVIYQYMDDLYVGSDLEIGQHR	A11	Walker *et al.* (1989)
359–383	DLEIGQHRTKIEELRQHLLRWGLTT	Bw60	Walker *et al.* (1989)
476–484	ILKEPVHGV	A2	Tsomides *et al.* (1991)
495–519	EIQKQGQGQWTYQIYQEPFKNLQTG	A11	Walker *et al.* (1989)
588–596	PLVKLWYQL	A2	Haas *et al.* (1995b)
648–673	AIYLALQDSGGLEVNIVTDSQYALGI	B14	Kalams *et al.* (1994)
681–691	ESELVNQIIEQ	A2	Haas *et al.* (1995b)
695–703	YLAWVPAHK	A2	Haas *et al.* (1995b)

[a]According to the HIV-1-LAI sequence.

1.2.4. CTL Epitopes in HIV-1 Nef

Studies of murine CTLs specific for cytomegalovirus demonstrated the potential protective value of CTLs that recognize viral proteins expressed early in the infectious cycle (Reddehase *et al.*, 1987). This observation has sparked interest in the early regulatory HIV proteins, such as Nef, Vif, Tat, or REV, as possible important targets for virus-specific cytotoxic effector cells. Among these accessory proteins, Nef is the most immunogenic for CTLs, HIV-1-LAI Nef being recognized by half of the infected individuals (Rivière *et al.*, 1989; Culmann *et al.*, 1989). Cytotoxic effector T cells recognizing distinct Nef epitopes are differentiated *in vivo* and present in lymphoid tissues from HIV-infected individuals at very high frequencies between 10^{-4} and 10^{-6} lymphocytes (Hadida *et al.*, 1992). The CTL epitopes are located in two major immunodominant regions in the center and in the COOH-terminus of the protein (amino acids 66–150 and 182–206, respectively) (Hadida *et al.*, 1992, 1995; Culmann *et al.*, 1989, 1991) (Table V). In these two regions a continuum of epitopes are recognized by CTLs in association with a variety of HLA molecules, including HLA-A1, -A2, -A3, -A11, -B7, -B8, -B17, -B18, -B35, -B52, and -B62. The B- and T-cell repertoires specific for Nef appear to differ since the central region, which is highly immunogenic for CTL, is poorly recognized by human and murine anti-Nef antibodies; these antibodies preferentially recognize the NH_2- and COOH-terminal portions of the molecule (Bahraoui *et al.*, 1990). The COOH-terminal CTL epitopes, limited by amino acids 182–206, overlap a major antibody-binding site and a Th site. This region may therefore be of use in developing an HIV vaccine (Hadida *et al.*, 1992). Nef-specific CTLs can also be primed *in vitro* from the naive peripheral T-cell compartment of seronegative healthy donors after appropriate stimulation with cells coexpressing HLA and Nef mole-

TABLE V. HLA Class I-Restricted CTL Epitopes in the HIV-1 Nef Protein

Amino acid numbering[a]	Sequences	HLA restricting elements	References
68–77	FPVTPPQVPLR	B7	Haas *et al.* (1995a)
66–80	VGFPVTPPQVPLRPMT	A1	Hadida *et al.* (1992)
73–82	QVPLRPMTYK	A3.1	Koenig *et al.* (1990)
73–82	QVPLRPMTYK	A3, A11, B35	Culmann *et al.* (1991)
84–91	AVDLSHFLK	A11	Culmann *et al.* (1994)
90–97	FLKEKGGL	B8	Culmann *et al.* (1994)
93–106	EKGGLEGLIHSQRR	A1	Hadida *et al.* (1992)
113–128	WIYHTQGYFPDWQNYT	A1	Hadida *et al.* (1992)
116–125	HTQGYFPDWQ	B57, B58	Culmann *et al.* (1994)
117–127	TQGYFPDWQNQ	B62	Culmann *et al.* (1994)
120–128	YFPDWQNYT	B37	Culmann *et al.* (1994)
126–138	NYTPGPGVRYPLT	A1, A11, B7, B18	Culmann *et al.* (1991)
134–141	RYPLTFGW	B27	Culmann *et al.* (1991)
132–147	GVRYPLTFGWCYKLVP	A1	Hadida *et al.* (1992)
135–143	YPLTFGWCY	B18	Culmann *et al.* (1994)
136–145	PLTFGWCYKL	A2	Haas *et al.* (1995a)
180–189	VLEWRFDSRL	A2	Haas *et al.* (1995a)
182–198	EWRFDSRLAFHHVAREL	A1, B8, B35	Hadida *et al.* (1995)
190–198	AFHHVAREL	A2, (A2.1, A2.2, A2.4) B52	Hadida *et al.* (1995)
190–206	AFHHVARELHPEYFKNC	A1	Hadida *et al.* (1992)

[a]According to the HIV-1-LAI sequence.

cules (Lucchiari *et al.*, 1994). Interestingly, CTLs specific for HIV-1 Gag, RT, and Nef are detectable in seronegative, PCR-negative individuals who are highly exposed to HIV (Rowland-Jones *et al.*, 1995; Langlade-Demoyen *et al.*, 1994), suggesting that a certain protection might be conferred by CTLs specific for Nef. Finally, SIV Nef-specific CTLs have also been found in macaques with a similar distribution of CTL epitopes and might confer partial protection against disease protection as shown in immunized macaques (A. Venet, personal communication; Bourgault *et al.*, 1994).

1.3. Repertoire Analysis of the HIV-Specific CTLs

Several studies of T-cell repertoire (TCR) showed a biased usage of the TCR variable regions by $CD8^+$ cells or CTLs, indicating that active oligoclonal responses do occur *in vivo*. An apparent restriction of the TCR Vβ segments in peripheral blood T cells or in tissue-infiltrating lymphocytes from HIV-infected individuals appears related to the $CD8^+$ cell subset (De Paoli *et al.*, 1993; Itescu *et al.*, 1993; Gorochov *et al.*, 1992). Such bias might be predominant at the time of primary infection in lymphoid tissues both in humans and in macaques (Chen *et al.*, 1995; Pantaleo *et al.*, 1994) and indicates the onset of an active oligoclonal primary T-cell response against HIV. Analysis of the hypervariable segments allows the mapping of CTL clones in various samples. Studies conducted by S. Wain-Hobson's group showed that a single CTL clone can expand simultaneously among various germinative centers and be over-represented at a given time point in the lymphoid tissue (Cheynier *et al.*, 1994). They also suggest that some T-cell clones are mobilized *in vivo* against highly conserved regions of HIV gene products since a single clone can coexist *in vivo* with highly diverse HIV variants. Studies from B. Walker's group showed that a single CTL clone directed against a gp41 epitope could be followed over several years in the peripheral blood lymphocytes despite constant antigenic stimulation (Kalams *et al.*, 1994). Moss *et al.* (1995) could also observe a switch in TCR usage reflecting the adaptation over time of the CTL repertoire. The estimated frequencies of usage of hypervariable regions by PBL of infected donors in the same studies led to extremely high frequencies for each CTL clone, representing between 02. and 1% of T cells. Despite the relative lack of precision of the method used in this study, such high frequencies, if confirmed, suggest that the number of $CD8^+$ T cells engaged against HIV might be considerably higher than previously suggested.

2. DYNAMICS OF HIV-SPECIFIC CYTOTOXIC T-CELL RESPONSES

2.1. Frequencies of HIV-Specific CTLs in Infected Individuals

The intensity of the HIV-specific CTL responses was assessed by analyzing the frequencies of CTL effectors or CTL precursors. Though results might vary, depending on the assays, the various limiting dilution analyses of CTL frequencies in infected individuals indicate high frequencies as compared to other viral infections. Indeed, effector CTLs reacting against a single LAI-encoded protein represent between 0.1 and 10 per 10^4 peripheral or tissular lymphocytes during the asymptomatic stages of HIV infection. Our studies conducted in infected tissues such as lung and lymphoid organs demonstrated that HIV-specific CTLs were present *in vivo* at high effector cell frequencies, ranging from 10^{-4}

to 10^{-6} cells for peptide-specific effector CTLs (Hadida *et a.*, 1992, 1995) and from 10^{-3} to 10^{-4} cells for protein-specific effector CTLs, at stages II and III of the disease (Hoffenbach *et al.*, 1989; Joly *et al.*, 1989). Given the fact that HIV-specific CTLs simultaneously recognize several conserved and nonconserved regions in the various HIV proteins, the cumulative frequencies of effector CTLs specific for HIV epitopes might represent an order of magnitude as high as $n \times 10^{-2}$ cells, both in the peripheral blood and in the infected organs. Therefore, the HIV-specific CTLs might represent a significant percentage of the $CD8^+$ cell expansion observed in HIV infection.

Those surprisingly high numbers of circulating virus-specific CTLs might be induced by the persistent replication of HIV in immunologically active tissues although the need for antigen in maintenance of a CTL memory is still a matter of debate (Hou *et al.*, 1994; Müllbacher, 1994). Indeed, the continuous viral replication now known to occur throughout the course of HIV infection strongly supports this hypothesis (Ho *et al.*, 1995; Wei *et al.*, 1995; Wain-Hobson, 1995; Pantaleo *et al.*, 1993). Alternatively, the capacity of HIV to infect antigen presenting cells such as macrophages or dendritic cells, though at low frequency (McIlroy *et al.*, 1995), might be responsible for persisting stimulation of CTL clones. An inverse correlation was reported between the frequencies of HIV gag-specific precursor CTLs and viral load, suggesting that high frequencies of CTLs might be associated with low levels of HIV replication in nonprogressors (Klein *et al.*, 1995). Nevertheless, the remarkably high CTL frequencies, though detectable at the site of an active HIV replication (Hadida *et al.*, 1992, 1995), are probably not sufficient enough to eradicate infected cells since viral replication persists. The recent report of a lack of protection conferred by clonal Gag-specific CTL response to a candidate vaccine in immunized macaques, illustrates the relative inefficiency of clonal CTL responses despite the very high frequencies generated in that model (Letvin, personal communication).

2.2. Evolution over Time of HIV-Specific Cytotoxic T-Cell Responses

Cytotoxic T-cell responses directed against HIV appear very early after the HIV primary infection, as soon as the first week postinoculation and before the appearance of specific antibodies (Koup *et al.*, 1994; Safrit *et al.*, 1994; Cooper *et al.*, 1988), while a strong bias in the early $CD8^+$ T-cell repertoire suggests that oligoclonal T cells initiate the immune responses to the homogeneous HIV isolates at the time of primary infection (Pantaleo *et al.*, 1994). The HIV-specific CTLs rapidly become polyclonal during the first month, recognizing the whole set of the HIV proteins (Lahmamedi *et al.*, 1995). Such early vigorous CTL responses are probably induced by the major initial burst of HIV replication and the high frequency of CTLs recognizing the accessory proteins Rev, Vif, and Tat at this stage might reflect the intense HIV production (F. Hadida, unpublished observations). It is generally accepted that HIV-specific CTLs are the major tools of the dramatic decrease of free and cell-associated HIV particles usually observed after seroconversion since the neutralizing antibodies appear only several weeks after the HIV invasion. In some cases, however, the initial viral burst is not controlled and patients progress rapidly toward AIDS despite the initial appearance of HIV-specific CTLs, as recently observed by our group (Hadida *et al.*, submitted for publication). The intensity and the efficacy of the host CTL response at primary infection might be a determinant of the further evolution of the disease, suggesting that the more efficient the initial immune response, the longer the asymptomatic stage of the disease will be.

These polyclonal CTL responses are maintained throughout the incubation period of AIDS. Recent descriptions of long-term asymptomatic (LTA) individuals or nonprogressors (LTNP) have suggested a prominent role of HIV-specific CTL responses in that apparent protection against disease progression, although there is not enough support for this hypothesis at present (Pantaleo *et al.*, 1995).

A progressive decrease in the frequencies of HIV-specific precursor CTLs has been associated with AIDS. Whether such decrease is the cause or the consequence of progression to AIDS remains to be determined. A decrease in precursor CTL frequencies might coincide with progression toward AIDS (Klein *et al.*, 1995; Carmichael *et al.*, 1993), though our group and others observed such a decline later on, with the onset of the opportunistic infections characteristic of full-blown AIDS (Hoffenbach *et al.*, 1989). Comparing primary HIV-specific CTL activity at stages II, III, and IV of the HIV disease, both in cross-sectional studies and in longitudinal studies, we observed a decreased effector CTL activity at stage IV while a $CD8^+$ cell infiltration persisted in infected organs (Joly *et al.*, 1989). These CTLs, however, remain inducible *in vitro* and are detectable easily after stimulation with autologous HIV-infected PHA blasts or appropriate peptides even in patients with $CD4^+$ counts below 200/mm^3 (Autran *et al.*, 1994).

Therefore, the loss of *in vivo* activity of CTLs directed against HIV appears to be correlated to disease progression. A variety of mechanisms have been proposed to account for the diminished efficiency of CTLs in the infected host. These mechanisms include: virus variants escaping to CTL control, CTL exhaustion, CTL anergy, and lack of T-cell help. To date none of these mechanisms appears as sufficient to explain by itself the loss of relative protection conferred by CTLs. Interestingly, the profile of the HIV antigen specificities recognized by CTLs is extremely stable with disease progression and not a single protein appears to be associated with protection or progression.

2.3. HIV-Specific CTL Responses: A Lost Race?

2.3.1. Does HIV Escape from CTLs by Mutations?

The rapid turnover of HIV and infected cells occurring from the primary infection to the full-blown AIDS generates HIV variants as a correlate of the high rate of transcription errors during virus cycles (Saag *et al.*, 1988). A number of stochastic events indeed activate HIV replication at various sites in the infected host, generating HIV quasispecies (Meyerhans *et al.*, 1989; Delassus *et al.*, 1992; Cheynier *et al.*, 1994). The coexistence of a highly mutating virus and of strong CTL responses has raised the question of a selective pressure maintained by CTLs upon virus mutations. The impressive collection of data reviewed above teaches us that the cytotoxic T cells specific for HIV antigens appear early after virus inoculation and probably control such primary infection, as they might play a role in controlling more or less the HIV replication afterwards, but eventually fail. Reasons for such a failure appear to be multifactorial. Indeed, the immune system not only has to build permanent lines of defense against chronic HIV replication but this has to be maintained in the context of a decreased T-helper cell function. Viruses can indeed mutate under selection by CTL pressure, as shown in the experimental model using lymphocytic choriomeningitis virus (LCMV), a murine RNA virus with a high mutation rate and an exclusive dependence on CTLs for control of early infection (Pircher *et al.*, 1990; Aebischer *et al.*, 1991). Mutations inducing alterations of the gp120 tertiary conformation might allow the HIV isolates derived after initial infection to lose their susceptibility to V3 loop-directed neutralization *in vitro* (Nara *et al.*, 1990). To date, however, studies assessing HIV escape from CTLs *in vivo* have yielded contradictory results.

Phillips *et al.* (1991) demonstrated fluctuations over time in a predominant HLA-B8-restricted Gag epitope. In HIV strains isolated several months later, sequence substitutions affected B8- but not B27-restricted Gag-epitope recognition in three patients. In contrast, in a similarly designed study, Meyerhans *et al.* (1991) sequenced Gag provirus from four patients with B27-restricted CTLs over a 14-month period and did not find similar results: a predominant form of the virus was found to persist over time in 75–95% of the sequences despite constant CTL recognition. A similar persistence of variants in the face of a constant CTL recognition was observed in the SIV–macaque model (Chen *et al.*, 1992). When analyzing CTLs directed at Nef epitopes, Couillin *et al.* (1994, 1995) reported an impaired CTL recognition of mutants in the HLA-A11- and -B18-restricted Nef epitopes. The genetic variations occurring at anchor positions prevented HLA-A11/peptide binding in this study. In contrast, by analyzing sequential changes in five HLA-A2- and -B7-restricted epitopes in four patients, we demonstrated the capacity of the CTL repertoire to simultaneously adapt to epitope variations over time and to eliminate corresponding variants, even in patients with CD4 counts below 200/mm^3 (Haas *et al.*, 1995a; G. Haas, unpublished observations; Autran *et al.*, 1995b). Remarkably, the rare mutations occurring at HLA-A2 anchor positions induced a switch in the epitope restriction from HLA-A2 to HLA-A3 giving an HLA-heterozygous host the opportunity to choose the proper HLA-antigen to maintain epitope variant recognition. In the same study, major variants also persisted in more conserved antigenic regions despite constant CTL recognition, as previously shown by Meyerhans *et al.*

Thus, the evidence to support the hypothesis that HIV mutations occur under selective pressure from CTLs is far from conclusive. Rather, the flexibility of the immune system in a genetically heterozygous host allows continuous expansion of variant-specific CTLs seemingly capable of limiting to some extent and for several years the number of HIV-variant-promoting cells. Such a constant chase occurring *in vivo* between variants does not, however, eradicate HIV and CTLs finally lose the race against HIV. According to Nowak's (1995) model, the heterogeneous HIV population might induce "strong" or "weak" epitopes and oscillations in CTL responses thereby reducing their efficiency in controlling the virus. Disease progression in that case should be the result of a progressive loss in the ability to activate new precursor CTLs. However, experimental evidence supporting such mathematical model remains very limited. Our observation that CTLs continue to adapt to virus variation even in AIDS patients argues against this hypothesis. The frequency of mutations appears even higher in slowly progressing donors (Wolinsky *et al.*, 1996). The exceptionally high polyclonality and intensity of the CTL responses against HIV antigens appears therefore as a host answer to the continuous production of large numbers of antigenic HIV variants, but might be only partially efficient at controlling the number of infected cells.

2.3.2. CTL Exhaustion?

A persistent specific and nonspecific hyperactivation of the immune system is observed throughout the course of the HIV infection and might be detrimental for a number of immune functions (Fauci, 1993). The ability of repeated antigenic exposure to induce apoptosis allows the immune system to control the intensity and the duration of specific immune responses (Glickstein and Huber, 1995). This might affect memory CTLs as a consequence of continuous exposure to antigenic stimulations. Peripheral clonal deletion can thereby result in loss of antiviral memory CTLs, as shown in the LCMV model (Moskophidis *et al.*, 1993). An enhanced Fas-dependent apoptosis can be observed in $CD8^+$ lymphocytes as well as in $CD4^+$ T cells from HIV-infected individuals (Katsikis *et al.*, 1995; Chia *et al.*, 1995; Lewis *et al.*, 1994; Gougeon *et al.*, 1992). The low bcl-2 expression which characterizes memory $CD8^+$ $CD45RO^+$ T cells during acute viral infections enhances susceptibility of these cells to activation-induced programmed cell death (Akbar *et al.*, 1993) and might therefore make memory HIV-specific CTLs more susceptible to apoptosis. The observation of decreasing frequencies of HIV gag-specific precursor CTLs has suggested that clonal deletion might occur among HIV-specific CTLs and induce losses in the CTL repertoire (Gotch *et al.*, 1990). As mentioned above, however, a particular CTL clone specific for HIV-1 gp41 or Gag can persist over time in a single patient (Kalams *et al.*, 1994; Moss *et al.*, 1995). When evaluating infected patients in the French cohort IMMUNOCO, we observed that CTL recognition of at least two HIV-1 LAI proteins remains detectable in most patients with CD4 counts between 100 and $200/mm^3$, after *in vitro* restimulation with autologous PHA-blasts and IL-2 (Autran *et al.*, 1994). We also reported that Nef epitope-specific CTLs remained detectable after permanent *in vivo* exposure to persistent antigens (Haas *et al.*, 1995a). These latter observations suggest that HIV-specific CTLs are not deleted *in vivo* but persist and even can be expanded *in vitro*, thereby fighting against the hypothesis of a clonal exhaustion induced by a chronic antigenic stimulation of memory $CD8^+$ CTLs specific for HIV.

2.3.3. CTL Anergy?

The decreased effector CTL activity observed in AIDS patients contrasts with the persistent differentiation of $CD8^+$ T cells in cytotoxic effector T cells in lymphoid organs. This suggest that HIV-specific effector CTLs might be anergized *in vivo* while a "reserve" of CTLs is still present (Devergne *et al.*, 1995; Tenner-Racz *et al.*, 1993). This CTL anergy occurs at a time when the $CD4^+$ T-cell anergy is massive and various mechanisms have been proposed to explain HIV-specific CTL lack of activity.

First, viral variations can affect not only the binding of peptides to HLA molecules but also the affinity of the peptide/MHC complex for the T-cell receptor. Such variants might act as antagonists or partial agonists of the original epitope inducing negative signaling through the TCR transduction pathways, resulting in clonal anergy. While this phenomenon can be elicited by designing peptide modifications (Gairin and Oldstone, 1992), natural viral variants also appear to induce antagonistic signals for CTLs, as recently suggested for HBV or HIV-Gag variants (Bertoletti *et al.*, 1994; Klenerman *et al.*, 1994, 1995). Some HIV variants might function as altered peptide ligands capable of stimulating the growth of specific CTLs but also of antagonizing CTL response to the original variant sequence. Whether a clonal anergy of HIV-specific CTLs does occur *in vivo* according to such mechanisms is uncertain and the physiopathological significance of antagonistic variants, while attractive, remains to be determined. If confirmed, such HIV epitope antagonists would induce a clonal CTL anergy restricted to some of the HIV antigens. However, a series of observations suggests that not only the CTL responses against HIV antigens might decrease but also the CTLs directed against a variety of viruses such as EBV or CMV

(Carmichael *et al.*, 1993) indicating that CTL anergy might be a global phenomenon in AIDS.

Continuous activation of the immune system is also capable of generating polyclonal T-cell anergy thus impairing CTL activity through several other mechanisms *in vivo*. We showed, along with the decreasing HIV-specific CTL activity, increasing numbers of *in vivo* activated $CD8^+$ T cells bearing the CD57 marker that act as potent inhibitors of CTL activity by enhancing the levels of cAMP in effector killer cells. This phenomenon enters a cytokine regulatory network since antagonized by IL-4 and IFN-γ and might be partly responsible for the progressive loss of killer cell activity *in vivo* (Sadat-Sowti *et al.*, 1991, 1994; Joly *et al.*, 1989). Other cell-surface alterations appear as consequences of T-cell activation and might be associated with low CTL responsiveness. The downmodulation of the CD28 molecule reported on $CD8^+$ T cells from HIV-infected individuals might be another mechanism for such activation-induced anergy (Vingerhoets *et al.*, 1985; Borthwick *et al.*,1994). Other $CD8^+$ cell-surface molecules might also assess deleterious activation processes or play a role in $CD8^+$ cell-decreasing activity such as CD38 (Hong-Nerng *et al.*, 1993). Giorgi and coauthors indeed showed that increased expression of CD38 combined to a decreased expression of HLA-DR on $CD8^+$ cells might result in decreased HIV-specific CTL activity since effector CTLs are mainly detectable in the $CD8^+DR^+CD38^{+/-}$ cell subpopulation (Hong-Nerng *et al.*, 1993). Finally, CTL anergy against HIV might be only one aspect of global immune disorders appearing with disease progression. In such a hypothesis, the ascension of HIV load preceding the onset of AIDS and concurrently with the loss of CTL activity would be interpreted as an "opportunistic" complication of the HIV infection.

2.3.4. Lack of T-Cell Help?

A T-helper cell function might be required for the *de novo* differentiation of precursor CTLs although CD4 knock-out mice can develop CTL responses (Matloubian *et al.*, 1994). The decreasing frequencies of precursor and effector CTLs in such chronic viral infection could be related to the progressive defect in Th1 cell functions and production of IL-2 which is observed with the asymptomatic stages (Shearer *et al.*, 1986). This should in theory limit the differentiation of new CTL precursors. In such a hypothesis, CTL precursors specific for new HIV variants would be unable to activate and differentiate *in vivo* (Phillips *et al.*, 1993). The loss of Th1 function might be paralleled by persistent Th2 cell differentiation and function among the residual $CD4^+$ T cells (Clerici *et al.*, 1992). Although the hypothesis of an increasing Th2 cell function remains highly debated (Fauci, 1993), evidence exists that Th2 cells are activated with HIV disease progression but that their function is impaired (Autran *et al.*, 1995a) and therefore does not result in increased Th2 cytokine production *in vivo*. The predominance of a Th2 cell function induced by helminthic infection has been shown to inhibit HIV-specific CTL activity (Actor *et al.*, 1993). The relevance of such phenomena for the *in vivo* decrease of CTL efficiency remains to be determined. In the meantime, one has to remember that the CTL repertoire can activate CTL precursors specific for new variants even at the time of $CD4^+$ Th1 cell defects. Such observation raises the question of the ability of $CD8^+$ T cells to mediate help for CTLs. Nevertheless, restoring a Th1 cell function *in vivo* appears as a major goal for immune therapies aimed at enhancing HIV-specific CTLs. Analysis of HIV-specific CTL responses in patients undergoing IL-2 treatment or future IL-12 therapies should help to answer this question (Kovacs *et al.*, 1995; McMahon *et al.*, 1994).

3. SIGNIFICANCE OF HIV-SPECIFIC CTLs: PROTECTION OR PATHOGENESIS?

The relevance of HIV-specific CTLs in protection against HIV infection remains to be determined: are HIV-specific CTLs beneficial or deleterious for the host? Such a key question has not been definitely answered. For a number of investigators, and myself, the weight of the evidence favors a partial protective role for HIV-specific CTLs, at least during the primary infection and the asymptomatic stages of the infection where they seem able to clear emerging HIV variants. On the contrary, HIV-specific CTLs might only be witnesses of a strong HIV antigenicity but their actual role in controlling the virus might be only minor (Coffin, 1995; Phillip, 1996).

3.1. Do HIV-Specific CTLs Confer Protection against Infection or Disease Progression?

Studies of immune control in other viral infections suggest that CTLs should play an important role in containing an HIV infection (Cannon *et al.*, 1988; Plata, 1985; Plata *et al.*, 1987b; Engers *et al.*, 1984; Greenberg *et al.*, 1981; Buchmeier *et al.*, 1980; Leclerc and Cantor, 1980). However, while CTLs can clear acute viral infections such as influenza, they only limit primary infection and control chronic retrovirus infections but do not eradicate the latter. Several reports have underlined links observed between some HLA haplotypes and HIV infection or evolution toward AIDS (Oksenhendler *et al.*, 1992; Fabio *et al.*, 1992; Kaslow *et al.*, 1990; Itescu *et al.* 1990), thereby suggesting the importance of an immune control of HIV. Seronegative but highly exposed individuals have also been shown to develop HIV-specific CTL responses which might play a role in their protection against HIV (Rowland-Jones *et al.*, 1995; Langlade-Demoyen *et al.*, 1994). Some HLA antigens in those individuals might favor induction of protective immune responses as shown in Nairobi prostitutes. Children born to seropositive mothers also display CTL responses that might protect them in some cases (Paul, 1995; Buseyne *et al.*, 1993a; Mcfarland *et al.*, 1993; Cheynier *et al.*, 1992). However, the role of CTLs in controlling HIV replication in the infected individual has not been established and immune parameters associated with CTL protection are still not fully understood. Polyclonality of HIV-specific CTL responses might be one of the parameters for protection against disease progression as recently suggested by our studies of CTLs from nonprogressors recognizing a mean number of 3.7 proteins from the LAI strain versus 2.5 proteins for progressors (B. Autran, unpublished data). The positive effect of polyclonality has been discussed by Nowak *et al.* (1995). Intensity of the CTL responses might be another parameter. Klein *et al.* (1995) reported an apparent relationship between high frequencies of Gag-specific CTLs and low viral load, though the temporal relationship between the two phenomena is not obvious. Similarly, studies of macaque models teach us that the intensity of CTL responses to SIV might indeed limit progression toward AIDS (Bourgault *et al.*, 1993).

If protective, the mechanisms by which CTL act *in vivo* might be multiple. The $CD8^+$ lymphocytes from HIV-infected individuals can inhibit HIV replication *in vitro*. Such antiviral activity might be mediated by cytolysis of infected cells (Tsubota *et al.*, 1989; Kannagi *et al.*, 1988, 1990), as assessed by the presence of cytolytic granules in $CD8^+$ T cells *in vivo* (Emilie *et al.*, 1995; Tenner-Racz *et al.*, 1993). Cytokine release also appears as an important protective mechanism for the antiviral $CD8^+$ cell activity which might be enhanced in long-term nonprogressors (Walker *et al.*, 1986; Brinchmann *et al.*, 1990; Mackewicz *et al.*, 1994; Levy, 1993; Cao *et al.*, 1995). The recent evidence for a role of chemokines such as RANTES, MIP-1α, MIP-1β, and IL-16 (Cocchi *et al.*, 1995; Baier *et al.*, 1995) might open new perspectives in the understanding of $CD8^+$ CTL-mediated protection against disease progression. The ability of cloned HIV-specific human CTLs to prevent HIV infection has also been reported in severe combined immunodeficiency (SCID) mice reconstituted with a human immune system (Van Kuyk *et al.*, 1995). However, an HTLV-1-specific CTL clone conferred the same protection indicating that CTL might act *in vivo* by releasing soluble mediators such as IFN-γ or other cytokines. Such an animal model also allows demonstration of protection conferred by neutralizing antibody specific for HIV (Safrit *et al.*, 1993), suggesting that the two arms of host immune responses can protect against HIV.

Finally, our recent description of a correlation between amplification of variant-specific CTLs and disappearance of the corresponding variants *in vivo* suggests that CTLs can limit to some extent the outgrowth of variants, thereby opening new perspectives aimed at reinforcing CTL activity against HIV-producing cells.

3.2. Are HIV-Specific CTLs Deleterious?

The persistence of virus-specific CTLs directed against chronic infections caused by nonpathogenic viruses may actually contribute to disease pathogenesis (Zinkernagel and Hengartner, 1994). The question of HIV pathogenicity for $CD4^+$ T cells remained open until several lines of evidence recently indicated that HIV is indeed responsible for an *in vivo* dramatic decrease of the $CD4^+$ T-cell half-life (Ho *et al.*, 1995; Wei *et al.*, 1995). Nevertheless, mechanisms responsible for such enhanced mortality of HIV-infected $CD4^+$ T cells might be indirect, involving CTL-mediated killing. Moreover, the property of virus-specific CTLs to act as "serial killers" might expose infected $CD4^+$ T cells to death by CTL killing more than by HIV cytopathogenicity. $CD8^+$ T cells frequently infiltrate tissues in HIV-infected patients. We evidenced tissular HIV-specific CTLs in lungs of patients with lymphocytic alveolitis, an HIV-related disorder observed before the onset of opportunistic infections (Guillon *et al.*, 1988). These alveolar $CD8^+$ CTLs mediate spontaneous cytotoxic activity against autologous alveolar macrophages (Autran *et al.*, 1988; Plata *et al.*, 1987b), and are strongly correlated with clinical and functional lung abnormalities (Meignan *et al.*, 1989; Guillon *et al.*, 1988). This suggests that the immune conflict occurring *in vivo* between CTLs and their targets might be deleterious for the organ function. An infiltration of $CD8^+$ T lymphocytes is also observed in various tissues, in parotids and salivary glands of HIV-infected individuals (Itescu *et al.*, 1990, 1993; Guillon *et al.*, 1986) and can even result in a polyclonal pseudo tumoral enlargement of lymphoid organs (Oksenhendler *et al.*, 1992). Such CD8 cell infiltration is associated first with some HLA haplotypes such as DR5 (Itescu *et al.*, 1990) or A1, B8, DR3 (Oksenhendler *et al.*, 1992) and second with either slow disease progression (Itescu *et al.*, 1990) or with rapid disease progression (Oksenhendler *et al.*, 1992). Effector CTLs present in tissues harbor high level of granules containing perforin and granzymes, the function of which is to kill target cells, but also produce high levels of various cytokines (Price *et al.*, 1995; Emilie *et al.*, 1990), while target cell death might release toxic products that participate in pathogenesis. $CD8^+$ lymphocytes and HIV-specific CTLs, infiltrating the white pulp and the germinal centers in lymph nodes of HIV-infected individuals (Devergne *et al.*, 1995; Tenner-Racz *et al.*, 1993; Emilie *et al.*, 1990, 1995) may partially control *in vivo* the high local viral burden (Hadida *et al.*, 1992, 1995; Cheynier *et al.*, 1994; Pantaleo *et al.*, 1993). They might also participate in the $CD4^+$ T-cell depletion and in the progressive disorganization of these tissues (Grant *et al.*, 1994). In all of these settings, HIV-specific CTLs may play a role in the immunopathogenesis of HIV infection.

Finally, the passive transfer of high doses of a Nef-specific CTL clone in a single recipient resulted in deterioration of the HIV disease (Koenig *et al.*, 1995). The lack of control in this clinical trial limits interpretation and the massive doses of IL-2 coinjected with the clone might have played a major role in the enhanced HIV replication observed in this patient. Similar passive transfers of cytotoxic T cells have also been performed in different clinical centers. These assays included either HIV-specific CTLs restimulated *in vitro* with HIV peptides, aimed at controlling HIV infection (Lieberman *et al.*, 1995), or PHA-activated nonspecific $CD8^+$ cells (Whiteside *et al.*, 1993; Ho *et al.*, 1993). In none of these cases was there a similar dramatic deterioration of HIV infection and host immune status, suggesting that, if efficient at all, those passive transfers of polyclonal cytotoxic T cells might not be harmful.

Therefore, a delicate dynamic balance probably exists between an efficient clearance of the major part of the HIV burden on the one hand and, on the other, an unavoidable pathogenicity of CTLs directed against HIV-infected cells.

4. CONCLUSION

The data summarized herein provide a general insight into HIV-specific T-cell responses: an early and unusually strong virus-specific $CD8^+$ T-cell immunity is detectable throughout the asymptomatic phase but fails to eliminate viral infection and to prevent the later general impairment of T-cell functions. Mechanisms leading to the breakpoint in T-cell protective immunity are probably multiple. While HIV-specific CTLs might be implicated in the pathogenesis of AIDS, we cannot exclude their protective role in the 7- to 10-year incubation period of AIDS. One of our main goals remains to better establish the ranges of the *in vivo* efficiency of the immune cytolytic responses to HIV during the course of the infection and, ultimately, the reasons for the progressive degradation of immune status.

Beyond the multiple factors capable of limiting CTL efficiency that were reviewed herein, virus-specific CTLs might be destined to lose the race against HIV simply because their activation always follows but never precedes the emergence of viruses during an established infection. A simple explanation for ultimate CTL failure would therefore be that the mathematical accumulation of HIV particles and variants with time is overwhelming the host CTL defenses that adapt, but too late, to the emergence of new HIV-replicating cells. A major goal is therefore to define immunodominant epitopes in very conserved regions of HIV in order to induce or to reinforce CTLs, capable fo reacting with some HIV antigens whatever the variants. At a time when our observations are felt to be instrumental for immune strategies aimed at amplifying CTL activity *ex vivo* or *in vivo*, these strategies have to be carefully devised and combined with efficient antiretroviral drugs. A series of observations provide a strong basis for therapeutic strategies based on the administration of cytokines such as IL-2 or IL-12 for an *in vivo* restimulation of a CTL repertoire adapted to HIV variation. An *in vivo* amplification of CTLs recognizing and controlling viral variants at advanced stages of the disease therefore appears feasible and might be useful for immunotherapy.

There is today a general agreement that virus-specific CTLs represent valuable tools for vaccine strategies. Adequate vaccines against HIV might play two roles: they could either prevent HIV infection in seronegative individuals or help to control an established infection. The prevention of a *de novo* infection usually requires high titers of neutralizing antibodies. Virus-specific CTLs are also required for an early elimination of infected cells and for the prevention of a rapid viral dissemination from cell to cell. The activation of antigen-specific $CD4^+$ T cells exposes T cells to an increased susceptibility to infection or lysis or to an enhanced virus replication and should therefore be avoided in vaccine strategies while MHC class I CTLs should be favored. HIV-specific class I-restricted CTLs therefore represent the best possible candidates for an active control of an established HIV infection. Efficient vaccines also require strong CTL memory and mucosal immune responses, two questions that remain unelucidated. Do we need persistent antigenic exposure and therefore a chronically replicating viral genome, or simply a massive initial antigenic exposure to get a long-lasting CTL memory? Can CTLs confer early protection against a sexually transmitted virus? These latter points are only examples of the unanswered questions in the quest of a protective CTL immunity against HIV.

ACKNOWLEDGMENTS. I would like to thank all of my colleagues participating in the studies mentioned herein and particularly Patrice Debré, Anne Hosmalin, Gaby Haas, and Fabienne Hadida for useful discussions and careful reading of the manuscript and Valérie Aquerreta for expert secretarial assistance.

REFERENCES

Achour, A., Picard, O., Zagury, D., Sarin, P. S., Gallo, R. C., Naylor, P. H., and Goldstein, A. L., 1990, Hgp-30, a synthetic analogue of human immunodeficiency virus (HIV) p17, is a target for cytotoxic lymphocytes in HIV-infected individuals, *Proc. Natl. Acad. Sci. USA* **87:**7045–7049.

Actor, J. K., Shirai, M., Kullberg, M. C., Buller, R. M., Sher, A., and Berzofsky, J. A., 1993, Helminth infection results in decreased virus-specific $CD8^+$ cytotoxic T cell and Th1 cytokine responses as well as delayed virus clearance, *Proc. Natl. Acad. Sci. USA* **90:**948–952.

Aebischer, T., Moskophidis, D., Hoffmann Rohrer, U., Zinkernagel, R. M., and Hengartner, H., 1991, In vitro selection of lymphocytic choriomeningitis virus escape mutants by cytotoxic T lymphocytes, *Proc. Natl. Acad. Sci. USA* **88:**11047–11051.

Akbar, A. N., Borthwick, N., Salmon, M., Gombert, W., Bofill, M., Shamsadeen, N., Pilling, D., Pett, S., Grundy, J. E., and Janossy, G., 1993, The significance of low bcl-2 expression by CD45RO T cells in normal individuals and patients with acute viral infections. The role of apoptosis in T cell memory, *J. Exp. Med.* **178:**427–438.

Autran, B., and Letvin, N. L., 1991, HIV epitopes recognized by cytotoxic T-lymphocytes, *AIDS* **5(Suppl 2):** S145–S150.

Autran, B., Mayaud, C. M., Raphael, M., Plata, F., Denis, M., Bourguin, A., Guillon, J.M., Debre, P., and Akoun, G., 1988, Cytotoxic T lymphocyte alveolitis in HIV infected patients, *AIDS* **2:**179–183.

Autran, B., Plata, F., and Debré, P., 1991, MHC-restricted cytotoxicity against HIV, *J AIDS* **4:**361–368.

Autran, B., Gomard, E., Rivière, Y., Bouley, J. M., Aboulker, J. P., Katlama, C., 1994, HIV-specific CTL responses and immunodominant reactivities in the French IMMUNOCO cohort, Int. Conf. on AIDS, Yokohama, Abstr.

Autran, B., Legac, E., Blanc, C., and Debré, P., 1995a, Th0/Th2 function of $CD4^+Cd7^-$ T lymphocyte subset in normal and HIV-seropositive individuals, *J. Immunol.* **154:**1408–1417.

Autran, B., Haas, G., Hadida, F., Plikat, U., Hosmalin, A., Meyerhans, A., Jung, G., Oksenhendler, E., Mayaud, C., Katlama, C., and Debré, P., 1995b, *Adaptation of the HIV-Specific CTL Repertoire with Disease Progression*, Editions INSERM, Série Focus.

Bahraoui, E., Yagello, M., Billaud, N. J., 1990, Immunogenicity of the HIV recombinant Nef gene product. Mapping of T-cell and B-cell epitopes in immunized chimpanzees, *AIDS Res. Hum. Retrovir.* **6:**1087–1097.

Baier, M., Albrecht, W., Bannert, N., Metzner, K., and Kurth, R., 1995, HIV suppression by interleukin-16, *Nature* **378:**563.

Baltimore, D., 1995, The enigma of HIV infection, *Cell* **82:**175–176.

Bertoletti, A., Sette, A., Chisari, F., Penna, A., Levrero, M., Decarli, M., Fiaccadori, F., and Ferrari, C., 1994, Natural variants of cytotoxic epitopes are T-cell receptor antagonists for antiviral cytotoxic T cells, *Nature* **369:**407–410.

Berzofsky, J. A., Pendleton, C. D., Clerici, M., Ahlers, J., Lucey, D. R., Putney, S. D., and Shearer, G. M., 1995, Construction of peptides encompassing multideterminant clusters of HIV envelope to induce in vitro T-cell responses in mice and humans of multiple MHC types, *J. Clin. Invest.* **88:**876.

Bevan, M. J., 1995, Antigen presentation to cytotoxic T lymphocytes in vivo, *J. Exp. Med.* **182:**639–641.

Borthwick, N. J., Bofill, M., Gombert, W. M., Akbar, A. N., Medima, E., Sagawa, K., Lipman, M. C., Johnson, M. A., and Janossy, G., 1994, Lymphocyte activation in HIV-1 infection. Functional defects of CD28 T cells, *Curr. Sci.* **8:**431–441.

Bourgault, I., Villefroy, P., Beyer, C., Aubertin, A. M., Levy, J. P., and Venet, A., 1993, Cytotoxic T-cell response and AIDS-free survival in simian immunodeficiency virus-infected macaques, *AIDS* **7:**S73–79.

Bourgault, I., Chirat, F., Tartar, A., Lévy, J. P., Guillet, J. G., and Venet, A., 1994, Simian immunodeficiency virus as a model for vaccination against HIV: Induction in rhesus macaques of Gag- or Nef-specific cytotoxic T lymphocytes by lipopeptides, *J. Immunol.* **52:**2530–2537.

Brinchmann, J., Gaudernack, G., and Vartdal, F., 1990, CD8+ T cells inhibit HIV replication in naturally infected CD4+ cells: Evidence for a soluble inhibitor, *J. Immunol.* **144:**2961–2969.

Buchmeier, M. J. R., Welsh, R. M., Dutko, F. J., and Oldstone, M. B. A., 1980, The virology and immunobiology of lymphocytic choriomeningitis virus: Clearance of virus *in vivo*, *Adv. Immunol.* **30:**275.

Buseyne, F., Blanche, S., Schmidt, D., Griscelli, C., and Rivière, Y., 1993a, Detection of HIV-specific cell-mediated cytotoxicity in the peripheral blood from infected children, *J. Immunol.* **150:**3569–3581.

Buseyne, F., McChesney, M., Porrot, F., Kovarik, S., Guy, B., and Rivière, Y., 1993b, Gag-specific cytotoxic T lymphocytes from human immunodeficiency virus type 1-infected individuals: Gag epitopes are clustered in three regions of the P24 Gag protein, *J. Virol.* **67(2):**694–702.

Buseyne, F., Janvier, G., Fleury, B., Schmidt, D., and Rivière, Y., 1994, Multispecific and heterogeneous recognition of the gag protein by cytotoxic T lymphocytes (CTL) from HIV-infected patients: Factors other than the MHC control the epitopic specificities, *Clin. Exp. Immunol.* **97(3):**353–360.

Cannon, M. J., Openshaw, P. J. M., and Askonas, B. A., 1988, Cytotoxic T cells clear virus but augment lung pathology in mice infected with respiratory syncitial virus, *J. Exp. Med.* **168:**1163–1168.

Cao, Y., Qin, L., Zhang, L., Safrit, J., and Ho, D. D., 1995, Virologic and immunologic characterization of long-term survivors of human immunodeficiency virus type 1 infection, *N. Engl. J. Med.* **332(4):**201–232.

Carmichael, A., Jin, X., Sissons, P., and Borysiewicz, L., 1993, Quantitative analysis of the human immunodeficiency virus type 1 (HIV-1)-specific cytotoxic T lymphocyte (CTL) response at different stages of HIV-1 infection: Differential CTL responses to HIV-1 and Epstein–Barr virus in late disease, *J. Exp. Med.* **177:** 249–256.

Chen, Z. W., Shen, L., Miller, M. D., Ghim, S. H., Hughes, A. L., and Letvin, N. L., 1992, Cytotoxic T lymphocytes do not appear to select for mutations in an immunodominant epitope of simian immunodeficiency virus gag, *J. Immunol.* **149:**4060–4066.

Chen, Z. W., Kou, Z. C., Lekutis, C., Shen, L., Zhou, D., Halloran, M., Li, J., Sodroski, J., Lee-Parritz, D., and Letvin, N. L., 1995, T cell receptor Vβ repertoire in an acute infection of rhesus monkeys with simian immunodeficiency viruses and a chimeric simian–human immunodeficiency virus, *J. Exp. Med.* **182:**21–31.

Chenciner, N., Michel, F., Dadaglio, G., Langlade-Demoyen, P., Hoffenbach, A., Leroux, A., Garcia-Pons, F., Rautmann, G., Guy, B., Guillon, J. M., Mayaud, C., Girard, M., Autran, B., Kieny, M. P., and Plata, F., 1989, Multiple subsets of HIV-specific cytotoxic T lymphocytes in mice and human, *Eur. J. Immunol.* **337:**743–745.

Cheynier, R., Langlade-Demoyen, P., Marescot, M. R., Blanche, S., Blondin, G., Wain-Hobson, S., Griscelli, C., Vilmer, E., and Plata, F., 1992, Cytotoxic T lymphocyte responses in the peripheral blood of children born to human immunodeficiency virus-1-infected mothers, *Eur. J. Immunol.* **22:**2111.

Cheynier, R., Henrichwark, S., Hadida, F., Pelletier, E., Oksenhendler, E., Autran, B., and Wain-Hobson, S., 1994, HIV and T cell expansion in splenic white pulps is accompanied by infiltration of HIV-specific cytotoxic T lymphocytes, *Cell* **78:**373–387.

Chia, W. K., Freedman, J., Li, X., Salit, I., Kardish, M., and Read, S. E., 1995, Programmed cell death induced by HIV type 1 antigen stimulation is associated with a decrease in cytotoxic T lymphocyte activity in advanced HIV type 1 infection, *AIDS Res. Hum. Retrovir.* **11:**249–256.

Choppin, J., Martinon, F., Connan, F., Gomard, E., and Levy, J. P., 1991, HLA-binding regions of HIV-1 proteins. A systematic study of viral proteins, *J. Immunol.* **147**:575–583.

Claverie, J. M., Kourilsky, P., Langlade-Demoyen, P., Chalufour-Prochnicka, A., Dadaglio, G., Tekaia, F., Plata, F., and Bougueleret, L., 1988, T-immunogenic peptides are constituted of rare sequences patterns. Use in the identification of T epitopes in the human immunodeficiency virus Gag protein, *Eur. J. Immunol.* **18**:1547–1553.

Clerici, M., Lucey, D. R., Zajac, R., Boswell, R. N., Gebel, H. M., Takahashi, H., Berzofsky, J. A., and Shearer, G. M., 1992, Detection of cytotoxic T lymphocytes specific for synthetic peptides of gp160 in HIV-seropositive individuals, *J. Immunol.* **146**:2214–2219.

Clerici, M., Hakim, F. T., Venzon, D. J., Blatt, S., Hendrix, C. W., Wynn, T. A., and Shearer, G. M., 1993, Changes in interleukin-2 and interleukin-4 production in asymptomatic human immunodeficiency virus-seropositive individuals, *J. Clin. Invest.* **91**:759.

Cocchi, F., DeVico, A. L., Garzino-Demo, A., Arya, S. K., Gallo, R. C., and Lusso, P., 1995, Identification of RANTES, MIP-1α, MIP-1β, as the major suppressive factors produced by CD8+ T cells, *Science* **270**:1811–1815.

Coffin, J. M., 1995, Lines drawn in epitope wars, *Nature* **375**:534–535.

Cooper, D. A., Tindall, B., Wilson, E., Imri, A. A., and Penny, R., 1988, Characterization of T lymphocyte responses during primary HIV infection, *J. Infect. Dis.* **157**:889–896.

Couillin, I., Culmann-Penciolelli, B., Gomard, E., Choppin, J., Levy, J. P., Guillet, J. G., and Saragosti, S., 1994, Impaired cytotoxic T lymphocyte recognition due to genetic variations in the main immunogenic regions of the human immunodeficiency virus 1 Nef protein, *J. Exp. Med.* **180**:1129–1134.

Couillin, I., Connan, F., Culmann-Penciolelli, B., Gomard, E., Guillet, J. G., and Choppin, J., 1995, HLA-dependent variations in human immunodeficiency virus Nef protein alter peptide/HLA binding, *Eur. J. Immunol.* **25**:728–732.

Cox, J. H., Yewdel, J. W., Eisenlohr, L. C., Johnson, P. R., and Bennink, J. R., 1990, Antigen presentation requires transport of MHC class I molecules from the endoplasmic reticulum, *Science* **247**:715.

Culmann, B., Gomard, E., Kieny, M. P., Guy, B., Dreyfus, F., Adrien-Gerard, H., Saimot, G., Sereni, D., and Levy, J. P., 1989, An antigenic peptide of the HIV-1 Nef protein recognized by cytotoxic T lymphocytes of seropositive individuals in association with different HLA-B molecules, *Eur. J. Immunol.* **12**:2382–2386.

Culmann, B., Gomard, E., Kieny, M. P., Guy, B., Dreyfus, F., Saimot, A. G., Sereni, D., Sicard, D., and Levy, J. P., 1991, Six epitopes reacting with human cytotoxic CD8+ cells in the central region of the HIV-1 Nef protein, *J. Immunol.* **146**:1465–1470.

Dadaglio, G., Leroux, A., Langlade-Demoyen, P., Bahraoui, E. M., Traincard, F., Fischer, R., and Plata, F., 1991, Epitope recognition of conserved HIV envelope sequences by human cytotoxic T lymphocytes, *J. Immunol.* **147**:2302–2309.

Dai, L. C., West, K., Littaua, R., Takahashi, H., and Ennis, F. A., 1992, Mutation of human immunodeficiency virus type 1 at amino acid 585 on gp41 results in loss of killing by CD8+ A24-restricted cytotoxic T lymphocytes, *J. Virol.* **66**:3151–3154.

De Groot, A. S., Clerici, M., Hosmalin, A., Hugues, S. H., Barnd, D., Hendrix, C. W., Houghten, R., Shearer, G. M., and Berzofsky, J. A., 1991, HIV reverse transcriptase T helper epitopes identified in mice and humans: Correlation with a cytotoxic T cell epitope, *J. Infect. Dis.* **164**:1058–1065.

Delassus, S., Cheynier, R., and Wain-Hobson, S., 1992, Inhomogenous distribution of human immunodeficiency virus type-1 genomes within an infected spleen, *J. Virol.* **66**:5642.

Del Val, M., Schlicht, H. J., Ruppert, T., Reddehase, M. J., and Koszinowski, U. H., 1991, Efficient processing of an antigenic sequence for presentation by MHC class I molecules depends on its neighboring residues in the protein, *Cell* **66**:1145–1153.

De Paoli, P., Caffau, C., D'andrea, M., Ceolin, P., Simonelli, C., Tirelli, U., and Santini, G., 1993, The expansion of CD8 lymphocytes using T cell receptor variable gene products during HIV infection, *Clin. Exp. Immunol.* **94(3)**:486–489.

Devergne, O., Raphael, M., Autran, B., Leger-Ravet, M. B., Coumbaras, J., Crevon, M. C., Galanaud, P., and Emilie, D., 1995, Intratumoral activation of CD8+ positive cytotoxic lymphocytes in acquired immunodeficiency syndrome lymphomas, *Hum. Pathol.* **26(3)**:284–290.

Dupuis, M., Kundu, S. K., and Merigan, T. C., 1995, Characterization of HLA-A *0201 restricted cytotoxic T cell epitopes in conserved regions of the HIV type 1 gp160 protein, *J. Immunol.* **155.4**:2232–2239.

Driscoll, J., and Finley, D., 1992, A controlled breakdown: Antigen processing and the turnover of viral proteins, *Cell* **68**:823–825.

Egan, M. A., Pavlat, W. A., Tartaglia, J., Paoletti, E., Weinhold, K. J., Clements, M. L., and Siliciano, R. F., 1995,

Induction of human immunodeficiency virus type 1 (HIV-1)-specific cytolytic T lymphocyte responses in seronegative adults by a nonreplicating, host-range-restricted canarypox vector (ALVAC) carrying the HIV-1MN env gene, *J. Infect. Dis.* **171**:1623–1627.

Emilie, D., Peuchmaur, M., Maillot, M. C., Crevon, M. C., Brousse, N., Delfraissy, J. F., Dormont, J., and Galanaud, P., 1990, Production of interleukins in human immunodeficiency virus-1 replicating lymph nodes, *J. Clin. Invest.* **86**:148–159.

Engers, H. D., La Haye, T., Sorenson, G. D., Glasebrook, A. L., Horvath, C., and Brunner, T. K., 1984, Functional activity in vivo of effector T-cell populations. Anti-tumor activity exhibited by syngeneic anti-Momulv-specific cytolytic T-cell clones, *J. Immunol.* **133**:1664–1670.

Fabio, G., Scorza, R., Lazzarin, A., Marchini, M., Zarantonello, M., D'arminio, A., Marchisio, P., Plebani, A., Luzzati, R., and Costigliola, D., 1992, HLA-associated susceptibility to HIV-1 Infection, *Clin. Exp. Immunol.* **87**:20–23.

Falk, K., Rotzschke, O., Stevanovic, S., Jung, G., and Rammensee, H. G., 1991, Allele specific motifs revealed by sequencing of self-peptides eluted from MHC molecules, *Nature* **351**:290–296.

Fauci, A. S., 1993, Multifactorial nature of human immunodeficiency virus disease: Implication for therapy, *Science* **262**:104.

Gairin, J. E., and Oldstone, M. B. A., 1992, Design of high-affinity major histocompatibility complex-specific antagonist peptides that inhibit cytotoxic T lymphocyte activity: Implications for control of viral disease, *J. Virol* **66**:6755–6762.

Glickstein, L. H., and Huber, B. T., 1995, Karoushi-death by overwork in the immune system, *J. Immunol.* **155**:522–524.

Gorochov, G., Autran, B., Debré, P., and Sigaux, F., 1992, Conservation of the TCR-V-beta chains repertoire in CD4+ T cells during progression of HIV infection, *VII Int. Conf AIDS, Amsterdam*, Abstr. ThA 1541.

Gotch, F. M., Nixon, D. F., Alp, N., Mcmichael, A. J., and Borysievicz, L. K., 1990, High frequency of memory and effector Gag-specific cytotoxic T lymphocytes in HIV seropositive individuals, *Int. Immunol.* **2**:707–712.

Gougeon, M. L., Olivier, R., Garcia, S., Guetard, D., Dragic, T., Dauguet, C., and Montagnier, L., 1992, Mise en évidence d'un processus d'engagement vers la mort cellulaire par apoptose dans les lymphocytes de patients infectés par le VIH, *C.R. Acad Sci.* **312**(III):529–537.

Grant, M. D., Smail, F. M., and Rosenthal, K. L., 1994, Cytotoxic T-lymphocytes that kill autologous CD4+ lymphocytes are associated with CD4+ lymphocyte depletion in HIV-1 infection, *J. Acq. Immune Defic. Syndr.* **7**:571–579.

Greenberg, P. D., Cheever, M. A., and Feffer, A., 1981, Eradication of disseminated murine leukemia by chemoimmunotherapy with cyclophosphamide and adoptively transferred immune syngeneic Lyt-1+2− lymphocytes, *J. Exp. Med.* **154**:952.

Guillon, J. M., Fouret, P., Mayaud, C., Picard, F., Raphael, M., Touboul, J. L., Chaunu, M. P., Hauw, J. J., and Akoun, G., 1986, Extensive T8-positive lymphocytic visceral infiltration in a homosexual man, *Am. J. Med.* **82**:655–661.

Guillon, J. M., Autran, B., Denis, M., Fouret, P., Plata, F., Mayaud, C., and Akoun, G., 1988, HIV-related lymphocytic alveolitis, *Chest* **94**:1264–1268.

Haas, G., David, R., Frank, R., Gausepohl, H., Devaux, C., Claverie, J. M., and Pierres, M., 1991, Identification of a major human immunodeficiency virus-1 reverse transcriptase epitope recognized by mouse CD4+ T lymphocytes, *Eur. J. Immunol.* **21**:1371–1377.

Haas, G., Debré, P., Dudoit, Y., Bonduelle, O., Katlama, C., Maier, B., Plikat, U., Meyerhans, A., Ihlenfeldt, H. G., Jung, G., and Autran, B., 1995a, Time course adaptation if HIV-1 Nef-specific CTL to epitope variations, *J. Cell. Biochem.* Abstr. Suppl. **21a**:142.

Haas, G., Hosmalin, A., Duntze, J., Samri, A., Magierowska, M., Katlama, C., Jung, G., Agut, H., Debré, P., and Autran, B., 1995b, Evolution of HIV-1 reverse transcriptase specific cytotoxic T cells (CTL) with disease progression and anti-retroviral therapy, *9th Int. Congr. Immunol.*, Abstr. 851, p. 144.

Hadida, F., Parrot, A., Kieny, M. P., Sadat-Sowti, B., Debré, P., and Autran, B., 1992, Carboxyl-terminal and central regions of HIV-1 Nef recognized by cytotoxic T lymphocytes from lymphoid organs, *J. Clin. Invest.* **89**:53–60.

Hadida, F., Haas, G., Zimmermann, N., Hosmalin, A., Spohn, R., Jung, R., Debré, P., and Autran, B., 1995, Cytotoxic T lymphocytes from lymphoid organs recognize an optimal HLA-A2 and -B52 restricted nonapeptide and several epitopes in the C-terminal region of HIV-1 Nef, *J. Immunol.* **154**:4174–4186.

Hammond, S. A., Obah, E., Stanhope, P., Monell, C. R., Strand, M., Robbins, F. M., Bias, W. B., Karr, R. W., Koenig, S., and Siliciano, R. F., 1991, Characterization of a conserved T cell epitope in HIV-1 gp41 recognized by vaccine-induced human cytolytic T cells, *J. Immunol.* **146**:1470–1479.

Hammond, S. A., Bollinger, R. C., Stanhope, P. E., Quinn, T. C., Schwartz, D., Clements, M. L., and Siliciano, R. F., 1992, Comparative clonal analysis of human immunodeficiency virus type 1 specific CD4+ and CD8+ cytolytic T lymphocytes isolated from seronegative humans immunized with candidate HIV-1 vaccines, *J. Exp. Med.* **176:**1531–1542.

Hammond, S. A., Johnson, R. P., Kalams, S. A., Waler, B. D., Takiguchi, M., Safrit, J. T., Koup, R. A., and Siliciano, F. R., 1995, An epitope-selective, transporter associated with antigen presentation (TAP)-1/2-independent pathway and a more general TAP-1/2 dependent antigen-processing pathway allow recognition of the HIV-1 envelope glycoprotein by CD8+ CTL, *J. Immunol.* **154:**6140–6156.

Ho, M., Armstrong, J., McMahon, D., Pazin, G., Huang, X. L., Rinaldo, C., Whiteside, T., Tripoli, C., Levine, C., and Moody, D., 1993, A phase 1 study of adoptive transfer of autologous CD8+ T lymphocytes in patients with acquired immunodeficiency syndrome (AIDS)-related complex or AIDS, *Blood* **81(8):**2093–2101.

Ho, D. D., Neumann, A. U., Perelson, A. S., Chen, W., Leonard, J. M., and Markowitz, M., 1995, Rapid turnover of plasma virions and CD4 lymphocytes in HIV-1 infection, *Nature* **373:**123–126.

Hoffenbach, A., Langlade-Demoyen, P., Vilmer, E., Dadaglio, G., Michel, F., Mayaud, C., Autran, B., and Plata, F., 1989, Very high frequencies of HIV specific cytotoxic T lymphocytes in humans, *J. Immunol.* **142:**452–456.

Hong-Nerng, H., Hultin, L. E., Mitsuyasu, R. T., Matud, J. I., Hausner, M. A., Bockstoce, D., Cheng-Cheng, C., O'Rourke, S., Taylor, J. M. G., and Giorgi, J. V., 1993, Circulating HIV-specific CD8+ cytotoxic T cells express CD38 and HLA-DR antigens, *J. Immunol.* **150:**70–79.

Hosmalin, A., Clerici, M., Houghten, R., Pendleton, C. D., Flexner, C., Lucey, D. R., Moss, B., Germain, R. N., Shearer, G. M., and Berzofsky, J. A., 1990, An epitope in human immunodeficiency virus 1 reverse transcriptase recognized by both mouse and human cytotoxic T lymphocytes, *Proc. Natl. Acad. Sci. USA* **87:**2344–2348.

Hou, S., Hyland, L., Ryan, K. W., Portner, A., and Doherty, P. C., 1994, Virus-specific CD8+ T-cell memory determined by clonal burst size, *Nature* **369:**652–654.

Itescu, S., Brancato, L. J., Buxbaum, J., Gregersen, P. K., Rizk, C. C., Croxson, T. S., Solomon, G. E., and Winchester, P., 1990, A diffuse infiltrative CD8 lymphocytosis syndrome in human immunodeficiency virus (HIV) infection: A host immune response associated with HLA-DR5, *Ann. Intern. Med.* **112:**3–10.

Itescu, S., Dalton, J., Zhang, H.-Z., and Winchester, R., 1993, Tissue infiltration in a CD8 lymphocytosis syndrome associated with human immunodeficiency virus-1 infection has the phenotypic appearance of an antigenically driven response, *J. Clin. Invest.* **91:**2216–2225.

Jassoy, C., Johnson, R. P., Navia, B. A., Worth, J., and Walker, B. D., 1992, Detection of a vigorous HIV-1-specific cytotoxic T lymphocyte response in cerebrospinal fluid from infected persons with AIDS dementia complex, *J. Immunol.* **149:**3113–3119.

Johnson, R. P., Trocha, A., Yang, L., Mazzara, G. P., Panicali, D. L., Buchanan, T. M., and Walker, B. D., 1991, HIV-1 Gag-specific cytotoxic T lymphocytes recognize multiple highly conserved epitopes, *J. Immunol.* **147:**1512–1519.

Johnson, R. P., Trocha, A., Buchanan, T. M., and Walker, B. D., 1992, Identification of overlapping HLA class I-restricted cytotoxic T cell epitopes in a conserved region of the human immunodeficiency virus type 1 envelope glycoprotein: Definition of minimum epitopes and analysis of the effects of sequence variation, *J. Exp. Med.* **175:**961–971.

Johnson, R. P., Hammond, S. A., Trocha, A., Siliciano, R. F., and Walker, B. D., 1994, Induction of a major histocompatibility complex class I restricted cytotoxic T lymphocyte response to a highly conserved region of human immunodeficiency virus type 1 gp 120 in seronegative humans immunized with a candidate HIV-1 vaccine, *J. Virol.* **68:**3145–3153.

Joly, P., Guillon, J. M., Mayaud, C., Plata, F., Theodorou, I., Denis, M., Debré, P., and Autran, B., 1989, Cell mediated suppression of HIV-specific cytotoxic T lymphocytes, *J. Immunol.* **143:**2193–2201.

Kalams, S. A., Johnson, R. P., Trocha, A. K., Dynan, M. J., Ngo, H. S., D'aquila, R. T., Kurnick, J. T., and Walker, B. D., 1994, Longitudinal analysis of T cell receptor (TCR) gene usage by human immunodeficiency virus 1 envelope-specific cytotoxic T lymphocyte clones reveals a limited TCR repertoire, *J. Exp. Med.* **179:**1261–1271.

Kannagi, M., Chalifoux, L. V., Lord, C. I., and Letvin, N. L., 1988, Suppression of simian immunodeficiency virus replication in vitro by CD8+ lymphocytes, *J. Immunol.* **140:**2237.

Kannagi, M., Masuda, T., Hattori, T., and Letvin, N. L., 1990, Interference with human immunodeficiency virus (HIV) replication by CD8+ cells in peripheral blood leukocytes of asymptomatic HIV carriers in vitro, *J. Virol.* **64:**3399–3406.

Kaslow, R. A., Dusquenoy, R., Vanraden, M., Kinglsey, L., Marrari, M., Friedman, H., Su, S., Saah, A. J., Detels,

R., and Phalr, J., 1990, A1, CW7, B8, DR3 HLA antigen combination associated with rapid decline of T-helper lymphocytes in HIV-1 infection, *Lancet* **335**:927–930.

Katsikis, P. D., Wunderlich, E. S., Smith, C. A., Herzenberg, L. A., and Herzenberg, L. A., 1995, Fas antigen stimulation induces marked apoptosis of T lymphocytes in human immunodeficiency virus-infected individuals, *J. Exp. Med.* **181**:2029–2036.

Klein, M. R., Van Baalen, C. A., Holwerda, A. M., Garde, K. S. R., Bende, R. J., Keet, I. P. M., Eeftinck-Schattenkerk, J. K. M., Osterhaus, A. D. M. E., Schuitemaker, H., and Miedema, F., 1995, Kinetics of Gag-specific cytotoxic T lymphocyte responses during the clinical course of HIV-1 infection: A longitudinal analysis of rapid progressors and long-term asymptomatics, *J. Exp. Med.* **181**:1365–1372.

Klenerman, P., Rowland-Jones, S., McAdam, S., Edwards, J., Daenke, S., Lailoo, D., Köppe, B., Rosenberg, W., Boyd, D., Edwards, A., Glangrande, P., Phillips, R. E., and McMichael, A. J., 1994, Cytotoxic T-cell activity antagonized by naturally occurring HIV-1 Gag variants, *Nature* **369**:403–410.

Klenerman, P., Meier, U. C., Phillips, R. E., and McMichael, A. J., 1995, The effects of natural altered peptide ligands on the whole blood cytotoxic T lymphocyte response to human immunodeficiency virus, *Eur. J. Immunol.* **25**:1927–1931.

Koenig, S., Earl, P., Powell, D., Pantaleo, G., Merli, S., Moss, B., and Fauci, A. S., 1988, Group specific major histocompatibility complex class I-restricted cytotoxic responses to human immunodeficiency virus 1 (HIV-1) envelope proteins by cloned peripheral blood T cells from an HIV-1 infected individual, *Proc. Natl. Acad. Sci. USA* **85**:8638–8642.

Koenig, S., Fuerst, T. R., Wood, L., Woods, R. M., Suzich, J. A., Jones, G. M., De La Cruz, V. F., Davey, R. T., Venkatesan, S., Moss, B., Biddison, W. E., and Fauci, A. S., 1990, Mapping the fine specificity of a cytolytic T cell response to HIV-1 Nef protein, *J. Immunol.* **145**:127–133.

Koenig, S., Conley, A. J., Brewah, Y. A., Jones, G. M., Leath, S., Boots, L. J., Davey, V., Pantaleo, G., Demarest, J. F., Carter, C., Wannebo, C., Yannelli, J. R., Rosenberg, S. A., and Lane, H. .C., 1995, Transfer of HIV-1 specific cytotoxic T lymphocytes to an AIDS patient leads to selection for mutant HIV variants and subsequent disease progression, *Nature Med.* **1(4)**:330–336.

Koup, R. A., 1994, Virus escape from CTL recognition, *J. Exp. Med.* **180**:779–782.

Koup, R. A., and Sullivan, J. L., 1989, Why high levels of virus-specific CTL persist in HIV-1 infected individuals, *Res. Immunol.* **140**:92–95.

Koup, R. A., Pikora, C. A., Luzuriaga, K., Brettler, D. B., Day, E. S., Mazzara, G. P., and Sullivan, J. L., 1991, Limiting dilution analysis of cytotoxic T lymphocytes to human immunodeficiency virus gag antigens in infected persons: In-vitro quantitation of effector cell populations with p17 and p24 specificities, *J. Exp. Med.* **176**:1593–1600.

Koup, R. A., Safrit, J. T., Cao, Y., Andrews, A., McLeod, G., Borkosky, W., Farthing, C., and Ho, D. D., 1994, Temporal association of cellular immune responses with the initial control of viremia in primary human immunodeficiency virus type 1 syndrome, *J. Virol.* **68**:4560–4655.

Kovacs, J. A., Baseler, M., Dewar, R. J., Vogel, S., Davey, R. T., Falloon, J., Polis, M. A., Walker, R. E., Steven, R., Salzman, N. P., Metcalf, J. A., and Masur, H., 1995, Increases in CD4 lymphocytes with intermittent course of interleukin-2 in patients with human immunodeficiency virus infection, *N. Engl. J. Med.* **332**:567–575.

Kundu, S. K., Katzenstein, D., Moses, L. E., and Merigan, T. C., 1992, Enhancement of human immunodeficiency virus (HIV)-specific CD4+ and CD8+ cytotoxic T-lymphocyte activities in HIV-infected asymptomatic patients given recombinant Gp160 vaccine, *Proc. Natl. Acad. Sci. USA* **89**:11204–11208.

Lahmamedi-Cherradi, S., Culmann-Penciolelli, B., Guy, B., Duong Ly, T., Goujard, C., Guillet, J. G., and Gomard, E., 1995, Different patterns of HIV-1-specific cytotoxic T lymphocyte activity after primary infection, *AIDS* **9**:421.

Langlade-Demoyen, P., Michel, F., Hoffenbach, A., Vilmer, E., Dadaglio, G., Garcia-Pons, F., Mayaud, C., Autran, B., Wain-Hobson, S., and Plata, F., 1988, Immune recognition of AIDS-virus antigens by human and murine cytolytic T lymphocytes, *J. Immunol.* **141**:1949–1956.

Langlade-Demoyen, P., Ngo-Giang-Huong, N., Ferchal, F., and Oksenhendler, E., 1994, Human immunodeficiency virus (HIV) Nef-specific cytotoxic T lymphocytes in non infected heterosexual contact of HIV-infected patients, *J. Clin. Invest.* **93**:1293–1297.

Lanzavecchia, A., Roosnek, E., Gregory, T., Berman, P., and Abrignani, S., 1988, T cells can present antigens such as HIV gp120 targeted to their own surface molecules, *Nature* **334**:530–533.

Leclerc, J. C., and Cantor, H., 1980, T cell-mediated immunity to oncorna-virus induced tumors. Ability of different T-cell sets to prevent tumor growth *in vivo*, *J. Immunol.* **124**:851.

Letvin, N. L., 1990, Animals models for AIDS, *Immunol. Today* **11**:322–326.

Levy, J. A., 1993, The transmission of HIV and factors influencing progression to AIDS, *Am. J. Med.* **95:**86–100.

Lewis, D. E., NgTang, D. S., Adu-Oppong, A., Schober, W., and Rodgers, J. R., 1994, Anergy and Apoptosis in CD8+ T cells from HIV-infected persons, *J. Immunol.* **53:**412–420.

Lieberman, J., Fabry, J. A., Kuo, M. C., Earl, P., Moss, B., and Skolnik, P. R., 1992, Cytotoxic T lymphocytes from HIV-1 seropositive individuals recognize immunodominant epitopes in gp160 and reverse transcriptase, *J. Immunol.* **148:**2738–2747.

Lieberman, J., Fabry, J. A., Shankar, P., Beckett, J., and Skolnik, P. R., 1995, Ex vivo expansion of HIV type-1 specific cytolytic T cells from HIV type 1-seropositive subjects, *AIDS Res. Hum. Retrovir.* **11:**257–271.

Littaua, R. A., Oldstone, M. B. A., Takeda, A., Debouck, C., Wong, J. T., Tuazon, C. U., Moss, B., Kievits, F., and Ennis, F. A., 1991, An HLA-C-restricted CD8+ cytotoxic T-lymphocyte clone recognizes a highly conserved epitope on human immunodeficiency virus type 1, *J. Virol* **65:**4051–4056.

Long, E. O., and Jacobson, S., 1989, Pathways of viral antigen processing and presentation to CTL: Defined by the mode of virus entry? *Immunol. Today* **10:**45–48.

Lucchiari, M., Niedermann, G., Leipner, C., Meyerhans, A., Eichmann, K., and Maier, B., 1994, Human immune response to HIV-1 Nef. I. CD45RO− T lymphocytes of non infected donors contain CTL-precursors at high frequency, *Int. Immunol.* **6:**1939–1948.

McChesney, M., Tanneau, F., Regnault, A., Sansonetti, P., Montagnier, L., Kieny, M. P., and Rivière, Y., 1990, Detection of primary cytotoxic T lymphocytes specific for the envelope glycoprotein of HIV-1 by deletion of the env-amino terminal signal sequence, *Eur. J. Immunol.* **20:**215–220.

Mcfarland, E. J., Curiel, T. J., Schoen, D. J., Rosandich, M. E., Schooley, R. T., and Kuritzkes, D. R., 1993, Cytotoxic T lymphocyte lines specific for human immunodeficiency virus type 1 gag and reverse transcriptase derived from a vertically infected child, *J. Infect. Dis.* **167:**719–723.

McIlroy, D., Autran, B., Cheynier, R., Wain-Hobson, S., Clauvel, J. P., Oksenhendler, E., Debré, P., and Hosmalin, A., 1995, Infection frequency of dendritic cell and CD4+ T lymphocytes in spleens of human immunodeficiency virus-positive patients, *J. Virol.* **69:**4737–4745.

Mackewicz, C. E., Ortega, H., and Levy, J. A., 1994, Effect of cytokines on HIV replication in CD4+ lymphocytes: Lack of identity with the CD8+ cell antiviral factor, *Cell Immunol.* **153:**329–343.

McMahon, D. K., Armstrong, J. A., Huang, X. L., Rinaldo, C. R., Gupta, P., and Whiteside, T. L., 1994, A phase I study of subcutaneous recombinant interleukin-2 in patients with advanced HIV disease while on zidovudine, *AIDS* **8:**59–66.

Matloubian, M., Concepcion, R. J., and Ahmed, R., 1994, CD4+ T cells are required to sustain CD8+ cytotoxic T cell responses during chronic viral infection, *J. Virol.* **68:**8056–8063.

Meignan, M., Guillon, J. M., Denis, M., Joly, P., Rosso, J., Carrette, M. F., Buad, L., Parquin, F., Plata, F., Debré, P., Akoun, G., Autran, B., and Mayaud, C., 1989, Increased lung epithelial permeability in HIV infected patients with isolated cytotoxic T lymphocytic alveolitis, *Am. Rev. Respir. Dis.* **40:**65–91.

Meyerhans, A., Cheynier, R., Abert, J., Seth, M., Kwok, S., Sninsky, J., Morfeld-Manson, L., Asjö, B., and Wain-Hobson, S., 1989, Temporal fluctuations in HIV quasi-species *in vivo* are not reflected by sequential HIV isolations, *Cell* **58:**901.

Meyerhans, A., Dadaglio, G., Vartanian, J. P., Langlade-Demoyen, P., Frank, R., Asjö, B., Plata, F., and Wain-Hobson, S., 1991, In vivo persistence of a HIV-1-encoded HLA-B27-restricted cytotoxic T lymphocyte epitope despite specific in vitro reactivity, *Eur. J. Immunol.* **21:**2637–2640.

Morrison, L. A., Lukacher, A. E., Braciale, V. L., Fan, D. P., and Braciale, T. J., 1986, Differences in antigen presentation to MHC class-I and class-II-restricted influenza virus specific cytolytic T lymphocyte clones, *J. Exp. Med.* **163:**903–921.

Moskophidis, D., Laine, E., and Zinkernagel, R. M., 1993, Peripheral clonal deletion of antiviral memory CD8+ T cells, *Eur. J. Immunol.* **23:**3306–3311.

Moss, B., and Flexner, C., 1987, Vaccinia virus expression vector, *Annu. Rev. Immunol.* **5:**305–324.

Moss, P. A. H., Rowland-Jones, S. L., Frodsham, P. M., McAdam, S., Giangrande, P., McMichael, A. J., and Bell, J. I., 1995, Persistent high frequency of human immunodeficiency virus-specific cytotoxic T cells in peripheral blood of infected donors, *Proc. Natl. Acad. Sci. USA* **92:**5773–5777.

Müllbacher, 1994, The long-term maintenance of cytotoxic T cell memory does not require persistence of antigen, *J. Exp. Med.* **179:**317–321.

Nara, P. L., Smit, N., Dunlop, W., Hatch, W., Merges, M., Waters, D., Kelliher, J., Gallo, R. C., Fischinger, P. J., Goudsmit, J. J., 1990, Emergence of viruses resistant to neutralization by V3-specific antibodies in experimental human immunodeficiency virus type 1 LIIB infection of chimpanzees, *J. Virol.* **64:**3779.

Nietfeld, W., Bauer, M., Fevrier, M., Maier, R., Holzwarth, B., Frank, R., Maier, B., Rivière, Y., and Meyerhans, A.,

1995, Sequence constraints and recognition by CTL of an HLA-B27-restricted HIV-1 gag epitope, *J. Immunol.* **54:**2188–2197.

Nixon, D. F., and McMichael, A. J., 1991, Cytotoxic T cell recognition of HIV proteins and peptides, *AIDS* **5:**1049–1059.

Nixon, D. F., Townsend, A. R. M., Elvin, J. G., Rizza, C. R., Gallwey, J., and McMichael, A. J., 1988, HIV-1 gag-specific cytotoxic T lymphocytes defined with recombinant vaccinia virus and synthetic peptides, *Nature* **336:**484–487.

Nowak, M. A., May, R. M., Phillips, R. E., Rowland-Jones, S., Lalloo, D., McAdam, S., Klenerman, P., Köppe, B., Sigmund, K., Bangham, C. R. M., and McMichael, A. J., 1995, Antigenic oscillations and shifting immunodominance in HIV-1 infections, *Nature* **375:**606–611.

Obst, R., Armandola, E. A., Jijenhuis, M., Momburg, F., and Hämmerling, G. J., 1995, TAP polymorphism does not influence transport of peptide variants in mice and humans, *Eur. J. Immunol.* **25:**2170–2176.

Pantaleo, G., Koenig, S., Baseler, M., Lane, H. C., and Fauci, A. S., 1990, Defective clonogenic potential of $CD8^+$ T lymphocytes in patients with AIDS, *J. Immunol.* **144:**1696–1705.

Oksenhendler, E., Autran, B., Gorochov, G., Dehaye, C., Rabian, C., D'agay, M. F., Malbec, D., Wolf, M., Uring-Lambert, B., Seligmann, M., and Clauvel, J. P., 1992, Hyper CD8 lymphocytosis and pseudotumoral splenomegaly in human immunodeficiency virus (HIV) infection: An immune hyperactivation syndrome associated with HLA-A1 B8 DR3, *Lancet* **340**:208–209.

Pantaleo, G., Graziosi, C., Demarest, J. F., Butini, L., Montroni, M., Fox, C. H., Orenstein, J. M., Kotler, D. P., and Fauci, A. S., 1993, HIV infection is active and progressive in lymphoid tissue during the clinically latent stage of disease, *Nature* **362:**355–358.

Pantaleo, G., Demarest, J. F., Soudeyns, H., Graziosi, C., Denis, F., Adeisberger, J. W., Borrow, P., Saag, M. S., Shaw, G. M., Sekaly, R., and Fauci, A. S., 1994, Major expansion of CD8+ T cells with a predominant Vβ usage during the primary immune response to HIV, *Nature* **370:**463–467.

Pantaleo, G., Menzo, S., Vaccarezza, M., Graziosi, C., Cohen, O. J., Demarest, J. F., Montefiori, D., Orenstein, J. M., Fox, C., Schrager, L. K., Margolick, J. B., Buchbinder, S., Giorgi, J. V., and Fauci, A., 1995, Studies in subjects with long-term nonprogressive human immunodeficiency virus infection, *N. Engl. J. Med.* **332:** 209–216.

Paul, W. E., 1995, Can the immune response control HIV infection? *Cell* **82:**177–182.

Phillips, R. E., Rowlands-Jones, S., Nixon, D., Gotch, F. M., Edwards, P., Ogulensi, A., Elvin, J. G., Rothbard, J. A., Rizza, C. R., and McMichael, A. J., 1991, Human immunodeficiency virus variants that escape cytotoxic T-cell recognition, *Nature* **354:**453–459.

Pircher, H., Moskophidis, D., Rohrer, U., Burki, K., and Hengartner, H., 1990, Viral escape by selection of cytotoxic T-cell resistant virus variants in vivo, *Nature* **346:**629–633.

Plata, F., 1985, Enhancement of tumor growth correlated with suppression of the tumor-specific cytolytic T lymphocyte response in mice chronically infected by Trypanosoma cruzi, *J. Immunol.* **134:**1312–1319.

Plata, F., Langlade-Demoyen, P., Abastado, J. P., Berbar, T., and Kourilsky, P., 1987a, Retrovirus antigens recognized by cytolytic T lymphocytes activate tumor rejection *in vivo*, *Cell* **48:**231.

Plata, F., Autran, B., Martins, L. P., Wain-Hobson, S., Raphael, M., Mayaud, C., Denis, M., Guillon, J. M., and Debré, P., 1987b, AIDS-virus specific cytotoxic T-lymphocytes in lung disorders, *Nature* **328:**348–351.

Plata, F., Dadaglio, G., Chenciner, N., Hoffenbach, A., Wain-Hobson, S., Michel, F., and Langlade-Demoyen, P., 1989, Cytotoxic T lymphocytes in HIV-induced disease: Implications for therapy and vaccination, *Immunodefic. Rev.* **1:**227–246.

Price, P., Johnson, R. P., Scadden, D. T., Jassoy, C., Rosenthal, T., Kalams, S., and Walker, B. D., 1995, Cytotoxic CD8+ T lymphocytes reactive with human immunodeficiency virus-1 produce granulocyte/macrophage colony-stimulating factor and variable amounts of interleukins 2,3 and 4 following stimulation with the cognate epitope, *Clin. Immunol. Immunopathol.* **74:**100–106.

Rammensee, H. G., Falk, K., and Rotzschke, O., 1993, Peptides naturally presented by MHC class I molecules, *Annu. Rev. Immunol.* **11:**213–244.

Reddehase, M. J., Mutter, W., Munch, K., Buring, H. J., and Kosinowski, U. H., 1987, CD8+ T lymphocytes specific for murine cytomegalovirus immediate-early antigens mediate protective immunity, *J. Virol.* **61:**3102.

Rivière, Y., Tanneau-Salvadori, F., Regnault, A., Lopez, O., Sansonetti, P., Guy, B., Kieny, M. P., Fournel, J. J., and Montagnier, L., 1989, Human immunodeficiency virus specific cytotoxic responses of seropositive individuals: Distinct types of effector cells mediate killing of targets expressing gag and env proteins, *J. Virol.* **63:**2270–2277.

Rowland-Jones, S., Sutton, J., Ariyoshi, K., Dong, T., Gotch, F., McAdam, S., Whitby, D., Sabally, S., Allimore,

A., Corrah, T., Takiguchi, M., Schultz, T., McMichael, A., and Whittle, H., 1995, HIV-specific cytotoxic T cells in HIV-exposed but uninfected Gambian women, *Nature Med.* **1:**59–64.

Saag, M. S., Hahn, B. H., Gibbsons, J., Li, Y., Parks, E. S., Parks, W. P., and Shaw, G. M., 1988, Extensive variation of immunodeficiency virus type 1 in vivo, *Nature* **334:**440–443.

Sadat-Sowti, B., Debré, P., Idziorek, T., Guillon, J. M., Hadida, F., Oksenhendler, E., Katlama, C., Mayaud, C., and Autran, B., 1991, A lectin-binding soluble factor released by CD8^{+} CD57^{+} lymphocytes from AIDS patients inhibits T cell cytotoxicity, *Eur. J. Immunol.* **21:**737.

Sadat-Sowti, B., Debré, P., Quint, L., Mollet, L., Hadida, F., Leblond, V., Bismuth, G., and Autran, B., 1994, An inhibitor of cytotoxic functions (I.C.F.) produced by CD8+CD57+ T lymphocytes from AIDS and immunosuppressed bone marrow recipients, *Eur. J. Immunol.* **24:**2882–2888.

Safrit, J. T., Fung, M. S., Andrews, C. A., Braun, D. G., Sun, W. N., Chang, T. W., and Koup, R. A., 1993, Hu-PBL-SCID mice can be protected from HIV-1 infection by passive transfer of monoclonal antibody to the principal neutralizing determinant of envelope gp120, *AIDS* **7:**15–21.

Safrit, J. T., Cao, Y., Andrews, C. A., Zhu, T., Ho, D. D., and Koup, R. A., 1994, Characterization of human immunodeficiency virus type 1-specific cytotoxic T lymphocyte clones isolated during acute seroconversion: Recognition of autologous virus sequences within a conserved immunodominant epitope, *J. Exp. Med.* **179:** 463–472.

Sawyer, L. A., Katzenstein, D. A., Hendry, R. M., Boone, E. J., Vujcic, L. K., Williams, C. C., Zeger, S. L., Saah, A. J., Rinaldo, C. J., and Phair, J. P., 1990, Possible beneficial effects of neutralizing antibodies and antibody-dependent, cell-mediated cytotoxicity in human immunodeficiency virus infection, *AIDS Res. Hum. Retrovir.* **6:**341–356.

Sethi, K. K., Naher, H., and Stroehman, N., 1988, Phenotypic heterogeneity of cerebrospinal fluid-derived HIV-specific and HLA-restricted cytotoxic T-cell clones, *Nature* **335:**178–181.

Shearer, G. M., Bernstein, D. C., Tung, K. S., Via, C. S., Redfield, R., Salahuddin, S. Z., and Gallo, R. C., 1986, A model for the selective loss of major histocompatibility complex self- restricted T cell immune response during the development of acquired immunodeficiency syndrome (AIDS), *J. Immunol.* **137:**2514.

Shirai, M., Pendleton, C. D., and Berzofsky, J. A., 1992, Broad recognition of cytotoxic T cell epitopes from the HIV-1 envelope protein with multiple class I histocompatibility molecules, *J. Immunol.* **148:**1657–1667.

Siliciano, R. F., Lawton, T., Knall, C., Karr, R. W., Berman, P., Gregory, T., and Reinherz, E. L., 1988, Analysis of host–virus interactions in AIDS with anti-gp 120 T-cell clones: Effect of HIV sequence variation and a mechanism for CD4+ cell depletion, *Cell* **54:**561–575.

Stanhope, P. E., Liu, A. Y., Pavlat, W., Pithia, P. M., Clemens, M. L., and Siliciano, R. F., 1993, An HIV-1 envelope protein vaccine elicits a functionally complex human CD4^{+} T cell response that includes cytolytic T lymphocytes, *J. Immunol.* **150:**4672–4686.

Takahashi, H., Cohen, J., Hosmalin, A., Cease, K. B., Houghten, R., Cornette, J., Delisi, C., Moss, B., Germain, R. N., and Berzofsky, J. A., 1988, An immunodominant epitope of the HIV gp160 envelope glycoprotein recognized by class I MHC molecule-restricted murine cytotoxic T lymphocytes, *Proc. Natl. Acad. Sci. USA* **85:**3105–3109.

Takahashi, H., Dai, L. C., Fuerst, T. R., Biddison, W. E., Earl, P. L., Moss, B., and Ennis, F. A., 1991, Specific lysis of human immunodeficiency virus type 1-infected cells by HLA-A3.1 restricted CD8^{+} cytotoxic T-lymphocyte clone that recognizes a conserved peptide sequence within the gp41 subunit of the envelope protein, *Proc. Natl. Acad. Sci. USA* **88:**1277–1280.

Takahashi, H., Nakagawa, Y., Pendleton, C. D., Houghten, R. A., Yokomuro, K., Germain, R. N., and Berzofsky, J. A., 1992, Induction of broadly cross-reactive cytotoxic T cells recognizing an HIV-1 envelope determinant, *Science* **255:**333–336.

Takeshita, T., Takahashi, H., and Kozlowski, S., 1995, Molecular analysis of the same HIV peptide functionally binding to both a class I and a class II MHC molecule, *J. Immunol.* **154:**1973–1986.

Tenner-Racz, K., Racz, P., Thome, C., Meyer, C. G., Anderson, P. J., Schlossman, S. F., and Letvin, N. L., 1993, Cytotoxic effector cell granules recognized by the monoclonal antibody Tia-1 are present in CD8+ lymphocytes in lymph nodes of human immunodeficiency virus-1-infected patients, *Am. J. Pathol.* **142:**1750–1758.

Townsend, A. R. M., Gotch, F. M., and Davey, J., 1985, Cytotoxic T cells recognize fragments of the influence nucleoprotein, *Cell* **42:**457–467.

Tsomides, T. J., Walker, B. D., and Eisen, H. N., 1991, An optimal viral peptide recognized by CD8+ T cells binds very tightly to the restricting class I major histocompatibility complex protein on intact cells but not to the purified class I protein, *Proc. Natl. Acad. Sci. USA* **88:**11276–11280.

Tsubota, H., Lord, C. I., Watkins, D. I., Morimoto, C., and Letvin, N. L., 1989, A cytotoxic T lymphocyte inhibits acquired immunodeficiency syndrome virus replication in peripheral blood lymphocytes, *J. Exp. Med.* **169**:1421–1434.

Tussey, L. G., Rowland-Jones, S., Zheng, T. S., Androlewicz, M. J., Creswell, P., Frelinger, J. A., and McMichael, A. J., 1995, Different MHC class I alleles compete for presentation of overlapping viral epitopes, *Immunity* **3**:66–77.

Van Baalen, C. A., Klein, M. R., Geretti, A. M., Keet, R. I. P. M., Miedema, F., Van Els, C. A. C. M., and Osterhaus, A. D. M. E., 1993, Selective *in vitro* expansion of HLA class I-restricted HIV-1 gag-specific CD8+ T cells: Cytotoxic T lymphocyte epitopes and precursor frequencies, *AIDS* **7**:781–786.

Van der Burg, S. H., Klein, M. R., van de Velde, C. J., Kast, W. M., Miedema, F., and Melief, C. J., 1995, Induction of a primary human cytotoxic T-lymphocyte response against a novel conserved epitope in a functional sequence of HIV-1 reverse transcriptase, *AIDS* **9**:121–127.

Van Kuyk, R., Torbett, B. E., Gulizia, R. J., Leath, S., Mosier, D. E., and Koenig, S., 1994, Cloned human CD8+ cytotoxic T lymphocytes protect human peripheral blood leukocyte-severe combined immunodeficient mice from HIV-1 infection by an HLA-unrestricted mechanism, *J. Immunol.* **53**:4826–4833.

Vingerhoets, J. H., Vanham, G. L., Kestens, L. L., Penne, G. G., Colebunder, R. L., Vandenbruaene, M. J., Goeman, J., Gigase, P. L., DeBoer, M., and Ceuppens, J. L., 1995, Increased cytolytic T lymphocyte activity and decreased B7 responsiveness are associated with CD28 down-regulation on CD8+ T cells from HIV-infected subjects, *Clin. Exp. Immunol.* **100(3)**:425–433.

Wain-Hobson, S., 1995, Virological mayhem, *Nature* **373**:102.

Walker, B. D., Chakrabarti, S., Moss, B., Paradis, T. J., Flynn, T., Durno, A. G., Blumberg, R. S., Kaplan, J. C., Hirsch, M. S., and Schooley, R. T., 1987, HIV-specific cytotoxic T lymphocytes in seropositive individuals, *Nature* **328**:345–348.

Walker, B. D., Flexner, C., Paradis, T. J., Fuller, T. C., Hirsch, M. S., Schooley, R. T., and Moss, B., 1988, HIV-1 reverse transcriptase is a target for cytotoxic T lymphocytes in infected individuals, *Science* **240**:64–66.

Walker, B. D., Birch-Limberger, K., Fischer, L., Yoong, B., Moss, B., and Schooley, R. T., 1989, Long-term culture and fine specificity cytotoxic T-lymphocyte clones reactive with human immunodeficiency virus type 1, *Proc. Natl. Acad. Sci. USA* **86**:9514–9517.

Walker, C. M., Moody, D. J., Stites, D. P., and Levy, J. A., 1986, CD8+ lymphocytes can control HIV infection in vitro by suppressing virus replication, *Science* **234**:1563–1565.

Walker, M. C., Walker, B. D., Mestecky, J., and Mathieson, B. J., 1994, Conference on advances in AIDS vaccine development—1993 summary: Cytotoxic T-cell immunity workshop, *AIDS Res. Hum. Retrovir.* **10(Suppl. 2)**: S177–S179.

Wei, W., Ghosh, S. K., Taylor, M. E., Johnson, V. A., Emini, E. A., Deutsch, P., Lifson, J. D., Bonhoeffer, S., Nowak, M. A., Hahn, B. H., Saag, M. S., and Shaw, G. M., 1995, Viral dynamics in human immunodeficiency virus type 1 infection, *Nature* **373**:117–122.

Weinhold, K. J., Lyerly, H. K., and Matthews, T. J., 1988, Cellular anti-gp 120 cytolytic reactivities in HIV-1 seropositive individuals, *Lancet* **1**:902–904.

Whiteside, T. L., Elder, E. M., Moody, D., Armstrong, J., Ho, M., Rinaldo, C., Huang, X., Torpey, D., Gupta, P., McMahon, D., *et al.*, 1993, Generation and characterization of ex vivo propagated autologous CD8+ cells used for adoptive immunotherapy of patients infected with human immunodeficiency virus, *Blood* **81**:2085–2092.

Wolinsky, S. M., Korber, B. T. M., Neumann, A. U., Daniels, M., Kunstman, K. J., Whetsell, A. J., Furtado, M. R., Cao, Y., Do, D. D., Safrit, J. T., and Koup, R. A., 1996, Adaptive evolution of human immunodeficiency virus-type 1 during the natural course of infection, *Science* **272**:537–542.

Zinkernagel, R. M., and Hengartner, H., 1994, T-cell-mediated immunopathology versus direct cytolysis by virus: Implications for HIV and AIDS, *Immunol. Today* **15**:262–268.

Zinkernagel, R. M., Dunlop, M. B. C., Blanden, R. V., Doherty, P. C., and Shreffler, D. C., 1976, H-2 compatibility requirement for virus-specific T-cell mediated cytolysis. Evaluation of the role of H-2 region and non H-2 genes in regulating immune response, *J. Exp. Med.* **144**:519–527.

CHAPTER 11

TYPE 1 AND TYPE 2 RESPONSES IN HIV INFECTION AND EXPOSURE

GENE M. SHEARER and MARIO CLERICI

1. INTRODUCTION

A fundamental principle of immune regulation resides in the concept that an immune response to antigenic stimulation is self-limiting. It is generally considered that such regulation is advantageous for the immunized individual, because downregulation of the immune response after the infecting organism or virus as been cleared or controlled may prevent the development of an autoimmune or immunopathologic condition. One might expect that chronic infections or chronic antigenic stimulation of the immune system would provide examples in which immune regulation would be replaced by a state of immune dysregulation. In fact, several examples indicating that chronic antigenic stimulation results in immune dysregulation have been described, including infections with parasites (Wynn and Cheever, 1995) and viruses (Griffin and Ward, 1993), as well as autoimmune conditions such as systemic lupus erythematosus (Via *et al.*, 1993). It has become clear that the immune system is regulated by cytokines, and in particular those that comodulate cell-mediated and antibody-mediated immunity (abbreviated CMI and Ab, respectively). Thus, cytokines can affect the strength, kinetics, and type of immune response generated following antigenic stimulation.

Mosmann and Coffman (1989) and their colleagues have published a series of papers demonstrating that clones of murine $CD4^+$ T cells express and produce distinct cytokine patterns such that one type of clone produces interferon-γ (IFN-γ) (termed Thl), and the other type of clone produces interleukin-4 (IL-4) (termed Th2). Additional complexities have since been discovered, including Th0 clones that produce both IFN-γ and IL-4; Th0 clones appear to be less differentiated than their Thl and Th2 relatives. It is generally considered that Thl and Th2 clones and their characteristic cytokines respectively enhance

GENE M. SHEARER • Experimental Immunology Branch, National Cancer Institute, National Institutes of Health, Bethesda, Maryland 20892. MARIO CLERICI • Cattedra di Immunologica, Università degli Studi di Milano, Milano, Italy.

Immunology of HIV Infection, edited by Sudhir Gupta. Plenum Press, New York, 1996.

the cellular and humoral arms of the immune system. However, such interpretations may be somewhat oversimplified, as help for production of certain subclasses of antibodies can be enhanced by IFN-γ, and IL-4 can augment cellular responses in certain situations (Mosmann and Coffman, 1989). Some years after the discovery of murine Thl and Th2 clones, the laboratory of Romagnani (1991) identified and isolated the first human Thl and Th2 clones. Thus, T cells from both species can be driven by culture conditions into Thl and Th2 clones.

$CD4^+$ Th clones have provided an important foundation that alerted immunologists to the concept that the cellular and humoral arms of the immune system have a tendency to counteract each other via cytokine regulation. Furthermore, investigation of clones continues to generate important insights into the intricate regulatory workings of the immune system. This clonal approach, however, does not take into consideration the interaction of immunoregulatory cytokines produced by the many different cell types operating in a dynamic and open system. For example, it has subsequently been found that cells other than $CD4^+$ T cells, including CD8+ T cells, B cells, and monocytes/macrophages, can produce regulatory cytokines, including IL-4 and IFN-γ (the benchmark Thl and Th2 cytokines) (Erard *et al.*, 1994; Maggi *et al.*, 1994a; Romagnani *et al.*, 1994; Burdin *et al.*, 1993). Because the process of cloning of T cells can eliminate important cytokine-producing cells that contribute to immune regulation and would therefore not necessarily reflect or approximate conditions seen in patients or healthy controls, we chose to focus on cytokine production of unfractionated peripheral blood mononuclear cells (PBMC) (Clerici and Shearer, 1994; Clerici *et al.*, 1989, 1993a, 1994a). We defined "type 1 cytokines" as those that provide potent help for cellular responses, and "type 2 cytokines" as those that mainly enhance humoral responses (Clerici and Shearer, 1994). Type 1 cytokines include IFN-γ, IL-2, IL-12, and IL-15; type 2 cytokines include IL-4, IL-5, IL-10, and IL-13 (see Fig. 1). Several of these cytokines exhibit cross-regulatory properties in that they not only enhance one arm of the immune system, but also downregulate the other arm (Mosmann and Coffman, 1989). The type 1 and type 2 terminology can also be used to describe cellular and antibody responses, respectively. Thus, a type 1 response describes a dominant cellular response, whereas a type 2 response describes a dominant antibody response.

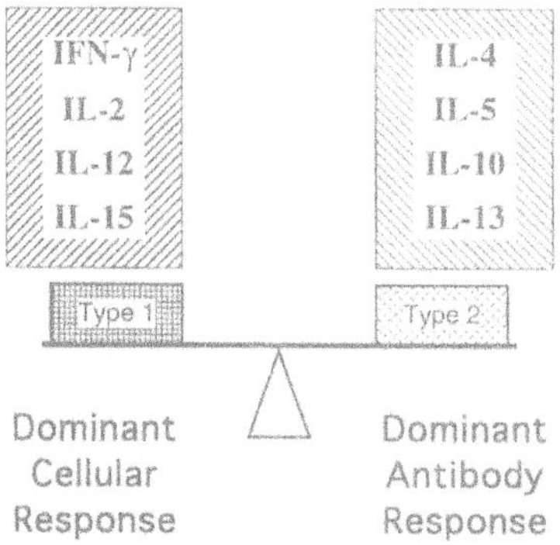

FIGURE 1. Type 1 and type 2 cytokines that modulate cellular and antibody responses.

2. TYPE 1 AND TYPE 2 RESPONSES IN AIDS PROGRESSION

An immunologic consequence of HIV infection is the loss of Th function in asymptomatic individuals, even before an appreciable decline in CD4 count is seen. This effect can be detected *in vitro* by loss of T-cell proliferation and reduced IL-2 and IFN-γ production (Clerici *et al.*, 1989; Miedema *et al.*, 1988; Giorgi *et al.*, 1987; Shearer *et al.*, 1986; Lane *et al.*, 1985), and *in vivo* by reduced ability to elicit delayed-type skin reactions (Blatt *et al.*, 1993). Furthermore, asymptomatic individuals exhibit evidence of B-cell activation and increases in certain classes of immunoglobulin (Lucey *et al.*, 1990; Mildvan *et al.*, 1982), as well as evidence of eosinophilia (Smith *et al.*, 1994; Fleury-Feith *et al.*, 1992). These observations suggest that immune dysregulation occurs prior to the characteristic drop in CD4 count, and raises the possibility that it may contribute to $CD4^+$ T-cell depletion. Based on the above findings, as well as our observations that mitogen-induced IL-4 and IL-10 levels are elevated in PBMC cultures from HIV^+ individuals (Clerici *et al.*, 1993a, 1994a), and the earlier report of Maggi *et al.* (1987) in AIDS patients, we suggested that HIV-associated immune dysregulation involves a shift from a dominant cellular to a dominant antibody response, with changes in the cytokine profile that promote and reflect such a shift (Clerici and Shearer, 1993, 1994) (Fig. 2). These findings have been verified at the clonal level by Meyaard *et al.* (1994), and in cultures of unfractionated PBMC from HIV^+ patients by Barcellini *et al.* (1994). However, not all studies agree with the type 1-to-type 2 shift (Maggi *et al.*, 1994a; Graziosi *et al.*, 1994). Nevertheless, recent studies indicate that $CD8^+$ T cells can produce Th2 cytokines that contribute to the shift toward a dominant antibody response and loss of cellular immunity (Maggi *et al.*, 1994a; Erard *et al.*, 1993). IL-12 is another cytokine that induces strong Th function and that is reduced in HIV^+ patients (Chehimi *et al.*, 1994). Addition of IL-12 to cultures of PBMC from HIV^+ patients can restore cellular immune function, including natural killer cell activity, IFN-γ production, and T-cell proliferation to recall antigens (Chehimi *et al.*, 1994; Clerici *et al.*, 1993b). Recent unpublished data indicate that the loss of IL-12 production and gene expression is paralleled by an increase in IL-10 production (C. Chougnet *et al.*, in press).

We view cytokine-induced immune dysregulation as a central component in the progression to AIDS. As shown in Fig. 3, the loss of IL-2 production and the increase in sustained IL-10 production may be a persistent feature of the type 1-to-type 2 shirt. The temporary increase in IL-4 production (Clerici and Shearer, 1993) appears to occur during the first year after HIV infection (Meroni *et al.*, 1996), and may initiate the type 1-to-2 shift.

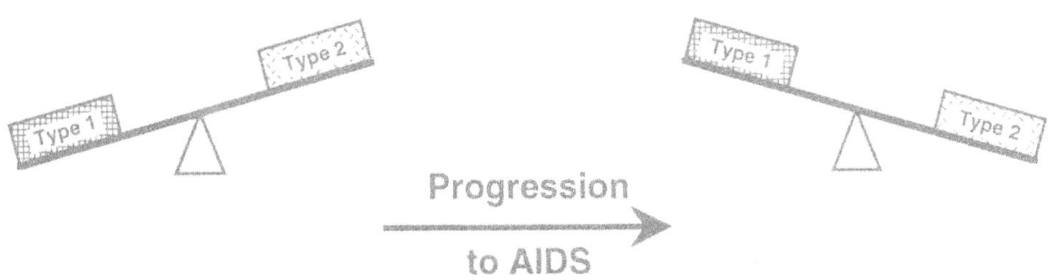

FIGURE 2. Progression toward AIDS involves a reduction in cellular immune activity and a reduction in one or more type 1 cytokines with an increase in one or more type 2 cytokines.

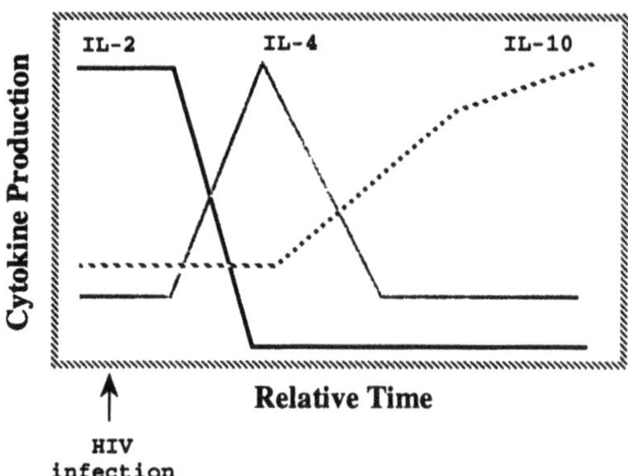

FIGURE 3. Progression toward AIDS involves a reduction in antigen- and mitogen-induced IL-2 production and an increase in antigen- and mitogen-induced IL-4 (transient) and IL-10 production.

The decline in CD4 production after approximately 1 year could be related to the finding that $CD4^+$ Th2 cells appear to be more easily infected with HIV than Th1 cells (Romagnani *et al.*, 1994). Therefore, HIV infection could induce selective viral cytopathic death of IL-4-producing Th2 cells, resulting in a less obvious type 1-to-type 2 shift than might be expected (Clerici and Shearer, 1994).

3. TYPE 1 AND TYPE 2 RESPONSES IN AIDS IMMUNOPATHOGENESIS

AIDS pathogenesis is an important but unresolved topic that is frequently divided into virus- and immune-mediated mechanisms. Although both may contribute to depletion of $CD4^+$ T cells, we limit our comments here to an immune-mediated model that is modulated by type 1 and type 2 cytokines. One unique features of HIV^+ individuals is that their PBMC contain a high percentage of activated T cells (Kestens *et al.*, 1994). Because activated T cells are susceptible to apoptotic death, it has been suggested that these activated T cells undergo extensive death by an apoptotic mechanism (Gougeon and Montagnier, 1993; Ameisen and Capron, 1991). Increased apoptotic death of T cells has been observed in both unstimulated (Meyaard *et al.*, 1992) and pan-T-cell-stimulated (Finkel and Banda, 1994; Clerici *et al.*, 1994c) cultures of HIV^+ patients' PBMC compared to death seen in cultures of PBMC from healthy donors or patients with lupus (Clerici *et al.*, 1994c). Although it can be argued whether unstimulated or stimulated PBMC more closely approximate the *in vivo* situation, several laboratories including ours have studied the increased percentage of apoptotic T-cell death seen after *in vitro* stimulation (Finkel *et al.*, 1995; Clerici *et al.*, 1994c; Finkel and Banda, 1994; Groux *et al.*, 1992). Stimulation with pan-T-cell activators such as anti-CD3 induces death in 40–60% of T cells that involves both the $CD4^+$ and $CD8^+$ subsets (Clerici *et al.*, 1994c). Furthermore, it has recently been shown that activation-induced death of T cells from HIV^+ children does not involve the T cells that are HIV-infected (Finkel *et al.*, 1995). In fact, most of the T cells that exhibited apoptotic nuclei were not HIV-infected.

We have studied both pan-T-cell-activated and antigen-induced cell death, and have found that anti-CD3 stimulation results in the death of both subsets, whereas stimulation with infectious influenza virus or with synthetic peptides of HIV envelope induces death that is selected for the $CD4^+$ subset (Clerici *et al.*, 1994c, in press; Clerici *et al.*, 1996). This latter model may more closely approximate the situation *in vivo*, as progression to AIDS involves CD4 depletion, and patients' immune systems are more likely to be stimulated with specific antigens than with pan-T-cell activators. We also observed that apoptotic death induced by either anti-CD3 or viral antigens is regulated by cytokines. The type 1 cytokines IL-2, IL-12, and IFN-γ reduced apoptotic T-cell death, as did antibodies against IL-4 and IL-10 (Clerici *et al.*, 1994b, 1996, in press). In contrast, IL-4 and IL-10, as well as antibodies against IL-12 did not prevent and in some patients increased T-cell death. Our most recent studies suggest that two of the effector molecules for antigen-stimulated apoptotic T-cell death are tumor necrosis factor-α and lymphotoxin (Clerici *et al.*, 1996).

As noted above, a unique feature of activation- or antigen-induced T-cell death is the fact that a high proportion of cells appears to be activated or primed to undergo death when stimulated, and an increase in the proportion of T cells expressing activation markers is seen in the PBMC of HIV^+ individuals (Kestens *et al.*, 1994). These activated cells exhibit extensive apoptotic death if stimulated in the presence of type 2 cytokines, but not in the presence of type 1 cytokines (Clerici *et al.*, 1994c). Some of the characteristics of T-cell death in PBMC of HIV^+ individuals that we briefly review here are illustrated in Fig. 4.

The model proposed is that $CD4^+$ T-cell activation, possibly resulting from an aberrant interaction between CD4 and gp120, primes a high proportion of $CD4^+$ T cells for apoptotic death (Finkel and Banda, 199; Ameisen and Capron, 1992). Antigenic stimulation in a type 2 cytokine environment results in a high proportion of dying cells. However, the death process can be rescued if antigenic stimulation occurs in a type 1 cytokine environment. This model is consistent with the IL-2 clinical trials of Kovacs *et al.* (1995) that showed stabilized or increased CD4 counts in HIV^+ patients with entry CD4 counts $> 300/\mu l$. Finally, if antigen-stimulated apoptotic death of $CD4^+$ T cells is a model relevant for the drop in the CD4 count in progression to AIDS, an understanding of the mechanism responsible for T-cell activation in HIV^+ individuals could provide a new strategic avenue for immune-based therapy.

4. TYPE 1 AND TYPE 2 RESPONSES IN AIDS THERAPY

As noted above, progression to AIDS and the loss of $CD4^+$ T cells is associated with a shift from a type 1 to a type 2 cytokine profile and replacement of a dominant cellular with a dominant antibody response. Therefore, consideration and emphasis should be given to cytokine-based therapy, with the aim being to restore a dominant cellular response and a type 1 cytokine profile (Fig. 5). As also noted above, intermittent IL-2 therapy appears to hold promise (Kovacs *et al.*, 1995). Because (1) IL-12 mRNA expression and production is reduced in the monocyte/macrophage population of HIV^+ individuals (Chehimi *et al.*, 1994; Clerici *et al.*, 1993c; Chougnet *et al.*, 1996), and (2) cellular responses and IFN-γ are increased in the cultures of PBMC from HIV^+ patients, this cytokine has recently been considered for AIDS therapy (Hall, 1995; Balter, 1995). However, IL-12 appears to have serious side effects in patients (Marshall, 1995).

Alternate strategies to intervention by direct cytokine infusion would be to treat patients with agents that either bypass a cytokine defect or induce endogenous cytokine

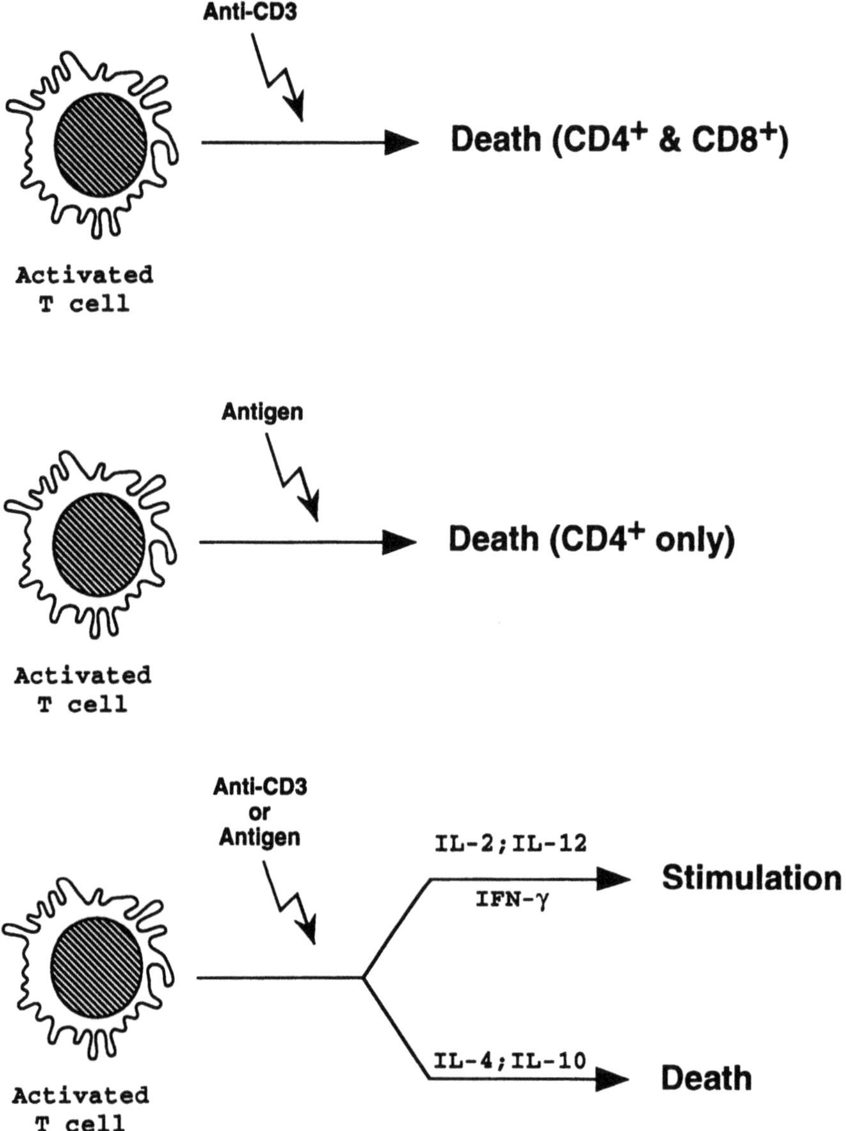

FIGURE 4. Some characteristics of anti-CD3- and antigen-stimulated apoptotic T-cell death.

production (Shearer, 1995). Such approaches might circumvent the toxic side effects associated with direct cytokine administration. A recent report investigated the effects of inoculating mice with small Schiff base-forming molecules to bypass costimulatory requirements (Rhodes *et al.*, 1995). The study demonstrated enhancement of cellular immune responses that were effective against viral infection and tumor growth. Endogenous cytokine production might be even more effective, because it offers the potential advantages of (1) cytokine self-regulation that could reduce cytokine toxicity, (2) a longer effective half-life, and (3) production of the cytokine in the primary lymphoid tissues, where helper and

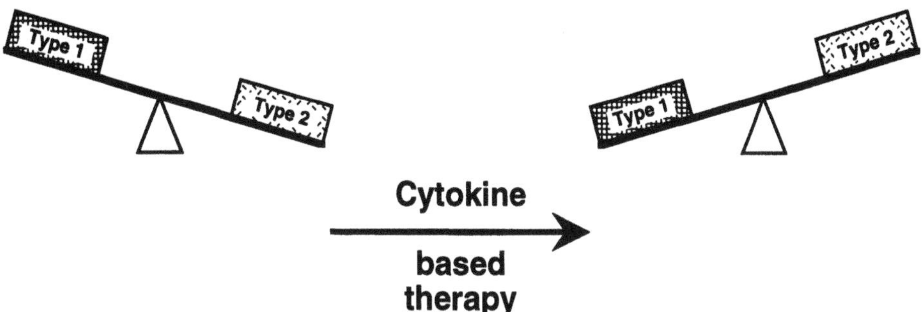

FIGURE 5. Objective of cytokine-based therapy.

effector components of the immune system communicate. This strategy, however, would require that some endogenous cytokine-producing potential remains intact in the patient. We reported an example of such an approach *in vitro*, using PBMC from HIV^+ individuals that produced IL-2 when stimulated with allogeneic cells but not when stimulated with influenza virus (Clerici *et al.*, 1990). Costimulation with allogenic cells plus influenza virus resulted in the generation of influenza-specific cytotoxic T lymphocytes, similar to the effect of exogenous IL-2. Thus, it is possible that HIV^+ patients who have lost the ability to respond to recall antigens but retain alloresponsive activity would benefit from allogenic leukocyte transfusions via alloantigen-driven help.

5. TYPE 1 AND TYPE 2 RESPONSES IN PREVENTING HIV INFECTION

If a strong cellular immune response and a dominant type 1 cytokine profile can prevent or delay progression of HIV-infected individuals to AIDS, it seems reasonable to question whether such immunity would also be protective against detectable infection (Fig. 6). During the past 8 years, several laboratories have reported the phenomenon that exposure to HIV can result in virus-specific T cellular immune activity without seroconversion or evidence of HIV infection (for review see Shearer and Clerici, 1996; Rowland-Jones and McMichael, 1995). This observation includes every exposed or at-risk category of individuals. The studies include unprotected heterosexual and homosexual individuals, newborns of HIV^+ mothers, intravenous drug users, and even accidental single needle-sticks. The positive cellular immune responses detected include HIV-stimulated T-cell proliferation, IL-2 production, and CD8-mediated cytolytic T-lymphocyte activity. In some studies, as many as 50–65% of exposed seronegative individuals exhibited cellular responses to HIV antigens. One study demonstrated that HIV-exposed seronegative individuals exhibit even stronger type 1 cytokine activity than the healthy, unexposed population (Barcellini *et al.*, 1995). These findings support the concept that strong cellular immune potential and a dominant type 1 cytokine profile is also protective against detectable HIV infection. However, it may be that a very low level of HIV infection accompanies protective cellular immunity, because the CD8-mediated, class I-restricted cytolytic activity reported should involve at least limited HIV infection (Pinto *et al.*, 1995; Langlade-Demoyen *et al.*, 1994; Rowland-Jones *et al.*, 1993). Support for cellular immune protection via low-dose live virus

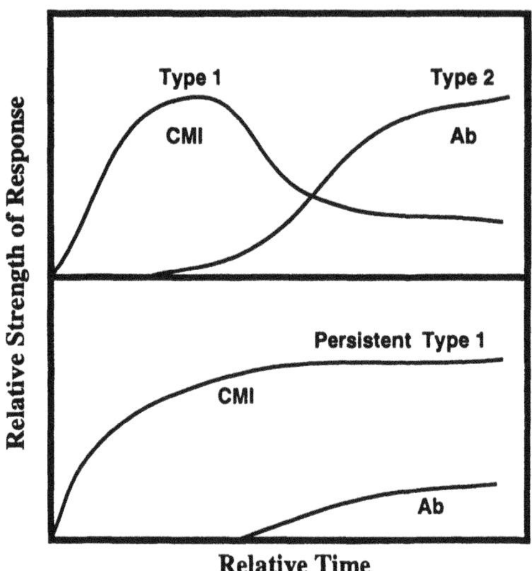

FIGURE 6. (Upper) Kinetics of typical biphasic dominant cellular (CMI) and antibody (Ab) responses after immunization or infection. (Lower) Model of dominant and persistent cellular (CMI) response that might be needed to maintain protective immunity against HIV infection and AIDS progression.

exposure (infection?) comes from the SIV macaque model in which inoculation of very low doses of live SIV protected against high infectious challenge doses (Clerici *et al.*, 1994b).

It can be argued that although potent cellular immunity and a dominant type 1 cytokine pattern may retard progression to AIDS, a strong cellular immune response does not appear to be protective against initial infection. However, long-term immune protection may require immunization prior to a first encounter with enough live virus to induce a productive infection, which is the purpose of prophylactic vaccination. Infected individuals actually exhibit a potent cellular response in the absence of neutralizing antibody, as evidenced by early HIV-specific CTL activity that heralds the impressive drop in viral load in the blood at the end of the acute infection phase (Koup and Ho, 1994). One can question why this initial "success" of cellular immunity over HIV does not eliminate the virus at the end of the acute phase. Several possibilities can be considered, including (1) the fact that the initial infection or exposure induces a primary immune response, giving the virus the edge, (2) the observation that after reduction of virus in the blood, surviving infectious virus homes to the germinal centers of lymph nodes (Pantaleo and Fauci, 1995), which may be immunologically privileged sites where protective cellular immune responses such as HIV-specific CTL may not be potent, or (3) the initial strong cellular response is compromised at the expense of an increasing antibody response (Salk *et al.*, 1993). These possibilities are not mutually exclusive, and all may contribute. It is noteworthy that Koup and Ho (1994) reported a reduction in HIV-specific CTL precursor frequency after acute HIV infection in one patient as antibody increased. Furthermore, Safrit and Koup (1995) observed a persistently high level of CTL precursors to Gag, Pol, and Env in three HIV^+ patients who did not develop antibodies during several months following HIV infection. This pattern contrasts with that of one patient who elicited antibodies and exhibited a reduction in CTL precursors specific for Gag and Env as the antibody response increased. It is possible that the increase in antibody production is accompanied by a decrease in CTL activity that is critical for keeping the virus in check. It is also possible that certain types of HIV-specific antibodies will enhance HIV infection (Levy, 1993).

These later findings are consistent with our type 1 versus type 2 model for resistance to HIV infection and progression to AIDS (Clerici and Shearer, 1993, 1994), and the suggestion that simultaneous optimization of the cellular and humoral arms of the immune system may be difficult because of the counteracting effects of cross-regulatory cytokines (Salk *et al.*, 1993). Figure 6 illustrates this model by showing a decline in CMI activity with increasing antibody, similar to the findings noted above (Safrit and Koup, 1995; Koup and Ho, 1994). The lower panel presents a model in which a high level of CMI activity persists at the expense of high antibody activity. It is our opinion that this persistent type 1 response is desirable for protecting against HIV infection, as well as for retarding AIDS progression. It should also be noted that HIV^+ long-term nonprogressors maintain strong HIV-specific CTL activity (Rinaldo *et al.*, 1995).

6. TYPE 1 AND TYPE 2 RESPONSES IN VACCINE DESIGN

If a strong cellular response and a dominant type 1 cytokine profile can protect against AIDS progression and HIV infection, serious consideration should be given to optimizing cellular immunity. Although it may be possible to concurrently maximize the cellular and antibody arms, this would not be the natural tendency of the immune system. We suggest that strategies be developed to determine the ways to optimize cellular immunity that is persistently strong. One such strategy would be to immunize with low doses of immunogen. It has been well established in murine studies that low-dose immunization can induce a strong cellular response without eliciting antibody production, whereas higher doses of the same immunogen preferentially induced strong antibody responses (Parish, 1972). This phenomenon has also been demonstrated in human volunteers who received different doses of an rgp160 candidate AIDS vaccine. Doses of rgp160 less than 80 μg induced cellular immune responses but no detectable antibodies; higher doses induced both cellular and antibody responses (Clerici *et al.*, 1991). This phenomenon is illustrated in Fig. 7. It could be argued that the higher doses of the vaccine induced both arms of the immune system, and one should take advantage of this. The issue here may be whether induction of antibody compromised the cellular component, thereby reducing the major cellular protective mechanism.

Another vaccine-related issue that should be considered was noted above in the surprisingly high proportion of exposed seronegative individuals who exhibited T cell immune activity against HIV antigens. Although this does not necessarily indicate infection, it does strongly suggest immunologic exposure and priming to HIV antigens. Seronegative, exposed, or at-risk volunteers have been recruited for vaccine trials. Large-scale trials of this type in the United States have been postponed because of lack of evidence that the gp120 vaccines that were to be used would be beneficial (Cohen, 1994). We emphasize that such vaccine trials should not be performed without also prescreening prospective vaccinees for cellular responses to HIV antigens, as well as the routine antibody screening. We expect that a significant proportion of such volunteers could be primed for cellular responses to HIV that would go undetected by serologic screening alone. Such individuals would be developing secondary immune response, while the investigators would consider

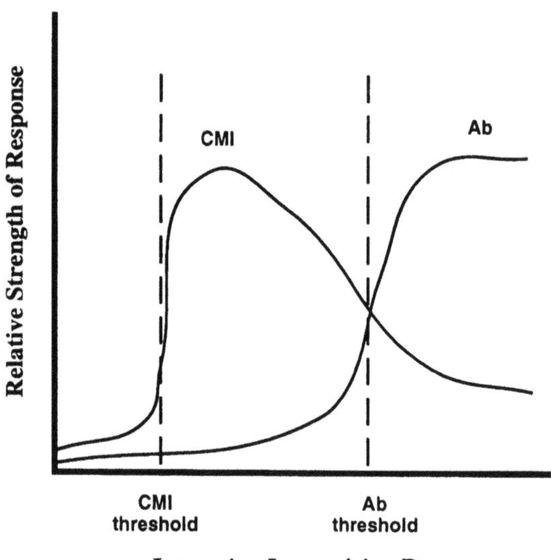

FIGURE 7. Effect of antigen dose on cellular (CMI) and antibody (Ab) responses.

them to be generating a primary response as the result of the vaccination. Having an unknown proportion of unidentified vaccinees receiving a primary immunization and another proportion receiving a booster immunization could confound interpretation of possibly protective immunity.

7. TYPE 1 AND TYPE 2 RESPONSES BEYOND HIV/AIDS

The immunologic evidence routinely used to test for exposure to and/or infection with viruses is serum antibodies against viral antigens. The results summarized above indicating that exposure and possibly low-level infection can induce cellular immune activity without eliciting antibodies raise the possibility that viruses other than HIV and SIV will yield similar findings. In fact, we have reported that seronegative, HTLV-1-exposed individuals can exhibit T-cell responses to the Tax peptide of HTLV-1 (Nishimura *et al.*, 1994). Other examples of viral exposure that do not result in seroconversion or detectable infection should also be tested for evidence of possible virus-specific cellular immunity. Studies of this type might indicate that cellular immunity is as protective or more so than humoral immunity for intracellular viruses. Such a finding might be helpful in redesigning vaccine strategies for which antibodies are either not protective or have only a limited protective effect.

REFERENCES

Ameisen, J.-C., and Capron, A., 1991, Cell dysfunction and depletion in AIDS: Programmed cell death hypothesis, *Immunol. Today* **12**:102–105.

Balter, M., 1995, Cytokines move from the margins to the spotlight, *Science* **268:**205–206.

Barcellini, W., Rizzardi, G. P., Borghi, M. O., Fain, C., Lazzarin, A., and Meroni, P. L., 1994, Thl and Th2 cytokine production by peripheral blood mononuclear cells from HIV-infected patients, *AIDS* **8:**757–762.

Barcellini, W., Rizzardi, G. P., Velati, C., Borghi, M. O., Fain, C., Lazzarin, A., and Meroni, P. L., 1995, In vitro production of type 1 and type 2 cytokines by peripheral blood mononuclear cells from high-risk HIV-negative intravenous drug users, *AIDS* **9:**691–694.

Blatt, S. P., Hendrix, C. W., Butzin, C. A., Freeman, T. M., Ward, W. W., Hensley, R. E., Melcher, G. P., Donovan, D. J., and Boswell, R. N., 1993, Delayed type hyper-sensitivity skin testing predicts progression to AIDS in HIV-infected patients, *Ann. Intern. Med.* **119:**177–184.

Burdin, N., Peronne, C., Banchereau, J., and Rousset, J., 1993, Epstein–Barr virus transformation induces B lymphocytes to produce human interleukin-10, *J. Exp. Med.* **177:**295–304.

Chehimi, J., Starr, S. E., Frank, L., D'Andrea, A., Ma, X., MacGregor, R. R., Sennelier, J., and Trinchieri, G., 1994, Impaired interleukin 12 production in human immunodeficiency virus-infected patients, *J. Exp. Med.* **179:**1361–1366.

Chougnet, C., Wynn, T. A., Clerici, M., Landay, A., Kessler, H., Rusnak, J., Melcher, G. P., Sher, A., and Shearer, G. M., 1996, Molecular analysis of decreased IL-12 production in HIV-infected individuals and in vitro reciprocal regulation of IL-10 and IL-12, *J. Infect. Dis.*, in press.

Clerici, M., and Shearer, G. M., 1993, A THl–TH2 switch is a critical step in the etiology of HIV infection, *Immunol. Today* **14:**107–111.

Clerici, M., and Shearer, G. M., 1994, The Thl/Th2 hypothesis of HIV infection: New insights, *Immunol. Today* **15:**575–581.

Clerici, M., Stocks, N. I., Zajac, R. A., Boswell, R. N., Lucey, D. R., Via, C. S., and Shearer, G. M., 1989, Detection of three distinct patterns of T helper cell dysfunction in asymptomatic, HIV-seropositive patients: Independence of $CD4^+$ cell numbers and clinical staging, *J. Clin. Invest.* **84:**1892–1899.

Clerici, M., Stocks, N. I., Zajac, R. A., Boswell, R. N., Via, C. S., and Shearer, G. M., 1990, Circumvention of defective CD4 T helper cell function in HIV-infected individuals by stimulation with HLA alloantigens, *J. Immunol.* **144:**3266–3271.

Clerici, M., Tacket, C. O., Via, C. S., Muluk, S. C., Berzofsky, J. A., and Shearer, G. M., 1991, Immunization with subunit HIV vaccine generates stronger T helper cell immunity than natural infection, *Eur. J. Immunol.* **21:**1345–1349.

Clerici, M., Hakim, F. T., Venzon, D. J., Blatt, S. P., Hendrix, C. W., Wynn, T. A., and Shearer, G. M., 1993a, Changes in interleukin-2 and interleukin-4 production in asymptomatic, human immunodeficiency virus-seropositive individuals, *J. Clin. Invest.* **91:**759–765.

Clerici, M., Sison, A. V., Berzofsky, J. A., Rakusan, T. A., Brandt, C. D., Ellaurie, M., Colie, C., Venzon, D. J., Sever, J. L., and Shearer, G. M., 1993b, Cellular immune factors associated with mother-to-infant transmission of HIV, *AIDS* **7:**1427–1432.

Clerici, M., Lucey, D. R., Berzofsky, J. A., Pinto, L. A., Wynn, T. A., Blatt, S. P., Dolan, M. J., Hendrix, C. W., Wolf, S., and Shearer, G. M., 1993c, Restoration of HIV-specific cell-mediated immune responses by interleukin-12 in vitro, *Science* **262:**1721–1724.

Clerici, M., Wynn, T. A., Berzofsky, J. A., Blatt, S. P., Hendrix, C. W., Sher, A., Coffman, R. L., and Shearer, G. M., 1994a, Role of interleukin-10 in T helper cell dysfunction in asymptomatic individuals infected with the human immuno-deficiency virus (HIV-1), *J. Clin. Invest.* **93:**768–775.

Clerici, M., Clark, E. A., Polacino, P., Axeberg, I., Kuller, L., Casey, N. I., Morton, W. R., Shearer, G. M., and Beneviste, R. E., 1994b, Induction of cellular immune response by subinfectious doses of SIV: Protection from virus challenge, *AIDS* **8:**1391–1395.

Clerici, M., Sarin, A., Coffman, R. A., Wynn, T. A., Blatt, S. P., Hendrix, C. W., Wolf, S., Shearer, G. M., and Henkart, P. A., 1994c, Type l/type 2 cytokine modulation of T cell programmed cell death as a model for HIV pathogenesis, *Proc. Natl. Acad. Sci. USA* **91:**11811–11815.

Cohen, J., 1994, U.S. panel votes to delay real-world vaccine trials, *Science* **264:**1839.

Clerici, M., Sarin, A., Berzofsky, J. A., Landay, A. L., Kessler, H. A., Hendrix, C. W., Blatt, S. P., Coffman, R. L., Henkart, P. A., and Shearer, G. M., 1996, Antigen-stimulated CD4+ cell death in HIV infection: Role of immunoregulatory cytokines and lymphotoxin, *AIDS*, in press.

Erard, F., Wild, M. T., Garciz-Sanz, J. A., and Legros, G., 1993, Switch of CD8 T cells to noncytokitic CD8-CD4- cells that make Th2 cytokines and help β cells, *Science* **260:**1802–1805.

Erard, F., Dunbar, P. R., and Le Gros, G., 1994, The IL-4-induced switch of CD8+ T cells to a TH2 phenotype and its possible relationship to the onset of AIDS, *Res. Immunol.* **145:**643–646.

Finkel, T. H., and Banda, N. K., 1994, Indirect mechanisms of HIV pathogenesis: How does HIV kill T cells? *Curr Opin. Immunol.* **6**:605–615.

Finkel, T. H., Tudor-Williams, G., Banda, N. K., Cotton, M. F., Curiel, T., Baba, T. W., Ruprecht, R. M., and Kupfer, A., 1995, Apoptosis occurs predominantly in bystander cells and not in productively infected cells of HIV- and SIV-infected lymph nodes, *Nature Med.* **1**:129–134.

Fleury-Feith, J., van Nheieu, J. T., Picard, C., Escudier, E., and Bernaudin, J. F., 1992, Bronchoalveolar lavage eosinophilia associated with *Pneumocystis carinii* pneumonitis in AIDS patients. Comparative study with non-AIDS patients, *Chest* **95**:1198–1201.

Giorgi, J. V., Fahey, J. L., Smith, D. C., Hultin, L. E., Cheng, H. L., Mitsuyasu, R. T., and Detels, R., 1987, Early effects of HIV on CD4 lymphocytes in vivo, *J. Immunol.* **138**:3725–3730.

Gougeon, M. L., and Montagnier, L., 1993, Apoptosis in AIDS, *Science* **260**:1269–1270.

Graziosi, C., Pantaleo, G., Gantt, K. R., Fortin, J.-P., Demarest, J. F., Cohen, O. J., Sekaly, R. P., and Fauci, A. S., 1994, Lack of evidence for the dichotomy of Thl and Th2 predominance in HIV-infected individuals, *Science* **265**:248–252.

Griffin, D. E., and Ward, B. J., 1993, Differential CD4 T cell activation in measles, *J. Infect. Dis.* **668**:275–281.

Groux, H., Monte, D., Bourrez, J. M., Capron, A., and Ameisen, J.-C., 1992, Activation-induced death by apoptosis in $CD4^+$ T cells from human immunodeficiency virus-infected asymptomatic individuals, *J. Exp. Med.* **175**:331–340.

Hall, S. S., 1995, IL-12 at the crossroads, *Science* **268**:1432–1434.

Kestens, L., Vanham, G., Vereecken, C., vandenBruaene, M., Vercauteren, G., Colbunders, R. L., and Gigase, P. L., 1994, Selective increase of activation antigens HLA-DR and CD38 on $CD4^+CD45RO^+$ T lymphocytes during HIV-1 infection, *Clin. Exp. Immunol.* **95**:436–441.

Koup, R. A., and Ho, D. D., 1994, Shutting down HIV, *Nature* **370**:416.

Kovacs, J. A., Baseler, M., Dewar, R. J., Vogel, S., Davey, R. T., Fallon, J., Polis, M. A., Walker, R. E., Stevens, R., Salzman, N. P., Metcalf, J. A., Masur, H., and Lane, H. C., 1995, Sustained increases in $CD4^+$ T lymphocytes in HIV-infected patients with intermittent continuous infusion interleukin-2 therapy: A preliminary report, *N. Engl. J. Med.* **332**:567–575.

Lane, H. C., Depper, J. M., Greene, W. C., Whalen, G., Waldmann, T. A., and Fauci, A. S., 1985, Qualitative analysis of immune function in patients with the acquired immunodeficiency syndrome: Evidence for selective defect in soluble antigen recognition, *N. Engl. J. Med.* **313**:79–84.

Langlade-Demoyen, P., Ngo-Giang-Huong, N., Ferchal, F., and Oksenhender, E., 1994, Human immunodeficiency virus (HIV) *nef*-specific cytotoxic T lymphocytes in noninfected heterosexual contacts of HIV-infected patients, *J. Clin. Invest.* **93**:1293–1297.

Levy, J. A., 1993, Pathogenesis of human immunodeficiency virus infection, *Microbiol. Rev.* **57**:183–289.

Lucey, D. R., Zajac, R. A., Melcher, G. P., Butzin, C. A., and Boswell, R. N., 1990, Serum IgE levels in 662 persons with human immunodeficiency virus infection: IgE elevation with marked depletion of CD4+ T-cells, *AIDS Res. Hum. Retrovir.* **6**:427–429.

Maggi, E., Macchia, D., Parronchi, P., Mazzetti, M., Ravina, A., Milo, D., and Romagnani, S., 1987, Reduced production of interleukin 2 and interferon gamma and enhanced helper activity for IgG synthesis by cloned CD4 T cells from patients with AIDS, *Eur. J. Immunol.* **17**:1685–1690.

Maggi, E., Mazzetti, M., Ravina, A., Manetti, R., DeCarli, M., Annunziato, F., Piccinni, M.-P., Carbonari, M., Presco, A. M., Del Prete, G., and Romagnani, S., 1994a, Ability of HIV to promote a TH1 to TH2 shift and to replicate preferentially in Th2 and Th0 cells, *Science* **265**:244–248.

Maggi, E., Giudizi, M. G., Biagiotti, R., Annunziato, F., Manetti, R., Piccinni, M.-P., Parronchi, P., Sampognaro, S., Giannarini, L., Zuccati, G., and Romagnani, S., 1994b, Th2-like CD8+ T cells showing B cell helper function and reduced cytotoxic activity in human immunodeficiency virus type 1 infection, *J. Exp. Med.* **180**:489–495.

Marshall, E., 1995, Cancer trial of interleukin-12 halted, *Science* **268**:1555.

Meroni, L., Trabattoni, D., Bolotta, C., Riva, C., Gori, A., Moroni, M., Villa, M. L., Clerici, M., and Galli, M., 1996, Evidence for type 2 cytokine production and lymphocyte activation in the early phases of HIV-1 infection, *AIDS* **10**:23–30.

Meyaard, L., Otto, S. A., Jonker, R. R., Mijnster, M. J., Keet, R. P. M., and Miedema, F., 1992, Programmed death of T cells in HIV-1 infection, *Science* **257**:217–219.

Meyaard, L., Otto, S. A., Keet, I. P. M., vanLier, R. A. W., and Miedema, F., 1994, Changes in cytokine secretion patterns of $CD4^+$ T-cell clones in human immunodeficiency virus infection, *Blood* **84**:4262–4268.

Miedema, F., Petit, A. J. C., Terpstra, F. G., Schattenkerk, J. K. M., DeWold, B. J. M., Roos, I. P. M., Lange, S. A., Danner, S. A., Goudsmit, J., and Schellekens, P. T., 1988, Immunologic abnormalities in human immunodeficiency virus (HIV)-infected asymptomatic homosexual men. HIV affects the immune system before CD4+ T helper cell depletion occurs, *J. Clin. Invest.* **82**:1908–1914.

Mildvan, D., Mathur, U., Enlow, R. W., Romain, P. L., Winchester, R. J., Colp, C., Singman, H., Adelsberg, B. R., and Spigland, I., 1982, Opportunistic infections and immune deficiency in homosexual men, *Ann. Intern. Med.* **96**:700–704.

Mosmann, T. R., and Coffman, R. L., 1989, Thl and Th2 cells: Different patterns of lymphokine secretion lead to different functional properties, *Annu. Rev. Immunol.* **7**:145–173.

Nishimura, M., Kedmode, A. G., Clerici, M., Shearer, G. M., Berzofsky, J. A., Uchiyawa, T., Witkor, S. Z., Pate, E., Maloney, B., Manns, A., Blattner, W., and Jacobson, S., 1994, Demonstration of HTLV-1 specific T cell responses from seronegative and PCR negative individuals exposed to HTLV-1, *J. Infect. Dis.* **170**:334–338.

Pantaleo, G., and Fauci, A. C., 1995, New concepts in the immunopathogenesis of HIV infection, *Annu. Rev. Immunol.* **13**:487–512.

Parish, C. R., 1972, The relationship between humoral and cell mediated immunity, *Transplant, Rev.* **13**:35–66.

Pinto, L. A., Sullivan, J., Berzofsky, J. A., Clerici, M., Kessler, H. A., Landay, A. L., and Shearer, G. M., 1995, Env-specific cytotoxic T lymphocyte responses in HIV seronegative health care workers occupationally exposed to HIV-contaminated body fluids, *J. Clin. Invest.* **96**:867–873.

Rhodes, J., Chen, H., Hall, S. R., Beesley, J. E., Jenkins, D. C., Collins, P., and Zheng, B., 1995, Therapeutic potentiation of the immune system by costimulatory Schiff-base-forming drugs, *Nature* **377**:71–75.

Rinaldo, C., Huang, X.-L., Fan, Z., Ding, M., Beltz, L., Logar, A., Panciali, D., Mazzara, G., Liebman, J., Cottrill, M., and Gupta, P., 1995, High levels of anti-human immunodeficiency virus type 1 (HIV-1) memory cytotoxic T-lymphocyte activity and low viral load are associated with lack of disease in HIV-1-infected long-term nonprogressors, *J. Virol.* **69**:5838–5842.

Romagnani, S., 1991, Human THI and TH2 subsets: Doubt no more, *Immunol. Today* **12**:256–258.

Romagnani, S., Maggi, E., and Del Prete, G., 1994, HIV can induce a THl to TH0 shift and preferentially replicates in CD4+ T-cell clones producing TH2-type cytokines, *Res. Immunol.* **145**:611–618.

Rowland-Jones, S. L., and McMichael, A., 1995, Immune responses in HIV-exposed seronegatives: Have they repelled the virus? *Curr. Opin. Immunol.* **7**:448–455.

Rowland-Jones, S. L., Nixon, D. F., Aldhous, M. C., Gotch, F., Aryoshi, K., Hallam, N., Kroll, K., Frobel, K., and McMichael, M., 1993, HIV-specific cytotoxic T-cell activity in HIV-exposed but uninfected infant, *Lancet* **341**:860–861.

Safrit, J. T., and Koup, R. A., 1995, The immunology of primary HIV infection: Which immune responses control HIV replication? *Curr. Opin. Immunol.* **7**:456–461.

Salk, J., Bretscher, P., Salt, P. L., Clerici, M., and Shearer, G. M., 1993, A strategy for prophylactic vaccination against HIV, *Science* **260**:1270–1272.

Shearer, G. M., 1995, Redirecting T-cell function, *Nature* **377**:16–17.

Shearer, G. M., and Clerici, M., 1996, Protective immunity against HIV infection: Has nature done the experiment for us? *Immunol. Today* **17**:21–24.

Shearer, G. M., Bernstein, D. C., Tung, K. S. K., Via, C. S., Redfield, R., Salihuddin, S. Z., and Gallo, R. C., 1986, A model for the selective loss of major histocompatibility complex self-restricted T cell immune responses during the developing of acquired immune deficiency syndrome (AIDS), *J. Immunol.* **137**:2514–2521.

Smith, K. J., Shelton, H. G., Drabick, J. J., McCarthy, W. F., Ledsky, R., and Wagner, K. F., 1994, Hyper-eosinophilia secondary to immune dysregulation in patients with HIV-1 disease, *Arch. Dermatol.* **130**: 119–121.

Via, C. S., Tsokos, G. C., Bermas, B. L., Clerici, M., and Shearer, G. M., 1993, T-cell-antigen-presenting cell interactions in human systemic lupus erythematosus: Evidence for heterogeneous expression of multiple defects, *J. Immunol.* **151**:3914–3922.

Wynn, T., and Cheever, A. W., 1995, Cytokine regulation of granuloma formation in schistosomiasis, *Curr. Opin. Immunol.* **7**:505 –511.

CHAPTER 12

HUMORAL IMMUNITY TO HIV-1

Lethal Force or Trojan Horse?

PETER L. NARA

1. INTRODUCTION

The emerging evidence that specific genomic clades of HIV-1 are improving their fitness for efficient transmission via mucosal surfaces, i.e., heterosexual routes (Cohen, 1995; Osborn, 1995; Mastro *et al.*, 1994), is disturbing and serves as an important backdrop for this book and a discussion of the role of humoral immunity. The evolution to improved fitness for mucosal transmission does not come as a surprise to those in the comparative lentivirus field, because the animal lentiviruses are as capable of broad transmission spectrum as one finds for enveloped RNA viruses (reviewed in Nara, 1988; Nara *et al.*, 1991). These viral pathogens can assume either a cell-free or a cell-associated state, as dictated by the social and reproductive behaviors of the species. Because of genomic plasticity, primitive retroviral ancestry, and likely evolution with the vertebrates' innate and adaptive immune systems, various aspects of humoral host defenses may have been exploited by the virus. Insights gained over the past few years now contribute to a more complete picture and understanding of so-called "humoral immunity," which includes both nonclonal, innate, or nonadaptive immune system and the clonal, acquired (i.e., specific), or adaptive immune system. Together, these complementary defense systems must communicate to protect infectious nonself from noninfectious self. This is accomplished through similar structural/functional forms of nonclonal and clonal inducible soluble host defense molecules (Janeway, 1992) by providing a continuous antimicrobial state during the period of initial infection and subsequent colonization of the host. These two defense systems now appear to be more inextricably linked in their induction than previously appreciated. Thus, depending on which effect or arms are activated, and in what order, may influence the establishment of conventional T- and B-cell-type immunity. This chapter is dedicated to outlining and

PETER L. NARA • Laboratory of Tumor Cell Biology, Division of Basic Sciences, National Cancer Institute, National Institutes of Health, Frederick, Maryland 21702.

Immunology of HIV Infection, edited by Sudhir Gupta. Plenum Press, New York, 1996.

highlighting some recent evidence demonstrating how HIV-1 may have evolved to reside in a niche that has at its beginnings the most primitive of humoral defenses, the nonadaptive acute-phase response and, at its end, adaptive immunity. The virus may have employed various host-specific soluble defense molecules of both systems, which can substitute for virus-encoded ligands while limiting the polyclonal nature and antigenic discretionary power of both the effector and memory components of the immune system. These immune-modulating characteristics of the virus have given HIV-1 the potential to be one of the most currently uncontrolled, successful, and deadly sexually transmitted disease pathogens to emerge from the so-called "tropical rain forest." With scientific insight and perseverance this agent should serve as an "immunologic Rosetta stone" and provide future scientists with a molecular probe to dissect the intricacies of our innate and acquired immune systems.

2. HIV-1 IN THE HUMORS

Human immunodeficiency virus type 1 (HIV-1) infection of humans represents a relatively recent successful introduction and/or adaptation of a very old RNA viral pathogen into the human host. The clinico-pathobiological spectrum and course of disease produced by this agent during the past 15 years are characteristic of an animal retrolentivirus (reviewed in Nara, 1989, 1991).

The fact that HIV-1 is capable of replicating and existing within as well as being transmitted between members of a given species as either a cell-free or a cell-associated state implies that this viral pathogen is well endowed with a broad repertoire of humoral survival strategies. Early selection pressure for survival as a cell-free viral pathogen during the early part of the epidemic involves the urogenital mucosal and hemolymphatic systems through repeated addictive and/or abnormal social behaviors, i.e., intravenous drug injection, and/or receptive anal intercourse principally associated with homosexuality, bisexuality, and/or multiple partner heterosexuality. Among persons engaged in these various behaviors, a high number of partners allowed in many cases for direct (parenteral) transmission, as evidenced by the rapidity and ease of its spread through the nation's and world's blood supplies. The introduction of the viral agent directly into the systemic humors of the body through injection violates a number of natural defense barriers designed to prevent invading opportunistic and pathogenic organisms from gaining access to the host.

Consideration of HIV-1 in the body's humor begins generally with the introduction of the cell-free virion onto a mucosal surface or directly into the hemolymphatic system. For the sake of the discussions here, cell-associated transmission, those infections occurring as the result of a donor cell carrying either actively replicating HIV-1 or a proviral genome capable of reactivation, will not be included. The hematogenous and lymphatic compartments represent in themselves rather hostile microenvironments that communicate directly with one another. HIV-1 is capable of being transmitted from these compartments in as little as a few days to as long as 8 or more years following parenteral inoculation. These colloidal-fluid body compartments are endowed with both immediate/early acting nonspecific host defenses and later-acting defenses (adaptive immune systems) which interfere with the colonization of the host by various pathogens. Viral pathogens successfully surviving in these hostile niches appear to have evolved both extra- and intracellular strategies which circumvent these antimicrobial effects as shown in Tables I and II (for a review see Marrack and Kappler, 1994; Gooding, 1992).

TABLE I. Host Defense-Evading Strategies of Viruses

- Produce overabundance of soluble receptors to "sponge up" or decoy antiviral cytokines
- Coat themselves with host-derived proteins
- Synthesize enzymes or their inhibitors to prevent antibody and/or complement effector activity
- Stimulate immune suppressive cytokines which in turn produce more cells for the virus to infect
- Synthesize complementary proteins to tie up immune recognition molecules (i.e., MHC I, II)
- Evolve mechanisms that serve to limit the full development of the host's available immunologic repertoire–deceptive imprinting

TABLE II. Virus-Specific Mechanisms for Circumventing Extracellular or Intracellular Host Innate and Acquired Immunity

Virus	Mechanism of action
Extracellular	
Vaccinia virus	Encodes a secreted protein, VCP, that binds C4b fragment of complement component C4 blocking classical pathway activation
Herpes viruses	
Saimiri	VCP-like protein
Simplex	C1 glycoprotein binds C3b fragment of complement component C3 and prevents both C'-mediated virus neutralization and cytolysis of infected cells
	Code for a pair of proteins gE and g1 that bind 1°C region of IgG, may protect from C' lysis and Fc uptake
Shope fibroma (poxviruses)	T2, a soluble form of the TNF receptor, competitvely blocks TNF from binding to infected cells
	Secrete and IL-1 binding protein B15R
Myxoma virus	Binds β_2-microglobulin, uses MHC 1 receptor, and interferes with neutralization
Human immunodeficiency virus type 1	Binding to plasma mannose binding protein (MBP), C' components (C36, C46, factor H, and properdin), fibronectin, heparin, chondroitin, keratin sulfate, plasma polyanions, and Ig may provide alternate entry into various organ-specific macrophages through other receptors
Intracellular	
Adenovirus	VA RNAs block IFN-induced autophosphorylation of double-stranded RNA-activated inhibitor (DAI)
	E3-14.7k, E-10/14.5k, and E18-19k interfere with TNF cytolysis in a post-receptor–ligand mechanism
	Synthesize an integral membrane protein, E3-gp 19k, that contains a C-terminal sequence which anchors it in the endoplasmic reticulum and binds to MHC 1, prevents MHC 1-mediated CTL activity
Epstein–Barr virus	Same as above
Shope fibroma virus	Secreted homologue of IFN-α receptor
Human immunodeficiency virus	Mechanisms unclear
Cowpox virus	Encodes a serpior-like protease inhibitor crmA that prevents cleavage of IL-1β to its active form
Cytomegalovirus	Produces and MHC 1 homolgue, UL18, binds β_2-microglobulin, a subunit of MHC 1 also necessary for MHC 1 transport
Retroviruses	P15e, a viral transmembrane envelope protein, inhibits IL-2-driven T-cell proliferation, monocyte chemotaxis, natural killer and B-cell activation by inhibiting signal transduction U1 a protien kinase C

One effective strategy for pathogens is to evolve molecular interactions with other bioactive molecules, i.e., proteases such as cathepsin, thrombin, trypsin, etc., as well as other proteins, lipoproteins, phospholipids, found in the various soluble or colloidal secretions and filtrates naturally present within the body (Table III). These resultant molecular interactions may be a prerequisite and/or facilitate entry into the host (Fig. 1).

Examples of the infectivity and tropism of viruses known to be altered by various physiological factors (Kumar *et al.*, 1984) include: human cytomegalovirus with β_2-microglobulin (Grundy *et al.*, 1987), murine retrovirus with serum lipoproteins (Kane *et al.*, 1979; Levy, 1975; Fischinger *et al.*, 1976), visna virus with sheep serum (Thormar *et al.*, 1979), vesicular stomatitis virus with fresh human serum (Thiry *et al.*, 1978), and caprine arthritis encephalitis virus with goat serum (Yilma *et al.*, 1985). The interactions could inhibit and/or enhance infectivity and alter cellular tropism. It is worthwhile noting that HIV-1 has been isolated in its infectious form from all of the body fluids listed in Table III (for a review see Levy, 1993). Very little information currently exists regarding this area of research in HIV-1. Because the virus has been reported to be transmitted and/or isolated from many of these special fluid compartments, further research is required into their biochemistry and their effect on the antigenic structure, determinants of cellular entry, tropism, and potential new targets for the induction of effective systemic and mucosal immunity.

Early retroviral history regarding this subject demonstrated that animal retroviruses from many species, including avian, rodent, and feline leukemia viruses in the family Retroviridae, could be destroyed by fresh human sera (Welsh *et al.*, 1975). This was later discovered to be mediated by complement (Cooper *et al.*, 1976). In the late 1970s, on the basis of these findings, it was assumed that these superior human "antiretroviral serum factors" were responsible for keeping the human race free of a similar viral scourge. However, members of both subfamilies of human oncoviruses (HTLV-1 and -2) and lentiviruses (HIV-1 and -2) were identified and linked to focal and pandemic disease, respectively, in humans and found resistant to human complement (Banapour *et al.*, 1986; Hoshino *et al.*, 1984). Paradoxically, it was discovered, based on earlier work, that the sera of other animals were capable of lysing and/or blocking infection of the human retroviruses including HIV-1 *in vitro*, appearing to be complement-dependent (Hosoi *et al.*, 1990).

To date, only three publications address the biology of the virus in the different bodily fluid environments listed in Table III. Generally, these three papers demonstrated that HIV-1 infectivity is enhanced in seminal, breast, blood plasma, and fecal fluids (H. Zhang *et al.*, 1993), vaginal fluid (Messaoudi *et al.*, 1994), and normal human plasma (Wu *et al.*, 1995). Enhanced infectivity resulted from a wide variety of specific biochemical effects inherent in

TABLE III. Colloidal Solutes, Secretions, and Filtrates *in Vivo* in Which HIV-1 May Be Present

Colloidal solutes	Secretions	Filtrates	Inflammatory
Blood plasma	Vaginal	Lymphatics	Transudates/exudates
Cerebrospinal fluid	Seminal	Urine	
Synovial fluid	Colostrum		
	Saliva		
	Lacrimal		

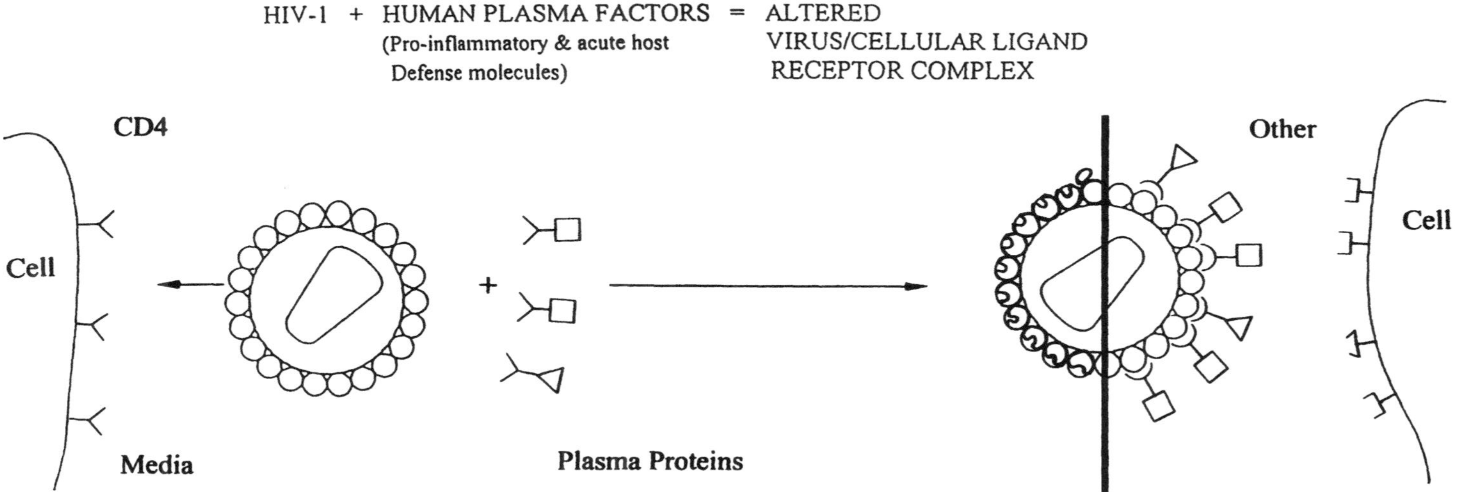

FIGURE 1. Proposed schematic of HIV-1 in blood plasma and/or other specialized bodily fluids. The solid line drawn through the virus indicates that one of two conditions could result from the interaction with fluid factors.

these fluids. Nascent intravirion DNA synthesis secondary to physiological concentrations of deoxyribonucleotide triphosphates and divalent cation accounted for the effect in the Zhang study, whereas a cathepsin-like protease was responsible in the Messaoudi study. Studies of HIV-1 infectivity and entry kinetics have only been done in tissue culture media containing low concentrations (10–20%) of fetal bovine/calf serum utilizing either established T-cell lines or PBMCs (Dimitrov *et al.*, 1992; Fernandez-Larsson *et al.*, 1992; Srivastava *et al.*, 1991; Nara, 1989a). Physiologic concentration of normal human plasma was found to enhance HIV-1 infectivity of primary isolates and significantly alter their entry kinetics (Wu *et al.*, 1995). Entry times for the enhanced fraction in both PBMCs and macrophages were increased from control values (in medium) of less than 1 hr to 1.5 to 14 hr in plasma. Given the differences in the density of the CD4 receptors between these two cell types, it appears that entry may be facilitated by other means. In addition, human plasma was found to increase the resistant infectious fraction following the attempted blocking of infection by neutralizing antibody and sCD4 as well as to alter the immunochemistry of the viral envelope (Nara *et al.*, 1995). Interestingly, the physiologic enhancement observed in PBMCs and macrophages was sensitive to fresh/frozen plasma and/or serum immediately derived from it and required divalent cation(s). Heat inactivation of the plasma resulted in a significant loss of enhancement of HIV-1 infectivity in PBMCs, but not in blood-derived macrophages. These results suggest that blood-derived factors in addition to serum-derived complement and cellular receptors may be involved. Complement factors involved with HIV-1 will be discussed in greater detail in another chapter.

Normal blood plasma, the largest of the specialized compartments, represents a much more complex and different biochemical milieu than serum (Fig. 2). Complex humoral amplification casade zymogens exist in plasma which are not found in serum. They initiate protective and restorative inflammatory networks. The interesting aspect of this innate "humoral amplification cascade pathway" otherwise known as the "contact/complement system" is how common activators such as Hageman factor (XII) can lead to one or more important inflammatory pathways such as kinin generation, complement activation and/or inhibition, fibrinolysis and/or coagulation (Fig. 2). Some examples of plasma factor(s) known to interact with HIV-1 and cells include both alternate and classical complement components (e.g., factor H, C3b, C4b, and properdin) with or without fibronectin, plasma acute-phase response proteins such as C-reactive protein, mannose-binding protein (MBP) and naturally occurring plasma polyanions, e.g., heparin, chondroitin sulfate, and keratin sulfate (Table IV) (reviewed by Dierich *et al.*, 1993; Stoiber *et al.*, 1995; Spear, 1993). In addition, another plasma protein, complement factor H, was recently found to directly bind to the C1 domain of HIV-1 gp120 and, in a CD4-dependent manner, to enhance heterologous syncytium formation (Pinter *et al.*, 1995). As a negative regulator to complement activation, factor H in the presence of these as yet undefined plasma factor(s) may stabilize and protect HIV-1 virions and infected cells from direct and/or phagocytic lysis. In addition, complement regulation is also mediated in seminal plasma by a membrane cofactor (CD46) along with decay-accelerating factor (DAF) and CD59 found bound to prostasomes present in the seminal plasma (Kitamura *et al.*, 1995; Hara *et al.*, 1993; Rooney *et al.*, 1993a,b). These factors are known to regulate complement activation, thereby preventing complement activation/lysis which could contribute to stability of infectious HIV-1 virions. These reports suggest that various factors including normal human plasma, specialized fluids of the body, and serum-derived complement may naturally promote HIV-1 infection rather than reinforcing the natural host defenses during the acute-phase response to primary infection.

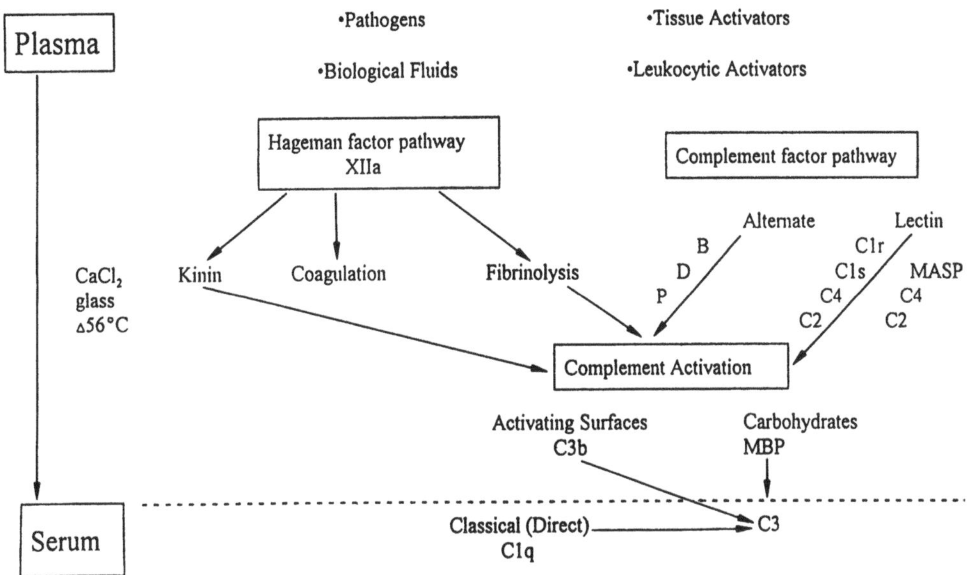

FIGURE 2. Overview of the humoral amplification system. Some factors found only in blood plasma are important in initiating various immediate/early acute-phase inflammatory responses important in host defense, repair, and healing. These factors would not be properly studied if conventional serum were used.

In theory, the viral envelope following interaction with plasma proteins may be modified to the oligomeric and/or monomeric conformation resulting in a glycoprotein with different structure, function, and antigenicity/immunogenicity. Alternatively, the subsequent interaction with plasma could lead to complementarity binding of various host-derived proteins from plasma or other bodily fluids, leading to a new host–virus ligand/receptor complex in addition to or in the absence of CD4 (Fig. 1). This type of humoral interaction would provide the virus a strategy to cloak its virus-specific ligand with host cellular determinants. This type of interaction would pose a significant problem for humoral-based immunity and is a successful strategy routinely employed by other metazoan obligate intracellular parasites (e.g., *Leishmania*, *Trypanosoma*, and *Toxoplasma*) (for

TABLE IV. Viral Envelope/Membrane-Associated Proteins Reported for HIV-1 Which Could Influence Infectivity, Tropism, and Neutralization

Viral envelope/membrane
HLA I, HLA II, LFA-1, β_2-microglobulin, CD46, CD55, CD59
Humoral component(s)
Clq, C3b, C4b, factor H, properdin, MBP, fibronectin, heparin, chondroitin sulfate, keratin sulfate, DAF

a review see Hall and Joiner, 1991). On the other hand, it represents what should be a conserved target for vaccine design.

3. AN OVERVIEW OF THE ACUTE-PHASE RESPONSE

Acute inflammation is an organism's normal homeostatic immediate physiological response to injury or infection. Its primary role is to maintain the integrity of the tissue by restricting damage to the injured site. Recently, significant advances have been made at the biochemical level defining the molecules and cascades (reviewed by Baumann and Gauldie, 1994). Also, some insight has been gained regarding the interplay of the innate humoral system with those microbial agents that live and survive in them. These observations have generally come from the bacterial.and parasite fields (Marrack and Kappler, 1994). Although some viral systems have been studied (i.e., herpesvirus, adenovirus, poxvirus, and some retroviruses; see Gooding, 1992, and Table II) in general, little is known about how these agents survive and thrive *in vivo* despite these host defenses. Because of their simplicity, viruses were not generally considered likely to trigger innate immunity or induce related costimulatory signals (Janeway, 1992).

The acute-phase response (APR) in inflammation may be divided into two phases. The first is the local response involving coagulation, kinin generation, phospholipid metabolism with vasodilation and cellular emigration. The second is the systemic response, including fever, leukocytosis, changes in the concentration of plasma heavy metals and increased levels of a number of hepatic derived proteins, and modifications to the amino acid pools (for a review see Baumann and Gauldie, 1994). In addition, endocrine changes accompanying the systemic phase include the increased levels of cortisol, glucagon, catecholamine, and thyroid hormones. The net sum of these acute changes results in a general increase in body metabolism, including protein catabolism, increased gluconeogenesis, and negative nitrogen balance. The systemic response is generally triggered by blood-borne mediators released from activated local tissue sources and includes products of phospholipid metabolism and polypeptide hormone-like mediators or cytokines. These have a broad range of physiological effects.

Tissue macrophages and peripheral blood monocytes are the cells most likely reported to initiate the process of inflammation, as they become activated on encounter with foreign organisms (Koj, 1985). Some of the earliest cytokines synthesized are the pleiomorphic actions of IL-1, IL-6, and TNF, which contribute generally to both local and systemic effects that mediate host defenses. In particular, IL-6 induces the synthesis of molecules from hepatocytes of the liver which can opsonize a wide variety of microbial pathogens (e.g., C-reactive protein, lipopolysaccharide-binding protein, collectins) thus rendering them susceptible in some cases for complement activation and possible elimination through phagocytosis.

The APR molecules are the functional equivalent of antibodies and one of the most ontologically early responses of the innate humoral system. One of the best studied and interesting of these molecules, known as the C-type or Ca^{2+}-dependent animal lectin superfamily (for a review see Holmskov *et al.*, 1994; Drickamer, 1988), seems to have evolved for the host to identify nonself, complex-carbohydrate-covered pathogens. The lectinlike molecules are found circulating in the blood plasma at a baseline level and undergo a rapid increase in concentration under specific conditions as part of the APR.

Functional studies indicate that MBP, a member of the plasma collecting family, is able to distinguish a wide array of bacterial oligosaccharides while maintaining selectivity, as collectins apparently do not recognize oligosaccharide side chains that decorate "self glycoproteins" (Ezekowitz, 1991). MBP is a multimeric protein in which promoters associate as trimers and six trimers form the multimer complex, resembling the first component of complement Clq in its overall structure (Malhotra *et al.*, 1990). Carbohydrate binding by MBP is a calcium-dependent reaction (Drickamer, 1988). Similar molecules are found in the abdominal cavities of echinoderms and cockroaches, and are rapidly upregulated in response to infectious challenge (Jomori and Natori, 1991; Giga *et al.*, 1987). In man, lectin-dependent alternate complement pathway activation, lymphocyte homing, phagocytosis of microorganisms, and clearance of senescent proteins are among the functions of various members of this expanding gene family and can be found in both blood plasma and pulmonary surfactant. The microbe–MBP collecting complex, should it form, can act as an opsinin and subsequently initiate the primary APR. This probably happens by directing the binding of the complexed virus/pathogen to one of the seven families of collecting receptors found on a diverse array of cells of the monocyte/macrophage lineage including those of the reticuloendothelial system. A calcium-dependent, Cls-like serine protease of normal human plasma was found to activate the early components of complement when in association with MBP (Matsushita and Fujita, 1992). This is intriguing in light of the earlier discussions of the calcium-dependent enhancing properties of plasma for HIV-1. In 1989, evidence was presented whereby high-mannose-type oligosaccharides with seven, eight, and nine mannose residues of the HIV-1 gp120 were recognized and bound MBP with high affinity (Larkin *et al.*, 1989). In the same year, MBP was reported to be elevated in the plasma of HIV-1-infected patients and when purified from the plasma was capable of inactivating HIV-1 infectivity *in vitro* (Ezekowitz *et al.*, 1989). In addition, the terminal mannose residues of the HIV-1 gp120, to be discussed later in this chapter, have also been found to bind to a type II cell-associated mannose-binding lectin domain of human macrophage mannose receptor and human placenta (Curtis *et al.*, 1992). This binding was reported to occur with even higher affinity than CD4–gp120. When viewed together, evidence is in favor of the envelope of HIV-1 interacting with a large array of other molecules of the host innate APR/defense system.

4. HIV-1: USURPING THE ACUTE-PHASE RESPONSE?

The previous discussion indicated the macrophage, particularly the Kupffer cells of the liver, to be the early and key player in the initiation of the APR. It is more than coincidental that all of the animal lentiviruses, including HIV-1, use these cells during the incubation phase to replicate and establish themselves in the host. In the natural lentiviral infection of horses, known as equine infectious anemia, a completely hematogenously transmitted virus localizes and replicates to high titers (i.e., 1.0×10^9 particles/ml) primarily in the liver Kupffer cells and splenic macrophages. At a teleologic level it is interesting to note that both pathogen and host target cell represent two of the oldest of the ancestral players in this primitive virus–host interaction. Manipulating, controlling, and usurping the humoral host defense during the APR would seem a prerequisite for extended survival and offer the pathogen a safe haven for chronic transmission. Early skewing of the Thl and 2 responses currently being studied in the fields of parasitic diseases such as leishmania and HIV-1 may have their origins in some of the pathways shared by both the innate and acquired host defense systems.

As previously discussed, the introduction of a pathogen into the host at some point in time generally results in either a local and/or systemic inflammatory reaction. Available clinical studies documenting what is believed to be the acute phase of HIV-1 infection (defined here as being the initial state of plasma-associated viremia) report a rather pronounced, systemic, virus-induced clinical sequela known as the "acute retroviral syndrome" (ARS) (reviewed in Feinberg, 1992). The clinical symptoms indicate that a wide array of these acute mediators are activated and contribute to the well-known clinical signs which include fever, malaise, arthralgia, night sweats, rash, and local and/or systemic lymphadenopathy. Despite the eventual clinical outcome of HIV-1 infection, the importance of the inflammatory response should not be underestimated in reestablishing homeostasis during ARS. Following a variable incubation period (averaging ~21 days), infection with HIV-1 generally leads to a period of intense viral replication which results in peak titers of virus particles (based on quantitative extrapolation from plasma RNA values) of approximately 10 logs 6–9, with infectivity titers reaching between 10 log 1 and 3.5 (Clark *et al.*, 1991; Daar *et al.*, 1991). This viremia is also accompanied by concomitant increases in the proviral content of the circulating PBMCs.

Very little has been published regarding the APR during primary HIV-1 infection (Nara *et al.*, 1995; Sinicco *et al.*, 1993; Roos *et al.*, 1992; Gaines *et al.*, 1990; von Sydow *et al.*, 1990) (Table V). This is related in part to the difficulty in identifying and obtaining the proper samples from those patients undergoing ARS, as numerous other acute viral pathogens can mimic the syndrome. It appears that some aspects of the APR to HIV-1 involving systemic cytokine measurements are expected while some others are not. In general, IFN-α, IL-1, IL-6, TNF-α, 5-neopterin, β^2-microglobulin, and soluble CD8 receptor appear to be elevated either transiently as in the case of IFN-α or persistently as in the case of TNFα. Absent or low concentrations of IL-2 have been reported (Nara *et al.*, 1995; Sinicco *et al.*, 1993), although these two studies reported different results for plasma IFN-γ. One report found elevated IFN-γ levels during acute HIV-1 infection (Sinicco *et al.*, 1993), while the other study found no detectable levels in ARS plasma (Nara *et al.*, 1995). Reasons for the differences were not addressed. Other cytokines that were not detected in the blood plasma included IL-4 and TNF-β. In the only study that measured the levels of MBP during ARS, elevated levels two- to sixfold over controls were observed for three of six patients between 4 and 16 days following the onset of symptoms (Nara *et al.*, 1995). The remaining three patients demonstrated either a subnormal elevation (two patients) or none at all. An interesting finding in this study was the inverse relationship between the highest and longest presence of IFN-α and subnormal levels of MBP and the rapid clinical progression of disease as measured by CDC staging criteria (Table V). The most rapidly advancing patient had the longest ARS period of clinical symptoms (i.e., 132 days), as well as the highest chronic levels of IFN-α and the lowest levels of MBP. No correlation was found between the decline in plasma virus titer as measured by either infectious titer and/or RNA copy and any of the cytokines (particularly IFN-α) otherwise known to effect viral replication. Although a strong direct correlation during ARS between the kinetics and levels of IFN-α in plasma and virus load was not found as measured by RNA particles, a slightly better correlation was observed for the slopes of the tissue culture infectious doses ($TCID_{50}$) in the plasma virus. A previous report suggested that IFN-α *in vitro* primarily reduced the infectivity of the virus and did not significantly reduce the number of particles (Hansen

TABLE V. Clincal/Virologic History and Acute-Phase Response Plasma Cytokine Determinations during HIV-1 Primary Infection

Patient ID	ΔCDC stage I–II	ΔCDC stage II–III	SX	Virus load QC-PCR ×10⁴ (RNA/ml)	MBP	Cytokines: IFN IU/ml α	IFN IU/ml γ	IL-1β	IL-2	IL-4	IL-6	TNF-α	TNF-β
Inme	42	<770	7	22–70(6/20)	↑↑↑[a]	80–160/E[b]	–	+[c]	+	+	+++	+++	–
Suma	13	>483 8		93–148(5/8)	↑↑	~80/E	–	+	–	–	–	++	–
Bori	14	>556 9		13–34(5/17)	↑↑	~80/E	–	++	+	–	–	+++	–
Hobr	28	>343	18	22–59(14/16)	NC	320–640/E	–	NT	NT	–	NT	+	NT
Weau	27	44–51	27	21–35(15/17)	↓	320–640/E	–	–	–	–	–	+++	–
Fash	31	31–132	132	217(17)	↓	320–640P	–	NT	NT	–	NT	+	NT

[a]↑↑↑ elevated 6× normal; ↑↑, elevated 2× normal; NC, no change; ↓, reduced between 2 and 10×.
[b]E, episodic production; P, persistent production.
[c]+, 0–5 indicated units; ++, 5–10 indicated units; +++, > 10 indicated units.

et al., 1992). This loss of infectivity was subsequently demonstrated to be secondary to the lack of incorporation of gp120 into the budding virions with significant retention in the infected cells (Hansen *et al.*, 1992). This finding is similar to what is observed clinically during ARS where it appears that the infectious particles undergo a rather rapid decline within a few weeks following the onset of clinical signs (Clark *et al.*, 1991).

Viral bioassays of the patients' plasma with two different viral assay systems revealed a very interesting result (Fig. 3). Although HIV-1 patients' plasma were capable of inactivating VSV effectively unit-for-unit as recombinant IFN-α, little to no antiviral effect was detected against HIV-1. Based on bioactivity, the IFN-α in the HIV-1-positive ARS patients' plasma was 10–100 times less potent than recombinant IFN-α at controlling HIV-1 replication *in vitro*. When anti-IFN-α antibody was used to test the specificity of the plasma IFN-α, a twofold level of enhancement of viral replication was observed at all virus titrations tested. These findings suggest that during ARS, enhancing factors are elaborated

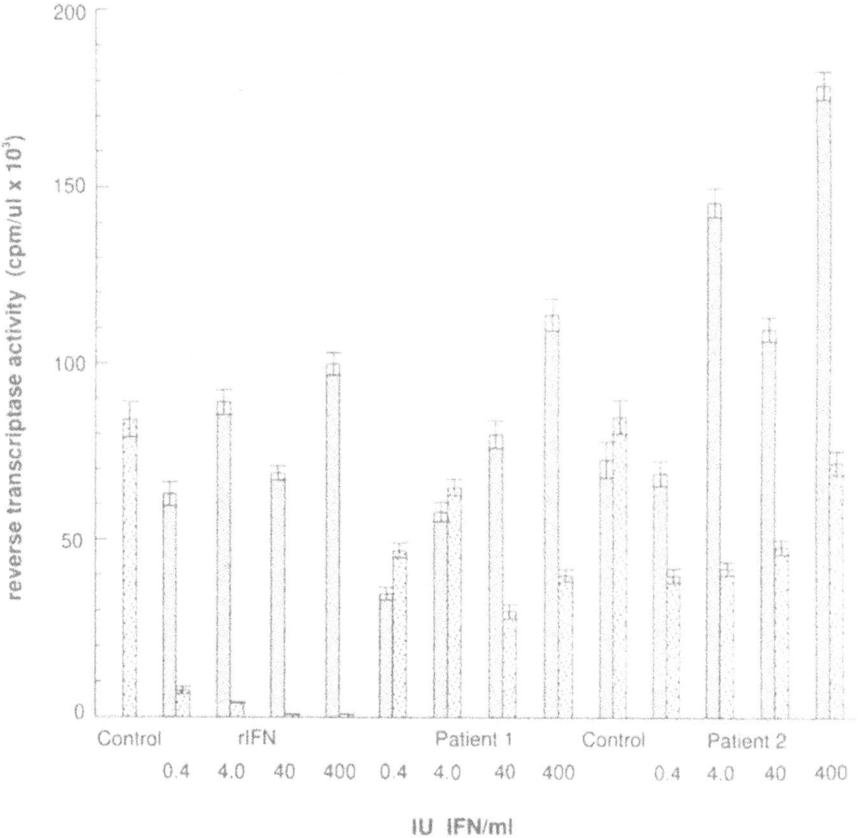

FIGURE 3. Enhancement of HIV-1 infection in primary human macrophages *in vitro* by plasma of two HIV-1 patients collected during the acute-phase response (pre-seroconversion). When compared to recombinant IFN (rIFN) at varying concentrations (stippled bars), marked inhibition of virus was observed whereas patients' IFN in plasma at identical concentrations failed to inhibit infection. The gray bars represent viral replication in the presence of IFN antibody.

in the plasma which appear to counteract the full antiviral properties of IFN-α. These patients both had elevated levels of MBP in their plasma. The possibility exists that this APR lectin-binding protein may provide an infectivity factor for the virus. When viewing the APR of humans during the ARS of HIV-1 infection, it appears that the absence of IL-2 and IFN-γ coupled to the elevated but less potent IFN-α, IL-6, TNF-α, and MBP responses are directed at subverting the innate humoral defenses (i.e., inactivating complement). This may lead to subsequent skewing the early Th-1 and Th-2 effector arms of both humoral and cell-mediated immunity. In combination, these abnormal immune patterns would serve the virus by downregulating class II MHC gene expression as well as limiting both NK cell activity and Th-1 activity. Poor or absent induction of IL-2, IL-2R, and IFN-γ has been reported to be related to activity of the HIV-1 envelope and/or other viral-encoded proteins (Tyring *et al.*, 1991; Oyaizu *et al.*, 1990) present in relatively high concentrations during primary viremia.

At the cellular level, the ARS is characterized in the first 1–2 weeks by a thrombocytopenia and lymphopenia generally caused by decreased $CD3^+$, $CD4^+$, $CD8^+$, NK cells and B cells which rebound as a lymphocytosis characterized by an increasing proportion of $CD8^+$ cells with some atypical lymphocytes, NK cells, and activated $CD38^+$ and $HLA\text{-}DR^+$ cells. No evidence for increased concentrations of serum immunoglobulins IgM, IgG, IgA was noted within the first few weeks of the ARS. Afterwards a gradual increase of IgG only was noted with the appearance of oligoclonal bands occurring in 50% of the eight sera studied (mean IgG serum level 10.5 g/liter) at 1–2 weeks after onset of symptoms, in 80% of 15 sera (mean IgG serum level 13.7 g/liter) and in 82% of 17 sera (mean IgG serum level 18.3 g/liter) (Gaines *et al.*, 1990).

5. WHY ALL THE COMPLEX CARBOHYDRATE?

The biochemistry of the HIV-1 envelope glycoprotein, when compared to other known glycoproteins, demonstrates an unusual degree of complex posttranslational glycosylation with both high-mannose and complex-type N-linked oligosaccharides (Leonard *et al.*, 1990; Geyer *et al.*, 1988; Mizuochi *et al.*, 1988). This high degree of carbohydrate on the gp120 may have lectinlike activity and bind to cellular glycoprotein oligosaccharides (Gattegno *et al.*, 1991) and sulfated galactocerebrosides (sulfatide) (Harouse *et al.*, 1991). In addition, it appears that approximately 14% of the complex-type N-linked oligosaccharides are sulfated (Shilatifard *et al.*, 1993). The reasons for sulfation of the gp120 are unclear, although this chemical modification could contribute to a more stable association of gp120 to the virus. It may also provide another means of entry to cells independent of CD4-independent entry into cells such as Kupffer cells of the liver (Fiete *et al.*, 1991) and highly venular endothelial cells (Imai *et al.*, 1991).

The relative conservation of a majority of these sites on the gp120/41 molecule may indicate an evolutionarily important function(s) for this carbohydrate. These functions may involve the protection of the viral glycoprotein from nonspecific proteolysis (which could occur in any of the various compartments previously mentioned) or direct the specific proteases to their molecular targets. In addition, virus-encoded complex high-mannose oligosaccharides affect the tertiary and quaternary structure of the monomers and oligomers.

Glycans may play a critical role in both the humoral and cell-mediated immune responses to viruses (Olofsson *et al.*, 1990; Huso *et al.*, 1988; Sjoblom *et al.*, 1987). During mutation and selection, sites can be added or lost resulting in antigenic variation and effectively masking or directing antibody responses to nonneutralizing sites (Alexander and Elder, 1984). Different cell-dependent glycosylation patterns (related to differences in posttranslational glycosylation modifications) (Mizuochi *et al.*, 1990) will result in different structural forms and may contribute to both differences in cell tropism and/or immune escape.

Recently, another interesting and more direct mechanism of immune diversion has been reported, namely a carbohydrate ligand-specific mechanism. Oligosaccharides such as lacto-*N*-fucopentose III which contain the Lewis × trisaccharide (a carbohydrate antigen) have the ability to induce IL-10 production by $B220^+$ cells through a ligand-specific mechanism directly leading to proliferation and downregulation of Th-1 cells (Velupilli and Harn, 1994). Another carbohydrate antigen, Ley, has been found to be upregulated during infection of lymphocytes and incorporated into the gp120. Antibodies raised to the carbohydrate Ley antigen have been found to be both neutralizing and enhancing depending on the cell type on which the assays were performed (Hansen *et al.*, 1990, 1991, 1993) and thus could contribute to the humoral "Trojan horse" argument made in this chapter.

In addition to the role of carbohydrate influencing a type Th-2 cytokine profile in B cells, the simplest explanation for the common appearance of the restricted antibody responses to an antigen such as gp120 is that of immune recognition of only very few epitopes. The precedents for this finding are innumerable, and are best exemplified by responses to simple haptens that are often associated with clonal focusing in the secondary responses, and by many antipolysaccharide responses in which three or fewer dominant clones are generally detected, because of a simple polymeric antigen structure that expresses few epitopes (reviewed in Silverman and Kohler, 1992). In support of this limited epitope hypothesis in HIV-1, Neurath *et al.* (1990) assessed reactivity with a large series of overlapping peptides covering the entire envelope, but found that only nine were recognized by sera from infected human donors. One possible explanation for the expression of only a limited number of protein epitopes is the significant degree of glycosylation present in the chemical structure of gp120, which may limit its recognition by T-helper lymphocytes (Benjoudad *et al.*, 1992). The envelope protein, gp120, is a protein antigen that requires T-helper activity to initiate the secretion of specific antibodies, and this requires recognition of the antigen in conjunction with MHC class II antigens after processing by antigen-presenting cells (APC). Carbohydrates have been shown to interfere with peptide presentation by APC (Botarelli *et al.*, 1991). Therefore, it is also plausible that the heavy glycosylation (55% of the molecular mass of gp120 is contributed by carbohydrates) may interfere with one or more of the following steps: (1) proteolytic degradation into peptides, (2) peptide binding to MHC, and (3) recognition of the MHC peptide complex by T lymphocytes. In support, recent data establish that glycosylation interferes with gp120 recognition by T-helper lymphocytes through a mechanism that probably encompasses either the second or third hypothesis. Evidence of this interference has also been reported by Hosmalin *et al.* (1991), who demonstrated an enhanced antibody response to gp160 in rhesus monkeys by priming with three immunodominant T-cell epitopes, all of which were from highly conserved and nonglycosylated regions of the envelope protein. While analogous antiprotein responses have not been widely described, Gerhard and co-workers (Kavaler *et al.*, 1990) have demonstrated that after immunization with influenza hemagglutinin, more than half of the clones recognize the CB determinant and utilize a single V_H–V_K gene pair that recurs in genetically identical mice. The immune response evoked by this virus was initially described as the phenomenon of "the original antigenic sin" whereby the primary encounter with the agent leads to a long-term anamnestic recall when the host is exposed to another influenza strain (Francis, 1953). This will be discussed in more detail in a later section of this chapter.

Host tolerance to most potential HIV-1 epitopes may also contribute to the clonal restriction of antibody responses. In particular, gp120 proteins present molecular features that are similar to many autologous proteins (see Table IV). In addition, the excessive glycosylation of the molecule with host carbohydrate could easily result in tolerance. Consequently, following exposure to this retroviral protein, there is an inability to evoke a specific immune response to the viral epitopes that resemble aspects of self-antigens. As such, Bjork (1991) has recently reviewed the evidence that molecular mimicry by HIV-1 or self proteins likely contributes to the impaired response.

6. THE ROLE OF VIRAL LIGAND gp120 SHEDDING?

Accumulating evidence indicates that shedding of soluble ligands and receptors may have evolved as a means to locally regulate various cellular functions. Shedding of surface proteins is observed with many cytokinelike receptors in the immune system (e.g., IL-2R, ICAMR, FcγR) and with a wide array of bacterial and metazoan pathogens (e.g., *Nisseria*, trypanosomes). In fact, recent studies have demonstrated that various chronic microbial pathogens produce soluble factors that are functional complements and/or mimic a number of important cytokines [e.g., IFN, TNF, IL-1, IL-10, β_2-microglobulin; reviewed in Marrack and Kappler (1994), Gooding (1992), and Table II]. The complex oligomeric subunit conformation of the gp120/41 in the viral envelope is thought to contain three or four monomers held together by various weak noncovalent bonds which seem to explain the relative instability of the oligomer as previously reported by numerous investigators (Schneider *et al.*, 1986; Gelderblom *et al.*, 1985). The spontaneous shedding of the gp120 from the viral envelope was later demonstrated to correlate directly with the loss of infectivity of the laboratory strains *in vitro* (Layne *et al.*, 1992). The biologic role of the spontaneous shedding of gp120 from the HIV-1 envelope is unknown at this time. Explanations include a laboratory artifact secondary to selection, growth, and adaptation of the virus for rapid replication in high-expressing CD4$^+$ transformed human cell lines (reviewed in Moore and Ho, 1995), modulation of various cytokine pathways (Clouse, 1991), as discussed earlier, autoregulation of infection (Layne and Dembo, 1992), and/or deceptive imprinting and decoying of the immune system (Kohler *et al.*, 1994; Nara *et al.*, 1993). The well-documented shedding of the gp120 of laboratory-adapted strains of HIV-1 leading to a direct loss of infectivity as well as enhanced neutralization by antibodies, sCD4, and a higher affinity for the CD4 receptor may be related to adaptation to replication in the artificial microenvironment of transformed human T-cell lines. Recently, however, a PBMC-tropic primary isolate was evaluated for its infectivity and spontaneous shedding half-life. Surprisingly, no loss of infectivity occurred over 72 hr of incubation at 37°C; however, the amount of virion-associated gp120 fell to background levels by 120 hours (Merges *et al.*, 1996). This is in stark contrast to a laboratory strain that demonstrated a complex biphasic decay curve where a direct correlation was observed between the loss of infectivity and spontaneous loss of gp120 from the virions (Layne *et al.*, 1992). In the Layne study, a residual low concentration of gp120 was observed to remain on the virion. It was speculated, and subsequently demonstrated, that a high concentration of $CD4^+$ cells, as would occur in a lymph node, would be sufficient to promote infection (Layne *et al.*, 1990, 1992). This was observed for other HIV-1 isolates in another study (Moore *et al.*, 1992). Both of these groups found that neutralization by either sCD4 or antibody followed a similar biphasic course. The greatest degree of resistance to neutralization occurred in acute harvest virus stocks (which had higher gp120 concentrations per virion) and with those infectious virions remaining after a period of spontaneous shedding (which had just measurable concentrations of gp120). In contrast to the preliminary primary isolate study, evidence exists for a macrophage-tropic primary isolate that sheds very little of its viral envelope over a 3- to 4-day period (Tsai *et al.*, 1996). Speculatively, the stability of the viral envelope during the early establishment of the infection by macrophagic-tropic variants would improve the chances for dissemination of the virus. An interesting aside regarding this point is the recent evidence that attenuated macrophage-tropic clones of SIV yielded a faster and broader neutralizing response and gave broader protection than observed with a lymphotropic clone (Clements *et al.*, 1995). After dissemination to the lymphoid-rich microenvironments of high $CD4^+$ lymphocytes as well as B-cell concentrations, large amounts of viral replication led to adaptive mutations for enhanced infection via the CD4 receptor and possibly a much less stable gp120 oligomer as discussed earlier.

7. IMMUNOLOGIC CONSEQUENCES OF SHEDDING

The high concentrations of soluble gp120, measured to be from 12 to 92 ng/ml in serum of asymptomatic and ARC patients (Oh *et al.*, 1992), would contribute to antigen saturation of the follicular dendritic cells with an irrelevant antigenic form. Another factor is the long half-life of monotonous homogenetic antigen (due in part to the protease-resistant nature of the heavily glycosylated molecule) either directly or secondarily after binding some of the multisubunit plasma lectins and complement components as discussed in Section 2. In addition to shed gp120 from the mature virion, virally infected cells have been shown to secrete soluble gp120 independent from cell surface gp120/41 dissociation in a monensin-insensitive pathway (Spies and Compans, 1993). The virus, deposited on follicular dendritic cells in follicular centers, would provide for chronic presentation and stimulation to B cells. Evidence that the soluble form of the gp120 presents an antigenically irrelevant immunogen to the humoral system was demonstrated when comparing the binding of a V3-specific murine monoclonal antibody to spontaneously shed soluble gp120 and native, infectious virions by a native particle suspension ELISA (Conley, 1993; Nara *et al.*, 1993). The V3 mAb demonstrated several orders of magnitude more binding to the shed gp120 than to the intact gp120 on virus particles. This suggested that the so-called immunodominant V3 neutralization epitope is more cryptic when assembled in the oligomeric conformation (Fig. 4). This finding was also observed for a primary isolate (Bou-Habib *et al.*, 1994). These findings, as well as the fact that V3 mAbs derived from mice following immunization with oligomeric forms of the gp160 are rare (Broder *et al.*, 1994) and the inability of antibodies to C1 and C5 to bind oligomeric and/or neutralize virus gp160 (reviewed by Moore and Ho, 1995), seem to support that the shed form of the HIV-1 envelope elicits a less than functional B-cell response. In a separate study, a general lack of potent neutralizing antibodies was disappointing despite good binding to the gp160 oligomer (Early *et al.*, 1994). The presenta-

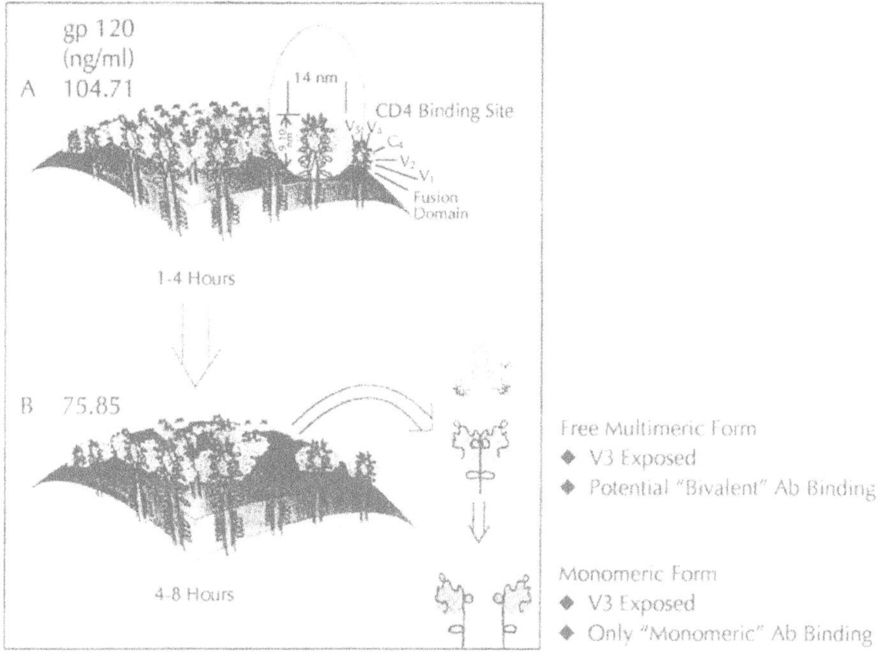

FIGURE 4. A proposed diagram of HIV-1 gp120 shedding and its relationship to V3-specific neutralizing IgG. The relative sizes of the virus surface, gp120 oligomers, dimers, monomers, and IgG are close approximations.

tion of this complex multimeric subunit made up of both host and virus-encoded proteins is speculated to be a major mechanism(s) responsible for the induction of deceptive immunity (Kohler *et al.*, 1992; Nara *et al.*, 1991).

8. THE EARLIEST ANTIBODY: TO WHAT AND WHAT FOR?

The previous discussion described the concept that the unique conformations of gp120/41 on the infectious virion particle are important in determining the specificity of neutralizing antibody. Recently, a more potent and broadly neutralizing human mAb, IgG1, was shown to recognize the oligomeric form of the viral envelope (Burton *et al.*, 1994). Another study utilizing oligomeric gp160 showed that antibodies could be detected earlier in seroconversion panels (Nair *et al.*, 1994) and may act as a more effective neutralizing response against primary isolates.

Knowledge of the humoral immune response following infection and establishment of HIV-1 infection is rather limited. The most controlled animal model studies utilizing HIV-1 were reported using a laboratory strain, HIV-1/IIIB (Nara *et al.*, 1990). This study demonstrated that the earliest antibody to be elicited was capable of neutralizing the most replication-competent viral subspecies found in the viral challenge inoculum given the chimpanzees. This response occurred generally within 4–6 weeks and always preceded antibodies capable of either precipitating gp120 and/or recognizing p24 by ELISA or

Western blot from the mixed viral lysate homologous viral strain. The strain-specific neutralizing response in naive animals generally increased in titer over the next 2–6 months after which a lower titer and more broadly neutralizing response arose. Based on this and other findings, evidence was provided that the earliest antibody response to HIV-1 was to the HIV-1 envelope and appeared to be a conformational antibody which was only detectable by either *in vitro* neutralization (Nara *et al.*, 1990), radioimmunoprecipitation (Manca *et al.*, 1987; Kitchen *et al.*, 1986), or EIA using gp160 and/or live cell immunofluorescence assay (Nair *et al.*, 1994; Race *et al.*, 1991). Recently, one study has reported on the antibody response during ARS using detergent-disrupted virus cultured from the patient's plasma and tested for binding by ELISA (Moore *et al.*, 1994). Serum anti-gp120 antibodies were first detected between 4 and 23 days after the decline of serum p24 and infectious virus in three patients undergoing the ARS. These antibodies were stated to be directed against conformational epitopes which included reactivity to the full-length autologous V3 peptide and were also capable of blocking autologous gp120/CD4 interactions better than heterologous gp120. However, the detergent used routinely in these assays by these authors could have disrupted the fine conformational epitopes of either protein or carbohydrate origins.

To further dissect the early antibody response to the complex oligomeric structure of the viral env during acute HIV-1 infection, the chimpanzee model was studied using plasmon resonance spectroscopy and oligomeric gp160 (Nara *et al.*, in preparation). High titers (1:100–1:1000) of previously undetected IgG binding antibodies were present in these sera some 2–4 weeks prior to those detected by neutralization. The nature of the binding antibody is currently under investigation and attention will focus initially on the role of the complex N-linked carbohydrate discussed previously. It is well known that antibody to carbohydrate may be generated in a T-independent manner and could be a strategy used by the virus for eliciting an initial opsonizing humoral response. This response could enhance viral infectivity during dissemination and uptake by Fc-facilitated mechanisms. This would effectively reduce the circulating titer early, as has been observed. The importance of looking for this type of antibody and the epitopes to which it is directed cannot be underestimated. If the viral envelope in its monomeric and/or oligomeric form elicits a predominance of binding rather than functional antibody, and considering other factors (e.g., viral genetic variation, the need for long-lived mucosal and systemic immunity), little to no efficacy can be expected of our early current recombinant envelope-based vaccine trials. The Phase I trial of an envelope-based vaccine is currently experiencing a number of infections in the vaccine arm. Breakthrough virus sequences in the V3 region in some cases are similar to those in which they were vaccinated (Kahn *et al.*, 1995). Further insight will have to await more study into the infected gp160 vaccines during the course of the trial.

9. NEUTRALIZATION OF HIV-1: JUST A MATTER OF GETTING THE RIGHT ANTIBODY?

When laboratory and primary isolates of HIV-1 are compared for their sensitivity to neutralization with both sCD4 and antibodies on an infectious unit basis, the primary isolates are generally significantly more resistant to blocking (Hanson, 1994; Matthews, 1994; Daar *et al.*, 1990). This finding seems to result from an array of different properties found between the two selected virus populations and the cells from which they are passaged and assayed (for a review see Moore and Ho, 1995). In summary, it appears that lentiviruses exhibit a significant degree of selection artifact to their entry properties, and therefore immunologic properties to Ab blocking of virus entry. On a macro scale, passage through transformed human T-cell lines selects for those HIV-1 variants most fit for high-affinity binding to the overexpressed CD4 molecules on the surface of the transformed human T cells. This appears to coincide with molecular/structural changes that allow for the more efficient entry into these cells via this receptor (Kabat *et al.*, 1994). These changes probably involve aspects of the transmembrane and possibly matrix proteins which are presumed to interact during entry (Dorfman *et al.*, 1994; Yu *et al.*, 1992). This modification for enhanced *in vitro* replication appears to be conferred as enhanced sensitivity to neutralizing antibody and sCD4. In addition, epigenetic factors such as the presence, or absence, of various host cell-type-specific proteins (e.g., HLA I, HLA II, LFA-1, β_2-microglobulin, CD46, CD55, CD59) (Montefiori *et al.*, 1994; Arthur *et al.*, 1993; Henderson *et al.*, 1987), posttranslational glycosylation, and efficiency of envelope glycoprotein incorporation (which secondarily determine the final quaternary functional structure) probably also contribute. The reader is reminded of the previous discussions pertaining to the additional humoral epigenetic factors found in the various bodily fluids in which the virus resides.

In relating the recent discussion of laboratory strain selection artifact for the CD4 molecule to the previous discussion of other humoral factors (e.g., plasma, lectin-binding proteins, complement components) which are most likely involved in the entry of primary isolates of HIV-1 *in vivo*, one finds significant differences between these selected populations of virus. Considering the structural specificities of the gp120 oligomers now are required to maintain a complementarity of binding not necessarily for the CD4 molecule, but to the previously discussed host plasma factors (e.g., lectin-binding proteins), the selection now will be for envelop structures that favor entry via these other ligand–receptor interactions, and possibly infecting macrophages and lymphocytes in very different ways. The apparent redundancy of entry for this virus is disturbing. Elucidating any additional *in vivo* mechanisms involved should become a significant priority in the humoral area of research.

From the previous discussion, one could conclude that very little evidence exists for neutralizing antibodies against primary isolates. In the few cases studied of early natural infections, evidence is reported both for and against the existence of neutralizing antibody being mounted to the early reisolated plasma virus over time (Moore *et al.*, 1994; Cheingsong-Popov *et al.*, 1991; Albert *et al.*, 1990). In one case, a number of reports exists indicating that primary isolates are sensitive to neutralization (Tsang *et al.*, 1994; Arendrug *et al.*, 1992; Montefiori *et al.*, 1991; Tremblay and Wainberg, 1990). Another report shows that late-stage patients' infectious plasma and reisolated virus were of similar sensitivity in *ex vivo* neutralization experiments using a human monoclonal antibody (Conley *et al.*, 1994). Generally the kinetics and titers of the primary neutralizing response reported in HIV-1-infected humans to date indicate a slow induction phase. In contrast to this slow development of homologous neutralization in humans, infection of chimpanzees with the HIV-1 primary isolate (DH012) resulted in the rapid development (8 to 12 weeks) of a high-titered, isolate-restricted neutralization (Bolognesi, 1994). This was consistent with the amount of time reported previously for chimpanzees infected with the laboratory strain HIV-1 IIIB (Nara *et al.*, 1990). Despite the high-titered (1:20,000) neutralization response to DH012, no neutralization was observed with the laboratory strains classified as more sensitive to neutralization, nor to other primary isolates. These findings suggest that cross neutralization is not simply a "titered effect." Also, V3 peptides derived from DH012 sequence were unable to compete with the neutralizing polyclonal sera for neutralization, whereas they did with serum from the HIV-1 IIIB-infected chimpanzee serum. This result indicates either that the DH012 V3 peptide was unable to faithfully mimic the structure of the V3 epitope on the virion or that the V3 epitope/peptide was not a major component of the neutralization response. In support of the latter hypothesis, another recent study used V3 sequences from infected patients to determine their role in primary isolate neutralization and concluded that these peptides were capable of competing for a greater percentage of neutralizing activity when tested against laboratory strains than for autologous isolates (VanCott *et al.*, 1995).

The critical aspect of studying primary virus/serum antibody interaction involves the ability to recover the actual virus that may have initialized the infection and immune response. If the infecting virus is not the one recovered, then by definition the isolate may be an escape mutant and will appear as described by some investigators as not capable of being neutralized for an extended period of time. This may not be as easy as it seems. Evidence for the rapidity by which antibody may select a viral population from a quasispecies has already been observed earlier (Nara *et al.*, 1990). In the chimpanzee studies where the viral quasispecies was characterized, the most replication-competent variant was shown to elicit the earliest neutralizing antibody but was never recovered from the animal, although it represented at least one-third of the viral inoculum. Future studies designed to investigate this relationship will have to minimally use virus isolated directly from the infected person's plasma as soon as possible to avoid further culture selection. Attempts should also be made to reisolate viruses from vaginal and seminal fluids as well as lymphoid organs during this very early phase.

10. DECEPTIVE IMPRINTING: "ORIGINAL ANTIGENIC SIN" GONE AWRY

Introduction of foreign antigens into the host either by vaccination or by infection in many cases leads to the production of specific antibody (Briles and Davie, 1980). Depending on the nature of the immunogen and the various pathways leading to B-cell activation, the clonality of the response is ultimately evoked by a given epitope. In most cases, antigens represent a broad array of epitopes, and consequently the antibody response is chemically heterogeneous and antigenically specific. Some multideterminant antigens (e.g., albumin, hen egg white lysozyme, HBV epitope, Cro Lac–gp41) result in an unequal response to some epitopes (Scheerlinck *et al.*, 1993; reviewed in Benjamin *et al.*, 1984). Given the potentially large B-cell repertoire in any given host, selective recognition of specific epitope by a limited population of B cells needs explanation to determine whether this restriction is related to the immunogen itself, or to host factors involved in its selection. Some antigens induce a less variable response, e.g., certain carbohydrate antigens, antigens with structural/functional homology to self (Table I), other antigens displaying a limited, highly ordered, or redundant number of immunodominant cross-reactive sites, more often with a unique steric presentation (i.e., streptococcal group A-variant cell wall) (Briles and Davie, 1980). For example, an animal immunized with one of these antigenic determinants and later exposed to a different, but structurally similar determinant responds to this second determinant by initially producing antibody (sometimes with a higher affinity) to the

TABLE VI. Immunological Imprinting

Normal imprinting	
	Induction of a polyclonal immune response with immunological memory, which protects againsts future infections
Original antigenic sin	
	Induction of an immune response by an antigen that elicits a long-term, cross-reactive memory resulting sometimes in protection. Considered on a populational level (e.g., influenza), a host protective phenomenon
Deceptive imprinting	
	Abnormal imprinting that limits the polyclonal nature of the immune response and characterized by immunodominant, cross-reactive epitopes leading to the loss of antigenic discretionary power at both the T- and B-cell effector and memory arms

original antigen, a phenomenon referred to as OAS (Table VI). In many cases, depending on the antigen concentration, continued boosting with the first or second antigen also elicits a normal primary response to the second antigen (Briles and Davie, 1980).

As mentioned previously, this OAS-like phenomenon was first described for an influenza viral infection of humans by Francis in 1953. Since then, OAS-like phenomena have been recognized, to influenza, in other virus families such as toga-, paramyxo-, and enteroviruses (Fenner *et al.*, 1974). Previously, this phenomenon has been considered (on a populational level) a beneficial immune response of the host (Angelova and Shuartsman, 1982). Providing various members of the population long-term, protective anamnestic immune responses to different strains of the virus would ensure that some members of the population are immune to viral agents constantly undergoing antigenic drift and shift. In general, the OAS phenomenon challenges the dogma of immunologic response specificity and the induction of its memory in a host where there may be sequential infections over time with two different, but antigenically related, strains of virus; or as it appears is the case with HIV-1 with the generation of such viruses during a "single" persistent viral infection. Evidence is mounting that a number of microbial pathogens including HIV-1 and other animal lentiviruses may have evolved to use it in a diversionary way (Table VII). By providing immunodominant epitopes capable of undergoing antigenic variation to the immune system, these pathogens appear to limit or fix the humoral and cell-mediated responses to the initial resident pathogen and thus the host seems unable to eliminate and/or control the agent. This type of host response is somewhat reminiscent of those described in the field of parasitology and tumor immunology some 25 years ago. The term *concomitant immunity*, *premunition*, and *heterotypic immunity* were coined to describe an immune response in a host whereby the resident pathogens or tumor cells were tolerated but pathogenic variants in the surrounding *transmission community* were susceptible. This prevented them from establishing a new infection in the same host (reviewed in Mitchell, 1991).

As mentioned earlier, the immunologic phenomenon of OAS was considered in the literature to be a type of protective host response in humans and rats infected with strains of influenza. Recently, however, Nara and colleagues have proposed data and a model of OAS which represents an immunopathogenic immune-diverting and evading strategy termed *deceptive imprinting* (Table VI) (Nara *et al.*, 1991). The nature of this phenomenon as modeled in HIV-1-infected chimpanzees is presented below based on previously published data.

TABLE VII. Pathogens Possibly Utilizing Deceptive Imprinting

	Location/name
Trypanosoma brucei	Variant/specific glycoprotein (VSG)
Borrelia recurrentis	Variable major protein (VMP)
Borrelia burgdorferi	
Neisseria	Pilins, minor outer membrane protein (OPA)
Giardia lamblia	Surface proteins
Plasmodium sp.	Circumsporite protein (CSP), schizant surface antigen (MSA1), erythrocyte surface
Salmonella	Surface proteins
Streptococci	Surface polysaccharides
Haemophilus influenzae	Capsular $type_b$ polysaccharide
Influenza	HA/neuraminidase
Herpesviruses	gB, gC, gE
Orthopoxviruses	Outer membrane proteins
Lentivirus	Envelope
Tumors	Emergence-associated tumor immunogen (EATI)

Chimpanzees previously immunized with immunoaffinity-purified homologous gp120 and challenged within weeks with the same virus stock elicited a rather robust anamnestic response capable of neutralizing at high titer both the homologous strain as well as those of divergent strains (~18% sequence different in the gp120). Viruses were reisolated from PBMCs of the immunized animals, and found to be completely neutralization resistant. Interestingly, when the genetic sequences of these viruses were determined, they were found to be only 1 to 5% divergent in the gp120 and completely identical in the V3 region to which the neutralizing response was directed (Nara *et al.*, 1990). The mechanism(s) by which this polyclonal antibody response was raised, to effectively neutralize a widely divergent strain (not previously seen by the animals' immune system), but incapable of neutralizing a genetically near-identical varient (with identical V3 sequence), is unknown and extremely important if one is to understand how to develop effective humoral immunogens against HIV-1. One potential explanation is that cross-reactive neutralizing antibodies are elicited that recognize epitopes present on these divergent strains. Why they are also not capable of neutralizing the closely related reisolated viruses remains unknown at this time. This phenomenon may depend on the virus since specific distant-site mutations (to the neutralization epitope) were found to occur in both the gp120 and gp41 molecules which conveyed some structural and/or functional alteration to the neutralization epitope itself thus making the neutralizing antibody ineffective (Back *et al.*, 1993; Nara *et al.*, 1990). In addition, the kinetics of the subsequent neutralizing response were determined for the early neutralization escape viruses and generally found to be slow to develop and of low titer, while the neutralizing titers to both the parental and divergent strains continued to increase to a plateau level after 6 months to 1 year. The explanation and name given to this immunologic phenomenon, briefly mentioned earlier in the chapter, was initially described as a form of "original antigenic sin" (Nara *et al.*, 1991), subsequently explained in terms of "clonal dominance" (Kohler *et al.*, 1992), and later refined to include other aspects related to the phenomenon and distinguish it as an immunopathogenic strategy is now termed "deceptive imprinting" (Kohler *et al.*, 1994).

In general, the model and the data suggest that antigenic variation of the virus envelope secondary to random mutation/selection theory provide for the continued presentation of either identical and/or cross-reactive pseudoneutralizing epitopes present on "escape variants." Continued clonal expansion of a limited functional B-cell repertoire restricts the subsequent complete development and/or functional maturation of the humoral response to other less immunodominant epitopes (for reviews see Müller *et al.*, 1992; Nara *et al.*, 1991). The initial immune clonal expansion seems to be initiated through a viral clonal expansion in both chimpanzees (Nara *et al.*, 1990) and humans (H. Zhang *et al.*, 1993; Zhu *et al.*, 1993; McNearney *et al.*, 1992; Pang *et al.*, 1992; Wolfs *et al.*, 1992) with saturation of follicular dendritic cells of the germinal centers with a genetically homogeneous HIV-1. The resulting immune response from the deceptive imprinting model predicts that an overt conality for specific and/or all structural viral antigens should exist. This immunologic mechanism effectively restricts or reduces the available T- and B-cell immune repertoire which functionally limits the polyclonal nature of the response while expanding a founder population of cross-reactive B and T cells. The signature of such an immune response is observed as a stable oligoclonal population of antibody (reviewed in Müller *et al.*, 1992) and clonality of the T-cell response to virus-encoded antigens. Recently, evidence has been reported that supports this model at the T cell level. Both limited V_β usage (Pantaleo *et al.*, 1994) during ARS and unusual oligoclonal TCR usage/expansions in later-stage patients of specific cytotoxic T cells over long periods of time have been reported during HIV-1 infection (Kalams *et al.*, 1994).

11. DECEPTIVE IMPRINTING: HYPERACTIVE B-CELL Ig-MEDIATED CONTROL OF T-CELL MODEL?

11.1. The B-Cell Problem

During HIV-1 infection there is a generalized abnormality of the B-cell compartment that persists during the transition from early HIV-1 infection to AIDS (Schnittman *et al.*, 1986). Circulating B cells are at a high level of activation, and *in vitro* mononuclear cell cultures have demonstrated both polyclonal activation and production of anti-HIV-1 antibodies (Martinez *et al.*, 1987; Briault *et al.*, 1988; Shirai *et al.*, 1992) and also that 26% of sera from HIV-infected individuals contain monoclonal IgG populations. McGrath and coworkers (Ng *et al.*, 1988) purified from the sera of an ARC patient an electrophoretic spike of oligoclonal Ig origin that had high titer binding activity (>1:100,000) to a variety of HIV epitopes ($p66^{pol}$, $p55^{gag}$, $p53^{pol}$, $p41^{gag}$, and $p24^{gag}$). Later IgG oligoclonal bands in HIV-1-infected patients were shown to be directed against HIV-1-specific determinants (Amadori *et al.*, 1990; reviewed in Amadori and Cheico-Bianchi, 1992). The striking finding regarding this oligoclonal activation is the spontaneous *in vitro* production of anti-HIV-1 antibody occurring in unstimulated PBMCs, bone marrow, lymph nodes, and cerebrospinal fluid cultures from HIV-1-infected patients. In general, the antibody is directed against the gp120, although antibody against Gag and Pol were reported (Amadori and Chieco-Bianchi, 1992). Paradoxically, this spontaneous B-cell activation is associated with a poor B-cell response to mitogens and antigens in terms of both proliferation and antibody response to recall antigens (Birx *et al.*, 1992; Lane *et al.*, 1983).

Isoelectric focusing (IEF) was used to evaluate the clonal diversity of B-cell responses, as this method is capable of identifying single clone products, i.e., spectrotypic patterns reflect the number of actively secreting specific B-cell clones. This approach has been used to study the antibody spectrotypes in the sera and in the cerebrospinal fluid of certain HIV-1-infected patients, and the detection of oligoclonal spectrotypes (characterized by a few clusters of bands) has been interpreted as evidence that during infection there are expansions of a limited number of B-cell clones. We have also employed IEF to evaluate the antibody responses of HIV-1-infected patients (reviewed in Müller *et al.*, 1992). In a longitudinal study, each patient (during 12–36 months of evaluation) maintained a stable characteristic spectrotype of anti-gp120 antibodies. Each spectrotype is a form of immune fingerprinting and indicates a rather continuous production over time. Therefore, clonal dominance or polyclonal restriction was consistently present over the course of the disease, regardless of clinical stage or the development of ARC and AIDS.

Studies in VH gene usage stress the qualitative abnormality of the humoral immune responses in seropositive patients. Maturation of VH3L genes, the largest in the B cell of genes, was found in some studies to be selectively depleted, suggesting that B cells from HIV-1-infected patients present a maturational arrest at the level of the germinal center. Further evidence for this was demonstrated more directly when it was observed that gp120 had Fab surface receptor-binding capacity for B cells similar to that of staphylococcal protein A (Berberian *et al.*, 1993). This binding demonstrated that between 20 and 40% of human peripheral B cells bind gp120 and lead to the induction and synthesis of Ig enriched in VH3 IgM *in vitro*. Although circumstantial, the gp120 molecule may behave like SpA which acts as a B-cell superantigen through specific interactions with B cells expressing VH3 heavy chain rearrangements (Silverman, 1994). For mechanisms on how both expansion and clonal depletion of VH3 occur in HIV-1-infected individuals, the reader is referred to a previous review (Müller *et al.*, 1992). Although both protein and carbohydrate-type antigens can elicit a clonally expanded population of B cells, molecular and serological approaches have shown that their selection of VH subfamily specificity can be very different. Some antigens, termed "conventional" such as *Haemophilus influenzae*, type B polysaccharide, use only two types of VH3 H chains preferentially. So-called "unconventional" antigens, however, such as staphylococcal protein A, have been found to bind both the Fcγ-binding site of the Ig framework structure and the Fab receptor on some IgM, IgG, IgA, and IgE expressing B cell surface molecules (Langone, 1982; Harboe and Folling, 1974; Inganas, 1981). These antigens do not appear to be limited to a small number of germline gene elements within the large VH3 family and elicit a B-cell superantigenic-like effect (reviewed in Silverman, 1994). A direct mechanism of B-cell activation via carbohydrate and/or protein on the gp120 could lead to the types of B-cell clonal expansions described above.

Mechanism(s) to reinforce the preferential expansion of B-cell clones just described, for a single antigen administration, would be that which on a second administration with a similar antigen suppresses and/or limits the antibody response. This type of phenomenon exists and is well known as "antigenic competition" (Albright *et al.*, 1970; Möller and Sjoberg, 1970; Waterston, 1970; Schechter, 1968; Radovick and Talmadge, 1967). Various mechanisms for this phenomenon have been demonstrated and/or proposed (Table VIII) to occur with various antigens from numerous sources (e.g., bacteria, plant and animal viruses, animal proteins, tumor antigens). In general, antigens capable of eliciting these types of responses share various immunochemical characteristics as presented in Table V. Recently, the phenomenon of antigenic competition with regard to MHC class II presentation has been

TABLE VIII. Proposed Mechanisms for Immunodominant Epitope-Mediated Suppression/Restriction

1. Consumption/exhaustion of "critical" cells or factors
2. Induction/activation of nonantigenspecific regulatory cells (e.g., NK cells)
3. Antibody-dependent epitope masking
4. Carrier-induced epitopic suppression (effector cell or idiotypic network)
5. Ig-mediated TGF-β CTL suppression
6. B-cell-driven T-cell diversification (superantigen-like effect)
7. "Unconventional" B-cell antigens (leading to VH expansion)

found to be dependent on the specificity of both the internalization and subsequent presentation (Kakiuchi *et al.*, 1995). Kittlesen *et al.* (1993) have suggested that the B-cell processing pathway for an endogenous antigen which is recognized by MHC class II-restricted T cells is different from that for exogenous antigen internalized nonspecifically, the latter being resistant to protein synthesis inhibitors and sensitive to antigenic competition (Kakiuchi *et al.*, 1990, 1991). Also, Lorenz *et al.* (1990) demonstrated the presentation of antigen internalized through the mannose receptor into macrophages resistant to competition by self proteins. Thus, antigens internalized through both the mannose receptor and a specific antigen receptor seem to be processed via similar pathways. The biochemical, biophysical, and immunochemical properties of shed and virion-associated gp120 make it a very good candidate for eliciting a direct B-cell clonal dominance and/or clonal dominance through one or more mechanisms associated with the phenomenon of antigenic competition.

11.2. The T-Cell Problem

What mechanism could help contribute to suppression or limit the polyclonal nature of the cytolytic T-cell response? Recently, Rowley and Stach (1993) and Stach and Rowley (1993) have demonstrated that IgG and TGF-β form complexes with macrophages through Fc receptors which localize at antigenic sites and play important roles in homeostasis of immunity by augmenting proliferation of already activated dominant lymphocyte clones (Coffman *et al.*, 1989), promoting isotope switching (Lin and Stavnezer, 1992; Kuruvilla *et al.*, 1991; Coffman *et al.*, 1989; Sonoda *et al.*, 1989), suppressing activation/proliferation of new specific antigen-reactive clones that may arise during ongoing immunity (Kuruvilla *et al.*, 1991). It seems remarkable that a mechanism of nonantigen-specific IgG-mediated suppression and/or regulation of CTL should exist. If it provides some protective mechanism in the immunity of pregnancy as has been speculated, it would have evolved as an important and conserved mechanism (Rowley and Stach, 1993). On the other hand, failure to develop both CTL-mediated and B-cell immunity to particular protective epitopes while expanding the response to other antigens expressed sequentially after a first or dominant immunization should be detrimental to individuals bearing immunogenic tumors or infected with organisms that give rise to variants expressing new or cross-reactive epitopes. The aforementioned discussion of newly discovered basic immunologic networks regulating the presentation of antigen to the immune system is providing a wealth of scientific opportunities to piece together an old phenomenon which may provide insights into the immunity of pregnancy, immunologic memory, how to develop new ways for promoting allograft survival in transplant recipients, and lastly, a means for the induction of more effective immunity to the class of currently "vaccine-resistant" microbes and tumor cells.

12. EPILOGUE

It appears from the previous discussion that the so-called "immune response" to HIV-1 is not all or none, but rather inefficient and semiprotective which may have a greater capacity for preventing superinfection than preventing initial infection and/or elimination of the resident virus. It also appears that various biochemical and immunochemical properties of the virus envelope as well as other structural/regulatory proteins have usurped early humoral host defense pathways which inadvertently help in establishing both the infection and diversion of the immune responses thus ensuring a chronic-active infective state. Infections that have some or all of the qualities of deceptive imprinting represent a diverse array of pathogens including tumor cells for which protective vaccines, based on the previously successful Jennerian model, have not been identified. Given the need for a new paradigm, some new questions for consideration are: (1) whether HIV-1 and other chronic-active pathogens (e.g., the metazoan parasites) exist because of a "semiprotective" host response which has as its basis a very poorly understood, yet fundamental immunologic mechanism that diverts the antigenic discretionary power of both the T and B cells at both the effector and memory cell level while limiting the polyclonal nature of the immune repertoire—probably through the induction of both viral promoting and restricting components; or (2) is the conventional immune response (i.e., humoral) and therefore antigenic variation in part or wholly an epiphenomenon secondary to some as yet not understood aspect of virus-mediated, autoregulatory mechanism(s) involving innate aspects of host defense which control levels of viral replication/expression through viral gene products like soluble gp120, Tat, and so forth? These in turn could regulate various cytokine pathways and cell signaling events which both limit and enhance virus and/or infected host cells when appropriate for transmission. Can vaccination schemes be found to induce these types of pathways?

Given the treatise on HIV-1 in the humors, it certainly seems plausible that this very old viral pathogen could have found a niche between our innate host defense system and our acquired immune systems. In light of the evidence that HIV-1 is not done evolving and sculpting itself for transmission in the human population, the knowledge, insight, and ability to raise and answer these important new questions in the very near future may mean the success or failure that prophylactic vaccination has to offer. The author hopes this chapter is novel enough in content to stimulate a fundamental rethinking of our current dogma and planning for future research and developments in the areas of immunoprophylactic and therapeutic medicine. Although the concepts presented here are not mutually exclusive, they represent potentially very different pathways.

ACKNOWLEDGMENTS. The author thanks Dr. Sherry Hand for the title; my working colleagues and staff of the Virus Biology Section, Drs. Robert Garrity and Wen-Po Tsai, for thoughtful discussion; Mr. Shawn Conley, Ms. Nancy Dunlop, and Mr. Michael Merges for their review of the chapter; and especially Ms. Susan Nelson for the needed administrative support to create such a document.

REFERENCES

Albert, J., Abrahamson, B., Nagy, K., Aurelius, E., Gaines, H., Nystrom, G., and Fenyo, E. M., 1990, Rapid development of isolate-specific neutralizing antibodies after primary HIV-1 infection and consequent emergence of virus variants which resist neutralization by autologous sera, *AIDS* **4(2):**107–112.

Albright, J. F., Omer, T. F., and Deitchman, J. W., 1970, Antigenic competition: Antigens compete for a cell occurring with limited frequency, *Science* **167:**196.

Alexander, S., and Elder, J. H., 1984, Carbohydrate dramatically influences immune reactivity of antisera to viral glycoprotein antigens, *Science* **226:**1325–1330.

Amadori, A., and Chieco-Bianchi, L., 1992, B cell activation and HIV infection: Protective or potentially detrimental response? *Int. Rev. Immunol.* **9:**15–24.

Amadori, A., Gallo, P., Zamarchi, R., Veronese, M. L., DeRossi, A., Wolf, D., and Chieco-Bianchi, L., 1990, IgG oligoclonal bands in sera of HIV-1 infected patients are mainly directed against HIV-1 determinants, *AIDS Res. Hum. Retrovir.* **6(5):**581–586.

Angelova, L. A., and Shvartsman, Y. S., 1982, Original antigenic sin to influenza in rats, *Immunology* **46:**183–188.

Arendrup, M., Nielsen, C., Hansen, J. E. S., Pedersen, C., Mathiesen, L., and Nielsen, J. O., 1992, Autologous HIV-1 neutralizing antibodies: Emergence of neutralization-resistant escape virus and subsequent development of escape virus neutralizing antibodies, *J. Acq. Immune Defic. Syndr.* **5:**303–307.

Arthur, L. O., Bess, J. W., Jr., Sowder, R. C., II, Benveniste, R. E., Mann, D. L., Chermann, J. C., and Henderson, L. E., 1992, Cellular proteins bound to immunodeficiency viruses: Implications for pathogenesis and vaccines, *Science* **258:**1935–1938.

Back, N. K. T., Smit, L., Schutten, M., Nara, P. L., Tersmette, M., and Goudsmit, J., 1993, Mutations in human immunodeficiency virus type 1 gp41 after sensitivity to neutralization by gp120 antibodies, *J. Virol.* **67:**6897–6902.

Banapour, B., Sernatinger, J., and Levy, J. A., 1986, The AIDS-associated retrovirus is not sensitive to lysis or inactivation by human sera, *Virology* **152:**268–271.

Baumann, H., and Gauldie, J., 1994, The acute phase response, *Immunol. Today* **15(2):**74–80.

Benjamin, D. C., Berzofsky, J. A., East, I. J., Gurd, F. N., Hannum, C., Leach, S. J., Margoliash, E., Michael, J. G., Miller, A., Prager, E. M., Reichlin, M., Sercarz, E. E., Smith-Gill, S. J., Todd, P. E., and Wilson, A. C., 1984, The antigenic structure of proteins: a reappraisal, *Annu. Rev. Immunol.* **2:**67–101.

Benjoudad, A., Gluckman, J.-C., Rochat, H., Montagnier, L., and Bahraoui, E., 1992, Influence of carbohydrate moieties on the immunogenicity of human immunodeficiency virus type 1 recombinant gp160, *J. Virol.* **66:**2473–2483.

Birx, D. L., Redfield, R. R., and Tosato, G., 1986, Defective regulation of Epstein–Barr virus infection in patients with acquired immunodeficiency syndrome (AIDS) or AIDS-related disorders, *N. Engl. J. Med.* **314:**874.

Bjork, R. L., Jr., 1991, HIV-1: Seven facets of functional molecular mimicry, *Immunol. Lett.* **28(2):**91–96.

Bolognesi, D. P., 1994, Humoral immune responses to primary HIV isolates: Implications for vaccine development, in: *Retroviruses of Human AIDS and Related Animal Diseases* (M. Girard and Dodet, B., eds.), Pasteur Merieux, France, pp. 285–291.

Botarelli, P., Houlden, B. A., Haighwood, N. L., Servig, C., Montagna, D., and Abrignani, S., 1991, N-glycosylation of HIV-gp120 may constrain recognition by T lymphocytes, *J. Immunol.* **147:**3128–3132.

Bou-Habib, D. C., Roderiquez, G., Oravecz, T., Berman, P. W., Lusso, P., and Norcross, M. A., 1994, Cryptic nature of envelope V3 region epitopes protects primary human immunodeficiency virus type 1 from antibody neutralization, *J. Virol.* **68:**6006–6013.

Briault, S., Courtois-Capella, M., Duarter, F., Aucouturier, P., and Preud'-Homme, J. L., 1988, Isotypy of serum monoclonal immunoglobulins in human immunodeficiency virus-infected adults, *Clin. Exp. Immunol.* **74(2):**182–184.

Briles, D. E., and Davie, J. M., 1980, Clonal nature of the immune response. II. The effect of immunization on clonal commitment, *J. Exp. Med.* **152:**151–160.

Broder, C. C., Earl, P. L., Long, D., Abedon, S. T., Moss, B., and Doms, R. W., 1994, Antigenic implications of human immunodeficiency virus type-1 envelope quaternary structure: Oligomeric-specific and -sensitive monoclonal antibodies, *Proc. Natl. Acad. Sci. USA* **91:**11699–11703.

Burton, D. R., Pyati, J., Koduri, R., Sharp, S. J., Thornton, G. B., Parren, P. W. H. I., Sawyer, L. S. W., Hendry, R. M., Dunlop, N., Nara, P. L., Lamacchia, M., Garratty, E., Stiehm, E. R., Bryson, Y. J., Cao, Y., Moore, J. P., Ho, D. D., and Barbas C. F., III, 1994, Efficient neutralization of primary isolates of HIV-1 by a recombinant human monoclonal antibody, *Science* **266:**1024–1027.

Cheingsong-Popov, R., Panagiotidi, C., Bowcock, S., Aronstam, A., Wadsworth, J., and Weber, J., 1991, Relation between humoral responses to HIV gag and env proteins at seroconversion and clinical outcome of HIV infection, *Lancet* **302:**23–26.

Clark, S. J., Saag, M. S., Decker, W. D., Cambell-Hill, S., Roberson, J. L., Veldkamp, P. J., Kappes, J. C., Hahn, B. H., and Shaw, G. M., 1991, High titers of cytopathic virus in plasma of patients with symptomatic primary HIV-1 infection, *N. Engl. J. Med.* **324:**954.

Clements, J. E., Montelaro, R. C., Zink, M. C., Amedee, A. M., Miller, S., Trichel, A. M., Jagerski, B., Hauer, D., Martin, L. N., Bohm, R. P., and Murphey-Corb, M., 1995, Cross-protective immune responses induced in rhesus macaques by immunization with attenuated macrophage-tropic simian immunodeficiency virus, *J. Virol.* **69;**2737–2744.

Coffman, R. L., Lebman, D. A., and Shrader, B., 1989, Transforming growth factor β specifically enhances IgA production by lipopolysaccharide-stimulated murine B lymphocytes, *J. Exp. Med.* **170:**1039.

Cohen, J., 1995, Differences in HIV strains may underlie disease patterns, *Science* **270:**30–31.

Conley, A. J., Gorny, M. K., Kessler, J. A., II, Boots, L. J., Ossorio-Costro, M., Koenig, S., Lineberger, D. W., Emeni, E. A., Williams, C., and Zolla-Pazner, S., 1994, Neutralization of primary human immunodeficiency virus type I isolates by the broadly reactive anti-V3 monoclonal antibody, 447-52D, *J. Virol.* **68:**6994–7000.

Conley, S. R., 1993, Native particle suspension ELISA (NPSE): A novel method for studying the immunochemistry of HIV-1 surface glycoproteins, Masters thesis, Hood College, pp. 1–58.

Cooper, N. R., Jensen, F. C., Welsh, R. M., and Oldstone, M. B. A., 1976, Lysis of RNA tumor viruses by human serum: Direct antibody independent triggering of the classical complement pathway, *J. Exp. Med.* **144:** 970–984.

Curtis, B. M., Scharnowske, S., and Watson, A. J., 1992, Sequence and expression of a membrane-associated C-type lectin that exhibits CD4-independent binding of human immunodeficiency virus envelope glycoprotein gp120, *Proc. Natl. Acad. Sci. USA* **89:**8356–8360.

Daar, E. S., Li, X. L., Moudgil, T., and Ho, D. D., 1990, High concentrations of recombinant soluble CD4 are required to neutralize primary human immunodeficiency virus type 1 isolates, *Proc. Natl. Acad. Sci. USA* **87:**6574–6578.

Daar, E. S., Moudgil, T., Meyer, R. D., and Ho, D. D., 1991, Transient high levels of viremia in patients with primary human immuno-deficiency virus type 1 infection, *N. Engl. J. Med.* **324:**961.

Dierich, M. P., Ebenbichler, C. F., Marschang, P., Füst, G., Thielens, N. M., and Arlaud, G. J., 1993, HIV and human complement: Mechanisms of interaction and biological implication, *Immunol. Today* **14:**435–440.

Dimitrov, D. S., Willey, R. L., Martin, M. A., and Blumenthal, R., 1992, Kinetics of HIV-1 interactions with sCD4 and CD4+ cells: Implications for inhibition of virus infection and initial steps of virus entry into cells, *Virology* **187:**398–406.

Dorfman, T., Mammano, F., Haseltine, W., and Gottlinger, G., 1994, Role of the matrix protein in the virion association of the human immunodeficiency virus type 1 envelope glycoprotein, *J. Virol.* **68:**1689–1696.

Drickamer, K., 1988, Two distinct classes of carbohydrate-recognition domains in animal lectins, *J. Biol. Chem.* **263:**9557–9560.

Earl, P. L., Broder, C. C., Long, D., Lee, S. A., Peterson, J., Chakrabarti, S., Dons, R. W., and Moss, B., 1994, Native oligomeric human immunodeficiency virus type 1 envelope glycoprotein elicits diverse monoclonal antibody reactivities, *J. Virol.* **68:**3015–3026.

Ezekowitz, R. A. B., Kuhlman, M., Groopman, J. E., and Byrn, R. A., 1989, A human serum mannose-binding protein inhibits *in vitro* infection by the human immunodeficiency virus, *J. Exp. Med.* **169:**185–196.

Ezekowitz, R. A. B., 1991, Ante-antibody immunity, *Curr. Biol.* **1:**60–62.

Feinberg, J., 1992, The acute HIV seroconversion syndrome, *Curr. Opin. Infect. Dis.* **5:**221.

Fenner, F., McAuslan, B. R., Mims, C. A., Sambrook, J., and White, D. O., eds., 1974, Pathogenesis: The immune response, in: *The Biology of Animal Viruses*, 2nd ed., Academic Press, London, pp. 417–418.

Fernandez-Larsson, R., Srivastava, K. K., Lu, S., and Robinson, H. L., 1992, Replication of patient isolates of human immunodeficiency virus type 1 in T cells: A spectrum of rates and efficiencies of entry, *Proc. Natl. Acad. Sci. USA* **89:**2223–2226.

Fiete, D., Srivastava, V., Hindsgaul, O., and Baenziger, J. U., 1991, A hepatic reticuloendothelial cell receptor specific for SO_4GalNAcβ1,4GlcNcβ1,2Manα that mediates rapid clearance of lutropin, *Cell* **67:**1103–1110.

Fischinger, P. J., Ihle, J. N., Bolognesi, D. P., and Schafer, W., 1976, Inactivation of murine xenotropic oncornavirus by normal mouse sera is not immunoglobulin-mediated, *Virology* **71:**346–351.

Francis, T., Jr., 1953, Influenza: New acquaintance, *Ann. Intern. Med.* **39:**203–221.

Gaines, H., vonSydow, M. A. E., vonStedingk, L. V., Biberfield, G., Böttiger, B., Hansson, L. O., Lundbergh, P.,

Sönnerborg, A. B., Wasserman, J., and Strannegård, Ö. O., 1990, Immunological changes in primary HIV-1 infection, *AIDS* **4**:995–999.

Gattegno, L., Sadeghi, H., Saffar, L., Bladier, D., Clerget-Raslain, B., Gluckman, J.-C., and Bahraoui, E., 1991, *N*-Acetyl-β-*D*-glucosaminyl-binding properties of the envelope glycoprotein of human immunodeficiency virus type 1, *Carbohydr. Res.* **213**:79–93.

Gelderblom, H. R., Reupke, H., and Pauli, G., 1985, Loss of envelope antigens of HTLV-III/LAV, a factor in AIDS pathogenesis? *Lancet* **2**:1016–1017.

Geyer, H., Holschback, C., Hunsmann, G., and Schneider, J., 1988, Carbohydrates of human immunodeficiency virus. Structures of oligosaccharides linked to the envelope glycoprotein 120, *J. Biol. Chem.* **263**:11760–11767.

Giga, Y., Atsushi, I., and Takahaski, K., 1987, The complete amino acid sequence of echinoiden, a lectin from the coelomic fluid of the sea urchin *Anthociadaris crassispina*, *J. Biol. Chem.* **262**:6197–6203.

Gooding, L. R., 1992, Virus proteins that counteract host immune defenses, *Cell* **71**:5–7.

Grundy, J. E., McKeating, J. A., Ward, P. J., Sanderson, A. R., and Griffiths, P. D., 1987, β_2 microglobulin enhances the infectivity of cytomegalovirus and when bound to the virus enables class I HLA molecules to be used as a virus receptor, *J. Gen. Virol.* **68**:793–803.

Hall, B. F., and Joiner, K. A., 1991, Strategies of obligate intracellular parasites for evading host defences, *Immunol. Today* **12(3)**:A22–A27.

Hansen, B. D., Nara, P. L., Maheshwari, R. K., Sidhu, G. S., Bernbaum, J. G., Hoekzema, D., Meltzer, M. S., and Gendelman, H. E., 1992, Loss of infectivity by progeny virus from alpha interferon-treated human immunodeficiency virus type 1-infected T cells is associated with defective assembly of envelope gp120, *J. Virol.* **66**:7543.

Hansen, J.-E. S., Clausen, H., Nielsen, C., Teglbjaerg, L. S., Hansen, L. L., Nielsen, C. M., Dabelsteen, E., Mathiesen, L., Hakomori, S., and Nielsen, J. O., 1990, Inhibition of human immunodeficiency virus (HIV) infection in vitro by anti-carbohydrate monoclonal antibodies: Peripheral glycosylation of HIV envelope glycoprotein gp120 may be a target for virus neutralization, *J. Virol.* **64**:2833–2840.

Hansen, J.-E. S., Nielsen, C., Clausen, H., Mathiesen, L. R., and Nielsen, J. O., 1991, Effect of monoclonal antibodies against carbohydrate epitopes of gp120 on HIV infection in a monocytic cell line (U937), *Antivir. Res.* **16**:233–242.

Hansen, J.-E. S., Sorensen, A. M., Arendrup, M., Olofsson, S., Nielsen, J. O., Janzek, E., Nielsen, C., and Loibner, H., 1993, Enhancement of retroviral infection in vitro by anti-Le^y IgG: Reversal by humanization of monoclonal mouse antibody, *APMIS* **101**:711–718.

Hanson, C. V., 1994, Measuring vaccine-induced HIV neutralization: Report of a workshop, *AIDS Res. Hum. Retrovir.* **10**:645–648.

Hara, T., Matsumoto, M., Fukumori, Y., Miyagawa, S., Hatanaka, M., Kinoshita, T., Seya, T., and Akedo, H., 1993, A monoclonal antibody against human decay-accelerating factor (DAF, CD55), D17, which lacks reactivity with semen-DAF, *Immunol. Lett.* **37(2,3)**:145–152.

Harboe, M., and Folling, I., 1974, Recognition of two distinct groups of human IgM and IgA based on different binding to staphylococci, *J. Immunol.* **3(4)**:471–482.

Harouse, J. M., Bhat, S., Spitalnik, L., Laughlin, M., Stefano, K., Silberberg, D. H., and Gonzalez-Scarano, F., 1991, Inhibition of entry of HIV-1 in neural cell lines by antibodies against galactosyl ceramide, *Science* **253**:320–323.

Henderson, L. E., Sowder, R., Copeland, T. D., Oroszlan, S., Arthur, L. O., Robey, W. G., and Fischinger, P. J., 1987, Direct identification of class II histocompatibility DR proteins in preparations of human T cell lymphotropic virus type III, *J. Virol.* **61(2)**:629–632.

Holmskov, U., Malhotra, R., Sim, R. B., and Jensenious, J. C., 1994, Collectins: Collagenous C-type lectins of the innate immune defense system, *Immunol. Today* **15(2)**:67–74.

Hoshino, H., Tanaka, H., Mina, M., and Okada, H., 1984, Human T-cell leukaemia virus is not lysed by human serum, *Nature* **310**:324–325.

Hosmalin, A., Nara, P. L., Zweig, M., Lerche, N. W., Cease, K. B., Gard, E. A., Markham, P. D., Putney, S., Daniel, M. D., and Desrosier, R. C., 1991, Priming with T helper cell epitope peptides enhances the antibody response to the envelope glycoprotein of HIV-1 in primates, *J. Immunol.* **146**:1667–1673.

Hosoi, S., Borsos, T., Dunlop, N., and Nara, P. L., 1990, Heat-labile, complement-like factor(s) of animal sera prevent(s) HIV-1 infectivity in vitro, *J. Acq. Immune Defic. Syndr.* **3**:366–371.

Huso, D. L., Narayan, O., and Hart, G. W., 1988, Sialic acids on the surface of caprine arthritis-encephalitis virus define the biological properties of the virus, *J. Gen. Virol.* **62**:1974–1980.

Imai, Y., Singer, M. S., Fennie, C., Lasky, L. A., and Rosen, S. D., 1991, Identification of a carbohydrate-based endothelial ligand for a lymphocyte homing receptor, *J. Cell Biol.* **113:**1213–1221.

Inganas, M., 1981, Comparison of mechanisms of interaction between protein A from Staphylococcus aureus and human monoclonal IgG, IgA, and IgM in relation to the classical FC gamma and the alternative F(ab′)2 epsilon protein A interactions, *J. Immunol.* **13:**434–352.

Janeway, C. A., Jr., 1992, The immune system evolved to discriminate infectious nonself from noninfectious self, *Immunol. Today* **13(1):**11–16.

Jomori, T., and Natori, S., 1991, Molecular cloning of cDNA for lipopolysaccharide-binding protein from the hemolymph of the American cockroach, *Periplaneta americana.* Similarity of the protein with animal lectins and its acute phase expression, *J. Biol. Chem.* **266:**13318–13323.

Kabat, D., Kozak, S. L., Wehrly, K., and Chesebro, B., 1994, Differences in CD4 dependence for infectivity of laboratory-adapted and primary patient isolates of human immunodeficiency virus type 1, *J. Virol.* **68:**2570–2577.

Kahn, J. O., Steimer, K. S., Baenziger, J., Duliege, A.-M., Feinberg, M., Elbeik, T., Chesney, M., Mucar, N., Chernoff, D., and Sinagil, F., 1995, Clinical, immunologic, and virologic observations related to human immunodeficiency virus (HIV) type 1 infection in a volunteer in an HIV-1 vaccine clinical trial, *J. Infect. Dis.* **171:**1343–1347.

Kakiuchi, T., Watanabe, M., Hozumi, N., and Nariuchi, H., 1990, Differential sensitivity of specific and nonspecific antigen-presentation by B cells to a protein synthesis inhibitor, *J. Immunol.* **145:**1653.

Kakiuchi, T., Takatsuki, A., Watanabe, M., and Nariuchi, H., 1991, Inhibition by brefeldin A of the specific B cell antigen presentation to MHC class II-restricted T cells, *J. Immunol.* **147:**3289.

Kakiuchi, T., Okada, Y., Kokuho, T., Gyotoku, Y., Mizucuchi, J., and Nariuchi, H., 1994, Differential sensitivity to antigenic competition in antigen-specific and -nonspecific antigen presentation by B cells, *Immunology* **193:** 84–97.

Kalams, S. A., Johnson, R. P., Trocha, A. K., Dynan, M. J., Ngo, H. S., D'Aquila, R. T., Kurnick, J. T., and Walker, B. D., 1994, Longitudinal analysis of T cell receptor (TCR) gene usage by human immunodeficiency virus 1 envelope-specific cytotoxic T lymphocyte clones reveals a limited TCR repertoire, *J. Exp. Med.* **179:**1261–1271.

Kane, J. P., Hardman, D. A., Dimpfl, J. C., and Levy, J. A., 1979, Apolipo-protein is responsible for neutralization of xenotropic type C virus by mouse serum, *Proc. Natl. Acad. Sci. USA* **76:**5957–5961.

Kavaler, J., Caton, A. J., Staudt, L. M., Schwartz, D., and Gerhard, W., 1990, A set of closely related antibodies dominates the primary antibody response to the antigenic site CB of the A/PR/8/34 influenza virus hemagglutinin, *J. Immunol.* **145:**2312–2321.

Kitamura, M., Namiki, M., Matsumiya, K., Tanaka, K., Matsumoto, M., Hara, T., Kiyohara, H., Okabe, M., Okuyama, A., and Seya, T., 1995, Membrane cofactor protein (CD46) in seminal plasma is a prostasome-bound form with complement regulatory activity and measles virus neutralizing activity, *Immunology* **84:**626–632.

Kitchen, L., Malone, G., Orgad, S., Barin, F., Zaizov, R., Ramot, B., Gazit, E., Kreiss, J., Leal, M., Wichmann, I., Martinowitz, U., and Essex, M., 1986, Viral envelope protein of HTLV-III is the major target antigen for antibodies in hemophiliac patients, *J. Infect. Dis.* **153:**788–790.

Kittlesen, D. J., Brown, L. R., Braciale, V. L., Sambrook, J. P., Gething, M.-J., and Braciale, T. J., 1993, Presentation of newly synthesized glycoproteins to $CD4^+$ T lymphocytes. An analysis using influenza hemoagglutinin transport mutants, *J. Exp. Med.* **177:**1021–1030.

Kohler, H., Goudsmit, J., and Nara, P., 1992, Clonal antibody dominance in HIV-1 infection: Cause for a limited and failing immune response to HIV-1 infection and vaccination, *J. Acq. Immune Defic. Syndr.* **5:**1158–1168.

Kohler, H., Muller, S., and Nara, P., 1994, Deceptive imprinting in the immune response against HIV-1, *Immunol. Today* **13:**475–478.

Koj, A., 1985, Acute-phase response to injury and infection: The roles of interleukin-1 and other mediators, in: *The Acute Phase Response to Injury and Infection* (A. H. Gordon and A. Koj, eds.), Elsevier, Publishers, Paris, Vol. 10, pp. 139–144.

Kumar, S., McKerlie, M. L., Albrecht, T. B., Goldman, A. S., and Baron, S., 1984, A broadly active viral inhibitor in human and animal organ extracts and body fluids, *Proc. Soc. Exp. Biol. Med.* **177:**104–111.

Kuruvilla, A. P., Shah, R., Hochwald, G. M., Liggitt, H. D., Palladino, M. A., and Thorbecker, G. J., 1991, Protective effect of transforming growth factor β1 on experimental autoimmune disease in mice, *Proc. Natl. Acad. Sci. USA* **88:**2918.

Lane, H. C., Masur, H., Edgar, L. C., Whalen, G., Rook, A. H., and Fauci, A. S., 1983, Abnormalities of B-cell activation and immunoregulation in patients with the acquired immunodeficiency syndrome, *N. Engl. J. Med.* **309:**453.

Langone, J. J., 1982, Protein A of Staphylococcus aureus and related immunoglobulin receptors produced by streptococci and pneumonococci, *Adv. Immunol.* **32**:157–252.

Larkin, M., Childs, R. A., Matthews, T. J., Thiel, S., Mizuochi, T., Lawson, A. M., Savill, J. S., Haslett, C., Diaz, R., and Teizi, T., 1989, Oligosaccharide-mediated interactions of the envelope glycoprotein gp120 of HIV-1 that are independent of CD4 recognition, *AIDS* **3**:793–798.

Layne, S. P., and Dembo, M., 1992, The auto-regulation model: A unified concept of how HIV regulates its infectivity, pathogenesis and persistence, *Int. Rev. Immunol.* **8**:1–32.

Layne, S. P., Merges, M. J., Dembo, M., Spouge, J. L., and Nara, P. L., 1990, HIV requires multiple gp120 molecules for CD4-mediated infection, *Nature* **346**:277–279.

Layne, S. P., Merges, M. J., Dembo, M., Spouge, J. L., Conley, S. R., Moore, J. P., Raine, J. L., Renz, H., Gelderbloom, H. R., and Nara, P. L., 1992, Factors underlying spontaneous inactivation and susceptibility to neutralization of human immunodeficiency virus, *Virology* **189**:695–714.

Leonard, C. K., Spellman, M. W., Riddle, L., Harris, R. J., Thomas, J. N., and Gregory, T. J., 1990, Assignment of intrachain disulfide bonds and characterization of potential glycosylation sites of type 1 recombinant human immunodeficiency virus envelope glycoprotein (gp120) expressed in Chinese hamster ovary cells, *J. Biol. Chem.* **265**:10373–10382.

Levy, J. A., 1975, Type C virus inhibitor associated with cells cultivated from New Zealand Black mice, *Persp. Virol.* **9**:207–214.

Levy, J. A., 1993, Pathogenesis of human immunodeficiency virus infection, *Microbiol. Rev.* **57**:183–289.

Lin, Y. A., and Stavnezer, J., 1992, Regulation of transcription of the germ-line Igα constant region gene by an ATF element and by novel transforming growth factor-β1 responsive elements, *J. Immunol.* **149**:2914.

Lorenz, R. G., Blum, J. S., and Allen, P. M., 1990, Constitutive competition by self proteins for antigen presentation can be overcome by receptor-enhanced uptake, *J. Immunol.* **144**:1600.

McKeating, J. A., Griffiths, P. D., and Grundy, J. E., 1987, Cytomegalovirus in urine specimens has host β_2 microglobulin bound to the viral envelope: A mechanism of evading the host immune response? *J. Gen. Virol.* **68**:785–792.

McNearney, T., Hornickova, Z., Markham, R., Birdwell, A., Arens, M., Saab, A., and Ratner, L., 1992, Relationship of human immunodeficiency virus type 1 sequence heterogeneity to stage of disease, *Proc. Natl. Acad. Sci. USA* **89**:10247–10251.

Malhotra, R., Thiel, S., Reid, K. B. M., and Sim, R., 1990, Human leukocyte Clq receptor binds other soluble proteins with collagen domains, *J. Exp. Med.* **172**:955–959.

Manca, N., Veronese, F. D., Ho, D. D., Gallo, R. C., and Sarngadharan, M. G., 1987, Sequential changes in antibody levels to the env and gag antigens in human immunodeficiency virus infected subjects, *Eur. J. Epidemiol.* **3**:96–102.

Marrack, P., and Kappler, J., 1994, Subversion of the immune system by pathogens, *Cell* **76**:323–332.

Martinez-Maza, O., Crabb, E., Mitsuyasu, R. T., Fahey, J. L., and Giorgi, J. V., 1987, Infection with the human immunodeficiency virus (HIV) is associated with an in vivo increase in B lymphocyte activation and immaturity, *J. Immunol.* **138**:3720– 3724.

Mastro, T. D., Satten, G. A., Nopkesorn, T., Sangkharomya, S., and Longini, I. M., 1994, Probability of female-to-male transmission of HIV-1 in Thailand, *Lancet* **343**:204–207.

Matsushita, M., and Fujita, T., 1992, Activation of the classical complement pathway by mannose-binding protein in association with a novel Cls-like serine protease, *J. Exp. Med.* **176**:1497–1502.

Matthews, T. J., 1994, Dilemma of neutralization resistance to HIV-1 field isolates and vaccine development, *AIDS Res. Hum. Retrovir.* **10**:631–632.

Merges, M. J., Layne, S. P., Spouge, J. L., Conley, S. R., Moore, J. P., and Nara, P. L., 1996, Antibody valency and reversibility, and the state of the virion determine in vitro efficacy of HIV-1 neutralization (submitted for publication).

Mesesaoudi, K. E., Englert, Y., Steens, M., Thiry, L., and Tieghem, N. V., 1994, HIV-1 infectivity enhanced by a cathepsin-like activity in vaginal secretions, *Arch. Int. Physiol. Biochim. Biophys.* **102**:217–223.

Mitchell, G. F., 1991, Co-evolution of parasites and adaptive immune responses, *Immunol. Today* **12(3)**:A2–5.

Mizuochi, T., Spellman, M. W., Larkin, M., Solomon, J., Basa, L. J., and Feizi, T., 1988, Carbohydrate structures of the human immunodeficiency virus (HIV) recombinant envelope glycoprotein gp120 produced in Chinese hamster ovary cells, *Biochem. J.* **254**:599–603.

Mizuochi, T., Matthews, T. J., Kato, M., Hamako, J., Titani, K., Solomon, J., and Feizi, T., 1990, Diversity of oligosaccharide structures on the envelope glycoprotein gp120 of human immunodeficiency virus 1 from the lymphoblastoid cell line H9, *J. Biol. Chem.* **265**:8519–8524.

Möller, G., and Sjoberg, O., 1970, Effect of antigenic competition on antigen-sensitive cells and on adoptively transferred immunocompetent cells, *Cell. Immunol.* **1:**110.

Montefiori, D. C., Zhou, J., Barnes, B., Lake, D., Hirsh, E. M., Masuho, Y., and Lefkowitz, L. B., Jr., 1991, Homotypic antibody responses to fresh clinical isolates of human immunodeficiency virus, *Virology* **182(2):**635–643.

Montefiori, D. C., Cornell, R. J., Zhou, J. Y., Zhou, J. T., Hirsch, V. M., and Johnson, P. R., 1994, Complement control proteins, CD46, CD55, and CD59, as common surface constituents of human and simian immunodeficiency viruses and possible targets for vaccine protection, *Virology* **205:**82–92.

Moore, J. P., Cao, Y., Ho, D. D., and Koup, R. A., 1994, Development of the anti-gp120 antibody response during seroconversion to human immunodeficiency virus type 1, *J. Virol.* **68:**5142–5155.

Moore, J. P., and Ho, D. D., 1995, HIV-1 neutralization: the consequences of viral adaptation to growth on transformed cells, *AIDS* **9:**S117–136.

Moore, J. P., McKeating, J. A., Huang, Y., and Ho, D. D., 1992, Virions of primary human immunodeficiency virus type 1 isolates resistant to soluble CD4 (sCD4) neutralization differ in sCD4 binding and glycoprotein gp120 retention from sCD4-sensitive isolates, *J. Virol.* **66:**235–243.

Müller, S., Nara, P., D'Amelio, R., Biselli, R., Gold, D., Wang, H., Köhler, H., and Silverman, G. J., 1992, Clonal patterns in the human immune response to HIV-1 infection, *Int. Rev. Immunol.* **9:**1–13.

Nair, B. C., Ford, G., Kalyanaraman, V. S., Zafari, M., Fang, C., and Sarngadharan, M. G., 1994, Enzyme immunoassay using native envelope glycoprotein (gp160) for detection of human immunodeficiency virus type 1 antibodies, *J. Clin. Microbiol.* **32(6):**1449–1456.

Nara, P. L., 1989a, HIV-1 neutralization: Evidence for rapid, binding/postbinding neutralization from infected human, chimpanzees, and gp120-vaccinated animals, in: *Vaccines 89* (R. A. Lerner, H. Ginsberg, R. M. Chanock, and F. Brown, eds.), Cold Spring Harbor Laboratory Press, Cold Spring Harbor, NY, pp. 137–144.

Nara, P., 1989b, The "AIDS" viruses of animals of man: Nonliving parasites of the immune system, in: *Los Alamos Science Magazine*, No. 18 (N. G. Cooper, ed.), Los Alamos National Laboratory, Los Alamos, NM, pp. 54–89.

Nara, P. L., and Goudsmit, J., 1990a, Neutralization-resistant variants of HIV-1 escape via the hypervariable immunodominant V3 region: Evidence for a conformational neutralization epitope, in: *Vaccines 90* (F. Brown, R. M. Chanock, H. Ginsberg, and R. A. Lerner, eds.), Cold Spring Harbor Laboratory Press, Cold Spring Harbor, NY, pp. 77–86.

Nara, P. L., and Goudsmit, J., 1991, Clonal dominance of the neutralizing response to the HIV-1 V3 epitope: Evidence for "original antigenic sin" during vaccination and infection in animals, including humans, in: *Vaccines 91* (R. A. Lerner, H. Ginsberg, R. M. Chanock, and F. Brown, eds.), Cold Spring Harbor Laboratory Press, Cold Spring Harbor, NY, pp. 51–58.

Nara, P. L., Smit, L., Dunlop, N., Natch, W., Merges, M., Waters, D., Kelliher, J., Gallo, R. C., Fischinger, P. J., and Goudsmit, J., 1990b, Emergence of viruses resistant to neutralization by V3-specific antibodies in experimental human immunodeficiency virus type 1 IIIB infection of chimpanzees, *J. Virol.* **64:**3779–3791.

Nara, P. L., Garrity, R. R., and Goudsmit, J., 1991, Neutralization of HIV-1: A paradox of humoral proportions, *FASEB J.* **5:**2437–2455.

Nara, P. L., Merges, M. J., Garrity, R. R., Conley, S., Minassian, A., Tsai, W.-P., Rimmelzwaan, G. F., Goudsmit, J., Muller, S., and Kohler, H., 1993, HIV-1: Decoying the host humoral immune system through immunologic and biophysical means, in: *Vaccines 93* (F. Brown, R. Chanock, H. Ginsberg, and R. Lerner, eds.), Cold Spring Harbor Laboratory Press, Cold Spring Harbor, NY, pp. 167–175.

Nara, P. L., Wu, S.-C., Merges, M., Spouge, J., 1995, Physiologic concentrations of human plasma alters the immunochemistry and increases the neutralization resistant fraction of HIV-1, in: *Dixieme Colloque Des Cent Gardes* (M. Girard and B. Dodet, eds.), Elsevier Publishers, Paris, France, pp. 117–125.

Neurath, A. R., Strick, N., and Lee, E. S. Y., 1990, B cell epitope mapping of human immunodeficiency virus envelope glycoproteins with long (19- to 36-residue) synthetic peptides, *J. Gen. Virol.* **71(1):**85–95.

Ng, V. L., Hwang, K. M., Reyes, G. R., Kaplan, L. D., Khayam-Bashi, H., Hadley, W. K., and McGrath, M., 1988, High titer anti-HIV antibody reactivity associated with a paraprotein spike in a homosexual male with AIDS related complex, *Blood* **71:**1397–1401.

Oh, S.-K., Cruikshank, W. W., Raina, J., Blanchard, G. C., Adler, W. H., Walker, J., and Kornfeld, H., 1992, Identification of HIV-1 envelope glycoprotein in the serum of AIDS and ARC patients, *J. Acq. Immune Defic. Syndr.* **5:**251–256.

Olofsson, S., Sjoblom, I., and Jeansson, S., 1990, Activity of herpes simplex virus type 1-specified glycoprotein C antigenic site epitopes reversibly modulated by peripheral fucose or galactose units of glycoprotein oligosaccharides, *J. Gen. Virol.* **71:**889–895.

Osborn, J. E., 1995, HIV: The more things change, the more they stay the same, *Nature Med.* **1**:991–993.

Oyaizu, N., Chirmule, N., Kalyanaraman, V. S., Hall, W. W., Good, R. A., and Pahwa, S., 1990, Human immunodeficiency virus type 1 envelope glycoprotein gp120 produces immune defects in CD4+ T lymphocytes by inhibiting interleukin 2 mRNA, *Proc. Natl. Acad. Sci USA* **87**:2379–2383.

Pang, S., Sclesinger, Y., Daar, E. S., Moudgil, T., Ho, D. D., and Chen, I. S. Y., 1992, Rapid generation of sequence variation during primary HIV-1 infection, *AIDS* **6**:453–460.

Pantaleo, G., Demarest, J. F., Soudeyns, H., Graziosi, C., Denis, F., Adelsberger, J. W., Borrow, P., Saag, M. S., Shaw, G. M., Sekaly, R. P., and Fauci, A. S., 1994, Major expansion of $CD8^+$ T cells with a predominant Vβ usage during the primary immune responses to HIV, *Nature* **370**:463–467.

Pinter, C., Siccardi, A. G., Longhi, R., and Clivio, A., 1995, Direct interaction of complement factor H with the C1 domain of HIV type 1 glycoprotein 120, *AIDS Res. Hum. Retrovir.* **11**:577–588.

Race, E. M., Ramsey, K. M., Lucia, H. L., and Cloyd, M. W., 1991, Human immunodeficiency virus elicits antibody not detected by standard tests: implications for diagnostics and viral immunology, **184**:716–722.

Radovick, J., and Talmadge, D. W., 1967, Antigenic competition: Cellular or humoral, *Science* **158**:512.

Rooney, I. A., Atkinson, J. P., and Krul, E. S., 1993a, Physiologic relevance of membrane attack complex inhibitory protein CD59 in human seminal plasma: CD59 is present on extracellular organelles (prostasomes), binds cell membranes, and inhibits complement-mediated lysis, *J. Exp. Med.* **177**:1409.

Rooney, I. A., Atkinson, J. P., Krul, E. S., Schonfeld, G., Polakoski, K., Saffitz, J. E., and Morgan, B. P., 1993b, Carriage of complement regulatory proteins by vesicles (prostasomes) in seminal plasma, *Mol. Immunol.* **30(1)**:47.

Roos, M. T. L., Lang, J. M. A., deGoede, R. E. Y., Coutinho, R. A., Schellekens, P. T. A., Miedema, F., and Tersmette, M., 1992, Viral phenotype and immune response in primary human immunodeficiency virus type 1 infection, *J. Infect. Dis.* **165**:427–432.

Rowley, D. A., and Stach, R. M., 1993, A first or dominant immunization. I. Suppression of simultaneous cytolytic T cell responses to unrelated alloantigens, *J. Exp. Med.* **178**:835–840.

Schechter, I., 1968, Antigenic competition between polypeptidyl determinants in normal and tolerant rabbits, *J. Exp. Med.* **127**:237.

Scheerlinck, J. Y., DeLeys, R., Saman, E., Brys, L., Geldhoff, A., and Bactselier, P. D., 1993, Redistribution of a murine humoral immune response following removal of an immunodominant B cell epitope from a recombinant fusion protein, *Mol. Immunol.* **30**:733–739.

Schneider, J., Kaaden, O., Copeland, T. D., Oroszlan, S., and Hunsmann, G., 1986, Shedding an interspecies type sero-reactivity of the envelope glycopolypeptide gp120 of the human immunodeficiency virus, *J. Gen. Virol.* **67**:2533–2538.

Schnittman, S., Lane, H., Higgins, S., Folks, T., 1986, Direct polyclonal activation of human B lymphocytes by the acquired immune deficiency syndrome virus, *Science* **233**:1084–1088.

Shilatifard, A., Merkle, R. K., Helland, D. E., Welles, J. L., Haseltine, W. A., and Cummings, R. D., 1993, Complex-type N-linked oligosaccharides of gp120 from human immunodeficiency virus type 1 contain sulfated *N*-acetylglucosamine, *J. Virol.* **67**:943–952.

Shirai, A., Cosentino, M., Leitman-Klinman, S. F., and Klinman, D. M., 1992, Human immunodeficiency virus infection induces both polyclonal and virus-specific B cell activation, *J. Clin. Invest.* **89(2)**:561–566.

Silverman, G. J., and Kohler, H., 1992, Clonal restriction in human antibody responses to infections, *Int. Rev. Immunol.* **9(1)**:1–57.

Silverman, G. J., 1994, Superantigens and the spectrum of unconventional B-cell antigens, *Immunologist* **2(2)**: 51–57.

Sinicco, A., Biglino, A., Sciandra, M., Forno, B., Pollono, A. M., Raiteri, R., and Gioannini, P., 1993, Cytokine network and acute primary HIV-1 infection, *AIDS* **7**:1167–1172.

Sjoblom, I., Lundstrom, M., Sjogren-Janson, E., Glorioso, C., Jeansson, S., and Olofsson, S., 1987, Demonstration and mapping of highly carbohydrate-dependent epitopes in the herpes simplex virus type 1 specific glycoprotein C, *J. Gen. Virol.* **68**:545–554.

Sonoda, E., Matsumoto, R., Hitoshi, Y., Ishil, T., Sugimoto, M., Araki, S., Tominaga, A., Yamaguchi, N., and Takatsu, K., 1989, Transforming growth factor β induces IgA production and acts additively with interleukin 5 for IgA production, *J. Exp. Med.* **170**:1415.

Spear, G. T., 1993, Interaction of non-antibody factors with HIV in plasma, *AIDS* **7**:1149–1157.

Spies, C. P., and Compans, R. W., 1993, Alternate pathways of secretion of simian immunodeficiency virus envelope glycoproteins, *J. Virol.* **67**:6535–6541.

Srivastava, K. K., Fernandez-Larsson, R., Zinkus, D. M., and Robinson, H. L., 1991, Human immunodeficiency virus type 1 NL4-3 replication in four T-cell lines: Rate and efficiency of entry, a major determinant of permissiveness, *J. Virol.* **65:**3900–3902.

Stach, R. M., and Rowley, D. A., 1993, A first or dominant immunization. II. Induced immunoglobulin carries transforming growth factor β and suppresses cytolytic T cell responses to unrelated alloantigens, *J. Exp. Med.* **178:**841–852.

Stadnyk, A. W., and Gauldie, J., 1991, The acute phase protein response during parasitic infection, *Immunol. Today* **12(3):**A7–A12.

Stoiber, H., Schneider, R., Janatova, J., and Dierich, M. P., 1995, Human complement proteins C3b, C4b, Factor H and properdin react with specific sites in gp120 and gp41, the envelope proteins of HIV-1, *Immunobiology* **193:**98–113.

Thiry, L., Clerc, J. C., Content, S., and Tack, L., 1978, Factors which influence inactivation of vesicular stomatitis virus by fresh human serum, *Virology* **87:**384–393.

Thormar, H., Wisniewski, H. M., and Lin, F. H., 1979, Sera and cerebro-spinal fluids from normal uninfected sheep contain a visna virus-inhibiting factor, *Nature* **279:**245–246.

Tremblay, M., and Wainberg, M. A., 1990, Neutralization of multiple HIV-1 isolates from a single subject by autologous sequential sera, *J. Infect. Dis.* **162:**735–737.

Tsai, W.-P., Conley, S. R., Kung, H. F., Garrity, R. R., Growth cycle studies of a primary isolate of HIV-1 reveal the dynamics of virus infectivity, replication rates and transmission in reciprocal primary cultures of blood-derived macrophages and peripheral blood mononuclear cells, (submitted).

Tsang, M. L., Evans, L. A., McQueen, P., Hurren, L., Byrne, C., Penny, R., Tindall, B., and Cooper, D. A., 1994, Neutralizing antibodies against sequential autologous human immunodeficiency virus type 1 isolates after seroconversion, *J. Infect. Dis.* **170(5):**1141–1147.

Tyring, S. K., Cauda, R., Tumbarello, M., Ortona, L., Kennedy, R. C., Chanh, T. C., and Kanda, P., 1991, Synthetic peptides corresponding to sequences in HIV envelope gp41 and gp120 enhance in vitro production of interleukin-1 and tumor necrosis factor but depress production of interferon-alpha, interferon-gamma and interleukin-2, *Viral Immunol.* **4(1):**33–42.

VanCott, T. C., Polonis, V. R., Loomis, L. D., Michael, N. L., Nara, P. L., and Birx, D. L., 1995, Differential role of V3-specific antibodies in neutralization assays involving primary and laboratory-adapted isolates of HIV type 1, *AIDS Res. Hum. Retrovir.* **11:**1379–1391.

Velupillai, P., and Harn, D. A., 1994, Oligosaccharide-specific induction of interleukin 10 production by B220+ cells from schistosome-infected mice: A mechanism for regulation of CD4+ T-cell subsets, *Proc. Natl. Acad. Sci. USA* **91:**18–22.

von Sydow, M., Sönnerborg, A., Gaines, H., and Strannegard, Ö., 1991, Interferon-alpha and tumor necrosis factor-alpha in serum of patients in various stages of HIV-1 infection, *AIDS Res. Hum. Retrovir.* **7:**375–380.

Waterston, R. H., 1970, Antigen competition: A paradox, *Science* **170:**1108.

Welsh, R. M., Cooper, N. R., Jensen, F. C., Oldstone, M. B. A., 1975, Human serum lyses RNA tumor viruses, *Nature* **257:**612–614.

Wolfs, T. F., Zwart, G., Bakker, M., and Gousmit, J., 1992, HIV-1 genomic RNA diversification following sexual and parenteral virus transmission, *Virology* **189:**103–110.

Wu, S.-C., Spouge, J. L., Conley, S. R., Tsai, W. P., Merges, M. J., Nara, P. L., 1995, Human plasma enhances the infectivity of primary human immunodeficiency virus type 1 isolates in peripheral blood mononuclear cells and monocyte-derived macrophages, *J. Virol.* **69:**6054–6062.

Yilma, T., Owens, S., and Adams, S. D., 1985, Preliminary characterization of a serum viral inhibitor in goats, *Am. J. Vet. Res.* **46(11):**2360–2362.

Yu, X., Yuan, X., Matsuda, Z., Lee, T.-H., and Essex, M., 1992, The matrix protein of human immunodeficiency virus type 1 is required for incorporation of viral envelope protein into mature virions, *J. Virol.* **66:**4966–4971.

Zhang, H., Zhang, Y., Spicer, T. P., Abbott, Z., Abbott, M., and Poiesz, B. J., 1993, Reverse transcription takes place within extracellular HIV-1 virions: Potential biological significance, *AIDS Res. Hum. Retrovir.* **9:**1286–1296.

Zhang, L. Q., MacKenzie, P., Cleland, A., Holmes, E. C., Leigh-Brown, A. J., and Simmonds, P., 1993, Selection for specific sequences in the external envelope protein of human immunodeficiency virus type 1 upon primary infection, *J. Virol.* **67:**3345–3356.

Zhu, T., Mo, H., Wang, N., Nam, D. S., Cho, Y., Koup, R. A., and Ho, D. D., 1993, Genotypic and phenotypic characterization of HIV-1 in patients with primary infection, *Science* **261:** 1179–1181.

Zwart, G., Back, N. K., Ramautarsing, C., Valk, M., van der Hoek, L., and Goudsmit, J., 1994, Frequent and early HIV-1MN neutralizing capacity in sera from Dutch HIV-1 seroconverters is related to antibody reactivity to peptides from the gp120 V3 domain, *AIDS Res. Hum. Retrovir.* **10:**245–251.

CHAPTER 13

AUTOIMMUNITY IN HIV

CHARLES S. VIA and ARIF R. SARWARI

1. INTRODUCTION

Autoimmunity has been referred to as a dyslexic process of self-recognition (Katz, 1993), that is, a disturbance in the ability to communicate such that the immune system is unable to properly "read" the markers on partner cells. Such communication is essential for immune reactions against foreign antigens to occur in a normal manner as well as for tolerance to occur following self-recognition. The role of viruses in the etiopathogenesis of human autoimmune disease has long been suspected but as yet unproven. However, recent evidence suggests that viruses may be involved in the pathogenesis of Sjogren's syndrome (Talal, 1991). If viruses do in fact play a role in inducing autoimmune disease, the mechanism(s) involved remain to be elucidated. In particular, it is not clear whether virus-induced autoimmunity is the result of a normal antiviral immune response that subsequently cross-reacts with self-antigens or whether viruses actually induce abnormal communication within the immune system such that self-antigens are misread as foreign.

With the advent of the human immunodeficiency virus (HIV) epidemic, there has been great interest in the role of retroviruses in the induction of autoimmune disease. Studies have shown that 30% of Sjogren's syndrome patients and 36% of patients with systemic lupus erythematosus (SLE) have serum antibodies to the p24 Gag protein of HIV-1 (Talal *et al.*, 1990a,b). Further, there is evidence that endogenous retroviral sequences are important in immunoregulation, suggesting that these sequences may also be important in the disordered immune regulation characteristic of Sjogren's syndrome and SLE (Talal *et al.*, 1992).

With the growing understanding of the immunopathogenesis of the acquired immunodeficiency syndrome (AIDS), the possibility of HIV-induced autoimmunity has been given increasing attention. A number of recent reviews have examined the evidence for HIV-related autoimmunity and the possible clinical relevance, if any (Edelman and Zolla-Pazner,

CHARLES S. VIA • Research Service, Baltimore VA Medical Center, and Division of Rheumatology and Clinical Immunology, University of Maryland School of Medicine, Baltimore, Maryland 21201. ARIF R. SARWARI • Division of Infectious Diseases, University of Maryland School of Medicine, Baltimore, Maryland 21201.

Immunology of HIV Infection, edited by Sudhir Gupta. Plenum Press, New York, 1996.

1989; Eales and Parkin, 1988; Schattner and Bentwich, 1993; Atlan *et al.*, 1994; Dalgleish, 1993). In this chapter we update the current literature, examine some of the suggested mechanisms of HIV-induced autoimmunity, and discuss parallels with some of the known murine models of autoimmune disease.

2. HUMORAL AUTOANTIBODIES IN HIV INFECTION

The wide variety of serum autoantibodies reported in patients infected with HIV is indeed remarkable, especially in the setting of an immunodeficiency state. For example, antibodies against T cells, B cells, erythrocytes, neutrophils, and platelets have been demonstrated in HIV-infected patients (Edelman and Zolla-Pazner, 1989; Eales and Parkin, 1988; Schattner and Bentwich, 1993; Atlan *et al.*, 1994; Dalgleish, 1993). Serum antibodies to many nuclear, cytoplasmic, and cell membrane antigens have been found by a variety of assays in HIV-seropositive patients. Positivity rates for antinuclear antigen (ANA) have ranged from 13 to 23% (Kopelman and Zolla-Pazner, 1988; Savige *et al.*, 1994) and have mostly been low titer. In one series, antihistone antibodies were found in 50% of HIV-positive cases, compared to 24% of seronegative male homosexuals and 5% of heterosexual controls (Argov *et al.*, 1991). Among those with lupuslike autoantibodies, lupuslike disease is uncommon (Edelman and Zolla-Pazner, 1989). More recently, it has been noted that there is extensive amino acid sequence homology between HIV-1 gp120/41 and over 33% of a U1RNA-associated 70-kDa splicing protein (Douvas and Takehana, 1994). The latter is a target of autoimmune anti-RNP antibodies in patients with mixed connective disease/overlap syndrome. The sequence homology between these two antigens suggest a role for antibody cross-reactivity in the pathogenesis of HIV-induced autoimmunity.

Rheumatoid factors and more often circulating immune complexes have also been noted in HIV-positive patients (Gupta and Licorish, 1984; Yu *et al.*, 1986; Solder *et al.*, 1990). However, their incidence is also increased in HIV-negative homosexuals and may reflect repeated exposure to multiple antigens (Euler *et al.*, 1985).

Antiphospholipid antibodies, usually determined as either anticardiolipin antibodies or "lupus-anticoagulant," are found in a large proportion of AIDS patients as well as in HIV-positive, asymptomatic male homosexuals (Daraco *et al.*, 1992; Stimmler *et al.*, 1989; Canoso and Zon, 1987; Cohen *et al.*, 1986). Detection rates may vary from 50% to as high as 93% of HIV-positive patients. The absence of these antibodies in HIV-negative homosexuals suggests a more direct link to HIV infection. However, the stage of disease does not appear to correlate with the presence of the antibody (Daraco *et al.*, 1992).

Antibodies directed against neural targets are being recognized with increasing frequency and are of considerable interest given the myriad of neurological findings associated with HIV infection. HIV-infected patients with serum antibodies recognizing an immunodominant portion of HIV-1 gp41 (amino acids 584–602) were shown to bind to the surface of human astrocytoma cells. A monoclonal antibody generated against this portion of gp41 was found to react with antigens expressed by astrocytes in human brain tissue and by various human astrocytoma cell lines (Spehar and Strand, 1994). A 100-kDa protein was identified as the target antigen of this monoclonal antibody. Similarly, monoclonal antibodies derived from the blood of three HIV-infected patients which bound to amino acids 644–664 were shown to cross-react with human astrocytes (Eddleston *et al.*, 1993). Since a major function of astrocytes is to maintain appropriate neuronal function, these data suggest that anti-HIV antibodies may play a role in AIDS dementia. Moreover, antibodies against myelin basic protein, the putative antigenic target in multiple sclerosis, have been reported in the sera and CSF of HIV-infected patients (Mathiesen *et al.*, 1989).

An intriguing observation is the presence of an increased incidence of gastric parietal cell antibodies among AIDS patients (Lake-Bakaar *et al.*, 1988). In that study, over 50% of AIDS patients demonstrated parietal cell antibodies compared to 2–4% of a matched healthy population. The AIDS patients also have markedly higher fasting gastric pH and lower stimulated gastric juice volume and acid output compared to controls. The significance and implications of these observations have yet to be determined.

3. RELATIONSHIP OF AUTOANTIBODIES TO DISEASE IN HIV INFECTION

A major unresolved question is whether any of the autoantibodies present in HIV-infected patients actually mediate clinically important disease or are merely markers of altered immune system function. Some autoantibodies have been associated more strongly with clinical disease than others. An etiologic role of antiplatelet antibodies in the pathogenesis of idiopathic thrombocytopenic purpura has been proposed (Karpatkin and Nardi, 1992). Similarly, autoantibodies against neuronal targets have been felt to be involved in the neuropsychological complications of AIDS (Kumar *et al.*, 1989). However, such causal associations remain difficult to prove. Furthermore, despite the presence of numerous autoantibodies associated with HIV infection, no clear correlation of any of these autoantibodies with clinical disease has been demonstrated thus far. Savige *et al.* (1994) have demonstrated that while the presence of ANA, ANCA, and anti-GBM antibodies was not uncommon in HIV-infected individuals, there was no association with the clinical manifestations of the corresponding autoimmune disease. In addition, there was no correlation with the immunologic status of the individual, or with survival. Similarly, the presence of antiphospholipid antibodies did not appear to be related to thromboembolic phenomenon. Lastly, some groups have failed to find evidence of the relevant autoantibodies in HIV-positive patients who have clinical symptoms suggestive of autoimmune mediated disease (Canoso and Zon, 1987; Solinger *et al.*, 1988; Berman *et al.*, 1988).

4. MECHANISMS OF AUTOIMMUNITY

Viral infections may theoretically induce autoimmunity through three broad, non-mutually exclusive mechanisms: virus-induced changes in host self-antigenic structures nonspecific polyclonal B-cell activation, antiviral antibodies which cross-react with self-antigens. While a comprehensive mechanistic understanding of HIV-induced autoimmunity is not yet at hand, evidence does exist to support these mechanisms.

Though autoantibodies are considered to be the hallmark of autoimmune disease, lymphocytes that produce autoantibodies are common and are part of the normal B-cell repertoire (Schattner, 1987; Madaio *et al.*, 1986). Nonspecific activation of these precursor B cells leads to the production of a variety of autoantibodies that are often transient, of low titer, frequently IgM, and of little clinical significance. This type of nonspecific B-cell activation could occur in response to infectious or noninfectious stimuli. Thus, it is possible that a portion of the humoral autoimmunity observed in HIV-infected patients may be the result of various cofactors observed in HIV-seropositive patients such as sexual practices, infection, drugs, and neoplasms. Additionally, HIV has been shown to be a polyclonal B-cell activator (Yarchoan *et al.*, 1986); thus, HIV by itself may account for the generation of autoantibodies. In this case, the autoantibodies described above may be no more than markers of the B-cell hyperactivity that precedes AIDS.

Harmful effects of reactive antiviral antibodies may be mediated through molecular mimicry or through the formation of antiidiotypic antibodies. HIV-infected individuals have been shown to exhibit antibodies to lymphocytes including antibodies against T and B cells (Pruzanski *et al.*, 1984), and to MHC-related epitopes (Golding *et al.*, 1988). The identification of specific antibodies against the CD4-bearing lymphocyte or to the CD4 molecule itself (Callahan *et al.*, 1992; Thiriart *et al.*, 1988) may have a more direct bearing on the pathogenesis of AIDS. Such antibodies probably arise as a result of an antiidiotypic response to anti-HIV antibodies (Ziegler and Stites, 1986) and may play a role in the progressive lymphoid cell depletions and dysfunction observed in AIDS. Infectivity of HIV is related to the ability of the outer envelope proteins, gp41/120, to bind to the CD4 molecule. Thus, these proteins must resemble to a certain extent the natural ligand for the CD4 molecule, a nonpolymorphic region on MHC class II. The antigen binding site of anti-HIV antibodies would be expected to resemble the CD4 molecule and to bind to MHC class II molecules. Further, antiidiotypic antibodies formed in response to anti-HIV antibodies would resemble MHC class II molecules and bind to CD4 molecules. In support of this hypothesis, antibodies directed against MHC class II molecules (Golding *et al.*, 1988) and CD4+ T cells (Callahan *et al.*, 1992; Thiriart *et al.*, 1988) have been demonstrated in HIV-infected patients. In addition, mice that have never been exposed to HIV have been reported to make antibodies to HIV gp120 following the injection of allogeneic cells and the development of anti-MHC antibodies (Kion and Hoffmann, 1991).

Anti-CD4 antibodies are thought to play a role in mediating the decline in $CD4^+$ T cells characteristic of AIDS. In a recent study (Muller *et al.*, 1994), 60% of HIV-infected patients exhibited anti-CD4 antibodies. These patients presented with significantly lower numbers of circulating $CD4^+$ T cells and the degree of antibody reactivity was negatively correlated with $CD4^+$ T-cell numbers. These workers also reported (Muller *et al.*, 1993) that greater than 90% of HIV-infected patients had increased levels of surface-bound Ig on $Cd4^+$ T cells and 72% had anti-CD4 antibodies in plasma. A highly significant correlation was found between surface Ig on $CD4^+$ T cells and plasma anti-CD4 antibody levels, suggesting that the majority of increased surface Ig in HIV-infected patients is of autoantibody in nature and is associated with $CD4^+$ T-cell depletion.

Although not all workers have observed a clear association between anti-CD4 antibody levels and $CD4^+$ T-cell depletion in HIV-infected patients, recent studies by Zagury *et al.* provide a mechanistic framework by which such an association could occur. These authors identified a pentapeptide, SLWDQ, which is required for the functioning of the CD4-MHC class II complex and is present on both HIV-1 gp120 and CD4 molecules (Zagury *et al.*, 1992, 1993); HIV-infected patients but not controls exhibited autoantibodies and cytotoxic T lymphocytes directed against autologous $CD4^+$ T cells carrying the SLWDQ peptide. Anti-CD4 SLWDQ antibodies were fond to strongly inhibit T-cell activation, leading these workers to postulate that these autoantibodies could contribute to the defective T-cell function seen in AIDS patients.

HIV-infected individuals have also been reported to exhibit another form of cross-reactive antibody formation involving recognition of IgG $F(ab)_2$ determinants. Susal *et al.* (1992) have demonstrated that patients with AIDS have significantly higher IgG antibodies to the $F(ab)_2$ portion of IgG than do HIV-positive patients without AIDs, HIV-negative patients, or cohorts. A striking inverse association was also noted between the level of anti-$F(ab)_2$ activity and the $CD4^+$ T-cell count. These authors (Susal *et al.*, 1993) also found a high degree of sequence homology between HIV-1, immunoglobulins, and the T-cell antigen receptor. Based on findings that the appearance of anti-Fab autoantibodies and attachment of gp120/immunoglobulin/complement complexes on $CD4^+$ T cells are associated with the decrease in numbers of $CD4^+$ T cells in HIV-infected patients, these authors hypothesize that cross-reactive anti-$F(ab)_2$ autoantibodies and circulating gp120 molecules are responsible for a destabilization of the immune network and the elimination of $CD4^+$ T cells. However, it cannot as yet be decided whether the decrease in $CD4^+$ cells is caused by anti-$F(ab)_2$ antibodies or whether the increase anti-$F(ab)_2$ antibodies is the consequence of an autoimmune dysregulation related to the loss of $CD4^+$ cells.

Additional potentially important homologies have been recognized, such as the common structural pattern in the sequences of the HIV-1 Nef proteins and the β-chain of HLA class II molecules (Vega *et al.*, 1990), the HIV envelope protein and interleukin-2 (Reither *et al.*, 1986) and the envelope protein gp120 and IgG CH1 domain (Solder *et al.*, 1990). The clinical significance of these homologies remains unknown. However, from the scientific evidence available, it is conceivable that the molecular mimicry between HIV-1 proteins and molecules important in immune response and regulation may lead to the generation of an autoimmune response directed at the immune system and resulting in compromised immune function.

5. SIMILARITIES BETWEEN HIV INFECTION AND MURINE MODELS OF AUTOIMMUNITY

As mentioned above, alloimmunization of mice results in antibodies which react with HIV gp120 which are thought to reflect anti-MHC antibodies which cross-react on HIV determinants as outlined above (Kion and Hoffmann, 1991). However, it has been noted that mice undergoing an *in vivo* allogeneic response (allogeneic effect) exhibit additional similarities to HIV-infected individuals (Katz, 1993). In particular, the parent-into-F_1 model of murine graft-versus-host disease results in defective T-cell function *in vitro* which is also observed in HIV-infected patients, humans with SLE, several murine models of SLE, and a murine model of AIDS (MAIDS) (Via and Shearer, 1988a,b; Clerici *et al.*, 1989; Via *et al.*, 1990, 1993). The *in vitro* T-cell defect common to these entities was manifested as defective proliferation and IL-2 production in response to MHC self-restricted antigens (e.g., tetanus, influenza, trinitrophenol) but a strong T-cell response to alloantigen. The ramifications of this T-cell defect are not completely understood, although recent work suggests that this T-cell defect occurs in the context of increased IL-4 and IL-10 (Th2) cytokine production (Bermas *et al.*, 1994; Clerici *et al.*, 1993, 1994; Clerici and Shearer, 1993; Rus *et al.*, 1995) which may inhibit *de novo* IL-2 (Th1) cytokine production *in vitro*. The significance of these observations is not to undermine HIV as the etiologic agent in AIDS pathogenesis but rather to underscore the notion that some of the immune alterations in HIV-infected individuals may represent common immunoregulatory disturbances which are HIV nonspecific. These observations indicate that therapeutic strategies may be of benefit which are not targeted specifically to HIV but rather are aimed at restoring the altered balance in cytokine production. If successful, such an approach might prove useful in other autoimmune conditions such as SLE.

REFERENCES

Argov, S., Schattner, A., Burstein, R., Handzel, Z. T., Shoenfeld, Y., and Bentwich, Z., 1991, Autoantibodies in male homosexuals and HIV infection, *Immunol. Lett.* **30**:31–36.

Atlan, H., Gersten, M. J., Salk, P. L., and Salk, J., 1994, Mechanisms of autoimmunity and AIDS: Prospects for therapeutic intervention, *Res. Immunol.* **145**:165–183.

Berman, A., Espinoza, L. R., Diaz, J. D., Aguilar, J. L., Rolando, T., Vasey, F. B., Germain, B. F., and Lockey, R. F., 1988, Rheumatic manifestation of human immunodeficiency virus infection, *Am. J. Med.* **85**:59–64.

Bermas, B. L., Petri, M., Goldman, D., Mittleman, B., Miller, M., Stocks, N., Via, C. S., and Shearer, G. M., 1994, T helper cell dysfunction in systemic lupus erythematosus (SLE): Relation to disease activity, *J. Clin. Immunol.* **14**:169–177.

Callahan, L. N., Roderiquez, G., Mallinson, M., and Norcross, M. A., 1992, Analysis of HIV-induced autoantibodies to cryptic epitopes on human CD4, *J. Immunol.* **149**:2194–2202.

Canoso, R. T., and Zon, L. I., 1987, Anticardiolipin antibodies associated with HTLV-III infection, *Br. J. Haematol.* **65**:495–498.

Clerici, M., and Shearer, G. M., 1993, A Th1→Th2 switch is a critical step in the etiology of HIV infection, *Immunol. Today* **14**:107–111.

Clerici, M., Stocks, N. I., Zajac, R. A., Boswell, R. N., Lucey, D. R., Via, C. S., and Shearer, G. M., 1989, Detection of three distinct patterns of T helper cell dysfunction in asymptomatic, human immunodeficiency virus-seropositive patients: Independence of CD4+ cell numbers and clinical staging, *J. Clin. Invest.* **84**:1892–1899.

Clerici, M., Hakim, F. T., Venzon, D. J., Blatt, S., Hendrix, C. W., Shearer, G. M., and Wynn, T. A., 1993, Changes in interleukin-2 and interleukin-4 production in asymptomatic, human immunodeficiency virus-seropositive individuals, *J. Clin. Invest.* **91**:759–765.

Clerici, M., Wynn, T. A., Berzofsky, J. A., Blatt, S. P., Hendrix, C. W., Sher, A., Coffman, R. L., and Shearer, G. M., 1994, Role of interleukin-10 in T helper cell dysfunction in asymptomatic individuals infected with the human immunodeficiency virus, *J. Clin. Invest.* **93**:768–775.

Cohen, A. J., Philips, T. M., and Kressler, C. M., 1986, Circulating coagulation inhibitors in the acquired immunodeficiency syndrome, *Ann. Intern. Med.* **104**:175–180.

Dalgleish, A. G., 1993, What is the role of autoimmunity in AIDS? *Autoimmunity* **15**:237–244.

Daraco, J. C., Gutierrez-Cebollada, J., Yazbeck, H., Berges, A., and Rubies-Prat, J., 1992, Anticardiolipin antibodies and acquired immunodeficiency syndrome: Prognostic marker or association with HIV infection? *Infection* **20**;140–142.

Douvas, A., and Takehana, Y., 1994, Cross-reactivity between autoimmune anti-U1 sn RNP antibodies and neutralizing epitopes of HIV-1 gp 120/41, *AIDS Res. Hum. Retrovir.* **10**:253–262.

Eales, L., and Parkin, J. M., 1988, Current concepts in the immunopathogenesis of AIDS and HIV infection, *Br. Med. Bull.* **44**:38–55.

Eddleston, M., de La Torre, J. C., Xu, J. Y., Dorfman, N., Notkins, A., Zolla-Pazner, S., and Oldstone, M. B., 1993, Molecular mimicry accompanying HIV-1 infection: human monoclonal antibodies that bind to gp 41 and to astrocytes, *AIDS Res. Hum. Retrovir.* **9**:939–944.

Edelman, A. S., and Zolla-Pazner, S., 1989, AIDS: A syndrome of immune dysregulation, dysfunction and deficiency, *FASEB J.* **3**:22–30.

Euler, H. H., Kern, P., Loffler, H., and Dietrich, H., 1985, Precipitable immune complexes in healthy homosexual men, acquired immune deficiency syndrome and the related lymphadenopathy syndrome, *Clin. Exp. Immunol.* **59**:267–275.

Golding, H., Robey, F. A., Gates, F. T., Linder, W., Beining, P. R., Hoffman, T., and Golding, B., 1988, Identification of homologous regions in human immunodeficiency virus 1 gp41 and human MHC class II beta 1 domain. I. Monoclonal antibodies against the gp 41-derived peptide and patient's sera react with native HLA class II antigens, suggesting a role for autoimmunity in the pathogenesis of acquired immune deficiency syndrome, *J. Exp. Med.* **167**:914–923.

Gupta, S., and Licorish, K., 1992, Circulating immune complex in AIDS [letter], *N. Engl. J. Med.* **310**:1530–1531.

Karpatkin, S., and Nardi, M., 1992, Autoimmune anti-HIV-1 gp 120 antibody with antiidiotype-like activity in sera and immune complex of HIV-1 related immunologic thrombocytopenia, *J. Clin. Invest.* **89**:356–364.

Katz, D. H., 1993, AIDS: Primarily a viral or autoimmune disease? *AIDS Res.* **9**:489–493.

Kion, T. A., and Hoffmann, G. W., 1991, Anti-HIV and anti-anti-MHC antibodies in alloimmune and autoimmune mice, *Science* **253**:1138–1140.

Kopelman, R. A., and Zolla-Pazner, S., 1988, Association of human immunodeficiency virus infection and autoimmune phenomena, *Am. J. Med.* **84**:82–88.

Kumar, M., Resnick, L., Loewenstein, D. A., Berger, J., and Eisdorfer, C., 1989, Brain-reactive antibodies and the AIDS dementia complex, *J. Acq. Immune Defic. Syndr.* **2**:469–471.

Lake-Bakaar, G., Quadros, E., Beidas, S., Eisakr, M., Tom, W., Wilson, D. E., Dincsoy, H. P., Cohen, P., and Straws, E. W., 1988, Gastric secretory failure in patients with the acquired immunodeficiency syndrome (AIDS), *Ann. Intern. Med.* **109**:502–504.

Madaio, M. P., Schattner, A., Schattner, M., and Schwartz, R. S., 1986, Lupus serum and normal human serum contain anti-DNA antibodies with the same idiotypic marker, *J. Immunol.* **137**:2535–2540.

Mathiesen, T., Sonnerborg, A. S., and Wahren, B., 1989, Detection of antibodies against myelin basic protein and increased level of HIV IgG antibodies and HIV antigen after stabilization of immune complexes in sera and CSF of HIV infected patients, *Viral Immunol.* **2**:1–9.

Muller, C., Kukel, S., and Bauer, R., 1993, Relationship of antibodies against CD4+ T cells in HIV-infected patients to markers of activation and progression: Autoantibodies are closely associated with CD4 cell depletion, *Immunology* **79**:248–254.

Muller, C., Kukel, S., and Bauer, R., 1994, Antibodies against $CD4^+$ lymphocytes in plasma of HIV-infected patients are related to CD4 cell depletion in vivo, *Immunol. Lett.* **41**:163–167.

Pruzanski, W., Jacobs, J., and Lorne, P., 1984, Lymphocytotoxic antibodies against peripheral blood B and T lymphocytes in homosexuals with AIDS and ARC, *AIDS Res. Hum. Retrovir.* **1**:211–220.

Reither, W. E., Blalock, J. E., and Brunck, T. K., 1986, Sequence homology between acquired immunodeficiency syndrome virus envelope protein and interleukin 2, *Proc. Natl. Acad. Sci. USA* **83**:9188–9192.

Rus, V., Svetic, A., Nguyen, P. H., Gause, W. C., and Via, C. S., 1995, Kinetics of Th1 and Th2 cytokine production during the early course of acute and chronic murine graft-versus-host disease: Regulatory role of donor CD8+ T cells, *J. Immunol.* **155**:2396–2406.

Savige, J. A., Chang, L., Horns, S., and Crowe, S. M., 1994, Anti-nuclear anti-neutrophil cytoplasmic and anti-glomerular basement membrane antibodies in HIV-infected individuals, *Autoimmunity* **18**:205–211.

Schattner, A., 1987, The origin of autoantibodies, *Immunol. Lett.* **14**:143–153.

Schattner, A., and Bentwich, Z., 1993, Autoimmunity in human immunodeficiency virus infection, *Clin. Aspects Autoimmun.* **5**:19–27.

Solder, B., Marschang, P., Wachter, H., Dierich, M. P., Nayyar, S., Lewin, I. V., and Stanworth, D. R., 1990, Antiviral antibodies in HIV (HTLV-III) infection possess autoantibody activity against CH1 domain determinant in human Ig4: Possible immunological consequences, *Immunol. Lett.* **23**:9–20.

Solinger, A. M., Adams, L. E., Freidman-Kien, A. E., and Hess, E. V., 1988, Acquired immune deficiency syndrome (AIDS) and autoimmunity—Mutually exclusive entities? *J. Clin. Invest.* **8**:32–42.

Spehar, T., and Strand, M., 1994, Cross-reactivity of anti-human immunodeficiency virus type 1 gp41 antibodies with human astrocytes and astrocytoma cell lines, *J. Virol.* **68**:6262–6269.

Stimmler, M. M., Quismorio, F. P., McGehee, F. P., Boylent, T., and Sharma, O. P., 1989, Anticardiolipin antibodies in acquired immunodeficiency syndrome, *Arch. Intern. Med.* **149**:1833–1835.

Susal, C., Daniel, V., Ober, H. H., Terness, P., Huth-Kuhne, A., Zimmerman, R., and Opelz, A., 1992, Striking inverse association of IgG-anti-Fabγ antibodies and CD4 cell counts in patients with acquired immunodeficiency syndrome (AIDS)/AIDS related complex, *Blood* **79**:954–957.

Susal, C., Kropelin, M., Daniel, V., and Opelz, A., 1993, Molecular mimicry between HIV-1 and antigen receptor molecules: A clue to the pathogenesis of AIS, *Vox Sang.* **65**:10–17.

Talal, N., 1991, Aids and Sjogren's syndrome, *Bull. Rheum. Dis.* **40**:6–8.

Talal, N., Dauphinee, M. J., Dang, H., Alexander, S. S., Hart, D. J., Garry, R. F., 1990a, Detection of serum antibodies to retroviral protein in patients with primary Sjogren's syndrome (autoimmune exocrinopathy), *Arthritis Rheum.* **33**:774–781.

Talal, N., Garry, R. F., Schur, P. H., Alexander, S., Dauphinee, M. J., Livas, J. H., Ballester, A., Takei, M., and Dang, H., 1990b, A conserved idiotype and antibodies to retroviral proteins in systemic lupus erythematosus, *J. Clin. Invest.* **85**:1866–1871.

Talal, N., Flescher, E., and Dang, H., 1992, Are endogenous retroviruses involved in human autoimmune disease? *J. Autoimmun.* **5(Suppl A)**:61–66.

Thiriart, C., Goudsmit, J., Schellekens, P., Barin, F., Zagury, D., de Wilde, M., and Bruck, C., 1988, Antibodies to soluble CD4 in HIV-1 infected individuals, *AIDS* **2**:345–350.

Vega, M. A., Guiso, R., and Smith, T. F., 1990, Autoimmune response in AIDS [letter], *Nature* **345**:26.

Via, C. S., and Shearer, G. M., 1988a, Functional heterogeneity of L3T4+ T cells in MRL-*lpr*/*lpr* mice: L3T4+ T cells suppress major histocompatibility complex-self-restricted L3T4+ T helper cell function in association with autoimmunity, *J. Exp. Med.* **168**:2165–2181.

Via, C. S., and Shearer, G. M., 1988b, T-cell interactions in autoimmunity—Insights from a murine model of graft-versus-host disease, *Immunol. Today* **9**:207–212.

Via, C. S., Morse, H. C., III, and Shearer, G. M., 1990, Altered immunoregulation and autoimmune aspects of HIV infection: Relevant murine models, *Immunol. Today* **11**:250–255.

Via, C. S., Tsokos, G. C., Bermas, B. L., Clerici, M., and Shearer, G. M., 1993, T cell-antigen-presenting cell interactions in human systemic lupus erythematosus, *J. Immunol.* **151**:3914–3922.

Yarchoan, R., Redfield, R. R., and Broder, S., 1986, Mechanisms of B cell activation in patients with acquired immunodeficiency syndrome and related disorders, *J. Clin. Invest.* **78**:439–447.

Yu, J. R., Lennett, E. T., and Karpatkin, S., 1986, Anti-F(ab′) antibodies in thrombocytopenic patients at risk for acquired immunodeficiency syndrome, *J. Clin. Invest.* **77**:1756–1761.

Zagury, J. F., Cantalloube, H., Bernard, J., Bizzini, B., Mornon, J. P., and Zagury, D., 1992, A striking identity between HIV-1 envelope glycoprotein gp120 and its CD4 receptor, *Lancet* **340**:483–484.

Zagury, J. F., Bernard, J., Achour, A., Astgen, A., Lachgar, A., Fall, L., Carelli, C., Issing, W., Mbika, J. P., Cantalloube, H., Picard, O., Gourbil, A., Guignon, J. M., Cozette, J., Faure, J. P., Biou, D., Carlotti, M., Callebaut, I., Mornon, J. P., Burny, A., Feldman, M., Bizzini, B., and Zagury, D., 1993, HIV-1 induced immune suppression may result from autoimmune disorders including anti-SLWDQ autoantibodies, *Biomed. Pharmacother.* **47**:93–99.

Ziegler, J. L., and Stites, D. P., 1986, Hypothesis: AIDS is an autoimmune disease directed at the immune system and triggered by a lymphotropic retrovirus, *Clin. Immunol. Immunopathol.* **41**:305–313.

CHAPTER 14

CYTOKINE CASCADES IN HIV INFECTION

GUIDO POLI and ANTHONY S. FAUCI

1. INTRODUCTION

Since the recognition of human immunodeficiency virus type 1 (HIV-1) as the causative agent of the acquired immunodeficiency syndrome (AIDS), the search to unravel the viral and cellular factors controlling its replicative ability has become an important goal of both basic and applied research. Cellular transcription factors, such as NF-κB, as well as viral proteins may activate HIV transcription in cells latently infected with HIV. In this regard, certain studies indicate that latent infection is the predominant virological state of infected cells *in vivo* (Embretson *et al.*, 1993), although a fraction of cells express virus in lymphoid organs throughout the entire course of disease (Pantaleo *et al.*, 1993). In addition, plasma viremia can be detected throughout the entire course of HIV disease (Piatak *et al.*, 1993). Furthermore, both HIV and $CD4^+$ T lymphocytes (the predominant target of HIV infection) rapidly turn over, particularly in the advanced stages of HIV disease. This has been ascertained from studies on patients treated with antiretroviral agents, including nucleoside analogues and inhibitors of HIV protease that can dramatically, but transiently, decrease circulating HIV until drug-resistant strains repopulate the plasma compartment (Wei *et al.*, 1995; Ho *et al.*, 1995). However, residual virus invariably is unaffected by antiretroviral agents, at least those currently in use. An important component of this residual HIV burden is in the form of integrated proviruses that exist in the latent state and are refractory to agents such as zidovudine that affect the preintegration steps of HIV replication (Perno *et al.*, 1989; Poli *et al.*, 1989). Thus, understanding the regulatory mechanisms controlling HIV replication in infected cells that are not actively expressing virus will be critical for the development of strategies aimed at eliminating or at least curtailing virus spread in the host.

In addition to infecting $CD4^+$ T lymphocytes, HIV can productively or latently infect cells belonging to the mononuclear phagocyte lineage, i.e., monocytes/macrophages. The biology of HIV infection in these latter cells is substantially different from that of $CD4^+$ T

GUIDO POLI • AIDS Immunopathogenesis Unit, DIBIT, San Raffaele Scientific Institute, 20127 Milan, Italy.
ANTHONY S. FAUCI • Laboratory of Immunoregulation, National Institute of Allergy and Infectious Diseases, National Institutes of Health, Bethesda, Maryland 20892.

Immunology of HIV Infection, edited by Sudhir Gupta. Plenum Press, New York, 1996.

cells, and has been described in detail elsewhere in this volume. Some important peculiarities of *in vitro* infected macrophages relative to CD4+ T lymphocytes can be summarized as follows (Poli and Fauci, 1992): (1) susceptibility to non-syncytium-inducing (NSI) strains of HIV; (2) absence or reduced cytopathicity, resulting in a sustained production of virus for several weeks of culture; (3) active production and accumulation of virions in intracytoplasmic vacuolar compartments (observed both *in vitro* and *in vivo*), resulting in a potential "Trojan horse" phenomenon whereby viral reservoirs are hidden from immune surveillance mechanisms and are refractory to certain antiviral agents (Biswas *et al.*, 1992; Gendelman *et al.*, 1988; Gartner *et al.*, 1986); (4) different anatomical distribution in that macrophages are the predominant infected cells in nonlymphoid tissue such as the brain, and contribute significantly to the pool of infected cells in important organs such as the lung and the liver.

A third class of cells has gained increasing attention because of their potential role in the pathogenesis of HIV disease; this group is represented by the multiple subtypes of dendritic cells, including epidermis-associated Langerhans cells (Tschachler *et al.*, 1987), the latter having been recently proposed to represent a key initial target cell for the E clade of HIV-1 that is the predominant HIV-1 subtype in Thailand (Cohen, 1995). A subset of circulating dendritic cells of bone marrow origin appears to be extremely sensitive to HIV infection (Patterson and Knight, 1987; Macatonia *et al.*, 1990) and another fraction of dendritic cells can adsorb and very efficiently transmit virions to naive CD4+ T cells (Weissman *et al.*, 1995a). Another class of cells that are distinct from bone marrow-derived dendritic cells are called *follicular dendritic cells*. These cells reside in the germinal centers of lymphoid tissue and are the predominant antigen-presenting cells to B lymphocytes. It has been demonstrated that these cells trap extracellular HIV virions on their cell surface and constitute an important viral reservoir (Pantaleo *et al.*, 1993; reviewed in Pantaleo *et al.*, 1994).

Thus, any rational approach to controlling HIV infection *in vivo* must take into account the different cell types that are targeted by the virus, and the peculiarity of the diverse biologies of HIV infection of these cell types. Studies on HIV pathogenesis over the past 10 years have indicated that when the HIV provirus integrates into the genome of its different target cells (predominantly T lymphocytes and macrophages), it becomes functionally dependent on a variety of cellular mechanisms that control the state of activation of the cell (Bukrinsky *et al.*, 1991; Zack *et al.*, 1990; Koyanagi *et al.*, 1988; Folks *et al.*, 1986, 1987). Under these circumstances, the functional network and cascades of cytokines, which homeostatically regulate and coordinate the different cellular components of the immune system, have become a subject of major interest in AIDS research. Up to the present time, at least three major areas of interface between HIV and the cytokine network have been identified: (1) HIV-induced dysregulation of cytokine production, (2) cytokine modulation of HIV replication, and (3) cytokines as important autocrine/paracrine growth factors for HIV-associated tumors, namely, Kaposi's sarcoma and B-cell lymphomas. This latter subject will not be further discussed herein, as it has been reviewed extensively by others (Ensoli *et al.*, 1992).

2. CYTOKINE CASCADES

2.1. Cytokine Cascades in Infected Individuals

A defect in the production of the T-cell growth factor interleukin 2 (IL-2) was described early in the AIDS epidemic and was explained in simplest terms by the impaired function of the immune system in HIV-infected individuals (Lane *et al.*, 1985; Murray *et al.*, 1984). This defect in IL-2 production was proposed as a partial explanation for the lack of proliferative responses to recall antigens and mitogens that was observed in these patients (Clerici and Shearer, 1993; Lane *et al.*, 1985). Defective production of IL-2 has been confirmed by several studies, including studies of cytokine gene expression in lymph node cells of HIV-infected individuals at various stages of disease (Graziosi *et al.*, 1994). More recently, a second cytokine important for T-cell activation, IL-12, has been found to be defective in HIV-infected individuals (Chehimi *et al.*, 1994). Of interest, *in vitro* HIV infection of $CD4^+$ T cells and macrophages has resulted in impaired production of IL-2 (Oyaizu *et al.*, 1990) and IL-1 (Chehimi *et al.*, 1994), respectively, supporting a direct role of the virus in the etiology of this aspect of immune dysfunction.

It is more complex and less clear whether class I (α, β) and II (γ) interferons (IFN) are decreased or increased during HIV infection. Increased levels of "acid-labile" IFN-α in HIV-infected individuals have been described in a number of studies analogous to certain autoimmune diseases, such as systemic lupus erythematosus and rheumatoid arthritis (Capobianchi *et al.*, 1992; Krown *et al.*, 1991; Rinaldo *et al.*, 1990). These findings have been interpreted as an indication of the presence of autoimmune pathogenic components in HIV disease. In contrast, defective production of acid-resistant IFN-α has been observed both in patients and as a consequence of *in vitro* infection (Gendelman *et al.*, 1990). Furthermore, IFN-α can effectively prevent HIV replication *in vitro* (Shirazi and Pitha, 1992; Poli *et al.*, 1989; Ho *et al.*, 1985) and has been administered with some success to HIV-infected individuals (Lane *et al.*, 1988).

High levels of IFN-γ, or of its related markers of cellular activation such as neopterin, have been observed in infected individuals (Buhl *et al.*, 1993; Krown *et al.*, 1991; Emilie *et al.*, 1990; Fuchs *et al.*, 1988; Lane *et al.*, 1985). However, the *in vitro* production of IFN-γ from PBMC or T cells isolated from these patients is usually not efficient (Lane *et al.*, 1985; Murray *et al.*, 1984). This apparent discrepancy is likely explained by the observation that *in vivo* production of IFN-γ is accounted for mostly by activated $CD8^+$ T lymphocytes infiltrating the hyperplastic germinal centers of lymph nodes (Emilie *et al.*, 1990). These findings also underscore the fact that conflicting information sometimes results when different anatomic compartments, such as peripheral blood and lymphoid organs, are studied.

IL-12 and IFN-γ are the cytokines selectively secreted by $CD4^+$ T-cell clones of the T-helper (Th)l type (Trinchieri, 1993; Sher *et al.*, 1992). Notwithstanding the high levels of IFN-γ production by $CD8^+$ T cells in lymph nodes of HIV-infected individuals, the defective production of these two cytokines has been used as an argument in support of a "shift" from a Thl- to a Th2-type pattern of cytokine secretion over the course of progression of HIV disease (Clerici and Shearer, 1993). This hypothesis is based on the observed predominance of Th2-related cytokines (IL-4 and IL-10) in the advanced stages of disease (Clerici and Shearer, 1993) and is supported by the defective expression of IL-12 observed both *in vitro* and *in vivo* after HIV infection (Chehimi *et al.*, 1994). The functional consequences of this shift in cytokine patterns are the predominance of a humoral response and, conversely, a loss of a presumably protective cell-mediated immune response. This theory is based largely on studies conducted in both animal and human $CD4^+$ T-cell clones secreting preferentially either Thl- or Th2-type cytokines and tipping the balance either in favor of or against one versus the other type of immune response. Susceptibility to or protection from parasitic infection in animal models has been achieved by influencing Thl- or Th2-dependent immune responses, for example, as a consequence of IL-4 or IL-12 administration, respectively (Trinchieri, 1993; Sher *et al.*, 1992). In HIV infection and

AIDS, the currently available information does not support either the existence of a clear-cut shift in Th1-to-Th2 pattern of cytokine secretion or a clear importance in the progression of HIV disease. For example, in one study, a Th1-to-Th0 (mixed patterns of HIV production) shift has been observed in T-cell clones derived from infected individuals (Maggi *et al.*, 1994). In another study, a PCR-based *ex vivo* study of cytokine expression in PBMC and lymph node cells found evidence of Th1 and Th2 patterns of cytokine secretion throughout the course of HIV disease without evidence of a shift in pattern associated with disease progression (Graziosi *et al.*, 1994). Similarly, defective production of the Th2-related cytokine IL-4 and/or loss of IL-4-producing cells has been independently observed in HIV-infected individuals (Re *et al.*, 1992). Furthermore, in the human system IL-10 cannot be considered as a cytokine selectively expressed by Th2 T-cell clones, as is the situation in mice. In humans, IL-10 is secreted by a number of T-cell and non-T-cell types not strictly related to Th1/Th2 immune responses. In this regard, $CD8^+$ T cells can secrete Th2 cytokines in patients with advanced HIV disease and a hyper-IgE syndrome associated with the virtual absence of $CD4^+$ T cells (Paganelli *et al.*, 1995; Manetti *et al.*, 1994).

Proinflammatory cytokines such as tumor necrosis factor-α (TNF-α) and IL-1β appear to be upregulated during both *in vivo* and *in vitro* HIV infection. *In vitro*, interaction of either HIV or its gp120 envelope with CD4 on the surface of macrophages has been demonstrated to induce the expression of TNF-α and IL-1β (Clouse *et al.*, 1989b; Merrill *et al.*, 1989; Folks *et al.*, 1987), suggesting that the increased levels of these cytokines detected in HIV-infected individuals may be the consequence of both viral replication and shedding of HIV envelope components. Furthermore, interaction of recombinant gp120 with a component of the B-cell surface other than CD4 (B lymphocytes do not express CD4) has resulted in increased production of TNF-α and IL-6 (Rieckmann *et al.*, 1991). This gp120-dependent upregulation of cytokine expression was observed selectively in B cells purified from HIV-infected individuals in that gp120 did not affect production of TNF-α or IL-6 from activated B cells obtained from healthy volunteers or from people with autoimmune diseases (Rieckmann *et al.*, 1991). Although the precise nature of the molecule interacting with gp120 on the B-cell surface was not defined, it is likely to be a cell surface immunoglobulin specific for gp120, based on previous observations that a large component of B-cell responses in HIV-infected individuals is directed toward HIV proteins (Amadori *et al.*, 1991).

Several investigators have described the presence of increased levels of proinflammatory cytokines in the plasma, cerebrospinal fluid, epithelial lining fluid of the lung, intestinal mucosa, and/or spontaneously secreted from PBMC or lung alveolar macrophages of HIV-infected individuals (Agostini *et al.*, 1995; Barcellini *et al.*, 1995; Aukrust *et al.*, 1994; Gallo *et al.*, 1994; McGowan *et al.*, 1994; Reka *et al.*, 1994; Krown *et al.*, 1991; Scott-Algara *et al.*, 1991; Honda *et al.*, 1990; Voth *et al.*, 1990). In addition, soluble receptors (R) for TNF and other cytokines have been found to be increased in the body fluids of infected individuals. Soluble cytokine receptors are usually present at concentrations 100- to 1000-fold higher on a molar basis than their related cytokines; they are currently being appreciated as important markers for monitoring inflammatory and infectious diseases (Barcellini *et al.*, 1995; Aukrust *et al.*, 1994; Pizzolo *et al.*, 1994; Scott-Algara *et al.*, 1991; Honda *et al.*, 1990). However, the biological role of soluble cytokine receptors remains to be fully elucidated. In contrast to their *in vitro* function as cytokine inhibitors (based on their ability to complex with their respective cytokine with a high affinity, thus preventing its biological function), *in vivo* they likely represent carrier molecules stabilizing and prolonging the half-life of cytokines. In addition to TNF-R, elevated concentrations of CD30, the soluble form of another member of the TNF-R family, have been described as a marker of HIV disease progression, independent of $CD4^+$ T-cell counts (Pizzolo *et al.*, 1994). In general, the increased levels of soluble cytokine receptors observed in HIV-infected individuals underlie a state of chronic cellular activation that is an important component of the pathogenesis of HIV disease (Fauci, 1993). Conversely, this state of chronic activation likely contributes to the state of persistent HIV replication, perpetuating a vicious cycle of activation and virus replication that propagates the progression of HIV disease (Fauci, 1993; see below).

2.2. Cytokine Cascades *in Vitro*

Isolation of HIV from infected individuals has been accomplished through cocultivation of their PBMC with allogeneic mitogen-stimulated PBMC (PHA blasts) maintained in IL-2-containing medium. In contrast, HIV does not spread efficiently in resting PBMC (Folks *et al.*, 1986). Furthermore, the addition to HIV-infected cell cultures of antibodies (Ab) that neutralize IFN-α was found to enhance viral replication (Markham *et al.*, 1986). These early findings had therefore already shed important light on certain aspects of HIV/host cell interaction. First, HIV requires activated cells in order to spread efficiently; IL-2 appeared to be an essential factor that positively regulated viral propagation. Next, certain host factors, such as IFN-α, either endogenously released or experimentally added to the cultures, could exert a negative effect on virus replication. Both of these points have been further confirmed and characterized.

Cell lines of T-lymphocytic and monocytic lineages that were chronically infected by HIV (such as ACH-2 and U1, respectively) have been important tools for the study of the relationship between various cytokines and the regulation of HIV expression. In this regard, among several recombinant or purified cytokines, TNF-α or TNF-β (also known as cachectin and lymphotoxin-α, respectively) induced HIV expression severalfold from an almost undetectable baseline to levels comparable to those achieved by stimulation by the phorbol ester PMA (Clouse *et al.*, 1989a; Folks *et al.*, 1989). The common denominator at the molecular level of both the PMA- and TNF-stimulatory effects on virus expression was soon identified as the cellular transcription factor NF-κB (Duh *et al.*, 1989; Griffin *et al.*, 1989; Osborn *et al.*, 1989). This transcription factor, which encompasses a large and complex family of molecules, resides in a latent form in the cytoplasm of a variety of cell types conjugated to an inhibitory molecule, termed I-κB (Siebenlist *et al.*, 1994). Cellular activation, such as that observed as a consequence of PMA or TNF stimulation, leads to the physical dissociation of I-κB from NF-κB, which exists in its prototypical form as a p50–p65 heterodimer complex. NF-κB migrates to the nucleus of the cell where it binds to specific consensus sequences present in the promoter regions of several cellular and viral genes, including HIV-1, HIV-2, and SIV. Binding of NF-κB leads to either initiation or potentiation of gene transcription (Siebenlist *et al.*, 1994). Thus, the interaction between TNF and TNF-R on the surface of an infected cell leading to activation of NF-κB and the enhancement of HIV replication via the binding of NF-κB to the promoter region of the viral long terminal repeat (LTR) has served as the paradigm of cytokine-mediated control of HIV replication. Recently, cross-linking of another member of the TNF-R family, CD30, whose soluble form is elevated in HIV-infected individuals (Pizzolo *et al.*, 1994), has been shown to activate HIV expression in the ACH-2 T-cell line through an NF-κB-mediated mechanism (Biswas *et al.*, 1995). Confirmatory evidence of an inductive effect of CD30 on HIV replication has been subsequently obtained in primary cells from HIV-infected individuals

(Maggi *et al.*, 1995). Other TNF-R family members which were expressed on the surface of these cells either were ineffective in inducing HIV expression, as was the case with CD27, or induced death in the absence of virus expression, as was the case with CD95 (Fas/Apo-1) (Biswas *et al.*, 1995; Kobayashi *et al.*, 1990). In a previous study, we had compared TNF-α and TNF-β to CD95 stimulation in U1 cells, and observed a similar dichotomy of effects (Biswas *et al.*, 1994). Synergistic and concomitant induction of virus expression and cell death was observed in U1 cells costimulated with TNF-α/-β and IFN-γ, with microscopic features of both apoptosis and necrosis, extending earlier observations in acutely infected cell lines (Matsuyama *et al.*, 1989). No substantial differences could be detected in infected U1 cells versus uninfected parental U937 cells, in that several uninfected clones of the latter cell line showed comparable sensitivity to either TNF- or CD95-mediated lysis in the presence or absence of IFN-γ (Biswas *et al.*, 1994). These studies indicate that apart from a certain degree of redundancy in terms of molecular pathways triggered by TNF and related molecules such as CD30 that lead to virus expression, other molecules and cytokines can affect HIV-infected cells with completely different outcomes, such as induction of cell death as is observed by cross-linking of CD95.

Other cytokines and factors capable of inducing HIV expression have been associated with activation of NF-κB. Among these, IL-1β was shown to activate NF-κB in a murine cell line (Osborn *et al.*, 1989). In contrast, we have not observed activation of NK-κB following IL-1α or IL-1β stimulation of the promonocytic U1 cell line, either alone or in combination with other cytokines or glucocorticoid hormones, although high levels of virus expression were observed under these conditions (Poli *et al.*, 1994). In the latter experiments, IL-1 appeared to induce virus expression predominantly by posttranscriptional mechanisms.

HIV replication in mononuclear phagocytes is influenced by a broader spectrum of cytokines compared to T lymphocytes. In addition to TNF-α, IL-1 and IL-6 exert inductive effects on both primary monocyte-derived macrophages (MDM) infected *in vitro* and in the chronically infected U1 cell line (Schuitemaker *et al.*, 1992; Poli *et al.*, 1990b). As mentioned above for IL-1, these molecules appear to affect predominantly posttranscriptional steps in the HIV life cycle in that accumulation of HIV mRNAs (as in the case of IL-1) or viral proteins and particles (as observed for IL-6) was not coupled with substantial changes at the transcriptional level (Koostra *et al.*, 1994; Poli *et al.*, 1990b). These observations were confirmed in costimulatory conditions, where IL-1 plus IL-6 or glucocorticoids induced levels of virion production comparable to or even greater than those observed after stimulation with TNF-α (Kinter *et al.*, unpublished observations). In addition, synergistic induction of virion production was observed in U1 cells costimulated with TNF-α and IL-6, and this effect was correlated with enhanced HIV transcription (Poli *et al.*, 1990b). Thus, complex molecular pathways appear to characterize the interaction between HIV and the cytokine network. In this scenario it is likely that the NF-κB-dependent pathway represents the best identified, but certainly not the exclusive, pathway through which cellular activation leads to increased virus expression.

An additional level of complexity is suggested by the observation that several cytokines do not exert unidimensional effects on virus replication; with certain cytokines dichotomous effects of induction or suppression can be seen as a function of the experimental conditions. In this regard, transforming growth factor-β (TGF-β), IFN-γ, IL-4, and IL-10 have been described as dichotomous regulators of virus replication (Table I). Primary MDM or U937 cells that had been stimulated with TGF-β prior to infection with HIV have shown

TABLE I. Cytokines and Cytokine-Related Molecules with Regulatory Effects on HIV Replication

Cytokine	Effects on[a] T cells	Effects on[a] Macrophages	References
IL-1 α/-β	α	α	1–4
IL-2	α	↔	2, 5, 6
IL-3	↔	α	1,7
IL-4	α	α↓	8, 9
IL-6	↔	α	2, 10
IL-10	↔	α↓	11–14
IL-12	α	↔	5, 8, 15
IL-13	↔	↓	16, 17
IFN-α/-β	↓	↓	18–23
IFN-γ	α↓	α↓	7, 24–20
TGF-β	α↓	α↓	27–29
GM-CSF	↔	α	1, 7
M-CSF	↔	α	30, 31
TNF-α/-β	α	α	2, 4, 24–26, 32–36
CD30 (ligand)	α	↔	37

[a]α, enhancement of HIV replication; ↓, suppression of HIV replication; ↔, not tested or no substantial effects have been reported.
1. Folks, T. M., 1987 2. Kinter, A. L., 1995a 3. Poli, G., 1994 4. Schuitemaker, H., 1992 5. Kinter, A. L., 1995b 6. Kovacs, J. A., 1995 7. Koyanagy, Y., 1988 8. Foli, A., 1995 9. Kazai, F., 1992 10. Poli, G., 1990b 11. Koostra, N. A., 1994 12. Saville, M. W., 1994 13. Weissman, D., 1994 14. Weissman, D., 1995b 15. Chehimi, J., 1994 16. Montaner, L. J., 1993 17. Mikovits, J. A., 1994 18. Gendelman, H. E., 1990 19. Ho, D. D., 1985 20. Markham, P. D., 1986 21. Poli, G., 1989 22. Shirazi, Y., & Pitha, P. M., 1992 23. Williams, G. J., & Colby, C. B., 1989 24. Biswas, P., 1992 25. Biswas, P., 1994 26. Vyakarnam, A., 1990 27. Lazdins, J. K., 1991 28. Poli, G., 1991 29. Poli, G., 1992 30. Gendelman, H. E., 1988 31. Gruber, M. F., 1995 32. Butera, S. T., 1993 33. Clouse, K. A., 1989a 34. Folks, T. M., 1989 35. Griffin, G. E., 1989 36. Poli, G., 1990a 37. Biswas, P., 1995.

substantial enhancement of virus production throughout several days of culture; in contrast, when TGF-β was added to the same MDM or U937 cultures approximately 1 week following infection, inhibition of virus production was observed (Poli *et al.*, 1991, 1992). Others have observed only inductive effects in MDM stimulated with TGF-β (Lazdins *et al.*, 1991). Effects similar to those induced by TGF-β were observed in MDM and U937 cultures treated with retinoic acid (RA), a well-known differentiating agent (Poli *et al.*, 1992). In the U937-derived chronically infected cell line U1, both TGF-β and RA profoundly suppressed HIV expression induced by PMA or cytokines including IL-1 and IL-6, but not TNF-α (Poli *et al.*, 1992), indicating a similarity of mechanisms of these agents in controlling HIV replication in mononuclear phagocytes.

A similar time-dependency of inductive or suppressive effects on HIV replication in MDM was reported for cells exposed to IFN-γ (Koyanagi *et al.*, 1988). A later study using U1 cells has shown that IFN-γ induces accumulation of HIV RNA, proteins, and virions, although it also exerted an apparent suppressive effect on virus expression in cells stimulated by PMA (Biswas *et al.*, 1992). However, this "inhibitory" effect was explained by a major effect exerted by IFN-γ in redirecting the predominant site of virion production from the cell surface to intracytoplasmic vacuoles (Biswas *et al.*, 1992). Thus, at least for IFN-γ in the U1 model system, the dichotomy of effects was only apparent and not real, and the net effect was, in fact, an upregulation of virus expression.

Opposite regulatory effects on HIV expression have also been described by different groups for IL-4 and IL-10 (Foli *et al.*, 1995; Koostra *et al.*, 1994; Mikovits *et al.*, 1994; Saville *et al.*, 1994; Kazazi *et al.*, 1992; Schuitemaker *et al.*, 1992; Novak *et al.*, 1990). In our experience, IL-10 could inhibit HIV production in MDM cultures at concentrations sufficient to cause a block of secretion of endogenous cytokines, including TNF-α and IL-6, whereas enhancement of virus production could be observed at lower concentrations of IL-10 (Weissman *et al.*, 1994, 1995b). In U1 cells, IL-4 and IL-10 do not directly affect virus production, but potently synergize with TNF-α or IL-1 in increasing virus production (Weissman *et al.*, 1995b).

Other molecules, such as IFN-α/-β, IL-13, and the IL-1 receptor antagonist (IL-1Ra), have been described as suppressors of virus replication in T cells and/or mononuclear phagocytes (Kinter *et al.*, 1995a; Mikovits *et al.*, 1994; Poli *et al.*, 1989, 1994; Montaner *et al.*, 1993; Shirazi and Pitha, 1992; Williams and Colby, 1989) and may represent the counterparts of clear-cut inductive cytokines, such as TNF-α and IL-1.

Therefore, it seems plausible that a hierarchy of cytokines may exist in which a few molecules, such as TNF-α and IL-1β, are capable of directly inducing virus replication, whereas several others, including IFN-γ, IL-4, IL-10, and TGF-β, act as positive or negative modulators depending on the cytokine milieu and/or the functional state of the infected cell. It is of interest to note that neither the Th1-related cytokine IFN-γ nor Th2-related cytokines such as IL-4 play an exclusively positive or negative role in the regulation of virus replication *in vitro*, adding complexity to the issue of the role of "cytokine profile" in the determination of the course of HIV disease.

2.3. Autocrine/Paracrine Regulation of HIV Replication

An important step in understanding how cytokines affect virus replication and the pathogenesis of HIV disease *in vivo* has been the demonstration of their ability to regulate HIV expression endogenously in an autocrine/paracrine manner. In this regard, autocrine/paracrine regulation by cytokines of tissue remodeling, wound repair, as well as chronic inflammation and tumorigenesis has been broadly demonstrated under a variety of conditions. AIDS-related neoplasma are associated with an abundant production of cytokines and related factors that are capable in turn of upregulating tumor growth (Ensoli *et al.*, 1992). In this regard, IL-6 may play a special role in that it is involved in the neoplastic growth of both B-cell lymphomas and Kaposi's sarcoma, the two most frequently observed neoplasma in HIV-infected individuals. Clinical trials aimed at interfering with the production of IL-6 are ongoing and have already shown some evidence of efficacy in terms of normalization of metabolic and immunologic parameters (Marfaing-Koka *et al.*, 1995). A variety of other mechanisms including production and uptake of HIV-1 Tat protein have been postulated to play a role in the establishment and growth of these tumors (Ensoli *et al.*, 1992), and in the induction of cytokines, such as IL-6 (Scala *et al.*, 1994) and TNF-β (Buonaguro *et al.*, 1994).

Early studies demonstrated that PMA stimulation of U1 and ACH-2 cell lines resulted in the secretion of TNF-α that preceded the production of HIV particles in the culture supernatants. In the same experiments, inhibition of the bioactivity of endogenously produced TNF-α by anti-TNF-α neutralizing Ab resulted in a substantial, although not complete, inhibition of HIV production (Poli *et al.*, 1990a). It was later demonstrated that the residual HIV-inductive activity of PMA (not dependent on TNF-α) was blocked by either TGF-β or RA (Poli *et al.*, 1991, 1992). More recently, it has also been observed that under certain experimental conditions, IL-10 can induce moderate levels of HIV in U1 cells. In this study, no detectable endogenous TNF-α was measured in the culture supernatants; however, increased expression of membrane-bound (mb) TNF-α as well as TNF-R-1, which appeared first on the cell surface and then was shed in the culture supernatants, was observed (Barcellini *et al.*, in press). Of note is the fact that mbTNF-α, which is expressed together with TNF-R on the surface of lung alveolar macrophages obtained from HIV-infected individuals (Agostini *et al.*, 1995), has previously been implicated in driving HIV replication in acutely infected U937 cells (Tadmori *et al.*, 1991); furthermore, mbTNF-α has been implicated as a major trigger of B-cell activation in HIV infection (Macchia *et al.*, 1993). Similar findings were also independently observed in the OM10.1 persistently infected promyelocytic cell line (Butera *et al.*, 1993).

We have also observed recently that activation of HIV expression in U1 cells by costimulation with granulocyte–macrophage colony-stimulating factor (GM-CSF) and lipopolysaccharide (LPS) derived from gram-negative microorganisms resulted in the induction of virus expression independently of TNF-α production (Goletti *et al.*, 1996) as previously reported by others (Pomerantz *et al.*, 1990). However, virus production under these culture conditions was demonstrated to depend on the secretion of endogenous IL-1β. Of note is the fact that antiinflammatory cytokines such as TGF-β, IL-4, and IL-13, but not IL-10, suppressed virus expression induced by GM-CSF plus LPS, and this effect was correlated with a substantial increase of endogenous IL-1Ra to levels sufficient to neutralize the endogenously produced IL-1β (Goletti *et al.*, 1996). Thus, in this *in vitro* system, modulation of the ratio between IL-1β and IL-1Ra concentrations by proinflammatory stimuli (GM-CSF and LPS) or antiinflammatory cytokines (TGF-β, IL-4, IL-13) was shown to directly upregulate, respectively, HIV expression.

Autocrine/paracrine regulation of HIV replication has been demonstrated to occur in primary MDM (Gruber *et al.*, 1995). Evidence of a positive regulatory role of TNF-α, TNF-β, and IFN-γ were previously shown in primary PBMC and purified $CD4^+$ T cells infected *in vitro* (Vyakarnam *et al.*, 1990). We have recently confirmed and extended these observations in primary PBMC stimulated in the presence of exogenous IL-2 in the absence of mitogenic stimulation. Under these conditions, replication of both T-cell-tropic, SI and macrophage-tropic, NSI strains of HIV was tightly regulated by endogenous cytokines, including TNF-α, IFN-γ, and IL-1β, as demonstrated by neutralization studies with specific mAb and IL-1Ra (Kinter *et al.*, 1995a). It should be emphasized that the only biological effect known for IL-1Ra is the selective competitive blockade of type 1 IL-1R (Dinarello and Thompson, 1991). Therefore, the inhibitory effects of IL-1Ra on HIV replication in PBMC must be the consequence of a selective inhibition of IL-1-mediated effects. In support of this hypothesis, similar findings were obtained by blocking type 1 IL-1R with specific mAb, whereas blockade of type 2 IL-1R did not result in any detectable effect (Kinter *et al.*, 1995a), consistent with the interpretation that type 2R act as "receptor decoys" or "deceptors" for IL-1 (Colotta *et al.*, 1994).

Autocrine/paracrine regulation of HIV replication by different endogenous cytokines, including TNF-α, IL-1β, IFN-γ, and cytokine antagonists such as IL-1Ra (Gruber *et al.*, 1995; Kinter *et al.*, 1995a,b; Weissman *et al.*, 1995b; Goletti *et al.*, 1996), is likely to be a component of the relentless ability of HIV to replicate in the HIV-infected host, justifying the design of strategies aimed at diminishing viral load and replication by modifying certain host factors such as the level of cellular activation and the secretion of endogenous cytokines. As described in detail elsewhere in this volume, cytokines such as IL-2 have entered the arena of experimental clinical trials on the basis of encouraging results, such as the ability to stably rescue $CD4^+$ T lymphocytes to near-normal or normal levels in asymptomatic subjects with $CD4^+$ T-cell counts greater than 200 cells/μl (Kovacs *et al.*, 1995). As expected, administration of IL-2 resulted in transient increases in viremia necessitating the concomitant administration of antiretroviral drugs. It has been observed that *in vitro* production of endogenous cytokines, such as TNF-α, are elevated following IL-2 administration (H. C. Lane, personal communication). Of interest, secretion of endogenous TNF-α in PBMC cultures established *ex vivo* from individuals treated with IL-2 appeared to mediate HIV replication, as indicated by the ability of anti-TNF-α mAb to block virus production (H. C. Lane, personal communication); these observations are similar to the results observed in an IL-2-dependent model of *in vitro* PBMC infection (Kinter *et al.*, 1995a). If these results are confirmed and fully validated, they will imply that HIV replication *in vivo* might be controlled by cytokines or cytokine antagonists in addition to antiretroviral agents. In this regard, targeting host factors such as cytokines may allow one to circumvent the extremely difficult problem of HIV drug resistance, which has now been experienced with virtually all antiretrovirals tested.

3. CYTOKINES, $CD8^+$ T CELLS, AND DENDRITIC CELLS

3.1. CD8-Dependent Nonlytic Suppression of HIV Replication

In addition to the killing of HIV-infected cells by an MHC-restricted cytolytic T-lymphocyte (CTL) mechanism, $CD8^+$ T cells have been described that are capable of exerting profound suppressive effects on HIV replication in $CD4^+$ T cells of infected individuals *in vitro* (reviewed by Blackbourn *et al.*, 1994). The suppressive effect has been described in both HIV and SIV infection, is independent of MHC restriction, can be mediated by activated $CD8^+$ T-cell-derived culture supernatants, and has recently been linked to C-C chemokines (Cocchi *et al.*, 1995) or IL-16 (Baier *et al.*, 1995). Evidence that the suppressive effect results from an inhibition of HIV transcription has been reported (Blackbourn *et al.*, 1994).

$CD8^+$ T-cell-dependent suppression of virus replication may account for the apparently larger number of latently infected cells that are present in different organs and body compartments compared to a much smaller fraction of cells (100:1) actively expressing HIV (Embretson *et al.*, 1993). In this regard, it is important to point out that infiltration of $CD8^+$ T cells in the germinal centers of lymph nodes has been described as a pathological hallmark of HIV infection (Emilie *et al.*, 1990). These cells are clearly activated, as indicated by their phenotype and by the high levels of cytokines, particularly IFN-γ, that they express (Graziosi *et al.*, 1994; Emilie *et al.*, 1990). Therefore, it is conceivable that these infiltrating $CD8^+$ T cells exert a nonlytic suppressive effect on infected $CD4^+$ T cells in the lymph node microenvironment. In support of this concept, it has recently been demonstrated that under conditions in which cultures are stimulated with IL-2 alone, HIV could be readily isolated from either PBMC or lymph node mononuclear cells (LNMC) of HIV-infected individuals only when the $CD8^+$ T cells were removed (Kinter *et al.*, 1995b). In the same studies, the effect of IL-2 was compared to that of IL-12 with regard to the $CD8^+$ T-cell-dependent suppressive effect on virus replication. Of interest is the fact that IL-2 exerted a profound enhancement of the $CD8^+$ T-cell-mediated suppressive effect which overcame its inductive activity on virus replication (Fig. 1); conversely, IL-12 increased virus replication [as also independently reported by others (Foli *et al.*, 1995)] even in the presence of $CD8^+$ T cells and did not appear to modulate efficiently the $CD8^+$ T-cell suppressive effect (Kinter *et al.*, 1995b). An attractive hypothesis is that IL-2-dependent enhancement of the $CD8^+$ T-cell-mediated suppressive effect may be a component of the effects observed in patients receiving intermittent infusions of IL-2. In these patients, as described in detail elsewhere in this volume, stable increase of $CD4^+$ T cells and only transient peaks of viremia in the absence of a substantial increased viral load have been reported (Kovacs *et al.*, 1995).

3.2. Dendritic Cells and HIV Infection

Although a separate chapter will discuss the role of dendritic cells (DC) in HIV infection, certain aspects of their role in the pathogenesis of HIV disease may be related to the modulation of their function by cytokines. In an *in vitro* model mimicking events potentially occurring in the paracortical region of the lymph nodes, peripheral blood-derived DC were pulsed with HIV and cocultured with purified resting $CD4^+$ T cells in the presence or absence of cytokines and anticytokine agents. T-cell-activating cytokines, such as IL-2, IL-4, and IL-12, increased HIV replication in these cocultures; in contrast, IL-10 blocked the endogenously produced IL-2 and DC-dependent antigen presentation resulting in inhibition of virus replication (Weissmann *et al.*, unpublished observations). In this model system, proinflammatory cytokines only moderately increased HIV replication (Weissmann *et al.*, unpublished observations). Therefore, a complex interplay may likely occur in

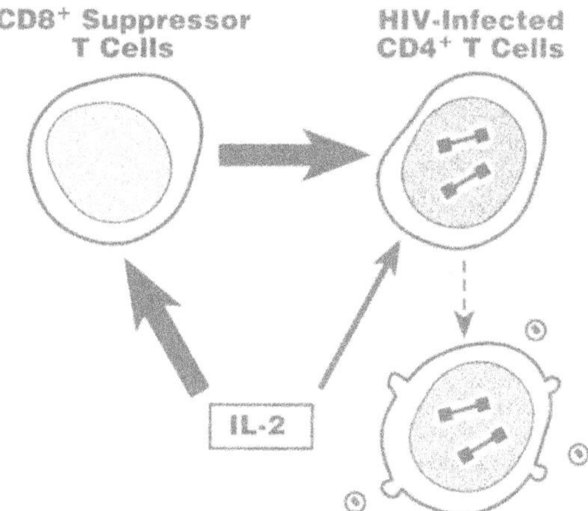

FIGURE 1. Effect of IL-2 on the $CD8^+$ T-cell suppressor phenomenon versus the induction of HIV expression. IL-2 is capable of inducing HIV replication in HIV-infected $CD4^+$ T cells; IL-2 also potentiates the $CD8^+$ T-cell nonlytic suppression of HIV replication in $CD4^+$ T cells. In HIV-infected individuals with competent $CD8^+$ T cells, the IL-2 induction of the $CD8^+$ T-cell suppressor phenomenon overrides *in vitro* the ability of IL-2 to induce the expression of HIV resulting in a net suppressor effect on HIV replication.

lymphoid organs such as lymph nodes where both $CD8^+$ T-cell-mediated and perhaps $CD8^+$ T-cell-independent suppressive signals compete with T-cell activation-dependent inductive effects on HIV replication. IL-2 appears to be a critical player in this scenario because of its ability to act potentially as both a direct and/or indirect positive and negative regulator of HIV replication.

4. CONCLUSIONS

Cytokines were originally used as simple growth factors for maintaining the viability of PBMC cultures during virus isolation or *in vitro* infection. Since then, an impressive amount of information has indicated that several cytokines may have a profound, direct or indirect, impact on the ability of HIV to replicate and on pathogenic mechanisms in HIV-infected individuals. Both proinflammatory cytokines, such as TNF-α and IL-1β, and immunoregulatory molecules, such as IL-2 and IL-12, are candidates for playing a major role in the pathogenesis of HIV infection. Selective cytokine inhibitors such as IL-1Ra or agents neutralizing TNF-α may become part of the armamentarium of therapeutic strategies aimed at the control of viral replication. Observations from both long-term nonprogressing infected individuals (Pantaleo *et al.*, 1995; Ho *et al.*, 1995) and macaques infected by *nef*-deleted SIV (Kestler *et al.*, 1991; Daniel *et al.*, 1992) suggest that a low viral burden and replication is associated, if not directly correlated, with a relatively nonpathogenic infection and perhaps even with protection from superinfection by more virulent strains of HIV. Manipulation of the cytokine network may represent a potentially important strategy in the control of HIV replication.

REFERENCES

Agostini, C., Zambello, R., Trentin, L., Cerutti, A., Enthammer, C., Facco, M., Milani, A., Sancetta, R., Garbisa, S., and Semenzato, G., 1995, Expression of TNF receptors by T cells and membrane TNF-α by alveolar macrophages suggests a role for TNF-α by regulation of the local immune responses in the lung of HIV-1 infected patients, *J. Immunol.* **154**:2928–2938.

Amadori, A., Zamarchi, R., Veronese, M. L., Panozzo, M., Barelli, A., Borri, A., Sironi, M., Colotta, F., Mantovani, A., and Chieco-Bianchi, L., 1991, B cell activation during HIV-1 infection, *J. Immunol.* **146**:57–62.

Aukrust, P., Liabakk, N. B., Muller, F., Lien, E., Espevik, T., and Froland, S. S., 1994, Serum levels of tumor necrosis factor-α (TNFα) and soluble TNF receptors in human immunodeficiency virus type 1 infection. Correlation to clinical, immunologic, and virologic parameters, *J. Infect. Dis.* **169**:420–424.

Baier, M., Werner, A., Bannert, N., Metzner, K., and Kurth, R., 1995, HIV suppression by interleukin-16. *Nature* (London) 1995; **378**:563.

Barcellini, W., Rizzardi, G. P., Marriott, B. J., Fain, C., Shattock, R. J., Meroni, P. L., Poli, G., and Dalgleish, A. G., IL-10-induced HIV-1 expression is mediated by the induction of both endogenous membrane bound TNF-α and TNF receptor type 1 in a latently infected promonocytic cell line (U1). *AIDS* (in press).

Barcellini, W., Rizzardi, G. P., Poli, G., Tambussi, G., Velati, C., Meroni, P. L., and Lazzarin, A., 1996, Cytokines and soluble receptor changes in the transition from primary to early chronic HIV type 1 infection, *AIDS Res. Hum. Retrovir.* **12**:325–330.

Biswas, P., Poli, G., Kinter, A. L., Justement, J. S., Stanley, S. K., Maury, W. J., Bressler, P., Orenstein, J. M., and Fauci, A. S., 1992, Interferon-γ modulates the expression of human immunodeficiency virus in persistently infected promonocytic cells by redirecting the production of virions to intracytoplasmic vacuoles, *J. Exp. Med.* **176**:739–750.

Biswas, P., Poli, G., Orenstein, J. M., and Fauci, A. S., 1994, Cytokine-mediated induction of human immunodeficiency virus (HIV) expression and cell death in chronically infected U1 cells: Do tumor necrosis factor alpha and gamma interferon selectively kill HIV-infected cells? *J. Virol.* **68**:2598–2604.

Biswas, P., Smith, C. A., Goletti, D., Hardy, E. C., Jackson, R. W., and Fauci, A. S., 1995, Cross-linking of CD30 induces HIV expression in chronically infected T cells, *Immunity* **2**:587–596.

Blackbourn, D. J., Mackewicz, C., Barker, E., and Levy, J. A., 1994, Human CD8+ cell non-cytolytic anti-HIV activity mediated by a novel cytokine, *Res. Immunol.* **145**:653–659.

Buhl, R., Jaffe, H. A., Holroyd, K. J., Borok, Z., Roum, J. H., Mastrangeli, A., Wells, F. B., Kirby, M., Saltini, C., and Crystal, R. G., 1993, Activation of alveolar macrophages in asymptomatic HIV-infected individuals, *J. Immunol.* **150**:1019–1028.

Bukrinsky, M. I., Stanwick, T. L., Dempsey, M. P., and Stevenson, M., 1991, Quiescent T lymphocytes as an inducible virus reservoir in HIV-1 infection, *Science* **254**:423–427.

Buonaguro, L., Buonaguro, F. M., Giraldo, G., and Ensoli, B., 1994, The human immunodeficiency virus type I Tat protein transactivates tumor necrosis factor beta gene expression through a TAR-like structure, *J. Virol.* **68**:2677–2682.

Butera, S. T., Roberts, B. D., and Folks, T. M., 1993, Regulation of HIV-1 expression by cytokine networks in a CD4+ model of chronic infection, *J. Immunol.* **150**:625–634.

Capobianchi, M. R., Mattana, P., Mercuri, F., Conciatori, G., Ameglio, F., Anke, H., and Dianzani, F., 1992, Acid lability is not an intrinsic property of interferon-alpha induced by HIV-infected cells, *J. Interferon Res.* **12**:431–438.

Chehimi, J., Starr, S. E., Frank, I., D'Andrea, A., Ma, X., MacGregor, R. R., Sennelier, J., and Trinchieri, G., 1994, Impaired interleukin-12 production in human immunodeficiency virus-infected patients, *J. Exp. Med.* **179**:1361–1366.

Clerici, M., and Shearer, G. M., 1993, A TH1→TH2 switch is a critical step in the etiology of HIV infection, *Immunol. Today* **14**:107–111.

Clouse, K. A., Powell, D., Washington, I., Poli, G., Strebel, K., Farrar, W., Barstad, P., Kovacs, J., Fauci, A. S., and Folks, T. M., 1989a, Monokine regulation of human immunodeficiency virus-1 expression in a chronically infected human T cell clone, *J. Immunol.* **142**:431–438.

Clouse, K. A., Robbins, P. B., Fernie, B., Ostrove, J. M., and Fauci, A. S., 1989b, Viral antigen stimulation of the production of human monokines capable of regulating HIV-1 expression, *J. Immunol.* **143**:470–475.

Cocchi, F., DeVico, A. L., Garzino-Demo, A., Arya, S. K., Gallo, R. C., and Lusso, P., 1995, Identification of RANTES, MIP-1α, and MIP-1β as the major HIV-suppressive factors produced by $CD8^+$ T cells. *Science* **270**:1811–1815.

Cohen, J., 1995, Differences in HIV strains may underlie disease patterns, *Science* **270**:30–31.

Colotta, F., Dower, S. K., Sims, J. E., and Mantovani, A., 1994, The type II "decoy" receptor: A novel regulatory pathway for interleukin-1, *Immunol. Today* **15**:562–566.

Daniel, M. D., Kirchhoff, F., Czajak, S. C., Sehgal, P. K., and Desrosiers, R. C., 1992, Protective effects of a live attenuated SIV vaccine with a deletion in the *nef* gene, *Science* **258**:1938–1941.

Dinarello, C. A., and Thompson, R. C., 1991, Blocking IL-1: Interleukin 1 receptor antagonist in vivo and in vitro, *Immunol. Today* **12**:404–410.

Duh, E. J., Maury, W. J., Folks, T. M., Fauci, A. S., and Rabson, A. B., 1989, Tumor necrosis α activates human immunodeficiency virus type 1 through induction of nuclear factor binding to the NF-κB sites in the long terminal repeat, *Proc. Natl. Acad. Sci. USA* **86**:5974–5978.

Embretson, J., Zupancic, M., Ribas, J. L., Burke, A., Racz, P., Tenner-Racz, K., and Haase, A. T., 1993, Massive covert infection of helper T lymphocytes and macrophages by HIV during the incubation period of AIDS, *Nature* **362**:359–362.

Emilie, D. M., Peuchmaur, M. C., Maillot, M. C., Crevon, N., Brousee, J. F., Delfraissy, J., Dormont, P., and Galanaud, P., 1990, Production of interleukins in human immunodeficiency virus-1-replicating lymph nodes, *J. Clin. Invest.* **86**:148–159.

Ensoli, B., Barillari, G., and Gallo, R. C., 1992, Cytokines and growth factors in the pathogenesis of AIDS-associated Kaposi's sarcoma, *Immunol. Rev.* **127**:147–155.

Fauci, A. S., 1993, Multifactorial nature of human immunodeficiency virus disease: Implications for therapy, *Science* **262**:1011–1018.

Foli, A., Saville, M. W., Baseler, M. W., and Yarchoan, R., 1995, Effects of the Th1 and Th2 stimulatory cytokines interleukin-12 and interleukin-4 on human immunodeficiency virus replication, *Blood* **85**:2114–2123.

Folks, T. M., Kelly, J., Benn, S., Kinter, A., Justement, J., Gold, J., Redfield, R., Sell, K., and Fauci, A. S., 1986, Susceptibility of normal human lymphocytes to infection with HTLVIII/LAV, *J. Immunol.* **136:**4049–4053.

Folks, T. M., Justement, J., Kinter, A., Dinarello, C. A., and Fauci, A. S., 1987, Cytokine-induced expression of HIV-1 in a chronically infected promonocyte cell line, *Science* **238:**800–802.

Folks, T. M., Clouse, K. A., Justement, J., Rabson, A., Duh, E., Kehrl, J. H., and Fauci, A. S., 1989, Tumor necrosis factor alpha induces expression of human immunodeficiency virus in a chronically infected T-cell clone, *Proc. Natl. Acad. Sci. USA* **86:**2365–2368.

Fuchs, D., Hansen, A., Reibnegger, G., Werner, E. R., Dierich, M. P., and Wachter, H., 1988, Neopterin as a marker for activated cell-mediated immunity: Application in HIV infection, *Immunol. Today* **9:**150–155.

Gallo, P., Sivieri, S., Rinaldi, L., Yan, X. B., Lolli, F., De Rossi, A., and Tavolato, B., 1994, Intrathechal synthesis of interleukin-10 (IL-10) in viral and inflammatory disease of the central nervous system, *J. Neurol. Sci.* **126:**49–53.

Gartner, S., Markovits, P., Markovitz, D. M., Kaplan, M. H., Gallo, R. C., and Popovic, M., 1986, The role of mononuclear phagocytes in HTLV-III/LAV infection, *Science* **233:**215–219.

Gendelman, H. E., Orenstein, J. M., Martin, M. A., Ferrua, C., Mitra, R., Phipps, T., Wahl, L. A., Lane, H. C., Fauci, A. S., Burke, D. S., Skillman, D., and Meltzer, M. S., 1988, Efficient isolation and propagation of human immunodeficiency virus on recombinant colony-stimulating factor 1-treated monocytes, *J. Exp. Med.* **167:** 1428–1441.

Gendelman, H. E., Friedman, R. M., Joe, S., Baca, L. M., Turpin, J. A., Dveksler, G., Meltzer, M. S., and Dieffenbach, C., 1990, A selective defect of interferon-α production in human immunodeficiency virus-infected monocytes, *J. Exp. Med.* **172:**1433–1442.

Goletti, D., Kinter, A. L., Hardy, E. C., Poli, G., and Fauci, A. S., 1996, Modulation of endogenous IL-1β and IL-1 receptor antagonist results in opposing effects on HIV expression in chronically infected monocytic cells. *J. Immunol.* **156:**3501–3508.

Graziosi, C., Pantaleo, G., Gantt, K. R., Fortin, J. P., Demarest, J. F., Cohen, O. J., Sekaly, R. P., and Fauci, A. S., 1994, Lack of evidence for the dichotomy of TH1 and TH2 predominance in HIV-infected individuals, *Science* **265:**248–252.

Griffin, G. E., Leung, K., Folks, T. M., Kunkel, S., and Nabel, G. J., 1989, Activation of HIV gene expression during monocyte differentiation by induction of NF-kappa B, *Nature* **339:**70–73.

Gruber, M. F., Weih, K. A., Boone, E. J., Smith, P. D., and Clouse, K. A., 1995, Endogenous macrophage CSF production is associated with viral replication in HIV-1-infected human monocyte-derived macrophages, *J. Immunol.* **154:**5528–5535.

Ho, D. D., Hartshorn, K. L., Rota, T. R., Andrews, C. A., Kaplan, J. C., Schooley, R. T., and Hirsch, M. S., 1985, Recombinant human interferon alpha-A suppresses HTLV-III replication in vitro, *Lancet* **1:**602–604.

Ho, D. D., Neumann, A. U., Perelson, A. S., Chen, W., Leonard, J. M., and Markowitz, M., 1995, Rapid turnover of plasma virions and CD4 lymphocytes in HIV-1 infection, *Nature* **373:**123–126.

Honda, M., Kitamura, K., Mizutani, Y., Oishi, M., Arai, M., Okura, T., Igarahi, K., Yasukawa, K., Hirano, T., Kishimoto, T., Mitsuyasu, R., Chermann, J.-C., and Tokunaga, T., 1990, Quantitative analysis of serum IL-6 and its correlation with increased levels of serum IL-2R in HIV-induced diseases, *J. Immunol.* **145:**4059–4064.

Kazazi, F., Mathijs, J. M., Chang, J., Malafiej, P., Lopez, A., Dowton, D., Sorrell, T. C., Vadas, M. A., and Cunningham, A. L., 1992, Recombinant interleukin 4 stimulates human immunodeficiency virus production by infected monocytes and macrophages, *J. Gen. Virol.* **73:**941–949.

Kestler, H. W., Ringler, D. J., Mori, K., Panicali, D. L., Sehgal, P. K., Daniel, M. D., and Desrosiers, R. C., 1991, Importance of the *nef* gene for maintenance of high virus loads and for development of AIDS, *Cell* **65:** 651–662.

Kinter, A. L., Poli, G., Fox, L., Hardy, E., and Fauci, A. S., 1995a, HIV replication in IL-2-stimulated peripheral blood mononuclear cells is driven in an autocrine/paracrine manner by endogenous cytokines, *J. Immunol.* **154:**2448–2459.

Kinter, A. L., Bende, S. M., Hardy, E. C., Jackson, R., and Fauci, A. S., 1995b, Interleukin-2 induces CD8-mediated suppression of HIV replication in CD4+ T cells and this effect overrides its ability to stimulate virus expression, *Proc. Natl. Acad. Sci. USA* **92:**10985–10989.

Kobayashi, N., Hamamoto, Y., Yamamoto, N., Ishii, A., Yonehara, M., and Yonehara, S., 1990, Anti-Fas monoclonal antibody is cytocidal to human immuno-deficiency virus-infected cells without augmenting viral replication, *Proc. Natl. Acad. Sci. USA* **87:**9620–9624.

Koostra, N. A., van'T Wout, A. B., Huisman, H. G., Miedema, F., and Schuitemaker, H., 1994, Interference of interleukin-10 with human immunodeficiency virus type 1 replication in primary monocyte-derived macrophages, *J. Virol.* **68**:6967–6975.

Kovacs, J. A., Baseler, M., Dewar, R. J., Vogel, S., Davey, R. T., Falloon, J., Polis, M. A., Walker, R. E., Stevens, R., Salzman, N. P., Metcalf, J. A., Masur, H. M., and Lane, H. C., 1995, Increases in CD4 T lymphocytes with intermittent course of interleukin-2 in patients with human immunodeficiency virus infection. A preliminary study, *N. Engl. J. Med.* **332**:567–575.

Koyanagi, Y., O'Brien, W. A., Zhao, J. Q., Golde, D. W., Gasson, J. C., and Chen, I. S. Y., 1988, Cytokines alter production of HIV-1 from primary mononuclear phagocytes, *Science* **241**:1673–1675.

Krown, S. E., Niedzwiecki, D., Bhalla, R., Flomenberg, B., Bundow, D., and Chapman, D., 1991, Relationship and prognostic value of endogenous interferon-α, β2-microglobulin, and neopterin serum levels in patients with Kaposi's sarcoma and AIDS, *J. Acq. Immun Defic. Syndr.* **4**:871–880.

Lane, H. C., Depper, J. M., Greene, W. C., Whalen, G., Waldmann, T. A., and Fauci, A. S., 1985, Qualitative analysis of immune function in patients with the acquired immunodeficiency syndrome. Evidence for a selective defect in soluble antigen recognition, *N. Engl. J. Med.* **313**:79–84.

Lane, H. C., Kovacs, J. A., Feinberg, J., Herpin, B., Davey, V., Walker, R., Deyton, L., Metcalf, J. A., Baseler, M., Salzman, N., Manischewitz, J., Quinnan, G., Masur, H., and Fauci, A. S., 1988, Anti-retroviral effects of interferon-α in AIDS-associated Kaposi's sarcoma, *Lancet* **2**:1218–1222.

Lazdins, J. K., Klimkait, T., Woods-Cook, K., Walker, M., Alteri, E., Cox, D., Cerletti, N., Shipman, R., Bilbe, G., and McMaster, G., 1991, In vitro effect of transforming growth factor-β on progression of HIV-1 infection in primary mononuclear phagocytes, *J. Immunol.* **147**:1201–1207.

Macatonia, S. E., Lau, R., Patterson, S., Pinching, A. J., and Knight, S. C., 1990, Dendritic cell infection, depletion and dysfunction in HIV-infected individuals, *Immunology* **71**:38–45.

Macchia, D., Almerigogna, F., Parronchi, P., Ravina, A., Maggi, E., and Romagnani, S., 1993, Membrane tumor necrosis factor-alpha is involved in the polyclonal B-cell activation induced by HIV-infected human T cells, *Nature* **363**:464–466.

McGowan, I., Radford-Smith, G., and Jewell, D. P., 1994, Cytokine gene expression in HIV-infected intestinal mucosa, *AIDS* **8**:1569–1575.

Maggi, E., Mazzetti, M., Ravina, A., Annunziato, F., De Carli, M., Piccinni, M. P., Manetti, R., Carbonari, M., Pesce, A. M., Del Prete, G., and Romagnani, S., 1994, Ability of HIV to promote to TH1 to TH0 shift and to replicate preferentially in TH2 and TH0 cells, *Science* **265**:244–248.

Maggi, E., Annunziato, F., Manetti, R., Biagiotti, R., Giudizi, M. G., Ravina, A., Almerigogna, F., Boiani, N., Alderson, M., and Romagnani, S., 1995, Activation of HIV expression by CD30 triggering in CD4+ T cells from HIV-infected individuals, *Immunity* **3**:251–255.

Manetti, R., Annunziato, F., Biagiotti, R., Giudizi, M. G., Piccinni, M. P., Giannarini, L., Sampognaro, S., Parronchi, P., Vinante, F., Pizzolo, G., Maggi, E., and Romagnani, S., 1994, CD30 expression by CD8+ T cells producing type 2 helper cytokines. Evidence for large numbers of CD8+ CD30+ T cell clones in human immunodeficiency virus infection, *J. Exp. Med.* **180**:2407–2411.

Marfaing-Koka, A., Aubin, J.-T., Grangeot-Keros, L., Portier, A., Benattar, C., Merrien, D., Agut, H., Aucouturier, P., Autran, B., Wijdened, J., Galanaud, P., and Emilie, D., 1996, In vivo role of IL-6 on the viral load and on immunological abnormalities of HIV-infected patients, *AIDS* (in press).

Markham, P. D., Salahuddin, S. Z., Veren, K., Orndorff, S. H., and Gallo, R. C., 1986, Hydrocortisone and some other hormones enhance the expression of HTLV-III, *Int. J. Cancer* **37**:67–72.

Matsuyama, T., Hamamoto, Y., Soma, G.-I., Mizuno, D., Yamamoto, N., and Kobayashi, N., 1989, Cytocidal effect of tumor necrosis factor on cells chronically infected with human immunodeficiency virus (HIV): Enhancement of HIV replication, *J. Virol.* **63**:2504–2509.

Merrill, J. E., Koyanagi, Y., and Chen, I. S. Y., 1989, Interleukin-1 and tumor necrosis factor-α can be induced from mononuclear phagocytes by human immunodeficiency virus type 1 binding to the CD4 receptor, *J. Virol.* **63**:4404–4408.

Mikovits, J. A., Meyers, A. M., Ortaldo, J. R., Minty, A., Caput, D., Ferrara, P., and Ruscetti, F. W., 1994, IL-4 and IL-13 have overlapping but distinct effects on HIV production in monocytes, *J. Leuk. Biol.* **56**:340–346.

Montaner, L. J., Doyle, A. G., Collin, M., Georges, H., James, W., Minty, A., Caput, D., Ferrara, P., and Gordon, S., 1993, Interleukin 13 inhibits human immunodeficiency virus type 1 production in primary blood-derived human macrophages in vitro, *J. Exp. Med.* **178**:743–747.

Murray, H. W., Rubin, B. Y., Masur, H., and Roberts, R. B., 1984, Impaired production of lymphokines and immune (gamma) interferon in the acquired immunodeficiency syndrome, *N. Engl. J. Med.* **310**:883–889.

Novak, R. M., Holzer, T. J., Kennedy, M. M., Heynen, C. A., and Dawson, G., 1990, The effect of interleukin 4 (BSF-1) on infection of peripheral blood monocyte-derived macrophages with HIV-1, *AIDS Res. Hum. Retrovir.* **6**:973–976.

Osborn, L., Kunkel, S., and Nabel, G. J., 1989, Tumor necrosis factor α and interleukin 1 stimulate the human immunodeficiency virus enhancer by activation of the nuclear factor kB, *Proc. Natl. Acad. Sci. USA* **86**:2336–2340.

Oyaizu, N., Chirmule, N., Kalyanaraman, V. S., Hall, W. W., Pahwa, R., Shuster, M., and Pahwa, S., 1990, Human immunodeficiency virus type 1 envelope glycoprotein gp120 produces immune defects in CD4+ T lymphocytes by inhibiting interleukin 2 mRNA, *Proc. Natl. Acad. Sci. USA* **87**:2379–2383.

Paganelli, R., Scala, E., Ansotegui, I. J., Ausiello, C. M., Halapi, E., Fanales-Belasio, E., D'Offizi, G., Mezzaroma, I., Pandolfi, F., Fiorilli, M., Cassone, A., and Aiuti, F., 1995, $CD8^+$ T lymphocytes provide helper activity for IgE synthesis in human immunodeficiency virus-infected patients with hyper-IgE, *J. Exp. Med.* **181**:423–428.

Pantaleo, G., Graziosi, C., Demarest, J. F., Butini, L., Montroni, M., Fox, C. H., Orenstein, J. M., Kotler, D. P., and Fauci, A. S., 1993, HIV infection is active and progressive in lymphoid tissue during the clinically latent stage of disease, *Nature* **362**:355–358.

Pantaleo, G., Graziosi, C., Demarest, J., Cohen, O., Vaccarezza, M., Gantt, K., Muro-Cacho, C., and Fauci, A. S., 1994, Role of lymphoid organs in the pathogenesis of human immunodeficiency virus (HIV) infection, *Immunol. Rev.* **140**:105–130.

Pantaleo, G., Menzo, S., Vaccarezza, M., Graziosi, C., Cohen, O. J., Demarest, J. F., Montefiori, D., Orenstein, J. M., Fox, C. H., Schrager, L. K., Margolik, J. B., Buchbinder, S., Giorgi, J. V., and Fauci, A. S., 1995, Studies in subjects with long-term nonprogressive human immunodeficiency virus infection, *N. Engl. J. Med.* **332**: 209–216.

Patterson, S., and Knight, S. C., 1987, Susceptibility of human peripheral blood dendritic cells to infection by human immunodeficiency virus, *J. Gen. Virol.* **68**:1177–1181.

Perno, C. F., Yarchoan, R., Cooney, D. A., Hartman, N. R., Webb, D. S., Hao, Z., Mitsuya, H., Dohns, D. G., and Broder, S., 1989, Replication of human immunodeficiency virus in monocytes. Granulocyte/macrophage colony-stimulating factor (GM-CSF) potentiates viral production yet enhances the antiviral effect mediated by 3′-azido-2′3′-dideoxythymidine (AZT) and other dideoxynucleoside congeners of thymidine, *J. Exp. Med.* **169**:933–951.

Piatak, M., Saag, M. S., Yang, L. C., Clark, S. J., Kappes, J. C., Luk, K. C., Hahn, B. H., Shaw, G. M., and Lifson, J. D., 1993, High levels of HIV-1 in plasma during all stages of infection determined by competitive PCR, *Science* **259**:1749–1754.

Pizzolo, G., Vinante, F., Morosato, L., Nadali, G., Chilosi, M., Gandini, G., Sinicco, A., Raiteri, R., Semenzato, G., Stein, H., and Perona, G., 1994, High serum levels of the soluble form of CD30 molecule in the early phase of HIV-1 infection as an independent predictor of progression to AIDS, *AIDS* **8**:741–745.

Poli, G., and Fauci, A. S., 1992, The role of monocyte/macrophages and cytokines in the pathogenesis of HIV infection, *Pathobiology* **60**:246–251.

Poli, G., Orenstein, J. M., Kinter, A., Folks, T. M., and Fauci, A. S., 1989, Interferon-α but not AZT suppresses HIV expression in chronically infected cell lines, *Science* **244**:575–577.

Poli, G., Kinter, A. L., Justement, J. S., Kehrl, J. H., Bressler, P., Stanley, S., and Fauci, A. S., 1990a, Tumor necrosis factor α functions in an autocrine manner in the induction of human immunodeficiency virus expression, *Proc. Natl. Acad. Sci. USA* **87**:782–785.

Poli, G., Bressler, P., Kinter, A., Duh, E., Timmer, W. C., Rabson, A., Justement, J. S., Stanley, S., and Fauci, A. S., 1990b, Interleukin 6 induces human immunodeficiency virus expression in infected monocytic cells alone and in synergy with tumor necrosis factor α by transcriptional and posttranscriptional mechanisms, *J. Exp. Med.* **172**:151–158.

Poli, G., Kinter, A. L., Justement, J. S., Bressler, P., Kehrl, J. H., and Fauci, A. S., 1991, Transforming growth factor β suppresses human immuno-deficiency virus expression and replication in infected cells of the monocyte/macrophage lineage, *J. Exp. Med.* **173**:589–597.

Poli, G., Kinter, A. L., Justement, J. S., Bressler, P., Kehrl, J. H., and Fauci, A. S., 1992, Retinoic acid mimics transforming growth factor β in the regulation of human immunodeficiency virus expression in monocytic cells, *Proc. Natl. Acad. Sci. USA* **89**:2689–2693.

Poli, G., Kinter, A. L., and Fauci, A. S., 1994, Interleukin 1 induces expression of the human immunodeficiency virus alone and in synergy with interleukin 6 in chronically infected U1 cells: Inhibition of inductive effects by the interleukin 1 receptor antagonist, *Proc. Natl. Acad. Sci. USA* **91**:108–112.

Pomerantz, R. J., Feinberg, M. B., Trono, D., and Baltimore, D., 1990, Lipopolysaccharide is a potent monocyte/macrophage-specific stimulator of human immunodeficiency virus type 1 expression, *J. Exp. Med.* **172:**253–261.

Re, M. C., Zauli, G., Furlini, G., Ranieri, S., and La Placa, M., 1992, Progressive and selective impairment of IL-3 and IL-4 production by peripheral blood CD4+ T-lymphocytes during the course of HIV-1 infection, *Virol. Immunol.* **5:**185–194.

Reka, S., Garro, M. L., and Kotler, D. P., 1994, Variation in the expression of human immunodeficiency virus RNA and cytokine mRNA in rectal mucosa during the progression of infection, *Lymphokine Cytokine Res.* **13:** 391–398.

Rieckmann, P., Poli, G., Fox, C. H., Kehrl, J. H., and Fauci, A. S., 1991, Recombinant gp120 specifically enhances tumor necrosis factor-alpha production and Ig secretion in B lymphocytes from HIV-infected individuals but not from seronegative donors, *J. Immunol.* **147:**2922–2297.

Rinaldo, C. R., Armstrong, J. A., Kingsley, L. A., Zhou, S., and Ho, M., 1990, Relation of alpha and gamma interferon levels to development of AIDS in homosexual men, *J. Exp. Pathol.* **5:**127–132.

Saville, M. W., Taga, K., Foli, A., Broder, S., Tosato, G., and Yarchoan, R., 1994, Interleukin-10 suppresses human immunodeficiency virus-1 replication in vitro in cells of the monocyte/macrophage lineage, *Blood* **83:**3591–3599.

Scala, G., Ruocco, M. R., Ambrosino, C., Mallardo, M., Giordano, V., Baldassarre, F., Dragonetti, E., Quinto, I., and Venuta, S., 1994, The expression of the interleukin 6 gene is induced by the human immuno-deficiency virus 1 TAT protein, *J. Exp. Med.* **179:**961–971.

Schuitemaker, H., Kootstra, N. A., Koppelman, M. H. G. M., Bruistein, S. M., Husiman, H. G., Tersmette, M., and Miedema, F., 1992, Proliferation dependent HIV-1 infection of monocytes occurs during differentiation into macrophages, *J. Clin. Invest.* **89:**1154–1160.

Scott-Algara, D., Vuillier, F., Marasescu, M., De Saint Martin, J., and Dighiero, G., 1991, Serum levels of IL-2, IL-1, TNF-α, and soluble receptor of IL-2 in HIV-1 infected patients, *AIDS Res. Hum. Retrovir.* **7:**381–386.

Sher, A., Gazzinelli, R. T., Oswald, I. P., Clerici, M., Kullberg, M., Pearch, E. J., Berzofsky, J. A., Mossman, T. R., James, S. L., and Morse, H. C., 1992, Role of T cell derived cytokines in the downregulation of immune responses in parasitic and retroviral infection, *Immunol. Rev.* **127:**183–204.

Shirazi, Y., and Pitha, P. M., 1992, Alpha interferon inhibits early stages of the human immunodeficiency virus type 1 replication cycle, *J. Virol.* **66:**1321–1328.

Siebenlist, U., Franzoso, G., and Brown, K., 1994, Structure, regulation and function of NF-kB, *Annu. Rev. Cell Biol.* **10:**405–455.

Tadmori, W., Mondal, D., Tadmori, I., and Prakash, O., 1991, Transactivation of human immunodeficiency virus type 1 long terminal repeats by cell surface tumor necrosis factor alpha, *J. Virol.* **65:**6425–6429.

Trinchieri, G., 1993, Interleukin-12 and its role in the generation of TH1 cells, *Immunol. Today* **14:**335–338.

Tschachler, E., Groh, V., Popovic, M., Mann, D. L., Konrad, K., Safai, B., Eron, L., DiMarzo Veronese, F., Wolff, K., and Stingl, G., 1987, Epidermal Langerhan's cells: A target for HTLV-III/LAV infection, *J. Invest. Dermatol.* **88:**233–237.

Voth, R., Rossol, S., Klein, K., Hess, G., Schutt, K. H., Schroder, H. C., Meyer Zum Buschenfelde, K. H., and Muller, W. E., 1990, Differential gene expression of IFN-α and tumor necrosis factor-α in peripheral blood mononuclear cells from patients with AIDS related complex and AIDS, *J. Immunol.* **144:**970–975.

Vyakarnam, A., McKeating, J., Meager, A., and Beverley, P. C., 1990, Tumour necrosis factors (α,β) induced by HIV-1 in peripheral blood mononuclear cells potentiate virus replication, *AIDS* **4:**21–27.

Wei, X., Ghosh, S. K., Taylor, M. E., Johnson, V. A., Emini, E. A., Deutsch, P., Lifson, J. D., Bonhoeffer, S., Nowak, M. A., Hahn, B. H., Saag, M. S., and Shaw, G. M., 1995, Viral dynamics in human immunodeficiency virus type 1 infection, *Nature* **373:**117–122.

Weissman, D., Poli, G., and Fauci, A. S., 1994, Interleukin 10 blocks HIV replication in macrophages by inhibiting the autocrine loop of TNF-α and IL-6 induction of virus, *AIDS Res. Hum. Retrovir.* **10:**1199–1206.

Weissman, D., Li, Y., Ananworanich, J., Zhou, L.-J., Adelsberg, J., Tedder, T. F., Baseler, M., and Fauci, A. S., 1995a, Three populations of cells with dendritic morphology exist in peripheral blood, only one of which is infectable with HIV 1, *Proc. Natl. Acad. Sci. USA* **92:**826–830.

Weissman, D., Poli, G., and Fauci, A. S., 1995b, IL-10 synergizes with multiple cytokines in enhancing HIV production in cells of monocytic lineage, *AIDS Res. Hum. Retrovir.* **9:**442–449.

Williams, G. J., and Colby, C. B., 1989, Recombinant human interferon-beta suppresses the replication of HIV and acts synergistically with AZT, *J. Interferon Res.* **9:**709–718.

Zack, J. A., Arrigo, S. J., Weitsman, S. R., Go, A. S., Haislip, A., and Chen, I. S. Y., 1990, HIV-1 entry into quiescent primary lymphocytes: Molecular analysis reveals a labile, latent viral structure, *Cell* **61:**213–222.

CHAPTER 15

MACROPHAGE FUNCTIONS IN HIV-1 INFECTION

SHARON M. WAHL, JAN M. ORENSTEIN,
and PHILLIP D. SMITH

1. INTRODUCTION

Human immunodeficiency virus type 1 (HIV-1) infects host cells through the CD4 molecule expressed on T lymphocytes and mononuclear phagocytes. CD4 recognition, binding, and internalization of HIV-1 precede viral replication in $CD4^+$ T cells, which subsequently undergo depletion leading to immunosuppression. Mononuclear phagocytes also are infected by HIV-1, but depletion is not an inevitable consequence of infection. This enables HIV-1-infected mononuclear phagocytes to contribute to AIDS pathogenesis by serving as a viral reservoir, as a mobile source of virus, and as an amplifier of immune dysfunction. In this chapter, we focus on the role of mononuclear phagocytes in HIV-1 infection and the consequences of monocyte/macrophage–virus interactions in compromising host defense. Monocyte cell lines have been used as models for HIV-1 infection because of the difficulty in obtaining primary cells, but these model systems have generated considerable controversy concerning tropism, viral replication, and chronicity. Therefore, we emphasize information from studies of primary cells of monocyte lineage *in vitro* and from analysis of these cells *in vivo* to develop a clearer picture of the contribution of mononuclear phagocytes to AIDS pathogenesis.

SHARON M. WAHL • Cellular Immunology, National Institute of Dental Research, National Institutes of Health, Bethesda, Maryland 20892. JAN M. ORENSTEIN • Department of Pathology, George Washington University Medical Center, Washington, D.C. 20037. PHILLIP D. SMITH • Department of Medicine, University of Alabama, School of Medicine, Birmingham, Alabama 35294.

Immunology of HIV Infection, edited by Sudhir Gupta. Plenum Press, New York, 1996.

2. HIV-1 INFECTION OF MONOCYTES *IN VITRO*

2.1. *In Vitro* Infection

HIV-1 is a complex pathogenic retrovirus with a 9.4-kb genome. The genome encodes a number of proteins necessary for transcription, integration, and expression, which precede the packaging, encapsulation, and release of progeny virions (Haseltine, 1991). Despite the large body of information on the molecular virology of HIV-1, the mechanism whereby HIV-1 infects and propagates itself in human mononuclear phagocytes in culture has not been fully elucidated, related in part to the genetic heterogeneity of HIV-1 and to varying susceptibility of the cellular hosts. However, mononuclear phagocytes express CD4 and, when exposed to macrophage-tropic HIV-1 isolates *in vitro*, bind, internalize, and support viral replication (Gartner *et al.*, 1986). Ultrastructural analysis has revealed HIV-1 in macrophage vacuoles derived from the Golgi apparatus (Orenstein *et al.*, 1988) and on the cell surface (Fig. 1A,B). Consistent with this morphologic evidence of viral infection, reverse transcriptase (RT) levels increase during viral replication and p24 antigen is released into the culture supernatants.

In addition to cell-specific viral tropism, important factors that influence monocyte/macrophage infection *in vitro* include the source of the donor cells, the level of cell maturation, possible subpopulation susceptibility, and presence of constitutive or exogenous cytokines. For example, interferon-α (IFN-α) consistently inhibits primary monocyte HIV-1 infection *in vitro*, whereas tumor necrosis factor-α (TNF-α) augments viral transcription, apparently through protein kinase C-dependent binding of NF-κB to a promoter region of the viral DNA long terminal repeat (Griffin *et al.*, 1989; Osborn *et al.*, 1989; Duh *et al.*, 1989; Koyanagi *et al.*, 1988). Other cytokines have variable and often opposing effects on viral expression (Table I) (reviewed in Poli and Fauci, 1994). Although continued investigation of the role of individual cytokines in these events may shed further light on the control of viral replication, viral expression is likely regulated by a network of cytokines.

2.2. Cellular Tropism

The cellular receptor for HIV-1 is CD4, a surface molecule recognized by the viral envelope glycoprotein gp120 (Dalgleish *et al.*, 1984; Klatzmann *et al.*, 1984) and expressed on mononuclear phagocytes and helper/inducer lymphocytes. Many isolates of HIV-1 can infect both lymphocytes and macrophages, but the initial isolate that infects an individual is often characterized by its propensity to infect monocyte-derived macrophages, whereas viruses isolated later in infection are genotypically more diverse and capable of infecting both T cells and macrophages (Zhu *et al.*, 1993; Schuitemaker *et al.*, 1992a). Although not universally accepted, cell-specific tropism has been associated with postbinding events involving the third hypervariable region (V3 loop) of the viral envelope glycoprotein gp120

FIGURE 1. Productive HIV-1 infection of peripheral blood monocytes *in vitro*. HIV replicating in cytoplasmic vacuoles (A) and on the plasma membrane (B) of cultured blood monocytes. Note the budding (arrows) and immature particles (arrowhead) on the convoluted plasma membrane. Magnification: A, × 11,500; B, × 32,000.

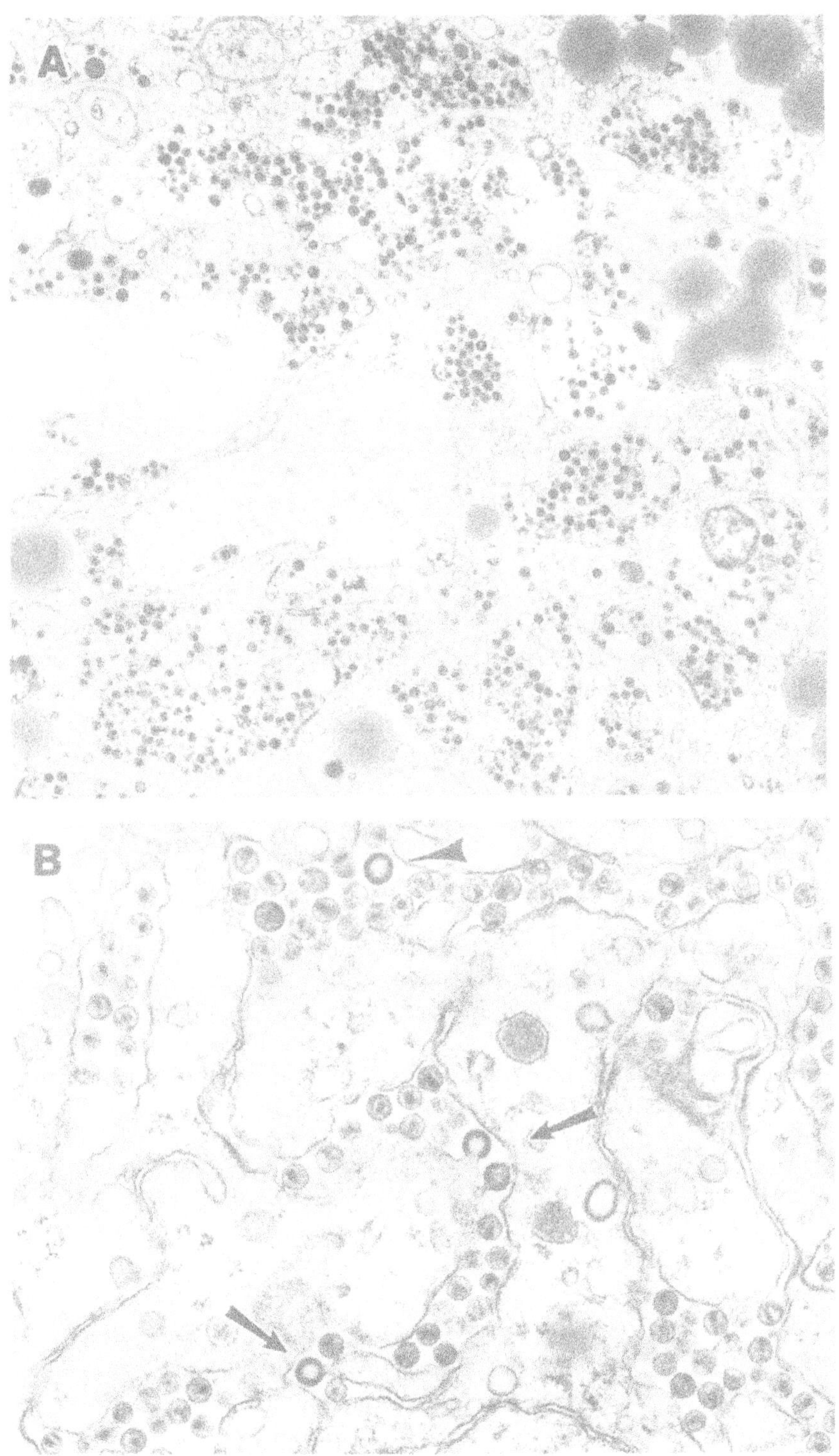
A
B

TABLE I. **Cytokine Regulation of Macrophage HIV-1 Expression *in Vitro***

Cytokine	HIV-1 expression[a]	References[b]
IL-1	↑	Osborn *et al.* (1989)
IL-3	↓	Koyanagi *et al.* (1988)
IL-4	↑↓	Schuitemaker *et al.* (1992b), Kazai *et al.* (1992), Novak *et al.* (1990)
IL-6	↑	Schuitemaker *et al.* (1992b), Poli *et al.* (1990)
GM-CSF	↑	Koyanagi *et al.* (1988), Perno *et al.* (1989)
M-CSF	↑⊖	Gendelman *et al.* (1988), Koyanagi *et al.* (1988), Crowe *et al.* (1994)
TNF-α/β	↑	Osborn *et al.* (1989), Vyakarnam *et al.* (1990), Poli *et al.* (1990)
IFN-α/β	↓	Meylan *et al.* (1993), Gendelman *et al.* (1990a), Kornbluth *et al.* (1989)
IFN-γ	↑↓⊖	Koyanagi *et al.* (1993), Kornbluth *et al.* (1989), Meylan *et al.* (1993), Fan *et al.* (1994)
IL-10	↑↓⊖	Weissman *et al.* (1994)
IL-13	↓	Montaner *et al.* (1993)
TGF-β	↑↓	Poli *et al.* (1991, 1992), Lazdins *et al.* (1991), Peterson *et al.* (1991)

[a]↑, increase; ↓, decrease; ⊖, no effect.

(Westervelt *et al.*, 1992a; O'Brien *et al.*, 1990; Shioda *et al.*, 1991; Hwang *et al.*, 1991). Distinct from the CD4 binding site (O'Brien *et al.*, 1990), the V3 loop appears to contain the principal neutralizing domain, to have a role in viral entry, and to determine cellular tropism (Bou-Habib *et al.*, 1994; Hwang *et al.*, 1991; Cann *et al.*, 1992; Skinner *et al.*, 1988). The basis for this cellular tropism may reside in specific amino acid residues of the V3 region (Chesebro *et al.*, 1992; DeJong *et al.*, 1992; Fouchier *et al.*, 1992) present in macrophage-tropic isolates, obtained during primary infections (Zhang *et al.*, 1993; McNearney *et al.*, 1992; Zhu *et al.*, 1993). Macrophage-tropic strains generally have a lower net negative charge and possess Iso-Glu or Iso-Asp at gp120 amino acids 317 and 318, whereas Lys or other positively charged amino acids may occur at this site in T-cell-tropic strains (Shioda *et al.*, 1991; Hwang *et al.*, 1991; Westervelt *et al.*, 1992b; Stamatos and Cheng-Mayer, 1993). In addition to the V3 loop, other regions of gp120 may influence cell tropism and viral phenotype (Westervelt *et al.*, 1992a; Brighty *et al.*, 1991; Willey *et al.*, 1989). Moreover, increased gp120 and spike density reflected by an increase in the gp120/p24 ratio have been associated with macrophage-tropic viruses (O'Brien *et al.*, 1994b) and may influence whether the virus is non-syncytium-inducing (NSI) and macrophage-tropic, or syncytium-inducing (SI) and T-cell-tropic (Tersmette *et al.*, 1988; Schuitemaker *et al.*, 1992; Roos *et al.*, 1992).

After viral gp120 engages the CD4 molecule, subsequent fusion of the cellular and viral membranes enables entry of the viral core into the host cell cytoplasm (Stein *et al.*, 1987). In macrophages, CD4 reportedly triggers a conformational change in gp120 that exposes V3 determinants which promote viral entry (O'Brien *et al.*, 1990; Werner and Levy, 1993; Sattentau and Moore, 1991). Postbinding viral entry may be aided by one or more cellular cofactors (Chesebro *et al.*, 1992; Dragic *et al.*, 1992), including fusin, heparan sulfate, HLA-1, CD44, and cellular proteases such as tryptase, the ectopeptidase dipeptidyl peptidase IV (CD26), or another molecule with an elastaselike binding motif (Feng *et al.*, 1996; Roderiquez *et al.*, 1995; Devaux *et al.*, 1990; Kido *et al.*, 1991; Patel *et al.*, 1993; Dukes *et al.*, 1995; Koito *et al.*, 1989; Callebaut *et al.*, 1993; McNeely *et al.*, 1995). Within the V3 loop is a proline-rich region that has been suggested to be a substrate for cellular proteases such as CD26 and may interact with and/or cleave gp120 after CD4 binding to facilitate viral entry (Callebaut *et al.*, 1993; Dalgleish, 1995). Support for CD26 as the HIV-1 cofactor is far from unanimous (Broder *et al.*, 1994; Patience *et al.*, 1994; Camerini *et al.*, 1994; Lazaro *et al.*, 1994; Alizon and Dragic, 1994; Morimoto *et al.*, 1994), but new studies suggest that CD26 expression correlates with susceptibility to macrophage-tropic, rather than T-cell-tropic, viral phenotypes (Oravecz *et al.*, 1995). Cleavage or modification of cellular protease-sensitive sites within the V3 domain may lead to conformational changes, enabling gp41 to fuse with the cell membrane for viral entry (Murakami *et al.*, 1991; Kido *et al.*, 1991; Clements *et al.*, 1991; Moore *et al.*, 1991; Werner and Levy, 1993).

2.3. Viral Entry and Replication

After the virus enters the host cell and is uncoated, reverse transcription is initiated to synthesize viral DNA and begin the HIV-1 life cycle. The initial postentry events include reverse transcription of the two copies of the single-stranded RNA genome utilizing viral tRNA–lysine primer, RT, and free nucleotides. Although both monocytes and lymphocytes express CD4 and are susceptible to HIV-1 infection, there are marked differences in how the virus commandeers these two cell types. Following internalization of the virus, the rate of HIV-1 production is dependent on the cell type and proliferative status. Initiation of reverse transcription of new viral DNA occurs within hours in both T cells and macrophages, yet the rate of accumulation of full-length reverse transcripts varies from 4 hr in proliferating lymphocytes to 24–48 hr in macrophages as determined by quantitative polymerase chain reaction (PCR) *in vitro* (Zack *et al.*, 1990; O'Brien *et al.*, 1994). Delayed reverse transcription in macrophages may be attributed to limited intracellular nucleotide pools (O'Brien *et al.*, 1994a; Terai and Carson, 1991) along with other yet to be defined cellular and viral factors.

Although quiescent lymphocytes are susceptible to viral binding, internalization, and retroviral reverse transcription, they do not support productive replication of virus until they proliferate (Zack *et al.*, 1990), at which time they integrate HIV-1 DNA. In contrast, macrophages integrate HIV-1 DNA in the absence of cell division and produce virus, albeit at an initially delayed rate (Weinberg *et al.*, 1991). Virion-derived nucleophilic proteins, including viral matrix protein (MA p17) and viral protein R (Vpr) associated with the preintegration complex, may facilitate nuclear targeting of HIV-1 DNA through the nuclear envelope in nondividing macrophages (Bukrinsky *et al.*, 1993; Heinzinger *et al.*, 1994). Recent studies have identified a specific nuclear localization signal (NLS) containing a stretch of lysine residues within MA p17 which is responsible for translocation of the preintegration complex into the nucleus (Bukrinsky *et al.*, 1993). Once the HIV-1 DNA is transported to the nucleus, it is integrated into host cell DNA and eventually transcribed to produce progeny virions.

Many features of productive HIV-1 infection in lymphocytes and macrophages are distinct. The virus replicates in $CD4^+$ lymphocytes by budding from the plasma membrane (Fig. 2). Infected lymphocytes exhibit cytopathic manifestations, undergo apoptosis, and are destroyed by HIV-specific cytotoxic T lymphocytes (CTL) (Meyaard *et al.*, 1992; Phillips *et al.*, 1994; Wain-Hobson, 1993; Zinkernagel and Hengartner, 1994). Over time, the virally mediated destruction of $CD4^+$ lymphocytes exceeds the regenerative capacity of the

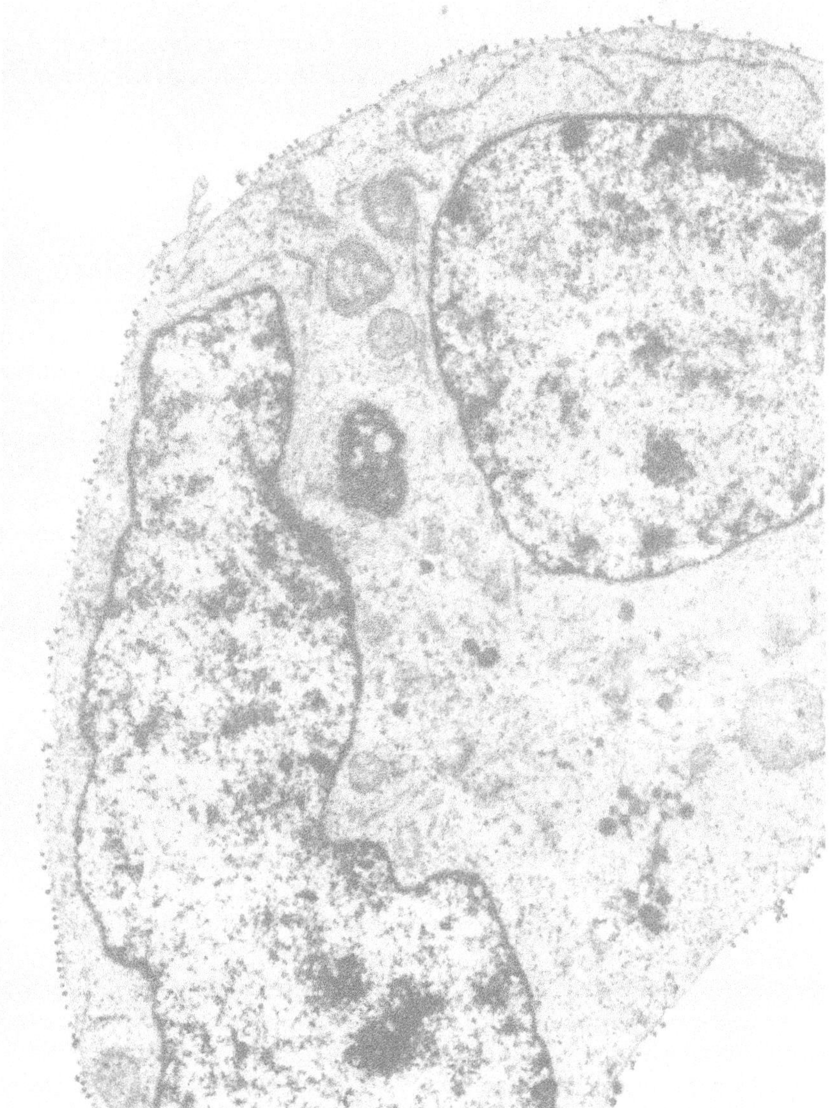

FIGURE 2. Productive HIV-1 infection of peripheral blood lymphocytes *in vitro*. Binucleated cultured lymphocyte with numerous budding virions present on the plasma membrane. ×49,000.

immune system, leading to a decline in the number of CD4+ lymphocytes and impaired defense mechanisms (Wei *et al.*, 1995; Ho *et al.*, 1995). On the other hand, when HIV-1 replicates in macrophages, either *in vivo* or *in vitro*, the virus accumulates intracellularly without inevitably killing the cell (Figs. 1, 3). HIV-1-infected macrophages contribute to viral persistence by serving as a reservoir for virus, disseminating the virus, and promoting immunosuppression. Importantly, the ability of macrophages to provide a safe haven for viral replication may be aided by the ability of macrophages to escape CTL activity. As a consequence of its furtive transport of the virus, the macrophage has commonly been referred to as the "Trojan horse" of HIV-1 immunopathogenesis.

3. *IN VIVO* HIV INFECTION OF MONONUCLEAR PHAGOCYTES

3.1. Primary Infection

Although cells of many lineages can be infected with HIV-1 *in vitro*, replication *in vivo* appears to be restricted to CD4+ bone marrow-derived cells, including T lymphocytes and mononuclear phagocytes (reviewed by Levy, 1993a). Even more specificity may reside in the preferential tropism of primary viral isolates, since the strains that are isolated from acutely infected individuals exhibit a macrophage-tropic phenotype, implicating macrophages as early cellular hosts (Zhu *et al.*, 1993; Schuitemaker *et al.*, 1992a). Later in disease, macrophages in the brain (Wahl *et al.*, 1991) and mucosa (Smith *et al.*, 1994) commonly support HIV-1 infection, when the frequency of infected monocytes in the peripheral blood is low (Schnittman *et al.*, 1989). This difference in the prevalence of HIV-1 -infected cells is consistent with evidence that the susceptibility to infection in the brain and mucosa increases during differentiation (Schuitemaker *et al.*, 1992b). Alternatively, the higher levels of infection may reflect the rapid exit of infected monocytes from the circulation into the tissues. Since the half-life of circulating monocytes is less than 2–3 days, these cells could enter the extravascular compartment, take up residence as tissue macrophages, and become potential sites of viral replication (Fig. 3).

3.2. Mucosal Transmission

Mucosal surfaces represent an important participant in the pathogenesis of HIV-1 infection. First, the mucosa is the site of HIV-1 entry into the host in heterosexual, homosexual, and vertical transmission (Fig. 4). Second, the mucosa likely contributes to the apparent selective entry of genotypically and phenotypically homogeneous minor variants of HIV-1 that are present in the transmitted inoculum. Third, as the largest lymphoid organ in the body, the mucosa is a rich source of CD4+ target cells. Fourth, because of its exposure to microbial products and the local production of certain cytokines, both of which are capable of activating HIV-1-infected cells to cause viral expression, the mucosa may also be the largest site of viral expression.

3.2.1. Mucosal Routes of Entry

Breaches in the columnar epithelium of mucosa caused by trauma, inflammation, or infection provide HIV-1 direct access to the underlying lymphoid cells and microcirculation

A

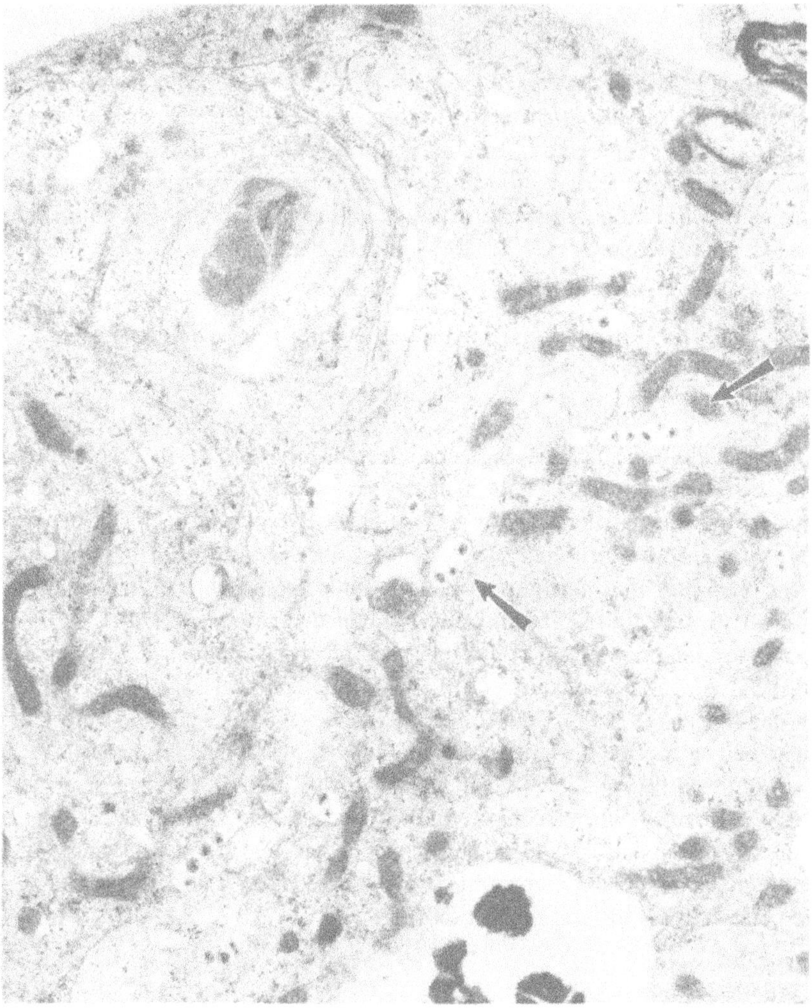

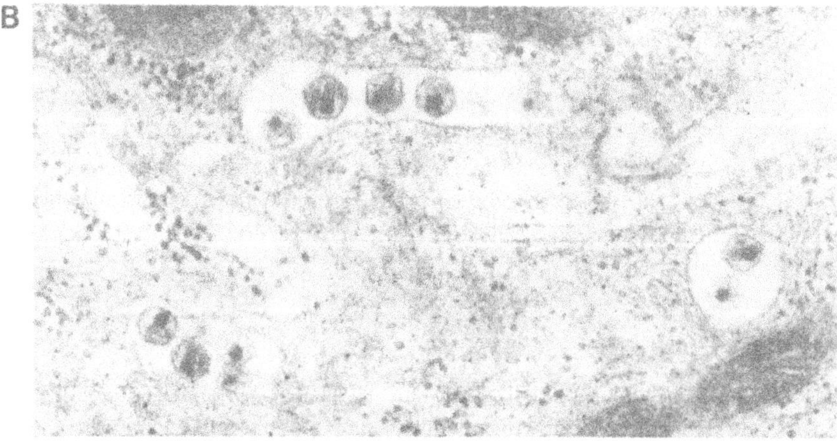

of the distal gastrointestinal tract (Smith *et al.*, 1994). Animal model studies (Amerongen *et al.*, 1991) suggest that M cells, which are specialized epithelial cells that transport macromolecules and certain microorganisms by a nondegradative process, may also be involved in the transcytotic delivery of intact virus to mononuclear cells in the underlying organized lymphoid structures (Peyer's patches in the small intestine and lymphoid aggregates in the rectum). Importantly, the highest density of lymphoid aggregates with overlying M cells is in the rectum (O'Leary and Sweeney, 1986), increasing the likelihood of contact between HIV-1 and M cells in homosexual transmission. Analogous to mucosal events in the rectum, disruption of the normal integrity of the cervicovaginal mucosa by trauma and infection likely facilitates HIV-1 entry into subepithelial tissues in the genital tract. However, mechanisms of transport of virus across the vaginal mucosa may differ from transport across the rectal mucosa, since the vagina is lined by squamous epithelium and does not contain M cells. Finally, in vertical transmission, the upper gastrointestinal tract mucosa likely serves as a conduit for viral entry through the swallowing of cell-free and cell-associated virus in infected amniotic fluid *in utero*, in cervical secretions and blood intrapartum, and in breast milk postpartum (Smith, 1995).

3.2.2. Mucosal Selection

Elucidation of the sequence of events involved in the selective transport of virus across the epithelium, the infection of underlying mucosal lymphoid cells, and the subsequent distribution of those cells to distant sites is critical for understanding HIV-1 pathogenesis and vaccine development. The importance of these early events is underscored by studies suggesting that the selection of virus-bearing specific env determinants occurs in the mucosa during the interval between exposure and seroconversion (Zhu *et al.*, 1993). As indicated above, HIV-1 isolated from acutely infected persons displays astonishing (>99%) genotypic homogeneity, whereas the transmitted (chronically infected) partner's virus is a mixture of genotypes (90–94% genetic similarity) (Zhu *et al.*, 1993). Among recent seroconverters, the degree of similarity is greatest in the V3 loop sequences, which are associated with macrophage tropism in primary viral isolates (Zhang *et al.*, 1993; Chesebro *et al.*, 1992). A similar selectivity in the transmission of viral genotypes appears to occur between an infected mother and her infant (Wolinsky *et al.*, 1992). In addition to genomic homogeneity, acutely acquired HIV-1 also appears to show homogeneity for the NSI phenotype (Zhu *et al.*, 1993; Roos *et al.*, 1992).

The apparent selection of genotypically and phenotypically similar minor variants has been investigated in female macaques infected intravaginally with SIV (Spira *et al.*, 1996). In this model, the first SIV-infected cells were located by *in situ* PCR exclusively in the lamina propria and showed the morphology (elongated, irregular processes) and phenotype (MHC class II molecule expression) of antigen-presenting cells. Thus, in the cervicovaginal mucosa, antigen-presenting cells, such as dendritic cells and possibly macrophages, likely play a critical role in the initial viral selection in heterosexual transmission.

FIGURE 3. Productive HIV-1 infection of a macrophage *in vivo*. (A) Portion of a macrophage in a stereotactic CNS biopsy from a patient with AIDS dementia complex. HIV-1 particles are present in numerous cytoplasmic vacuoles (e.g., arrows), paralleling the distribution of replicating HIV-1 in macrophages *in vitro* (Fig. 1) (× 16,000). (B) Higher magnification (× 52,000) shows three of the vacuoles evident in the lower left of panel A.

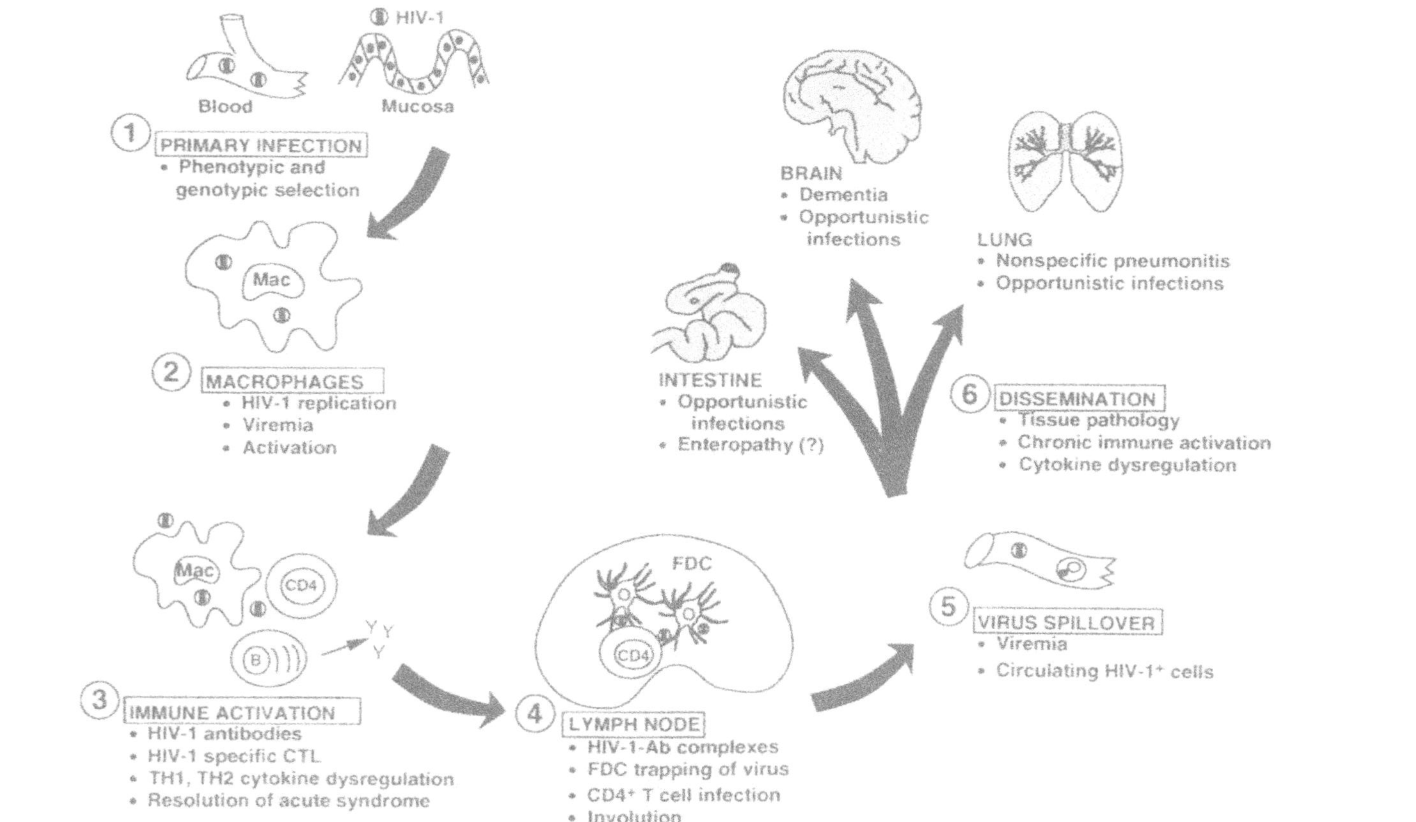

FIGURE 4. Macrophage function in HIV-1 pathogenesis. (1) Transmission of HIV-1 by blood or through mucosal sites results in primary infection with genotypic and phenotypic selection of macrophage-tropic variants (2). HIV-1 replication and antigen processing trigger a cellular and humoral immune response (3). HIV-1-specific antibodies (Ab) complexed with the virus adhere to follicular dendritic cells (FDC) in lymph nodes or lymphoid aggregates in the mucosa where trafficking $CD4^+$ cells become infected (4). Viral replication within the germinal centers contributes to dissolution of lymph node architecture and the release of virions within cells and as free virus (5). Dissemination of the virus to distant tissue sites predisposes to opportunistic pathogens and tissue pathology (6).

The distribution of HIV-1-infected mononuclear cells to distant mucosal sites by either random or homing mechanisms accounts for the presence of infected cells in mucosa throughout the gastrointestinal tract, including the rectum and colon (Fox *et al.*, 1990), ileum (Harriman *et al.*, 1989), duodenum (Ullrich *et al.*, 1989; Jarry *et al.*, 1990), and esophagus (Smith *et al.*, 1993, 1994). Besides acting as a reservoir for HIV-1-infected cells, the gastrointestinal tract mucosa is also a site of HIV-1 expression by infected mucosal macrophages. The level of HIV-1 mRNA-expressing cells in the mucosa of AIDS patients with enteric infections is reportedly greater (Smith *et al.*, 1994) than the apparent frequency of cells reported to express viral RNA in lymph nodes (Harper *et al.*, 1986), and may reflect the local abundance of stimuli such as bacterial products (J. L. Ho *et al.*, 1995), herpes group viruses (Gendelman *et al.*, 1986; Mosca *et al.*, 1987), inflammation (S. Wahl and J. Orenstein, in preparation), and cytokines (Smith *et al.*, 1994) capable of activating macrophages and thereby upregulating viral transcription.

3.3. Immune Activation

After entry into the lamina propria, HIV-1 encounters a rich abundance of $CD4^+$ target macrophages and lymphocytes (Smith, 1994, 1995). Infection of these resident cells undoubtedly occurs through the $CD4^+$-mediated mechanism described above. HIV-1-infected cells in the lymphoid aggregate could be distributed to mucosal sites throughout the body by the receptor-mediated homing mechanism that normally directs antigen-stimulated lymphocytes from the lymphoid aggregate via the lymphatics and systemic circulation to mucosa throughout the body (Picker and Butcher, 1992). Cell-free and donor cell-associated virus that enters the microcirculation via mucosal breaks is likely distributed randomly to nonmucosal sites. Regardless of the route of viral entry, HIV-1 is disseminated to the lymphoid elements and initiates a specific immune response (Koup *et al.*, 1994).

With the production of HIV-1-specific antibodies, viral immune complexes form, adhere to, and are filtered by follicular dendritic cells (FDC) in the germinal centers of peripheral lymph nodes and mucosal lymphoid aggregates for presentation to $CD4^+$ lymphocytes as they traffic through these areas (Fig. 4). Lymph nodes and other components of the lymphoreticular system appear to serve as the primary reservoir and site of replication of HIV-1 (Pantaleo *et al.*, 1993; Embretson *et al.*, 1993; Fox *et al.*, 1991; Weissman *et al.*, 1995). In gut-associated lymphoid tissue (GALT), preliminary analysis reveals that activated germinal centers in lymphoid aggregates display the same dendritic cell uptake of HIV-1 observed in peripheral lymph nodes (P. Smith and J. Orenstein, in preparation). In contrast, the diffuse GALT (lamina propria) appears to contain fewer $HIV\text{-}1^+$ cells. In lymph node germinal centers, virions are associated with the labyrinth of FDC processes (Fig. 5), presumably coated with complement and attached to FDC complement receptors (Lund *et al.*, 1995), where they remain infectious (Heath *et al.*, 1995). Virus appears to remain on the FDC exterior, since budding from FDC, which would indicate productive infection, is rarely observed *in vivo*. Viral particles can occasionally be identified in lymph node macrophages within lymph node tissue sections and in cell suspensions of lymph nodes (Fig. 6). The paucity of lymphocytes in these locations with HIV-1 budding from their membranes is striking. Despite demonstration of productively infected $CD4^+$ cells in lymph nodes and spleen by *in situ* hybridization (Fox *et al.*, 1991), to our knowledge, there is no published documentation of HIV-1 budding from lymphocytes in these locations, or in fact, in any other tissue or organ from an HIV-1-infected patient. This morphological assessment

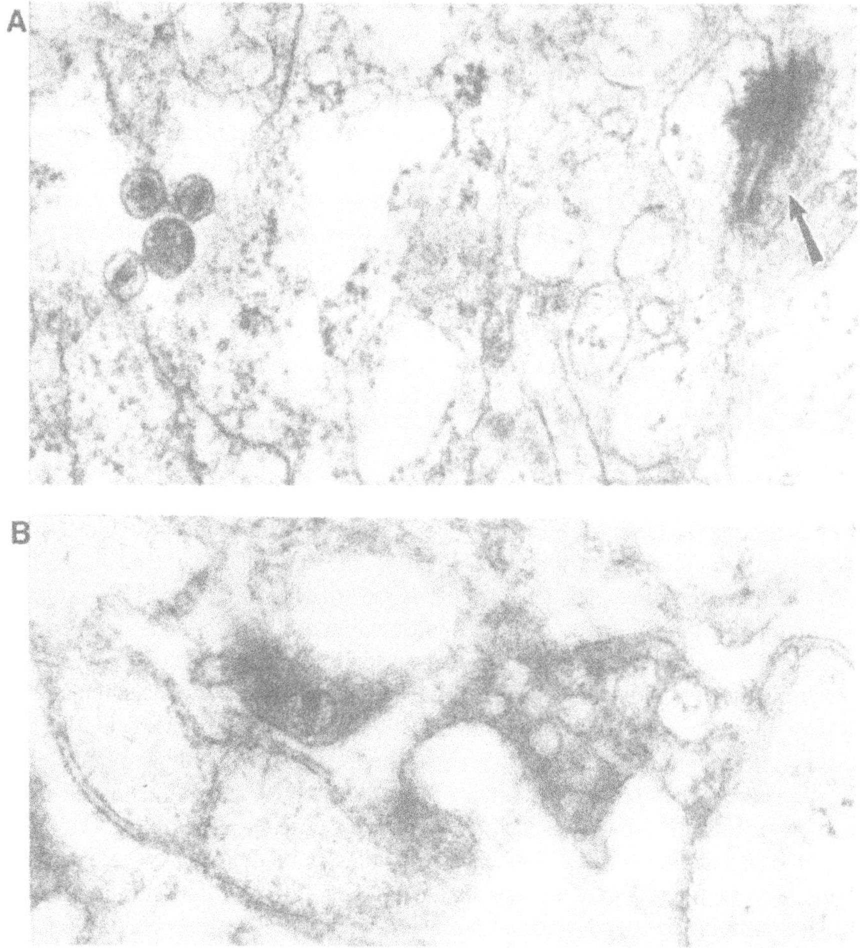

FIGURE 5. HIV-1 trapping by follicular dendritic cells. (A) HIV-1 particles associated with follicular dendritic cell processes in a hyperplastic germinal center. Evident is a rare cluster of four viral particles (× 58,000). Note the complicated processes, desmosome (arrow in A), and dense matrix material (B; × 63,000).

likely reflects the relative rarity of the event and the complexities of ultrastructural detection. Infrequently, degenerating lymphocytes with clear budding particles have been observed in hyperplastic lymph node cell suspensions (Fig. 7), but not in tissue sections. However, within these tissues, viral replication, infection, immune activation, and cell turnover presumably occur continuously with the production of prodigious numbers of virions.

Days to weeks after inoculation, an acute flulike illness occurs in 30–70% of acutely infected persons. This acute HIV-1 syndrome is accompanied by high-titer viremia (Daar *et al.*, 1991; Clark *et al.*, 1991). After 1 to 3 weeks, seroconversion and a cytotoxic lymphocyte response (Koup *et al.*, 1994) occurs, heralding a decline in the viremia

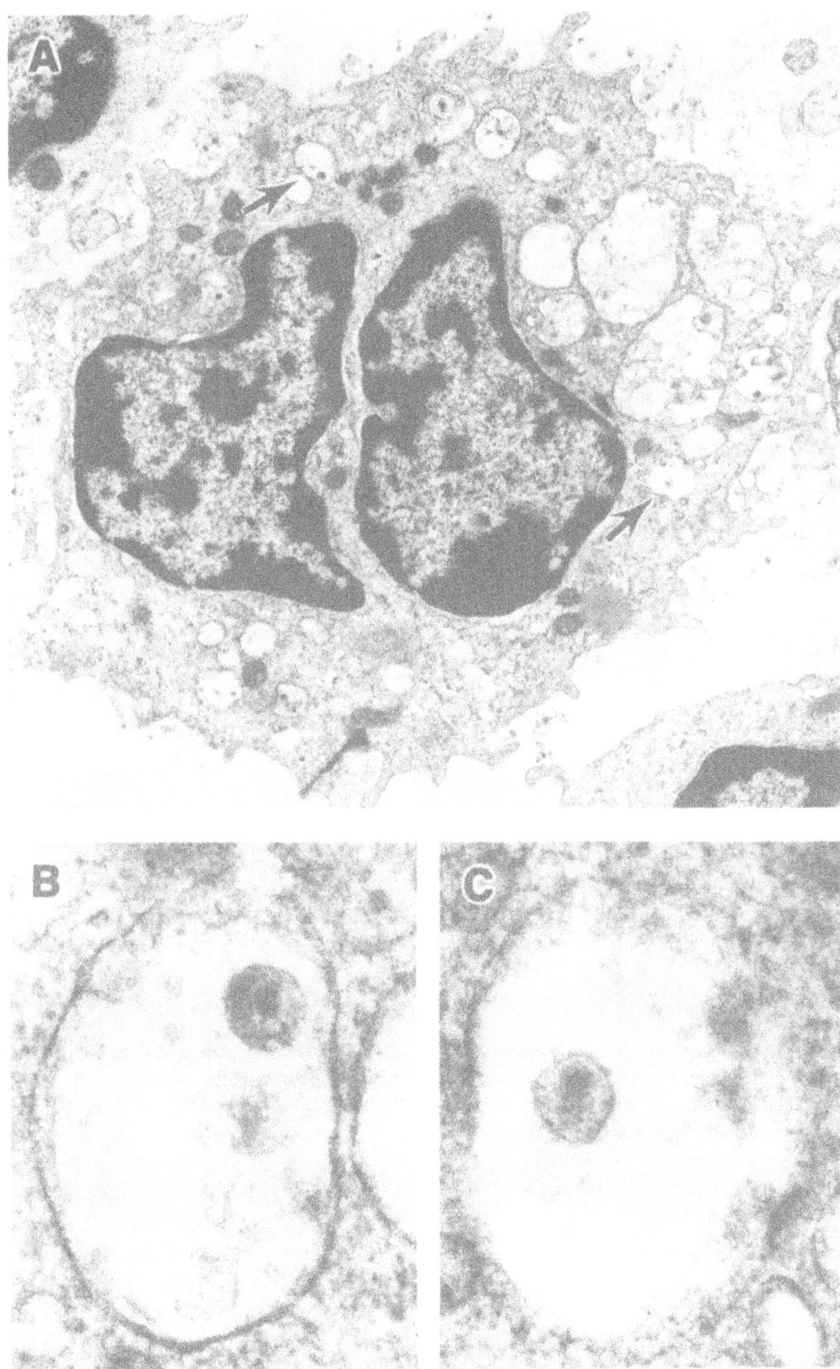

FIGURE 6. Isolated lymph node macrophages express HIV-1. (A) Macrophage in lymph node suspension from a patient with lymphadenopathy syndrome (LAS) contains many lysosomes and vacuoles, two of which contain mature HIV-1 particles (arrows) (× 11,500). (B,C) Enlarged vacuoles from A; × 110,000.

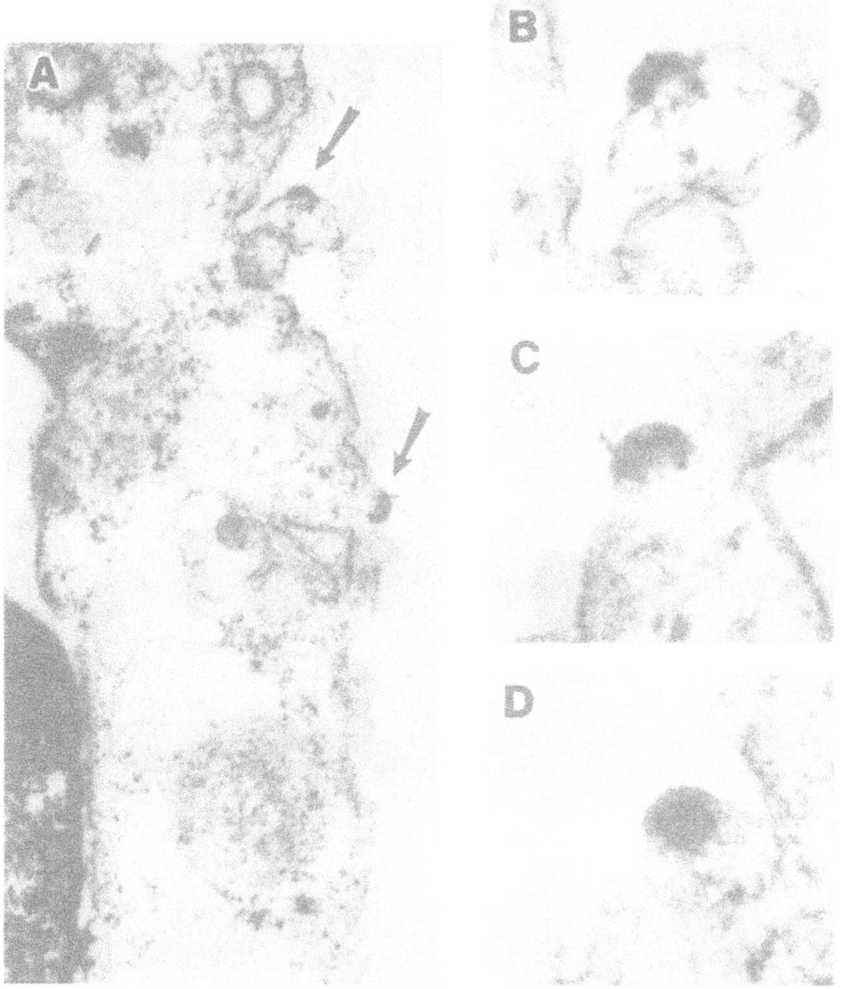

FIGURE 7. Isolated lymph node lymphocytes with budding HIV-1. (A) Portion of degenerating lymphocyte with budding HIV-1 identified in a cell suspension prepared from the lymph node of an individual with AIDS. Two particles are budding from this cell (A, arrows; × 15,000) and are magnified in B and C (× 135,000). (D) Budding virus from an additional lymph node cell (× 135,000).

and resolution of the acute syndrome. That proinflammatory cytokines mediate this syndrome is suggested by *in vitro* studies showing that the virus itself can induce IL-1 and TNF-α (Table II).

A variable 8- to 10-year period between acute HIV-1 syndrome and the development of clinical AIDS (Schragger *et al.*, 1994) was previously thought to correspond to viral latency, but recent evidence indicates that during this period, systemic HIV-1 infection is active and progressive, leading to destructive involution of lymph node centers (Pantaleo *et al.*, 1993; Embretson *et al.*, 1993). In parallel, organized lymphoid structures in the gastrointestinal tract mucosa also appear to undergo progressive destruction during this period (P. Smith

TABLE II. HIV-1 Infection Alters Primary Macrophage Cytokine Profiles[a]

Cytokine	HIV-1 infection *in vitro*	HIV-1 *in vivo*	References
IL-1	↑↓⊖	↑⊖	Twigg *et al.* (1992), Merrill *et al.* (1989), Gupta *et al.* (1987), Roy *et al.* (1988), Valentin *et al.* (1992, Weiss *et al.* (1989), Molina *et al.* (1990b)
IL-6	↑⊖	↑⊖	Nakajima *et al.* (1989), Honda *et al.* (1990), Gan *et al.* (1991), Poli *et al.* (1990), Molina *et al.* (1990), Breen *et al.* (1990b)
TNF-α	↑⊖	↑⊖	Merrill *et al.* (1989), Munis *et al.* (1990), Dezube *et al.* (1992), Lahdevitra *et al.* (1988), Wright *et al.* (1988), Roux-Lombard *et al.* (1989), Israel-Biet *et al.* (1991), Molina *et al.* (1990a,b), Mintz *et al.* (1989), Manbondzo *et al.* (1991), Voth *et al.* (1990), Vyakarnam *et al.* (1990), Valentin *et al.* (1992)
IL-8	↑	NE	Tiemessen *et al.* (1995)
IL-10	↑	↑	Akridge *et al.* (1994), Clerici *et al.* (1993)
IL-12	↓	NE	Chehimi *et al.* (1994)
TGF-β	↑	↑	Kekow *et al.* (1990), Allen *et al.* (1991), Wahl *et al.* (1991), Lotz and Seth (1993)
IFN-α/β	↑↓	↑↓	Szebeni *et al.* (1991), Krown *et al.* (1991), Gendelman *et al.* (1990b), Voth *et al.* (1990), Lau and Livesey (1989)
IFN-γ	NE	↑	Fuchs *et al.* (1989), Emilie *et al.* (1990)
M-CSF	↑	↑	Gruber *et al.* (1995)

[a]↑, increase; ↓, decrease; ⊖, no effect; NE, no evidence.

et al., in preparation). As the follicular dendritic system is compromised and unable to successfully filter out the virus, HIV-1 spills out into the circulation (Fig. 4), exposing additional target populations to the virus and accounting for the increased viremia apparent later in HIV-1 disease (Wei *et al.*, 1995; D. D. Ho *et al.*, 1995). This production of 10^7—10^9 virions per day with transport of the virions from the extravascular spaces into the plasma is associated with rapidly emerging mutant drug-resistant forms (Wei *et al.*, 1995; Ho *et al.*, 1995).

Viral turnover studies with HIV-1 protease inhibitors show that the half-life of plasma virus and virus-producing $CD4^+$ cells is approximately 2 days (Ho *et al.*, 1995; Wei *et al.*, 1995). The absolute number of $CD4^+$ T cells and the ratio of T4/T8 cells in the mucosa parallel the decline in the circulation (Rodgers *et al.*, 1986), and likely involve a dynamic process of continuous rounds of viral replication and $CD4^+$ cell depletion. Since mucosal $CD4^+$ helper cells play a central role in IgA B-cell differentiation, the selective depletion of these cells, together with a relative increase in suppressor $CD8^+$ T cells (Strober, 1992) and disturbance in local regulatory cytokines (Steffen *et al.*, 1993; Kotler *et al.*, 1993), cause dysregulation of the production of secretory IgA, the predominant Ig at mucosal surfaces (Janoff *et al.*, 1995; Kozlowski *et al.*, 1995). In conjunction with altered nonspecific mucosal defense mechanisms (reviewed in Smith, 1995), this impaired local immune function predisposes the host to the acquisition of a wide array of viral, bacterial, parasitic, and fungal opportunistic pathogens and to B-cell lymphomas in the gastrointestinal tract and other tissues.

The natural history and progression of HIV-1 infection appear to be dependent on the rate of replication of virus, viral load, host genetics, environmental factors, including other

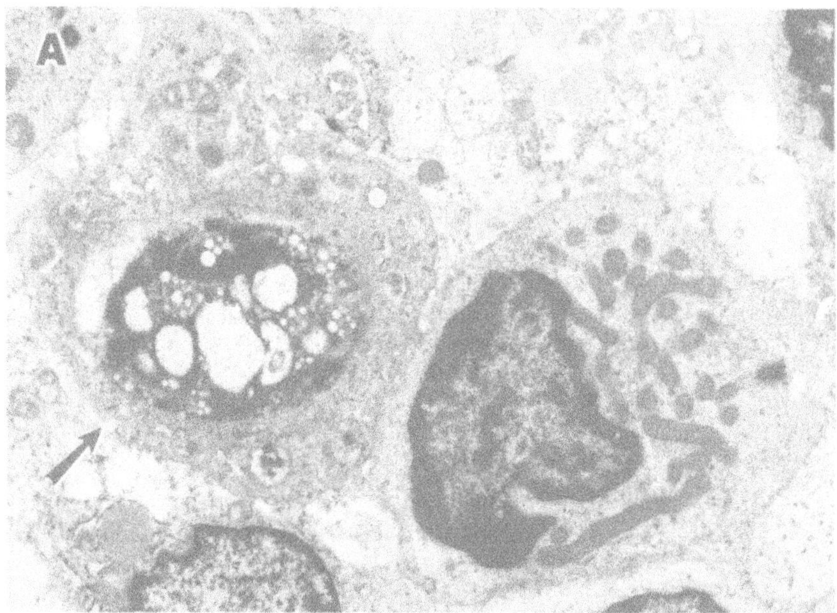

FIGURE 8. Phagocytosis of a productively infected apoptotic lymphocyte. (A) Macrophage (arrow) in the lamina propria of a colonic biopsy from an AIDS patient contains an apoptotic cell, possibly a lymphocyte, with a virion budding from the surface (B). The macrophage is in intimate association with lymphocytes. A, × 8600; B, × 104,000.

viral infections (CMV), and subversion of host defense mechanisms. By late-stage disease, systemic immune compromise is well advanced. An increase in SI T-cell variants is thought to represent a harbinger of an impending decline in $CD4^+$ T cells and rapid progression to AIDS (Tersmette *et al.*, 1988; Koot *et al.*, 1992; Schuitemaker *et al.*, 1992a).

3.4. Cellular Transmission

During HIV-1 infection of lymphoid cells, the expression of viral proteins on the host cell surfaces marks these cells as targets for HIV-1-specific CTL (Tenner-Racz *et al.*, 1993; Cheynier *et al.*, 1994; Zinkernagel and Hengartner, 1994; Koup *et al.*, 1994) and rapid destruction, whereas mononuclear phagocytes which can produce new virions furtively within intracellular vacuoles (Orenstein *et al.*, 1988) avoid CTL recognition. As $CD4^+$ lymphocytes are destroyed by cytotoxic and/or apoptotic pathways, rapid phagocytosis of these cells has been suggested as a mechanism for carrying virus into macrophages. At the ultrastructural level, apoptotic lymphocytes with budding HIV-1 particles have been identified within macrophages (Fig. 8). Lymphocyte apoptosis, which may be triggered by gp120, Fas, oxidant stress, accumulation of nonintegrated viral DNA, and CTLs (Zinkernagel and Hengartner, 1994; Terai *et al.*, 1991; Schwartz *et al.*, 1994; Laurent-Crawford *et al.*, 1993; Amendola *et al.*, 1994; Kornbluth, 1994; Petito and Roberts, 1995) undoubtedly contributes to the T-cell decline that eventually follows HIV-1 infection. Whether phagocytosis of lymphocytes that contain viral particles (Fig. 8) or linear nonintegrated retroviral DNA

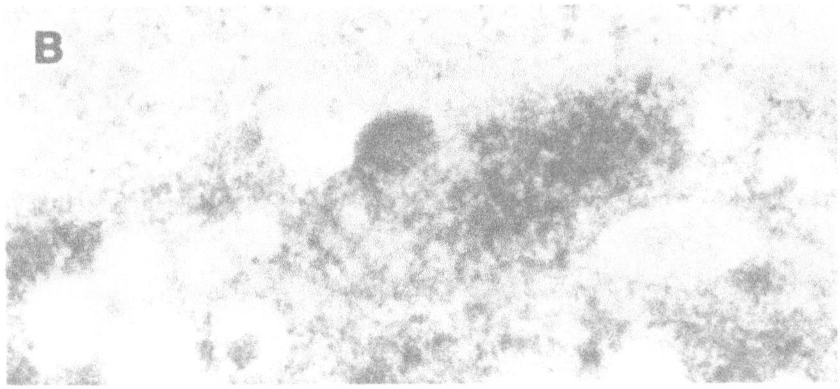

FIGURE 8. (*Continued*)

results in transfer of infection is speculative (Kornbluth, 1994), but retroviral DNA has been shown to resist endonuclease digestion (Weller *et al.*, 1980). As part of a preintegration complex, viral DNA could be transported to the phagocytic cell nucleus, become integrated, and initiate production of new virions.

Besides infection through the CD4 route and the potential for viral transfer during apoptosis, viral entry may be facilitated through receptors for the Fc (FcR) portion of immunoglobulins (Ig) expressed on phagocytic cells. The expression of Fc for IgG (FcγR) on the surface of monocytes and other immune cells may play a critical role in the immunopathogenesis of HIV-1 infection. Of the three members of the FcγR family on monocytes, FcγRIII, which are elevated on monocytes in seropositive individuals (Allen *et al.*, 1991), have been proposed as a route of antibody-dependent enhancement of HIV-1 infectivity involving internalization of HIV-1 antibody complexes (Homsy *et al.*, 1989). Alternatively, IgG-sensitized viral particles that are bound to FcγRIII could facilitate HIV-1–CD4 interaction, possibly amplified by complement (Lund *et al.*, 1995). In addition to FcγR and complement receptors, recent studies emphasize further the complexity of the potential pathways of viral entry. Serum IgA from HIV-1-seropositive patients augments HIV-1 infection of peripheral blood monocytes and lamina propria macrophages in culture, suggesting that Fcα receptors may also contribute to the infection process (Janoff *et al.*, 1995; Kozlowski *et al.*, 1995). Although requiring further investigation, the disproportionate balance between neutralizing and enhancing virus-specific antibodies must be factored into the host response to HIV-1, not only at the level of infection, but also in vaccine development (Morens, 1994).

4. FUNCTIONAL CONSEQUENCES OF MACROPHAGE HIV-1 INFECTION

4.1. Early Immune Deficits

Infection of CD4$^+$ T cells and macrophages by HIV-1 initiates a sequence of cellular events that results in a progressive loss of immune function, which is generally considered the consequence of T-cell depletion. However, recent evidence indicates that during the clinically asymptomatic phase of HIV-1 infection, when macrophage-tropic isolates of the NSI phenotype predominate and before substantial T-cell loss, antigen-specific responses are compromised (Pantaleo and Fauci, 1995). These observations suggest that the early immune deficit may be related to the ability of HIV-1 to alter the capacity of macrophages to function as antigen-presenting cells (Meyaard *et al.*, 1993). Accessory cell function appears to be altered despite the apparent absence of cytopathicity. Subsequently, as lymphocyte-tropic SI variants emerge, $CD4^+$ T cells are depleted and the entire immune system is compromised.

4.2. Opportunistic Infections

In immunocompetent persons, infections are controlled or eliminated by intact cell-mediated and humoral defense mechanisms. In HIV-1-infected persons, however, severe immunosuppression predisposes the host to increased susceptibility and complications from an array of reactivated and newly acquired opportunistic pathogens. Many of these pathogens are common species of organisms that are normally controlled by macrophages, pointing in AIDS patients to a dysfunction in macrophage microbicidal activity and not the emergence of hypervirulent or unique strains of pathogens (Crowe *et al.*, 1991; Whelan *et al.*, 1990). Analyses of biopsy and autopsy specimens from patients with AIDS demonstrate widespread dissemination of opportunistic pathogens, including *Cryptococcus neoformans, Mycobacterium avium* complex, and *Histoplasma capsulatum*. Surprisingly, these organisms accumulate within tissue macrophages (Fig. 9), indicating that macrophage dysfunction does not occur at the level of phagocytic uptake. Although several early studies suggested that FcγR-mediated monocyte functions might be defective in patients with AIDS (Capsoni *et al.*, 1992; Kent *et al.*, 1994; Pos *et al.*, 1992; Estevez *et al.*, 1986), there appears to be little correlation between defects in such functions and the expression of Fcγ surface receptors (Allen *et al.*, 1991).

Tissue macrophages in HIV-1-infected persons often engorge themselves with fungi, bacteria, or protozoa, yet the organisms do not undergo lysosomal digestion (Fig. 9) and may even replicate within the ruptured cell. Studies of the mechanism(s) responsible for the inability of macrophages to degrade and clear organisms have failed to define the etiology of this dysfunction. Reports of aberrant production of reactive oxygen intermediates, cytokines, and enzymes have generally been negated by conflicting data from other studies (Baldwin *et al.*, 1990; Eales *et al.*, 1987; Dukes *et al.*, 1993; Newman *et al.*, 1993; Chaturvedi *et al.*, 1995). Nevertheless, the survival of microorganisms within macrophage phagocytic vacuoles suggests impaired production of microbicidal products.

The defective containment of opportunistic pathogens by macrophages in HIV-1-infected persons is likely multifactorial. Impaired microbicidal activity could be related to HIV-1 itself, altered signaling induced by gp120–CD4 interaction (S. M. Wahl *et al.*, 1989; L. M. Wahl *et al.*, 1989), or interaction with products from infected cells that can modulate molecular and biochemical functions of uninfected macrophages. Early evidence suggested that a deficit in T-cell-derived cytokines, such as IFN-γ, limited the ability of mononuclear phagocytes to function at full capacity (Murray *et al.*, 1984). Reduced levels of T-cell-derived activation signals for microbicidal and tumoricidal activities would presumably impair macrophage killing of certain microorganisms. Unfortunately, the administration of IFN-γ or GM-CSF to AIDS patients does not induce adequate immune enhancement (Pennington *et al.*, 1986; Pluda *et al.*, 1990).

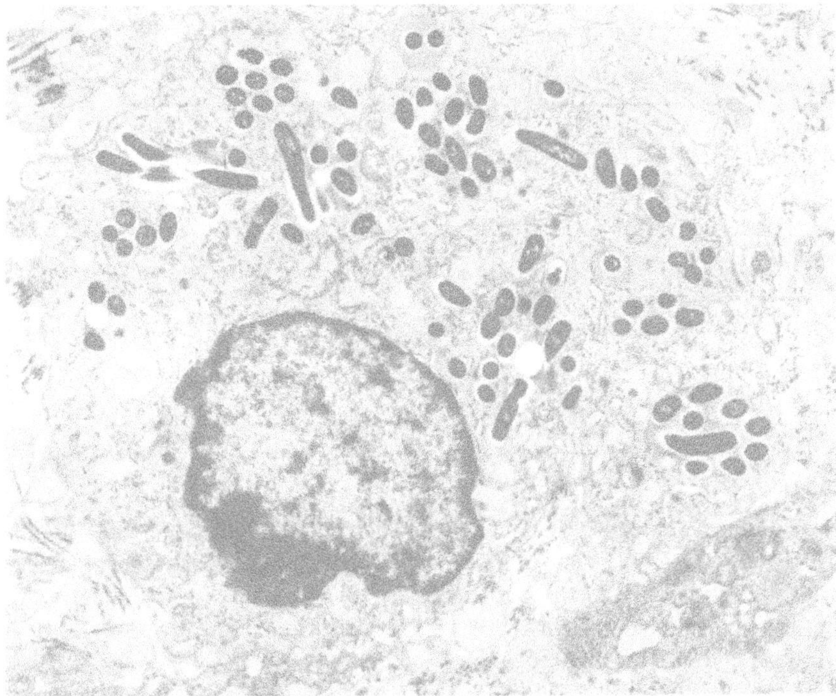

FIGURE 9. Macrophages fail to digest pathogens. Macrophage from a lymph node from an AIDS patient which contains numerous intact typical mycobacteria consistent with *Mycobacterium avium* complex (× 72,000).

4.3. Thl and Th2 Cytokines

The altered mononuclear cell response to antigenic stimuli and microorganisms characteristic of HIV-1-infected persons may be associated with a shift in the relative production of Thl (IFN-γ, IL-2) to Th2 (IL-10, IL-4) cytokines (Clerici and Shearer, 1994; Diaz-Mitoma *et al.*, 1995; Clerici *et al.*, 1994), emergence of a Th0 cytokine profile (Romagnani *et al.*, 1994; Graziosi *et al.*, 1994) and/or aberrant production of monocyte-derived cytokines (Table II). The network of cytokines regulating cell function(s) *in vivo* is complex. For example, enhanced production of IL-10 by monocytes after HIV-1 infection (Akridge *et al.*, 1994; Clerici *et al.*, 1994) may induce a tolerant, nonresponsive state through inhibition of Thl cytokines and an increase in IL-4, the latter cytokine being a powerful inhibitor of monocyte microbicidal activity and cytokine production (Wong *et al.*, 1992, 1993). Elevations in IL-10, together with a corresponding decrease in IL-12 (Chehimi *et al.*, 1994; Clerici *et al.*, 1993), could provide negative regulatory pressure on the entire immune system.

The mechanism(s) by which HIV-1 alters monocyte-produced cytokines is somewhat enigmatic, since the virus has been shown to induce both decreased and increased cytokine production *in vitro* (Table II). Moreover, the results of *in vitro* studies may not be relevant to *in vivo* events, since cytokine levels in HIV-1-seropositive persons vary widely (Table II), reflecting different stimulation protocols, varying stages of disease in the study population, administration of potentially stimulatory drugs, and the presence of opportunistic infections. Importantly, cytokines produced in a particular tissue may not be detectable in plasma

TABLE III. Macrophages as Antiviral Targets

Agent	Target	Active in acute/ chronic infected cells	References
DAB-IL-2	IL-2R	A/C	Finberg *et al.* (1991)
AZT, ddC, ddI	RT		Perno *et al.* (1988), Szebeni *et al.* (1989, 1990a,b), Weinstein *et al.* (1991)
AZT, ddC in liposomes	RT in phagocytic cells	A	Szebeni *et al.* (1990b)
Tat inhibitors	Tat	A	Dunne *et al.* (1994), Perno *et al.* (1994)
Anti-NLS drugs	NLS	A	Dubrovsky *et al.* (1995)
Protease inhibitors	HIV protease	A/C	Bugelski *et al.* (1994)
IFN-α	Multiple	A	Perno *et al.* (1994)
Antisense Rev	Rev	A	Perno *et al.* (1994)
SLPI	Internalization	A	McNeely *et al.* (1995), Wahl *et al.* (1995)

and yet profoundly affect local immunoregulation, virus production, and pathology. In summary, HIV-1 appears capable of exploiting the cytokine network of the host cell to promote its replication, but in the process causes its own virologic demise through the loss of host cells and impaired immune function which enables opportunistic pathogens to emerge.

Another cytokine that appears to contribute to HIV-1-induced immunosuppression is transforming growth factor-β (TGF-β). This regulatory cytokine is a potent inhibitor of many immunologic functions (Wahl, 1992, 1994; McCartney-Francis and Wahl, 1994), including the production of microbicidal products such as reactive oxygen intermediates and nitric oxide (reviewed in Wahl, 1992, 1994), which are normally operative against opportunistic pathogens prevalent in AIDS. Enhanced levels of TGF-β have been reported in cell cultures and sera from patients with AIDS (Kekow *et al.*, 1990; Allen *et al.*, 1991; Lotz and Seth, 1993; Wahl *et al.*, 1991). That mononuclear phagocytes are a potential source of the elevated TGF-β levels in these patients is supported by observations that HIV-1 infection of monocytes *in vitro* and brain macrophages *in situ* (Kekow *et al.*, 1990; Allen *et al.*, 1991; Wahl *et al.*, 1991) augmented TGF-β gene expression and secretion. TGF-β, in turn, may regulate viral replication (Poli *et al.*, 1992). Mechanistically, the HIV-1 Tat protein, a ligand for CD26 (Gutheil *et al.*, 1994) and a potent transactivator of HIV-1 transcription, has been identified as a stimulus for TGF-β synthesis (Lotz and Seth, 1993). By this pathway, HIV-1 could initiate a potential cyclic response in which viral induction of TGF-β would influence viral replication, and then induce further TGF-β synthesis and secretion, thereby amplifying immune dysfunction (McCartney-Francis *et al.*, 1990).

4.4. Pathogenesis

Despite the vast literature on the molecular characterization of HIV-1 replication in cultured cells (Haseltine, 1991) and more recently in the host (D. D. Ho *et al.*, 1995; Wei *et al.*, 1995; Wain-Hobson, 1995), HIV-1 pathogenicity is poorly understood. Still debated is the relative contribution of HIV-1-induced cytopathic effects versus immune-mediated mechanisms to disease pathogenesis (Pantaleo and Fauci, 1995). In this context, several lines of evidence indicate that monocyte dysfunction, in addition to the selective depletion of $CD4^+$ lymphocytes, contributes to the pathogenesis of AIDS. First, in the initial state of infection, macrophage-tropic HIV-1 variants may initiate aberrant immune function (Mosier and Sieburg, 1994; Meyaard *et al.*, 1993), possibly through deficient production of IL-12, a key macrophage-derived cytokine that regulates cell-mediated immune reactions (Chehimi *et al.*, 1994; Clerici and Shearer, 1994). Second, numerous proinflammatory functions of mononuclear phagocytes, including chemotaxis to inflammatory stimuli (Smith *et al.*, 1984; S. M. Wahl *et al.*, 1989), cytotoxicity (Bender *et al.*, 1988), Fc receptor-mediated activities (Allen *et al.*, 1991), and secretion of inflammatory mediators (Table II), are altered in patients with AIDS. Third, higher numbers of HIV-1-infected macrophages have been identified in tissues such as the brian, lungs, and gastrointestinal mucosa where inflammatory changes are prominent (Ho *et al.*, 1989; Wahl *et al.*, 1991; Sierra-Madero *et al.*, 1994; Smith, 1994).

Virological and immunologic events in the brains of HIV-1-infected persons illustrate dynamic pathological processes. A prominent feature of central nervous system (CNS) disease in HIV-1 infection is the accumulation of HIV-1 in perivascular mononuclear cell infiltrates in the brain (Ho *et al.*, 1989; Wahl *et al.*, 1991; Koenig *et al.*, 1986) which implicates an acute recruitment process. Increased expression of adhesion molecules (Birdsall *et al.*, 1994) and the release of chemotactic signals such as TGF-β by HIV-1-infected cells could direct such an extravascular migration (Wahl *et al.*, 1991, 1993). Once contact with brain microvascular endothelial cells has been established, viral replication is facilitated in local macrophages (Gilles *et al.*, 1995). In the CNS, the virus can be abundant and is associated with mononuclear and multinucleated microglial cells, replicating from the plasma membrane and into Golgi vacuoles. Despite the fusogenic effect of HIV-1 on $CD4^+$ cells and macrophages *in vitro*, only infected macrophages in the CNS of patients with AIDS-dementia complex (ADC) have been shown to form syncytia *in vivo* (J. Orenstein, unpublished observations). HIV-1 can be readily visualized in the brain and spinal cord of patients with ADC and vacuolar myelopathy, linking productive viral replication within macrophages to tissue pathology. As the primary host for HIV-1, and a source of cytokines, nitric oxide, eicosanoids, and other neurotoxic substances (Dawson *et al.*, 1993; Merrill and Chen, 1991; Wahl *et al.*, 1991; Morganti-Kossmann *et al.*, 1992), macrophages may orchestrate the neuropathology and neurological manifestations characteristic of AIDS (Nottet and Gendelman, 1995). Thus, tissue damage in the brain and other tissues, such as gastrointestinal mucosa (Smith, 1995), reflects the consequences of HIV-1 infection and chronic activation of local lymphoid cells unable to eliminate the antigenic stimulus (Ascher and Sheppard, 1988; Pantaleo and Fauci, 1995). Although HIV-1 may not be cytopathic for mononuclear phagocytes, the ability of the virus to infect these cells, disseminate to vital organs, and modulate macrophage effector functions implicates a fundamental role for these cells in tissue pathology.

5. MACROPHAGES AS TARGETS FOR ANTIVIRAL THERAPY

5.1. Reverse Transcriptase Inhibitors

Virus-encoded RT catalyzes the replication of single-stranded viral RNA to yield double-stranded DNA required for integration of HIV-1 genome into host DNA. Early studies suggested that nucleoside analogues, including the RT inhibitors 3′-azido-3′-deoxythymidine [zidovudine (AZT)],2′,3′-dideoxyinosine (ddI), and 2′,3′-dideoxycytidine (ddC), which inhibit HIV-1 replication in $CD4^+$ T cells, were less effective in inhibiting viral replication in monocytes (Richman *et al.*, 1987). Subsequent studies demonstrated that viral replication in monocytes was susceptible to these and other inhibitors (Perno *et al.*, 1988; Szebeni *et al.*, 1989, 1990b) (Table III). However, RT and protease inhibitors may be only transiently effective (Mitsuya and Yarchoan, 1994). With the rapid emergence of drug-resistant viral mutations (Wei *et al.*, 1995; D. D. Ho *et al.*, 1995), viral inhibition is not sustained. Consequently, multidrug antiviral therapy must be employed to ameliorate the inexorable progression of HIV-1 disease.

5.2. Endogenous Inhibitors

Endogenous inhibitors and mechanisms of innate host immunity likely participate in defense against HIV-1. In repeatedly exposed, but uninfected persons, as well as infected long-term nonprogressors (Sheppard *et al.*, 1993; Levy, 1993a,b), putative endogenous inhibitors may win the battle against the virus. Consequently, there is intense interest in defining whether potentially unique mechanisms of resistance occur in these subsets of persons.

Recent studies have shown that certain mucosal sites appear to possess an endogenous inhibitor of HIV-1 that could influence viral transmission. In this connection, the virtual absence of documented oral transmission of HIV-1 appears to reflect the presence of an inhibitor, known as secretory leukocyte protease inhibitor (SLPI), in the oral cavity (McNeely *et al.*, 1995; Wahl *et al.*, 1995). Produced by mucosal cells within salivary glands, SLPI's previously defined primary function concerned its potent antiprotease activity against human neutrophil elastase, cathepsin G, and other serine proteases. SLPI, a non-glycosylated polypeptide with a molecular mass of 12 kDa, recently was shown to inhibit HIV-1 infection of monocytes *in vitro*. At physiologic concentrations, it inhibited the appearance of RT and p24 antigen expression in human monocyte/macrophage cell cultures exposed to the virus (McNeely *et al.*, 1995). The protein consists of two homologous cysteine-rich domains, both of which are required for antiviral activity. SLPI does not interact with purified viral components, including gp120, gp160, or aspartyl protease, but appears to inhibit HIV-1 replication by acting on the monocyte primarily, although perhaps not exclusively, during internalization of virus.

Similar to recombinant soluble CD4, which competitively inhibits HIV-1 binding, SLPI's inhibitory activity requires that it only be present when the virus binds to the target cell. Unlike CD4, however, SLPI binds specifically and with high affinity to a cell surface receptor thereby blocking early entry events (McNeely *et al.*, submitted). The inhibition of HIV-1 entry by SLPI (McNeely *et al.*, 1995) is consistent with a gp120 V3 loop interaction by a CD26-like molecule characteristic of macrophage-tropic viruses (Oravecz *et al.*, 1995). Determining the mechanism of action of SLPI may provide further insight into how HIV-1 is internalized. Moreover, if the inhibition of HIV-1 entry by SLPI is shown to be related to cell-derived molecules and processes, such molecules and targets could be exploited as targets for anti-HIV-1 therapy.

5.3. Targeting Activation Markers

5.3.1. IL-2 Receptors

Targeting other cell-associated, rather than virally encoded, molecules has provided new strategies for antiretroviral therapy. Macrophages exposed to HIV-1 and/or gp120 *in vitro* show phenotypic and functional activation (L. M. Wahl *et al.*, 1989; S. M. Wahl *et al.*, 1989, 1991; Finberg *et al.*, 1991; Allen *et al.*, 1990, 1991), mirroring the activation of circulating monocytes from HIV-1-infected persons (Allen *et al.*, 1990, 1991; Wahl *et al.*, 1991; Trial *et al.*, 1995). The expression of activation markers could provide appropriate targets for selective drug delivery. In this regard, the expression of IL-2 receptor α chain (CD25), present shortly after exposure to HIV-1 and before viral replication, suggested a potential target for specific and early elimination of infected monocytes through the cytotoxic action of IL-2 toxin conjugates (Finberg *et al.*, 1991). DAB-IL-2 is a genetically engineered IL-2 conjugate that contains diphtheria toxin (DT) in which the DT receptor binding domain is replaced with human IL-2 sequences. This fusion toxin selectively binds to and thereby eliminates cells bearing high-affinity IL-2R by catalyzing NAD-dependent ADP ribosylation of eukaryotic elongation factor 2 to inhibit protein synthesis (Finberg *et al.*, 1991). Since the toxin conjugates bind only to activated and/or HIV-1-infected, IL-2R-bearing monocytes and lymphocytes, these populations are deleted. The potential to selectively target HIV-1-infected IL-2R$^+$ monocytes, as well as T cells, early in HIV-1 infection has provided the basis for initiating clinical trials with this agent in patients with AIDS.

5.3.2. Fc Receptors

The expression of FcγRIII (CD16), which is normally associated with monocyte activation and maturation (Welch *et al.*, 1990), is also associated with HIV-1 infection (Allen *et al.*, 1991). On phagocytic cells, Fc receptors function to bind the Fc region of immunoglobulins to promote phagocytosis of antigen–antibody complexes and antibody-dependent cellular cytotoxicity. Whereas monocytes from normal individuals generally express only two members of the FcγR family, FcγRI (CD64) and FcγRII (CD32), the identification of CD16$^+$ monocytes in AIDS patients may provide another venue for targeting selected cell populations. Although there is no direct evidence that CD16$^+$ cells bear HIV-1, such cells may be influenced by the chronic immune activation associated with HIV-1 infection. Fc receptors, which play a critical role in the phagocytic activity of monocyte-macrophages, could also be exploited for antiviral and cytotoxic agents. In this regard, antibody-conjugated liposomes have been used effectively as a vehicle to deliver antiviral agents to macrophages in culture (Szebeni *et al.*, 1990b).

5.4. Nuclear Localization Signals

New evidence indicates that HIV-1 replicates in nondividing macrophages by virtue of a specific nuclear localization signal (NLS) within the viral matrix protein (MA p17) (Bukrinsky *et al.*, 1993). NLS enables transport of the HIV-1 preintegration complex into the nucleus where integration of DNA and viral replication occur. In dividing T cells, disruption of the nuclear membrane during mitosis enables interaction between cellular genomic DNA and viral preintegration complexes, whereas in nondividing monocytes viral replication depends on an active, energy-dependent translocation of the complex through the nuclear membrane into the nucleus (Bukrinsky *et al.*, 1993). The viral preintegration complex includes MA p17 together with viral RNA, DNA, and viral protein R(Vpr) (Heinzinger *et al.*, 1994). Since transport into the nucleus relies on the NLS within MA p17, this sequence could be targeted to block nuclear translocation. Indeed, mutations in the MA p17 signal attenuate viral replication in monocytes (Heinzinger *et al.*, 1994), as do compounds that bind and inactivate the NLS. Arylene bis(methyl ketone) compounds have been shown to target NLS and inhibit HIV-1 replication in human monocytes by interrupting nuclear importation of viral DNA (Dubrovsky *et al.*, 1995). Interestingly, these compounds are ineffective in proliferating lymphocytes, emphasizing the potential for targeting antiviral therapy to monocyte-macrophages, microglia and other nondividing cells of the mononuclear phagocytic lineage.

The integration of HIV-1 into the host cell genome, the rapid emergence of viral mutants, and the ability of the virus to cloister itself within macrophages underscore the complexity of problems that must be overcome in designing antiviral agents. Thus, a combination of therapeutic approaches will be required to inhibit the virus and reconstitute the host immune system, and such approaches will need to target monocytes and macrophages. Although targeting a single population has limitations, adjunctive therapy focusing on the unique features of this crucial cell has substantial merit. Designing therapies that exploit our evolving knowledge of the phenotypic, biochemical, and molecular modifications of mononuclear phagocytes coupled with the use of direct antiviral agents may uncover additional targeting strategies.

ACKNOWLEDGMENTS. The authors are indebted to Kiki Angelis for assistance in manuscript preparation and illustrations. J.M.O. was supported, in part, by NIDR contract DE-12585 and P.D.S. by NIDR contract DE-42600, NIAID contract NOI 45218, and NIDDK grant 47322.

REFERENCES

Akridge, R. E., Oyafuso, L., and Reed, S. G., 1994, Interleukin 10 is induced during HIV-1 infection and is capable of decreasing viral replication in human macrophages, *J. Immunol.* **153:**5782–5789.

Alizon, M., and Dragic, T., 1994, CD26 antigen and HIV fusion? [Technical Comments] *Science* **264:**1161–1162.

Allen, J. B., McCartney-Francis, N., Smith, P. D., Simon, G., Gartner, S., Wahl, L. M., Popovic, M., and Wahl, S. M., 1990, Expression of IL-2 receptors by monocytes from patients with acquired immune deficiency syndrome and induction of monocyte IL-2 receptors by human immunodeficiency virus-1 *in vitro, J. Clin. Invest.* **85:**192–199.

Allen, J. B., Wong, H. L., Guyre, P., Simon, G., and Wahl, S. M., 1991, Circulating FcγRIII positive monocytes in AIDS patients with elevated levels of transforming growth factor β, *J. Clin. Invest.* **87:**1773–1779.

Amendola, A., Lombardi, G., Oliverio, S., Colizzi, V., and Piacentini, M., 1994, HIV-1 gp120-dependent induction of apoptosis in antigen-specific human T cell clones is characterized by 'tissue' transglutaminase expression and prevented by cyclosporin A, *FEBS* **339:**258–264.

Amerongen, H. M., Weltzin, R., Farnet, C. M., Michetti, P. L., Haseltine, W. A., and Neutra, M. R., 1991, Transepithelial transport of HIV-1 by intestinal M cells: A mechanism for transmission of AIDS, *J. Acq. Immune Defic. Syndr.* **4:**1773–1779.

Ascher, M. S., and Sheppard, H. W., 1988, AIDS as immune system activation, a model for pathogenesis, *Clin. Exp. Immunol.* **73:**165–167.

Baldwin, G. C., Fleischmann, J., Chung, Y., Koyanagi, Y., Chen, I. S. Y., and Golde, D. W., 1990, Human immunodeficiency virus causes mononuclear phagocyte dysfunction, *Proc. Natl. Acad. Sci. USA* **87:**3933–3937.

Bender, B. S., Davidson, B. L., Kline, R., Brown, C., and Quinn, T. C., 1988, Role of mononuclear phagocyte system in the immunopathogenesis of human immunodeficiency virus infection and the acquired immunodeficiency syndrome, *Rev. Infect. Dis.* **10:**1142–1154.

Birdsall, H. H., Trial, J., Hallum, J. A., de Jong, A. L., Green, L. K., Bandres, J. C., Smole, S. C., Laughter, A. H., and Rossen, R. D., 1994, Phenotypic and functional activation of monocytes in HIV-1 infection: Interactions with neural cells, *J. Leuk. Biol.* **56:**310–317.

Bou-Habib, D. C., Roderiquez, G., Oravecz, T., Berman, P. W., Lusso, P., and Norcross, M. A., 1994, Cryptic nature of envelope V3 region epitopes protects primary M-tropic human immunodeficiency virus type I from antibody neutralization, *J. Virol.* **68:**6006–6013.

Breen, E. C., Rerzai, A. R., Nakajima, K., Beall, G. N., Mitsuyasu, R. T., Hirano, T., Koshimoto, T., and Martinez-Maza, O., 1990, Infection with HIV is associated with elevated IL-6 levels and production, *J. Immunol.* **144:** 480–484.

Brighty, D. W., Rosenberg, M., Chen, I. S. Y., and Ivey-Hoyle, M., 1991, Envelope proteins from clinical isolates of human immunodeficiency virus type 1 that are refractory to neutralization by soluble CD4 possess high affinity for the CD4 receptor, *Proc. Natl. Acad. Sci. USA* **88:**7802–7805.

Broder, C. C., Nussbaum, O., Gutheil, W. G., Bachovchin, W. W., and Berger, E. A., 1994, CD26 antigen and HIV fusion? [Technical Comments] *Science* **264:**1156–1159.

Bugelski, P. J., Kirsh, R., and Hart, T. K., 1994, HIV protease inhibitors: Effects on viral maturation and physiologic function in macrophages, *J. Leuk. Biol.* **56:**374–380.

Bukrinsky, M. I., Haggerty, S., Dempsey, M. P., Sharova, N., Adzhubel, A., Spitz, L., Lewis, P., Goldfarb, D., Emerman, M., and Stevenson, M., 1993, A nuclear localization signal within HIV-1 matrix protein that govens infection of non-dividing cells, *Nature* **365:**666–669.

Callebaut, C., Krust, B., Jacotot, E., and Hovanessian, A. G., 1993, T cell activation antigen, CD26, as a cofactor for entry of HIV in $CD4^+$ cells, *Science* **262:**2045–2050.

Camerini, D., Planelles, V., and Chen, I. S., 1994, CD26 antigen and HIV fusion? [Technical Comments] *Science* **264:**1160–1161.

Cann, A. J., Churcher, M. J., Boyd, M., O'Brien, W., Zhao, J. Q., Zack, J., and Chen, I. S., 1992, The region of the envelope gene of human immunodeficiency virus type-1 responsible for determination of cell tropism, *J. Virol.* **66:**305–309.

Capsoni, F., Minonzio, F., Ongari, A. M., Rizzardi, G. P., Lazzarin, A., and Zanussi, C., 1992, Monocyte-derived macrophage function in HIV-infected subjects: In vitro modulation by rIFN-gamma and rGM-CSF, *Clin. Immunol. Immunopathol.* **62:**176–182.

Chaturvedi, S., Frame, P., and Newman, S. L., 1995, Macrophages from human immunodeficiency virus-positive persons are defective in host defense against, *Histoplasma capsulatum, J. Infect. Dis.* **171:**320–327.

Chehimi, J., Starr, S. E., Frank, I., D'Andrea, A., Ma, X., MacGregor, R. R., Sennelier, J., and Trinchieri, G., 1994, Impaired interleukin 12 production in human immunodeficiency virus-infected patients, *J. Exp. Med.* **179:** 1361–1366.

Chesebro, B., Wehrly, K., Nishino, J., and Perryman, S., 1992, Macrophage-tropic human immunodeficiency virus isolates from different patients exhibit unusual V3 envelope sequence homogeneity in comparison with T-cell-tropic isolates: Definition of critical amino acids involved in cell tropism, *J. Virol.* **66:**6547–6554.

Cheynier, R., Henrichwark, S., Hadida, F., Pelletier, E., Oksenhendler, E., Autran, B., and Wain-Hobson, S., 1994, HIV and T cell expansion in splenic white pulp is accompanied by infiltration of HIV-specific cytotoxic T lymphocytes, *Cell* **78:**373–387.

Clark, S. J., Saag, M. S., Decker, W. D., Campbell-Hill, S., Roberson, J. L., Veldkamp, P. J., Kappes, J. C., Hahn, B. H., and Shaw, G. M., 1991, High titers of cytopathic virus in plasma of patients with symptomatic primary HIV-1 infection, *N. Engl. J. Med.* **324:**954–960.

Clements, G. J., Prince-Jones, M. J., Stephens, P. E., Sutton, C., Schultz, T. F., Clapham, P. R., McKeating, J. A., McClure, M. O., Thomson, S., Marsh, M., Kay, J., Weiss, R. A., and Moore, J. P., 1991, The V3 loops of the HIV-1 and HIV-2 surface glycoproteins contain proteolytic cleavage sites: A possible function in viral fusion? *AIDS Res. Hum. Retrovir.* **7:**3–16.

Clerici, M., and Shearer, G. M., 1994, The Thl-Th2 hypothesis of HIV infection: New insights, *Immunol. Today* **15:**575–581.

Clerici, M., Lucey, D. R., Berzofsky, J. A., Pinto, L. A., Wynn, T. A., Blatt, S. P., Dolan, M. J., Hendrix, C. W., Wolf, S. F., and Shearer, G. M., 1993, Restoration of HIV-specific cell-mediated immune responses by interleukin-12 in vitro, *Science* **262:**1721–1724.

Clerici, M., Synn, T. A., Berzofsky, J. A., Blatt, S. P., Hendrix, C. W., Sher, A., Coffman, R. L., and Shearer, G. M., 1994, Role of interleukin-10 in T helper cell dysfunction in asymptomatic individuals infected with the human immunodeficiency virus, *J. Clin. Invest.* **93:**768–775.

Crowe, S. M., Carlin, J. B., Stewart, K. I., Lucas, C. R., and Hoy, L. F., 1991, Predictive value of CD4 lymphocyte numbers for the development of opportunistic infections and mallignancies in HIV-infected persons, *J. Acq. Immune Defic. Syndr.* **4:**770–776.

Crowe, S. M., Vardaxis, N. J., Kent, S. J., Maerz, A. L., Hewish, M. J., McGrath, M. S., and Mills, J., 1994, HIV infection of monocyte-derived macrophages in vitro reduces phagocytosis of Candida albicans, *J. Leuk. Biol.* **56:**318–327.

Daar, E. S., Moudgil, T., Meyer, R. D., and Ho, D. D., 1991, Transient high levels of viremia in patients with primary human immunodeficiency virus type 1 infection, *N. Engl. J. Med.* **324:**961–964.

Dalgleish, A., 1995, HIV and CD26, *Nature Med.* **1:**881.

Dalgleish, A. G., Beverly, P. C. L., Clapham, P. R., Crawford, D. H., Greaves, M. F., and Weiss, R. A., 1984, The CD4 (T4) antigen is an essential component of the receptor for the AIDS retrovirus, *Nature* **312:**763–767.

Dawson, V. L., Dawson, T. M., Uhl, G. R., and Snyder, S. H., 1993, Human immunodeficiency virus type 1 coat protein neurotoxicity mediated by nitric oxide in primary cortical cultures, *Proc. Natl. Acad. Sci. USA* **90:** 3256–3259.

De Jong, J. J., Goudsmit, J., Keulen, W., Klaver, B., Krone, W., Tersmette, M., and De Ronde, T., 1992, Human immunodeficiency viruses type-1 chimeric for the envelope V3 domain are distinct in syncytium formation and replication capacity, *J. Virol.* **66:**757–765.

Devaux, C., Boucraut, J., Poirier, G., Corbeau, P., Rey, F., Benkirane, M., Perarnau, B., Kourilsky, F., and Chermann, J. C., 1990, Anti-β2-microglobulin monoclonal antibodies mediate a delay in HIV-1 cytopathic effect on MT4 cells, *Res. Immunol.* **141:**357–372.

Dezube, B., Pardee, A. B., Beckett, L. A., Ahlers, C. M., Ecto, L., Allen-Ryan, J., Anisowicz, A., Sager, R., and Crumpacker, C. S., 1992, Cytokine dysregulation in AIDS: In vivo expression of mRNA of tumor necrosis factor α and its correlation with that of the inflammatory cytokine GRO, *J. Acq. Immune Defic. Syndr.* **5:**1099–1104.

Diaz-Mitoma, F., Kumar, A., Karimi, S., Kryworuchko, M., Daftarian, P., Creery, W. D., Filion, L. G., and Cameron, W., 1995, Expression of interleukin (IL)-10, IL-4 and interferon-γ in unstimulated and mitogen stimulated peripheral blood lymphocytes from HIV seropositive patients, *Clin. Exp. Immunol.* **102:**31–39.

Dragic, T., Charneau, P., Clavel, F., and Alizon, M., 1992, Complementation of murine cells for human immunodeficiency virus envelope/CD4-mediated fusion in human/murine heterokaryons, *J. Virol.* **66:**4794–4802.

Dubrovsky, L., Ulrich, P., Nuovo, G. J., Manogue, K. R., Cerami, A., and Bukrinsky, M., 1995, Nuclear localization signal of HIV-1 as a novel target for therapeutic intervention, *Mol. Med.* **1:**217–230.

Duh, E. J., Maury, W. J., Folks, T. M., Fauci, A. S., and Rabson, A. B., 1989, Tumor necrosis factor alpha activates human immunodeficiency virus type 1 through induction of nuclear factor binding to the NF-κB sites in the long terminal repeat, *Proc. Natl. Acad. Sci. USA* **86:**5974–5978.

Dukes, C. S., Matthews, T. J., and Weinberg, J. B., 1993, Human immunodeficiency virus type 1 infection of human monocytes and macrophages does not alter their ability to generate on oxidative burst, *J. Infect. Dis.* **168:**459–462.

Dukes, C., Yu, Y., Rivadeneira, E. D., Sauls, D. L., Liao, H. X., Haynes, B. F., and Weinberg, J. B., 1995, Cellular CD44S as a determinant of HIV-1 infection and cellular tropism, *J. Virol.* **69:**4000–4005.

Dunne, A. L., Siregar, H., Mills, J., and Crowe, S. M., 1994, HIV replication of chronically infected macrophages is not inhibited by the Tat inhibitors Ro-5-3335 and Ro-24-7429, *J. Leuk. Biol.* **56:**369–373.

Eales, L.-J., Moshtael, O., and Pinching, J., 1987, Microbicidal activity of monocyte derived macrophages in AIDS and related disorders, *Clin. Exp. Immunol.* **67:**227–235.

Embretson, J., Zupancic, M., Ribas, J. L., Burke, A., Racz, P., Tenner-Racz, K., and Haase, A. T., 1993, Massive covert infection of helper T lymphocytes and macrophages by HIV during the incubation period of AIDS, *Nature* **362:**359–362.

Emilie, D. M., Peuchmaur, M. C., Maillot, M. C., Crevon, N., Brousee, J. F., Delfraissy, J., Dormont, P., and Galanaud, P., 1990, Production of interleukins in human immunodeficiency virus-1-replicating lymph nodes, *J. Clin. Invest.* **86:**148–159.

Estevez, M. E., Ballart, I. J., Diez, R. A., Planes, N., Scaglione, C., and Sen, L., 1986, Early defect of phagocytic cell function in subjects at risk for acquired immunodeficiency syndrome, *Scand. J. Immunol.* **24:**215–221.

Fan, S. X., Turpin, J. A., Aronovitz, J. R., and Meltzer, M. S., 1994, Interferon-γ protects primary monocytes against infection with human immunodeficiency virus type 1, *J. Leuk. Biol.* **56:**362–368.

Feng, Y., Broder, C. C., Kennedy, P. E., and Berger, E. A., 1996, HIV-1 entry cofactor: Functional cDNA cloning of a seven-transmembrane, G protein-coupled receptor, *Science* **272:**872–877.

Finberg, R. W., Wahl, S. M., Allen, J. B., Soman, G., Strom, T. B., Murphy, J. R., and Nichols, J. C., 1991, Selective elimination of HIV-1 infected cells using an IL-2 receptor specific cytotoxin, *Science* **252:**1703–1705.

Fouchier, R. A. M., Groenink, M., Kootstra, N. A., Tersmette, M., Huisman, H. G., Miedema, F., and Schuitemaker, H., 1992, Phenotype-associated sequence variation in the third variable domain of the human immunodeficiency virus type 1 gp120 molecule, *J. Virol.* **66:**3183–3187.

Fox, C. H., Kotler, D. P., Tierney, A. T., Wilson, C. S., and Fauci, A. S., 1989, Detection of HIV-1 RNA in lamina propria of patients with AIDS and gastrointestinal disease, *J. Infect. Dis.* **159:**467–471.

Fox, C. H., Tenner-Racz, K., Racz, P., Firpo, A., Rizzo, P. A., and Fauci, A. S., 1991, Lymphoid germinal centers are reservoirs of human immunodeficiency virus type 1 RNA, *J. Infect. Dis.* **164:**1051–1057.

Fuchs, D., Hausen, A., Reibnegger, G., Werner, E. R., Werner-Felmayer, G., Dierich, M. P., Wachter, H., 1989, Interferon-γ concentrations are increased in sera from individuals infected with human immunodeficiency virus type 1, *J. Acq. Immune. Defic. Syndr.* **2:**158–162.

Gan, H., Ruef, C., Hall, B. F., Tobin, E., Remold, H. G., and Mellors, J. W., 1991, Interleukin-6 expression in primary macrophages infected with human immunodeficiency virus-1 (HIV-1), *AIDS Res. Hum. Retrovir.* **7:**671.

Gartner, S., Markovitz, P., Markovitz, D. M., Kaplan, M. H., Gallo, R. C., and Popovic, M., 1986, The role of mononuclear phagocytes in HTLV-III/LAV infection, *Science* **233:**215–219.

Gendelman, H. E., Phelps, W., Feigenbaum, L., Ostrove, J. M., Adachi, A., Howley, P. M., Khoury, G., and Ginsberg, H. S., 1986, Transactivation of the human immunodeficiency virus long terminal repeat sequence by DNA viruses, *Proc. Natl. Acad. Sci. USA* **83:**9759–9763.

Gendelman, H. E., Orenstein, J. M., Martin, M. A., Ferruca, C., Mitra, R., Phipps, T., Wahl, L. A., Lane, H. C., Fauci, A. S., Burke, D. S., Skillman, D., and Meltzer, M. S., 1988, Efficient isolation and propagation of human immunodeficiency virus on recombinant colony-stimulating factor-1 treated monocytes, *J. Exp. Med.* **167:**1428–1441.

Gendelman, H. E., Baca, L. M., Turpin, J., Kalter, D. C., Hansen, B., Orenstein, J. M., Dieffenbach, C., Friedman, R. M., and Meltzer, M. S., 1990a, Regulation of HIV replication in infected monocytes by interferon α: Mechanisms for viral restriction, *J. Immunol.* **145:**2669–2677.

Gendelman, H. E., Friedman, R. M., Joe, S., Baca, L. M., Turpin, J., Dveskler, G., Meltzer, M. S., and Dieffenbach, C., 1990b, A selective defect of interferon-α production in human immunodeficiency virus-infected monocytes, *J. Exp. Med.* **172:**1433–1442.

Gilles, P. N., Lathey, J. L., and Spector, S. A., 1995, Replication of macrophage-tropic and T-cell-tropic strains of human immunodeficiency virus type 1 as augmented by macrophage–endothelial cell contact, *J. Virol.* **69:**2133–2139.

Graziosi, C., Pantaleo, G., Gantt, K. R., Fortin, J. P., Demarest, J. F., Cohen, O. J., Sekaly, R. P., and Fauci, A. S., 1994, Lack of evidence for the dichotomy of TH1 and TH2 predominance in HIV-infected individuals, *Science* **265:**248–252.

Griffin, G. E., Leung, K., Folks, T. M., Kunkel, S., and Nabel, G. J., 1989, Activation of HIV gene expression during monocyte differentiation by induction of NF-kappa B, *Nature* **339:**70–73.

Gruber, M. F., Weih, K. A., Boone, E. J., Smith, P. D., and Clouse, K. A., 1995, Endogenous macrophage CSF production is associated with viral replication in HIV-1-infected human monocyte-derived macrophages, *J. Immunol.* **154:**5528–5535.

Gupta, S., Vayuvegula, B., Ruhling, M., and Thorton, M., 1987, Interleukin 1 and interleukin 2 production in the acquired immunodeficiency syndrome (AIDS) and AIDS-related complex, *J. Clin. Immunol.* **22:**113–116.

Gutheil, W. G., Subramanyam, M., Flentke, G. R., Sanford, D. G., Munoz, E., Huber, B. T., and Bachovchin, W. W., 1994, Human immunodeficiency virus 1 Tat binds to dipeptidyl aminopeptidase IV (CD26): A possible mechanism for Tat's immunosuppressive activity, *Proc. Natl. Acad. Sci. USA* **91:**6594–6598.

Harper, M. E., Marselle, L. M., Gallo, R. C., and Wong-Staal, F., 1986, Detection of lymphocytes expressing human T-lymphocyte virus type-III in lymph nodes and peripheral blood from infected individuals by in situ hybridization, *Proc. Natl. Acad. Sci. USA* **83:**772–776.

Harriman, G. R., Smith, P. D., Horne, M. K., Fox, C. H., Koenig, S., Lack, E. E., Lane, H. C., and Fauci, A. S., 1989, Vitamin B12 malabsorption in patients with acquired immunodeficiency syndrome, *Arch. Intern. Med.* **149:**2039–2041.

Haseltine, W. A., 1991, Molecular biology of the human immunodeficiency virus type 1, *FASEB J.* **5:**2349–2360.

Heath, S., Tow, G., Taw, J. O., Szakal, A. K., and Burton, G. F., 1995, Follicular dendritic cells and human immunodeficiency virus infectivity, *Nature* **377:**740–744.

Heinzinger, N. K., Bukrinsky, M. I., Haggerty, S. A., Ragland, A. M., Lee, M.-A., Kewalramani, V., Gendelman, H. E., Ratner, L., Stevenson, M., and Emerman, M., 1994, The Vpr protein of human immunodeficiency virus type 1 influences nuclear localization of viral nucleic acids in non-dividing host cells, *Proc. Natl. Acad. Sci. USA* **91:**7311–7315.

Ho, D. D., Bredsen, D. E., Vinters, H. V., and Daar, E. S., 1989, The acquired immunodeficiency syndrome (AIDS) dementia complex, *Ann. Intern. Med.* **111:**400–410.

Ho, D. D., Neumann, A. U., Perelson, A. S., Chen, W., Leonard, J. M., and Markowitz, M., 1995, Rapid turnover of plasma virions and CD4 lymphocytes in HIV-1 infection, *Nature* **373**:123–126.

Ho, J. L., He, S., Hu, A., Geng, J., Basile, F. G., Almeida, G. B., Saito, A. Y., Laurence, J., and Johnson, W. D., 1995, Neutrophils from human immunodeficiency virus (HIV)-seronegative donors induce HIV replication from HIV-infected patients' mononuclear cells and cell lines: An *in vitro* model of HIV transmission facilitated by *Chlamydia trachomatis*, *J. Exp. Med.* **181**:1493–1505.

Homsy, J., Meyer, M., Tateno, M., Clarkson, S., and Levy, J. A., 1989, The Fc and not CD4 receptor mediates antibody enhancement of HIV infection in human cells, *Science* **244**:1357–1360.

Honda, M., Kitamura, K., Mizutani, Y., Oishi, M., Arai, M., Okura, T., Igarahi, K., Yasukawa, K., Hirano, T., Kishimoto, T., Mitsuyasu, R., Chermann, J.-C., and Tokunaga, T., 1990, Quantitative analysis of serum IL-6 and its correlation with increased levels of serum IL-2R in HIV-induced diseases, *J. Immunol.* **145**:4059–4064.

Hwang, S. S., Boyle, T. J., Lyerly, H. K., and Cullen, B. R., 1991, Identification of the envelope V3 loop as the primary determinant of cell tropism in HIV-1, *Science* **253**:71–74.

Israel-Biet, D., Cadranel, J., Beldjord, K., Andrieu, J. M., Jeffrey, A., and Even, P., 1991, Tumor necrosis factor production in HIV-seropositive subjects, *J. Immunol.* **147**:490–494.

Janoff, E. N., Wahl, S. M., Thomas, K., and Smith, P. D., 1995, Modulation of human immunodeficiency virus type 1 infection of human monocytes by IgA, *J. Infect. Dis.* **172**:855–858.

Jarry, A., Cortez, A., Rene, E., Muzeau, F., and Brousse, N., 1990, Infected and immune cells in the gastrointestinal tract of AIDS patients, An immunohistochemical study of 127 cases, *Histopathology* **16**:133–140.

Kazazi, F., Mathijs, J. M., Chang, J., Malafiej, P., Lopez, A., Dowton, D., Sorrell, T. C., Vadas, M. A., and Cunningham, A. L., 1992, Recombinant interleukin 4 stimulates human immunodeficiency virus production by infected monocytes and macrophages, *J. Gen. Virol.* **73**:941–949.

Kekow, J., Wachsmann, W., McCutchan, J. A., Cronin, M., Carson, D. A., and Lotz, M., 1990, Transforming growth factor beta and noncytopathic mechanisms of immunodeficiency in human immunodeficiency virus infection, *Proc. Natl. Acad. Sci. USA* **87**:8321–8325.

Kent, S. J., Stent, G., Sonza, S., Hunter, S. D., and Crowe, S. M., 1994, HIV-1 infection of monocyte-derived macrophages reduces Fc and complement receptor expression, *Clin. Exp. Immunol.* **95**:450–454.

Kido, H., Fukotomi, A., and Katunuma, N., 1991, Tryptase TL2 in the membrane of human $T4^+$ lymphocytes is a novel binding protein of the V3 domain of HIV-1 envelope glycoprotein gp120, *FEBS Lett.* **286**:2233–236.

Klatzmann, C., Champagne, E., Chamaret, S., Gruest, J., Guetard, D., Hercend, T., Gluckman, J.-C., and Montagnier, L., 1984, T-lymphocyte T4 molecule behaves as the receptor for human retrovirus LAV, *Nature* **312**:767–768.

Koenig, S., Gendelman, H. E., Orenstein, J. M., Dal Canto, M. C., Pezeshkpour, G. H., Yungbluth, M., Janotta, R., Aksamit, A., Martin, M. A., and Fauci, A. S., 1986, Detection of AIDS virus in macrophage in brain tissue from AIDS patients with encephalopathy, *Science* **233**:1089.

Koito, A., Hattori, T., Murakami, T., Matsushita, S., Maeda, Y., Yamamoto, T., and Takatsuki, K., 1989, A neutralizing epitope of human immunodeficiency virus type 1 has homologous amino acid sequences with the active site of intra-alpha-trypsin inhibitor, *Int. Immunol.* **1**:613–618.

Koot, M., Vos, A. H. V., Keet, R. P. M., DeGoede, R. E. Y., Dercksen, W., Terpstra, F. G., Coutinho, R. A., Miedema, F., and Tersmette, M., 1992, HIV-1 biological phenotype in long term infected individuals, evaluated with an MT-2 cocultivation assay, *AIDS* **6**:49–54.

Kornbluth, R. S., 1994, Significance of T cell apoptosis for macrophages in HIV infection, *J. Leuk. Biol.* **56**:247–256.

Kornbluth, R. S., Oh, P. S., Munis, J. R., Cleveland, P. H., and Richman, D. D., 1989, Interferons and bacterial lipopolysaccharide protect macrophages from productive infection of human immunodeficiency virus in vitro, *J. Exp. Med.* **169**:1137–1151.

Kotler, D. P., Reka, S., and Clayton, F., 1993, Intestinal mucosal inflammation associated with human immunodeficiency virus infection, *Dig. Dis. Sci.* **38**:1119–1127.

Koup, R., Safrit, J., Cao, Y., Andres, C., McLeod, G., Borkowsky, G., Farthing, C., and Ho, D., 1994, Temporal association of cellular immune responses with the initial control of viremia in primary human immunodeficiency virus type 1 syndrome, *J. Virol.* **68**:4659–4665.

Koyanagi, Y., O'Brien, W. A., Zhao, J. Q., Golde, D. W., Gasson, J. C., and Chen, I. S. Y., 1988, Cytokines alter production of HIV-1 from primary mononuclear phagocytes, *Science* **241**:1673–1675.

Kozlowski, P. A., Black, K. P., Shen, L., and Jackson, S., 1995, High prevalence of serum IgA HIV-1 infection-enhancing antibodies in HIV-infected persons, *J. Immunol.* **154**:6163–6173.

Krown, S. E., Niedzwiecki, D., Bhalla, R. B., Flomenberg, B., Bundow, D., and Chapman, D., 1991, Relationship and prognostic value of endogenous interferon-α, β2-microglobulin, and neopterin serum levels in patients with Kaposi's sarcoma and AIDS, *J. Acq. Immune Defic. Syndr.* **4**:871–880.

Lahdevitra, J., Maury, C. P. J., Teppo, A. M., and Repo, H., 1988, Elevated levels of circulating cachectin/tumor necrosis factor in patients with acquired immunodeficiency syndrome, *Am. J. Med.* **85**:289–291.

Lau, A. S., and Livesey, J. F., 1989, Endotoxin induction of tumor necrosis factor is enhanced by acid-labile interferon-α in acquired immunodeficiency syndrome, *J. Clin. Invest.* **84**:738–743.

Laurent-Crawford, A. G., Krust, B., Riviere, Y., Desgranges, C., Muller, S., Kieny, M. P., Dauguet, C., and Hovanessian, A. G., 1993, Membrane expression of HIV envelope glycoproteins triggers apoptosis in CD4 cells, *AIDS Res. Hum. Retrovir.* **9**:761–773.

Lazaro, I., Naniche, D., Signoret, N., Bernard, A. M., Marguet, D., Klatzmann, D., Dragic, T., Alizon, M., and Sattentau, Q., 1994, Factors involved in entry of the human immunodeficiency virus type 1 into permissive cells: Lack of evidence of a role for CD26, *J. Virol.* **68**:6535–6546.

Lazdins, J. K., Klimkait, T., Woods-Cook, K., Walker, M., Alteri, E., Cox, D., Cerletti, N., Shipman, R., Bilbe, G., and McMaster, G., 1991, In vitro effect of transforming growth factor-β on progression of HIV-1 infection in primary mononuclear phagocytes, *J. Immunol.* **147**:1201–1207.

Levy, J., 1993a, Pathogenesis of human immunodeficiency virus infection, *Microbiol. Rev.* **57**:183–289.

Levy, J., 1993b, HIV pathogenesis and long-term survival, *AIDS* **7**:1401–1410.

Lotz, M., and Seth, P., 1993, TGF-β and HIV infection, *Ann. N.Y. Acad. Sci.* **685**:501–511.

Lund, O., Hansen, J., Sorensen, A. M., Mosekilde, E., Nielsen, J. O., and Hansen, J. E. S., 1995, Increased adhesion as a mechanism of antibody-dependent and antibody-independent complement-mediated enhancement of human immunodeficiency virus infection, *J. Virol.* **69**:2393–2400.

McCartney-Francis, N., and Wahl, S. M., 1994, TGF-β: A matter of life and death, *J. Leuk. Biol.* **55**:401–409.

McCartney-Francis, N., Mizel, D., Wong, H., Wahl, L. M., and Wahl, S. M., 1990, TGF-β regulates production of growth factor and TGF-β by human peripheral blood monocytes, *Growth Factors* **4**:27–35.

McNearney, T., Hornickova, Z., Markham, R., Birdwell, A., Arens, M., Saah, A., and Ratner, L., 1992, Relationship of human immunodeficiency virus type 1 sequence heterogeneity to state of disease, *Proc. Natl. Acad. Sci. USA* **89**:10247–10251.

McNeely, T. B., Dealy, M., Dripps, D. J., Orenstein, J. M., Eisenberg, S. P., and Wahl, S. M., 1995, Secretory leukocyte protease inhibitor: A human saliva protein exhibiting anti-HIV-1 activity in vitro, *J. Clin. Invest.* **96**:456–464.

Manbondzo, A., Le Naour, R., Raoul, H., Clayette, P., Lafuma, C., Barré-Sinoussi, Cayre, Y., and Dormont, D., 1991, In vitro infection of macrophages by HIV: Correlation with cellular activation, synthesis of tumor necrosis factor alpha and proteolytic activity, *Res. Virol.* **142**:205.

Merrill, J. E., and Chen, I. S., 1991, HIV-1, macrophages, glial cell, and cytokines in AIDS nervous system disease, *FASEB J.* **5**:2391–2397.

Merrill, J. E., Koyanagi, Y., and Chen, I. S. Y., 1989, Interleukin-1 and TNF-α can be induced from mononuclear phagocytes by human immunodeficiency virus type 1 binding to the CD4 receptor, *J. Virol.* **63**:4404–4408.

Meyaard, L., Otto, S. A., Jonker, R. R., Mijnster, M. J., Keet, R. P. M., and Miedema, F., 1992, Programmed death of T cells in HIV-1 infection, *Science* **257**:217–219.

Meyaard, L., Schuitemaker, H., and Miedema, F., 1993, T-cell dysfunction in HIV infection: Anergy due to defective antigen presenting cell function, *Immunol. Today* **14**:161–164.

Meylan, P. R. A., Guatelli, J. C., Munis, J. R., Richman, D. D., and Kornbluth, R. S., 1993, Mechanisms for the inhibition of HIV replication by interferons-α, -β, -γ in primary macrophages, *Virology* **193**:138–148.

Mintz, M., Rapaport, R., Oleske, J. M., Connor, E. M., Koenigsberger, M. R., Denny, T., and Epstein, L. G., 1989, Elevated serum levels of tumor necrosis factor are associated with progressive encephalopathy in children with acquired immunodeficiency syndrome, *Am. J. Dis. Child.* **143**:771–774.

Mitsuya, H., and Yarchoan, R., 1994, Development of antiretroviral therapy for AIDS and related disorders, in: *Textbook of AIDS Medicine* (S. Broder, T. C. Merigan, and D. Bolognesi, eds.), Williams & Wilkins, Baltimore, pp. 721–742.

Molina, J.-M., Scadden, D. T., Byrn, R., Dinarello, C., and Groopman, J. E., 1990a, Production of tumor necrosis factor α by monocytic cells infected with human immunodeficiency virus, *J. Clin. Infect.* **144**:970–975.

Molina, J. M., Scadden, D. T., Amirault, C., Woon, A., Vannier, E., Dinarello, C. A., and Groopman, J. E., 1990b, Human immunodeficiency virus does not induce interleukin 1, interleukin 6, or tumor necrosis factor α in mononuclear cells, *J. Virol.* **64**:2901–2906.

Montaner, L. J., Doyle, A. G., Collin, M., Georges, H., James, W., Minty, A., Caput, D., Ferrar, P., and Gordon, S.,

1993, Interleukin 13 inhibits human immunodeficiency virus type 1 production in primary blood-derived human macrophages in vitro, *J. Exp. Med.* **178**:743–747.

Morens, D. M., 1994, Antibody-dependent enhancement of infection and the pathogenesis of viral disease, *Clin. Infect. Dis.* **19**:500–512.

Moore, J. P., McKeating, J. A., Norton, W. A., and Sattentau, Q. J., 1991, Direct measurement of soluble CD4 binding to human immunodeficiency virus type 1 virions: gp120 dissociation and its implications for virus-cell binding and fusion reactions and their neutralization by soluble CD4, *J. Virol.* **65**:1133–1140.

Morganti-Kossmann, M. C., Kossmann, T., and Wahl, S. M., 1992, Cytokines and neuropathology, *Trends Pharmacol.* **13**:286–290.

Morimoto, C., Lord, C. I., Zhang, C., Duke-Cohan, J. S., Letvin, N. L., and Schlossman, S. F., 1994, Role of CD26/dipeptidyl peptidase IV in human immunodeficiency virus type 1 infection and apoptosis, *Proc. Natl. Acad. Sci. USA* **91**:9960–9964.

Mosca, J. D., Bednarik, D. P., Faj, N. B. K., Rosen, C. A., Sodroski, J. G., Haseltine, W. A., and Pitha, P. M. V., 1987, Herpes simplex virus type-1 can reactivate transcription of latent human immunodeficiency virus, *Nature* **325**:67–70.

Mosier, D., and Sieburg, H., 1994, Macrophage-tropic HIV: Critical for AIDS pathogenesis? *Immunol. Today* **15**:332– 339.

Munis, J. R., Richman, D. D., and Kornbluth, R. S., 1990, Human immunodeficiency virus-1 infection of macrophages in vitro neither induces tumor necrosis factor (TNF)/cachectin gene expression or alters TNF/cachectin induction by lipopolysaccharide, *J. Clin. Invest.* **85**:591–596.

Murakami, T., Hattori, T., and Takatsuki, K., 1991, A principal neutralizing domain of human immunodeficiency virus type 1 interacts with proteinase-like molecule(s) at the surface of Molt-4 clone 8 cells, *Biochim. Biophys. Acta* **1079**:279–284.

Murray, H. W., Rubin, B. Y., Masur, H., and Roberts, R. B., 1984, Impaired production of lymphokines and immune (gamma) interferon in the acquired imunodeficiency syndrome, *N. Engl. J. Med.* **310**:883–889.

Nakajima, K., Martinez-Maza, O., Hirano, T., Breen, E. C., Nishanian, P. G., Salazar-Gonzalez, J. F., Fahey, J. L., and Kishimoto, T., 1989, Induction of IL-6 (B cell stimulatory factor-2/IFN-β2) production by HIV, *J. Immunol.* **142**:531.

Newman, G. W., Kelley, T. G., Gan, H., Kandil, O., Newman, M. J., Pinkston, P., Rose, R. M., and Remold, H. G., 1993, Concurrent infection of human macrophages with HIV-1 and Mycobacterium avium results in decreased cell viability, increased M. avium multiplication and altered cytokine production, *J. Immunol.* **151**:2261–2272.

Nottet, H. S., and Gendelman, H. E., 1995, Unraveling the neuroimmune mechanisms for the HIV-1-associated cognitive/motor complex, *Immunol. Today* **16**:441.

Novak, R. M., Holzer, T. J., Kennedy, M. M., Heynen, C. A., and Dawson, G., 1990, The effect of interleukin 4 (BSF-1) on infection of peripheral blood monocyte-derived macrophages with HIV-1, *AIDS Res. Hum. Retrovir.* **6**:973–976.

O'Brien, W. A., Koyanagi, Y., Namazi, A., Zhao, J.-Q., Diagne, A., Idler, K., Zack, J. A., and Chen, I. S. Y., 1990, HIV-1 tropism for mononuclear phagocytes can be determined by regions of gp120 outside the CD4-binding domain, *Nature* **348**:69–73.

O'Brien, W. A., Namazi, A., Kalhor, H., Mao, S.-H., Zack, J. A., and Chen, I. S., 1994a, Kinetics of human immunodeficiency virus type 1 reverse transcription in blood mononuclear phagocytes are slowed by limitations of nucleotide precursors, *J. Virol.* **68**:1258–1263.

O'Brien, W. A., Mao, S.-H., Cao, Y., and Moore, J. P., 1994b, Macrophage and T-cell tropic HIV-1 strains differ in their susceptibility to neutralization by soluble CD4 at different temperatures, *J. Virol.* **68**:5264–5269.

O'Leary, A. D., and Sweeney, E. C., 1986, Lymphoglandular complexes in the colon: Structure and distribution, *Histopathology* **10**:267–283.

Oravecz, T., Roderiquez, G., Koffi, J., Wang, J., Ditto, M., Bou-Habib, D. C., Lusso, P., and Norcross, M. A., 1995, CD26 expression correlates with entry, replication and cytopathicity of monocytotropic HIV-1 strains in a T-cell line, *Nature Med.* **9**:919.

Orenstein, J. M., Meltzer, M. S., Phipps, T., and Gendelman, H. E., 1988, Cytoplasmic assembly and accumulation of human immunodeficiency virus type 1 and 2 in recombinant human colony-stimulating factor-1-treated human monocytes: An ultrastructural study, *J. Virol.* **62**:2578–2586.

Osborn, L., Kunkel, S., and Nabel, G. J., 1989, Tumor necrosis factor α and interleukin 1 stimulate the human immunodeficiency virus enhancer by activation of the nuclear factor kB, *Proc. Natl. Acad. Sci. USA* **86**:2336–2340.

Pantaleo, G., and Fauci, A., 1995, New concepts in the immunopathogenesis of HIV infection, *Annu. Rev. Immunol.* **13**:487–512.

Pantaleo, G., Graziosi, C., Demarest, J. F., Butini, L., Montroni, M., Fox, C. H., Orenstein, J. M., Kotler, D. P., and Fauci, A. S., 1993, HIV infection is active and progressive in lymphoid tissue during the clinically latent stage of disease, *Nature* **362**:355–358.

Patel, M., Yanagishita, M., Roderiquez, G., Bou-Habib, D. C., Oravecz, T., Hascall, V. C., and Norcross, M. A., 1993, Cell-surface heparin sulfate proteoglycan mediates HIV-1 infection of T-cell lines, *AIDS Res. Hum. Retrovir.* **9**:167–174.

Patience, C., McKnight, A., Clapham, P. R., Boyd, M. T., Weiss, R. A., and Schulz, T. F., 1994, CD26 antigen and HIV fusion? [Technical Comments] *Science* **264**:1156–1162.

Pennington, J. E., Groopman, J. E., Small, G. J., Laubenstein, L., and Finberg, R., 1986, Effect of intravenous recombinant gamma-interferon on the respiratory burst of blood monocytes from patients with AIDS, *J. Infect. Dis.* **153**:609–612.

Perno, C. F., Yarchoan, R., Cooney, D. A., Hartman, N. R., Gartner, S., Popovic, M., Hao, Z., Gerrard, T. L., Wilson, Y. A., Johns, D. G., and Broder, S., 1988, Inhibition of human immunodeficiency virus (HIV-1/HTLV-III_{BaL}) replication in fresh and cultured human peripheral blood monocyte/macrophages by azidothymidine and related 2′,3′-dideoxynucleosides, *J. Exp. Med.* **168**:1111.

Perno, C. F., Yarchoan, R., Cooney, D. A., Hartman, N. R., Webb, D. S., Hao, Z., Mitsuya, H., Dohns, D. G., and Broder, S., 1989, Replication of human immunodeficiency virus in monocytes. Granulocyte/macrophage colony-stimulating factor (GM-CSF) potentiates viral production yet enhances the antiviral effect mediated by 3′-azido-2′,3′-dideoxythymidine (AZT) and other dideoxynucleoside congeners of thymidine, *J. Exp. Med.* **169**:933–951.

Perno, C. F., Aquaro, S., Rosenwirth, B., Balestra, E., Peichl, P., Billich, A., Villani, N., and Calio, R., 1994, In vitro activity of inhibitors of late stages of the replication of HIV in chronically infected macrophages, *J. Leuk. Biol.* **56**:381–386.

Peterson, P. K., Gekkar, G., Chao, C. C., Schut, R., Molitor, T. W., and Balfour, H. H., 1991, Cocaine potentiates HIV-1 replication in human peripheral blood mononuclear cell cocultures, *J. Immunol.* **146**:81–84.

Petito, C. K., and Roberts, B., 1995, Evidence of apoptotic cell death in HIV encephalitis, *Am. J. Pathol.* **146**:1121–1130.

Phillips, A. N., Sabin, C. A., Elford, J., Bofill, M., Emery, V., Griffiths, P. D., Janossy, G., and Lee, C. A., 1994, Viral burden in HIV infection, *Nature* **367**:124.

Picker, L. J., and Butcher, E. C., 1992, Physiological and molecular mechanisms of lymphocyte homing, *Annu. Rev. Immunol.* **10**:561–591.

Pluda, J. M., Yarchoan, R., McAtee, N., Smith, P. D., Thomas, R., Oette, D., Maha, M., Wahl, S. M., Myers, C., and Broder, S., 1990, A feasibility study using an alternating regimen of azidothymidine (AZT) and recombinant granulocyte–macrophage colony stimulating factor (GM-CSF) in patients with severe human immunodeficiency virus (HIV) infection and leukopenia, *Blood* **76**:463–472.

Poli, G., and Fauci, A. S., 1995, The role of cytokines in the pathogenesis of HIV disease, in: *Human Cytokines: Their Role in Human Disease and Therapy* (B. B. Aggarwal and R. K. Puri, eds.), Blackwell, Oxford.

Poli, G., Pressler, P., Kinter, A., Duh, E., Timmer, W. C., Rabson, A., Justement, J. S., Stanley, S., and Fauci, A. S., 1990, Interleukin 6 induces human immunodeficiency virus expression in infected monocytic cells alone and in synergy with tumor necrosis factor α by transcriptional and posttranscriptional mechanisms, *J. Exp. Med.* **172**:151–158.

Poli, G., Kinter, A. L., Justement, J. S., Bressler, P., Kehrl, J. H., and Fauci, A. S., 1992, Retinoic acid mimics transforming growth factor β in the regulation of human immunodeficiency virus expression in monocytic cells, *Proc. Natl. Acad. Sci. USA* **89**:2689–2693.

Pos, O., Stevenhagen, A., Meenhorst, P. L., Kroon, F. P., and van Furth, R., 1992, Impaired phagocytosis of Staphylococcus aureus by granulocytes and monocytes of AIDS patients, *Clin. Exp. Immunol.* **88**:23–28.

Richman, D. D., Kornbluth, R. S., and Carson, D. A., 1987, Failure of dideoxynucleosides to inhibit human immunodeficiency virus replication in cultured human macrophages, *J. Exp. Med.* **166**:1144–1149.

Roderiquez, G., Oravecz, T., Yanagishita, M., Bou-Habib, D. C., Mostowski, H., and Norcross, M. A., 1995, Mediation of human immunodeficiency virus type 1 binding by interaction of cell surface heparan sulfate proteoglycans with the V3 region of envelope gp 120–gp41, *J. Virol.* **69**:2233–2239.

Rodgers, V. D., Fassett, R., and Kagnoff, M. F., 1986, Abnormalities in intestinal mucosal T cells in homosexual populations including those with lymphadenopathy syndrome and acquired immunodeficiency syndrome, *Gastroenterology* **90**:552–558.

Romagnani, S., Del Prete, G., Manetti, R., Ravina, A., Annunziato, F., De Carli, M., Mazzetti, M., Piccinni, M.-P., D'Elios, M. M., Parronchi, P., Sampognaro, S., and Maggi, E., 1994, Role of TH-1/TH-2 cytokines in HIV infection, *Immunol. Rev.* **140:**73–92.

Roos, M. T. L., Lange, J. M. A., De Goede, R. E. Y., Coutinho, R. A., Schellekens, P. T. A., Miedema, F., and Tersmette, M., 1992, Virus phenotype and immune response in primary human immunodeficiency virus type 1 (HIV-1) infection, *J. Infect. Dis.* **165:**427–432.

Roux-Lombard, P., Modoux, C., Cruchaud, A., and Dayer, J.-M., 1989, Purified blood monocytes from HIV 1-infected patients produce high levels of TNFα and IL-1, *Clin. Immunol. Immunopathol.* **50:**374–384.

Roy. S., Fitz-Gibbon, L., Poulin, L., and Wainberg, M. A., 1988, Infection of human monocytes/macrophages by HIV-1: Effect on secretion of IL-1 activity, *Immunology* **64:**233.

Sattentau, Q. J., and Moore, J. P., 1991, Conformational changes induced in the human immunodeficiency virus envelope glycoprotein by soluble CD4 binding, *J. Exp. Med.* **174:**407–415.

Schnittman, S. M., Psallidopoulas, M. C., Lane, H. C., Thompson, L., Baseler, M., Massari, F., Fox, C. H., Salzman, N. P., and Fauci, A. S., 1989, The reservoir for HIV in human peripheral blood is a T cell that maintains expression of CD4, *Science* **245:**305–308.

Schragger, L. K., Young, J. M., Fowler, M. G., Mathison, B. J., and Vermund, S. T., 1994, Long-term survivors of HIV-1 infection: Definitions and research challenges, *AIDS* **8(Suppl. 1):**S95–S108.

Schuitemaker, H., Koot, M., Kootstra, N. A., Dereckson, M. W., De Goede, R. E. Y., Van Steenwijk, R. P., Lange, J. M. A., Eeftink Schattenkerk, J. K. M., Miedema, F., and Tersmette, M., 1992a, Biological phenotype of human immunodeficiency virus type 1 clones at different states of infection: Progression of disease is associated with a shift from monocytotrophic to T-cell-tropic virus population, *J. Virol.* **66:**1354–1360.

Schuitemaker, H., Kootstra, N. A., Koppelman, M. H. G., Bruistein, S. M., Huisman, H. G., Tersmette, M., and Miedema, F., 1992b, Proliferation dependent HIV-1 infection of monocytes occurs during differentiation into macrophages, *J. Clin. Invest.* **89:**1154–1160.

Schwartz, O., Alizion, M., Heard, J. M., and Danos, O., 1994, Impairment of T cell receptor-dependent stimulation in $CD4^+$ lymphocytes after contact with membrane-bound HIV-1 envelope glycoprotein, *Virology* **198:** 360–365.

Sheppard, H. W., Lang, W., Ashcer, M. S., Vittinghoff, E., and Winkelstein, W., 1993, The characterization of non-progressors: Long-term HIV-infection with stable $CD4^+$ T-cell levels, *AIDS* **7:**1159–1166.

Shioda, T., Levy, J. A., and Cheng-Mayer, C., 1991, Macrophage and T cell-line tropisms of HIV-1 are determined by specific regions of the envelope gp120 gene, *Nature* **349:**167–169.

Sierra-Madero, J. G., Toossi, Z., Hom, D. L., Finegan, C. K., Hoenig, E., and Rich, E. A., 1994, Relationship between load of virus in alveolar macrophages from human imunodeficiency virus type-1 infected persons, production of cytokines and clinical status, *J. Infect. Dis.* **169:**18–27.

Skinner, M. A., Langlois, A. J., McDanal, C. B., McDougal, J. S., Bolognesi, D. P., and Matthews, T. J., 1988, Neutralizing antibodies to an immunodominant envelope sequence do not prevent gp120 binding of CD4, *J. Virol.* **62:**4195–4200.

Smith, P. D., 1994, Mucosal immunopathophysiology of HIV infection, in: *Handbook of Mucosal Immunology* (P. L. Ogra, J. Mestecky, M. E. Lamm, W. Stober, J. R., McGhee, and J. Bienenstock, eds.), Academic Press, San Diego, pp. 719–728.

Smith, P. D., 1995, Intestinal infections of HIV-1 disease, in: *Infections of the Gastrointestinal Tract* (M. J. Blaser, P. D. Smith, J. I. Ravdin, H. B. Greenberg, and R. L. Guerrant, eds.), Raven Press, New York, pp. 483–498.

Smith, P. D., Ohura, K., Masur, H., Lane, H. C., Fauci, A. S., and Wahl, S. M., 1984, Monocyte–macrophage function in the acquired immune deficiency syndrome: Defective chemotaxis, *J. Clin. Invest.* **74:**2121–2128.

Smith, P. D., Eisner, M. S., Manischewitz, J. F., Gill, V. J., Masur, H., and Fox, C. H., 1993, Esophageal disease in AIDS is associated with pathologic processes rather than mucosal human immunodeficiency virus type 1, *J. Infect. Dis.* **167:**547–552.

Smith, P. D., Fox, C. H., Masur, H., Winter, H. S., and Alling, D. W., 1994, Quantitative analysis of mononuclear cells expressing human immunodeficiency virus type 1 RNA in esophageal mucosa, *J. Exp. Med.* **180:**1541–1546.

Spira, A. I., Marx, P. A., Patterson, B. K., Mahoney, J., Koup, R. A., Wolinsky, S. M., and Ho, D. D., 1996, Cellular targets of infection and route of viral dissemination following an intravaginal inoculation of SIV into rhesus macaques, *J. Exp. Med.* **183:**215–225.

Stamatos, L., and Cheng-Mayer, C., 1993, Evidence that the structural conformation of envelope gp120 affects human immunodeficiency virus type 1 infectivity, host range, and syncytium-forming ability, *J. Virol.* **67:**5635–5639.

Steffen, M., Reinecker, H. C., Petersen, J., Doehn, C., Pfluger, I., Voss, A., and Raedler, A., 1993, Differences in cytokine secretion by intestinal mononuclear cells, peripheral blood monocytes and alveolar macrophages from HIV-infected patients, *Clin. Exp. Med.* **91**:30–36.

Stein, G., Gowda, S., Lifson, J., Penhallow, R., Bensch, K., and Engelman, E., 1987, pH independent HIV entry into CD4$^+$ positive T cell via virus envelope fusion to the plasma membrane, *Cell* **49**:659–668.

Strober, W., 1992, Mechanisms of mucosal immunity in relation to AIDS, *Ann. Intern. Med.* **116**:63–77.

Szebeni, J., Wahl, S. M., Popovic, M., Wahl, L. M., Gartner, S., Fine, R. L., Skaleric, U., and Weinstein, J. N., 1989, Dipyridamole potentiates the inhibition of 3′-azido-3′-deoxythymidine and other dideoxynucleosides of human immunodeficiency virus replication in monocyte/macrophages, *Proc. Natl. Acad. Sci. USA* **86**:3842–3846.

Szebeni, ., Wahl, S. M., Schinazi, R. F., Popovic, M., Gartner, S., Wahl, L. M., Weislow, O. S., Betageri, G., Fine, R. L., Dahlberg, J. E., Hunter, E., and Weinstein, J. N., 1990a, Dipyridamole potentiates the activity of zidovudine and other dideoxynucleosides against HIV-1 in cultured cells, *Ann. N.Y. Acad. Sci.* **616**:613–616.

Szebeni, J., Wahl, S. M., Wahl, L. M., Gartner, S., Popovic, M., Parker, R., Black, C. D., and Weinstein, J. N., 1990b, Inhibition of HIV-1 in monocyte/macrophage cultures by 2′,3′-dideoxycytidine-5′-triphosphate, free and in liposomes, *AIDS Res. Hum. Retovir.* **6**:691–702.

Szebeni, J., Dieffenbach, C., Wahl, S. M., Venkateshan, C. N., Yeh, A., Wahl, L. M., Peterfy, M., Friedman, R. M., and Weinstein, J. N., 1991, Induction of interferon-α by human immunodeficiency virus type-1 in human monocyte–macrophage cultures *J. Virol.* **12**:61–74.

Tenner-Racz, K., Racz, P., Thome, C., Meyer, C. G., Anderson, P. J., Schlossman, S. F., and Letvin, N. L., 1993, Cytotoxic effector cell granules recognized by the monoclonal antibody TIA-1 are present in CD8+ lymphocytes in lymph nodes of human immunodeficiency virus-1-infected patients, *Am. J. Pathol.* **142**:1750.

Terai, C., and Carson, D. A., 1991, Pyrimidine nucleotide and nucleic acid synthesis in human monocytes and macrophages, *Exp. Cell Res.* **193**:375–381.

Terai, C., Kornbluth, R. S., Pauza, C. D., Richman, D. D., and Carson, D. A., 1991, Apoptosis as mechanism of cell death in cultured T lymphoblasts acutely infected with HIV-1, *J. Clin. Invest.* **87**:1710–1715.

Tersmette, M., De Goede, R. E. Y., Al, B. J. M., Winkel, I. N., Gruter, R. A., Cuypers, H. T. M., Huisman, H. G., and Miedema, F., 1988, Differential syncytium-inducing capacity of human immunodeficiency virus isolates: Frequent detection of syncytium-inducing isolates in patients with acquired immunodeficiency syndrome (AIDS) and AIDS-related complex, *J. Virol.* **62**:2026–2032.

Tiemessen, C. T., Meddows-Taylor, S., and Martin, D. J., 1995, Regulation of interleukin-8 gene expression in HIV-1 and mycobacterial infection, *9th Int. Congr. Immunol.*

Trial, J., Birdall, H. H., Hallum, J. A., Crane, M. L., Rodriguez-Barradas, M. C., deJong, A. L., Kirshnan, B., Lacke, C. E., Figdor, C. G., and Rosen, R. D., 1995, Phenotypic and functional changes in peripheral blood monocytes during progression of human immunodeficiency virus infection, *J. Clin. Invest.* **95**:1690–1701.

Twigg, H. L., Iwamoto, G. K., and Soliman, D. M., 1992, Role of cytokines in alveolar macrophage accessory cell function in HIV-infected individuals, *J. Immunol.* **149**:1462–1469.

Ullrich, R., Zeitz, M., Heise, W., L'age, M., Hoffken, G., and Riecker, E. O., 1989, Small intestinal structure and function in patients infected with human immunodeficiency virus (HIV): Evidence for HIV-induced enteropathy, *Ann. Intern. Med.* **111**:15–21.

Valentin, A., Albert, J., Svenson, S. B., and Åsjo, B., 1992, Blood-derived macrophages produce IL-1, but not TNF-α, after infection with HIV-1 isolates from patients at different stages of disease, *Cytokine* **4**:185–191.

Voth, R., Rossol, S., Klein, K., Hess, G., Schutt, K. H., Schroder, H. C., Meyer Zum Buschenfelde, K. H., and Muller, W. E., 1990, Differential gene expression of IFN-α and tumor necrosis factor-α in peripheral blood mononuclear cells from patients with AIDS related complex and AIDS, *J. Immunol.* **144**:970–975.

Vyakarnam, A., McKeating, J., Meager, A., and Beverley, P. C., 1990, Tumour necrosis factors (α,β) induced by HIV-1 in peripheral blood mononuclear cells potentiate virus replication, *AIDS* **4**:21–27.

Wahl, L. M., Corcoran, M. L., Pyle, S. W., Arthur, J. D., Harel-Bellaw, A., and Farrar, W. L., 1989, Human immunodeficiency virus glycoprotein (gp120) induction of monocyte arachidonic acid metabolites and interleukin 1, *Proc. Natl. Acad. Sci. USA* **86**:621–625.

Wahl, S. M., 1992, TGF-β in inflammation. A cause and a cure, *J. Clin. Immunol.* **12**:61–74.

Wahl, S. M., 1994, Transforming growth factor β: The good, the bad and the ugly, *J. Exp. Med.* **180**:1587–1590.

Wahl, S. M., Allen, J. B., Gartner, S., Orenstein, J. M., Chenoweth, D. E., Popovic, M., Arthur, L. O., Farrar, W. L., and Wahl, L. M., 1989, Human immunodeficiency virus and its envelope glycoprotein down-regulate chemotactic ligand receptors and chemotactic function of peripheral blood monocytes, *J. Immunol.* **142**:3553–3559.

Wahl, S. M., Allen, J. B., McCartney-Francis, N., Morganti-Kossmann, M. C., Kossmann, T., Ellingsworth, L., Mergenhange, S. E., and Orenstein, J. M., 1991, Transforming growth factor beta. A potential macrophage and astrocyte-derived mediator of CNS dysfunction in AIDS, *J. Exp. Med.* **173:**891–899.

Wahl, S. M., Allen, J. B., Weeks, B. S., Wong, H. L., and Klotman, P. E., 1993, TGF-β enhances integrin expression and type IV collagenase secretion in human monocytes, *Proc. Natl. Acad. Sci. USA* **90:**4577–4581.

Wahl, S. M., McNeely, T. B., and Eisenberg, S. P., 1995, A SLPI defense against HIV, *NIH Catalyst* **3:**8–9.

Wain-Hobson, S., 1993, Viral burden in AIDS, *Nature* **366:**22.

Wain-Hobson, S., 1995, Virological mayhem, *Nature* **373:**102.

Wei, X., Ghosh, S. K., Taylor, M. E., Johnson, V. A., Emini, E. A., Deutsch, P., Lifson, J. D., Bonhoeffer, S., Nowak, M. A., Hahn, B. H., Saag, M. S., and Shaw, G. M., 1995, Viral dynamics in human immunodeficiency virus type 1 infection, *Nature* **373:**117–122.

Weinberg, J. B., Matthews, T. J., Cullen, B. R., and Malim, M. H., 1991, Productive human immunodeficiency virus type 1 (HIV-1) infection of nonproliferating human monocytes, *J. Exp. Med.* **174:**1477–1482.

Weinstein, J. N., Bunow, B., Welslow, O. S., Schinazi, R. F., Wahl, S. M., Wahl, L. M., and Szebeni, J., 1991, Synergistic drug combinations in AIDS therapy: Dipyridamole–azidothymidine in particular and principles of analysis in general, *Ann. N.Y. Acad. Sci.* **616:**367–384.

Weiss, L., Laeffner-Cavaillon, N., Laude, M., Gilquin, J., and Kazatchkine, M. D., 1989, HIV infection is associated with the spontaneous production of interleukin-1 in vivo and with abnormal release of IL-1-alpha in vitro, *AIDS* **3:**695–699.

Weissman, D., Poli, G., and Fauci, A. S., 1994, Interleukin-10 blocks HIV replication in macrophages by inhibiting the autocrine loop of TNF-α and IL-6 induction of virus, *AIDS Res. Hum. Retrovir.* **10:**1199–1206.

Weissman, D., Li, Y., Orenstein, J. M., and Fauci, A. S., 1995, Both a precursor and a mature population of dendritic cells can bind HIV, *J. Immunol.* **155:**4111–4117.

Welch, G., Wong, H., and Wahl, S. M., 1990, Selective induction of FcγRIII on human monocytes by transforming growth factor-β, *J. Immunol.* **144:**3444–3448.

Weller, S. K., Joy, A. E., and Temin, H. M., 1980, Correlation between cell killing and massive second-round superinfection by members of subgroups of avian leukosis virus, *J. Virol.* **33:**494–506.

Werner, A., and Levy, J. A., 1993, Human immunodeficiency virus type 1 envelope gp120 is cleaved after incubation with recombinant soluble CD4, *J. Virol* **67:**2566–2574.

Westervelt, P., Trowbridge, D. B., Epstein, L. G., Blumberg, B. M., Li, Y., Hahn, B. H., Shaw, G. M., Price, R. W., and Ratner, L., 1992a, Macrophage tropism determinants of human immunodeficiency virus type 1 in vivo, *J. Virol.* **66:**2577–2582.

Westervelt, P., Henkel, T., Trowbridge, D. B., Orenstein, J., Heuser, J., Gendelman, H. E., and Ratner, L., 1992b, Dual regulation of silent and productive infection in monocytes by distinct human immunodeficiency virus type 1 determinants, *J. Virol.* **66:**3925–3931.

Whelan, W. L., Kirsch, D. R., Kwon-Chung, K. J., Wahl, S. M., and Smith, P. D., 1990, Candida albicans in patients with the acquired immunodeficiency syndrome: Absence of a novel or hypervirulent strain, *J. Infect. Dis.* **162:**513–518.

Willey, R. L., Ross, E. K., Buckler-White, A. J., Theodore, T. S., and Martin, M. A., 1989, Functional interactions of constant and variable domains of human immunodeficiency virus type 1 gp120, *J. Virol.* **63:**3595–3600.

Wolinsky, S., Wike, C., Korber, B., Hutto, C., Parks, W. I., Rosenblum, L., Kunstman, K., Furtado, M., and Munoz, J., 1992, Selective transmission of human immunodeficiency virus type-1 from mother to infant, *Science* **255:**1134–1137.

Wong, H., Lotze, M. T., Wahl, L. M., and Wahl, S. M., 1992, Administration of recombinant IL-4 to humans regulates gene expression, phenotype and function in circulating monocytes, *J. Immunol.* **148:**2118–2125.

Wong, H., Costa, G. L., Lotze, M. T., and Wahl, S. M., 1993, Interleukin-4 differentially regulates monocyte IL-1 family gene expression and synthesis *in vitro* and *in vivo*, *J. Exp. Med.* **177:**775–781.

Wright, S. C., Jewett, A., Nitsuyasu, R., and Bonavida, B., 1988, Spontaneous cytotoxicity and tumor necrosis factor production by peripheral blood monocytes from aids patients, *J. Immunol.* **141:**99–104.

Zack, J. A., Arrigo, S. J., Weitsman, S. R., Go, A. S., Haislip, A., and Chen, I. S. Y., 1990, HIV-1 entry into quiescent primary lymphocytes: Molecular analysis reveals a labile, latent viral structure, *Cell* **61:**213–222.

Zhang, I. Q., Mackenzie, P., Cleland, A., Holmes, E. C., Leigh-Brown, A. J., and Simmonds, P., 1993, Selection for specific sequences in the external envelope protein of HIV-1 upon primary infection, *J. Virol.* **67:**3345–3356.

Zhu, T., Mo, H., Wang, N., Nam, D. S., Cao, Y., Koup, R. A., and Ho, D. D., 1993, Genotypic and phenotypic characterization of HIV-1 in patients with primary infection, *Science* **261:**1179–1181.

Zinkernagel, R. M., and Hengartner, H., 1994, T-cell-mediated immunopathology versus direct cytolysis by virus: Implications for HIV and AIDS, *Immunol. Today* **15:**262–268.

CHAPTER 16

DENDRITIC CELL FUNCTIONS IN HIV INFECTION

STELLA C. KNIGHT

1. INTRODUCTION

The pathological effects of HIV-1 center around the loss of T cells and cell-mediated immunity. Deficiencies in proliferative responses of T cells are identified early in infection (Clerici *et al.*, 1989) and losses in both naive and memory populations of $CD4^+$ T cells occur during disease progression (Schnittman *et al.*, 1990; Van Noesel *et al.*, 1990; Rabin *et al.*, 1995; Roederer *et al.*, 1995). Most studies have focused on mechanisms for direct loss of T-cell populations. However, T-cell proliferation is dependent on specialized antigen-presenting cells (APC); alteration of T-cell populations secondary to changes in APC may therefore occur in HIV infection and increasing evidence points to the importance of these specialized APC in the development of the immunological changes initiated by the virus. The bone marrow-derived dendritic cells (DC) are involved in all aspects of T-cell development from the shaping of the T-cell populations within the thymus, the stimulation of naive T cells which have not yet encountered antigens, and the expansion of memory and effector T-cell populations. Follicular dendritic cells (FDC), which are possibly derived *in situ* within the lymphoid follicles, stimulate memory B-cell populations. The DC and FDC and their acquisition and presentation of antigens thus shape the development of immune responses and the balance between cellular and humoral immunity (Knight and Stagg, 1993; Knight, 1993). This review will describe the interaction of HIV with DC and the evidence suggesting that this is pivotal to the type of immunological changes seen within the T-cell populations.

2. MATURATION AND PROPERTIES OF DENDRITIC CELLS

Some essential aspects of DC biology are summarized here and further details and references can be found in other reviews (Knight, 1993; Knight and Stagg, 1993). DC are

STELLA C. KNIGHT • Imperial College School of Medicine, Antigen Presentation Research Group, Northwick Park Institute for Medical Research, Harrow HA1 3UJ, United Kingdom.

Immunology of HIV Infection, edited by Sudhir Gupta. Plenum Press, New York, 1996.

derived from precursors in the bone marrow, are present in peripheral blood, and have been identified in small numbers in all tissues of the body except the brain (Hart and Fabre, 1981). The bone marrow derivation of DC in humans was confirmed by the *in vitro* production of DC from individual CD34$^+$ stem cells under the influence of granulocyte–macrophage colony-stimulating factor (GM-CSF) and tumor necrosis factor-alpha (TNF-α). DC also share a stem cell with macrophages (mϕ) since joint colonies of DC and mϕ were derived from individual stem cells (Reid *et al.*, 1990, 1992). A small number of stem cells were also found in normal peripheral blood.

Large numbers of DC can now be derived from peripheral blood "stem cells" by maturation with cytokines. Although the original studies on derivation of DC from bone marrow stem cells indicate that cells could be committed to the DC lineage early in their life history at around the same time that the macrophage and granulocyte lineages separate, there is still much speculation that DC can be derived from blood "monocytes." Large numbers of DC can certainly be derived from transiently adherent mononuclear cells by growth with cytokines (Caux *et al.*, 1992; Sallusto and Lanzavecchia *et al.*, 1994). Derivation from transiently adherent cells was also an early method for preparation of mouse DC (Steinman *et al.*, 1979). A major problem lies with the difficulty in identifying the large mononuclear cells which may already be distinct and will give rise to the different mature cell types (Knight *et al.*, 1986), but the question as to the precise point in their common lineage that the mϕ and DC separate remains to be determined.

DC at different stages of maturity can also be isolated from peripheral blood (Patterson *et al.*, 1991; Thomas *et al.*, 1993; Weissman *et al.*, 1995) where the estimates of their numbers range from the usually quoted figure of 0.3–1% to a higher figure (around 2%). The former figures are based on purification and identification of DC on the basis of cell surface markers (van Voorhis *et al.*, 1982; Young and Steinman, 1988). This requires exclusion of cells bearing markers of other cells and may underestimate the actual numbers. The latter figure is based on partial purification and morphological assessment which may in turn overestimate the numbers since some mϕ can take on a veiled, DC-like morphology (Knight *et al.*, 1986).

DC from peripheral blood enter the spleen directly (Austyn *et al.*, 1988). Like the majority of DC in peripheral blood, splenic DC require a period of *in vitro* culture before they can be separated on the basis of their low buoyant density. During this culture period, changes in MHC class II molecules and adhesion molecules occur with an increase in the capacity to stimulate T-cell proliferation (Dai and Streilein, 1993; Kleijmeer *et al.*, 1995). DC also enter the thymus and may be involved in shaping the T-cell repertoire and particularly in the deletion of self-reactive T cells (Benson *et al.*, 1987). DC are present in small numbers in virtually all tissues of the body (Hart and Fabre, 1981) and the most widely studied of these cell types is the Langerhans cells of the skin. These tissue-specific DC show some capacity to phagocytose particles and are specialized at acquiring and processing antigens which may also occur via endocytotic mechanisms. On culture, Langerhans cells can mature into potent APC and may show a reduction in the capacity to process some antigens (Schuler and Steinman, 1985; Kampgen *et al.*, 1991). This maturation generally takes place when DC leave the tissue and, particularly after exposure to antigen, they travel as veiled cells in the afferent lymph to the lymph nodes and may become the interdigitating cells of the T-dependent areas. Naive T cells which have not yet encountered antigen home preferentially to the lymphoid tissues and are not generally found within other tissues, so that the property of DC in acquiring antigen and carrying it to the lymph nodes where they are able to cluster and activate naive T cells is of particular importance in the generation of primary immune responses. The unique property of DC in clustering naive T cells nonspecifically distinguishes them from macrophages and other APC which can only cluster T cells responsive to the antigen they carry. DC do not generally leave lymph nodes in the efferent lymphatics and may end their life within the lymph nodes. Cell death may occur perhaps by destruction by NK cells (Shah *et al.*, 1985). Our own studies have shown that mouse DC exposed to influenza virus or human DC exposed to HIV can become targets for lysis by specific cytotoxic T cells (CTL) (Freeman, Macatonia, Askonas, and Knight, unpublished observations), raising the possibility of a role for CTL-mediated pathology (Zinkernagel, 1988).

In conclusion, DC have a specialized life history and properties on maturation that allow them to distribute to different tissues, acquire antigens, travel to the lymph nodes, and focus the development of immune responses within these draining lymph nodes by stimulation of naive T cells. Within the lymph nodes and in peripheral tissues the DC can stimulate expansion of memory T cells. Both the development of protective immune responses against HIV and against other antigens and any unusual patterns of responsiveness will thus be dependent on properties of these bone marrow-derived DC.

3. BONE MARROW STEM CELLS

The question as to whether $CD34^+$ bone marrow stem cells are infected in HIV-infected individuals is controversial with many papers claiming to find the virus and others saying that there is no infection (M. C. Ree *et al.*, 1994). Ongoing studies are examining the derivation of DC from stem cells in bone marrow in HIV infection. Normal numbers of DC which retain the function of stimulating T-cell proliferation have been derived from bone marrow stem cells when taken from an asymptomatic donor. However, very few cells identifiable as DC have been derived from bone marrow samples from AIDS patients and the small numbers of cells isolated failed to stimulate T-cell proliferation (Gilmour, Helbert, Reid, Pinching, and Knight, unpublished observations). Infection and lack of function of these latter cells was seen even when the bone marrow cells were cultured in the presence of AZT, which suggests that the cells from which they were derived were infected. Further studies will be required, but it appears that reduction in the capacity to produce DC from bone marrow stem cells occurs with the development of disease. *In vitro* infection of DC generated from stem cells was not seen by electron microscopy, although particles were found at the cell membrane (Zucker-Franklin *et al.*, 1995). However, virus infection was detected by PCR (Gilmour, Elsley, Patterson, and Knight, unpublished).

4. PERIPHERAL BLOOD

4.1. Infection of DC

4.1.1. *In Vitro* Studies

Two early reports described involvement of peripheral blood DC. One of the papers found that there were fewer large MHC class II-positive low-density cells in the peripheral blood in HIV-infected patients and that these cells also showed a lower capacity to stimulate allogeneic mixed leukocyte reaction (Eales *et al.*, 1988). It was later shown that this reflected a loss of DC numbers (Macatonia *et al.*, 1990) although other authors have questioned this loss of DC and even reported an increase in cells labeling with CD1a (H. J. Ree *et al.*, 1994;

Hsia *et al.*, 1995). The other paper showed formally that peripheral blood DC could be productively infected with HIV-1 (Patterson and Knight, 1987); electron microscope studies showed that DC, securely identified from their morphology, had viruses attached to or budding from their membranes after 5–10 days' culture with the IIIB strain of virus. It was later shown that only the cells with what is believed to be a more mature phenotype were productively infected; the majority peripheral blood population (type 1 DC) with short projections were never found to have productive viral infection but the more mature cells (type 2 DC) with their larger bulbous projections and the very occasional veiled DC (type 3) more typical of afferent lymph veiled DC, showed infection (Patterson *et al.*, 1991; Blom *et al.*, 1993). Other studies also indicate that only a subpopulation of DC can be infected with HIV-1 *in vitro* (Weissman *et al.*, 1995) and this again may be related either to the maturational state of the DC or to their heterogeneity.

The cell populations used to show infection of the DC in the early studies were only partially purified cells containing many mϕ. Another group finding "explosive" *in vitro* infection of DC with a variety of strains of HIV cultured DC in the presence of "conditioned medium" (Langhoff *et al.*, 1991, 1993). In each case the presence of cytokines in the medium may influence maturation and infection. Addition to peripheral blood DC of GM-CSF and TNF-α during the exposure to HIV increased the infection level of the DC from around one provirus copy per 100 cells to a situation where there were more proviral copies than cells at the end of the 5- to 10-day culture. Many DC may be nonproductively infected and only become productively infected as they mature (Patterson *et al.*, 1991, 1995; Macatonia *et al.*, 1992b). For some time, there was considerable controversy about the capacity of DC to be infected with HIV and some studies suggested that infection of DC was rare *in vitro* (Cameron *et al.*, 1992b). However, highly purified cells were used which were also depleted of $CD2^+$ cells; a proportion of DC, possibly those that are more mature, express CD2 (Patterson, Roberts, and Knight, unpublished). The expression of CD4 on DC isolated from peripheral blood decreases with the period of culture and it was also found that the separation procedures used by the authors who obtained little infection, were long enough for the CD4 to have been lost from the cell surface before the addition of the virus (O'Doherty *et al.*, 1993). The infection of peripheral blood DC was shown to be largely dependent on CD4 by some authors (Patterson *et al.*, 1995) but to be independent of CD4 by others (Chehimi *et al.*, 1993a). The question as to whether HIV may enter DC through different receptor molecules requires further study, although preliminary reports suggest that some strains may infect Langerhans cells by a CD4-independent route (Essex, 1995). Most authors agree that DC infected with HIV remain viable, leaving them able either to act as a reservoir of virus which can be passed on to other cells, particularly clustering T cells, or alternatively, alteration of DC function may occur as a result of exposure to the virus.

When DC are added to T cells in culture, there is a spectrum of possible effects on the function of T cells probably related to the level of infection and this will be discussed in the next section. However, two groups show increasing proportions of cells with productive infection in mixed DC–T-cell cultures even in the presence of dideoxyadenosine or AZT (Macatonia *et al.*, 1989; Cameron *et al.*, 1994a). In one instance where infected cells were identified immunohistochemically and the virus by *in situ* hybridization, the increased infection was largely in DC populations (Macatonia *et al.*, 1989); perhaps the cytokine production from the T cells caused DC maturation. In the other case the infection was described in activated T cells (Cameron *et al.*, 1994a). In either situation, DC associated with T cells provide a milieu for productive infection. Studies aimed at identifying the mechanism of carriage of virus by DC in the absence of infection showed that trypsinizing did not remove viral particles, indicating that the virus most likely had been internalized. The virus may be maintained in some internal vacuoles within the cells. The capacity of DC which were not themselves productively infected to transfer live HIV acquired *in vitro* to T cells was lost after 2 hr, suggesting breakdown of the virus under these conditions (Cameron *et al.*, 1994a).

In conclusion, HIV may be taken up into DC by two separate mechanisms. First, it may be acquired in vacuoles and degraded and processed by these APC. Under these circumstances, there may be a transition phase during which the virus can be transmitted to other DC and to T cells that are clustered around them and this effect may not be prevented by the presence of AZT. Alternatively, there may be uptake and infection of the DC. Uptake may occur by a CD4-dependent or -independent mechanism and the infection may only be apparent as the cells mature. Three consequences of acquisition or infection of DC with HIV-1 have been described and will be considered in Section 4.2.

4.1.2. *In Vivo* Studies

As for the controversy about the infection of DC *in vitro*, there have also been varied results on infection *in vivo*. Some studies report little evidence for infection of DC from HIV-infected patients (Cameron *et al.*, 1992a; Hsia *et al.*, 1995). However, other studies using cells cultured for just 24 hr before separation on metrizamide gradients found a higher proportion of DC than of other cells infected. This was shown in initial studies with partially purified cells. Contaminating cells (T cells, B cells, NK cells, macrophages) were labeled histochemically and large irregularly shaped cells which did not label for any of these markers were shown to be the cells predominantly positive by *in situ* hybridization for HIV-1 (Macatonia *et al.*, 1990). DC have also been separated by removal of cells labeling with T cells, B cells, NK cells, and macrophage markers so that less than 2% of the cell population had any of these markers as assessed by flow cytometry. These studies confirm the high level of infection of DC since proviral copy numbers often exceeded the numbers of possible contaminating cells (Patterson *et al.*, 1994). The proportion of DC infected was also shown to increase with progression of the patients to AIDS. There is continuing controversy concerning the purity of DC used in such studies. However, experiments using Rauscher leukemia virus in mice show that this highly immunosuppressive retrovirus infects increasing numbers of DC during progression of disease (Gabrilovich *et al.*, 1993, 1994). In these studies, positive identification of DC using specific markers was possible and such work adds evidence supporting the susceptibility of DC to infection with retroviruses. Studies with the retrovirus, human T-cell leukemia virus type 1, also showed susceptibility of human DC to infection since a similar proportion of DC and of T cells was found to be infected in the blood of patients who were asymptomatic or who had tropical spastic paraparesis (Macatonia *et al.*, 1992a).

4.2. Functional Consequence of Exposure to HIV

4.2.1. Stimulation of Protective Immune Responses

DC exposed *in vitro* to HIV at a low dose or for a short period of time can stimulate primary proliferative and cytotoxic T-cell responses directed at the virus. Such studies confirmed that DC but not macrophages are able to stimulate primary T-cell responses to viruses and provide an opportunity for using this stimulation system for identifying primary

T-cell epitopes of HIV which might be useful in vaccine development. One primary T-cell epitope stimulating the development of T cells cytotoxic for virus-infected target cells in individuals with different histocompatibility antigens was identified. This peptide was not a target epitope for CTL stimulated by the whole virus in primary *in vitro* responses (Macatonia *et al.*, 1991), which suggests that epitopes not normally dominant might be exploited by immunization with such peptides. DC exposed to peptide antigens are able to produce specific responses *in vivo* (Takahashi *et al.*, 1993). The presence in HIV-seropositive but asymptomatic individuals of both $CD4^+$ and $CD8^+$ memory T cells able to recognize HIV or T-cell epitopes of the virus, indicates that protective immune responses are initially generated *in vivo* (Wahren *et al.*, 1989). The presence of CTL able to kill virus-infected target cells without the necessity of restimulation of the peripheral blood T cells with the antigen is indicative of the persistent presence of virus and stimulation of immune responses (Nixon and McMichael, 1991). Higher than normal levels of antibody are also present in HIV-positive patients and there is evidence implicating the DC in the persistent stimulation of antibody production. T cells plus B cells from asymptomatic individuals produce little antibody to the virus when depleted of APC. Adding back to the cultures the DC causes stimulation of antibody production (Roberts *et al.*, 1994a). The assumption is that this occurs by DC stimulating T-cell help for the B-cell population although this may not necessarily be the case since direct clustering of B cells around DC has been observed (Gabrilovich and Knight, unpublished). These results again suggest that the virus is persisting and continuing to stimulate CTL and B-cell activity. This contrasts sharply with the reduction in the capacity of these DC to stimulate T-cell proliferation (see Section 4.2.3).

4.2.2. Transmission of Virus from DC to T Cells

DC exposed to HIV *in vitro* under conditions where there is a low-level infection with the virus (see Section 4.1) can cause T-cell stimulation as described in Section 4.2.1. The proliferating T cells may then show infection with virus (Cameron *et al.*, 1992b, 1994b; Ayehunie *et al.*, 1994; Tsunetsugu-Yokota *et al.*, 1995). Under conditions where the DC themselves become infected, there may be lower levels of T-cell stimulation and consequently lower numbers of T cells become infected (Macatonia *et al.*, 1989). The transmission of virus from DC to T cells has been proposed as one mechanism by which T-cell infection and destruction could occur in HIV infection (Macatonia *et al.*, 1989; Cameron *et al.*, 1992b, 1994b).

4.2.3. Altered Signaling via DC

Stimulation by DC of many different $CD4^+$ T-cell responses is reduced. Non-T cells taken from peripheral blood of patients with HIV infection were originally shown to cause reduced levels of stimulation of autologous T cells. The autologous mixed leukocyte reaction is known to be stimulated by DC and may largely represent the ongoing presentation of environmental antigens to T cells. This lower autologous stimulation in HIV infection was shown formally to be related to reduced stimulation of T cells by DC (Roberts *et al.*, 1994b). This contrasts with the high levels of stimulation of antibody production and CTL (Section 4.2.1). An unusually low level of allogeneic mixed leukocyte reactivity (MLR) was stimulated by mononuclear cells from HIV-infected patients (Eales *et al.*, 1988). Further studies showed that this was the result of a block in the capacity of DC to stimulate these responses and this block was seen even when secondary infection of T cells was prevented (Macatonia *et al.*, 1989, 1990). The blocking effects of HIV on DC function can be seen when DC are exposed to a high dose of HIV *in vitro*; as the dose of virus increases, DC lose the capacity to stimulate responses both to the HIV itself and to other antigens (Knight *et al.*, 1993; Chehimi *et al.*, 1993b; Knight, 1994). DC, even from asymptomatic individuals, show a reduced capacity to stimulate recall responses in autologous memory T cells (Macatonia *et al.*, 1992b). In parallel studies, it was observed that macrophages could present the same recall antigens to T cells and initiate normal proliferative responses. In early HIV infection, the T-cell populations (both naive and memory) were, therefore, able to give normal proliferative responses, the macrophages could also present antigen normally, and the defect was located within the DC population. As patients move from the asymptomatic stage into AIDS, the T cells fail to respond normally to allogeneic normal DC, showing that with progression to disease a defect in T cells is now seen in addition to a defect in DC (Macatonia *et al.*, 1992b). In order to dissect the contributions of the different cell types from infected patients, the analysis could be made more easily using twins discordant for HIV infection. There are a variety of studies on twins, but since they fail to dissect the DC from the mϕ in identifying primary and secondary stimulation, they are difficult to interpret; some have shown a defect in antigen presentation, whereas others have failed to do so (Hofmann *et al.*, 1986; Rich *et al.*, 1988; Clerici *et al.*, 1990; Blauvelt *et al.*, 1995).

5. TISSUE-SPECIFIC DC

5.1. Langerhans Cells

A reduction in the level of ATPase and of MHC class II within the skin was the first indication that Langerhans cells (LC) are targets of HIV infection (Belsito *et al.*, 1994). Many subsequent papers have shown infection of LC on *in vitro* and *in vivo* exposure to HIV (Oxholm *et al.*, 1986; Tschachler *et al.*, 1987; Rappersberger *et al.*, 1988; Dreno *et al.*, 1988; Zambruno *et al.*, 1991; Berger *et al.*, 1992; Giannetti *et al.*, 1993; Cimarelli *et al.*, 1994; Henry *et al.*, 1994). As with the studies on peripheral blood, this has been a controversial area with a number of papers reporting little or no infection of these cells (Kanitakis *et al.*, 1989, 1991; Kalter *et al.*, 1991; von Stemm *et al.*, 1993). Essex (1995) reports that some strains of HIV found in Africa may preferentially infect LC and possibly by a CD4-independent mechanism. Strain variations in the susceptibility of LC could account for some of the differences within the literature. However, despite the variable results the evidence is overwhelming that LC can become infected. Perhaps the most convincing evidence has been obtained in cells isolated from epidermal cells in the skin; around 1% of the LC isolated from cadaveric skin of AIDS patients were infected (Cimarelli *et al.*, 1994). It may be that the techniques that use immunohistochemistry and *in situ* hybridization, where most of the controversy has arisen, may be less sensitive for identifying HIV within the skin.

There have been few functional studies of LC isolated from patients infected with HIV. A major study described a functional defect in the capacity of the LC to stimulate allogeneic MLR. A deficiency in the primary stimulation of T cells is evident but the authors failed to see a defect in the stimulation of secondary responses in autologous T cells. The latter were secondary to changes in the T-cell populations (Blauvelt *et al.*, 1995). Although there are differences in the experimental details, these are very close to the studies of Macatonia *et al.*

(1992b) in peripheral blood cells. Thus, it seems that DC function and particularly the unique function of stimulating naive T cells is reduced on HIV infection.

The LC from skin when exposed to HIV *in vitro* and mixed with T cells were shown to cluster and become "explosive" sites of HIV replication (Cameron *et al.*, 1992a; Ayehunie *et al.*, 1994). The clustered cells formed syncytia and these expressed both LC and T-cell markers. In the syncytia, the T cells involved were believed to be resting T cells and this supports the view that on exposure to higher amounts of HIV, the DC are unable to stimulate T-cell activation. Infection, syncytium formation, and destruction of both DC and T cells may result. This could account for the reduced numbers of DC in the skin reported by some authors.

5.2. DC at Mucosal Surfaces

The initial sites of exposure to HIV are frequently the mucosal surfaces within the genital tract. The presence of a potentially susceptible population of DC expressing CD4 which are present in the superficial areas of the epithelium in the foreskin of men and in the cervicovaginal epithelium in women makes these a likely target for the primary infection. The fact that there are measurable T-cell-mediated responses in HIV infection indicates that the antigens are most likely to have been acquired by these cells at the site of infection and transported to the draining lymph nodes and immune responses initiated via that route. Further studies will be required to assess the relevance of actual infection of DC and transmission of virus to other cells which may occur via this route of entry. The paucity of DC in the superficial epithelial cells of oral mucosa may explain the lack of transmission by oral exposure to virus (Hussein and Lehner, 1995).

Intestinal lamina propria cells were studied histochemically and a loss of DC in all clinical stages of disease was found (Lim *et al.*, 1993) which indicates that there may be deficiencies in mucosal immunity at that site. Reduced numbers of DC in peripheral blood, skin, and gut have thus been reported.

5.3. DC in the Heart

During progression to AIDS there is increasing infection in many tissues of the body (Donaldson *et al.*, 1995). Fifteen patients with HIV infection underwent endomyocardial biopsy; five of these patients had cardiovascular symptoms. Cardiac myocytes and DC were prepared by individual cell microdissection, the proviral sequences amplified in 15–20 cells of each type, and infection levels assessed (Rodriguez *et al.*, 1991). There was no evidence that symptomatic HIV cardiomyopathy was a consequence of virus in myocardial cells since a similar proportion in each group showed infection. DC were somewhat more numerous in the myocardium of symptomatic patients, and HIV was detected in almost all samples, raising the possibility of a role for DC infection in the development of disease.

5.4. Lymphoid Tissues

5.4.1. Thymus

Early CD1a$^+$ thymocytes as well as more mature thymic lymphocytes are susceptible to HIV infection. However, the CD1a$^+$ DC may also become infected as evidenced by studies of thymic cells from infants with rapidly fatal HIV infection (Valentin *et al.*, 1994). Abnormal morphology of thymic DC has also been reported during the early course of simian immunodeficiency virus infection (Muller *et al.*, 1993). Since DC and epithelial cells within the thymus are involved in the selection and maturation of T cells within the thymus (Boyd and Hugo, 1991), alterations within these cells may lead to abnormal selection of T cells. Reported loss of naive T cells in HIV infection (Rabin *et al.*, 1995; Roederer *et al.*, 1995) might have its origins in abnormalities within the thymic DC population.

5.4.2. Spleen and Lymph Nodes

In the spleen the viral load in isolated DC was reported to be tenfold lower than that in T cells, despite the expression of high levels of CD4 in the DC (McIlory *et al.*, 1995). In all of the *in vitro* infection studies comparing the level of DC and T-cell infection, one factor to be considered is the life span of these different cell types. DC are believed to proceed through the developmental pathway relatively quickly compared with T cells. Comparisons between numbers of infected T cells and DC may, therefore, underestimate the rate of infection of DC. The functional studies of splenic DC showed that these cells, even from AIDS patients, still function to stimulate allogeneic MLR. The spleen may, therefore, be one of the few sites where maturing functional DC may be found in AIDS. Within the splenic white pulp the localization of compartments containing single HIV genotypes suggests local dissemination (Cheynier *et al.*, 1994). The potency of DC in transmitting virus to T cells even when they show relatively little or no infection themselves but merely carry the virus (Cameron *et al.*, 1994a) means that they could easily form clusters of T cells and transmit the virus within individual areas. A single DC may cluster and activate large numbers of T cells attached to long veiled processes.

Within the lymph nodes PCR techniques have generally found very low numbers of interdigitating DC to be infected. However, Nuovo *et al.* (1994) using PCR-amplified *in situ* hybridization showed that some DC and T cells were infected. Within asymptomatic individuals, a high proportion of cells showed latent infection and more productive infection was seen in patients with AIDS.

6. FOLLICULAR DENDRITIC CELLS

This chapter is not concerned specifically with follicular DC (FDC) in the B-cell follicles. However, it is clear that HIV and antibody complexes located on the FDC occur in large quantities and early in HIV infection (Pantaleo *et al.*, 1993). Some FDC may become infected particularly in later infection (Armstrong and Horne, 1984). There are also reports that active virus which is infective may be recovered from FDC after exposure to virus treated with what was believed to be "neutralizing" antibody (Heath *et al.*, 1995). This means that FDC could act as a source of virus to infect cells passing through the lymph nodes. Late in HIV infection, there is loss of follicular structure. This could be a consequence of T-cell loss since the presence of T cells is required to maintain follicular structure. Stimulation via the FDC may be important in the maintenance and persistence of high levels of antibody in HIV-infected individuals and the loss of follicular structures may contribute to the loss of protective immunity late in infection.

7. EFFECTS OF TREATMENT

During AZT treatment of AIDS patients there is a transient rise in DC numbers in peripheral blood into the normal range. The reduction in viral load changes from around one provirus copy per 100 cells to one per 5000 cells and this decrease in proportion of DC infected is maintained for up to 20 months. Improved capacity to stimulate allogeneic T-cell proliferation is also seen as long as 15 months after treatment (Gompels *et al.*, 1996). These effects on DC may thus mirror more closely the beneficial effects of the therapy than measurement of direct effects on T cells.

The lack of cell-mediated immune responses in HIV infection may be mirrored by a loss in Thl cytokines such as interleukin 12 (IL-12). IL-12 is also reported to reverse defects in T-cell proliferation *in vitro* (Clerici *et al.*, 1993). Treatment of RLV-infected mice with IL-12 reversed the defect in T-cell stimulation by DC and, in parallel, restored the capacity to generate delayed hypersensitivity to contact sensitizer in the mice (Williams *et al.*, 1996). Improvement in the function of DC thus goes hand in hand with improvement in systemic immune activity.

8. CONCLUSIONS

DC may acquire, process, and present HIV antigens to produce T-cell stimulation resulting in the development of specific memory T cells, CTL, and antibody production. During activation of T cells, virus acquired by DC, even in the absence of productive infection of the DC, may be transmitted to the activated T cells; the latter can become productively infected. However, DC themselves are also targets for infection with HIV which may be acquired by CD4-dependent or -independent mechanisms and may be influenced by the strain of virus and the stage of maturity of the DC. DC may become productively infected as they mature, particularly in the presence of T cells or under the influence of maturational cytokines. Infection of DC has been seen in blood, skin, myocardium, and lymphoid tissues of HIV-seropositive individuals, are present in genital mucosal surfaces, and may be possible targets for primary infection.

In contrast to the stimulatory effects on T cells of DC exposed for a short time to HIV *in vitro*, increasing the time of exposure to virus can result in a block in the ability of DC to stimulate T-cell proliferation. This affects not only the response to HIV itself but also to others antigens. *In vivo*, reduced numbers of DC with a lower capacity to stimulate T-cell proliferation are found in DC from blood and skin of infected individuals and the dysfunction is most apparent in the blocked stimulation of naive T cells. The DC may not only fail to stimulate T cells but also show increasing infection which can lead to syncytium formation and death. Increasing infection of DC and failure to generate functional DC from stem cells is associated with progression to AIDS. AZT therapy in AIDS patients and IL-12 treatment of mice infected with an immunosuppressive retrovirus, can reverse defects in DC function in addition to improving cellular immunity, raising the hope that therapy aimed at restoring DC function may be beneficial.

REFERENCES

Armstrong, J. A., and Horne, R., 1984, Follicular dendritic cells and virus like particles in AIDS related lymphadenopathy, *Lancet* **2:**370–372.

Austyn, J. M., Kupiec-Weglinski, J. W., Hankins, D. F., and Morris, P. J. 1988, Migration patterns of dendritic cells in the mouse. Homing to T-cell dependent areas of spleen and binding within marginal zone, *J. Exp. Med.* **167**:646–651.

Ayehunie, S., Bruzzese, A. M., Groves, R. W., Kupper, T. S., and Langhoff, E., 1994, HIV-1 transmission by mucosal Langerhans cells, blood dendritic cells and monocytes in vitro, *Reg. Immunol.* **6(1–2)**:105–111.

Belsito, D. V., Sanchez, M. R., Baer, R. L., Valentine, F., and Thorbecke, G. J., 1984, Reduced Langerhans cell la antigen and ATPase activity in patients with the acquired immunodeficiency syndrome, *N. Engl. J. Med.* **310**:1279–1282.

Benson, M. T., Buckley, G., Jenkinson, E. J., and Owen, J. J. T., 1987, Survival of deoxyguanosine-treated fetal thymus allografts is prevented by priming with dendritic cells, *Immunology* **60**:593–596.

Berger, R., Gartner, S., Rappersberger, K., Foster, C. A., Wolff, K., and Stingl, G., 1992, Isolation of human immunodeficiency virus type 1 from human epidermis: Virus replication and transmission studies, *J. Invest. Dermatol.* **99**:271–277.

Blauvelt, A., Clerici, M., Lucey, D. R., Steinberg, S. M., Yarchoan, R., Walker, R., Shearer, G. M., and Katz, S. I., 1995, Functional studies of epidermal Langerhans cells and blood monocytes in HIV-infected person, *J. Immunol.* **154**:3506–3515.

Blom, J., Nielsen, C., and Rhodes, J. M., 1993, An ultrastructural study of HIV-infected human dendritic cells and monocytes/macrophages, *APMIS* **101(9)**:672–680.

Boyd, R. L., and Hugo, P., 1991, Towards an integrated view of thymopoiesis, *Immunol. Today* **12**:71–78.

Cameron, P. U., Forsum, U., Teppler, H., Granelli-Piperno, A., and Steinman, R. M., 1992a, During HIV-1 infection most blood dendritic cells are not productively infected and can function normally in clonal expansion of $CD4^+$ T cells, *Clin. Exp. Immunol.* **88**:226–236.

Cameron, P. U., Freudenthal, P. S., Barker, J. M., Gezelter, S., Inaba, K., and Steinman, R. M., 1992b, Dendritic cells exposed to human immunodeficiency virus-1 transmit a vigorous cytopathic infection to $CD4^+$ cells, *Science* **257**:383–386.

Cameron, P. U., Lowe, M. G., Crowe, S. M., O'Doherty, U., Pope, M., Gezelter, S., and Steinman, R. M., 1994a, Susceptibility of dendritic cells to HIV-1 infection *in vitro, J. Leuk. Biol.* **56**:257–265.

Cameron, P. U., Pope, M., Gezelter, S., Barker, J. M., and Steinman, R. M., 1994b, Infection and apoptotic cell death of $CD4^+$ T cells during an immune response to HIV-1-pulsed dendritic cells, *AIDS Res. Hum. Retrovir.* **10**:61–71.

Caux, C., Dezutter-Dambuyant, C., Schmitt, D., and Banchereau, J., 1992, GM-CSF and TNF-alpha cooperate in the generation of dendritic Langerhans cells, *Nature* **360**:258–261.

Chehimi, J., Prakash, K., Shanmugam, V., Collman, R., Jackson, S. J., Bandyopadhyay, S., and Starr, S. E., 1993a, CD4-independent infection of human peripheral blood dendritic cells with isolates of human immunodeficiency virus type 1, *J. Gen. Virol.* **74**:1277–1285.

Chehimi, J., Prakash, K., Shanmugam, V., Jackson, S. J., Bandyopadhyay, S., and Starr, S. E., 1993b, In-vitro infection of peripheral blood dendritic cells with human immunodeficiency virus-1 causes impairment of accessory functions, *Adv. Exp. Med. Biol.* **329**:521–526.

Cheynier, R., Henrichwark, S., Hadida, F., Pelletier, E., Oksenhendler, E., Autran, B., and Wain-Hobson, S., 1994, HIV and T cell expansion in splenic white pulp is accompanied by infiltration of HIV-specific cytotoxic T lymphocytes, *Cell* **78**:373–387.

Cimarelli, A., Zambruno, G., Marconi, A., Girolomoni, G., Bertazzoni, U., and Giannetti, A., 1994, Quantitation by competitive PCR of HIV-1 proviral DNA in epidermal Langerhans cells of HIV-infected patients, *J. Acq. Immune Defic. Syndr.* **7**:230–235.

Clerici, M., Stocks, N. I., Zajac, R. A., Boswell, R. N., Lucey, D. R., Via, C. S., and Shearer, G. M., 1989, Detection of three distinct patterns of T helper cell dysfunction in asymptomatic, human immunodeficiency virus-seropositive patients. Independent of $CD4^+$ cell numbers and clinical staging, *J. Clin. Invest.* **84**:1892–1899.

Clerici, M., Stocks, N. I., Zajac, R. A., Boswell, R. N., and Shearer, G. M., 1990, Accessory cell function in asymptomatic human immunodeficiency virus-infected patients, *Clin. Immunol. Immunopathol.* **54**:168–173.

Clerici, M., Lucey, D. R., Berzofsky, J. A., Pinto, L. A., Wynn, R. A., Blatt, S. P., Dolan, M. J., Hendrix, C. W., Wolf, S. F., and Shearer, G. M., 1993, Restoration of HIV-specific cell-mediated immune responses by interleukin-12 *in vitro*, *Science* **262**:1721–1724.

Dai, R., and Streilein, J. W., 1993, *In vitro* culture allows splenic dendritic cells to reach their full potential for T cell activation, *Reg. Immunol.* **5**:269–278.

Donaldson, Y. K., Bell, J. E., Ironside, J. W., Brettle, R. P., Robertson, J. R., Busuttil, A., and Simmonds, P., 1994, Redistribution of HIV outside the lymphoid system with onset of AIDS, *Lancet* **343**:383–385.

Dreno, B., Milpied, B., Bignon, J. D., Stalder, J. F., and Litoux, P., 1988, Prognostic value of Langerhans cells in the epidermis of HIV patients, *Br. J. Dermatol.* **118**:481–486.

Eales, L.-J., Farrant, J., Helbert, M., and Pinching, A. J., 1988, Peripheral blood dendritic cells in persons with AIDS and AIDS-related complex: Loss of high intensity class II antigen expression and function, *Clin. Exp. Immunol.* **B71:**423–427.

Essex, M., 1995, HIV Langerhans' cell tropism: Implications for vaccine design, Proceedings of 10th Cent Gardes Meeting, October.

Gabrilovich, D. I., Roberts, M. S., Harvey, J. J., Botcherby, M., Bedford, P. A., and Knight, S. C., 1993, Effects of murine leukemia viruses on the function of dendritic cells, *Eur. J. Immunol.* **23:**2932–2938.

Gabrilovich, D. I., Patterson, S., Harvey, J. J., Woods, G. M., Elsley, W., and Knight, S. C., 1994, Murine retrovirus induces defects in the function of dendritic cells at early stages of infection, *Cell. Immunol.* **158:**167–181.

Giannetti, A., Zambruno, G., Cimarelli, A., Marconi, A., Negroni, M., Girolomoni, G., and Bertazzoni, U., 1993, Direct detection of HIV RNA in epidermal Langerhans cells of HIV-infected patients, *J. Acq. Immune Defic. Syndr.* **6:**329–333.

Gompels, M., Patterson, S., Roberts, M. S., Pinching, A. J., and Knight, S.C., 1996, Increase in dendritic cell numbers, their function and the proportion uninfected during AZT therapy (in preparation).

Hart, D. N. J., and Fabre, J. W., 1981, Demonstration and characterization of Ia-positive dendritic cells in the interstitial connective tissues of rat heart and other tissues but not brain, *J. Exp. Med.* **153:**347–361.

Heath, S. L., Tew, J. G., Tew, J. G., Szakal, A. K., and Burton, G. F., 1995, Follicular dendritic cells and human immunodeficiency virus infectivity, *Nature* **377:**740–744.

Henry, M., Uthman, A., Ballaun, C., Stingl, G., and Tschachler, E., 1994, Epidermal Langerhans cells of AIDS patients express HIV-1 regulatory and structural genes, *J. Invest. Dermatol.* **103:**593–596.

Hofmann, B., Odum, N., Jakobsen, B. K., Plats, P., Ryder, L. P., Nielsen, J. O., Gerstoft, J., and Sveigaard, A., 1986, Immunologic studies in the acquired immunodeficiency syndrome. II. Active suppression or intrinsic defect investigated by mixing AIDS cells with HLA-DR identical normal cells, *Scand. J. Immunol.* **23:**669–678.

Hsia, K., Tsia, V., Zvaifler, N. J., and Spector, S. A., 1995, Low prevalence of HIV-1 proviral DNA in peripheral blood monocytes and dendritic cells from HIV-1 infected individuals, *AIDS* **9(4):**398–399.

Hussein, L. A., and Lehner, T., 1995, Comparative investigation of Langerhans' cells and potential receptors for HIV in oral, genitourinary and rectal epithelia, *Immunology* **85:**475–484.

Kalter, D., Greenhouse, C. J. J., Orenstein, J. M., Schnittman, S. M., Gendelman, H. E., and Meltzer, M. S., 1991, Epidermal Langerhans cells are not principal reservoirs of virus in HIV disease, *J. Immunol.* **146:**3396–3404.

Kampgen, E., Koch, N., Koch, F., Stoger, P., Heufler, C., Schuler, G., and Romani, N., 1991, Class II major histocompatibility complex molecules of murine dendritic cells: Synthesis, sialylation of invariant chain, and antigen processing capacity are down-regulated upon culture, *Proc. Natl. Acad. Sci. USA* **88:**3014–3018.

Kanıtakis, J., Marchand, C., Su, H., Thivolet, J., Zambruno, G., Schmitt, D., and Gazzolo, L., 1989, Immunohistochemical study of normal skin of HIV-infected patients shows no evidence of infection of epidermal Langerhans cell by HIV, *AIDS Res. Hum. Retrovir.* **5:**293–302.

Kanitakis, J., Escaich, S., Trepo, C., and Thivolet, J., 1991, Detection of human immunodeficiency virus-DNA and RNA in the skin of HIV-infected patients using the polymerase chain reaction, *J. Invest. Dermatol.* **97:**91–96.

Kleijmeer, M.-J., Ossevoort, M. A., Van Veen, C. J. H., van Hellemond, J. J., Neefjes, J. J., Kast, W. M., Melief, C. J. M., and Geuze, H. J., 1995, MHC II compartments and the kinetics of antigen presentation in activated mouse spleen dendritic cells, *J. Immunol.* **154:**5715–5725.

Knight, S. C., 1993, Dendritic cells, in: *Clinical Aspects of Immunology*, 5th ed. (P. J. Lachmann, D. K. Peters, R. S. Rosen, and M. J. Walport, eds.), Blackwell, Oxford, pp. 481–504.

Knight, S. C., 1994, Infection of dendritic cells with HIV-1, *AIDS Res. Hum. Retrovir.* **10:**1591–1595.

Knight, S. C., and Stagg, A. J., 1993, Antigen presenting cell types, *Curr. Opin. Immunol.* **5:**374–382.

Knight, S. C., Farrant, J., Bryant, A., Edwards, A. J., Burman, A., Lever, A., Clarke, J., and Webster, A. D. B., 1986, Non-adherent, low-density cells from human peripheral blood contain dendritic cells and monocytes, both with veiled morphology, *Immunology* **57:**595–603.

Knight, S. C., Macatonia, S. E., and Patterson, S., 1993, Infection of dendritic cells with HIV-1: Virus load regulates stimulation and suppression of T cell activity, *Res. Virol.* **144:**75–80.

Langhoff, E., Terwillinger, E. R., Box, H. J., Kalland, K. H., Poznansky, M. C., Bacon, O. M., and Haseltine, W. A., 1991, Replication of human immunodeficiency virus type 1 in primary dendritic cell cultures, *Proc. Natl. Acad. Sci. USA* **88:**7998–8002.

Langhoff, E., Kalland, K. H., and Hazeltine, W. A., 1993, Early molecular replication of human immunodeficiency virus type 1 in cultured blood derived T helper dendritic cells, *J. Clin. Invest.* **91:**2721–2726.

Lim, S. G., Condez, A., and Poulter, L. W., 1993, Mucosal macrophage subsets of the gut in HIV: Decrease in antigen-presenting cell phenotype, *Clin. Exp. Immunol.* **92(3):**442–447.

Macatonia, S., Lau, R., Patterson, S., Pinching, A. J., and Knight, S. C., 1990, Dendritic cell infection, depletion and dysfunction in HIV infected individuals, *Immunology* **71**:38–45.

Macatonia, S. E., Patterson, S., and Knight, S. C., 1989, Suppression of immune responses by dendritic cells infected with HIV, *Immunology* **67**:285–289.

Macatonia, S. E., Patterson, S., and Knight, S. C., 1991, Primary proliferative and cytotoxic T cell responses to HIV induced *in vitro* by human dendritic cells, *Immunology* **74**:399–406.

Macatonia, S., Gompels, M., Pinching, A. J., Patterson, S., and Knight, S., 1992a, Antigen presentation by macrophages but not by dendritic cells in human immunodeficiency virus (HIV) infection, *Immunology* **75**:576–581.

Macatonia, S. E., Cruickshank, J. K., Rudge, P., and Knight, S. C., 1992b, Dendritic cells from patients with tropical spastic paraparesis are infected with HTLV-1 and stimulate autologous lymphocyte proliferation, *AIDS Res. Hum. Retrovir.* **8**:1699–1706.

McIlroy, D., Autran, B., Cheynier, R., Wain-Hobson, S., Clauvel, J.-P., Oksenhendler, E., Debre, P., and Hoswalin, A., 1995, Infection frequency of dendritic cells and $CD4^+$ T lymphocytes in spleens of human immunodeficiency virus-positive patients, *J. Virol.* **69**:4734–4745.

Muller, J. G., Krenn, V., Czub, C., Stahl-Henning, C., Coulibaly, C., Hunsmann, G., Kneitz, C., Kerkau, T., Rethwilm, A., terMeulen, V., and Muller-Hermelink, H. K., 1993, Alteration of thymus cortical epithelium and interdigitating dendritic cells but no increase of thymocyte cell death in the early course of simian immunodeficiency virus infection, *Am. J. Pathol.* **143**:699–713.

Nixon, D. F., and McMichael, A. J., 1991, Cytotoxic T-cell recognition of HIV proteins and peptides, *AIDS* **5**:1049–1059.

Nuovo, G. J., Becker, J., Burk, M. W., Margiotta, M., Fuhrer, J., and Steigbigel, R. T., 1994, In situ detection of PCR-amplified HIV-1 nucleic acids in lymph nodes and peripheral blood in patients with asymptomatic HIV-1 infection and advanced stage AIDS, *J. Acq. Immune Defic. Syndr.* **7**:916–923.

O'Doherty, U., Pang, M., Steinman, R. M., Cameron, P. U., Kopeloff, I., Swiggard, W., Pope, M., and Bhardwaj, N., 1993, Dendritic cells freshly isolated from human blood express CD4 and mature into typical immunostimulatory dendritic cells after culture in monocyte-conditioned medium, *J. Exp. Med.* **178**:1067–1078.

Oxholm, P., Helweg-Larsen, S., and Permin, H., 1986, Immunohistological skin investigations in patients with the acquired immune deficiency syndrome, *Acta Pathol. Microbiol. Immunol. Scand.* **94**:113–116.

Pantaleo, G., Graziosi, C., Demarest, J. F., Butini, L., Montroni, M., Fox, C. H., Orenstein, J. M., Kotlier, D. P., and Fauci, A. S., 1993, HIV infection is active and progressive in lymphoid tissue during the clinically latent stage of disease, *Nature* **362**:355–358.

Patterson, S., and Knight, S. C., 1987, Susceptibility of human peripheral blood dendritic cells to infection by human immunodeficiency virus, *J. Gen. Virol.* **68**:1177–1181.

Patterson, S., Gross, J., Bedford, P., and Knight, S. C., 1991, Morphology and phenotype of dendritic cells from peripheral blood and their productive infection with human immunodeficiency virus type 1, *Immunology* **72**:361–367.

Patterson, S., Roberts, M. S., English, N. R., Macatonia, S. E., Gompels, M. N., Pinching, A. J., and Knight, S. C., 1994, Detection of HIV DNA in peripheral blood dendritic cells of HIV-Infected individuals, *Res. Virol.* **145**:171–176.

Patterson, S., Gross, J., English, N., Stackpoole, A., Bedford, P., and Knight, S. C., 1995, CD4 expression on dendritic cells and their infection by human immunodeficiency virus, *J. Gen. Virol.* **76**:1155–1163.

Rabin, R. L., Roederer, M., Maldonado, Y., Petro, A., Herzenberg, L. A., and Hess, L. A., 1995, Altered representation of naive and memory CD8 T cell subsets in HIV-infected children, *J. Clin. Invest.* **95(5)**:2054–2060.

Rappersberger, K., Gartner, S., Schenk, P., Stingl, G., Groh, V., Tschachler, E., Mann, D. L., Wolff, K., Konrad, K., and Popovic, M., 1988, Langerhans cells are an actual site of HIV-1 replication, *Intervirology* **29**:185–194.

Ree, H. J., Liau, S., Yancovitz, S. R., Qureshi, M. N., Khan, A. A., and Teplitz, C., 1994, The number of CD1a+ large low-density cells with dendritic cell features is increased in the peripheral blood of HIV+ patients, *Clin. Immunol. Immunopath.* **70(3)**:190–197.

Ree, M. C., Furlini, G., Zauli, G., and La Placa, M., 1994, Human immunodeficiency virus type 1 (HIV-1) and human hematopoietic progenitor cells, *Arch. Virol.* **137**:1–23.

Reid, C. D., Fryer, P. R., Clifford, C., Kirk, A., Tikerpae, J., and Knight, S. C., 1990, Identification of hematopoietic progenitors of macrophages and dendritic Langerhans cells (DL-CFU) in human bone marrow and peripheral blood, *Blood* **76**:1139–1149.

Reid, C. D., Stackpoole, A., Meager, A., and Tikerpae, J., 1992, Interactions of tumor necrosis factor with granulocyte–macrophage colony-stimulating factor and other cytokines in the regulation of dendritic cell growth *in vitro* from early bipotent CD34+ progenitors in human bone marrow, *J. Immunol.* **149:**2681–2688.

Rich, E. A., Toossi, Z., Fujiwara, H., Hanigosky, R., Lederman, M. M., and Ellner, J. J., 1988, Defective accessory function of macrophages in human immunodeficiency virus-related disease syndromes, *J. Lab. Clin. Med.* **112:**174–181.

Roberts, M., Gompels, M., Pinching, A. J., and Knight, S. C., 1994a, Dendritic cells persistently stimulate antibody responses to HIV in seropositive individuals, *AIDS* **8:**1097–1101.

Roberts, M., Gompels, M., Pinching, A. J., and Knight, S. C., 1994b, Dendritic cells from HIV-1 infected individuals show reduced capacity to stimulate autologous T-cell proliferation, *Immunol. Lett.* **43(1–2):** 39–43.

Rodriguez, E. R., Nasim, S., Hsia, J., Sandin, R. L., Ferreira, A., Hilliard, B. A., Ross, A. M., and Garrett, C. T., 1991, Cardiac myocytes and dendritic cells harbor human immunodeficiency virus in infected patients with and without cardiac dysfunction: Detection by multiplex, nested, polymerase chain reaction in individually microdissected cells from right ventricular endomyocardial biopsy tissue, *Am. J. Cardiol.* **68:**1511–1519.

Roederer, M., Dobbs, J. G., Anderson, M. T., Rajau, P. A., Herzenberg, L. A., and Herzenberg, L. A., 1995, CD8 naive T cell counts decrease progressively in HIV infected adults, *J. Clin. Invest.* **95(5):**2061–2066.

Sallusto, F., and Lanzavecchia, A., 1994, Efficient presentation of soluble antigen by cultured human dendritic cells is maintained by granulocyte/macrophage colony-stimulating factor plus interleukin 4 and downregulated by tumor necrosis factor alpha, *J. Exp. Med.* **179:**1109–1118.

Schnittman, S. M., Lane, H. C., Greenhouse, J., Justement, J. S., Baseler, M., and Fauci, A. S., 1990, Preferential infection of CD^{4+} memory T cells by human immunodeficiency virus type 1: Evidence for a role in the selective T-cell functional defects observed in infected individuals, *Proc. Natl. Acad. Sci. USA* **87:**6058–6062.

Schuler, G., and Steinman, R. M., 1985, Murine epidermal Langerhans cells mature into potent immunostimulatory dendritic cells *in vitro*, *J. Exp. Med.* **161:**526–546.

Shah, P. D., Gilbertson, S. M., and Rowley, D. A., 1985, Dendritic cells that have interacted with antigen are targets for natural killers, *J. Exp. Med.* **162:**625–636.

Steinman, R. M., Kaplan, G., Witmer, M. D., and Cohn, Z. A., 1979, Identification of a novel cell type in peripheral lymphoid organs of mice. V. Purification of spleen dendritic cells, maintenance *in vitro*, and new surface markers of dendritic cells, *J. Exp. Med.* **149:**1–16.

Takahashi, H., Nakagawa, Y., Yokomuro, K., and Berzofsky, J. A., 1993, Induction of $CD8^{+}$ cytotoxic T lymphocytes by immunization with syngeneic irradiated HIV-1 envelope derived peptide-pulsed dendritic cells, *Int. Immunol.* **5(8):**849–857.

Thomas, R., Davis, L. S., and Lipsky, P. E., 1993, Isolation and characterization of human peripheral blood dendritic cells, *J. Immunol.* **150:**821–834.

Tschachler, E., Groh, U., Popovic, M., Mann, D. L., Konrad, K., Safai, B., Eron, L., diMarzo Veronese, F., Wolff, K., and Stingl, G., 1987, Epidermal Langerhans cells: A target for HTLV-III/LAV infection, *J. Invest. Dermatol.* **88:**233–237.

Tsunetsugu-Yokota, Y., Akagawa, K., Kimoto, H., Suzuki, K., Iwasaki, M., Yasuda, S., Hausser, G., Hultgren, C., Meyerhans, A., and Takemolri, T., 1995, Monocyte-derived cultured dendritic cells are susceptible to human immunodeficiency virus infection and transmit virus to resting T cells in the process of nominal antigen presentation, *J. Virol.* **69:**4544–4547.

Valentin, H., Nugeyre, M.-T., Vuillier, F., Boumsell, L., Schmid, M., Barre-Sinoussi, B., and Pereira, R. A., 1994, Two subpopulations of human triple-negative thymic cells are susceptible to infection by human immunodeficiency virus type 1 *in vitro*, *J. Virol.* **68:**3041–3050.

Van Noesel, C. J. M., Gruters, R. A., Terpstra, F. G., Shellekens, P. A., van Lier, R. A. W., and Miedema, F., 1990, Functional and phenotypic evidence for a selective loss of memory T cells in asymptomatic HIV-infected men, *J. Clin. Invest.* **86:**293–299.

Van Voorhis, W. C., Hair, L. S., Steinman, R. M., and Kaplan, G., 1982, Human dendritic cells: Enrichment and characterization from peripheral blood, *J. Exp. Med.* **155:**1172–1187.

Von Stemm, A. M. R., Ramsauer, J., Tenner-Racz, K., Schmidt, H. F., Gigli, I., and Racz, P., 1993, Langerhans cells and interdigitating cells in HIV infection, *Adv. Exp. Med. Biol.* **329:**539–544.

Wahren, B., Rosen, J., Mathiesen, T., and Wigzell, H., 1989, Common and unique T cell epitopes of HIV-1, *J. Acq. Immune Defic. Syndr.* **2:**448–456.

Weissman, D., Li, Y., Ananworanich, J., Zhou, L. J., Adelsberger, J., Tedder, T. F., Baseler, M., and Fauci, A. S., 1995, Three populations of cells with dendritic morphology exist in peripheral blood, only one of which is infectable with human immunodeficiency virus type 1, *Proc. Natl. Acad. Sci. USA* **92:**826–830.

Williams, N., Harvey, J. J., Booth, R. F. G., Knight, S.C., 1996, Interleukin-12 restores dendritic cell function and cell mediated immunity in retrovirus infected mice (in preparation).

Young, J. W., and Steinman, R. M., 1988, Accessory cell requirements for the mixed leukocyte reaction and polyclonal mitogens, as studied with a new technique for enriching blood dendritic cells, *Cell. Immunol.* **111**:167–182.

Zambruno, G., Mori, L., Marconi, A., Mongiardo, N., De Rienzo, B., Bertazzoni, U., and Giannetti, A., 1991. Detection of HIV in epidermal Langerhans cells of HIV-infected patients using the polymerase chain reaction, *J. Invest. Dermatol.* **96**:979–982.

Zinkernagel, R. M., 1988, Virus-triggered AIDS: A T-cell mediated immunopathology? *Immunol. Today* **9**: 370–371.

Zucker-Franklin, D., Fraig, M., and Grusky, G., 1995, Interaction of human immunodeficiency virus type 1, human T-cell leukemia/lymphoma virus type I (HTLV-I), and HTLV-II with in vitro-generated dendritic cells, *Clin. Diagn. Lab. Immunol.* **2(3)**:343–348.

CHAPTER 17

NATURAL KILLER CELLS IN HIV INFECTION

BENJAMIN BONAVIDA and ANAHID JEWETT

1. INTRODUCTION

Natural killer (NK) cells were originally defined functionally as a lymphocyte subpopulation that spontaneously lysed tumor cells, virally infected cells, and, in some instances, normal cells (Trinchieri, 1989, 1995). It is generally thought that NK cells represent a first line of defense against certain infectious agents and tumor growth. NK cells differ from T or B cells as they do not express known TCR or Ig receptor for antigen. Unlike T cells, NK cells kill target cells in a non-MHC-restricted fashion.

NK maturation can occur in the absence of a functional thymus but NK cells share with T cells a number of properties including the expression of CD7 and CD2 antigens and effector functions such as cytolytic activity and cytokine production. These shared properties support the notion that T and NK cells may belong to the same or related lineages. Indeed, evidence exists suggesting that functional NK and/or T lymphocytes can be derived from immature cell precursors present in embryonic liver or thymus of mice and are included in a small fraction of cells expressing the CD45 antigen (Sanchez *et al.*, 1993). Precursors that are capable of undergoing *in vitro* differentiation toward mature NK cells are present in the immature $CD3^-CD4^-CD8^-$ thymocyte subset isolated from the postnatal thymus. Further, polyclonal or clonal populations can be isolated from human thymus which express phenotypic and functional features that are intermediate between T and NK cells (Poggi and Minagari, 1995). Phenotypically, NK cells are characterized by the expression of low-affinity receptors for IgG (CD16) and the NCAM homologous CD56 antigen. In addition, NK cells are characterized by typical cytoplasmic azurophilic granules [large granular lymphocytes (LGL)].

Recently, several studies have been reported on the characterization of surface receptors on NK cells that are implicated in the mechanism of NK killing. An inverse relationship

BENJAMIN BONAVIDA and ANAHID JEWETT • Department of Microbiology and Immunology, University of California School of Medicine, Los Angeles, California 90095.

Immunology of HIV Infection, edited by Sudhir Gupta. Plenum Press, New York, 1996.

was generally found between the expression of class I MHC on target cells and their susceptibility to killing by NK cells. This has led to the discovery of receptors on NK cells that recognize class I MHC and the existence of an NK cell repertoire (Bottino *et al.*, 1995). Several NK receptors have been discovered and these have been shown to serve as inhibitory receptors or activating receptors. Bottino *et al.* (1995) have identified inhibitory receptors on NK cells that recognize HLA class I molecules and this recognition generates a negative signal that inhibits NK cytotoxicity, thus resulting in target cell protection from lysis. Recognition of HLA class I is mediated by clonally distributed receptors a few of which have been identified and cloned. Further, other receptors may serve as activators when the inhibitory pathway is not engaged. While these activating receptors have not yet been identified, a specific receptor has been defined on NK cells, the Fc receptor CD16, through which NK cells mediate antibody-dependent cellular cytotoxicity (ADCC). As in humans, NK cells from the mouse also express receptors that recognize class I MHC and this recognition prevents the lysis of the target cells (Yokoyama *et al.*, 1995; Bennett *et al.*, 1995). Thus, the above evidence strongly suggests that NK cells eliminate target cells because they fail to express certain MHC class I products adequately.

While NK cells can be activated by various stimuli, recognition of class I MHC provides a negative inhibitory signal. However, NK cells in class I-deficient mice fail to reject autologous cells, and such NK cells thus acquired a state of tolerance. Raulet *et al.* (1995) propose that one or more mechanism might be involved in NK tolerance, namely: (1) specific clonal elimination of potentially autoaggressive NK sets, (2) specific anergy of the potentially autoaggressive NK set, and (3) potentially autoaggressive NK cells might be altered to eliminate their autoaggression while retaining their lytic potential. Such mechanisms are currently being examined by these authors. Jewett and Bonavida (1996) have demonstrated that NK cells can undergo a stage of split anergy following interaction with target cells: a subset is programmed for cell death and another subset is functionally anergic for cytotoxicity but can be activated for proliferation and cytokine production (see below for details).

NK cells kill by various mechanisms. Most notably, following interaction with target cells, degranulation takes place. In these granules, several factors are present such as perforin and granzymes (Shi *et al.*, 1992). Perforin kills target cells by necrosis via induction of pores on the target cell membrane. Through the pores, granzyme penetrates the cells and can induce apoptosis. This mechanism of killing is rapid. Another mechanism of NK killing reported in the mouse is through the Fas ligand on NK cells and the Fas receptor on target cells (Arase *et al.*, 1994). This Fas–Fas ligand killing induces apoptosis and takes place within 2–6 hr. Also, NK cells secrete TNF-α on activation and can kill TNF-α-sensitive target cells and killing is achieved by either necrosis or apoptosis. A fourth cytotoxic mechanism implicates a specific NK cytotoxic factor (NKCF) that is distinct from TNF-α and perforin (Wright and Bonavida, 1982). However, the molecular identity of this factor has not been determined.

Although NK cells have been primarily defined by their cytolytic activity, they also perform many other functions. NK cells are potent producers of cytokines such as TNF-α, IFN-γ, GM-CSF, and IL-3 (Trinchieri, 1995). *In vivo*, NK cells play an important role in fighting infections by secretion of cytokines like IFN-γ long before T-cell activation takes place and the T cells secrete their own cytokines. IFN-γ activates phagocytic cells for phagocytosis of microorganisms. The induction of cytokine production by NK cells is mediated by various nonspecific stimuli (immune complexes, target cells, microorganisms). Further, other cytokines produced by T cells and macrophages, such as IL-2, IFN-α, TNF-α,

IL-1, and IL-12, can also activate NK cells and phagocytic cells and thus both cells play a central role in innate resistance to certain microorganisms. An important new cytokine, IL-12, has been identified which is a potent stimulator of IFN-γ secretion from NK cells and B cells. Phagocytic cells, dendritic cells, and Langerhans cells are major producers of IL-12 on infection. Thus, IL-12 activates NK cells for IFN-γ secretion which then activates macrophages. IL-12 also acts on T cells for enhanced generation of CTL. Further, NK cells play a direct early role in IL-12 mediated induction of T-helper cells type 1 through secretion of IFN-γ in antigen-specific adaptive immunity (Trinchieri, 1995).

2. NK CELLS IN HIV INFECTION

2.1. Loss of NK Cytotoxic Function, Number, and Modification of NK-Specific Surface Markers

Several reports in the literature have demonstrated that NK cytotoxic function is depressed in HIV-infected individuals and this function deteriorates as a function of disease progression. Depressed NK functional activity has been observed in asymptomatic and symptomatic HIV-infected individuals and profound NK cell functional deficiency has been reported in AIDS (Plaeger-Marshall *et al.*, 1987; Liu and Janeway, 1990; Bonavida *et al.*, 1986; Voth *et al.*, 1988). The reported low NK cell numbers and their decreased functioning may contribute to the susceptibility of HIV-infected subjects to HIV-related opportunistic infections, Kaposi's sarcoma, and lymphomas. The role of NK cells in the pathogenesis of HIV infection, however, remains unknown and has been poorly investigated.

The reported deficiencies in NK numbers and function in HIV-infected individuals are primarily based on the identification and enumeration of circulating NK cells by the NK-associated surface markers CD16 and CD56. The majority of peripheral blood lymphocytes that mediate NK cytotoxic activity in healthy adult donors express both the CD16 and CD56 cell surface molecules (Lanier *et al.*, 1986). Routinely, the frequency of circulating levels of NK cells has been obtained using a single surface marker like CD16 or CD56; in some instances, both markers are used simultaneously. Using these two NK surface markers, a decrease in NK cell number has been reported in HIV-infected individuals (Landay *et al.*, 1990; Margolick *et al.*, 1991). Using the CD56 marker, most studies reported a decrease in both the percentage and the absolute number of NK cells in HIV-infected individuals (Vuillier *et al.*, 1988; Mansour *et al.*, 1990). Clearly, studies determining the frequency of NK cells on the basis of CD16 and/or CD56 expression might be misleading since NK cells in HIV$^+$ individuals exhibit significant downmodulation of the CD16 and CD56 markers, and such a population will not be accounted for in the estimated overall NK cell number.

In a recent study, we examined the expression of both CD16 and CD56 surface markers in HIV-infected individuals (Hu *et al.*, 1995). Three-color flow cytometry was used to examine the relationship between CD4$^+$ cell numbers and the numbers of circulating NK cells defined by expression of the CD16 and/or CD56 molecules in control uninfected subjects and in adults infected with the human immunodeficiency virus type 1 (HIV). The HIV-infected donors had a broad range of CD4$^+$ cell levels, thereby making it possible to correlate the degree of NK cell numerical deficiency with progressive stages of HIV-mediated disease including AIDS. The number and percentage of CD16$^+$CD56$^+$ NK cells, the subset that comprises more than 90% of the NK cells in normal adults, was profoundly decreased in HIV disease even in subjects with high CD4$^+$ cell levels. Meanwhile, the number of $CD16^{dim/+}CD56^{-}$ cells, an NK population that is rare in normal adults, was elevated (median of 20/mm^3 in uninfected controls and 64/mm^3 in early HIV disease). Furthermore, not only were many NK cells in HIV-infected subjects negative for expression of the CD56 molecule by FACS analysis, but the majority also expressed reduced levels of the CD16 molecule. Some $CD56^{+}$ cells and virtually all $CD56^{-}$ cells were $CD16^{dim}$. Functional studies on FACS-sorted cells revealed little NK or ADCC activity in the $CD16^{dim}CD56^{-}$ cell population (Hu *et al.*, 1995). The mechanisms underlying the phenotypic changes and decrease in NK cell frequency are not clear but our studies suggest strongly that these alterations are mediated primarily by interaction of naive NK cells with target cells (see Section 2.3).

We have previously proposed a model of NK cytotoxic function in which the NK cells bind to the target and trigger the cytotoxic mechanism through the secretion of cytotoxic factors (Wright and Bonavida, 1982). Further, it is now clear that cytotoxicity by NK cells can be mediated by degranulation of granules containing perforin and granzyme, both of which contribute to target cell lysis (Shi *et al.*, 1992). In a previous study, we reported that, unlike NK cells from normal individuals, NK cells from HIV-infected individuals were functionally depressed and this depression was caused in part by failure of the target cells to trigger the release of cytotoxic factors from the effector NK cells (Bonavida *et al.*, 1986). However, the NK cells were not devoid of cytotoxic factors since activation by IL-2 stimulated the secretion of cytotoxic factors but in quantities much less than in control NK cells. These studies thus established one mechanism of inactivation by which NK cells from HIV^{+} individuals may lack appropriate receptors that signal activation of degranulation.

2.2. ADCC Function in the Absence of NK Cytotoxicity

NK cells can mediate cytotoxicity against NK-resistant target cells by ADCC through the trigger of the FcR (CD16) on NK cells and binding of antibody-coated target cells. The same individual cell mediates both cytotoxic functions (Bradley and Bonavida, 1982). ADCC function by HIV-derived NK cells was examined and was found to be active although the same population was deficient in NK cytotoxicity. These studies demonstrated that the CD16 FcR on NK cells is functional and is independent of the NK trigger receptor for direct cytotoxicity. Further, these studies corroborated the findings above that suggested that the lytic machinery is not completely abolished in NK cells from HIV^{+} individuals. These studies prompted us to propose that ADCC may function *in vivo* since all of the components for the ADCC function are present, namely, the effector cells, the anti-HIV antibody, and HIV or HIV products coating target cells like $CD4^{+}$ T cells. We tested this hypothesis and indeed demonstrated *in vitro* NK-ADCC against autologous HIV-coated $CD4^{+}$ T cells. This finding suggests that NK cells may play a role in the elimination of both infected and normal viral peptide-coated $CD4^{+}$ T lymphocytes and thus participate in the pathogenesis of AIDS (see details in Section 3).

2.3. Induction of NK Anergy and Apoptosis

2.3.1. "Split Anergy" by Normal NK Cells following Interaction with Target Cells

Incubation of NK cells with twice the number of K562 target cells and their dissociation after a period of as short as 30 min renders the NK cells inactive for cytotoxic function.

However, addition of IL-2 or IFN-α to the inactive population of NK cells for a period of 4 hr increased their cytotoxic potential. Cell surface receptor modulation on the inactive NK cell population was evident when NK cells were incubated with K562 target cells overnight. There was a significant decrease in CD16, CD56, and CD2 surface expression whereas CD11b and CD69 surface expression were significantly increased (Jewett and Bonavida, 1996). Two-color analysis for CD16 and CD56 surface expression on NK cells inactivated by K562 target cells revealed a significant decrease in the number of double-positive $CD16^+$ $CD56^+$ NK cells and an increase in $CD16^{dim}CD56^{dim}$, $CD16^{dim}CD56^+$, and $CD16^-CD56^-$ subpopulations.

The above studies with unfractionated NK cells suggested that the anergy observed was likely restricted by the NK–target conjugate subset. In order to establish whether the inactivation was restricted to a particular subpopulation, we examined the cytotoxic activity of the purified and cell-sorted NK–target conjugates, the NK free subset, and the unfractionated NK cells. The cytotoxic activity of the conjugate fraction was lower than either the free NK subset or the unfractionated NK cells. The addition of IL-2 increased the cytotoxic activity of the NK free fraction although IL-2 treatment of the conjugate population had considerably less cytotoxic activity when compared to IL-2-treated free cells or IL-2-treated unfractionated NK cells (Jewett and Bonavida, 1995). Single-cell analyses corroborated the ^{51}Cr cytotoxic studies. The frequency of the killer cells as determined by propidium iodide (PI) uptake in the target was also decreased in IL-2-treated and untreated conjugates as compared to either the free or the unfractionated NK population. In contrast to the cytotoxic function, the conjugate subpopulation secreted higher levels of IFN-γ and TNF-α and proliferated in response to IL-2 relative to either the free NK or unfractionated NK cells. Table I provides a summary of the surface phenotypic and functional differences among unfractionated NK free, and conjugate subsets of NK cells in the absence and presence of IL-2 an IFN-α.

Analysis of the levels of DNA fragmentation in the free and conjugate subsets of NK cells established that the conjugate subset had the highest hypodiploid DNA population. To

TABLE I. Summary of Function and Surface Expression for CD Antigens and Receptors on Normal and Activated NK Subsets

	Unfractionated NK			Free			Conjugate		
	Control	IL-2	IFN-α	Control	IL-2	IFN-α	Control	IL-2	IFN-α
^{51}Cr release	+++[a]	+++++	++++	++	++++	+++	+	++	++
CD69	+	++	++	++	+++	+++	+++	++++	++++
CD25	−	+	−	−	++	−	+	+++	+
CD11b	±	±	++	±	±	++	++	++	++
CD38	+	+	+	+	+	+	++	++	++
CD16	++	+++	+++	++	+++	+++	+	++	++
CD54	+	+++	+	++	+++	++	++	++	++
TNFR (p75)	−	++	−	−	++	−	±	+	+
IFN-γ secretion	−	++	++	−	++	++	++	+++	+++
TNF-α secretion	−	++	−	−	++	−	++	+++	++
Proliferation	−	+++	−	−	+++	−	+	++++	+

[a]+++, high; ++,average; +, low; −, no activity.

further understand the mechanism of inactivation in the NK conjugate subset, the K562 target cells were dissociated from the NK cells and these NK were sorted out by flow cytometry. The dissociated NK conjugates had higher cytotoxic function than the nondissociated NK conjugates. Dissociated conjugates, inversely, lost the ability to secrete cytokines and proliferate when compared to nondissociated conjugates. As previously mentioned, the phenotype of the inactivated NK cells was found to be $CD16^{dim}$ $CD56^{+}$, $CD16^{dim}$ $CD56^{-}$, and $CD16^{-}CD56^{-}$, phenotypic properties reminiscent of those observed in NK cells from HIV infection (see below).

NK cell inactivation as a consequence of their interaction with sensitive target cells has been reported by us and others and several potential mechanisms have been proposed (Abrams and Brahmi, 1988; Xiao and Brahmi, 1989; Jewett and Bonavida, 1996). In our studies, as a consequence of their interaction with either NK-sensitive K562 target cells or ADCC target cells, the FCRγIII CD16 receptor is downmodulated. Although a direct causal relationship between CD16 downmodulation and induction of inactivation and anergy has yet to be established, several lines of evidence point to the importance of this receptor in induction of NK cell inactivation and its role in programmed death of NK cells. In fact, our studies with normal NK cells and NK from HIV-infected individuals showed that sorted $CD16^{-}CD56^{\pm}$ cells were functionally anergic and further that the $CD16^{-}CD56^{-}$ population underwent programmed cell death (Jewett *et al.*, 1996).

2.3.2. Induction of Apoptosis and Anergy in NK Cells Mediating ADCC with gp120-Coated T Cells

NK cells undergo both anergy and apoptosis following interaction with normal or infected target cells. Highly purified NK cells obtained from HIV-seronegative donors were cultured with gp120-coated autologous $CD4^{+}$ T lymphocytes in the presence and absence of anti-HIV antiserum and incubated overnight to induce antibody-dependent NK cell cytotoxicity (ADCC). The NK samples were then subjected to the 4-hr ^{51}Cr release assay to assess their cytotoxic function against K562 target cells. Relative to control samples, a significant inhibition of NK function was observed in the samples where ADCC had taken place. Likewise, a significant increase in the percentage of fragmented DNA was observed in the ADCC samples when compared to control samples.

We then tested peripheral blood lymphocytes (PBL) for functional inactivation of NK cells following ADCC. PBL samples were incubated with gp120 in the absence and presence of anti-HIV antiserum. After overnight incubation, the cytotoxic functions of the ADCC samples, as well as control samples, were determined in a 4-hr assay using ^{51}Cr-labeled K562 target cells. PBL samples that mediated ADCC had considerably less cytotoxic function when compared to control samples. Likewise, the percentage of fragmented DNA was significantly greater in the ADCC samples than in control samples. The same results were obtained when gp120-coated $CD4^{+}$ CEM and Jurkat T cells were used as ADCC targets. The addition of IL-2 to the ADCC samples in the 4-hr ^{51}Cr release assay increased the cytotoxic activity of NK cells relative to baseline cytotoxicity. The percentage of dead cells in the ADCC samples was further analyzed using two different methods, namely, trypan dye exclusion and PI uptake. Using both methods, a significant increase in the percentage of dead cells was observed in the ADCC samples when compared to control samples. It is of interest to note that addition of anti-HIV antiserum to NK from one HIV-infected patient mediated a significant increase in the number of dead cells as determined by PI uptake. This increase might reflect the increase in HIV-infected T cells in this patient.

The high percentage of dead cells and cells undergoing DNA fragmentation in ADCC may be a reflection of depletion of both NK effector cells and T cells serving as target cells. To obtain the percentage of dead cells for each subpopulation, NK cells were FITC-labeled after purification and reconstituted with gp120-coated target cells in the absence and presence of anti-HIV antiserum. After overnight incubation, the level of DNA fragmentation and the percentage of cells that had lost forward angle light scatter were calculated by using two parameters of log green fluorescence and forward angle scatter. It was found that a significant number of both NK cells and T cells in the mixed lymphocyte population had decreased in size and showed high levels of DNA fragmentation in the ADCC samples. NK cells incubated with gp120-coated CEM target cells in the presence of anti-HIV antiserum showed increased levels of DNA fragmentation in both the NK cells and the CEM targets. These experiments indicated a total loss of both NK and T lymphocytes in the ADCC samples. Table II summarizes the properties of the NK cells following ADCC.

2.3.3. Anergy of NK from HIV-Infected Individuals

The number and percentage of $CD16^+$ $CD56^+$ NK cells which comprises 90% of the NK cells in normal adults is profoundly decreased in HIV-seropositive individuals, while the number of $CD16^{dim}$ $CD56^-$ and $CD16^{dim}$ $CD56^+$ NK cells is increased. Some $CD56^+$ cells and virtually all $CD56^-$ cells were $CD16^{dim}$. By analogy to our *in vitro* results, these *in vivo* studies suggest that NK cells in HIV-infected subjects interact with target cells, possibly HIV-infected cells. Although functional and phenotypic analyses of the $CD16^{dim}$ $CD56^-$ NK subset in HIV individuals show depressed NK and ADCC (Jewett *et al.*, 1996), the surface expression of CD69 is elevated in the $CD16^{dim}CD56^-$ cells relative to the $CD16^+CD56^+$ cells. Secretion of IFN-γ and TNF-α was significantly depressed in the presence of PMA and calcium ionophore in the $CD16^{dim}$ $CD56^-$ NK subset when compared to the $CD16^+$ $CD56^+$ NK subset. Furthermore, unlike the $CD16^+$ $CD56^+$ NK subset, the $CD16^{dim}$ $CD56^-$ NK subset did not proliferate in the presence of IL-2. The $CD16^{dim}CD56^-$ subset was found to have a higher percentage of fragmented DNA in the presence and absence of dexamethasone when compared to the $CD16^+$ $CD56^+$ NK cells (Jewett *et al.*,

TABLE II. Properties of Normal NK Cells after Interaction with the ADCC Target Cells

Properties	Control	Anti-HIV serum	gp120	gp120 and anti-HIV
CD16	+++	+++	+++	−
CD56	+++	+++	+++	+
CD69	−	−	−	+++
Cytotoxicity	+++	++	+++	+
TNF-α secretion	−	−	−	+++
IFN-γ secretion	−	−	−	+++
Fas	−	−	−	+++
DNA fragmentation	−	−	−	+++
Recovery	+++	+++	+++	++

TABLE III. Properties of NK Subsets Sorted from HIV-Seropositive Donors

	$CD16^+CD56^+$	$CD16^{dim/+}CD56^-$
K562 cytotoxicity	+++	+
ADCC	+++	+
TNF-α secretion	+++	−
IFN-γ secretion	+++	−
Proliferation by IL-2	+++	−
CD69	+	++
Fas mRNA	−	++
Hypodiploid DNA	−	++

1996). Furthermore, the $CD16^{dim}$ $CD56^-$ subpopulation had higher levels of Fas mRNA as determined by RT-PCR. Table III summarizes the properties of NK subsets from HIV-infected individuals. Altogether, these studies indicate that the $CD16^+CD56^+$ NK subset undergoes a series of functional and phenotypic differentiation in the presence of K562 or HIV target cells which results in loss of cytotoxic function, proliferation, cytokine secretion, and death of the NK cells.

2.4. Depletion of $CD4^+$ T Lymphocytes by NK-Mediated ADCC

Indeed, we found that NK effector cells can mediate ADCC against HIV-coated $CD4^+$ tumor target cells (Katz *et al.*, 1987), autologous $CD4^+$ T-cell blasts (Katz *et al.*, 1987; Hober *et al.*, 1995), and gp120-coated circulating $CD4^+$ T lymphocytes (Jewett and Bonavida, 1966).

The findings demonstrate that AIDS effector cells can mediate lysis of CEM ($CD4^+$ T-cell line) coated with HIV protein in the presence of HIV-specific antibody. Lysis was specific, as non-HIV-coated CEM or the addition of HIV-negative serum resulted in no lysis. We then examined HIV-coated peripheral blood-derived $CD4^+$ T lymphocytes as targets in ADCC. We demonstrated that, in the presence of HIV-specific antibody, HIV-coated $CD4^+$ T lymphocytes serve as targets for ADCC by NK effector cells from HIV^+ patients. The lytic activity obtained with AIDS effector cells was comparable to that obtained with normal effector cells. These results demonstrate that AIDS effector cells can mediate ADCC against HIV-coated $CD4^+$ T lymphocytes and suggest that ADCC may play a role *in vivo* in elimination of $CD4^+$ T cells and the pathogenesis of AIDS.

NK cells after interaction with gp120-coated cells in the presence of anti-HIV antiserum lose their CD16 surface receptor significantly. This loss of CD16 is accompanied by a decrease in CD56 surface expression and an increase in CD69, CD25, and CD96 surface expression. On the other hand, the level of $CD3^+$ $CD4^+$ T cells is significantly decreased in the ADCC samples relative to control samples. In contrast to the $CD3^+CD4^+$ T cells, the frequency of $CD3^+CD8^+$ cells is significantly increased in ADCC samples indicating a specific loss or depletion of $CD4^+$ cells in the original $CD3^+$ T-cell population. Along with $CD3^+$ $CD4^+$, a subpopulation of $CD3^+CD4^-$ cells has been noted to occur as a consequence of ADCC indicating that either masking or downmodulation of $CD4^+$ cell surface receptor in ADCC had taken place.

NK cells were coincubated with gp120-coated CEM and autologous T cells in the presence of anti-HIV antigen overnight. Supernatants were recovered from the control and ADCC samples and subjected to a sensitive and specific IFN-γ and TNF-α ELISA assay. It was found that samples of ADCC contained significantly higher levels of IFN-γ and TNF-α when compared to control samples. These results indicated a functional split anergy in NK cells mediating ADCC.

Eight different anti-HIV antisera obtained from different HIV-seropositive donors when added to the recipient NK cells with gp120-coated Jurkat cells mediated varying degrees of ADCC activity. Likewise, when these different HIV antisera were tested in PBL samples, each mediated a different level of cell loss from the pool of the lymphocytes indicating differences in the levels of ADCC antibodies among HIV-seropositive donors.

The ability to induce ADCC is not restricted to NK cells since monocytes/macrophages alone were capable of lysing gp120- coated target cells in the presence of anti-HIV antibody (Wright *et al.*, 1988; Jewett and Bonavida, 1990a,b; Hober *et al.*, 1995). We have previously shown that monocytes from HIV-seropositive individuals have increased spontaneous cytotoxicity and ADCC relative to HIV-seronegative donors. Furthermore, we have also shown that monocytes obtained from normal donors are capable of lysing gp120-coated autologous $CD3^+$ T cells indicating that this subpopulation, similar to the NK cells, can contribute to the destruction of $CD4^+$ T lymphocytes in HIV-seropositive individuals.

3. GENERAL MODEL FOR THE ROLE OF NK CELLS IN THE PATHOGENESIS OF AIDS

NK cells have been shown to play an important role in first-line defense against viral infections, microbial infections, and cancer as well as regulation of both nonspecific and specific immune responses via the secretion of cytokines. Therefore, it is anticipated that they may also play an important role in HIV infection. Based on our studies and those of others, we propose the following model in which NK cells are implicated in the pathogenesis of AIDS (see Fig. 1).

Initially, following infection, NK cells will kill virally infected cells and also release cytokines like IFN-γ which in turn will activate the phagocytic system and subsequently the immune response. However, with time, the proportion of NK cells that respond to infection is much greater than that of newly recruited NK cells. NK cells that respond and interact with target cells become inactivated and a fraction undergoes apoptosis while the majority remains anergic and shows a decrease in both CD16 and CD56 markers. With disease progression, the number of $CD16^+CD56^+$ NK cells decreases as a result of apoptosis and the majority of NK cells become anergic and exhibit $CD16^-CD56^\pm$ markers. Further, NK cells participate directly in the destruction of both infected and noninfected HIV peptide-coated autologous $CD4^+$ T cells. Our studies clearly demonstrate that NK cells kill gp120-coated peripheral $CD4^+$ T lymphocytes in the presence of anti-HIV serum by an ADCC mechanism. Both gp120 and/or HIV peptide expression on normal $CD4^+$ T cells *in vivo* will render them susceptible targets for NK ADCC. Thus, with disease progression related to ADCC, the number of $CD4^+$ T cells decreases and at the same time the NK cells are rendered anergic and undergo phenotypic changes as well as some undergo apoptosis. At a later stage of disease progression, there is an overall decrease in the frequency of both circulating NK cells and $CD4^+$ T cells and acquisition of the immunodeficiency syndrome.

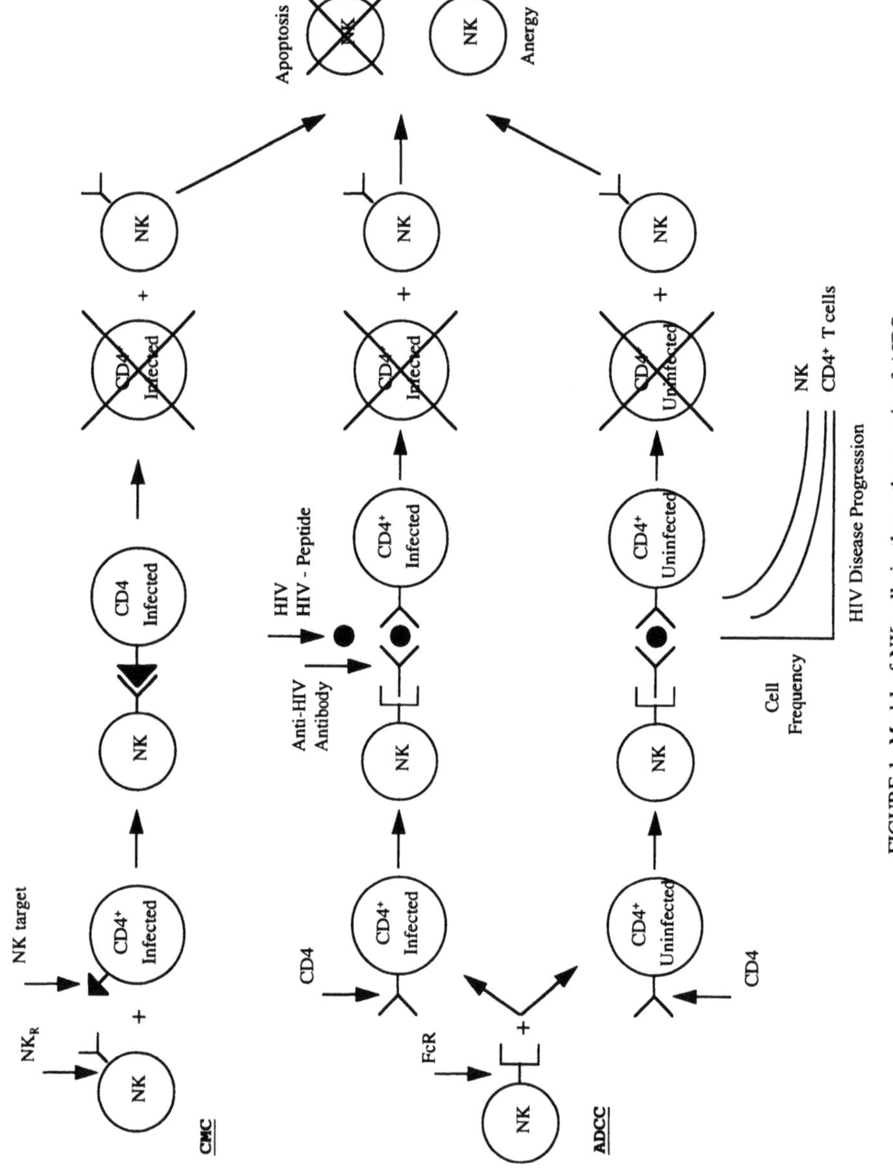

FIGURE 1. Model of NK cells in the pathogenesis of AIDS.

Thus, both the decline and/or inactivation of NK and CD4$^+$ T cells are key players in the pathogenesis of AIDS.

4. CONCLUDING REMARKS

While several mechanisms have been postulated to explain the loss of noninfected CD4$^+$ T lymphocytes during HIV infection, the above findings clearly demonstrate an intricate role of NK cells in the process of depletion of both infected and noninfected CD4$^+$ T lymphocytes. Clearly, the depletion of normal and infected CD4$^+$ T cells by NK cells, either directly or through ADCC, is a dynamic process with extreme outcomes. Initially, the NK cells protect the host by elimination of infected cells and maintain surveillance against spreading of the virus with concurrent inactivation of NK cells. There is replenishment of both fresh NK cells through the bone marrow and through maturation of precursor cells and the same for CD4$^+$ T lymphocytes. As infection progresses, the balance shifts toward an increase in NK and CD4$^+$ cell elimination that are not replenished, resulting in progressive decrease in both cell numbers. Subsequently, the viral infection takes over and immunodeficiency increases, resulting in overt clinical manifestations of AIDS.

While cytotoxicity by NK cells is one of their important functions, cytokine synthesis and regulation of the phagocytes and immune system by NK cells are also affected and thus amplify the immunosuppression. Clearly, clinical interventions are warranted to prevent both NK and normal CD4$^+$ T-cell depletion and thus preventing NK inactivation and/or apoptosis.

ACKNOWLEDGMENTS. The authors acknowledge the support from the UCLA AIDS Institute and from the American Association for Aids Research. The research assistance of Dr. Marta Cavalcanti and Dr. Xiao-Hu Gan is appreciated. The secretarial assistance of Ms. Samantha Nguyen and Ms. Jackie Tran is also appreciated.

REFERENCES

Abrams, S. I., and Brahmi, A., 1988, Target cell directed NK inactivation and concomitant loss of NK and antibody dependent cellular cytotoxicity activities, *J. Immunol.* **140**:290.

Arase, H., Arase, N., Kobayashi, Y., Nishimura, Y., Yonchara, S., and Onoe, K., 1994, Cytotoxicity of fresh NK 1.1$^+$ T cell receptor $\gamma\beta^+$ thymocyte population associated with intact Fas antigen expression on the target, *J. Exp. Med.* **180**:423.

Bennett, M., Yu, L., Y. Y., Stoneman, E., Rembecki, R. M., Porunelloor, A. M., Lindahl, K. F., and Kumar, V., 1995, Hybrid resistance: Negative and positive signalling of murine natural killer cells, *Sem. Immunol.* **7**:121.

Bonavida, B., Katz, J. D., and Gottlieb, M. S., 1986, Mechanism of defective NK cell activity in patients with acquired immunodeficiency syndrome (AIDS) and AIDS-related complex. I. Defective trigger on NK cells for NKCF production by target cells and partial restoration by IL-2, *J. Immunol.* **137**:1157.

Bottino, C., Vetale, M., Pende, R., Biassoni, R., and Moretta, A., 1995, Receptors for HLA class I molecules in human NK cells, *Semin. Immunol.* **7**:67.

Bradley, T. P., and Bonavida, B., 1982, Mechanism of cell-mediated cytotoxicity at the single cell level. IV. Natural killing and antibody dependent cellular cytotoxicity can be mediated by the same human effector cell as determined by the two target conjugate assay, *J. Immunol.* **129**:2260.

Hober, D., Jewett, A., and Bonavida, B., 1995, Lysis of uninfected HIV-1 gp120-coated peripheral blood-derived T lymphocytes by monocyte-mediated antibody-dependent cellular cytotoxicity, *FEMS Immunol. Med. Microbiol.* **10**:83–92.

Hu, P. F., Hultin, L. E., Hultin, P., Hausner, M. A., Hirji, K., Jewett, A., Bonavida, B., Detels, R., and Giorgi, J. V., 1995, CD16$^+$ CD56$^+$ NK cell numerical deficiency and the presence of CD16^{dim} CD56$^-$ NK cells with low lytic activity suggest NK cells are continuously inactivated in HIV-infected donors, *J. Acq. Immune Defic. Syndr.* **10**:331–340.

Jewett, A., and Bonavida, B., 1990a, Peripheral blood monocytes derived from HIV+ individuals mediated antibody dependent cellular cytotoxicity (ADCC), *Clin. Immunol. Immunopathol.* **54**:192.

Jewett, A., and Bonavida, B., 1990b, Antibody dependent cellular cytotoxicity (ADCC) against HIV-coated target cells by peripheral blood monocytes from HIV seropositive and seronegative individuals, *J. Immunol.* **145**:4065.

Jewett, A., and Bonavida, B., 1995, Target-induced anergy of natural killer cytotoxic function is restricted to the NK-target conjugate subset, *Cell. Immunol.* **160**:91.

Jewett, A., and Bonavida, B., 1996, Target-induced inactivation and cell death in a subset of human natural killer cells, *J. Immunol.* **156**:907–915.

Jewett, A., Cavalcanti, M., and Bonavida, B., 1996, Depletion of NK cells of uninfected CD4 T lymphocytes is concomitant with functional inactivation/apoptosis of NK cells in HIV-infected individuals, in preparation.

Katz, J. D., Mitsuyasu, R., Gottlieb, M. S., Lebow, L. T., and Bonavida, B., 1987, Mechanism of defective NK cell activity in patients with acquired immuno deficiency syndrome (AIDS) and AIDS-related complex. II. Normal antibody dependent cellular cytotoxicity (ADCC) mediated by effector cells defective in natural killer (NK) cytotoxicity, *J. Immunol.* **139**:55.

Landay, A., Ohlsson-Wilhelm, B., and Giorgi, J. V., 1990, Application of flow cytometry to the study of HIV infection, *AIDS* **4**:479.

Lanier, L. L., Le, A. M., Civin, C. L., Loken, M. R., and Phillips, J. H., 1986, The relationship of CD16 (LEU-11) and LEU-19 (NKH-1) antigen expression on human peripheral blood NK cells and cytotoxic T lymphocytes, *J. Immunol.* **136**:4480.

Liu, Y., and Janeway, C. A., Jr., 1990, Interferon-γ plays an initial role in induced cell death of effector T cells. A possible third mechanism of self-tolerance, *J. Exp. Med.* **172**:1735.

Mansour, I., Doinel, C., and Rouger, P., 1990, CD16$^+$ NK cells decrease in all stages of HIV infection through a selective depletion of the CD16$^+$ CD8$^+$ CD3$^-$ subset, *AIDS Res. Hum. Retrovir.* **6**:1451.

Margolick, J. B., Scott, E. R., Odaka, N., and Saah, A. J., 1991, Flow cytometric analysis of gamma delta T cells and natural killer cells in HIV-1 infection, *Clin. Immunol. Immunopathol.* **58**:126.

Plaeger-Marshall, S., Spina, C. A., Giorgi, J. V., Mitsuyasu, R., Worlfe, P., Gottlieb, M., and Beall, G., 1987, Alteration in cytotoxic and phenotypic subsets of natural killer cells in acquired immune deficiency syndrome (AIDS), *J. Clin. Immunol.* **7**:16.

Poggi, A., and Minagari, M. C., 1995, Development of human NK cells from the immature cell precursors, *Semin. Immunol.* **7**:61.

Raulet, D. H., Correa, I., Corral, L., Dorfman, J., and Wu, M. F., 1995, Inhibitory effects of class I molecules on murine NK cells: Specificity and self-tolerance, *Semin. Immunol.* **7**:103.

Sanchez, M., Spits, H., Lanier, L. L., and Phillips, J. H., 1993, Human natural killer cell committed thymocytes and their relation to the T cell lineage, *J. Exp. Med.* **178**:1857.

Shi, L., Krant, R. P., Aebersold, R., and Greenberg, A. H., 1992, A natural killer cell granule protein that induces DNA fragmentation and apoptosis, *J. Exp. Med.* **175**:553.

Trinchieri, G., 1989, Biology of natural killer cells, *Adv. Immunol.* **47**:187.

Trinchieri, G., 1995, Natural killer cells wear different hats: Effector cells of innate resistance and regulatory cells of adoptive immunity and of hematopoiesis, *Semin. Immunol.* **7**:83.

Voth, R., Rossol, S., Graff, E., Laubenstein, H. P., Schroder, H. C., Muller, W. E., Meyer Zum Buschenfelde, K. H., and Hess, B., 1988, Natural killer activity as a prognostic parameter in the progression to AIDS, *J. Infect. Dis.* **157**:851.

Vuillier, F., Bianco, N. E., Montagnier, L., and Digitiero, G., 1988, Selective depletion of low-density CD8$^+$, CD116$^+$ lymphocytes during HIV infection, *AIDS Res. Hum. Retrovir.* **4**:121.

Wright, S. C., and Bonavida, B., 1982, Studies on the mechanism of natural killer (NK) cell-mediated cytotoxicity (CMC). I. Release of cytotoxic factors specific for NK sensitive target cells (NKCF) during co-culture of NK effector cells with NK target cells, *J. Immunol.* **129**:433.

Wright, S. C., Jewett, A., Mitsuyasu, R., and Bonavida, B., 1988, Spontaneous cytotoxicity and TNF production by peripheral blood monocytes from AIDS patients, *J. Immunol.* **141**:99.

Xiao, J., and Brahmi, Z., 1989, Target cell directed inactivation of LAK cells, *Cell. Immunol.* **122**:295.

Yokoyama, W. M., Daniels, B. F., Seaman, W. E., Hunziker, R., Margulies, D. H., and Smith, H. R. C., 1995, A family of murine NK cell receptors specific for target cells MHC class I molecules, *Semin. Immunol.* **7**:89.

CHAPTER 18

HIV AND COMPLEMENT

MANFRED P. DIERICH, HERIBERT STOIBER,
and YING-HUA CHEN

1. HISTORY OF INTERACTION OF RETROVIRUSES AND COMPLEMENT

Avian, feline, murine, and simian RNA tumor viruses are inactivated and lysed by human serum (Fuchs *et al.*, 1988). Activation of complement occurs in the absence of antibody and is initiated by direct binding of Clq (Sölder *et al.*, 1988) to the transmembrane protein of Moloney leukemia virus (Sölder *et al.*, 1989a). Human complement was therefore considered to be the natural defense mechanism against RNA tumor viruses. In this respect it came as a big surprise when human T-cell lymphotropic virus 1, HTLV-1, and later on HIV-1 and HIV-2 were discovered. While human serum inactivated animal retroviruses, it obviously did not do so in the case of human retroviruses. We therefore undertook experiments to elucidate the relationship between human retroviruses and human complement.

2. MECHANISM OF HIV AND COMPLEMENT INTERACTION

During early stages of infection, when specific antibodies are not yet available, complement is an important defense mechanism of the immune system against different pathogens. In normal human serum, infection with HIV results in activation of the complement system (Dierich *et al.*, 1993). All HIV strains, including HIV-1, HIV-2 lab strains and primary isolates tested so far, consume complement activity in human serum (Marschang *et al.*, 1993; Sölder *et al.*, 1988, 1989a). Responsible for this activation is a direct and antibody-independent interaction of Clq, a subcomponent of the Cl complex, with the transmembrane glycoprotein of HIV (Ebenbichler *et al.*, 1991), leading to deposition of C3 fragments on the virus. Detailed analysis using overlapping peptides revealed that the immunodominant region of gp41 (aa 598–609, LGIWGCSGKLIC) is the main Clq binding

MANFRED P. DIERICH, HERIBERT STOIBER, and YING-HUA CHEN • Institute for Hygiene, Leopold-Franzens University, and Ludwig-Boltzmann Institute for AIDS Research, A-6010 Innsbruck, Austria.
Immunology of HIV Infection, edited by Sudhir Gupta. Plenum Press, New York, 1996.

site (Ebenbichler *et al.*, 1991); an intact cysteine bridge, forming a loop, is critical for the interaction (Thielens *et al.*, 1993). In addition, two further regions around aa 526–538 in the fusion region and aa 625–655, C-terminal to the immunodominant site, contribute to the gp41-C1q binding (Stoiber *et al.*, 1994). The binding to gp41 in C1q, which is dependent on calcium ions (Stoiber *et al.*, 1995a), appears to be located at the junction between the collagenlike stem and the globular heads; probably all three chains of C1q are involved (Thielens *et al.*, 1993). In addition to gp41, gp120, the surface unit of HIV, also exhibits complement activating capacity *in vitro* (Süsal *et al.*, 1994; Fuchs *et al.*, 1993). In the latter case, the interaction appears to be indirect: gp120 binds mannose binding protein (Ezekowitz *et al.*, 1989) and consecutively C1r and C1s. In comparison with gp41, gp120 seems to require higher concentrations of serum.

3. MECHANISM OF INTERACTION BETWEEN HIV-INFECTED CELLS AND COMPLEMENT

In contrast to free virus, which activates the classical pathway of the complement system, HIV-infected cells can induce both the classical as well as the alternative pathway of the complement cascade (Marschang *et al.*, 1994). Further differences were observed regarding the degree of complement activation. HIV-infected cells, but not free virus, differ in their ability to activate the complement system (Marschang *et al.*, 1993). Interestingly, the activation of the complement cascade correlates with the ability of the immunodominant loop of gp41 to bind C1q, which underlines the important role of gp41 in this context (Marschang *et al.*, 1993). Therefore, shedding of gp120 from the gp41–gp120 complex on HIV-infected cells by soluble CD4 increases complement activation (P. Marschang *et al.*, manuscript in preparation), which is also observed after the addition of HIV-specific antibodies (June *et al.*, 1991; Bakker *et al.*, 1992; Spear *et al.*, 1993). Both the antibody-dependent and -independent complement activation leads to deposition of C3 fragments on HIV-infected cells and thereby to increased adherence to complement receptor-positive cells (Sölder *et al.*, 1989b). Depending on the circumstances, an enhancement of HIV infection (Reisinger *et al.*, 1990; Larcher *et al.*, 1990; Boyer *et al.*, 1991, 1992; Delibrias *et al.*, 1993; June *et al.*, 1991) or elimination of infected cells, e.g., by NK cells (Yefenof *et al.*, 1991), is observable.

4. MULTIMIMICRY BETWEEN THE HIV ENVELOPE AND COMPLEMENT PROTEINS

Many viral proteins share epitopes with proteins of the host (Oldstone, 1987). These homology regions are used by viruses in different ways. Via these regions some viruses are able to bind to cellular receptors, as shown for EBV (Cooper, 1911). Other viral particles use such regions to survive in the host (Oldstone, 1987). For example, the vaccinia virus mimics motifs of C4bp, a negative regulator of the complement cascade; possibly it is thereby protected from complement-mediated lysis (Kotwal and Moss, 1988). In HIV-1, both envelope glycoproteins mimic a large variety of epitopes also found on human proteins (Santis *et al.*, 1994; Douvas and Takehana, 1994; Golding *et al.*, 1988; Reiher *et al.*, 1988; Lee *et al.*, 1987; Garry, 1990; Wu *et al.*, 1989; Yamada *et al.*, 1991; Sölder *et al.*, 1989c;

Brenneman *et al.*, 1988; Stricker *et al.*, 1987; Naylor *et al.*, 1987; Zagury *et al.*, 1993). Recently we reported similarities between HIV envelope and human complement proteins. Viral gp120 shares homology with properdin, C4bp (Stoiber *et al.*, 1995a,b, 1996), and Clq (Stoiber *et al.*, 1994). Antibodies, induced by viral gp 120 or vaccination with a high dose of recombinant gp120, react not only with the viral protein, but also with these complement molecules (Stoiber *et al.*, 1996). This might reduce complement activity. Furthermore Clq is known to be involved in the clearance of immune complexes (Schifferli *et al.*, 1986). Autoantibodies reacting with Clq might contribute to the presence of high amounts of immune complexes, found in HIV-positive sera (Morrow *et al.*, 1986; Carini *et al.*, 1987; Stoiber *et al.*, 1994). On the other hand, gp41 shares four regions of homology with human C3 (Stoiber *et al.*, 1995b). Anti-gp41 antibodies, isolated by affinity chromatography from HIV-infected individuals, recognize C3 in ELISA and in fluid phase. The consequences of these cross-reactions are presently under investigation in our lab, but an effect of the HIV-induced autoantibodies on the regular functions of these complement proteins is conceivable. In general, antibodies induced by gp120 and gp41 can cross-react with different human proteins, affect their biological functions, and contribute to the disease process in HIV-infected individuals (Morrow *et al.*, 1991).

5. RESISTANCE OF HIV TO COMPLEMENT-MEDIATED LYSIS

The C3 homology regions in gp41 mentioned above function like activated C3. Properdin or complement factor H (CFH), which are well-known interaction partners of activated C3 *in vivo* (Ross, 1986), bind also to the C3 homology regions in gp41 (Pinter *et al.*, 1995; Stoiber *et al.*, 1995a,b). The biological consequence of the properdin binding is not known, but the effect of factor H binding is well characterized. CFH in serum functions as a negative regulator of the complement cascade. CFH destabilizes the C3 convertase and acts as a cofactor for cleavage of C3b into iC3b (Ross, 1986). iC3b is an opsonin, but it cannot participate in the complement cascade. Therefore, both effects of CFH result in downregulation of the complement activation sequence. The same effect, namely, to protect the host cell against complement-mediated destruction, is also induced by membrane-anchored proteins such as decay accelerating factor (DAF, CD55), membrane cofactor protein (MCP, CD59), complement receptor type 1 (CR1, CD35), or homologous restriction factor (HRF) (Morgan and Meri, 1994). These proteins protect cells, but no invading microorganisms which usually lack these membrane-anchored proteins (Fig. 1).

During the budding process, HIV induces protrusions of the host cell plasma membrane and finally detaches, enveloped by the membrane, from the infected cells. Therefore, besides the viral gp120–gp41 complex, membrane-anchored host proteins are also found on the viral surface, such as MHC class I and II proteins which by far outnumber the gp120–gp41 complexes (Gelderblom *et al.*, 1987; Meerloo *et al.*, 1992; Arthus *et al.*, 1992; Orentas and Hildreth, 1993). DAF is also present on HIV derived from PBMC or H9 cells (Marschang *et al.*, 1995). Depending on the cell line used for infection, various amounts of CD59 are also present (Saifuddin *et al.*, 1995b) on free HIV. DAF at the level of the alternative and classical pathway C3- and C5-convertase and CD59 at the terminal complement or membrane attack complex inhibit complement activity. The protection of HIV against human complement-mediated destruction by DAF and CD59 is only partial (Marschang *et al.*, 1995; Saifuddin *et al.*, 1995b). For resistance against complement, additional

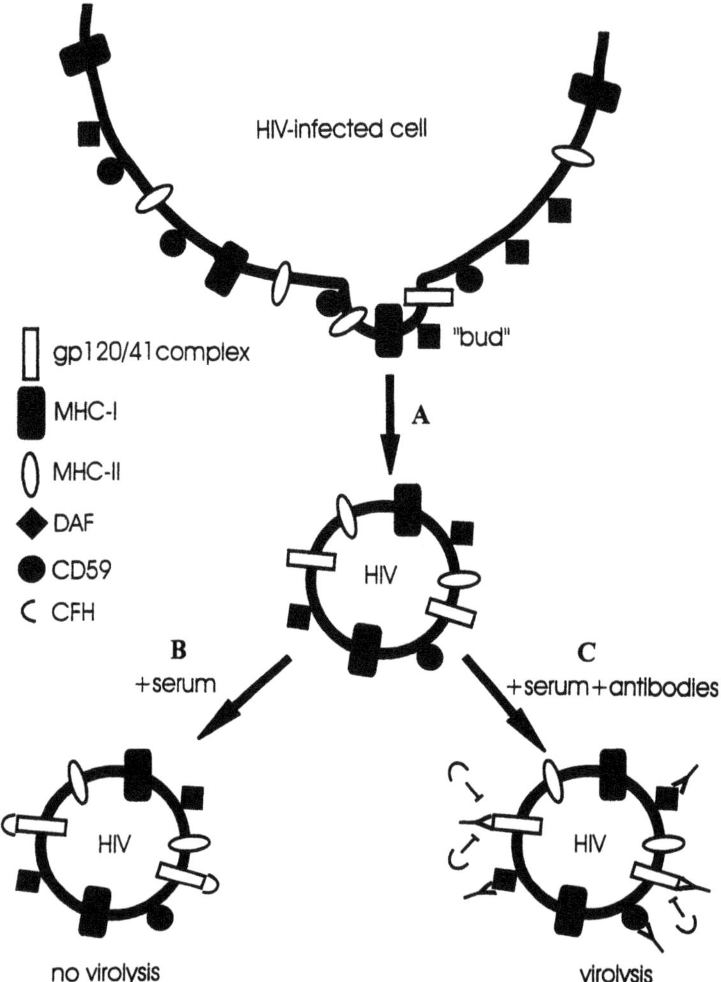

FIGURE 1. (A) The budding viral particle takes with it membrane of the host cell and membrane-anchored proteins. Therefore, present on free HIV are not only the viral proteins gp41 and gp120, but also host molecules, such as MHC class I, MHC class II, or complement control proteins (DAF, CD59). (B) In the presence of human serum, CFH is secondarily attached onto the viral surface. Therefore, HIV is protected against complement-mediated virolysis, and in spite of activation, the complement system is unable to destroy HIV. (C) When the activity of DAF and CD59 is blocked by mAb, and the binding of CFH is prevented by gp41-specific antibodies (symbolized by ⊥), the protection of HIV vis-à-vis human complement is abolished. Activated complement is then able to lyse HIV with high efficiency.

factors are required, namely, CFH. The role of CFH in this context was identified using 8E5 cells, chronically infected with HIV, and different viral isolates (Stoiber *et al.*, 1995c). 8E5 cells were incubated with serum, depleted of factor H by affinity chromatography, and with immunoglobulines purified from HIV-positive sera. The resulting very efficient destruction of the infected cells could be brought down to background levels by the addition of increasing amounts of factor H. The effect of factor H on free virus was investigated using the lab-strain HIV IIIB and primary isolates from Rwanda, Thailand, and Innsbruck. The poor lysis of lab strains and primary isolates in the presence of HIV-specific antibodies in normal human serum (Spear *et al.*, 1990; Stoiber *et al.*, 1996) increases up to around 50% in the case of IIIB and is around 30% in the case of primary isolates when the activity of DAF is blocked by monoclonal antibodies. Incubation of HIV-1 with serum from a patient with factor H deficiency results in lysis of 70 to 85% of available virus. Combination of a factor H-deficient serum and antibodies against DAF leads to nearly total destruction of different HIV strains. Using monoclonal antibody 2F5 to block the binding of CFH to gp41 2F5 (Purtscher *et al.*, 1994) results in around 50% destruction of free virus, which was incubated with normal human serum in the presence of physiological amounts of factor H (Stoiber *et al.*, 1996).

Retroviruses derived from animal cells are covered with the cell membrane of their specific host and carry on their surface species-specific membrane-anchored proteins. The strong species specificity of molecules, which regulate complement activity, now protects viruses against complement-mediated destruction when incubated with serum from its host. However, using sera of other species as complement resource, these viral particles will be destroyed. Therefore, human serum is able to lyse animal retroviruses (Welsh *et al.*, 1975). On the other hand, animal sera destroy human retroviruses, like HIV or HTLV-1, very efficiently (Fuchs *et al.*, 1988; Hosoi *et al.*, 1990; Spear *et al.*, 1991). These results clearly demonstrate the risks of HIV-into-animal models.

6. FOLLICULAR LOCALIZATION OF HIV

The biological importance of coating HIV with C3 fragments is particularly evident in the case of small amounts of HIV (Reisinger *et al.*, 1990). Here it can be demonstrated particularly well that complement mediates attachment of HIV to complement receptor-positive cells. It is suggested that complement-mediated adherence is the basis for the follicular localization of HIV since follicular dendritic cells are unique in that they carry CR1, CR3, and CR2. This suggestion is based on the observations that, on the one hand, isolated follicular dendritic cells, bind HIV very efficiently due to complement on HIV (Joling *et al.*, 1993) and, on the other hand, that follicular localization of antigens was demonstrated more than 20 years ago to depend on complement (Dukor *et al.*, 1970).

Presently, it is generally accepted that the amount of virus during the initial infection is critical for the final outcome of the disease. From the standpoint of complement, it is conceivable that because of opsonization by complement, small amounts of virus are directed to complement receptor-positive cells, including follicular dendritic cells as well as monocytes, macrophages, and tissue dendritic cells. Although large amounts of virus are overflowing also into a cell compartment such as lymphocytes carrying only small amounts of complement receptors, it is possibly critical that because of the presence of complement, HIV is directed to the compartment of antigen-presenting cells, while infection of lymphocytes may be a less important aspect.

7. EVIDENCE FOR COMPLEMENT-MEDIATED BINDING OF HIV-1 AND UPTAKE INDEPENDENTLY OF CD4

Cellular uptake of HIV-1 is initiated by binding of the envelope protein gp120 to its cellular receptor CD4 followed by an irreversible fusion of the virus with the cell membrane (McClure *et al.*, 1988; Stein *et al.*, 1987; Gallaher, 1987). Several studies have indicated that the binding and uptake of HIV-1 could be mediated by other cellular proteins, such as complement receptors (CRs), Fc receptors, galactosyl ceramide, or gp41 binding proteins, with or without dependence on CD4 (reviewed in Levy, 1993).

Complement activation by HIV-1 or HIV-infected cells leads to covalent binding of C3 (C3b, C3a, C3d) on the stimulating agent and then to binding of these complement-carrying entities on cells that express receptors for the third component of complement (C3) (Sölder *et al.*, 1989a; Thieblemont *et al.*, 1993; Boyer *et al.*, 1991; Delibrias *et al.*, 1993; June *et al.*, 1991; Fischer *et al.*, 1991; DePanfilis *et al.*, 1990; Moutefiori *et al.*, 1992). Of the various complement receptors CR1 (C3b receptor, CD35), CR3 (iC3b receptor, CD11b + CD18), and CR2 (C3d receptor, CD21), different cells express different combinations, namely, B lymphocytes: (CR1, CR2 in high concentrations; T lymphocytes: CR2, CR1 in low number; human erythrocytes: CR1; follicular dendritic cells: CR1, CR3, CR2; Langerhans cells: CR3. The infection with complement-treated HIV of U937 (human premonocyte cell line) in comparison to buffer-treated HIV was greatly enhanced (Sölder *et al.*, 1989b). This complement-dependent enhancement of HIV infection is dependent on CR3 (Sölder *et al.*, 1989b; Reisinger *et al.*, 1990). Interestingly, antibodies against CR3 partially inhibited this infection (Sölder *et al.*, 1989b; Larcher *et al.*, 1990). In this system, anti-CD4 antibodies could also partially inhibit HIV infection, suggesting that CR3 together with CD4 may mediate the virus uptake.

The complement-dependent enhancement of HIV infection was also observed for $CR2^+$ B lymphoblastoid cells (Raji) (Boyer *et al.*, 1992; Gras and Dormont, 1991) and for $CR2^+$ T cells (MT2) (Boyer *et al.*, 1991) independent of CD4. It has been demonstrated that at least 30% of the peripheral blood T cells ($CD4^+$ and $CD8^+$ subsets) are $CR2^+$ (June *et al.*, 1992; Fischer *et al.*, 1991), suggesting that these T cells may also become infected in a complement-dependent manner. Correspondingly, a decrease in $CR2^+$ cells in the $CD4^+$ T-cell compartment of HIV-1-infected individuals has been observed (June *et al.*, 1992). Besides loss of $CR2^+CD4^+$ T cells, downmodulation of CR2 expression could also be an explanation (Larcher *et al.*, 1990).

Recently, it was observed that treatment with human complement also increased binding of HTLV-1 to CR^+ HPB-ALL cells as judged by provirus formation (4- to 8-fold increase) and p24 production (5- to 10-fold increase). Heat inactivation or EDTA treatment of complement blocked this increased binding. Anti-CR2 antibody significantly blocked binding of complement-treated HTLV-1 to these cells (Saifuddin *et al.*, 1995a).

Binding of recombinant soluble $gp41_{IIIB}$ (rsgp41, aa 539–684) (Chen *et al.*, 1992, 1993a,b; Ebenbichler *et al.*, 1993) or of the immunosuppressive peptide (IS-P, aa 583–599) of HIV-1 $gp41_{IIIB}$ (Qureshi *et al.*, 1990; Henderson and Qureshi, 1993; Denner *et al.*, 1993, 1995) to human T-cell lines H9 and MT4 (Chen *et al.*, 1992; Ebenbichler *et al.*, 1993; Qureshi *et al.*, 1990; Henderson and Qureshi, 1993), B-cell line Raji (Chen *et al.*, 1993a), and premonocytic cell lines U937 and HL60 (Chen *et al.*, 1993b; Ebenbichler *et al.*, 1993; Henderson and Qureshi, 1993), as well as to human peripheral blood lymphocytes and monocytes (Denner *et al.*, 1995; Chen *et al.*, 1993c, 1995) was demonstrated. Like HIV-1 gp41, HIV-2 transmembrane glycoprotein gp36 binds human peripheral blood lymphocytes and monocytes (Chen *et al.*, 1995). Several cellular proteins in cell solutes were identified as putative cellular receptor(s) for HIV-1 gp41 (Chen *et al.*, 1992, 1993a,b, 1995; Ebenbichler *et al.*, 1993; Qureshi *et al.*, 1990; Henderson and Qureshi, 1993; Denner *et al.*, 1993, 1995) and HIV-2 gp36 (Chen *et al.*, 1995). Using rsgp41 or IS-P, different proteins were immunoprecipitated or blotted as putative gp41 receptor proteins by Chen *et al.* (1992, 1993a,b,

1995), Ebenbichler *et al.* (1993), Qureshi and Henderson (1990), Henderson *et al.* (1993), and Denner *et al.* (1993, 1995). Whether these membrane proteins are related to complement components or complement regulating proteins is unknown. Several investigations indicated that HIV-1 gp41, particularly its IS domain, plays an important role in HIV pathogenicity (virus uptake and syncytium formation). Antibodies to IS domain isolated from AIDS patient sera and mAb to IS peptide could inhibit syncytium formation (Vanini *et al.*, 1993; Ebersold *et al.*, 1992). Antibodies against the similar domains in SIV gp32 (transmembrane protein) could protect macaques from SIV infection (Shafferman *et al.*, 1991; Lewis *et al.*, 1993). These inhibitions of cell fusion and SIV infection may be based on the blocking of the binding site in HIV-1 gp41 and SIV gp32. Besides gp41, IS peptide conjugated to a carrier protein could also inhibit the cytopathic effect of HIV-1 on human MT4 cells (Denner *et al.*, 1994), and anti-p80 (p80 is one of three IS-P binding proteins identified by Henderson and colleagues, in Henderson *et al.*, 1993). antisera at a 1:40 dilution could inhibit 95% of HIV-1 infection (Henderson *et al.*, 1993). This inhibition of virus replication may be related to blocking of a secondary receptor or to inhibition of target cell proliferation preventing virus replication.

The collaboration between gp120/CD4 interaction and/or C3 fragment on HIV/CRs interaction, on the one hand, and gp41 binding proteins, on the other hand ("primary" and "secondary" receptors), is not understood presently.

8. IMMUNE COMPLEXES AND COMPLEMENT

Several investigations demonstrated that circulating immune complexes, not only core–anticore but also envelope–antienvelope immune complexes, are present in the sera of HIV-infected patients (Carini *et al.*, 1987a,b, 1989; Lin *et al.*, 1988; Ujhelyi *et al.*, 1987; Schupbach *et al.*, 1984; Ellaurie *et al.*, 1990). Whether these complexes are modified by complement in HIV-positive individuals has not been investigated. This seems to be an important question, since in 1975 Nussenzweig and colleagues observed that immune precipitates were solubilized by serum (Miller *et al.*, 1973; Miller and Nussenzweig, 1974, 1975), via C3 activation and deposition of C3 fragments on the complexes causing disruption of some of the Ag and Ab binding bonds (Takahashi *et al.*, 1976, 1977, 1978).

9. UNSOLVED ASPECTS

Although the relationship between HIV and human complement has been clarified in some important aspects, it is still unclear why, for example, normal B cells carry complement receptors in large quantity and yet are not infected by HIV. It is of interest to note that B lymphoblastoid cells like the Raji cell line can be infected well by HIV-1 opsonized with C3. The normal B cell obviously does not provide the proper environment for productive HIV infection.

Nothing is known about HIV infection of complement receptor-positive mesangium cells. During primary viremia, large amounts of virions are detected in the peripheral blood. Does this virus carry complement or is it unable to activate the complement system? T lymphoblastoid cells infected with different lab strains and primary isolates of HIV-1 and HIV-2 are different with respect to their capacity to activate the complement system. The difference is related to a difference in exposure of gp41 sites binding C1q. What determines the different behavior of the various viral strains? This is the more surprising as these viruses in their isolated form all activate complement well. These are just some of the questions that remain to be solved.

Finally, our present knowledge suggests that efforts will be worthwhile to try to overcome the intrinsic resistance of HIV to human complement. In principle this problem appears to be solved. The proper therapeutic use of the recently gained knowledge is now the challenge ahead of us.

REFERENCES

Arthus, L. O., Bess, J. W., Sowder, R. C., Benveniste, R. E., Mann, D. L., Chermann, J. C., and Henderson, L. E., 1992, Cellular proteins bound to immunodeficiency viruses: Implications for pathogenesis and vaccines, *Science* **258:**1935–1938.

Bakker, L. J., Nottet, H. S. L. M., Vos, N. M., Graaf, L., Van Strijp, J. A. G., Visser, M. R., and Verhoef, J., 1992, Antibodies and complement enhance binding and uptake of HIV-1 by human monocytes, *AIDS* **6:**35–41.

Boyer, V., Desgranges, C., Trabaud, M. A., Fischer, E., and Kazatchkine, M. D., 1991, Complement mediates human immunodeficiency virus type 1 infection of a human T cell line in a CD4- and antibody-independent fashion, *J. Exp. Med.* **173:**1151–1158.

Boyer, V., Delibrias, C., Noraz, N., Fischer, E., Kazatchkine, M. D., and Desgranges, C., 1992, Complement receptor type 2 mediates infection of the human CD4-negative Raji B-cell line with opsonized HIV, *Scand J. Immunol.* **26:**879–883.

Brenneman, D. E., Westbrook, G. L., Fitzgerald, S. P., Ennist, D. L., Elkins, K. L., Ruff, M. R., and Pert, C. B., 1988, Neuronal cell killing by the envelope protein of HIV and its prevention by vasoactive intestinal peptide, *Nature* **335:**639–642.

Carini, C., D'Amelio, R., Mezzaroma, I., and Aiuti, F., 1987a, Detection and characterization of circulating immune complexes in HIV-related diseases, *Diagn. Clin. Immunol.* **5:**135–139.

Carini, C., Mezzaroma, I., Scano, G., D'Amelio, R., Matricardi, P., and Aiuti, F., 1987b, Characterization of specific immune complexes in HIV-related disorders, *Scand. J. Immunol.* **26:**21–28.

Carini, C., Perricone, R., and Fratazzi, C., 1989, Complement activation is associated with the presence of specific human immunodeficiency virus (HIV)–anti-HIV immune complexes in patients with acquired immunodeficiency syndrome-related complex or lymphoadenopathy syndrome, *Scand J. Immunol.* **30:**347–353.

Chen, Y. H., Ebenbichler, C., Vornhagen, R., Schulz, T. F., Böck, G., Steindl, F., Katinger, H., and Dierich, M. P., 1992, HIV-1 gp41 contains two sites for interaction with several proteins on the helper T-lymphoid cell line, H9, *AIDS* **6:**533–539.

Chen, Y. H., Böck, G., Vornhagen, R., Steindl, F., Katinger, H., and Dierich, M. P., 1993a, HIV-1 gp41 binding to human peripheral blood mononuclear cells occurs preferentially to B lymphocytes and monocytes, *Immunobiology* **188:**323–329.

Chen, Y. H., Böck, G., Vornhagen, R., Steindl, F., Katinger, H., and Dierich, M. P., 1993b, HIV-1 gp41 binds to several proteins on the human B cell line, Raji, *Mol. Immunol.* **30:**1159–1163.

Chen, Y. H., Böck, G., Vornhagen, R., Steindl, F., Katinger, H., and Dierich, M. P., 1993c, The human monocyte cell line U937 binds HIV-1 gp41 by proteins 37, 45, 49, 62 and 92 kDa, *Immunol. Lett.* **37:**41–45.

Chen, Y. H., Christiansen, A., Böck, G., and Dierich, M. P., 1995, HIV-2 transmembrane protein gp36 like HIV-1 gp41 binds human lymphocytes and monocytes, *AIDS* **9:**1193–1194.

Cooper, N. R., 1991, Complement evasion strategies of microorganisms, *Immunol. Today* **12:**327–331.

Delibrias, C. C., Kazatchkine, M. D., and Fischer, E., 1993, Evidence for the role of CR1 (CD35), in addition to CR2 (CD21), in facilitating infection of human T cells with opsonized HIV, *Scand. J. Immunol.* **38:**183–189.

Denner, J., Vogel, T., Norley, S., Ennen, J., and Kurth, R., 1993, The immunosuppressive (ISU-) peptide of HIV-1: Binding to lymphocyte surface proteins, *J. Can. Res. Clin. Oncol.* **119(S1):**S28 (10/104).

Denner, J., Norley, S., and Kurth, R., 1994, The immunosuppressive peptide of HIV-1: Functional domains and immune response in AIDS patients, *AIDS* **8:**1063–1072.

Denner, J., Vogel, T., Norley, S., Hoffmann, A., and Kurth, R., 1995, The immunosuppressive (ISU-) peptide of HIV-1: Binding proteins on lymphocytes detected by different methods, *J. Can. Res. Clin. Oncol.* **121(S1):**S35 (11/128).

De-Panfilis, G., Soligo, D., Manara, G. C., Ferrari, C., Torresain, C., and Zucchi, A., 1990, Human normal-resting epidermal Langerhans cells do express the type 3 complement receptor, *Br. J. Dermatol.* **122:**127–136.

Dierich, M. P., Ebenbichler, C. F., Marschang, P., Füst, G., Thielens, N. M., and Arlaud, G. J., 1993, HIV and human complement: Mechanisms of interaction and biological implications, *Immunol. Today* **14:**435–440.

Douvas, A., and Takehana, Y., 1994, Cross-reactivity between autoimmune anti-U1 snRNP antibodies and neutralizing epitopes of HIV-1 gp120/41, *Aids Res. Hum. Retrovir.* **10:**253–262.

Dukor, P., Bianco, G., and Nussenzwej, V., 1970, Tissue localization of lymphocytes bearing a membrane receptor for antigen-antibody-complement complexes, *Proc. Natl. Acad. Sci (USA)* **67:**991–997.

Ebenbichler, C. F., Thielens, N. M., Vornhagen, R., Marschang, P., Arlaud, G. J., and Dierich, M. P., 1991, Human immunodeficiency virus type 1 activates the classical pathway of complement by direct C1 binding through specific sites in the transmembrane glycoprotein gp41, *J. Exp. Med.* **174:**1417–1424.

Ebenbichler, C. F., Röder, C., Vornhagen, R., Ratner, L., and Dierich, M. P., 1993, Cell surface proteins binding to recombinant soluble HIV-1 and HIV-2 transmembrane proteins, *AIDS* **7:**489–495.

Ebersold, A., Boyer, V., and Klasse, P. J., 1992, Human and murine monoclonal antibodies directed against a conserved sequence from gp41 (aa583–599) of human immunodeficiency virus type 1, *Res. Virol.* **143:** 179–191.

Ellaurie, M., Calvelli, T., and Rubinstein, A., 1990, Immune complexes in pediatric human immunodeficiency virus infection, *Am. J. Dis. Child.* **144:**1207–1209.

Ezekowitz, R. R., Kuhlman, M., Groopman, J. E., and Byrn, B. A., 1989, A human serum mannose-binding protein inhibits in vitro infection by the human immunodeficiency virus, *J. Exp. Med.* **169:**185–196.

Fischer, E., Delibrias, C., and Kazatchkine, M. D., 1991, Expression of CR2 (the C3dg/EBV receptor, CD21) on normal human peripheral blood T lymphocytes, *J. Immunol.* **146:**865–869.

Fuchs, D., Hausen, A., Reibnegger, G., Werner, E. R., Dierich, M. P., and Wachter, H., 1988, Neopterin as a marker for activated cell-mediated immunity, *Immunol. Today* **9:**150–155.

Fuchs, D., Zangerle, R., Artner-Dworzak, E., Weiss, G., Fritsch, P., Tilz, G. P., Dierich, M. P., and Wachter, H., 1993, Association between immune activation, changes of iron metabolism and anaemia in patients with HIV infection, *Eur. J. Haematol.* **50:**90–94.

Gallaher, W. R., 1987, Detection of a fusion peptide sequence in the transmembrane protein of human immunodeficiency virus, *Cell* **50:**327–328.

Garry, R. F., 1990, Extensive antigenic mimicry by retrovirus capsid proteins, *AIDS Res. Hum. Retrovir.* **12:**1361–1362.

Gelderblom, H. R., Reupke, H., Winkel, T., Kunze, R., and Pauli, G., 1987, MHC-antigens: Constituents of the envelopes of human and simian immunodeficiency virus, *Z. Naturforsch.* **42c:**1328–1334.

Golding, H., Robey, F. A., Gates, F. T., III, Linder, W., Beining, P. R., Hoffmann, T., and Golding, B., 1988, Identification of homologous regions in human immunodeficiency virus I gp41 and human MHC class II 1 domain, *J. Exp. Med.* **167:**914–923.

Gras, G. S., and Dormont, D., 1991, Antibody-dependent and antibody-independent complement-mediated enhancement of human immunodeficiency virus type 1 infection in a human, Epstein–Barr virus-transformed B-lymphocytic cell line, *J. Virol.* **65:**541–545.

Henderson, L. A., and Qureshi, M. N., 1993, A peptide inhibitor of human immunodeficiency virus infection binds to novel human cell surface polypeptides, *J. Biol. Chem.* **268:**15291–15297.

Hosoi, S., Borsos, T., Dunlop, N., and Nara, P. L., 1990, Heat-labile, complement-like factor(s) of animal sera prevent(s) HIV-1 infectivity in vitro, *AIDS* **3:**366–371.

Joling, P., Bakker, L. J., Van Strijp, J. A. G., Meerloo, T., de Graaf, L., Dekker, M. E. M., Goudsmit, J., Verhoef, J., and Schuurman, H.-J., 1993, Binding of human immunodeficiency virus type-1 to follicular dendritic cells in vitro is complement dependent, *J. Immunol.* **150:**1065–1073.

June, R. A., Schade, S. Z., Bankowski, M. J., Kuhns, M., McNamara, A., Lint, T. F., Landay, A. L., and Spear, G. T., 1991, Complement and antibody mediate enhancement of HIV infection by increasing virus binding and provirus formation, *AIDS* **5:**269–274.

June, R. A., Landay, A. L., Stefanik, K., Lint, T. F., and Spear, G. T., 1992, Phenotypic analysis of complement receptor 2+ T lymphocytes: Reduced expression on CD4+ cells in HIV-infected persons, *Immunology* **75:**59–65.

Kotwal, G. J., and Moss, B., 1988, Vaccinia virus encodes a secretory polypeptide structurally related to complement control proteins, *Nature* **325:**176–178.

Larcher, C., Schulz, T. F., Hofbauer, J., Hengster, P., Romani, N., and Wachter, H., 1990, Expression of the C3d/EBV receptor and of other cell membrane surface markers is altered upon HIV-1 infection of myeloid, T, and B cells, *J. Acq. Immune Defic. Syndr.* **3:**103–108.

Lee, M. R., Ho, D. D., and Gurney, M. E., 1987, Functional interaction and partial homology between human immunodeficiency virus and neuroleukin, *Science* **237**:1047–1051.

Levy, J. A., 1993, Pathogenesis of human immunodeficiency virus infection, *Microbiol. Rev.* **57**:183–289.

Lewis, M. G., Elkins, W. R., and McCutchan, F. E., 1993, Passively transferred antibodies directed against conserved regions of SIV envelope protect macaques from SIV infection, *Vaccine* **11**:1347–1355.

Lin, R. Y., Wildfeuer, O., Franklin, M. M., and Candido, K., 1988, Hypocomplementenia and human immunodeficiency virus infection, *Int. Arch. Allergy Appl. Immunol.* **87**:40–46.

McClure, M. O., Marsh, M., and Weiss, R. A., 1988, Human immunodeficiency virus infection of CD4 bearing cells occurs by a pH independent mechanism, *EMBO J.* **7**:513–518.

Marschang, P., Gürtler, L., Tötsch, M., Thielens, N. M., Arlaud, G. J., Hittmair, A., Katinger, H., and Dierich, M. P., 1993, HIV-1 and HIV-2 isolates differ in their ability to activate the complement system on the surface of infected cells, *AIDS* **7**:903–910.

Marschang, P., Ebenbichler, C. F., and Dierich, M. P., 1994, HIV and complement: Role of the complement system in HIV infection, *Int. Arch. Allergy Appl. Immunol.* **103**:113–117.

Marschang, P., Sodroski, J., Würzner, R., and Dierich, M. P., 1995, Decay-accelerating factor (CD55) protects human immunodeficiency virus type 1 from inactivation by human complement, *Eur. J. Immunol.* **25**:285–290.

Meerloo, T., Parmentier, H. K., Osterhaus, A. D. M. E., Goudsmit, J., and Schuurman, H. J., 1992, Modulation of cell surface molecules during HIV-1 infection of H9 cells. An immunoelectron microscopy study, *AIDS* **6**:1105–1116.

Miller, G. W., and Nussenzweig, V., 1974, Complement as a regulator of interactions between immune complexes and cell membranes, *J. Immunol.* **113**:464–469.

Miller, G. W., and Nussenzweig, V., 1975, A new complement function: Solubilization of antigen–antibody aggregates, *Proc. Natl. Acad. Sci. USA* **72**:418–422.

Miller, G. W., Saluk, P. H., and Nussenzweig, V., 1973, Complement-dependent release of immune complexes from the lymphocyte membrane, *J. Exp. Med.* **138**:495–507.

Montefiori, D. C., Zhou, J., and Shaff, D. I., 1992, CD4-dependent binding of HIV-1 to the B lymphocyte receptor CR2 (CD21) in the presence of complement and antibody, *Clin. Exp. Immunol.* **90**:383–389.

Morgan, B. P., and Meri, S., 1994, Membrane proteins that protect against complement lysis, *Springer Semin. Immunopathol.* **15**:369–396.

Morrow, W. J. W., Wharton, M., Stricker, R. B., and Levy, J. A., 1986, Circulating immune complexes in patients with acquired immune deficiency syndrome contain the AIDS-associated retrovirus, *Clin. Immunol. Immunopathol.* **40**:515–524.

Morrow, W. J. W., Isenberg, D. A., Sobol, R. E., Stricker, R. B., and Kieber-Emmons, T., 1991, AIDS virus infection and autoimmunity: A perspective of the clinical, immunological, and molecular origins of the autoallergic pathologies associated with HIV disease, *Clin. Immunol. Immunopathol.* **58**:163–180.

Naylor, P. H., Naylor, C. W., Badamchian, M., Wada, S., Goldstein, A. L., Wang, S. S., Sun, D. K., Thornton, A. H., and Sarin, P. S., 1987, Human immunodeficiency virus contains an epitope immunoreactive with thymosin α_1 and the 30-amino acid synthetic p17 group-specific antigen peptide HGP-30, *Proc. Natl. Acad. Sci. USA* **84**:2951–2955.

Oldstone, M. B. A., 1987, Molecular mimicry and autoimmune disease, *Cell* **50**:819–820.

Orentas, R. J., and Hildreth, J. E. K., 1993, Association of host cell surface adhesion receptors and other membrane proteins with HIV and SIV, *AIDS Res. Hum. Retrovir.* **9**:1157–1165.

Pinter, C., Siccardi, A. G., Lopalco, L., Longhi, R., and Clivio, A., 1995, HIV glycoprotein 41 and complement factor H interact with each other and share functional as well as antigenic homology, *AIDS Res. Hum. Retrovir.* **11**:971–980.

Purtscher, M., Trkola, A., Gruber, G., Buchacher, A., Predl, R., Steindl, F., Tauer, C., Berger, R., Barrett, N., Jungbauer, A., and Katinger, H., 1994, A broadly neutralizing human monoclonal antibody against gp41 of human immunodeficiency virus type 1, *AIDS Res. Hum. Retrovir.* **10**:1651–1658.

Qureshi, N. M., Coy, D. H., Garry, R. F., and Henderson, L. A., 1990, Characterization of a putative cellular receptor for HIV-1 transmembrane glycoprotein using synthetic peptides, *AIDS* **4**:553–558.

Reiher, W. E., Blalock, J. F., and Brunck, T. K., 1988, Sequence homology between acquired immunodeficiency syndrome virus envelope protein and interleukin 2, *Proc. Natl. Acad. Sci. USA* **85**:9188–9192.

Reisinger, E. C., Vogetseder, W., Berzow, D., Köfler, D., Bitterlich, G., Lehr, H. A., Wachter, H., and Dierich, M. P., 1990, Complement-mediated enhancement of HIV-1 infection of the monoblastoid cell line U 937, *AIDS* **4**:961–965.

Ross, G. D., ed., 1986, *Immunobiology of the Complement System*, Academic Press, New York, pp. 197–212.

Saifuddin, M. Landay, A. L., Ghassemi, M., Patki, C., and Spear, G. T., 1995a, HTLV-1 activates complement leading to increased binding to complement receptor-positive cells, *AIDS Res. Hum. Retrovir.* **11:**1115–1122.

Saifuddin, M., Parker, C. J., Peeples, M. E., Gorny, M. K., Zolla-Pazner, S., Ghassemi, M., Rooney, I. A., Atkinson, J. P., and Spear, G. T., 1995b, Role of virion-associated glycosylphosphatidylinositol-linked proteins CD55 and CD59 in complement resistance of cell line-derived and primary isolates of HIV-1, *J. Exp. Med.* **182:**501–509.

Santis, C., Lopalco, L., Robbioni, P., Longhi, R., Rappocciolo, G., Siccardi, A. G., and Beretta, A., 1994, Human antibodies to immunodominant C5 region of HIV-1 gp120 cross-react with HLA class I on activated cells, *AIDS Res. Hum. Retrovir.* **102:**157–162.

Schifferli, J. A., Yin, C., and Peters, D. K., 1986, The role of complement and its receptor in the elimination of immune complexes, *N. Engl. J. Med.* **315:**488–495.

Schupbach, J., Kalyanaraman, V. S., Sarngadharan, M. G., Bunn, P. A., Blayney, D. W., and Gallo, R. C., 1984, Demonstration of viral antigen p24 in circulating immune complexes of two patients with human T-cell leukaemia/lymphoma virus (HTLV) positive lymphoma, *Lancet* **1:**302–305.

Scott, M. E., Landay, A. L., Lint, T. F., and Spear, G. T., 1993, In vivo decrease in the expression of complement receptor 2 on B cells in HIV-infection, *AIDS* **7:**37–41.

Shafferman, A., Jahrling, P. B., and Benveniste, R. E., 1991, Protection of macaques with a simian immunodeficiency virus envelope peptide vaccine based on conserved human immunodeficiency virus type 1 sequences, *Proc. Natl. Acad. Sci. USA* **88:**7126–7130.

Sölder, B. M., Schulz, T. F., Hengster, P., Larcher, C., Bitterlich, G., Eigentler, A., Löwer, J., Kurth, R., Wachter, H., and Dierich, M. P., 1988, HIV and HIV-infected cells activate the complement system, *Immunobiology* **178:**69.

Sölder, B., Marschang, P., Wachter H., Dierich, M. P., Nayyar, S., Lewin, I. V., and Stanworth, D. R., 1989a, Antiviral antibodies in HIV (HTLV-III) infection possess auto-antibody activity against a CH1 domain determinant in human IgG: Possible immunological consequences, *Immunol. Lett.* **23:**9–20.

Sölder, B., Reisinger, E. C., Köfler, D., Bitterlich, G., Wachter, H., and Dierich, M. P., 1989b, Complement receptors: Another port of entry for HIV, *Lancet* **2:**271–272.

Sölder, B., Schulz, T. F., Hengster, P., Löwer, J., Larcher, C., Bitterlich, G., Kurth, R., Wachter, H., and Dierich, M. P., 1989c, HIV and HIV-infected cells differentially activate the human complement system independent of antibody, *Immunol. Lett.* **22:**135–146.

Spear, G. T., Sullivan, B. L., Landay, A. L., and Lint, T. F., 1990, Neutralization of human immunodeficiency virus type 1 by complement occurs by viral lysis, *J. Virol.* **64:**5869–5873.

Spear, G. T., Sullivan, B. L., Takefman, D. M., Landay, A. L., and Lint, T. F., 1991, Human immunodeficiency virus (HIV)-infected cells and free virus directly activate the classical complement pathway in rabbit, mouse and guinea-pig sera, activation results in virus neutralization by virolysis, *Immunology* **73:**377–382.

Spear, G. T., Takefman, D. M., Sullivan, B. L., Landay, A. L., and Zolla-Pazner, S., 1993, Complement activation by human monoclonal antibodies to human immunodeficiency virus, *J. Virol.* **67:**53–59.

Stein, B., Gowda, S., Lifson, J., Penhallow, R., Bensch, K., and Engelmann, E., 1987, pH independent HIV entry into CD4-positive T cells via virus envelope fusion to the plasma membrane, *Cell* **49:**659–668.

Stoiber, H., Thielens, N. M., Ebenbichler, C. F., Arlaud, G. J., and Dierich, M. P., 1994, The envelope glycoprotein of HIV-1 gp120 and human complement protein Clq bind to the same peptides derived from three different regions of gp41, the transmembrane glycoprotein of HIV-1, and share antigenic homology, *Eur. J. Immunol.* **24:**294–300.

Stoiber, H., Ebenbichler, C. F., Schneider, R., Janatova, J., and Dierich, M. P., 1995a, Interaction of several complement proteins with gp120 and gp41, the two envelope glycoproteins of HIV-1, *AIDS* **9:**19–26.

Stoiber, H., Ebenbichler, C. F., Thielens, N. M., Arlaud, G. J., and Dierich, M. P., 1995b, HIV-1 rsgp41 depends on calcium for binding of human Clq but not for binding of gp120, *Mol. Immunol.* **5:**371–374.

Stoiber, H., Schneider, R., Janatova, J., and Dierich, M. P., 1995c, Human complement proteins C3b, C4b, factor H and properdin react with specific sites in gp120 and gp41, the envelope proteins of HIV-1, *Immunobiology* **193:**98–113.

Stoiber, H., Pinter, C., Siccardi, A. G., Clivio, A., and Dierich, M. P., 1996, Efficient destruction of HIV in human serum by inhibiting the protective action of complement factor H and decay accelerating factor (DAF, CD55), *J. Exp. Med.* **183:**307–310.

Stricker, R. B., McHugh, T. M., Moody, D. J., Morrow, W. J. W., Stites, D. P., Shuman, M. A., and Levy, J. A., 1987, An AIDS-related cytotoxic antoantibody reacts with a specific antigen on stimulated CD4+ T cells, *Nature* **327:**710–713.

Süsal, C., Kirschfink, M., Kröpelin, M., Daniel, V., and Opelz, G., 1994, Complement activation by recombinant HIV-1 glycoprotein gp120, *J. Immunol.* **152**:6028.

Takahashi, M., Czop, J., Ferreira, A., and Nussenzweig, V., 1976, Mechanism of solubilization of immune aggregates by complement. Implications for immunopathology, *Transplant Rev.* **32**:121–139.

Takahashi, M., Tack, B. F., and Nussenzweig, V., 1977, Requirements for the solubilization of immune aggregates by complement. Assembly of a factor B-dependent C3-convertase on the immune complexes, *J. Exp. Med.* **145**:86–100.

Takahashi, M., Takahashi, S., Brade, V., and Nussenzweig, V., 1978, Requirements for the solubilization of immune aggregates by complement. The role of the classical pathway, *J. Clin. Invest.* **62**:349–358.

Thieblemont, N., Haeffner-Cavaillon, N. A., Ledur, A., L'Age-Stehr, J., Ziegler-Heitbrock, H. W. L., and Kazatchkine, M. D., 1993, CR1 (CD35) and CR3 (CD11b/CD18) mediate infection of human monocytes and monocytic cell lines with complement-opsonized HIV independently of CD4, *Clin. Exp. Immunol.* **92**: 106–113.

Thielens, N. M., Bally, I. M., Ebenbichler, C. F., Dierich, M. P., and Arlaud, G. J., 1993, Further characterization of the interaction between the C1q subcomponent of human C1 and the transmembrane envelope glycoprotein gp41 of HIV-1, *J. Immunol.* **151**:6583–6592.

Ujhelyi, E., Buki, B., Salavecz, V., Banhegyi, D., Horvath, A., Furst, G., and Hollan, S. R., 1987, A simple method for detecting HIV antibodies hidden in circulating immune complexes, *AIDS* **1**:161–165.

Vanini, S., Longhi, R., Lazzarin, A., Vigo, E., Siccardi, A. G., and Viale, G., 1993, Discrete regions of HIV-1 gp41 defined by syncytia-inhibiting affinity-purified human antibodies, *AIDS* **7**:167–174.

Welsh, R. M., Cooper, N. R., Jensen, F. C., and Oldstone, M. B. A., 1975, Human serum lyses RNA tumour viruses, *Nature* **257**:612–614.

Wu, A. F., Wood, C., and Wu, T. T., 1989, Possibility of HIV gp41 and thymosin beta-4 sharing the same antigenic epitope, *AIDS* **3**:319–320.

Yamada, M., Zurbriggen, A., Oldstone, M. B. A., and Fujinami, R. S., 1991, Common immunologic determinant between human immunodeficiency virus type 1 gp41 and astrocytes, *J. Virol.* **65**:1370–1376.

Yefenof, E., Asjö, B., and Klein, E., 1991, Alternative complement pathway activation by HIV infected cells: C3 fixation does not lead to complement lysis but enhances NK sensitivity, *Int. Immunol.* **3**:395–401.

Zagury, J. F., Bernhard, J., Achour, A., Astgen, A., Lachgar, A., Fall, L., Carelli, C., Issing, W., Mbika, J. P., Picard, O., Carlotti, M., Callebaut, I., Mornon, J. P., Burny, A., Feldman, M., Bizzini, B., and Zagury, D., 1993, Identification of CD4 and major histocompatibility complex functional peptide sites and their homology with oligopeptides from human immunodeficiency virus type 1 glycoprotein gp120: Role in AIDS pathogenesis, *Proc. Natl. Acad. Sci. USA* **90**:7573–7577.

CHAPTER 19

POLYMORPHONUCLEAR LEUKOCYTE FUNCTION IN HIV

SHYH-DAR SHYUR and HARRY R. HILL

1. THE POLYMORPHONUCLEAR LEUKOCYTE

The phagocytic system belongs to the nonspecific immune system, which includes polymorphonuclear leukocytes (e.g., neutrophils, eosinophils) and mononuclear phagocytes (e.g., circulating monocytes, tissue macrophages, and fixed macrophages). The major phagocytic functions include adherence to endothelium and aggregation, emigration or diapedesis, chemotaxis and random motility, attachment, phagocytosis, degranulation, and microbicidal activity. Neutrophils are the first line of defense against bacterial invasion of the surface barriers; they appear in the inflammatory focus within a few hours. The differentiation and maturation of neutrophils in the bone marrow requires about 2 weeks. This process can be divided into two phases. The first week of neutrophil development is a proliferative phase with cell division. The cells of the myeloid series evolve from the myeloblast to promyelocyte and then to the myelocyte. During this process neutrophils develop their various cytoplasmic granules. Then a maturation phase follows during the second week with no cell division. During this phase neutrophils mature from metamyelocytes to band forms and then to the segmented neutrophils (Gallin, 1993). The recruitment of neutrophils to sites of inflammation is initiated by the local production of bacterium-derived attractants, inflammatory cytokines, and other host-derived factors. These factors will initiate rolling of neutrophils along the endothelium, which is mediated by members of the selectin family. The selectin family include E- and P-selectin, which are expressed on the surface of activated endothelial cells, and L-selectin, which is constitutively expressed on neutrophils. The carbohydrate ligands for E- and P-selectin are sialyl-Lewis X, which is the basic defect in leukocyte adhesion deficiency type II, an abnormality that reflects a general defect in fucose metabolism (Lowe *et al.*, 1990) within the cell-surface

SHYH-DAR SHYUR • Department of Pediatrics, Mackay Memorial Hospital, Taipei, Taiwan, Republic of China. HARRY R. HILL • Divisions of Clinical Pathology and Clinical Immunology and Allergy, Departments of Pathology and Pediatrics, University of Utah School of Medicine, Salt Lake City, Utah 84132.
Immunology of HIV Infection, edited by Sudhir Gupta. Plenum Press, New York, 1996.

glycoproteins and glycolipids of the neutrophil. E- and P-selectin are thought to mediate a common step in the recruitment of neutrophils, eosinophils, monocytes, and a subclass of T cells to sites of inflammation or tissue injury. The expression of leukocyte adhesion surface glycoproteins, or integrins, including CD11a/CD18 (LFA-1), CD11b/CD18 (Mac-1), and CD11c/CD18 (p150/95) are then upregulated which is essential for firm attachment to the endothelium, chemotaxis, and ingestion of complement-coated particles. Neutrophils must be able to adhere to the vascular endothelium, detect and migrate toward a chemical stimulus (chemotaxis) before they can phagocytize and kill the ingested microorganism. The initial phase of this microbicidal activity may be dependent on lysosomal factors contained within granules; the late phase is dependent on the respiratory oxidative response and activation of the myeloperoxidase (MPO)–H_2O_2–halide system. The phagocytic system is responsible for defense against extracellular bacterial invasion in association with opsonins (e.g., antibodies, complement, and some acute-phase proteins).

If there is a defect in the number or function of the cells of the phagocytic system, both congenital and acquired disorders, the incidence of pyogenic bacterial infections will markedly increase. If the defect involves mainly neutrophils, the patients usually suffer from recurrent pyogenic surface or tissue infections including impetigo, furunculosis, abscesses, cutaneous candida infections, otitis media, and pneumonia.

Finally, it must be mentioned that PMNs also exhibit the following activities. Interferonlike substances can be released by neutrophils which result in the inhibition of virus replication. Neutrophils have been shown to mediate antibody-dependent cellular cytotoxicity (ADCC) against tumors and viruses in infected cells, especially in the presence of cytokines such as the interferons and granulocyte–monocyte and granulocyte colony-stimulating factors. MPO, H_2O_2, and chloride form an antimicrobial system in PMN effective against a variety of microorganisms. Normal human PMN, when stimulated with phorbol myristate acetate or opsonized zymosan, are viricidal to HIV-1. MPO released during degranulation reacts with H_2O_2 formed by the respiratory burst to oxidize chloride to hypochlorous acid which is toxic to HIV-1. It is possible that the viricidal effect of stimulated PMN may have a role in host defense against HIV-1 (Klebanoff and Coombs, 1992). On the other hand, viral infections can also cause dysregulation of neutrophil function.

2. HIV INFECTION

Acquired immunodeficiency syndrome (AIDS) caused by the human immunodeficiency retrovirus (HIV) has become one of the most important medical problems since initial reports in 1981 (Gottlieb *et al.*, 1981; Masur *et al.*, 1981; Siegal *et al.*, 1981).

Initially, it was believed to be a disease process limited to homosexual men, but soon it was realized that this infection does not have any limitation among different races, life-styles, or socioeconomic conditions. In the early 1980s, absence of "safe sex" practices and transmission through blood and blood products led to identification of the affected population as the so-called "four-Hs": homosexuals, hemophiliacs, Haitians, and other "high-risk" individuals (which included intravenous drug users, bisexual individuals, and individuals having sex with those exhibiting AIDS or at risk for HIV infection) (Schiff and Harville, 1996). Acquisition of HIV requires contact with infected blood, tissue, or body fluid from an HIV-infected individual so that the infected material can enter the circulation (Jones *et al.*, 1989).

Infants and children were later found to develop signs of HIV infection and AIDS. Pediatric AIDS (PAIDS) comprises about 1 to 2% of all AIDS patients. Approximately 80 to 90% of PAIDS patients acquired their HIV infection during the perinatal period (Katz and Wilfert, 1989; CDC, 1989). The rate of transmission from HIV-infected mothers to their infants is about 24 to 35% (European Collaborative Study, 1988; Blanche *et al.*, 1989). Approximately 80% of PAIDS patients have a parent with established AIDS or AIDS-related complex or one who belongs to a high-risk group (Cowan *et al.*, 1984). There exists a large difference in the manifestations and disease course between congenital or perinatal HIV-infected infants and that in adults or older children who become infected. The differences in infant HIV infection and AIDS from that of older patients include a shorter latency before the onset of AIDS, a greater degree of earlier immune system dysfunction, an increased incidence of recurrent infection with encapsulated bacterial, lymphoid interstitial pneumonitis (LIP), increased incidence of CNS disease (including poor developmental attainment or loss of developmental milestones), failure to thrive, multiple opportunistic infections, absence of Kaposi's sarcoma, lower incidence of lymphoma, and greater degree of hypergammaglobulinemia (MaWhinney *et al.*, 1993). Recurrent otitis media, sinusitis, skin infection, pneumonia, sepsis, and meningitis are common bacterial infections in PAIDS. The most frequent pathogens are *Streptococcus pneumoniae*, *Haemophilus influenzae*, *Staphylococcus aureus*, and *Salmonella*. Opportunistic infection caused by *Pneumocystis carinii* is very common in HIV-infected patients and causes a high mortality rate in these individuals. The majority of infants infected with HIV exhibit signs of AIDS by 9 to 12 months of age.

After entering the body, HIV primarily invades $CD4^+$ helper-inducer T cells by binding of the viral envelope protein gp120 to the T-cell CD1 receptor. Other cells can be infected by HIV including ones of the monocyte–macrophage lineage, CNS cells, and EB virus-infected B cells (Ho *et al.*, 1987).

Diagnosis of AIDS should be considered in the presence of risk factors for HIV infection or compatible clinical manifestations and evidence of T- and B-cell immunodeficiency (usually manifested by lymphopenia, depletion of $CD4^+$ helper-inducer cells, alteration of the Th/Ts ratio, functional abnormalities of T-cell immunity, polyclonal hypergammaglobulinemia, and poor antibody responses). The presence of HIV infection is suggested by the detection of anti-HIV antibody using enzyme immunoassay (ELISA) and immunoblotting (Western blot). Confirmation of infection in the infant is based on detection of HIV p24 core antigen by ELISA, detection in the patient's leukocytes of HIV proviral DNA using the polymerase chain reaction (Laure *et al.*, 1988; Rogers *et al.*, 1989), or by viral culture.

Management of patients with AIDS includes the use of antimicrobial prophylaxis or therapy for bacterial and fungal infections; aerosolized pentamidine (Leoung *et al.*, 1990) and/or TMP-SMX (Fischl *et al.*, 1988) for *P. carinii* pneumonia. Adjunctive steroid therapy in moderate to severe *P. carinii* pneumonia is useful in improving survival and decreasing the frequency of respiratory failure (Bozzette *et al.*, 1990; Gagnon *et al.*, 1990). Corticosteroids are also of value in the treatment of lymphoid interstitial pneumonitis (Charytan *et al.*, 1985). Administration of IVIG is useful in preventing recurrent bacterial and viral infections (Calvelli and Rubinstein, 1986). Dideoxynucleosides [zidovudine

(AZT), zalcitabine (ddC), didanosine (ddI)] are promising new agents for the management of HIV-1 infections. AZT, a thymidine analogue activated by cellular kinase, is incorporated into HIV DNA by reverse transcriptase and results in HIV DNA chain termination. This agent is useful for improving immunologic abnormalities and clinical symptoms and decreasing opportunistic infections and mortality rate and is of particular benefit in patients with encephalopathy (Pizzo *et al.*, 1988; Fischl *et al.*, 1987). In patients intolerant of AZT, ddC was comparable to ddI in terms of slowing progression of disease, and slightly better in prolonging survival. ddI, like AZT and ddC, also suppresses the circulating levels of p24, and induces an increase in CD4 counts (Cooley *et al.*, 1990). Combination of the above antiretroviral drugs may be used to achieve synergy, prevent resistance, and take advantage of different toxicity profiles (Landor, 1993). Additional immunomodulators currently under study include interferons, interleukins, colony-stimulating factors, CD4 immunoadhesins, CD4 immunotoxins (Ammann, 1990), recombinant CD4 (Letvin *et al.*, 1992), and various trials on different prophylactic and therapeutic AIDS vaccines (Walker and Fast, 1994).

3. POLYMORPHONUCLEAR LEUKOCYTE FUNCTIONS IN HIV INFECTION

HIV-associated immunodeficiency has become the most significant cause of acquired immunodeficiency in both adults and children. A variety of immunologic defects are detected both early and late in HIV infection. Various immunologic changes in the $CD4^+$ T-cell subset occur, but the principal defect is a marked lowering of circulating $CD4^+$ cells.

HIV can enter the susceptible $CD4^+$ cells via the binding of the gp120 surface envelope glycoprotein to the CD4 surface marker through endocytosis (Maddon *et al.*, 1986). But other studies also confirmed that HIV infection of cells can occur by direct fusion of the HIV envelope with the host cell membrane (Bedinger *et al.*, 1988; Hoxie *et al.*, 1988; Maddon *et al.*, 1988).

It has been shown from the study of concomitant infection with sexually transmitted *Chlamydia trachomatis* in HIV-infected individuals that HIV replication can be triggered by contact of HIV-infected cells with PMNs, by the generation of reactive oxygen intermediates (ROIs), and by soluble factors such as TNF-α and IL-6 (Ho *et al.*, 1995).

The possibility that bone marrow precursor cells can be infected with HIV was suggested by the following studies (Rosenberg and Fauci, 1989). Hematologic abnormalities, including leukopenia, anemia, thrombocytopenia, and myelodysplasia, have been found in the majority of AIDS patients under study (Delacretaz *et al.*, 1987; Spivak *et al.*, 1984). The myelodysplastic changes in HIV infection suggest involvement of hematopoietic progenitor cells in HIV infection (Schneider and Picker, 1985). Analysis of the proliferative capacity of granulocyte–macrophage (GM) progenitor cells from HIV-infected individuals reveals a significant inhibition of growth as compared to controls (Leiderman *et al.*, 1987).

Further studies supporting the hypothesis that the hematological abnormalities in AIDS are the result of HIV infection of bone marrow cells are summarized as follows:

1. HIV-1 RNA is present in myeloid precursor cells from bone marrow samples of AIDS patients (Busch *et al.*, 1986). The expression of HIV-1 in myeloid precursors, as detected by *in situ* hybridization of bone marrow from patients with AIDS,

suggests the possibility of infection and direct suppression of the functional integrity of mature myeloid elements by HIV-1 *in vivo.*

2. The experiments reported by Donahue *et al.* (1987) suggest that bone marrow progenitor cells for monocytes and macrophages may be infected by HIV and may be resistant to its cytopathic effects.
3. Direct evidence for HIV infection of bone marrow progenitor cells was obtained by Folks *et al.* (1988). Myeloid progenitor cells were highly purified from normal human bone marrow by positive immunoselection with high-affinity monoclonal antibodies (CD34) linked to magnetic beads. After exposure *in vitro* to HIV-1, these myeloid progenitor cells were shown to be infected with HIV-1.

In addition to infection of bone marrow myeloid precursor cells, HIV also infects peripheral PMNs directly. HIV DNA was detected by the polymerase chain reaction technique in PMNs in 11 of 37 (29.7%) HIV-infected patients. A detectable level of HIV DNA in PMNs was more common in symptomatic than asymptomatic HIV-infected patients (46.7 and 18.2%, respectively; $p < 0.05$). HIV DNA in PMNs was detected most frequently in patients with recurrent bacterial pneumonia or *P. carinii* pneumonia. An association between HIV DNA in PMNs and a low CD4/8 ratio as well as high levels of immunoglobulins in the sera was noted. Detectable HIV DNA was found more frequently in patients with neutropenia than in those with a normal level of neutrophils in peripheral blood (44.4 and 28.0%, respectively; $p < 0.05$). These data suggest that infection of PMNs by HIV may be associated with PMN impairment during HIV infection (Gabrilovich *et al.*, 1993).

Neutropenia has been reported among HIV-infected patients (Minchinton and Frazer, 1985; Murphy *et al.*, 1985). It has been estimated to occur in 20 to 40% of AIDS patients and in 22% of patients with persistent generalized lymphadenopathy. Antineutrophil antibodies (Murphy *et al.*, 1985) and deposition of immune complexes (Ras and Anderson, 1986) on the cell surface have been implicated in the cause of neutropenia in HIV-infected individuals. Neutropenia is more common in patients with AIDS and opportunistic infections.

Functional PMN defects in patients with HIV infection have also been described as follows:

3.1. Altered Adhesion Molecule Expression and Actin Polymerization

PMNs from patients with HIV infection appear to be activated *in vivo*, as demonstrated by increased expression of the adhesion molecule CD11b/CD18, reduced L-selectin antigen expression, increased actin polymerization, and increased H_2O_2 production. The alterations described were present in symptomatic patients with $CD4^+$ cell counts greater than 500/μl and did not increase with progression of the disease. Stimulation by bacterial *N*-formyl peptides showed dysregulation of L-selectin shedding and decreased H_2O_2 production after *ex vivo* priming with TNF-α or IL-8. These latter impairments, which correlated with a decrease in $CD4^+$ lymphocyte numbers and with IL-8 and IL-6 plasma levels, could contribute to the increased susceptibility of HIV-infected patients to bacterial infections (Elbim *et al.*, 1994).

3.2. Decreased Chemotaxis

Neutrophils from patients with AIDS-related complex (ARC) demonstrate significantly less chemotactic activity compared to controls. Sera from patients with AIDS and

Kaposi's sarcoma (KS) or with ARC have been reported to significantly inhibit chemotaxis of neutrophils from controls (Ellis *et al.*, 1988). Both the monocyte/macrophage lineage as well as granulocytes exhibit decreased chemotaxis, possibly related to a decreased expression of chemotactic receptors due to HIV or HIV proteins. HIV infection likely causes defective PMN chemotaxis which then increases susceptibility to recurrent bacterial infections in these patients (Ciaffoni *et al.*, 1991).

3.3. Decreased Phagocytosis

Defective phagocytic uptake has also been demonstrated in HIV-infected patients in a study by Ellis *et al.* (1988), while Boros *et al.* (1990) showed decreased FcγRIII expression on PMNs from HIV-infected patients. FcγRIII on neutrophils is a phosphatidylinositol glycan (PIG)-anchored protein that can be released from cells by activation with chemotactic peptides. In patients with AIDS and ARC and in HIV-1-positive intravenous drug abusers, a substantial population (25%) of neutrophils do not stain with the anti-FcγRIII mAb 3G8. This non-FcγRIII-bearing population was largely absent (3%) in HIV-1-negative control individuals. The presence of the Fc gamma RIII-negative neutrophil population may be related to altered function leading to common bacterial infections in advanced AIDS.

3.4. Altered Respiratory Burst Activity

Sonnerborg and Jarstrand (1986) have studied respiratory burst activity by neutrophils in patients with HIV infection. PMN chemiluminescence (CL) and intracellular enzyme activity were both depressed in HIV-infected patients at all stages of infection. PMN phagocytosis in the presence of serum was reduced in the early stage of HIV infections (LAS) but was in the normal range in AIDS patients. The appearance of recurrent upper respiratory tract infections was associated with reduced PMN CL. The most pronounced changes in PMN activity were observed in patients with severe, recurrent bacterial pneumonias and *P. carinii* pneumonia. A lower level of PMN activity was found in patients with rapidly progressing infection toward AIDS than in patients with a relatively stable course of infection. Thus, it was suggested that PMN CL may be regarded as a predictive factor for the progression of HIV infection (Gabrilovich *et al.*, 1994).

Superoxide production by PMNs, both nonstimulated and stimulated with zymosan particles in the presence of normal serum, was similar in normal controls, asymptomatic infections, and patients with AIDS. The serum from 65% of asymptomatic patients infected with HIV induced an increase in stimulated superoxide production by normal and patients' PMN, while the serum from 50% of AIDS patients induced a diminution. These effects did not appear to be related to complement (C3) and circulating immune complex levels; instead, they suggest that PMN of HIV-seropositive patients do not have an intrinsic dysfunction but that serum factor(s) may affect the normal oxidative activity of these cells depending on the stage of HIV infection (Pieri and Orsilles, 1994).

3.5. Decreased Bacterial Killing

Roilides and colleagues demonstrated defects in PMN bactericidal activity in HIV-1-infected patients (Roilides *et al.*, 1990) and that a relative deficiency of G-CSF is associated with a reduction in PMN bactericidal effect (Roilides *et al.*, 1991). Antineutrophil antibodies also have been found to cause a decrease in PMN bacterial killing (Klaassen *et al.*, 1992;

Murphy *et al.*, 1988). The induction of antileukocyte Ab occurs in the absence of allostimulation after HIV infection. HIV infection may enhance preexisting class II and antileukocyte responses in allostimulated individuals (Riera *et al.*, 1992).

3.6. Decreased Antibody-Dependent Cellular Cytotoxicity

PMN play an important role in host defense against bacterial and certain fungal infections. PMN are effectors in antibody-dependent cellular cytotoxicity (ADCC) against a variety of tumor and nontumor target cells. Significantly decreased ADCC was observed in patients with both AIDS and ARC. Deficient PMN-mediated ADCC in HIV infection might play a role in the increased predisposition to bacterial and certain opportunistic infections and perhaps in the spread of HIV infection (Kinne and Gupta, 1989).

Other PMN functions such as aggregation, adherence, and degranulation, as measured by β-glucuronidase release, were normal in HIV patients (Ellis *et al.*, 1988).

In conclusion, neutrophil abnormalities vary among patients in different stages of HIV infection. Impaired PMN function may contribute to the onset of certain life-threatening bacterial and fungal infections in HIV-infected patients.

4. MANAGEMENT OF PMN DEFECTS IN HIV-INFECTED PATIENTS

Treatment with antiretroviral dideoxynucleosides (AZT, ddC, and ddI) can enhance certain preexisting defective PMN functions (e.g., bactericidal capacity) in HIV-1-infected patients (Roilides *et al.*, 1990).

G-CSF not only increases the absolute number of neutrophils but also may improve neutrophil function. The importance of this therapeutic agent in combined quantitative and qualitative neutrophil abnormalities, best characterized by HIV infection and AIDS, should be emphasized. Roilides *et al.* (1991) evaluated the *in vitro* effects of rhG-CSF on neutrophil function from normal donors and patients with HIV infection. G-CSF (1000 to 4000 units/ml) caused a dose-dependent increase in bacterial killing and phagocytosis by normal neutrophils. HIV-1-infected neutrophils demonstrated defective bacterial killing compared to controls that could be corrected by G-CSF treatment. A word of caution is in order, however, as a similar cytokine (GM-CSF) increased HIV viral expression in macrophages *in vitro*. There are no documented increases in p24 antigen levels or HIV recovery from cultured lymphocytes with either GM-CSF or G-CSF exposure *in vitro* (Miles *et al.*, 1991).

Patients with defective PMN chemotactic or microbicidal activity who suffered repeated tissue infections often respond to antimicrobial prophylaxis with agents such as trimethoprim–sulfamethoxazole. Perhaps the use of this agent to prevent *P. carinii* infection helps to decrease infections related to PMN malfunction in HIV patients. The other useful agent in chronic granulomatous disease and perhaps Job's syndrome of hyper-IgE and recurrent infections is IFN-γ. To our knowledge this has not been used to combat infections in HIV patients to date.

REFERENCES

Ammann, A. J., 1990, Biologic and immunomodulating factors in the treatment of pediatric acquired immunodeficiency syndrome, *Pediatr. Infect. Dis. J.* **9**:894–904.

Bedinger, P., Moriarty, A., von Borstel, S. C., 2d, Donovan, N. J., Steimer, K. S., and Littman, D. R., 1988, Internalization of the human immunodeficiency virus does not require the cytoplasmic domain of CD4, *Nature* **334:**162–165.

Blanche, S., Rouzioux, C., Moscato, M. G., Veber, F., Mayaux, M.-J., Jacomet, C., Tricoire, J., De Ville, A., Vial, M., Pirtion, G., De Cropy, A., Douard, D., Robin, M., Courpotin, C., Ciraru-Vigneron, N., Le Deist, F., and Griscelli, C., 1989, A prospective study of infants born to women seropositive for human immunodeficiency virus type 1, *N. Engl. J. Med.* **320:**1643–1648.

Boros, P., Gardos, E., Bekesi, G. I., and Unkeless, J. C., 1990, Change in expression of Fc gamma RIII (CD16) on neutrophils from human immunodeficiency virus-infected individuals, *Clin. Immunol. Immunopathol.* **54:** 281–289.

Bozzette, S. A., Sattler, F. R., Chiu, J., Wu, A. W., Gluckstein, D., Kemper, C., Bartok, A., Niosi, J., Abramson, I., Coffman, J., Bughlett, C., Loya, R., Cassons, B., Akil, B., Meng, T.-C., Boylen, C. T., Nielsen, D., Richman, D. D., Talles, J. G., Leedom, J., McCutchan, A., and The California Collaborative Treatment Group, 1990, A controlled trial of early adjunctive treatment with corticosteroids for Pneumocystis carinii pneumonia in the acquired immunodeficiency syndrome, *N. Engl. J. Med.* **323:**1451–1457.

Busch, M., Beckstead, J., Gantz, D., and Vyas, G., 1986, Detection of human immunodeficiency virus infection of myeloid precursors in bone marrow samples from AIDS patients, *Blood* **68(Suppl.):**122A.

Calvelli, T. A., and Rubinstein, A., 1986, Intravenous gammaglobulin in infant acquired immunodeficiency syndrome, *Pediatr. Infect. Dis.* **5(Suppl. 3):**S207–S210.

Centers for Disease Control, 1989, *HIV/AIDS* Surveillance Report, August, pp. 8–9.

Charytan, M., Krieger, B. Z., Wiznik, A., Bernstein, L., Silverman, B., and Rubenstein, A., 1985, Treatment of AIDS associated lymphoid interstitial pneumonitis with intravenous gammaglobulin and prednisone, *Pediatr. Res.* **19(4 part 2):**401A.

Ciaffoni, S., Roata, C., Turrini, A., Gandini, A., Crocco, I., Mazzi, R., Malena, M., Luzzati, R., and Aprili, G., 1991, Chemotaxis deficiency in patients with HIV infection, *Boll. Ist. Sieroter. Milan.* **70:**433–437.

Cooley, T. P., Kunches, L. M., Saunders, C. A., Ritter, J. K., Perkins, C. J., McLaren, C., McCaffrey, R. P., and Liebman, H. A., 1990, Once-daily administration of 2′,3′-dideoxyinosine (ddI) in patients with the acquired immunodeficiency syndrome or AIDS-related complex: Results of a Phase I trial, *N. Engl. J. Med.* **332:**1340–1345.

Cowan, M. J., Hellmann, D., Chudwin, D., Wara, D. W., Chang, R. S., and Ammann, A. J., 1984, Maternal transmission of acquired immune deficiency syndrome, *Pediatrics* **73:**382–386.

Delacretaz, F., Perey, L., Schmidt, P. M., Chave, J. P., and Costa, J., 1987, Histopathology of bone marrow in human immunodeficiency virus infection, *Virchows Arch. A* **411:**543–551.

Donahue, R. E., Johnson, M. M., Zon, L. J., Clark, S. C., and Groopman, J. E., 1987, Suppression of in vitro haematopoiesis following human immunodeficiency virus infection, *Nature* **326:**200–203.

Elbim, C., Prevot, M. H., Bouscarat, F., Franzini, E., Chôllet-Martin, S. Hakim, J., and Gougerot-Pocidalo, M. A., 1994, Polymorphonuclear neutrophils from human immunodeficiency virus-infected patients show enhanced activation, diminished fMLP-induced L-selectin shedding, and an impaired oxidative burst after cytokine priming, *Blood* **84:**2759–2766.

Ellis, M., Gupta, S., Galant, S., Hakim, S., VandeVen, C., Toy, C., and Cairo, M. S., 1988, Impaired neutrophil function in patients with AIDS or AIDS-related complex: A comprehensive evaluation, *J. Infect. Dis.* **158:** 1268–1276.

European Collaborative Study, 1988, Mother-to-child transmission of HIV infection, *Lancet* **2:**1039–1043.

Fischl, M. A., Richman, D. D., Grieco, M. H., Gottlieb, M. S., Volberding, P. A., Laskin, O. R., Loodom, J. M., Groopman, J. R., Mildvan, D., Schooley, R. T., Jackson, G. G., Durack, D. T., King, D., and Group T. A. C. W., 1987, The efficacy of azidothymidine (AZT) in the treatment of patients with AIDS and AIDS-related complex: A double-blind, placebo-controlled trial, *N. Engl. J. Med.* **317:**185–191.

Fischl, M. A., Dickinson, G. M., and La Voie, L., 1988, Safety and efficacy of sulfamethoxazole and trimethoprim chemoprophylaxis for Pneumocystis carinii pneumonia in AIDS, *J. Am. Med. Assoc.* **259:**1185–1189.

Folks, T. M., Kessler, S. W., Orenstein, J. M., Justement, J. S., Jaffe, E. S., and Fauci, A. S., 1988, Infection and replication of HIV-1 in purified progenitor cells of normal human bone marrow, *Science* **242:**919–922.

Gabrilovich, D. I., Vassilev, V., Nosikov, V. V., Serebrovskaya, L. V., Ivanova, L. A., and Pokrovsky, V. V., 1993, Clinical significance of HIV DNA in polymorphonuclear neutrophils from patients with HIV infection, *J. Acq. Immune Defic. Syndr.* **6:**587–591.

Gabrilovich, D. I., Ivanova, L., Serebrovskaya, L., Shepeleva, G., and Pokrovsky, V. V., 1994, Clinical significance of neutrophil functional activity in HIV infection, *Scand. J. Infect. Dis.* **26:**41–47.

Gagnon, S., Boota, A. M., Fischl, M. A., Baier, H., Kirksey, O. W., and La Voie, L., 1990, Corticosteroids as adjunctive therapy for severe Pneumocystis carinii pneumonia in the acquired immunodeficiency syndrome: A double-blind, placebo-controlled trial, *N. Engl. J. Med.* **323:**1444–1450.

Gallin, J. I., 1993, Inflammation, in: *Fundamental Immunology*, 3rd ed. (W. E. Paul, ed.), Raven Press, New York, pp. 1015–1032.

Gottlieb, M. S., Schroff, R., Schanker, H. M., Weisman, J. D., Fan, P. T., Wolf, R. A., and Saxon, A., 1981, Pneumocystis carinii pneumonia and mucosal candidiasis in previously healthy homosexual men: Evidence of a new acquired cellular immunodeficiency, *N. Engl. J. Med.* **305:**1425–1431.

Ho, D. D., Pomerantz, R. J., and Kaplan, J. C., 1987, Pathogenesis of infection with human immunodeficiency virus, *N. Engl. J. Med.* **317:**278–286.

Ho, J. L., He, S., Hu, A., Geng, J., Basile, F. G., Almeida, M. G., Saito, A. Y., Laurence, J., and Johnson, W. D., Jr., 1995, Neutrophils from human immunodeficiency virus (HIV)-seronegative donors induce HIV replication from HIV-infected patients' mononuclear cells and cell lines: An in vitro model of HIV transmission facilitated by Chlamydia trachomatis, *J. Exp. Med.* **181:**1493–1505.

Hoxie, J. A., Rackowski, J. L., Haggarty, B. S., and Gaulton, G. N., 1988, T4 endocytosis and phosphorylation induced by phorbol esters but not by mitogen or HIV infection, *J. Immunol.* **140:**786–795.

Jones, D., Adinolfi, A., and Galli, H., eds., 1989, *Care of the Patient with HIV Infection*, Health Sciences Consortium, Chapel Hill.

Katz, S. L., and Wilfert, C. M., 1989, Human immunodeficiency virus infection of newborns, *N. Engl. J. Med.* **320:**1687–1688.

Kinne, T. J., and Gupta, S., 1989, Antibody-dependent cellular cytotoxicity by polymorphonuclear leukocytes in patients with AIDS and AIDS-related complex, *J. Clin. Lab. Immunol.* **30:**153–156.

Klaassen, R. J. L., Goldschmeding, R., Dolman, K. M., Viekke, A. B. J., Weigel, H. M., Eeftinek Schattenkerk, J. K. M., Mulder, J. W., Westedt, M. L., and Von Dem Borne, A. E. G. K. R., 1992, Anti-neutrophil cytoplasmic autoantibodies in patients with symptomatic HIV infection, *Clin. Exp. Immunol.* **87:**24–30.

Klebanoff, S. J., and Coombs, R. W., 1992, Viricidal effect of polymorphonuclear leukocytes on human immunodeficiency virus-1: Role of the myeloperoxidase system, *J. Clin. Invest.* **89:**2014–2017.

Landor, M., 1993, Drug therapy for human immunodeficiency virus infection, *Ann. Allergy* **71:**341–351.

Laure, F., Courgnaud, V., Rouzioux, C., Blanche, S., Veber, F., Burgard, M., Jacomet, C., Griscelli, C., and Brechot, C., 1988, Detection of HIV 1 DNA in infants and children by means of the polymerase chain reaction, *Lancet* **2:**538–541.

Leiderman, I. Z., Greenberg, M. L., Adelsberg, B. R., and Siegal, F. P., 1987, A glycoprotein inhibitor or in vitro granulopoiesis associated with AIDS, *Blood* **70:**1267–1272.

Leoung, G. S., Feigal, D. W., Jr., Montgomery, A. B., Corkery, K., Wardlaw, L., Adams, M., Busch, D., Gordon, S., Jacobson, M. A., Volberding, P. A., Abrams, D., and The San Francisco County Community Consortium, 1990, Aerosolized pentamidine for prophylaxis against Pneumocystis carinii pneumonia: The San Francisco Community prophylaxis trial, *N. Engl. J. Med.* **323:**769–775.

Letvin, N. L., Chen, Z. W., Yamamoto, H., and Watanabe, M., 1992, Active immune therapy for the treatment of HIV infections, *AIDS Res. Hum. Retrovir.* **8:**1499.

Lowe, J. B., Stoolman, L. M., Nair, R. P., Larsen, R. D., Berhend, T. L., and Marks, R. M., 1990, Elam-1-dependent cell adhesion to vascular endothelium determined by a transfected human fucosyltransferase cDNA, *Cell* **63:**475–484.

Maddon, P. J., Dalgleish, A. G., McDougal, J. S., Clapham, P. R., Weiss, R. A., and Axell, R., 1986, The T4 gene encodes the AIDS virus receptor and is expressed in the immune system and the brain, *Cell* **47:**333–348.

Maddon, P. J., McDougal, J. S., Clapham, P. R., Dalgleish, A. G., Jamal, S., Weiss, R. A., and Axel, R., 1988, HIV infection does not require endocytosis of its receptor, CD4, *Cell* **54:**865–874.

Masur, H., Michelis, M. A., Green, J. B., Greene, J. B., Onorato, I., Stouwe, R. A., Holzman, R. S., Wormser, G., Brettman, L., Lange, M., Murray, H. W., and Cunningham-Rundles, S., 1981, An outbreak of community-acquired Pneumocystis carinii pneumonia: Initial manifestation of cellular immune dysfunction, *N. Engl. J. Med.* **305:**1431–1438.

MaWhinney, S., Pagano, M., and Thomas, P., 1993, Age at AIDS diagnosis for children with perinatally acquired HIV, *J. Acq. Immune Defic. Syndr.* **6:**1139–1144.

Miles, S. A., Golde, D. W., and Mitsuyasu, R. T., 1991, The use of hematopoietic hormones in HIV infection and AIDS-related malignancies, *Hematol. Oncol. Clin. North Am.* **5:**267–280.

Minchinton, R. M., and Frazer, I., 1985, Idiopathic neutropenia in homosexual men [letter], *Lancet* **1:** 936–937.

Murphy, M. F., Metcalfe, P., Waters, A. H., Lynch, D. C., Cheingsong-Popov, R., Carne, C., and Weller, I. V. D., 1985, Immune neutropenia in homosexual men [letter], *Lancet* **1**:217–218.

Murphy, P. M., Lane, H. C., Fauci, A. S., and Gallin, J. I., 1988, Impairment of neutrophil bactericidal capacity in patients with AIDS, *J. Infect. Dis.* **158**:627–630.

Pieri, E., and Orsilles, M. A., 1994, Effect of serum from HIV-infected subjects on superoxide production by polymorphonuclear neutrophils, *APMIS* **102**:427–431.

Pizzo, P. A., Eddy, J., Falloon, J., Balis, F. M., Murphy, R. P., Moss, H., Wolters, P., Brouwers, P., Jarosinski, P., Rubin, M., Broder, S., Yarchoan, R., Brunetti, A., Maha, M., Nusinoff-Lehrman, S., and Poplack, D. G., 1988, Effect of continuous intravenous infusion of zidovudine (AZT) in children with symptomatic HIV infection, *N. Engl. J. Med.* **319**:889–896.

Ras, G. J., and Anderson, R., 1986, An in vitro study of oral therapeutic doses of co-trimoxazole and erythromycin sterate in abnormal polymorphonuclear leukocyte migration, *J. Antimicrob. Chemother.* **17**:185–193.

Riera, N. E., Galassi, N., de la Barrera, S., Rickard, E., Muchinik, G., Perez-Bianco, R., and de Bracco, M. M., 1992, Anti-leukocyte antibodies as a consequence of HIV infection in HIV+ individuals, *Immunol. Lett.* **33**: 99–104.

Rogers, M. F., Ou, C. Y., Rayfield, M., Thomas, P. A., Schoenbaum, E. E., Abrams, R., Krasinski, K., Selwyn, P. A., Moore, J., Kaul, A., Grimm, K. T., Bamji, M., Schochetman, G., and The New York City Collaborative Study of Maternal HIV Transmission and Montefiore Medical Center HIV Perinatal Transmission Study Group, 1989, Use of the polymerase chain reaction for early detection of the proviral sequences of human immunodeficiency virus in infants born to seropositive mothers, *N. Engl. J. Med.* **320**:1649–1654.

Roilides, E., Venzon, D., Pizzo, P. A., and Rubin, M., 1990, Effects of antiretroviral dideoxynucleosides on polymorphonuclear leukocyte function, *Antimicrob. Agents Chemother.* **34**:1672–1677.

Roilides, E., Walsh, T. J., Pizzo, P. A., and Rubin, M., 1991, Granulocyte colony-stimulating factor enhances the phagocytic and bactericidal activity of normal and defective human neutrophils, *J. Infect. Dis.* **163**:579–583.

Rosenberg, Z. F., and Fauci, A. S., 1989, The immunopathogenesis of HIV infection, *Adv. Immunol.* **47**:377–431.

Schiff, R. I., and Harville, T. O., 1996, Primary and secondary immunodeficiency diseases, in: *Allergy, Asthma, and Immunology from Infancy to Adulthood*, 3rd ed. (C. W. Bierman, D. S. Pearlman, G. G. Shapiro, and W. W. Busse, eds.), Saunders, Philadelphia, pp. 20–54.

Schneider, D. R., and Picker, L. J., 1985, Myelodysplasia in the acquired immune deficiency syndrome, *Am. J. Clin. Pathol.* **84**:144–152.

Siegal, F. P., Lopez, C., Hammer, G. S., Brown, A. E., Kornfeld, S. J., Gold, J., Hassett, J., Hirschman, S. Z., Cunningham-Rundles, C., Adelsberg, B. R., Parham, D. M., Siegal, M., Cunningham-Rundles, S., and Armstrong, D., 1981, Severe acquired immunodeficiency in male homosexuals manifested by chronic perinatal ulceration herpes simplex lesions, *N. Engl. J. Med.* **305**:1439–1444.

Sonnerborg, A., and Jarstrand, C., 1986, Nitroblue tetrazolium (NBT) reduction by neutrophilic granulocytes in patients with HTLV-III infection, *Scand. J. Infect. Dis.* **18**:101–103.

Spivak, J. L., Bender, B. S., and Quinn, T. C., 1984, Hermatologic abnormalities in the acquired immune deficiency syndrome, *Am. J. Med.* **77**:224–228.

Walker, M. C., and Fast, P. E., 1994, Clinical trials of candidate AIDS vaccines, *AIDS* **8(Suppl. 1)**:S213–S236.

CHAPTER 20

MUCOSAL IMMUNITY IN HIV INFECTION

HERMAN F. STAATS and JERRY R. McGHEE

1. INTRODUCTION

The mucosal immune system consists of T and B lymphocytes and accessory cells that function to protect the human body from pathogens and toxins that enter the host via the mucosal surfaces. One major pathogen is human immunodeficiency virus (HIV), the causative agent of the acquired immunodeficiency syndrome (AIDS). By the year 2000, an estimated 35–40 million people will be infected with HIV worldwide (Chin, 1991). The most common mode of transmission of HIV is via sexual contact where HIV-infected cells or possibly cell-free HIV initiate infection at the mucosal surfaces of the vagina or the rectum (Milman and Sharma, 1994). Based on studies performed in the simian immunodeficiency virus (SIV) model, it appears that HIV infection of newborns may be initiated at the mucosal surfaces of the alimentary canal after swallowing HIV during birth (Baba *et al.*, 1994, 1995). *In vitro* studies suggest that cells residing in mucosal tissues may be the first cells to become infected with HIV after exposure at the mucosal surface (Batman *et al.*, 1994). The mucosal immune system is therefore in a pivotal position to play a key role in resistance to as well as contribute to the morbidity associated with HIV infection. This chapter will introduce basic concepts of T-helper cell regulation of the mucosal antibody response, followed by a discussion of the effects of HIV infection on the mucosal immune system and conclude with current strategies being employed to prevent HIV infection at mucosal surfaces.

2. OVERVIEW OF THE MUCOSAL IMMUNE SYSTEM

To appreciate the impact that HIV infection has on mucosal immunity and the impact that mucosal immunity may have on HIV infection, it is necessary to understand certain

HERMAN F. STAATS • Department of Medicine and Center for AIDS Research, Duke University Medical Center, Durham, North Carolina 27710. JERRY R. McGHEE • Immunobiology Vaccine Center, Department of Microbiology, University of Alabama at Birmingham, Birmingham, Alabama 35294.

Immunology of HIV Infection, edited by Sudhir Gupta. Plenum Press, New York, 1996.

unique structural and functional features of the mucosal immune system. This system consists of both distinct and organized lymphoid compartments, such as the Peyer's patches (PP) of the gastrointestinal (GI) tract which comprise the gut-associated lymphoreticular tissue (GALT) and the tonsils and adenoids in the nasopharyngeal region of the upper respiratory tract (URT), which together with bronchus-associated tissues (BALT) in experimental animals are sometimes collectively termed *mucosa-associated lymphoreticular tissue* (MALT). The mucosal immune system also contains a diffuse network of lymphoid cells in the lamina propria regions of the GI, upper respiratory and the genitourinary tracts as well as in exocrine glands. Thus, tissues of the mucosal immune system can be usefully divided into two functionally distinct regions, the inductive sites (MALT) of organized lymphoid tissue and the more diffuse effector tissues (Fig. 1) (McGhee *et al.*, 1992; Mestecky and McGhee, 1987). The PP represent the inductive sites for the GI tract and the tonsils appear to be the inductive site for the URT (Bernstein, 1992; Kuper *et al.*, 1992; McGhee *et al.*, 1992; Mestecky and McGhee, 1987). It is in the inductive site that antigens from the environment are first encountered by lymphoid cells of the mucosal immune system and where initial antigen-specific B- and T-cell activation occurs. Antigen-specific B and T lymphocytes then leave the inductive sites via lymphatic drainage, circulate via the blood, and home to effector sites where actual antigen-specific responses occur [i.e., T-cell help for antibody production as well as cytotoxic T-lymphocyte (CTL) killing of virus-infected cells]. After mucosal immunization, antigen-specific lymphocytes may home to the original site of contact with antigen as well as to distant mucosal effector tissues. This observation has led to the term *common mucosal immune system* (reviewed in Mestecky *et al.*, 1994; McGhee *et al.*, 1992; Mestecky and McGhee, 1987).

2.1. Inductive Sites: Organized Mucosa-Associated Lymphoreticular Tissues

The inductive site of the mucosal immune system that typically receives the most attention is the PP of the small intestine and this chapter will be no exception. The PP consists of both T- and B-cell-enriched areas [the latter of which contains a high percentage of surface IgA-positive ($sIgA^+$) B cells] as well as antigen-presenting cells (APCs) necessary for the induction of specific immune responses (Fig. 1). Covering the PP is a specialized epithelium, namely, the follicle-associated epithelium (FAE) (Kato and Owen, 1994). The FAE contains a variety of cells including specially differentiated epithelial cells known as *microfold* or in abbreviated form simply as *M cells*, as well as columnar epithelial cells and lymphoid cells, the latter of which has led some to use the term *lymphoepithelium*. The dome M cell plays a crucial role in the initial phase of induction of mucosal immune responses by sampling antigens from the lumen of the gut and transporting the antigen intact to the underlying APCs for initiation of the immune response. In addition to its role of transporting antigen to the inductive environment of the PP, the M cell is also a portal of entry for many infectious agents including *Salmonella typhi*, *Yersinia enterocolitica*, *Vibrio cholerae*, *Shigella*, reovirus types 1 and 3, poliovirus, and HIV (reviewed in Kato and Owen, 1994). M cells have been identified in the FAE of the PP as well as in the nasal- and bronchus-associated lymphoreticular tissues (NALT and BALT) in rats (Morin *et al.*, 1994; Kuper *et al.*, 1992) and appear to be a feature of mucosal inductive sites.

2.1.1. Peyer's Patch T Cells

The T cells present in the parafollicular region of the PP are mature and $> 97\%$ express the $\alpha\beta$ T-cell receptor (TCR) (McGhee *et al.*, 1992; Mestecky and McGhee, 1987),

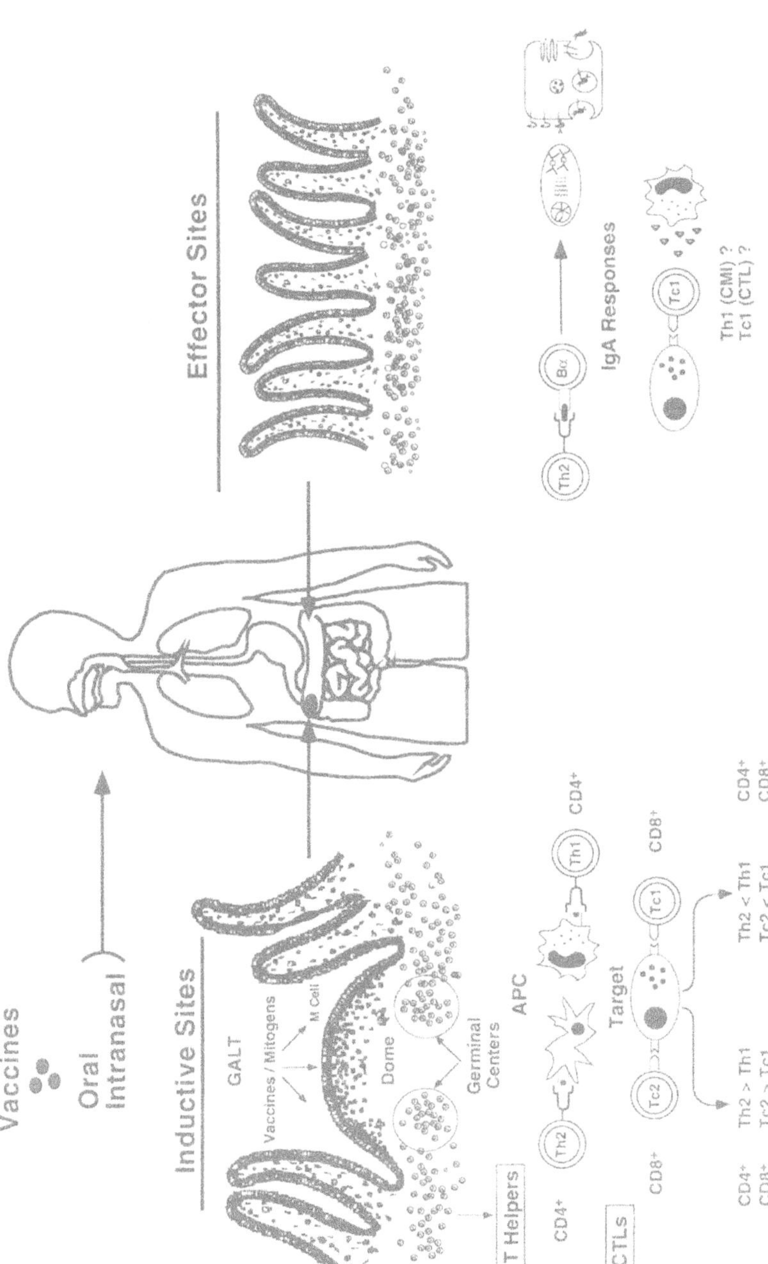

FIGURE 1. Current ideas regarding mucosal immunoregulation, mucosal inductive sites, and the concept of CD4$^+$ Th1- and Th2-type immune responses. Most mucosal vaccines are given either intranasally or orally, and following uptake in the inductive tissues, i.e., Peyer's patches (as shown), the adjuvant or carrier system can influence the nature of CD4$^+$ Th-cell responses, which in turn regulate CD4$^+$ T-cell-mediated immunity as well as the isotype/subclass of mucosal versus serum antibody responses. It is thought that initial induction is followed by homing effector sites (intestinal lamina propria as shown) of CD4$^+$ Th-cell subsets, CD8$^+$ precursor CTLs, and sIgA$^+$ B cells for ultimate mucosal and systemic antibody synthesis via the Common Mucosal Immune System.

while a small subset, which remains poorly characterized, expresses a γδ TCR. The $CD3^+CD4^+CD8^-$ helper T (Th) cells make up approximately 50–60% of αβ TCR^+ T cells in the parafollicular regions, while the remaining $CD3^+CD4^-CD8+$ T cells are precursors of CTLs. The first evidence that PP T cells regulate IgA biosynthesis came from the observation that Con A-stimulated murine PP T cells induced IgA production, while splenic T cells, similarly treated, suppressed IgA, IgG, and IgM synthesis, implying that the PP contain T cells that regulate IgA responses (Elson *et al.*, 1979).

2.1.1a. Early Studies. T-cell cloning studies in the early 1980s provided evidence for two distinct types of regulatory T cells. One type of T-cell clone induced surface IgM-positive ($sIgM^+$) B cells to switch to $sIgA^+$ (Kawanishi *et al.*, 1983a,b), whereas a second group of antigen-specific [sheep erythrocytes (SRBC)] Th cells preferentially supported IgA responses (Kiyono *et al.*, 1982, 1984). The PP switch T-cell (Tsw) clones, when added to $sIgM^+sIgA-$ B-cell cultures, induced increases in $sIgA^+$ cells but did not induce IgA secretion (Kawanishi *et al.*, 1983a,b). It was subsequently shown that Tsw cells were autoreactive and presumably arose in the unique PP microenvironment (Kawanishi *et al.*, 1985). On the other hand, clones of Th cells from SRBC-fed mice supported IgA anti-SRBC responses in $sIgA^+$ (but not $sIgA^-$) B-cell cultures (Kiyono *et al.*, 1984). These PP Th-cell clones expressed Fc receptors for IgA (FcαR) (Kiyono *et al.*, 1985). Other studies have further shown that the FcαR is usually associated with Th2- but not Th1-type cells (Fig. 1) (Sandor *et al.*, 1990). Evidence for Tsw cells in human mucosal immunity has also been presented. For example, a patient with mycosis fungoides/Sezary-like syndrome provided transformed T cells which were used to show that $sIgM^+$ B cells, when incubated with this malignant T-cell line, underwent switches to IgG and IgA (Mayer *et al.*, 1985, 1986). T-cell clones from human appendix provided preferential help for B-cell-derived IgA (Benson and Strober, 1988).

2.1.1b. The Modern Era. Clonal populations of Th cells can now be subdivided into at least two subsets, Th1 and Th2, based on unique profiles of cytokines produced and major functions in host immune responses (Mosmann *et al.*, 1986). The cytokine milieu present during T-cell activation and subsequent differentiation into clonal populations is important in determining the ultimate T-cell subset phenotype. For example, the presence of IL-12 and IL-4 may direct $CD4^+$ Th-cell development down a Th1 or Th2 pathway, respectively, while later in development interferon-γ (IFN-γ) and IL-10 can reinforce Th1 or Th2 phenotype expansion (Seder and Paul, 1994). It is well established that Th1 cells secrete IL-2, IFN-γ, and tumor necrosis factor-β (TNF-β) and function in T-cell-mediated immunity (CMI) for protection against intracellular bacteria and possible viruses. Th1 cells also provide limited help for B-cell responses and the IFN-γ produced supports IgG2a synthesis in mice (Mosmann and Coffman, 1989). The Th2 cells preferentially secrete IL-4, IL-5, IL-6, IL-10 (Fiorentino *et al.*, 1989) and IL-13 and provide effective help for B-cell responses, in particular for IgG1, IgE, and IgA synthesis (Street and Mosmann, 1991).

Studies from our group (Beagley *et al.*, 1988, 1989, 1991; Fujihashi *et al.*, 1991) and by others (Harriman *et al.*, 1988; Lebman and Coffman, 1988; Bond *et al.*, 1987; Coffman *et al.*, 1987; Murray *et al.*, 1987) have shown that two Th2 cytokines, e.g., IL-5 and IL-6, are of particular importance for inducing $sIgA^+$ B cells to differentiate into IgA-producing plasma cells. In this regard, IL-6 induced strikingly high IgA responses *in vitro* in both mouse (Beagley *et al.*, 1988, 1989, 1991) and human (Fujihashi *et al.*, 1991) systems, and mice with targeted disruption of the IL-6 gene showed greatly reduced numbers of IgA plasma cells (Ramsay *et al.*, 1994). Interestingly, vaccinia virus vector expressing hemagglutinin (HA) of influenza and rIL-6 could restore mucosal IgA anti-HA responses in IL-$6^{-/-}$ mice (Ramsay *et al.*, 1994). One would predict from these observations that higher frequencies of Th2 cells may occur in mucosal effector sites (e.g., the intestinal lamina propria and the salivary glands) and indeed this has been shown by studies from our group (Mega *et al.*, 1992; Taguchi *et al.*, 1990).

In order to more precisely understand the role of mucosal adjuvants and vectors for induction of secretory IgA (S-IgA) and serum antibody responses, we have assessed antigen-specific $CD4^+$ Th1- and Th2-type cells and cytokines for regulation of CMI and humoral [serum isotypes, IgG subclasses, and mucosal (S-IgA) antibody] responses. In general, we have used two classes of mucosal vaccine delivery systems, i.e., in the first oral administration of protein vaccine is done with cholera toxin (CT) as adjuvant, which induce mucosal S-IgA as well as serum antivaccine and anti-CT-B antibody responses. Recombinant *Salmonella* vectors are also excellent oral vaccine carriers and induce brisk mucosal S-IgA as well as serum antibody responses, and for comparison with vaccine given with oral adjuvants, we have used r*S. typhimurium* BRD 847 (*aro* A^-,*aro* D^-) expressing the C fragment of tetanus toxin (r*Salmonella*–Tox C). We initially found that mice given oral CT as adjuvant developed vaccine protein and CT-B-specific $CD4^+$ Th cells producing the cytokines IL-4 and IL-5, clearly associating mucosal S-IgA responses with a helper Th2 phenotype (Xu-Amano *et al.*, 1993, 1994). More careful analysis of serum antibody isotypes showed that CT indeed induced selective Th2-type responses associated with marked increases in total (up to 100-fold) and antigen-specific IgE and IgG1 and IgG2b antibody responses (Marinaro *et al.*, 1995).

We have also characterized $CD4^+$ Th-cell subsets and antibody isotype responses in mice orally immunized with r*Salmonella*–Tox C (expressing fragment C) under regulation of a *Nir B* promoter, a system previously shown to induce protective serum anti-TT antibodies (Chatfield *et al.*, 1992). Oral r*Salmonella*–Tox C elicited strong systemic IgG2a and IgG2b anti-TT antibody responses along with mucosal S-IgA (VanCott *et al.*, 1995, 1996a). Further, splenic and PP $CD4^+$ T cells restimulated *in vitro* with TT-coated latex beads selectively produced Th1-type cytokines and IFN-γ and IL-2 as well as the Th2 cytokine IL-10. IL-6 was elevated in MØ but not in T cells of mice orally immunized with r*Salmonella*–Tox C (VanCott *et al.*, 1996a).

We have now extended our studies with the model oral antigens r*Salmonella*–Tox C and TT plus CT as adjuvant to IFN-γ and IL-4 knockout (IFN-$\gamma^{-/-}$ and IL-$4^{-/-}$) mice, which exhibit defective Th1- and Th2-cell pathways, respectively (Dalton *et al.*, 1993; Kopf *et al.*, 1993; Kühn *et al.*, 1991). Oral immunization of IFN-$\gamma^{-/-}$ mice with TT plus CT as adjuvant resulted in mucosal S-IgA and serum IgG1, IgG2b, and IgE antibodies which were comparable to normal IFN-$\gamma^{+/+}$ mice (VanCott *et al.*, 1996b). Analysis of PP and splenic $CD4^+$ Th cells showed that antigen-specific T cells were of Th2 type. Of interest was our finding that oral immunization of IFN-$\gamma^{-/-}$ mice with r*Salmonella*–Tox C also resulted in good mucosal S-IgA and serum IgG1 and IgG2b anti-TT antibody responses (VanCott *et al.*, 1996b). Cytokine profiles of TT-specific $CD4^+$ Th cells showed a characteristic Th2-type (VanCott *et al.*, 1996b). These results suggest that oral immunization of IFN-$\gamma^{-/-}$ mice with either Th2- or Th1-inducing regimen results in significant mucosal S-IgA responses, and indicate that this isotype develops in the absence of IFN-γ.

Recent studies have shown that CT fails to induce adjuvant responses in IL-$4^{-/-}$ mice, suggesting that this Th2 cytokine is of central importance in mucosal adjuvanticity (Marinaro *et al.*, 1995; Vajdy *et al.*, 1995; Okahashi *et al.*, 1996). Thus, it was of interest to compare antibody responses in IL-$4^{-/-}$ mice given r*Salmonella*–Tox C versus TT plus CT as adjuvant. In this study, we found that oral r*Salmonella*–Tox C induced brisk TT-specific mucosal S-IgA as well as serum IgG2a responses (Okahashi *et al.*, 1996). Interestingly, oral TT with CT also resulted in serum IgG2a anti-TT antibodies; however, mucosal S-IgA was restricted to CT-B responses in this system (Okahashi *et al.*, 1996). Analysis of TT-specific $CD4^+$ Th cells showed that r*Salmonella*–Tox C rapidly induced Th1 as well as Th2 cells selectively producing IL-6 and IL-10. A similar Th-cell profile was noted when CT-B-specific $CD4^+$ T cells were assessed. These results show that IL-4 (and IL-5) are not essential for induction of mucosal S-IgA responses, but do point to the likely possibility that IL-6 and IL-10 are required (Okahashi *et al.*, 1996).

2.1.2. Peyer's Patch B Cells

Distinct B-cell follicles occur beneath the PP dome region and these exhibit active germinal centers where presumed $sIgM^+$ B cells undergo isotype switching to $sIgA^+$ B cells. Up to 60–70% of the $sIgA^+$ B cells in PP are associated with the germinal centers (Butcher *et al.*, 1982; Jones and Cebra, 1974). Current dogma suggests that isotype switching is mediated by increased accessibility of specific switch regions to recombinase (Lutzker and Alt, 1988; Stavnezer-Nordgren and Sirlin, 1986; Yancopoulos *et al.*, 1986) and the switch itself is preceded by transcription of this region, e.g., the formation of sterile transcripts (Lutzker *et al.*, 1988; Stavnezer *et al.*, 1988).

Two major cytokines, i.e., IL-4 and TGF-β, have clearly been shown to induce $sIgM^+$ B cells to switch to downstream isotypes. TGF-β is a 25-kDa protein which has ambivalent properties, i.e., stimulation of cell growth and differentiation as well as suppression of lymphocyte proliferation (Sporn *et al.*, 1986). Despite these suppressive properties, studies have shown that addition of TGF-β to LPS-triggered mouse B-cell cultures led to increased IgA synthesis (Lebman *et al.*, 1990a; Coffman *et al.*, 1989; Sonada *et al.*, 1986), an effect that could be enhanced by IL-2 (Lebman *et al.*, 1990a) or IL-5 (Sonada *et al.*, 1989). Molecular analysis showed that TGF-β induced $sIgM^+ \rightarrow sIgA^+$ B-cell switches, and the actual switch was preceded by production of sterile α transcripts (Lebman *et al.*, 1990b). Additional studies showed that TGF-β also induced $\mu \rightarrow \alpha$ switches in human B-cell cultures triggered with *Branhamella catarrhalis* (Islam *et al.*, 1991). Further, TGF-β induced B-cell switches to both α1 and α2, which were preceded by Ia region sterile transcripts (Nilsson *et al.*, 1991). In addition, anti-CD40 stimulation of tonsillar B cells together with TGF-β in the presence of IL-10 induced significant IgA synthesis (DeFrance *et al.*, 1992). It was also shown that Cα1 transcripts were induced by B-cell mitogen plus TGF-β, while Cα2 transcripts were induced by TGF-β together with IL-10, perhaps implying that switches to IgA2 are more T cell and cytokine dependent (Kitani and Strober, 1994). Elegant studies have provided direct evidence that somatic mutations occur during germinal center (GC) responses, a time when the antigen-specific B cells form high-affinity Ig receptors (Liu *et al.*, 1992). Presumably, isotype switches to IgA take place in PP GC; however, direct demonstration of this is also lacking.

2.1.3. Peyer's Patch Antigen-Presenting Cells

All three major types of APCs also occur in significant numbers in the various PP regions (Fig. 1). Macrophages, including both classical and tingible body types associated with uptake of apoptotic cells, are found in the dome region and GC, respectively. The T-cell zones are enriched in dendritic cells (DC), which have been shown in functional assays to form clusters with $CD4^+$ T cells that are adept in supporting IgA synthesis (Spalding *et al.*, 1983, 1984). No studies have addressed the role of APCs in the three major PP regions, i.e., the dome, T or B zones after M cell uptake, and especially whether the B cells (some of which express MHC class II) can function in this capacity.

The role of persistent antigen could be important for the generation of $sIgA^+$ B and $CD4^+$ Th-cell responses in PP. In this regard, it is well established that follicular dendritic cells (FDC) in B-cell areas can retain native antigen, usually via antigen–antibody complexes (Szakal *et al.*, 1989; Tew *et al.*, 1980). The slow release of these complexes may be important for stimulation and expansion of antigen-specific B-cell clones (Tew *et al.*, 1990; Szakal *et al.*, 1989). The PP contains FDC, and these cells may serve a similar role in this IgA inductive site; however, more studies will be required to determine the possible role for persistent antigen and IgA immune complexes in these mucosal inductive sites. Antigen trapped by FDC (as immune complexes) is released in the form of *i*mmune *c*omplex-*c*oated bodies (iccosomes). Specific GC B cells find iccosomes remarkably palatable and endocytose them. Iccosomal antigen is then processed with great efficiency and is presented to T cells. It would be tempting to postulate that orally encountered antigens are endocytosed into the PP via M cells in native form. The antigen, or possibly IgA immune complexes, may associate with FDC in the GC and release iccosomes for prolonged periods. This slow release may be sufficient to allow selective induction of antigen-specific $CD4^+$ Th and $sIgA^+$ B cells in the PP. A second encounter with antigen would result in expansion of $CD4^+$ Th cells and increased IgA responses in mucosal effector tissues.

The APCs in mucosal inductive sites may also be involved in dissemination of HIV infection. This point is well illustrated by a recent study that showed large amounts of HIV–immune complexes localized on FDCs (Heath *et al.*, 1995). Further, it would appear that FDCs may convert already neutralized HIV back to an infectious form, since immune HIV-neutralizing antibody complexes in antibody excess together with FDC resulted in infectious virions (Heath *et al.*, 1995).

2.2. Mucosal Effector Tissues

Effector sites for mucosal immune responses include the lymphoid cells in the lamina propria (LP) regions of the GI, the upper respiratory, and reproductive tracts as well as secretory glandular tissue such as mammary, salivary, and lacrymal glands (McGhee *et al.*, 1992). In addition, most evidence suggests that the lymphocytes that reside in the epithelium [i.e., the intraepithelial lymphocytes (IELs)] also serve as effector cells; however, it has been difficult to precisely define IEL functions.

Effector mechanisms employed to protect mucosal surfaces include CTLs, and effector $CD4^+$ Th cells for CMI (Th1) and for S-IgA antibody (Th2) responses (Kilian and Russell, 1994; London, 1994). Indeed, both CTL and S-IgA responses have been associated with protection against infection at mucosal surfaces and both may be important for resistance to or, more importantly, prevention of mucosal infection with infectious agents, including HIV (Staats *et al.*, 1994). Less is known regarding protective $CD4^+$ Th1–CMI responses; however, mucosal CMI would appear to be especially important in prevention of HIV infection.

The LP of the GI tract has been reasonably well studied, and some have estimated that

$> 10^{10}$ IgA plasma cells occur per meter of human small intestine (Brandtzaeg, 1989). Further, the LP contains large numbers of LP B and T lymphocytes (LPLs) and up to 60% of LPLs are T cells (McGhee *et al.*, 1992). In mucosal effector tissues, antigen uptake and presentation also occurs; however, important differences are noted. For example, vaccine antigen may be endocytosed by epithelial cells, and in certain situations the epithelial cells themselves can express class II MHC (Mayer and Shlien, 1987) and process antigen with subsequent association of immunogenic peptides with MHC class II. It is tempting to suggest that this type of presentation leads to suppression or anergy, and this may represent a major function of the epithelial cells in response to food antigens. It is known that some responses occur; however, this may be diminished by the presence of anergic T cells which cannot provide help for what could become an exaggerated mucosal S-IgA response. The induction of anergic T cells could result from an inappropriate delivery of signal 2 (B7-1/B7-2) by epithelial cells, which prevent an appropriate delivery by "normal" mucosal APCs. In other situations, intact proteins can transverse tight junctions, and in this instance intact vaccine antigen could trigger B- and T-cell responses. For example, $sIgA^+$ B cells may bind antigen and through endocytotic pathways process and present peptides, together with MHC class II, to Th cells. Macrophages in LP regions could also serve this function for more complex antigens. The simplest scenario would be that presentation by class II $sIgA^+$ B cells expressing B7-1/B7-2 to Th cells, expressing the coreceptor CD28, allows full activation of Th2 cells with IL-4, IL-5, IL-6, and IL-10 cytokine release. IgA-committed $sIgA^+$ B cells would receive CD40–CD40L second signals from activated Th2 cells and derived cytokines (IL-4, IL-5, IL-6, and IL-10) for subsequent B-cell proliferation and differentiation into IgA-producing plasma cells with specificity for the mucosal antigen.

2.3. Secretory IgA: Structure and Function

S-IgA responses are unique to mucosal surfaces and external secretions and are rarely if ever induced by parenteral immunization, whereas immunization (or infection) by a mucosal route (e.g., intranasal, oral, rectal, vaginal) frequently induces S-IgA responses (Staats *et al.*, 1996; Lehner *et al.*, 1994). In humans, serum IgA is predominantly detected as a monomer whereas S-IgA found in mucosal secretions is di-, tri-, or tetrameric (polymeric) (Underdown and Mestecky, 1994). The S-IgA antibody molecule contains two additional polypeptides, a J chain and secretory component (SC), in addition to immunoglobulin heavy and light chains. The J chain is produced by the IgA-producing plasma cell and is associated with polymeric IgA. Epithelial cells found in mucosal glandular tissues or that line mucosal surfaces of the GI and respiratory tracts produce polymeric immunoglobulin receptors (pIgR) or SC (Brandtzaeg *et al.*, 1994). Polymeric IgA interacts with pIgR (SC) at the basolateral surface of $pIgR^+$ epithelial cells, becomes internalized, is transported through the cell, and after enzymatic cleavage of the pIgR, is released onto the mucosal surface as S-IgA. The extracellular region of pIgR that remains associated the S-IgA is better known as SC. In addition to mediating transport across epithelial cells, the presence of SC may increase the resistance of S-IgA to proteolytic enzymes found in mucosal secretions (Kraehenbuhl and Neutra, 1992; Mestecky and McGhee, 1987; Brown *et al.*, 1970). The estimated daily synthesis of IgA (systemic and secretory) is 66 mg/kg and exceeds the production of all other Ig isotypes (Conley and Delacroix, 1987; Mestecky and McGhee, 1987). The need for a response of such magnitude becomes apparent when one considers that the mucosal surfaces comprise the largest area of the body in contact with potential pathogens and that constant production of mucosal antibody is required to combat the continual loss of S-IgA into mucosal secretions.

It should be indicated that in humans two IgA subclasses occur, i.e., IgA1 and IgA2. Careful immunohistochemical analysis of IgA1- and IgA2-producing cells in different compartments of human mucosal effector tissues has revealed that two distinct patterns of IgA plasma cell subclasses occur in the respiratory and upper digestive tracts when compared with the lower GI tract. Thus, IgA1-producing B-cell blasts and plasma cells are predominant (up to 80–90%) in the nasal and gastric mucosa and the small intestine, including the duodenum and jejunum (Brandtzaeg, 1994; Kett *et al.*, 1986). In contrast, IgA2-secreting cells are present in higher frequency in the ileum of the small intestine and in the large intestinal mucosa, including the colon and rectum (Brandtzaeg, 1994; Kett *et al.*, 1986). It should be noted that bacteria that cause diarrheal diseases, e.g., enterotoxigenic *E. coli* and *V. cholerae*, selectively colonize the ileum of the small intestine. It is likely that both IgA1 and IgA2 antibacterial antibodies would be induced in these situations and both subclasses may provide effective host immunity.

Transport of S-IgA across epithelial surfaces to external secretions where antigen-specific S-IgA interacts with potential pathogens and inhibits their interaction with the host may be the most important protective mechanism provided by S-IgA. This protective mechanism is referred to as *immune exclusion*. Passive transfer studies in mice using antigen-specific monoclonal IgA have provided evidence that antigen-specific IgA alone was able to protect against intranasal infection with influenza (Renegar and Small, 1991), intestinal infection with *V. cholerae* (Lee *et al.*, 1994; Winner *et al.*, 1991), or *Salmonella typhimurium* (Michetti *et al.*, 1992), as well as gastric infection with *Helicobacter felis* (Czinn *et al.*, 1993). In fact, passive transfer of anti-*S. typhimurium* IgA provided protection against oral challenge with virulent organisms but was unable to prevent infection when the organisms were injected intraperitoneally, suggesting that the mechanism for protection at a mucosal surface does not correlate with protection from a systemic challenge (Michetti *et al.*, 1992). Passive transfer of IgA that resulted in high titers of serum IgA (suggestive of high levels of IgA at mucosal surfaces) prevented infection in mice orally challenged with *S. typhimurium* whereas all mice with low serum IgA titers were infected. Antigen-specific S-IgA responses may therefore provide a means to totally prevent infection, or at least greatly reduce the size of the infectious inoculum by pathogens that infect via a mucosal route. Therefore, S-IgA responses may play a crucial role in prevention of mucosal infection with HIV or opportunistic pathogens in persons already infected with HIV.

2.4. The Female and Male Reproductive Tracts Are Part of the Mucosal Immune System

The fact that the most common route of HIV infection is via sexual contact brings to mind the following central question: Are the female and male reproductive tracts part of the mucosal immune system? The answer is clearly yes. Plasma cells producing IgA are located in the endo- and ectocervix, Fallopian tubes, and vagina of women at reproductive ages (Kutteh and Mestecky, 1994). Further, IgA plasma cells in the female reproductive tract are positive for J chain and SC, thereby suggesting that the plasma cells produce polymeric IgA (pIgA) and that the pIgA could be actively transported to the surface of the female reproductive tract via the SC transport pathway. Cervical mucus predominantly contains pIgA while vaginal fluid contains comparable amounts of pIgA and monomeric IgA. The relative contribution of pIgA (or S-IgA) and monomeric IgA to the total vaginal IgA varies with the time of the menstrual cycle (Hocini *et al.*, 1995). Vaginal secretions also contain serum-derived IgG that may play a role in host protection at this site (Hocini *et al.*, 1995). The female reproductive tract may therefore be classified as an effector arm of the mucosal immune system and may play an active role in prevention of sexually transmitted HIV and other sexually transmitted diseases.

Immunohistological studies of the reproductive tract of the female rhesus macaque have provided evidence that the lower female reproductive tract has the cellular components found typically in mucosal inductive sites (Miller *et al.*, 1992b). The epithelium of the vagina and ectocervix contains Langerhans cells while the endocervix contains dendritic cells. In addition to serving as potent APC for the induction of immune responses, Langerhans cells may serve as the initial cell infected with HIV (or SIV in monkeys) after sexual contact with an infected partner (see below). The submucosal layers of the female reproductive tract contain $CD4^+$ and $CD8^+$ T lymphocytes, macrophages, and B cells. Lymphoid nodules containing macrophages, $CD4^+$ and $CD8^+$ T cells, and Langerhans cells are detectable in the macaque vagina and ectocervix suggesting that the female reproductive tract has the cellular components required for the induction of a mucosal immune response. Further studies with human samples are needed to determine if similar features are found in humans.

The male reproductive tract is populated with lymphoid cells and also has characteristics of an effector tissue of the mucosal immune system. Human urethral epithelium contains S-IgA which may play a role in protecting the host from potential pathogens, including HIV (Perra *et al.*, 1994). Studies using a murine model have found that the male urethral epithelium contains Langerhans cells and macrophages while the urethral mucosa contains both $CD4^+$ and $CD8^+$ lymphocytes (Quayle *et al.*, 1994). Plasma cells producing IgA have not been detected in the urethra, suggesting that IgA or S-IgA detected in the male urethra is derived from a source outside of this particular tissue.

3. INFECTION WITH HIV AT MUCOSAL SURFACES

Epidemiological data from HIV-infected persons indicate that up to 75–80% of all cases of HIV infection worldwide are acquired by heterosexual transmission (Mestecky and Jackson, 1994). SIV infection of rhesus macaques has proven to be a reliable model for human HIV infection and disease. Studies performed in this model have provided evidence that infection may occur after exposure to cell-free SIV by the vaginal and urethral routes in female and male rhesus macaques, respectively (Miller *et al.*, 1989, 1994a; Marx *et al.*, 1993). Indeed, the reproductive tract of male rhesus macaques chronically infected with SIV contains cells infected with SIV and may serve as the source of infectious SIV responsible for transmitting SIV during sexual contact (Miller *et al.*, 1994b). In addition to transmission of HIV (SIV) by genital contact, recent studies have indicated that neonatal rhesus macaques may be infected with SIV by the oral route (Baba *et al.*, 1994, 1995). Therefore, studies performed in the rhesus macaque model provide experimental evidence that SIV (HIV) may be transmitted by sexual contact or oral exposure to SIV (HIV).

The first cells to become infected with HIV at mucosal surfaces are likely to be cells residing in mucosal tissues. Although there are reports suggesting that vaginal and colonic epithelial cells may be infected with HIV (Furuta *et al.*, 1994), studies with intestinal explant cultures provide evidence that after exposure to HIV, lymphocytes and macrophages become infected, whereas epithelial cells do not (Batman *et al.*, 1994). The reproductive tract of the female rhesus macaque contains Langerhans and dendritic cells, as well as $CD4^+$ and $CD8^+$ lymphocytes (Miller *et al.*, 1992b). Although no studies have been performed with a primate model, the murine penile foreskin contained few T lymphocytes and macrophages, but numerous Langerhans cells (Quayle *et al.*, 1994). The Langerhans cell is a prime target for HIV infection at mucosal surfaces (Blauvelt and Katz, 1995), and after mucosal Langerhans cells become infected with HIV, they may transmit this infection to T cells in regional lymph nodes. Indeed, recent studies have provided evidence that HIV-infected Langerhans cells are more efficient than T cells in transmitting HIV to activated T cells (Ayehunie *et al.*, 1995). Therefore, the human male and female reproductive tracts may contain cells such as macrophages and Langerhans cells that are susceptible to HIV infection. These target cells are located in anatomical sites that may permit them to become infected with HIV after sexual contact with an infected partner. After the Langerhans cells and/or macrophages become infected with HIV, they may very efficiently disseminate the infection to T cells in regional lymph nodes where HIV infection may then spread throughout the body.

4. EFFECTOR FUNCTIONS FOR IgA ANTI-HIV ANTIBODIES

4.1. IgA Neutralizes HIV Infection *in Vitro*

As previously mentioned, HIV most commonly initiates infection at the mucosal surfaces of the host and several studies have provided evidence that S-IgA is able to prevent viral or bacterial infection at mucosal surfaces. However, a central question remains: Will S-IgA anti-HIV prevent infection at mucosal surfaces? A variety of studies have been performed to determine if IgA anti-HIV isolated from HIV-infected persons has neutralizing capabilities *in vitro*. Sera from HIV-infected individuals known to contain HIV-1 neutralizing activity were screened for the presence of IgA anti-HIV by ELISA (Burnett *et al.*, 1994). The sera containing IgA were then depleted of IgG and assayed for the ability to neutralize HIV *in vitro*. Anti-HIV sera depleted of IgG but containing IgA anti-HIV antibodies were able to neutralize the ability of HIV-1_{MN} to infect CEM cells. Depletion of IgA1 abrogated the neutralizing activity in IgG- depleted, IgA-containing sera, suggesting that IgA anti-HIV was responsible for the neutralizing activity (Burnett *et al.*, 1994). Unfortunately, the neutralizing epitope recognized by IgA anti-HIV antibody was not determined in this study.

The ability of IgG anti-HIV versus IgA anti-HIV antibodies to neutralize HIV *in vitro* has also been compared (Kozlowski *et al.*, 1994). Anti-HIV IgA isolated from the serum of HIV-seropositive persons neutralized HIV-1 infection in a susceptible T-cell line *in vitro*. Although IgA anti-HIV antibodies neutralized HIV-1 *in vitro*, the neutralization activity of IgA was not as potent as that of IgG. The decreased neutralizing activity of IgA was associated with a decreased proportion of HIV- and V3-specific antibodies within purified IgA fractions as compared to the proportion of specific antibodies detected within purified IgG fractions. IgA produced by polyclonally activated B cells may dilute the HIV-specific IgA and therefore decrease the specific neutralizing activity of purified IgA (Kozlowski *et al.*, 1994). S-IgA antibodies induced by vaccination have been shown to have HIV-1 neutralizing activity. For example, oral immunization of mice with a macromolecular, multicomponent peptide vaccine candidate VC1 and cholera toxin (CT) as a mucosal adjuvant induced S-IgA antibody responses capable of neutralizing HIV-1_{IIIB}, HIV-1_{SF2}, and HIV-1_{MN} (Bukawa *et al.*, 1995) (see section below). This vaccine candidate was composed of peptides corresponding to V3 primary neutralizing determinants (PND), a CD4 binding site, and a Gag region. Therefore, IgA anti-HIV antibodies induced by natural infection or by vaccination can neutralize HIV infection *in vitro*.

4.2. IgA also Enhances HIV Infection *in Vitro*

IgA may also enhance HIV infection. Within a group of 20 seropositive persons, IgA purified from the serum of 14 HIV-infected individuals was able to enhance HIV infection of U937 promyelomonocytic cells (Kozlowski *et al.*, 1995). When IgG was assayed for the ability to enhance infection, only 7 of the 20 tested were able to enhance infection. Additionally, when enhancing IgA was mixed with physiologic concentrations of non-enhancing IgG, enhancement of HIV infection was not observed, suggesting that IgG may be able to block the enhancing effect of IgA *in vivo* in locations where IgG is abundant (Kozlowski *et al.*, 1995). However, at mucosal sites where IgA is more prominent, enhancing IgA may play a role in the initiation and/or dissemination of HIV infection. Purified IgA isolated from the serum of HIV-1-infected persons, but not uninfected controls, modestly enhanced HIV-1_{BAL} infection of primary human blood monocytes and intestinal LP mononuclear cells (Janoff *et al.*, 1995). Preincubation of monocytes with nonimmune IgA but not IgG blocked the IgA-mediated enhancement of HIV infection, suggesting that an IgA receptor could account for this enhancement. Further studies are warranted to identify the epitope recognized by enhancing IgA antibodies and to determine if vaccine-induced S-IgA anti-HIV antibodies are beneficial or detrimental to the host.

5. EFFECT OF HIV INFECTION AND AIDS ON THE MUCOSAL IMMUNE SYSTEM

5.1. IgA Hypergammaglobulinemia

As infection with HIV progresses and AIDS develops, a variety of problems associated with the mucosal immune system occur. One problem associated with HIV infection has been the development of hypergammaglobulinemia (Fig. 2) (Lyamuya *et al.*, 1994). Although it is clear that IgA hypergammaglobulinemia exists in persons infected with HIV, whether the increased IgA is serum derived or related to mucosal sources remains controversial (Quesnel *et al.*, 1994b; Kozlowski and Jackson, 1992; Vincent *et al.*, 1992) (Fig. 2). In one study, IgA hypergammaglobulinemia was found early in infection and remained throughout the disease progression and did not correlate with CD4 counts (Kozlowski and Jackson, 1992). The ratio of IgA1 to IgA2 was not found to be altered and there were no increases in the amount of pIgA detected in the serum of HIV-infected persons, suggesting that the IgA hypergammaglobulinemia was related to an increase in serum IgA and not to increases in mucosal IgA production. In support of this conclusion, total serum IgA was found to be increased while salivary S-IgA levels were decreased in HIV-positive patients with $CD4^+$ T-cell counts < 60 cells/μl (Muller *et al.*, 1991). In this study, both increased

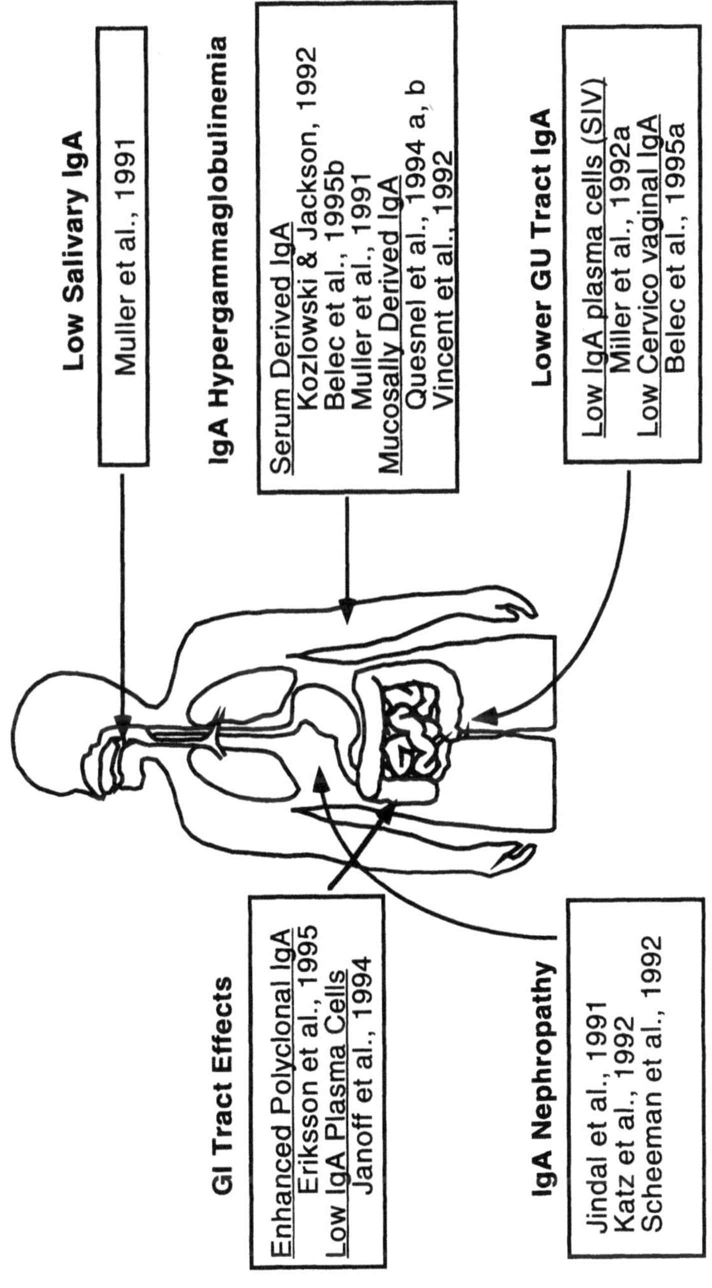

FIGURE 2. Effects of HIV infection and AIDS on the mucosal immune system.

serum IgA and decreased salivary S-IgA levels were associated with reduced CD4$^+$ T-cell counts. Others have also reported increased serum IgA levels with decreased local production of cervicovaginal IgA in women with AIDS (Belec *et al.*, 1995b).

Evidence also exists that the increased serum IgA concentrations observed in HIV-infected persons are associated with increased amounts of S-IgA (Quesnel *et al.*, 1994a,b; Vincent *et al.*, 1992). The concentrations of S-IgA detected in HIV-infected persons was significantly increased over those observed in age- and sex-matched controls (Quesnel *et al.*, 1994b) (Fig. 2). The sera from patients with IgA hypergammaglobulinemia were found to have an increased amount of IgA reactive with the dietary antigen gliadin whereas no increased antigliadin IgG activity was noted. In contrast, no increased IgA reactivity to cytomegalovirus or tetanus toxoid (to represent nonmucosal, systemic vaccine antigens) was observed. The increased presence of IgA specific for mucosal but not parenteral antigens supports the notion that IgA hypergammaglobulinemia is caused by increased IgA production in the mucosal compartment. Similar results were found with serum samples from HIV-infected children (Quesnel *et al.*, 1994a). Based on these observations, the authors concluded that the IgA hypergammaglobulinemia observed with HIV infection may be associated with a dysregulated mucosal IgA response spilling over into the systemic compartment (Quesnel *et al.*, 1994a,b) (Fig. 2). Others have also found that serum from HIV-infected patients contained increased amounts of S-IgA as well as S-IgM although no increase in free SC was observed (Vincent *et al.*, 1992).

In addition to the contrasting results reported for the origin of IgA observed in HIV-infected patients with IgA hypergammaglobulinemia, there are also contradictory reports on the frequency of Ig-secreting cells at mucosal sites of HIV-infected persons. Increased numbers of Ig-secreting cells of the IgG, IgA, and IgM isotypes were detected in the intestinal mucosa of HIV-infected persons (Eriksson *et al.*, 1995). When antibody-secreting cells (ASC) were assayed for specificity to HIV gp160 and the irrelevant antigens keyhole limpet hemocyanin (KLH) and dog serum albumin (DSA), there was an increase in the number of gp160, KLH, and DSA ASC in the intestinal mucosa of HIV-infected when compared with seronegative individuals. Increased numbers of ASC specific for gp160, KLH, and DSA were detected in HIV-infected patients who were either asymptomatic or symptomatic. Only increased numbers of gp160 ASC were detected in patients with AIDS, suggesting that with progression to AIDS, the polyclonal B-cell activation diminishes. The route of infection did not seem to be associated with the increased numbers of Ig-secreting cells detected in the intestinal mucosa of HIV-infected individuals since there was no detectable difference in the results obtained from patients infected with HIV via sexual contact or by exposure to contaminated needles. The observation that there are increased numbers of antigen-specific as well as polyclonally activated Ig-secreting cells in the intestinal mucosa lends support to the idea that mucosal IgA responses contribute to the IgA hypergammaglobulinemia associated with HIV infection. The numbers of IgA plasma cells in the intestinal LP has also been reported to be decreased in HIV infection (Janoff *et al.*, 1994) (Fig. 2). Additionally, the decrease in IgA plasma cells was specifically associated with a decrease in the IgA2 subclass. This group also reported that the amount of tetanus toxoid-specific IgG in the duodenal fluids was increased in HIV-infected patients when compared with seronegative controls, implying that serum IgG responses transudate to the GI tract during HIV infection. No differences in the numbers of IgG plasma cells in the intestinal LP between HIV-infected and seronegative controls were observed. SIV infection of rhesus macaques is also associated with a decreased frequency of IgG and IgA plasma cells in the female reproductive tract (Miller *et al.*, 1992a). Further studies are warranted to determine the source of IgA in HIV-infected patients with IgA hypergammaglobulinemia and to determine if there is a polyclonal activation of ASC in the intestinal LP. Additional information such as CD4$^+$ T-cell levels in the peripheral blood, route of infection with HIV, and recent immunization status should help determine if mucosally derived IgA is responsible for the IgA hypergammaglobulinemia observed in HIV-infected patients.

5.1.1. Increased IL-6 Expression in HIV Infection

IL-6 has a variety of immunological functions, one of which involves the induction of membrane sIgA$^+$ B cells to terminally differentiate into IgA-secreting plasma cells (Lebman and Coffman, 1994; Beagley *et al.*, 1989). Although the source of IgA in HIV-infected persons with IgA hypergammaglobulinemia remains controversial, increased production of IL-6 observed with HIV infection may be partly responsible for the elevated serum IgA (Gurram *et al.*, 1994; Reka *et al.*, 1994; Rautonen *et al.*, 1991). Elevated serum IL-6 in HIV-infected children correlated with increased serum IgG and IgA levels (Rautonen *et al.*, 1991). Increased serum IL-6 also correlated with increased serum concentrations of IL-4 and TNF-α, although no correlations were found between IL-4 or TNF-α concentrations and serum Ig levels. Significantly increased expression of IL-5 and IL-6 mRNA in the rectal LP of HIV-infected persons has also been reported (Reka *et al.*, 1994). Indeed, IL-5 has also been shown to be involved in the enhancement of IgA secretion from sIgA$^+$ B cells (Lebman and Coffman, 1994; Beagley *et al.*, 1988; Murray *et al.*, 1987). *In vitro* studies have found that the addition of the HIV-1 Tat protein to uninfected peripheral blood mononuclear cells (PBMC) increased the production of IL-6, IgG, IgA, and IgM (Rautonen *et al.*, 1994) Although all Ig isotypes were increased by the addition of Tat to PBMCs, the production of IgA was increased most by the presence of Tat. The increased production of IgG and IgA by PBMC was the result of Tat-induced production of IL-6 since the addition of neutralizing anti-IL-6 monoclonal antibodies abrogated the increased production of IgG and IgA. Therefore, the release of Tat protein during HIV infection may induce the production of IL-6 which in turn enhances IgA synthesis.

5.1.2. Decreased FcαR Expression

As indicated above, several plausible explanations for the increased serum concentrations of IgA in HIV-infected persons can be set forth; one major reason would be that peripheral blood monocytes and neutrophils from HIV-1-infected patients express significantly fewer IgA Fc receptors (FcαR) than monocytes or neutrophils from uninfected controls (Grossetete *et al.*, 1995). Decreased FcαR expression may result in an impaired clearance of IgA immune complexes from the circulation of HIV-infected individuals and therefore lead to an overall increase in the serum concentrations of IgA.

5.1.3. IgA Nephropathy

IgA nephritis is another IgA-related problem observed in HIV-infected patients (Fig. 2) (Katz *et al.*, 1992; Schoeneman *et al.*, 1992; Jindal *et al.*, 1991). Nephropathy is a problem commonly associated with HIV infection and although the exact cause of nephropathy in HIV-infected individuals is not known, the fact that HIV-infected patients with nephropathy have been found to have greatly elevated serum IgA levels (Katz *et al.*, 1992; Schoeneman *et al.*, 1992; Jindal *et al.*, 1991), circulating immune complexes containing IgA (Katz *et al*, 1992; Schoeneman *et al.*, 1992), and renal biopsy showing deposition of IgA (Schoeneman *et al.*, 1992; Jindal *et al.*, 1991) suggests that the elevated concentrations of IgA may be the cause of nephropathy observed in HIV-infected individuals. Further studies are warranted to discern the cause of IgA hypergammaglobulinemia and IgA nephritis observed in HIV-infected persons. Regulation of the IgA hypergammaglobulinemia associated with HIV infection may provide a means to prevent the nephropathy associated with HIV infection.

5.2. IgA Responses to Opportunistic Pathogens and to Common Vaccines

HIV infection of humans eventually leads to decreased levels of circulating $CD4^+$ T cells and this loss of $CD4^+$ T cells plays a central role in the development of the immunodeficient state associated with HIV infection and AIDS. Associated with the immunodeficient state is infection of the host with opportunistic pathogens that ordinarily do not pose a threat to immunocompetent individuals. Since most infectious agents first interact with the host at a mucosal surface, the ability of the HIV-infected host to undergo a mucosal immune response to infectious agents or their products is of interest. Although mucosal secretions (e.g., salivary, vaginal, intestinal) are the samples of choice for the analysis of mucosal immune responses, serum IgA has been analyzed as an indicator of mucosal IgA responses. CMV infection is common in the general population and reinfection or reactivation of latent virus is associated with a number of clinically significant infections in AIDS patients. Sera from HIV-seronegative controls did not contain detectable levels of IgA anti-CMV antibodies while sera from HIV-infected individuals at various stages of disease contained anti-CMV IgA (Levy *et al.*, 1991). The fact that the HIV-seropositive individuals were positive for anti-CMV IgA, while HIV-seronegative persons were not may be related to increased exposure to CMV in the test population; however, it also indicates that infection with HIV did not inhibit the development of an IgA response to CMV. This finding suggests that the mucosal immune system is indeed functioning in HIV-infected individuals. Sera from HIV-infected persons with or without obvious symptoms of crytosporidiosis had elevated levels of serum anti-*Cryptosporidium* IgA when compared with healthy HIV-seronegative controls (Kassa *et al.*, 1991). Finally, serum anti-*Cryptococcus neoformans* (CN) IgA antibodies were significantly elevated in persons infected with HIV when compared with HIV-seronegative controls, although IgA anti-CN antibodies were detected in both HIV-infected and uninfected individuals (Deshaw and Pirofski, 1995). The fact that HIV-infected persons have elevated levels of pathogen-specific serum IgA may be the result of increased exposure to the specific pathogen (caused by increased exposure of the pathogen in the environment or due to deficiencies in other host resistance mechanisms that would normally keep the pathogen in check), or alternatively, to polyclonal B-cell activation. Regardless of the eliciting agent, these observations support the conclusion that HIV infection *per se* does not inhibit the induction of IgA responses to mucosal pathogens.

To better answer the basic question—Are mucosal immune responses to specific pathogens increased or decreased with HIV infection and disease?—the level of salivary IgA anti-*Candida albicans* was determined in HIV-infected individuals, persons with AIDS, and HIV-seronegative individuals (Coogan *et al.*, 1994). Anti-*C. albicans* IgA, including both IgA1 and IgA2, were significantly increased in the parotid saliva of HIV-infected and AIDS patients when compared with controls. There was no change in the IgA1/IgA2 ratio in either HIV-positive group when compared with controls. The findings of this study suggest that the mucosal immune system is functioning to defend against the mucosal pathogen *C. albicans*. It would be interesting to determine if mucosal CMI to *C. albicans* was also intact. However, the fact that other defects in the immune system of HIV-infected persons may allow *C. albicans* to infect and persist, whereas immunocompetent persons would not become infected, may be associated with higher levels of anti-*C. albicans* antibodies in the salivary secretions. Regardless, HIV-infected persons appear to be able to undergo pathogen-specific mucosal immune responses to encountered pathogens. Parameters such as total IgG, IgM, and IgA concentrations (in the sample being monitored), $CD4^+$ T-cell counts in peripheral blood, prior history of exposure to antigen, and immune responses (humoral and/or cellular) to unrelated control antigens will help determine if the assessed immune responses are related to polyclonal activation of the immune system or to a normally regulated immune response. Careful monitoring of immune parameters will be necessary to determine if mucosal immune responses to mucosal immunogens/pathogens are impaired in HIV-infected individuals.

Immunization with known amounts of vaccine antigen has been used to determine if HIV infection is associated with decreased immune responses to specific antigen. Intramuscular injection with a pneumococcal polysaccharide vaccine induced comparable numbers of polysaccharide-specific IgG and IgA ASC in HIV-seronegative individuals and two groups of HIV-infected patients, those with $CD4^+$ T-cell counts < 300/ml or those with $\geqslant 300$/ml (Carson *et al.*, 1995). Although IgG and IgA ASC frequencies were comparable between HIV-negative and -positive individuals, the numbers of antigen-specific IgM ASCs were significantly lower in both groups of HIV-infected persons when compared with seronegative individuals. When serum antivaccine IgG, IgM, and IgA responses were monitored, immunization was associated with significantly increased levels of vaccine-specific antibody of all classes in both control and HIV-infected subjects. Even though immunization was associated with increased levels of specific antibody in HIV-infected persons, the postimmunization levels of IgM and IgA were significantly lower than those observed in HIV-negative control individuals. This study has thus raised an important question: Does HIV infection impair all immune responses or just *de novo* immune responses? The observation that HIV infection was associated with significantly decreased, vaccine-specific IgM ASC (but not IgG or IgA ASC) suggests that a defect exists in the induction of *de novo* immune responses but not memory responses (Carson *et al.*, 1995). However, postvaccination serum levels of both IgM and IgA were significantly lower in HIV-infected persons relative to control subjects. Collectively, these results suggest that there may be a defect in *de novo* immune responsiveness that is associated with lower increases in antibody titers to specific vaccine proteins while memory responses remain intact. As HIV infection progresses and the number of $CD4^+$ T cells decreases, the memory response may also decrease.

The previously mentioned study (Carson *et al.*, 1995) found that vaccine-specific IgA responses did increase after vaccination by the intramuscular route. However, the intramuscular route is not an ideal mode of immunization for the detection of mucosal immune responses. The orally administered whole-cell/CT-B cholera vaccine was used to determine if HIV infection affected immune responses to specific antigens delivered by a mucosal route (Lewis *et al.*, 1994). Oral immunization with the whole-cell/CT-B cholera vaccine increased serum anti-CT IgG and IgA titers in HIV-negative controls as well as two groups of HIV-infected persons with $CD4^+$ T-cell counts of 752 and 186 cells/μl, respectively. In contrast, oral immunization of a group of HIV-infected persons with 52 $CD4^+$ T cells/μl did not result in an increased titer of serum IgG or IgA antitoxin. Therefore, it appears that HIV-infected persons are able to respond to antigens delivered by the oral route even when $CD4^+$ T-cell counts are reduced. However, when $CD4^+$ T-cell counts dropped to 52 cells/μl, immune responses to orally delivered antigens were not detected. An important point to consider is that the HIV-positive groups with 752 and 186 $CD4^+$ cells/μl were Kenyans who may have had prior environmental exposure to CT (and therefore enhanced responsiveness to the oral vaccine) while the HIV-negative control and HIV-positive group with 52 $CD4^+$ cells/μl were residents of the United Kingdom who would be less likely to have received environmental exposure to cholera or related bacterial toxins. Therefore, further studies with mucosal immunization and immune responses are warranted in persons infected with HIV at various stages of the disease to determine the status of the mucosal immune system during HIV infection. although further work is needed in this area, this study provides encouraging results that in HIV-positive patients with moderately advanced disease, the oral route of immunization is functional and may be used to induce mucosal immune responses that may protect the host from opportunistic pathogens.

5.3. Mucosal Ig Levels after HIV Infection

The aforementioned studies provided evidence that HIV-infected persons were able to undergo vaccine/pathogen-specific mucosal immune responses. To determine if HIV infection affected the production of mucosal IgA, the concentration of total IgA in mucosal secretions was measured (Fig. 2). The total concentrations of cervicovaginal IgA including both IgA1 and IgA2 subclasses were increased in HIV-infected women in early stages of disease (CDC stages II and III) and in persons with AIDS (Belec *et al.*, 1995b). However, the level of albumin in cervicovaginal secretions was also significantly elevated in persons with AIDS. Calculations based on total IgA and albumin in serum and cervicovaginal secretions found that the relative coefficient of excretion (RCE) for IgA, IgA1, and IgA2 was significantly decreased (suggesting decreased local production of IgA) in HIV-infected individuals. Therefore, although the total level of IgA was increased with HIV infection, this elevation was likely caused by high levels of serum IgA transudating into the cervicovaginal secretions and not related to locally produced mucosal IgA. Additional studies reported that both total IgG and IgA in addition to albumin concentrations in cervicovaginal secretions were increased in HIV-infected women (Belec *et al.*, 1995a). When the RCE was calculated for IgG in HIV-infected women, it was found to be greater than the RCE observed for healthy controls and indicated increased mucosal production while the RCE for IgA was less than observed for healthy controls and suggested decreased local production of IgA. Studies with SIV-infected rhesus macaques support these findings (Miller *et al.*, 1992a). For example, normal cervical and vaginal tissue contained Ig-secreting cells (ISC) of the IgA, IgG, and IgM isotype with IgA-secreting cells accounting for 45–75% of all ISCs whereas IgG and IgM were equal among the remaining ISCs. After SIV infection, the numbers of IgA and IgG ISCs decreased to $< 5\%$ of total ISC detected in the cervix and vagina. Collectively, these findings suggest that the production of IgA in the female reproductive tract is impaired following infection with HIV.

HIV infection has also been reported to be associated with a decreased detection of both secretory and total IgA in parotid saliva (Muller *et al.*, 1991). Decreased salivary IgA, comprised of decreases in both IgA1 and IgA2 subclasses, was associated with decreased CD4$^+$ T-cell counts in peripheral blood. However, others have reported no differences in the level of total IgA in saliva of HIV-infected persons with or without *Streptococcus pneumoniae* bacteremia when compared with HIV-seronegative persons with or without *S. pneumoniae* (Opstad *et al.*, 1995). In addition, previously mentioned studies showed that salivary IgA specific for *C. albicans* was increased in HIV-infected persons relative to HIV-seronegative controls (Coogan *et al.*, 1994). It may be that mucosal Ig responses are intact while specific defects in mucosal cell-mediated or systemic immunity are responsible for increased infections via the mucosal route (Opstad *et al.*, 1995). Indeed, studies suggest there may be a decrease in the number of cells in the gut that are able to serve as APC (Lim *et al.*, 1993) and this defect in mucosal APC function may reduce T-cell responses to specific pathogens. The question remains: Are the increased opportunistic infections characteristic of AIDS associated with defects in the mucosal immune system (humoral or cellular immunity) or are these infections the result of a defect in systemic immunity secondary to decreased CD4$^+$ T-cell help which allows pathogens to go unchecked after penetrating the mucosal barrier? As previously mentioned, further studies that evaluate mucosal immune responses in HIV-infected persons should also monitor CD4$^+$ T-cell levels in peripheral blood, exposure to infectious agents, immunization history, and total and antigen-specific mucosal Ig antibody levels to standardize the results as much as possible and make comparisons to other work possible.

5.4. IgA as a Prognostic Indicator

The observation that IgA hypergammaglobulinemia (see Section 5.1) is one of the earliest immunological abnormalities associated with HIV infection has led several groups to determine if serum IgA levels are able to serve as prognostic indicators for a decrease in CD4$^+$ T-cell counts and progression to AIDS (Anonymous, 1994; Phillips *et al.*, 1993; Quesnel *et al.*, 1993; Schwartlander *et al.*, 1993). A significant correlation was found to exist between the disappearance of IgA specific for the p68 subunit of reverse transcriptase and either a CD4$^+$ T-cell count < 400/ml peripheral blood or a total IgA serum level of over 4.25 g/liter (Quesnel *et al.*, 1993). Determinations of total serum IgA, β_2-microglobulin, and erythrocyte sedimentation rate (ESR) were all found to improve the predictive value of CD4$^+$ T-lymphocyte counts for determining the time to development of AIDS in HIV-infected patients (Schwartlander *et al.*, 1993). Serum IgA was the only parameter to correlate with time to AIDS in patients with CD4$^+$ T-lymphocyte counts $> 500/\mu l$. The addition of serum IgA determinations, serum β_2-microglobulin levels, and ESR added to value of CD4$^+$ T-lymphocyte counts alone as concerned the prediction of time to the development of AIDS in patients with CD4$^+$ T-lymphocyte counts $< 500/\mu l$. A score created using CD8$^+$ lymphocyte counts and serum IgA levels (CD8/IgA score) was able to significantly predict the future occurrence of low CD4$^+$ T-lymphocyte counts and AIDS in a study that followed HIV-infected hemophiliacs from soon after seroconversion to up to 8½ years (Phillips *et al.*, 1993). Utilizing a data base derived from 1744 patients infected with HIV, elevated serum IgA and β_2-microglobulin levels were associated with an increased risk of progression to AIDS (Anonymous, 1994). Although it remains to be determined if elevated serum IgA levels observed in persons infected with HIV are related to defects in the systemic or mucosal IgA humoral compartments, elevated serum IgA levels may prove to be a clinically important prognostic indicator for progression to AIDS after infection with HIV.

6. VACCINES TO PREVENT HIV INFECTION MUST CONSIDER MUCOSAL IMMUNITY

HIV is most commonly transmitted via a mucosal route and opportunistic pathogens associated with AIDS such as *Candida albicans*, *Cryptosporidium* sp., and *Cryptococcus neoformans* likely initiate infection at mucosal surfaces of the host. The fact that the natural mechanism for HIV transmission is via contact at the mucosal surface and the fact that opportunistic pathogens associated with AIDS infect the host at mucosal surfaces imply that HIV infection and possibly infection with opportunistic pathogens may be prevented by the appropriate mucosal immune response. A variety of experimental approaches are currently being investigated for the development of vaccines that induce both systemic and mucosal immune responses to HIV (Table I). Although the immune responses required for prevention of HIV infection are not known, there is evidence suggesting that CTL responses may be required for protection against HIV infection (De Maria *et al.*, 1994; Koup *et al.*, 1994; Rowland-Jones *et al.*, 1993). For the purposes of this chapter, only those vaccination strategies that have been shown to induce mucosal immune responses will be discussed and the reader is referred to other chapters for discussion of parenteral vaccines.

One HIV vaccine strategy for the induction of anti-HIV mucosal immune responses is the use of peptide immunogens representing regions of HIV glycoproteins that contain immunogenic epitopes that correspond to Th, neutralizing B-cell, or CTL epitopes. Oral immunization with the B1M-P3C synthetic lipopeptide (corresponding to amino acids 308–331 of HIV-1 gp120 covalently coupled to the lipophilic group P3C) was found to induce serum IgG and IgA (1:1020 and 1:80 titers, respectively) and salivary IgA antipeptide antibody responses as well as splenic antipeptide and anti-HIV gp160 CTL responses

TABLE I. Summary of HIV-1 Vaccine Protocols in Humans, November 1988 to the Present

Vaccine formulaton	Company sponsor	Phase I/Phase II
1. Live recombinant *Vaccinia*–$gp160_{IIIB}$	Bristol/Oncogen	Nov. 88–Jan. 92
2. A. $rgp160_{IIIB}$ from r*Vaccinia*	IMMUNO-AG	Dec. 90–July 91
B. $rgp160_{IIIB}$ in HIV^+ (asymptomatic) people		July 92–Feb. 93
3. rgp120 + MTE adjuvant in MF59 emusion	BIOCINE	Jan. 91–Nov. 91
4. A. $rgp120/HIV\text{-}1_{IIIB}$	Genentech	March 91–June 91
B. $rgp120/HIV\text{-}1_{IIIB}$ + $rgp120/HIV\text{-}1_{MN}$		March 92–July 92
C. $rgp120_{MN}$ + alum/QS 21		May 93–Nov. 93
D. $rgp120_{MN}$ + alum in HIV^+ pregnant women		March 93–Jan. 95
5. A. V3 loop (octamer) "crown"	UBI Peptides	Feb. 93–June 93
B. Multivalent peptide		Feb. 94–July 94
C. Oral version		June 94–Present
D. Parenteral V3 peptide followed by oral boost with V3 branched peptide in microspheres		May 95–Present
6. Live recombinant canarypox–$gp160_{MN}$	Merieux/Connaught	May 93–June 94
ALVAC-MN expressing env/gag/pol $gp120_{MN}$		May 95–Present
7. p24-virus-like particle (VLP) (oral or rectal boost after IM vaccine)	British Biotechnology	May 95–Present
8. Live recombinant *Vaccinia* expressing env/gag/pol	Therion	April 94–July 94
9. rgp160 in HIV^+ pregnant women	MicroGeneSys	March 93–March 94
		Total ~ 1754 (April 30, 1995)

(Nardelli *et al.*, 1994). The ability of the IgG or IgA antibody responses to neutralize HIV infectivity was not determined. Oral immunization with a macromolecular multicomponent peptide vaccine with or without CT as a mucosal adjuvant induced serum and fecal antipeptide IgG and IgA responses (Bukawa *et al.*, 1995). Serum IgG titers peaked at 1:256 while fecal IgA titers reached a maximum of 1:2048. This macromolecular, multicomponent peptide antigen composed of HIV-1 peptides from the third variable region of gp120, a CD4 binding site, and a Gag region induced anti-HIV-1 secretory IgA responses that were able to neutralize HIV-1_{IIIB}, HIV-1_{SF2}, and HIV-1_{MN} *in vitro*. The ability of this immunization protocol to induce anti-HIV IgA in the female reproductive tract was not determined.

We have recently shown that the C4/V3 peptide T1SP10MN(A) which contains a Th epitope, a neutralizing B-cell epitope, and a CTL epitope from HIV-1 gp120 was able to induce serum HIV-1_{MN} neutralizing antibody responses when intranasally administered with CT (Staats *et al.*, 1996). In addition to high-titered serum IgG responses (1:131,072 in BALB/c mice and 1:524,288 in C57BL/6 mice), vaginal antipeptide IgG and IgA responses were also induced. Vaginal antipeptide antibody responses were associated with SC, suggesting that the anti-HIV IgA responses represented polymeric IgA that was locally produced and transported across the mucosal epithelium to the vaginal surface.

The observation that anti-HIV sera may easily neutralize laboratory-adapted strains of HIV but not primary isolates of HIV suggests that anti-HIV antibody responses may not be the optimal immune response to prevent HIV infection. Further studies with HIV peptide immunogens will be required to determine if the immune responses induced are able to protect against mucosal challenge with HIV with particular attention given to the induction of virus-specific CTL responses. Circumstantial evidence suggests that HIV-specific CTL may be able to protect against infection with HIV (De Maria *et al.*, 1994). Short peptides (10–15 amino acids in length) that represent CTL epitopes from HIV gp120 are able to induce CTL responses *in vivo* (Nehete *et al.*, 1995; Sastry *et al.*, 1992). Therefore, it may be possible to induce HIV-specific CTL responses in the systemic compartment as well as mucosal sites by mucosal immunization with HIV CTL peptides.

The use of viral vectors that express portions of the HIV genome has been investigated as an antigen delivery system to induce systemic and mucosal anti-HIV immune responses. Recombinant adenoviruses expressing HIV-1_{IIIB} gp160 or the entire Gag protein used to intranasally immunize chimpanzees induced serum anti-HIV antibody responses as determined by ELISA and neutralization assay (Lubeck *et al.*, 1994). Intranasal immunization with the recombinant adenoviruses was able to induce serum HIV neutralizing antibody responses although the responses were quite low ($\leq$ 1:40). However, serum neutralizing antibody responses increased up to 1:640 one month after intramuscular boosting with gp160 subunit vaccine.

With regard to the induction of mucosal immunity, intranasal immunization with recombinant adenoviruses induced salivary, nasal, and vaginal IgG responses with low IgA responses in salivary and nasal secretions with no IgA responses detected in vaginal or rectal secretions at any time tested. All IgG responses detected in mucosal secretions increased after the intramuscular boosting with the gp160 subunit and likely represent transudation of serum IgG into mucosal secretions. The induction of CTL responses to HIV was not determined in this study. Poliovirus is also being investigated as a mucosal HIV vaccine vector with encouraging results (Morrow *et al.*, 1994). Although the use of recombinant viruses as HIV vaccine vectors is theoretically very attractive because of the ability to induce both humoral and cell-mediated immune responses in both systemic and mucosal sites, further studies are needed to determine the immunization protocols required to induce immune responses of the desired magnitude and characteristics.

Recombinant bacterial vectors are also being investigated as HIV mucosal vaccine delivery vehicles. A prime candidate for a recombinant bacterial vector to deliver HIV antigens to the mucosal immune system is BCG. BCG, classically used to immunize against tuberculosis, is the most widely used vaccine in the world, is associated with a low occurrence of serious side effects, and can be engineered to express foreign antigens (Stover *et al.*, 1991). Recombinant BCG expressing a region of HIV-1 gp120 induced $CD8^+$ CTL responses when administered by the subcutaneous route (Kameoka *et al.*, 1994). Induction of CTL responses was not inhibited by preexisting immunity to BCG, indicating that the use of recombinant BCG as an HIV vaccine vector in persons previously immunized with BCG will be feasible. Oral immunization with recombinant BCG was able to induce both T-cell and antibody responses against an expressed foreign antigen, suggesting that oral immunization with BCG vectors expressing HIV antigens may induce mucosal and systemic immunity to HIV (Lagranderie *et al.*, 1993).

The true test of HIV mucosal vaccine strategies will be to determine if they are able to prevent infection of sexually transmitted HIV. The fact that no suitable animal model exists using HIV has made the use of the SIV model a critical component of HIV vaccine development. SIV infection of rhesus macaques results in a similar clinical presentation as human AIDS and provides researchers with a model to test immunization strategies for the ability to induce protective immunity against SIV. Intramuscular (i.m.) immunization with microencapsulated SIV followed by oral or intratracheal (i.t.) boosting was able to prevent vaginal infection with SIV (Marx *et al.*, 1993). After two vaginal challenges with SIV, 4 of 4 control animals, 4 of 4 orally immunized only, and 1 of 1 i.m. immunized animal were infected while only 1 of 3 i.m.–oral and 2 of 3 i.m.–i.t. immunized macaques were infected. Although performed with few monkeys, the data suggest that the combination of systemic (i.m.) and mucosal immunization may be the key to preventing vaginal infection with SIV. The protective correlate in this study is not known, but protection did not correlate with vaginal anti-SIV IgA responses and immune responses against the host cells used to grow the SIV challenge stocks were not ruled out as a protective mechanism (Marx *et al.*, 1993).

The SIV model has also been used to evaluate mucosal immunization with viruslike particles composed of SIV p27 and the p1 protein of the yeast retrotransposon Ty coupled to the B subunit of CT (p27:Ty-VLP/CT-B) (Lehner *et al.*, 1992). Vaginal followed by oral immunization with p27:Ty-VLP/CT-B induced anti-p27 IgG and IgA in vaginal secretions and serum, and lymphocyte proliferative responses in the blood, spleen, genital, and iliac/paraortic lymph nodes. Similar results were obtained in male rhesus macaques immunized urethrally and then boosted orally with p27:Ty-VLP/CT-B (Lehner *et al.*, 1994). When i.m. immunization with p27:Ty-VLP was compared to urethral followed by oral boosting with p27:Ty-VLP/CT-B, all three macaques immunized by the mucosal route had detectable anti-p27 IgG and IgA in both urine and seminal fluid whereas i.m. immunized monkeys had no urine or seminal fluid IgA and only one i.m. immunized animals had seminal fluid IgG. This illustrates the repeated observation that systemic immunization rarely if ever induces S-IgA responses. IgA responses induced by urethral immunization contained both J chain and SC, suggesting that the IgA was polymeric in nature and transported to the mucosal surface by SC. As previously observed with vaginal–oral immunization with p27:Ty-VLP/CT-B (Lehner *et al.*, 1992), urethral–oral immunization of male rhesus macaques induced antigen-specific proliferative responses in the blood, spleen, and several regional lymph nodes (Lehner *et al.*, 1994). Intramuscular immunization with p27:Ty-VLP/CT-B resulted in detectable lymphocyte proliferative responses in the blood and spleen only, suggesting that in addition to the induction of S-IgA responses, mucosal immunization induces antigen-specific lymphocyte responses in regional lymph nodes in addition to central sites such as the spleen. Mucosal challenge studies with SIV are required to determine if vaginal–oral or urethral-oral immunization with p27:Ty-VLP/CT-B induces protective immunity to SIV.

7. CONCLUSIONS

Infection with HIV most commonly occurs via a mucosal surface. Lymphoid cells and S-IgA antibodies of the mucosal immune system may represent the first line of immune cells and molecules to come in contact with the virus. In so doing, T and B cells and S-IgA antibodies of the mucosal immune system are in a position to play a pivotal role in the dissemination of HIV throughout the host as well as to prevent HIV infection altogether. HIV infection and its associated immunodeficiency result in a variety of defects in the mucosal immune system including IgA hypergammaglobulinemia, polyclonal mucosal B-cell activation, decreased production of S-IgA at mucosal sites, and increased susceptibility to opportunistic pathogens that infect at mucosal surfaces. The development of vaccines that induce the appropriate mucosal immune response(s) may prove to be beneficial in preventing sexual transmission of HIV as well as mucosal infection with opportunistic pathogens.

ACKNOWLEDGMENTS. We are most grateful to Ms. Wendy Jackson for editorial assistance as well as preparation of figures and the manuscript. We also thank members of our Immunobiology Vaccine Center for critical reading and constructive comments. Our research mentioned herein was supported by U.S. Public Health Service grants DE 04217, AI 18958, DK 44240, DE 09837, DE 08228, AI 35544, AI 35932, AI 30366, AI 35351, DMID NIAID Contract AI 15128 and AIDS NIAID Contract NO1 AI 45209, and Z P30 AI 28662 from the Veterans Administration Research Center on AIDS and HIV infection.

REFERENCES

Anonymous, 1994, Immunologic markers of AIDS progression: Consistency across five HIV-infected cohorts, *AIDS* **8:**911–921.

Ayehunie, S., Groves, R. W., Bruzzese, A. M., Ruprecht, R. M., Kupper, T. S., and Langhoff, E., 1995, Acutely infected Langerhans cells are more efficient than T cells in disseminating HIV type 1 to activated T cells following a short cell–cell contact, *AIDS Res. Hum. Retrovir.* **11:**877–884.

Baba, T. W., Koch, J., Mittler, E. S., Greene, M., Wyand, M., Penninck, D., and Ruprecht, R. M., 1994, Mucosal infection of neonatal rhesus monkeys with cell-free SIV, *AIDS Res. Hum. Retrovir.* **10:**351–357.

Baba, T. W., Jeong, Y. S., Penninck, D., Bronson, R., Greene, M. F., and Ruprecht, R. M., 1995, Pathogenicity of live, attenuated SIV after mucosal infection of neonatal macaques, *Science* **267:**1820–1825.

Batman, P. A., Fleming, S. C., Sedgwick, P. M., MacDonald, T. T., and Griffin, G. E., 1994, HIV infection of human fetal intestinal explant cultures induces epithelial cell proliferation, *AIDS* **8:**161–167.

Beagley, K. W., Eldridge, J. H., Kiyono, H., Everson, M. P., Koopman, W. J., Honjo, T., and McGhee, J. R., 1988, Recombinant murine IL-5 induces high rate IgA synthesis in cycling IgA-positive Peyer's patch B cells, *J. Immunol.* **141:**2035–2042.

Beagley, K. W., Eldridge, J. H., Lee, F., Kiyono, H., Everson, M. P., Koopman, W. J., Hirano, T., Kishimoto, T., and

McGhee, J. R., 1989, Interleukins and IgA synthesis. Human and murine interleukin 6 induce high rate IgA secretion in IgA-committed B cells, *J. Exp. Med.* **169:**2133–2148.

Beagley, K. W., Eldridge, J. H., Aicher, W. K., Mestecky, J., DiFabio, S., Kiyono, H., and McGhee, J. R., 1991, Peyer's patch B cells with memory cell characteristics undergo terminal differentiation within 24 hours in response to interleukin-6, *Cytokine* **3:**107–116.

Belec, L., Dupre, T., Prazuck, T., Tevibenissan, C., Kanga, J. M., Pathey, O., Lu, X. S., and Pillot, J., 1995a, Cervicovaginal overproduction of specific IgG to human immunodeficiency virus (HIV) contrasts with normal or impaired IgA local response in HIV infection, *J. Infect. Dis.* **172:**691–697.

Belec, L., Meillet, D., Gaillard, O., Prazuck, T., Michel, E., Ekome, J. N., and Pillot, J., 1995b, Decreased cervicovaginal production of both IgA1 and IgA2 subclasses in women with AIDS, *Clin. Exp. Immunol.* **101:** 100–106.

Benson, E. B., and Strober, W., 1988, Regulation of IgA secretion by T cell clones derived from the human gastrointestinal tract, *J. Immunol.* **140:**1874–1882.

Bernstein, J. M., 1992, Mucosal immunology of the upper respiratory tract, *Respiration* **59(Suppl. 3):**3–13.

Blauvelt, A., and Katz, S. I., 1995, The skin as target, vector, and effector organ in human immunodeficiency virus disease, *J. Invest. Dermatol.* **105(1 Suppl.):**S122–S126.

Bond, M. W., Shrader, B., Mosmann, T. R., and Coffman, R. L., 1987, A mouse T cell product that preferentially enhances IgA production. II. Physiochemical characterization, *J. Immunol.* **139:**3691–3696.

Brandtzaeg, P., 1994, Distribution and characterization of mucosal immunoglobulin-producing cells, in: *Handbook of Mucosal Immunology* (P. L. Ogra, J. Mestecky, M. E. Lamm, S. Warren, J. R. McGhee, and J. Bienenstock, eds.), Academic Press, San Diego, pp. 251–262.

Brandtzaeg, P., Krajci, P., Lamm, M. E., and Kaetzel, C. S., 1994, Epithelial and hepatobiliary transport of polymeric immunoglobulins, in: *Handbook of Mucosal Immunology* (P. L. Ogra, J. Mestecky, M. E. Lamm, S. Warren, J. R. McGhee, and J. Bienenstock, eds.), Academic Press, San Diego, p. 113.

Brown, W. R., Newcomb, R. W., and Ishizaka, K., 1970, Proteolytic degradation of exocrine and serum immunoglobulins, *J. Clin. Invest.* **49:**1374–1380.

Bukawa, H., Sekigawa, K. I., Hamajima, K., Fukushima, J., Yamada, Y., Kiyono, H., and Okuda, K., 1995, Neutralization of HIV-1 by secretory IgA induced by oral immunization with a new macromolecular multicomponent peptide vaccine candidate, *Nature Med.* **1:**681–685.

Burnett, P. R., VanCott, T. C., Polonis, V. R., Redfield, R. R., and Birx, D. L., 1994, Serum IgA-mediated neutralization of HIV type 1, *J. Immunol.* **152:**4642–4648.

Butcher, E. C., Rouse, R. V., Coffman, R. L., Nottenburg, C. N., Hardy, R. R., and Weissman, I. L., 1982, Surface phenotype of Peyer's patch germinal center cells: Implications for the role of germinal centers in B cell differentiation, *J. Immunol.* **129:**2698–2707.

Carson, P. J., Schut, R. L., Simpson, M. L., O'Brien, J., and Janoff, E. N., 1995, Antibody class and subclass responses to pneumococcal polysaccharides following immunization of human immunodeficiency virus-infected patients, *J. Infect. Dis.* **172:**340–345.

Chatfield, S. N., Charles, I. G., Makoff, A. J., Oxer, M. D., Dougan, G., Pickard, D., Slater, D., and Fairweather, N. F., 1992, Use of the *nirB* promoter to direct stable expression of heterologous antigen in *Salmonella* oral vaccines strains: development of a single dose oral tetanus vaccine. *Biotechnology* **10:**888–892.

Chin, J., 1991, Global estimates of HIV infection and AIDS cases, *AIDS* **5(Suppl. 2):**557–561.

Coffman, R. L., Shrader, B., Carty, J., Mosmann, T. R., and Bond, M. W., 1987, A mouse T cell product that preferentially enhances IgA production. I. Biologic characterization, *J. Immunol.* **139:**3685–3690.

Coffman, R. L., Lebman, D. A., and Shrader, B., 1989, Transforming growth factor β specifically enhances IgA production by lipopolysaccharide-stimulated murine B lymphocytes, *J. Exp. Med.* **170:**1039–1044.

Conley, M. E., and Delacroix, D. L., 1987, Intravascular and mucosal immunoglobulin A: Two separate but related systems of immune defense? *Ann. Intern. Med.* **106:**892–899.

Coogan, M. M., Sweet, S. P., and Challacombe, S. J., 1994, Immunoglobulin A (IgA), IgA1, and IgA2 antibodies to *Candida albicans* in whole and parotid saliva in human immunodeficiency virus infection and AIDS, *Infect. Immun.* **62:**892–896.

Czinn, S. J., Cai, A., and Nedrud, J. G., 1993, Protection of germ-free mice from infection by *Helicobacter felis* after active oral or passive IgA immunization, *Vaccine* **11:**637–642.

Dalton, D. K., Pitts-Meek, S., Keshav, S., Figari, I. S., Bradley, A., and Steward, T. A., 1993, Multiple defects of immune cell function in mice with disrupted interferon-γ genes, *Science* **259:**1739–1742.

DeFrance, T., Vanbervliet, B., Briére, F., Durand, I., Rousset, F., and Banchereau, J., 1992, Interleukin 10 and transforming growth factor β cooperate to induce anti-CD40-activated naive human B cells to secrete immunoglobulin A, *J. Exp. Med.* **175**:671–682.

De Maria, A., Cirillo, C., and Moretta, L., 1994, Occurrence of human immunodeficiency virus type 1 (HIV-1)-specific cytolytic T cell activity in apparently uninfected children born to HIV-1-infected mothers, *J. Infect. Dis.* **170**:1296–1299.

Deshaw, M., and Pirofski, L. A., 1995, Antibodies to the *Cryptococcus neoformans* capsular glucuronoxylomannan are ubiquitous in serum from HIV^+ and HIV^- individuals, *Clin. Exp. Immunol.* **99**:425–432.

Elson, C. O., Heck, J. A., and Strober, W., 1979, T-cell regulation of murine IgA synthesis, *J. Exp. Med.* **149**: 632–643.

Eriksson, K., Kilander, A., Hagberg, L., Norkrans, G., Holmgren, J., and Czerkinsky, C., 1995, Virus-specific antibody production and polyclonal B-cell activation in the intestinal mucosa of HIV-infected individuals, *AIDS* **9**:695–700.

Fiorentino, D. F., Bond, M. W., and Mosmann, T. R., 1989, Two types of mouse T helper cell. IV. Th2 clones secrete a factor that inhibits cytokine production by Thl clones, *J. Exp. Med.* **170**:2081–2095.

Fujihashi, K., McGhee, J. R.,'Lue, C., Beagley, K. W., Taga, T., Hirano, T., Kishimoto, T., Mestecky, J., and Kiyono, H., 1991, Human appendix B cells naturally express receptors for an respond to interleukin 6 with selective IgAl and IgA2 synthesis, *J. Clin. Invest.* **88**:248–252.

Furuta, Y., Eriksson, K., Svennerholm, B., Fredman, P., Horal, P., Jeansson, S., Vahlne, A., Holmgren, J., and Czerkinsky, C., 1994, Infection of vaginal and colonic epithelial cells by the human immunodeficiency virus type 1 is neutralized by antibodies raised against conserved epitopes in the envelope glycoprotein gp120, *Proc. Natl. Acad. Sci. USA* **91**:12559–12563.

Grossetete, B., Viard, J. P., Lehuen, A., Bach, J. F., and Monteiro, R. C., 1995, Impaired Fc alpha receptor expression is linked to increased immunoglobulin A levels and disease progression in HIV-1-infected patients, *AIDS* **9**:229–234.

Gurram, M., Chirmule, N., Wang, X. P., Ponugoti, N., and Pahwa, S., 1994, Increased spontaneous secretion of interleukin 6 and tumor necrosis factor alpha by peripheral blood lymphocytes of human immunodeficiency virus-infected children, *Pediatr. Infect. Dis. J.* **13**:496–501.

Harriman, G. R., Kunimoto, D. Y., Elliott, J. F., Paetkau, V., and Strober, W., 1988, The role of IL-5 in IgA B cell differentiation, *J. Immunol.* **140**:3033–3039.

Heath, S. L., Tew, J. G., Tew, J. G., Szakal, A. K., and Burton, G. F., 1995, Follicular dendritic cells and human immunodeficiency virus infection, *Nature* **377**:740–744.

Hocini, H., Barra, A., Belec, L., Iscaki, S., Preudhomme, J. L., Pillot, J., and Bouvet, J. P., 1995, Systemic and secretory humoral immunity in the normal human vaginal tract, *Scand. J. Immunol.* **42**:269–274.

Islam, K. B., Nilsson, L., Sideras, P., Hammarström, L., and Smith, C. I. E., 1991, TGF-β1 induces germ-line transcripts of both IgA subclasses in human B lymphocytes, *Int. Immunol.* **3**:1099–1160.

Janoff, E. N., Jackson, S., Wahl, S. M., Thomas, K., Peterman, J. H., and Smith, P. D., 1994, Intestinal mucosal immunoglobulins during human immunodeficiency virus type 1 infection, *J. Infect. Dis.* **170**:299–307.

Janoff, E. N., Wahl, S. M., Thomas, K., and Smith, P. D., 1995, Modulation of human immunodeficiency virus type 1 infection of human monocytes by IgA, *J. Infect. Dis.* **172**:855–858.

Jindal, K. K., Trillo, A., Bishop, G., Hirsch, D., and Cohen, A., 1991, Crescentic IgA nephropathy as a manifestation of human immune deficiency virus infection, *Am. J. Nephrol.* **11**:147–150.

Jones, P. P., and Cebra, J. J., 1974, Restriction of gene expression in B lymphocytes and their progeny. III. Endogenous IgA and IgM on the membranes of different plasma cell precursors, *J. Exp. Med.* **140**:966–976.

Kameoka, M., Nishino, Y., Matsuo, K., Ohara, N., Kimura, T., Yamazaki, A., Yamada, T., and Ikuta, K., 1994, Cytotoxic T lymphocyte response in mice induced by a recombinant BCG vaccination which produces an extracellular alpha antigen that fused with the human immunodeficiency virus type 1 envelope immunodominant domain in the V3 loop, *Vaccine* **12**:153–158.

Kassa, M., Comby, E., Lemeteil, D., Brasseur, P., and Ballet, J. J., 1991, Characterization of anti-Cryptosporidium IgA antibodies in sera from immunocompetent individuals and HIV-infected patients, *J. Protozool.* **38**:179S–180S.

Kato, T., and Owen, R. L., 1994, Structure and function of intestinal mucosal epithelium, in: *Handbook of Mucosal Immunology* (P. L. Ogra, J. Mestecky, M. E. Lamm, S. Warren, J. R. McGhee, and J. Bienenstock, eds.), Academic Press, San Diego, p. 11.

Katz, A., Bargman, J. M., Miller, D. C., Guo, J. W., Ghali, V. S., and Schoeneman, M. J., 1992, IgA nephritis in HIV-positive patients: A new HIV-associated nephropathy? *Clin. Nephrol.* **38**:61–68.

Kawanishi, H., Saltzman, L., and Strober, W., 1983a, Mechanisms regulating IgA class-specific immunoglobulin production in murine gut-associated lymphoid tissues. I. T cells derived from Peyer's patches that switch sIgM B cells to sIgA B cells *in vitro*, *J. Exp. Med.* **157**:433–450.

Kawanishi, H., Saltzman, L., and Strober, W., 1983b, Mechanisms regulating IgA class-specific immunoglobulin production in murine gut-associated lymphoid tissues. II. Terminal differentiation of postswitch sIgA-bearing Peyer's patch B cells, *J. Exp. Med.* **158**:649–669.

Kawanishi, H., Ozato, K., and Strober, W., 1985, The proliferative response of cloned Peyer's patch switch T-cells to syngeneic and allogeneic stimuli, *J. Immunol.* **134**:3586–3591.

Kett, K., Brandtzaeg, P., Radl, J., and Haaijman, J. F., 1986, Different subclass distribution of IgA-producing cells in human lymphoid organs and various secretory tissues, *J. Immunol.* **136**:3631–3635.

Kilian, M., and Russell, M. W., 1994, Function of mucosal immunoglobulins, in: *Handbook of Mucosal Immunology* (P. L. Ogra, J. Mestecky, M. E. Lamm, S. Warren, J. R. McGhee, and J. Bienenstock, eds.), Academic Press, San Diego, p. 127.

Kitani, A., and Strober, W., 1994, Differential regulation of Cα1 and Cα2 germ-line and mature mRNA transcripts in human peripheral blood B cells, *J. Immunol.* **153**:1466–1477.

Kiyono, H., McGhee, J. R., Mosteller, L. M., Eldridge, J. H., Koopman, W. J., Kearney, J. F., and Michalek, S. M., 1982, Murine Peyer's patch T-cell clones. Characterization of antigen-specific helper T cells for immunoglobulin A responses, *J. Exp. Med.* **156**:1115–1130.

Kiyono, H., Cooper, M. D., Kearney, J. F., Mosteller, L. M., Michalek, S. M., Koopman, W. J., and McGhee, J. R., 1984, Isotype-specificity of helper T cell clones. Peyer's patch Th cells preferentially collaborate with mature IgA B cells for IgA responses, *J. Exp. Med.* **159**:798–811.

Kiyono, H., Mosteller-Barnum, L. M., Pitts, A. M., Williamson, S. I., Michalek, S. M., and McGhee, J. R., 1985, Isotype-specific immunoregulation: IgA binding factors produced by Fcα receptor$^+$ T cell hybridomas regulate IgA responses, *J. Exp. Med.* **161**:731–747.

Kopf, M., LeGros, G., Bachmann, M., Lamers, M. C., Bluethmann, H., and Köhler, G., 1993, Disruption of the murine IL-4 gene blocks Th2 cytokine responses, *Nature* **362**:245–248.

Koup, R. A., Safrit, J. T., Cao, Y., Andrews, C. A., McLeod, G., Borkowsky, W., Farthing, C., and Ho, D. D., 1994, Temporal association of cellular immune responses with the initial control of viremia in primary human immunodeficiency virus type 1 syndrome, *J. Virol.* **68**:4650–4655.

Kozlowski, P. A., and Jackson, S., 1992, Serum IgA subclasses and molecular forms in HIV infection: Selective increases in monomer and apparent restriction of the antibody response to IgA1 antibodies mainly directed at *env* glycoproteins, *AIDS Res. Hum. Retrovir.* **8**:1773–1780.

Kozlowski, P. A., Chen, D., Eldridge, J. H., and Jackson, S., 1994, Contrasting IgA and IgG neutralizing capacities and responses to HIV type 1 gp120 V3 loop in HIV-infected individuals, *AIDS Res. Hum. Retrovir.* **10**:813–822.

Kozlowski, P. A., Black, P. B., Shen, L., and Jackson, S., 1995, High prevalence of serum IgA HIV-1 infection-enhancing antibodies in HIV-infected persons. Masking by IgG, *J. Immunol.* **154**:6163–6173.

Kraehenbuhl, J. P., and Neutra, M. R., 1992, Molecular and cellular basis for immune protection of mucosal surfaces, *Physiol. Rev.* **72**:853–879.

Kühn, R., Rajewsky, K., and Müller, W., 1991, Generation and analysis of interleukin-4 deficient mice, *Science* **254**:707–710.

Kuper, C. F., Koornstra, P. J., Hameleers, D. M. H., Biewenga, J., Spit, B. J., Duijvestijn, A. M., van Breda Vriesman, P. J. C., and Sminia, T., 1992, The role of nasopharyngeal lymphoid tissue, *Immunol. Today* **13**: 219–224.

Kutteh, W. H., and Mestecky, J., 1994, Secretory immunity in the female reproductive tract, *Am. J. Reprod. Immunol.* **31**:40–46.

Lagranderie, M., Murray, A., Gicquel, B., Leclerc, C., and Gheorghiu, M., 1993, Oral immunization with recombinant BCG induces cellular and humoral immune responses against the foreign antigen, *Vaccine* **11**: 1283–1290.

Lebman, D. A., and Coffman, R. L., 1988, The effects of IL-4 and IL-5 on the IgA responses by murine Peyer's patch B cell subpopulations, *J. Immunol.* **141**:2050–2056.

Lebman, D. A., and Coffman, R. L., 1994, Cytokines in the mucosal immune system, in: *Handbook of Mucosal Immunology* (P. L. Ogra, J. Mestecky, M. E. Lamm, J. R. McGhee, S. Warren, and J. Bienenstock, eds.), Academic Press, San Diego, p. 243.

Lebman, D. A., Lee, F. D., and Coffman, R. L. 1990a, Mechanism for transforming growth factor β and IL-2 enhancement of IgA expression in lipopolysaccharide-stimulated B cell cultures, *J. Immunol.* **144**:952–959.

Lebman, D. A., Lee, F. D., and Coffman, R. L., 1990b, Molecular characterization of germ-line immunoglobulin A transcripts produced during transforming growth factor type β-induced isotype switching, *Proc. Natl. Acad. Sci. USA* **87:**3962–3966.

Lee, C. K., Weltzin, R., Soman, G., Georgakopoulos, K. M., Houle, D. M., and Monath, T. P., 1994, Oral administration of polymeric immunoglobulin A prevents colonization with *Vibrio cholerae* in neonatal mice, *Infect. Immun.* **62:**887–891.

Lehner, T., Bergmeier, L. A., Panagiotidi, C., Tao, L., Brookes, R., Klavinskis, L. S., Walker, P., Walker, J., Ward, R. G., Hussain, L., Gearing, A. J. H., and Adams, S. E., 1992, Induction of mucosal and systemic immunity to a recombinant simian immunodeficiency viral protein, *Science* **258:**1365–1369.

Lehner, T., Tao, L., Panagiotidi, C., Klavinskis, L. S., Brookes, R., Hussain, L., Meyers, N., Adams, S. E., Gearing, A. J., and Bergmeier, L. A., 1994, Mucosal model of genital immunization in male rhesus macaques with a recombinant simian immunodeficiency virus p27 antigen, *J. Virol.* **68:**1624–1632.

Levy, E., Margalith, M., Sarov, B., Sarov, I., Rinaldo, C. R., Detels, R., Phair, J., Kaslow, R., Ginzburg, H., and Saah, A. J., 1991, Cytomegalovirus IgG and IgA serum antibodies in a study of HIV infection and HIV related diseases in homosexual men, *J. Med. Virol.* **35:**174–179.

Lewis, D. J., Gilks, C. F., Ojoo, S., Castello-Branco, L. R., Dougan, G., Evans, M. R., McDermott, S., and Griffin, G. E., 1994, Immune response following oral administration of cholera toxin B subunit to HIV-1-infected UK and Kenyan subjects, *AIDS* **8:**779–785.

Lim, S. G., Condez, A., and Poulter, L. W., 1993, Mucosal macrophage subsets of the gut in HIV: Decrease in antigen-presenting cell phenotype, *Clin. Exp. Immunol.* **92:**442–447.

Liu, Y.-J., Johnson, G. D., Gordon, J., and MacLennan, I. C. M., 1992, Germinal centers in T-cell dependent antibody responses, *Immunol. Today* **13:**17–21.

London, S. D., 1994, Cytotoxic lymphocytes in mucosal effector sites, in: *Handbook of Mucosal Immunology* (P. L. Ogra, J. Mestecky, M. E. Lamm, S. Warren, J. R. McGhee, and J. Bienenstock, eds.), Academic Press, San Diego, p. 325.

Lubeck, M. D., Natuk, R. J., Chengalvala, M., Chanda, P. K., Murthy, K. K., Murthy, S., Mizutani, S., Lee, S. G., Wade, M. S., Bhat, B. M., Dheer, S. K., Eichberg, J. W., Davis, A. R., and Hung, P. P., 1994, Immunogenicity of recombinant adenovirus–human immunodeficiency virus vaccines in chimpanzees following intranasal administration, *AIDS Res. Hum. Retrovir.* **10:**1443–1449.

Lutzker, S., and Alt, F. W., 1988, Structure and expression of germ line immunoglobulin G2b transcripts, *Mol. Cell. Biol.* **8:**1849–1852.

Lutzker, S., Rothman, P., Pollock, R., Coffman, R. L., and Alt, F. W., 1988, Mitogen and IL-4 regulated expression of germ-line IgG2b transcripts: Evidence for directed heavy chain class switching, *Cell* **53:**177–184.

Lyamuya, E. F., Maselle, S. Y., and Matre, R., 1994, Serum immunoglobulin profiles in asymptomatic HIV-1 seropositive adults and in patients with AIDS in Dar es Salaam, Tanzania, *East Afr. Med. J.* **71:**24–28.

McGhee, J. R., Mestecky, J., Dertzbaugh, M. T., Eldridge, J. H., Hirasawa, M., and Kiyono, H., 1992, The mucosal immune system: From fundamental concepts to vaccine development, *Vaccine* **10:**75–88.

Marinaro, M., Staats, H. F., Hiroi, T., Jackson, R. J., Coste, M., Boyaka, P. N., Okahashi, N., Yamamoto, M., Kiyono, H., Bluethmann, H., Fujihashi, K., and McGhee, J. R., 1995, Mucosal adjuvant effect of cholera toxin in mice results from induction of T helper 2 (Th2) cells and IL-4, *J. Immunol.* **155:**4621–4629.

Marx, P. A., Compans, R. W., Gettie, A., Staas, J. K., Gilley, R. M., Mulligan, M. J., Yamschikov, G. V., Chen, D., and Eldridge, J. H., 1993, Protection against vaginal SIV transmission with microencapsulated vaccine, *Science* **260:**1323–1327.

Mayer, L., and Shlien, R., 1987, Evidence for function of Ia molecules on gut epithelial cells in man, *J. Exp. Med.* **166:**1471–1483.

Mayer, L., Posnett, D. N., and Kunkel, H. G., 1985, Human malignant T-cells capable of inducing an immunoglobulin class switch, *J. Exp. Med.* **161:**134–144.

Mayer, L., Kwan, S. P., Thompson, C., Ko, H. S., Chiorazzi, N., Waldmann, T., and Rosen, F., 1986, Evidence for a defect in "switch" T cells in patients with immunodeficiency and hyperimmunoglobulin M, *N. Engl. J. Med.* **314:**409–413.

Mega, J., McGhee, J. R., and Kiyono, H., 1992, Cytokine- and Ig-producing cells in mucosal effector tissues: Analysis of IL-5 and IFN-γ producing T cells, T cell receptor expression, and IgA plasma cells from mouse salivary gland-associated tissues, *J. Immunol.* **148:**2030–2039.

Mestecky, J., and Jackson, S., 1994, Reassessment of the impact of mucosal immunity in infection with the human immunodeficiency virus (HIV) and design of relevant vaccines, *J. Clin. Immunol.* **14:**259–272.

Mestecky, J., and McGhee, J. R., 1987, Immunoglobulin A (IgA): Molecular and cellular interactions involved in IgA biosynthesis and immune response, *Adv. Immunol.* **40:**153–245.

Mestecky, J., Abraham, R., and Ogra, P. L., 1994, Common mucosal immune system and strategies for the development of vaccine effective at the mucosal surface, in: *Handbook of Mucosal Immunology* (P. L. Ogra, J. Mestecky, M. E. Lamm, S. Warren, J. R. McGhee, and J. Bienenstock, eds.), Academic Press, San Diego, p. 357.

Michetti, P., Mahan, M. J., Slauch, J. M., Mekalanos, J. J., and Neutra, M. R., 1992, Monoclonal secretory immunoglobulin A protects mice against oral challenge with the invasive pathogen *Salmonella typhimurium*, *Infect. Immun.* **60**:1786–1792.

Miller, C. J., Alexander, N. J., Sutjipto, S., Lackner, A. A., Hendrickx, A. G., Gettie, A., Lowenstine, L. J., Jennings, M., and Marx, P. A., 1989, Genital mucosal transmission of simian immunodeficiency virus: Animal model for heterosexual transmission of human immunodeficiency virus, *J. Virol.* **63**:4277–4284.

Miller, C. J., Kang, D. W., Marthas, M., Moldoveanu, Z., Kiyono, H., Marx, P., Eldridge, J. H., Mestecky, J., and McGhee, J. R., 1992a, Genital secretory immune response to chronic simian immunodeficiency virus (SIV) infection: A comparison between intravenously and genitally inoculated rhesus macaques, *Clin. Exp. Immunol.* **88**:520–526.

Miller, C. J., McChesney, M., and Moore, P. F., 1992b, Langerhans cells, macrophages and lymphocyte subsets in the cervix and vagina of rhesus macaques, *Lab. Invest.* **67**:628–634.

Miller, C. J., Marthas, M., Torten, J., Alexander, N. J., Moore, J. P., Doncel, G. F., and Hendrickx, A. G., 1994a, Intravaginal inoculation of rhesus macaques with cell-free simian immunodeficiency virus results in persistent or transient viremia, *J. Virol.* **68**:6391–6400.

Miller, C. J., Vogel, P., Alexander, N. J., Nandekar, S., Hendrickx, A. G., and Marx, P. A., 1994b, Pathology and localization of simian immunodeficiency virus in the reproductive tract of chronically infected male rhesus macaques, *Lab. Invest.* **70**:255–262.

Milman, G., and Sharma, O., 1994, Mechanisms of HIV/SIV mucosal transmission, *AIDS Res. Hum. Retrovir.* **10**:1305–1312.

Morin, M. J., Warner, A., and Fields, B. N., 1994, A pathway for entry of reoviruses into the host through M cells of the respiratory tract, *J. Exp. Med.* **180**:1523–1527.

Morrow, C. D., Porter, D. C., Ansardi, D. C., Moldoveanu, Z., and Fultz, P. N., 1994, New approaches for mucosal vaccines for AIDS: Encapsidation and serial passages of poliovirus replicons that express HIV-1 proteins on infection, *AIDS Res. Hum. Retrovir.* **10(Suppl. 2)**:S61–S66.

Mosmann, T. R., and Coffman, R. L., 1987, Two types of mouse helper T-cell clone, *Immunol. Today* **8**:223–227.

Mosmann, T. R., and Coffman, R. L., 1989, Thl and Th2 cells: Different patterns of lymphokine secretion lead to different functional properties, *Annu. Rev. Immunol.* **7**:145–173.

Mosmann, T. R., Cherwinski, H., Bond, M. W., Giedlin, M. A., and Coffman, R. L., 1986, Two types of murine helper T cell clone. 1. Definition according to profiles of lymphokine activities and secreted proteins, *J. Immunol.* **136**:2348–2357.

Muller, F., Froland, S. S., Hvatum, M., Radl, J., and Brandtzaeg, P., 1991, Both IgA subclasses are reduced in parotid saliva from patients with AIDS, *Clin. Exp. Immunol.* **83**:203–209.

Murray, P. D., McKenzie, D. T., Swain, S. L., and Kagnoff, M. F., 1987, Interleukin 5 and interleukin 4 produced by Peyer's patch T-cells selectively enhance immunoglobulin A expression, *J. Immunol.* **139**:2669–2674.

Nardelli, B., Haser, P. B., and Tam, J. P., 1994, Oral administration of an antigenic synthetic lipopeptide (MAP-P3C) evokes salivary antibodies and systemic humoral and cellular responses, *Vaccine* **12**:1335–1339.

Nehete, P. N., Casement, K. S., Arlinghaus, R. B., and Sastry, K. H., 1995, Studies on *in vivo* induction of HIV-1 envelope-specific cytotoxic T lymphocytes by synthetic peptides from the V3 loop region of HIV-1 IIIB gp120, *Cell. Immunol.* **160**:217–223.

Nilsson, L., Islam, K. B., Olaffsson, O., Zalcberg, I. I., Samakoulis, C., Hammarström, L., Smith, C. I. E., and Sideras, P., 1991, Structure of TGF-β1 induced human immunoglobulin Cα1 and Cα2 germ-line transcripts, *Int. Immunol.* **3**:1107–1115.

Okahashi, N., Yamamoto, M., VanCott, J. L., Chatifield, S. N., Roberts, M., Bluethmann, H., Hiroi, T., Kiyono, H., and McGhee, J. R., 1996, Mucosal immunity in IL-4 knockout mice: Oral administration of recombinant *Salmonella* or cholera toxin elicits $CD4^+$ Th2 cells producing IL-6 and IL-10 and IgA responses, *Infect. Immun.* **64**:1516–1525.

Opstad, N. L., Daley, C. L., Thurn, J. R., Rubins, J. B., Merrifield, C., Hopewell, P. C., and Janoff, E. N., 1995, Impact of Streptococcus pneumoniae bacteremia and human immunodeficiency virus type 1 on oral mucosal immunity, *J. Infect. Dis.* **172**:566–570.

Perra, M. T., Turno, F., and Sirigu, P., 1994, Human urethral epithelium: Immunohistochemical demonstration of secretory IgA, *Arch. Androl.* **32**:227–233.

Phillips, A. N., Sabin, C. A., Elford, J., Bofill, M., Lee, C. A., and Janossy, G., 1993, CD8 lymphocyte counts and serum immunoglobulin A levels early in HIV infection as predictors of CD4 lymphocyte depletion during 8 years of follow-up, *AIDS* **7**:975–980.

Quayle, A. J., Pudney, J., Munoz, D. E., and Anderson, D. J., 1994, Characterization of T lymphocytes and antigen-presenting cells in the murine male urethra, *Biol. Reprod.* **51**:809–820.

Quesnel, A., Pozzetto, B., Moja, P., Grattard, F., Lucht, F. R., Touraine, J. L., Gaudin, O. G., and Genin, C., 1993, Prognostic value of serum immunoglobulin A antibodies to *pol* gene products during HIV-1 infection, *Clin. Exp. Immunol.* **91**:237–240.

Quesnel, A., Moja, P., Blanche, S., Griscelli, C., and Genin, C., 1994a, Early impairment of gut mucosal immunity in HIV-1-infected children, *Clin. Exp. Immunol.* **97**:380–385.

Quesnel, A., Moja, P., Lucht, F., Touraine, J. L., Pozzetto, B., and Genin, C., 1994b, Is there IgA of gut mucosal origin in the serum of HIV-1 infected patients? *Gut* **35**:803–808.

Ramsay, A. J., Husband, A. J., Ramshaw, I. A., Bao, S., Matthaei, K. I., Kohler, G., and Kopf, M., 1994, The role of interleukin-6 in mucosal IgA antibody responses *in vivo*, *Science* **264**:561–563.

Rautonen, J., Rautonen, N., Martin, N. L., Philip, R., and Wara, D. W., 1991, Serum interleukin-6 concentrations are elevated and associated with elevated tumor necrosis factor-alpha and immunoglobulin G and A concentrations in children with HIV infection, *AIDS* **5**:1319–1325.

Rautonen, J., Rautonen, N., Martin, N. L., and Wara, D. W., 1994, HIV type 1 Tat protein induces immunoglobulin and interleukin 6 synthesis by uninfected peripheral blood mononuclear cells. *AIDS Res. Hum. Retrovir.* **10**:781–785.

Reka, S., Garro, M. L., and Kotler, D. P., 1994, Variation in the expression of human immunodeficiency virus RNA and cytokine mRNA in rectal mucosa during the progression of infection, *Lymphokine Cytokine Res.* **13**: 391–398.

Renegar, K. B., and Small, P., 1991, Passive transfer of local immunity to influenza virus infection by IgA antibody, *J. Immunol.* **146**:1972–1978.

Rowland-Jones, S. L., Nixon, D. F., Aldhous, M. C., Gotch, F., Ariyoshi, K., Hallam, N., Kroll, J. S., Froebel, K., and McMichael, A., 1993, HIV-specific cytotoxic T-cell activity in an HIV-exposed but uninfected infant, *Lancet* **341**:860–861.

Sandor, M., Gajewski, T., Thorson, J., Kemp, J. D., Fitch, F. W., and Hoover, R. G., 1990, $CD4^+$ murine T cell clones that express high levels of immunoglobulin binding belong to the interleukin-4 producing T helper cell type 2 subset, *J. Exp. Med.* **171**:2171–2176.

Sastry, K. J., Nehete, P. N., Venkatnarayanan, S., Morkowski, J., Platsoucas, C. D., and Arlinghaus, R. B., 1992, Rapid *in vivo* induction of HIV-specific $CD8^+$ cytotoxic T lymphocytes by a 15-amino acid unmodified free peptide from the immunodominant V3-loop of GP120, *Virology* **188**:502–509.

Schoeneman, M. J., Ghali, V., Lieberman, K., and Reisman, L., 1992, IgA nephritis in a child with human immunodeficiency virus: A unique form of human immunodeficiency virus-associated nephropathy? *Pediatr. Nephrol.* **6**:46–49.

Schwartlander, B., Bek, B., Skarabis, H., Koch, J., Burkowitz, J., and Koch, M. A., 1993, Improvement of the predictive value of $CD4^+$ lymphocyte count by beta 2-microglobulin, immunoglobulin A and erythrocyte sedimentation rate. The Multicentre Cohort Study Group, *AIDS* **7**:813–821.

Seder, R. A., and Paul, W. E., 1994, Acquisition of lymphokine-producing phenotype by $CD4^+$ T cells, *Annu. Rev. Immunol.* **12**:635–637.

Sonoda, E., Matsumoto, R., Hitoshi, Y., Ishii, T., Sugimoto, M., Araki, S., Tominaga, A., Yamaguchi, N., and Takatsu, K., 1989, Transforming growth factor β induces IgA production and acts additively with interleukin 5 for IgA production, *J. Exp. Med.* **170**:1415–1420.

Spalding, D. M., Koopman, W. J., Eldridge, J. H., McGhee, J. R., and Steinman, R., 1983, Accessory cells in murine Peyer's patch: I. Identification and enrichment of function and dendritic cells, *J. Exp. Med.* **157**:1646–1659.

Spalding, D. M., Williamson, S. I., Koopman, W. J., and McGhee, J. R., 1984, Preferential induction of polyclonal IgA secretion by murine Peyer's patch dendritic cell–T cell mixtures, *J. Exp. Med.* **160**:941–946.

Sporn, M. B., Roberts, A. B., Wakefield, L. M., and Assoian, R. K., 1986, Transforming growth factor β: Biologic function and chemical structure, *Science* **233**:532–534.

Staats, H. F., Jackson, R. J., Marinaro, M., Takahashi, I., Kiyono, H., and McGhee, J. R., 1994, Mucosal immunity to infection with implications for vaccine development, *Curr. Opin. Immunol.* **6**:572–583.

Staats, H. F., Nichols, W. G., and Palker, T. J., 1996, Mucosal immunity to HIV-1: Systemic and vaginal antibody responses after intranasal immunization with the HIV-1 C4/V3 peptide T1SP10MN(A), *J. Immunol.* (in press).

Stavnezer, J., Radcliffe, G., Lin, Y. C., Nietupski, J., Berggren, L., Sitia, R., and Severinson, E., 1988, Immunoglobulin heavy-chain switching may be directed by prior induction of transcripts from constant-region genes, *Proc. Natl. Acad. Sci. USA* **85**:7704–7708.

Stavnezer-Nordgren, J., and Sirlin, S., 1986, Specificity of immunoglobulin heavy chain switch correlates with activity of germ-line heavy chain genes prior to switching, *EMBO J.* **5**:95–102.

Stover, C. K., de la Cruz, V. F., Fuerst, T. R., Burlein, J. E., Benson, L. A., Bennett, L. T., Bansal, G. P., Young, J. F., Lee, M. H., Hatfull, G. F., Snapper, S. B., Barletta, R. G., Jacobs, W. R., Jr., and Bloom, B. R., 1991, New use of BCG for recombinant vaccines, *Nature* **351**:456–460.

Street, N. E., and Mosmann, T. R., 1991, Functional diversity of lymphocytes due to secretion of different cytokine patterns, *FASEB J.* **5**:171–177.

Szakal, A. K., Kosco, M. H., and Tew, J. G., 1989, Microanatomy of lymphoid tissue during humoral immune responses. Structure function relationships, *Annu. Rev. Immunol.* **7**:91–109.

Taguchi, T., McGhee, J. R., Coffman, R. L., Beagley, K. W., Eldridge, J. H., Takatsu, K., and Kiyono, H., 1990, Analysis of Th1 and Th2 cells in murine gut-associated tissues. Frequencies of $CD4^+$ and $CD8^+$ T cells that secrete IFN-γ and IL-5, *J. Immunol.* **145**:68–77.

Tew, J. G., Phipps, R. P., and Mandel, T. E., 1980, The maintenance and regulation of humoral immune response. Persisting antigen and the role of follicular antigen-binding dendritic cells as accessory cells, *Immunol. Rev.* **53**:175–201.

Underdown, B. J., and Mestecky, J., 1994, Mucosal immunoglobulins, in: *Handbook of Mucosal Immunology* (P. L. Ogra, J. Mestecky, M. E. Lamm, S. Warren, J. R. McGhee, and J. Bienenstock, eds.), Academic Press, San Diego, p. 79.

Vajdy, M., Kosco-Vilbois, M. H., Kopf, M., Köhler, G., and Lycke, N., 1995, Impaired mucosal immune responses in interleukin 4-targeted mice. *J. Exp. Med.* **181**:41–53.

VanCott, J. L., Staats, H. F., Pascual, D. W., Roberts, M., Chatfield, S., Yamamoto, M., Carter, P. B., Kiyono, H., and McGhee, J. R., 1996a, Regulation of mucosal and systemic antibody responses by T helper cell subsets, macrophages and derived cytokines following oral immunization with live recombinant *Salmonella*, *J. Immunol.* **156**:1504–1514.

VanCott, J. L., Pascual, D. W., Hone, D. M., Chatfield, S. N., Roberts, M., Fujihashi, K., Kiyono, H., and McGhee, J. R., 1996b, A novel approach to insure safety and immunogenicity of live oral *Salmonella* vaccine vectors, *Immunity* (submitted for publication).

Vincent, C., Cozon, G., Zittoun, M., Mellquist, M., Kazatchkine, M. D., Czerkinsky, C., and Revillard, J. P., 1992, Secretory immunoglobulins in serum from human immunodeficiency virus (HIV)-infected patients, *J. Clin. Immunol.* **12**:381–388.

Winner, L., 3d, Mack, J., Weltzin, R., Mekalanos, J. J., Kraehenbuhl, J.-P., and Neutra, M. R., 1991, New model for analysis of mucosal immunity: Intestinal secretion of specific monoclonal immunoglobulin A from hybridoma tumors protects against *Vibrio cholerae* infection, *Infect. Immun.* **59**:977–982.

Xu-Amano, J., Kiyono, H., Jackson, R. J., Staats, H. F., Fujihashi, K., Burrows, P. D., Elson, C. O., Pillai, S., and McGhee, J. R., 1993, Helper T cell subsets for immunoglobulin A responses: Oral immunization with tetanus toxoid and cholera toxin as adjuvant selectively induces Th2 cells in mucosa-associated tissues, *J. Exp. Med.* **178**:1309–1320.

Xu-Amano, J., Jackson, R. J., Fujihashi, K., Kiyono, H., Staats, H. F., and McGhee, J. R., 1994, Helper Th1 and Th2 cell responses following mucosal or systemic immunization with cholera toxin, *Vaccine* **12**:903–911.

Yancopoulos, G. D., DePinho, R. A., Zimmerman, K. A., Lutzker, S. G., Rosenberg, N., and Alt, F. W., 1986, Secondary genomic rearrangement events in pre-B cells. V_HDJ_H replacement by a LINE-1 sequence and directed class switching, *EMBO J.* **5**:3259–3266.

CHAPTER 21

THE PUTATIVE ROLE OF HIV-1 ENVELOPE PROTEINS IN THE NEUROIMMUNOLOGY AND NEUROPATHOLOGY OF CNS AIDS

PRASAD KOKA and JEAN E. MERRILL

1. INTRODUCTION

Cells of the immune and central nervous systems communicate or interact with each other through proinflammatory cytokines (Benveniste, 1994; Black, 1994; Williams *et al.*, 1994). There also exist parallels between the immune and central nervous systems in human immunodeficiency virus type 1 (HIV-1)-mediated secondary effects possibly triggered among others by cytokines leading to pathological abnormalities. In the immune system, although the T-helper cells are affected by the direct infection with HIV-1, other subsets of cells or their function are also altered by the virus, despite the lack of infection of these other cell subsets by the virus. These include the CD8-positive suppressor T cells whose numbers are diminished and/or their cytotoxic function reduced indirectly by the virus (Ho *et al.*, 1993; Watret *et al.*, 1993). Similarly, the ability of B lymphoid cells to provide help to T cells is also affected, although HIV-1 does not productively infect B lymphoid cells (Maggi *et al.*, 1994). Analogously, in the central nervous system (CNS), the blood-borne macrophages infected with the virus carry the virus across the blood–brain barrier to fuse with and infect microglial cells in the brain, and spread the infection to parenchymal microglial cells *in vivo*. While this gives rise to white matter pathology, the neurons in the gray matter of the CNS are not infected by the virus. But the damage done to oligodendrocytes and neurons is again indirect as for non-CD4 cells in the immune system and can occur even in the absence of viral infection of these cells and by interactions between viral envelope proteins and glial cells in the CNS.

Although CD4 is not expressed in parenchymal microglial cells, the virus is able to

PRASAD KOKA • Division of Hematology–Oncology, Department of Medicine, University of California, Los Angeles, California 90095. JEAN E. MERRILL • Department of Immunology, Berlex Biosciences, Richmond, California 94804.
Immunology of HIV Infection, edited by Sudhir Gupta. Plenum Press, New York, 1996.

infect these cells *in vivo* but not *in vitro* as determined in primary mixed glial cultures by polymerase chain reaction (PCR) (Koka *et al.*, 1995a). However, the virus- or its envelope protein (gp160)-mediated effects of cytokine and nitric oxide (NO) induction from these glial cells are evident from experimental studies carried out in our and other laboratories. Therefore, receptors other than CD4 are likely to be involved in viral interactions with glial cells in the CNS to produce pathology in the brain.

In the CNS, it has been shown that gp120 alone is sufficient to trigger pathology in the absence of other viral proteins, both *in vivo* in rodent brains and *in vitro* in primary cultures of glial cells and/or neurons (Brenneman *et al.*, 1994). Envelope protein sequences comparing 430 nucleotides including V3 loop and flanking regions derived from brains of HIV-1-infected demented and nondemented individuals were analyzed for differences in amino acid residues and were found to be significant and possibly associated with the clinical disposition of dementia (Power *et al.*, 1994). It is proposed that the likely mediators of these neuropathological abnormalities in CNS AIDS include the cytokines among other unidentified neurotoxic factors. Abnormal cytokine receptor patterns on neurons were observed when their dendritic processes were labeled with interleukin-1β (IL-1β) and transforming growth factor-β (TGF-β) in human brain neocortex cross sections (Masliah *et al.*, 1994). Cytokines, neurotransmitters, and other excitatory amino acids inducible by HIV-1 may act in coordination to affect cellular metabolic processes of the nervous system even in the absence of productive viral infection and thereby give rise to white and gray matter pathology. This chapter discusses the neuropathology mediated by the HIV-1 envelope proteins possibly through inducement of immune dysregulation in the CNS of HIV-1-infected brains.

2. CNS AIDS: WHITE AND GRAY MATTER PATHOLOGY AND MECHANISMS OF INDUCTION OF NEUROPATHOGENESIS

The CNS AIDS dementia complex which has recently been termed the *HIV-1-associated cognitive-motor complex* is a result of important clinical manifestations in HIV-1-infected brains (Syndulko *et al.*, 1994). The neurological symptoms can occur independently of or precede opportunistic infections arising from immunodeficiency in HIV-1-infected individuals. These symptoms include fever, loss of memory, cognitive and motor dysfunction, and cachexia. The neuropathological conditions associated with HIV-1 infection in the CNS (HIV-1 encephalitis) include microglial nodule formation, astrogliosis, multinucleated giant cell formation, infiltration of blood-derived macrophages, myelin pallor, and damage to or reduction in neurons in some gray matter areas.

A multitude of factors are suggested to be involved in the HIV-1-associated dementia or cognitive-motor complex including the role of HIV-1 envelope glycoprotein (gp160), cellular NO and quinolinic acid mediating cytokine action through altered blood–brain barrier permeability, and the release of arachidonic acid metabolites (Power and Johnson, 1995). An experimental model was proposed for HIV-induced neuropathogenesis involving the action of HIV-activated macrophages resulting in immunologically relevant molecules being produced and functioning as neurotoxins (Gendelman *et al.*, 1994; Lipton, 1994a,b; Epstein and Gendelman, 1993; Tyor *et al.*, 1993a). These toxic substances include the cytokines, IL-1β and tumor necrosis factor-α (TNF-α), and eicosanoids, quinolinate, and NO, which can further activate uninfected macrophages. As a result, glutamate release or decreased glutamate reuptake can occur (Lipton, 1994a). A mechanism involving the activation of voltage-dependent calcium channels and *N*-methyl-D-aspartate (NMDA) receptor-operated channels was proposed (Lipton, 1994a) which may induce NO synthase and NO production presumably by astrocytes (Brosnan *et al.*, 1994), which can be toxic to oligodendrocytes and neurons. Direct infection of the CNS was suggested to play a role in HIV-1-induced neuropathology (Tornatore *et al.*, 1994a; Atwood *et al.*, 1993). HIV-1 infection of astroglial cells revealed the presence of tat-, rev-, and nef-specific mRNAs which were reactivated with IL-1 and TNF-α (Tornatore *et al.*, 1994a,b). HIV-1 infection of astrocytes was proposed to lead to neuronal dysfunction involving dysregulation of growth factors and neurotransmitters and also promote increased permeability of blood–brain barrier (Blumberg *et al.*, 1994). The neurological abnormalities of behavior and pathology described in AIDS brains were also reproduced in rodent model systems *in vivo* and *in vitro* by the HIV-1 envelope glycoprotein (gp120) alone (Brenneman *et al.*, 1994; Hill *et al.*, 1993), suggesting the involvement of secondary substances because of susceptibility to reversal of these neurological abnormalities.

Oligodendrocytes themselves are not known to be infected by HIV-1. HIV-1 infection appears to result in alterations in oligodendrocytes and expression of glial fibrillary acid protein (GFAP) (Pulliam *et al.*, 1993; Weis *et al.*, 1993; Esiri *et al.*, 1991). However, the numbers of oligodendrocytes increase with mild myelin damage and decrease with severe myelin damage in CNS AIDS (Esiri *et al.*, 1991). The HIV-1-induced neuronal damage occurs in the absence of direct viral infection of neurons (Everall *et al.*, 1993) implicating the production and role of secondary factors or neurotoxins such as cytokines produced by fusion between infiltrating blood-derived HIV-1-infected macrophages and brain-derived microglial cells, or by direct interaction between the HIV-1-infected macrophages and microglial cells, or by direct interaction between the HIV-1 envelope proteins circulating in the brain with glial cells. Supporting evidence for these observations is derived not only from experiments on human glial cells lacking expression of CD4 but also from rodent glial cells wherein the species-specific CD4 antigen is essentially nonhomologous to human CD4.

3. INFILTRATION OF HIV-1 ACROSS THE BLOOD–BRAIN BARRIER AND AGE-DEPENDENT INFECTION OF GLIAL CELLS AND NEUROPATHOGENESIS

Although the mechanism of HIV-1 infiltration into and infection of the CNS is not proven, it is presumed that HIV-1 infection of CD4-positive T lymphocytes and macrophages and endothelial cells leads to activation of these cells, and these circulating, activated cells can then infiltrate the blood–brain barrier (Blumberg *et al.*, 1994; Georgsson, 1994; Hurwitz *et al.*, 1994; Moses and Nelson, 1994). Fusion may then occur between the HIV-1-infected macrophages from the blood and brain-derived macrophages and microglia at the blood–brain barrier. The cytokines or other toxic factors secreted by activated or glial cells likely create lesions facilitating the crossing of the blood–brain barrier (Georgsson, 1994). The observation that multinucleated giant cells consist of cells of the monocyte/macrophage lineage and also HIV-specific proteins (Hurwitz *et al.*, 1994) support the role of HIV-1-mediated cytokines in fusions of infected cells to cross the blood–brain barrier.

There are differences in viral infectivity and pathology when human brains of different ages are exposed to HIV-1 *in vivo*. Infection in fetal brain is difficult to detect even by the most sensitive techniques such as PCR or *in situ* hybridization and virus has rarely been isolated from these brains. Furthermore, fetal brain infection was minimal and either latent or defective. The clinical disease is more severe in children than in adults (Vazeux *et al.*, 1992; Sharer *et al.*, 1990) in contrast to the levels of virus present in their brain tissue. It is suggested that maternally acquired HIV-1 infection in children would lead to better cognitive abilities than were previously expected correlating with levels of CD4-positive cells which are predicted to be indicators of future educational achievement based on studies performed on 33 children born before 1985 (Tardieu *et al.*, 1995). Subgenomic HIV-1 or its products were more easily detected in neonatal than fetal brain. Nonetheless, infectivity of neonatal brains is less than that of adult brains. Some of the correlates of early disease in adults, such as gliosis, compare with those in children, but some other correlates of neonates occur late in adults (e.g., encephalopathy). With respect to myelination, it is delayed in pediatric AIDS (Dickson *et al.*, 1989). Very late disease in adults showed some demyelination in the optic nerve and spinal cord as well as neuronal loss (Levy, 1993; Budka, 1991; Kure *et al.*, 1991).

The primary cell type infected *in vivo* by HIV-1 is the macrophage lineage microglial cell (Perry *et al.*, 1994; Tardieu and Janabi, 1994; Levy, 1993; Budka, 1991). In *in vitro* human cultures, astroglioma cell lines or primary fetal astrocytes have been shown to demonstrate very low levels of HIV-1 infection. The infections were usually nonproductive, or defective and did not lead to *in vitro* cytopathicity. In human adult brain, macrophages and microglia were shown to fuse and die after *in vitro* infection by a macrophage-tropic strain of HIV-1 (Watkins *et al.*, 1990). Microglia from adult brain showed productive HIV-1 infection (Lee *et al.*, 1993b). Recently, Hatch *et al.* (1994) detected HIV-1 infection of human fetal primary glial cultures *in vitro*. They detected gp41 and p24 antigens of HIV-1 in infected microglia and astrocytes and also detected viral DNA by PCR and viral RNA in the cytoplasm of CNS by *in situ* hybridization. When human fetal microglia were infected *in vitro*, either a low-level (20%) or no infection was observed (Peudenier *et al.*, 1993; Lee *et al.*, 1993b). When infection occurred, CD4 was not involved and there was no pathology other than syncytium formation (Lee *et al.*, 1993b). It is therefore likely that a non-CD4 receptor exists for HIV-1 entry into brain cells.

There are not many published studies on the HIV-1 infection of primary cultures of human glia and the data are not always in agreement. Koka *et al.* (1995a) examined the infectivity of HIV-1 in these cells. An additional reason for examining the viral infection of glial cells is that the gp160-induced cytokine production from these glial cells may be causing pathology in the CNS even in the absence of a productive viral infection (Koka *et al.*, 1995a). Neither HIV-1 strain NL4-3 (T cell-tropic) nor JR-CSF (macrophage-tropic) ever produced infection in any cultures. HIV-1 JR-FL and recombinant NFN-SX produced no infection in fetal brain cultures and neonatal cultures were infected at low levels and only if cells were in medium containing interleukin 3 (IL-3), granulocyte–macrophage colony-stimulating factor (GM-CSF), and macrophage colony-stimulating factor (M-CSF) designated as CYTO medium. Adult tissue, cultured either in CYTO or in GCT (giant cell tumor supernatant), was also not infected. Despite a lack of infection, some morphological changes occurred in fetal cultures exposed to virus (Koka *et al.*, 1995a), suggesting that a productive viral infection is not required for pathological changes mediated by either HIV-1 or its encoded proteins such as the envelope region gp160.

4. ELEVATION AND PATHOLOGICAL ROLE OF CYTOKINES IN BRAINS OF HIV-1-INFECTED INDIVIDUALS

Because pathology occurs in cells not infected with virus, it is likely that cytokines and/or other toxic molecules (secondary factors) are indirectly at work in CNS AIDS (Merrill and Martinez-Maza, 1993). Cytokines and HIV-1 interact in a pernicious cycle of events in CNS AIDS patients (Merrill, 1992). Cytokines such as IL-1 and TNF-α maintain normal physiological functions within the healthy brain. When these cytokines are elevated during inflammatory disease, they may cause neuropathological damage (Feuerstein *et al.*, 1994; Merrill and Martinez-Maza, 1993; Budka, 1989, 1991; Price *et al.*, 1988).

During disease and trauma, both IL-1 and TNF-α have been associated with white matter lesions, astrogliosis, and vascular changes (Hofman *et al.*, 1986, 1991; Martin *et al.*, 1988; Grau *et al.*, 1987). The number and size of astrocytes contributing to astrogliosis were found to be controlled by IL-1 and TGF-β (de Cunha *et al.*, 1993). Multinucleated giant cell formation is probably induced by leukocyte function-associated antigen-1 (LFA-1) and intercellular adhesion molecule type 1 (ICAM-1) (Hussian *et al.*, 1989; McInnes and Rennick, 1988; Poli *et al.*, 1993; Thornhill *et al.*, 1990; Valentin *et al.*, 1990). Depending on the cell type, ICAM-1 is upregulated by IL-1 and TNF-α (Hurwitz *et al.*, 1994; Jurgensen *et al.*, 1990; Campbell *et al.*, 1989; Dustin *et al.*, 1988) and LFA-1 is induced by IL-3 and/or IL-4 (Frendl and Beller, 1990; Elliott *et al.*, 1990; Rousset *et al.*, 1989). The expression of ICAM-1 on neurons and astrocytes was upregulated by IL-1α, TNF-α, and interferon-γ (IFN-γ) (Hery *et al.*, 1995). It was found that monocytes adhered to both of these cell types and the adhesion was inhibited by monocyte-specific anti-CR3 and neuron-specific anti-ICAM-1 monoclonal antibodies. The adhesion also increased the production of IL-1 and TNF-α from monocytes. TNF-α and TGF-β both upregulate the expression of the chemoattractant protein-1 in astrocytes which may recruit and activate monocytes present at inflammatory sites (Hurwitz *et al.*, 1995), such as those occurring at the blood–brain barrier. Thus, there is a cycle of cytokine-induced adhesion promoting further cytokine production in monocytes. This is also consistent with the model of Gendelman *et al.* (1994) and the adhesion of HIV-infected monocytes/macrophages to astrocytes and neurons may be deleterious to CNS and cause neuronal loss although they are not directly infected by HIV-1. A decreased IL-4 and IL-10 production late in HIV-1 infection may cause increased macrophage function and activity (Tyor *et al.*, 1995). IL-6 may also induce fusion through induction of ICAM-1 (Kurihara *et al.*, 1990). Since IL-1β, IL-6, and TNF-α are elevated *in vivo* in serum, plasma, and cerebrospinal fluid (CSF) and *in vitro* in cultured monocyte supernatants in AIDS patients (Merrill and Chen, 1991), it is likely that these cytokines are responsible for pathological and clinical abnormalities in CNS AIDS. IL-1β inhibits long-term potentiation in the CA3 region of mouse hippocampus leading to inhibition of learning and memory (Katsuki *et al.*, 1990), a cognitive dysfunction associated with CNS AIDS. Multinucleated giant cells (syncytia induced by HIV-1) induced in HIV-1-associated dementia patients decreased on treatment with antiretroviral agents, supporting this as a pathological consequence of HIV-1 infection and mediated by the cytokines (Glass *et al.*, 1993).

The levels of these cytokines were found to be elevated by HIV-1 infection, in serum, CSF, and brain tissue of AIDS patients (Vitkovic *et al.*, 1995; Merrill and Martinez-Maza, 1993). TNF-α levels were found to be elevated in CNS AIDS brain tissue with significantly higher amounts in brains of demented compared to nondemented HIV-positive patients (Wesselingh *et al.*, 1993, 1994; Achim *et al.*, 1993; Glass *et al.*, 1993; Tyor *et al.*, 1992,

1993b) as measured by the intracerebral cytokine mRNA expression in patients with AIDS dementia (Wesselingh *et al.*, 1994). The brain macrophages and microglia in AIDS patients were found to produce higher levels of TNF-α (Tyor *et al.*, 1995). Levels of TNF-α were correlated with spinal cord vacuolar myelopathy and brain encephalitis (Tyor *et al.*, 1992). IL-1 is also elevated in CNS AIDS tissue (Vitkovic *et al.*, 1995).

Using a combination of techniques, including immunohistochemistry for cytokines and *in situ* hybridization for HIV-1, cytokines were detected in HIV-1-infected fixed brains. For example, TGF-β staining was demonstrated in both HIV-1-negative astrocytes and HIV-1-positive microglia in areas of white matter pathology (Wahl *et al.*, 1991). *In situ* hybridization was performed on biopsy specimens to detect IL-1β, IL-6, IL-2, and IFN-γ in lymph nodes from AIDS patients (Emilie *et al.*, 1990). The findings of HIV induction of IL-1, TNF-α, and IL-6 in macrophages and glia are interesting since all three of these cytokines upregulate HIV-1 replication in T cells or macrophages (Levy, 1993; Merrill and Martinez-Maza, 1993; Poli *et al.*, 1990). IL-4 and TNF-α were found to upregulate the HIV-1 mRNA on HIV-1 infection of U-937 cells (Naif *et al.*, 1994). Anti-TNF-α antibodies inhibited HIV-1 replication in virus-infected glial cultures (Wilt *et al.*, 1995). The mechanism for TNF-α stimulation of HIV-1 seems to be promoted through the binding of the transcription factor NF-κB (p50/p65) to the HIV-1 long terminal repeat (Atwood *et al.*, 1994). This could then produce a continuous cycle of pathology and infection within the brain.

The unknown factors that cause secondary pathological events such as changes in myelin in white matter and the loss of neurons in gray matter are not yet understood, but may include elevated levels of cytokines released from brain macrophages and glial cells on HIV-1 infection. It is proposed that the cytokine TNF-α, secreted by microglia, causes apoptotic death of oligodendrocytes in HIV-1 infection (Wilt *et al.*, 1995). TNF-α caused apoptosis in SK-N-MC human neuroblastoma cells that were differentiated to a neuronal phenotype but not in undifferentiated cells (Talley *et al.*, 1995). Since oligodendrocytes and neurons are not infected by HIV-1 (Sharpless *et al.*, 1992; Budka, 1989, 1991), these pathological changes suggest indirect toxicities as the result of exposure to virus. Since cells do not need to be infected to be damaged in CNS AIDS, it is likely the virus may interact with glial cells at the cell surface to induce neurotoxic intermediates some of which, like cytokines, indirectly cause neuropathology.

5. INDUCTION OF CYTOKINES AND NEUROPATHOLOGY IN GLIAL CELLS CAUSED BY THE ENVELOPE PROTEINS OF HIV-1

The cytokines IL-1 and TNF-α were found to be inducible in peripheral blood mononuclear cells and brain glial cells by both live and heat-inactivated HIV-1 (Pulliam *et al.*, 1994; Merrill *et al.*, 1989, 1992). The heat-inactivated virus was, in fact, a stronger inducer than live HIV-1 (Merrill *et al.*, 1992), suggesting that denatured virions express epitopes or domains not exposed in intact virus and that viral infection is not necessary for induction of cytokines. Recombinant gp41 and gp160 produced significant levels of IL-1 and TNF-α from the glial cells. Yeung *et al.* (1995) found that recombinant gp120SF2 induced IL-6 and TNF-α in primary human brain cultures as determined by ELISA and RT-PCR, and showing chromatin condensation of neural cells at longer incubation duration. Binding of antibodies to immunogenic HIV-1 envelope glycoprotein (env), gp160, epitopes suggested that the V3 loop of gp120 and the fusion domain of gp41 were putative inducing sites for cytokine induction by glial cells (Merrill *et al.*, 1992). However, binding of antibodies to gp120/gp41 may induce conformational changes exposing other formerly inaccessible, gp120 or gp41 epitopes which then may bind to cells (Moore *et al.*, 1993, 1994; Kang *et al.*, 1993; Hwang *et al.*, 1992). Since binding of antibodies may alter the conformational structure of gp120/gp41 and thereby the immunogenic domains of the envelope protein, a different strategy was employed to fine map the gp120/gp41 interactions with glia (Koka *et al.*, 1995b). Serial truncations of gp160 from the carboxy-terminus, as expressed through vaccinia virus vectors, were shown to retain their tertiary and posttranslational structure when recombinant viruses were constructed between the vaccinia vector and HIV-1 gp160 (Earl *et al.*, 1991). However, truncation may result in loss of conformational epitopes and residues (Kang *et al.*, 1993; Moore *et al.*, 1993; Earl *et al.*, 1991). Koka *et al.* (1995b) also employed as part of the mapping strategy studies nonglycosylated peptides of gp120/gp41 in conjunction with the serially deleted mutants to determine whether IL-1 and TNF-α were induced by linear or conformational epitopes.

As expected, the full-length gp160 of env:vaccinia virus recombinant vPE16 (851 amino acids) or vPE17 (747 amino acids) produced maximal levels of IL-1 and vPE16 produced maximal levels of TNF-α from mixed rat glial cells compared to other truncation mutants (Koka *et al.*, 1995b). The results suggested that the V3 loop of gp120 is critical for IL-1 production, but not the V3 loop linear peptide. Linear peptides of gp120 in the region V4–C4 were strong inducers of IL-1, but the absence of V4–C4 conformational domains was not important for IL-1 induction. When the env:vaccinia virus recombinant proteins were used to determine the effect of serial deletions of gp160 on TNF-α production, it was found that the carboxy-terminus region, V4–C5, of gp120 and the gp41 were found to be critical. Linear peptides of the V3 loop, C5 of gp120, and the ectodomain of gp41 were strong inducers of TNF-α with almost a full length of gp41 being the maximum inducer of TNF-α. Antibody inhibition of env regions confirmed these findings. Further, the cytokine induction by these env proteins was upregulated at the mRNA level.

The strategy of using serial truncations of env proteins expressed via recombinant vaccinia viruses was also utilized to study cytokine induction by human fetal, neonatal, and adult mixed glial cells (Koka *et al.*, 1995a). The human glial cells were first precultured either in an unknown cocktail of GCT medium or in a medium containing IL-3, GM-CSF, and M-CSF (CYTO). Recently, Lee *et al.* (1994) found that GM-CSF and M-CSF both promote proliferation of human fetal and adult microglia and that GM-CSF is a stronger proliferating agent than M-CSF by more than fivefold on fetal glia and twofold on adult glia and that they also act in synergy. CYTO medium produced more IL-1 and TNF-α than did GCT in fetal and neonatal cells, but the adult cells did better in GCT medium than did fetal or neonatal cells (Koka *et al.*, 1995a). Full-length gp160 vaccinia virus recombinant (vPE16) and gp41 alone were better inducers of IL-1 than those recombinants with deletions in gp41. The V3 loop also was important for IL-1 induction. When heat-inactivated virus strains were used, the macrophage-tropic strain was significantly better than the T-cell-tropic strain at IL-1 induction in all fetal, neonatal, and adult glial cells that were precultured in CYTO.

In contrast to medium/cofactor-dependent differences seen in IL-1 induction, TNF-α induction was the same in GCT and CYTO medium in fetal, neonatal, and adult cultures in response to env:vaccinia recombinants truncated to 635 amino acids or less. Neonatal glial cells produced significantly more TNF-α than did adult or fetal cells, which were not significantly different from each other. In fetal, neonatal, and adult cultures, it is suggested that gp41 is important in TNF-α production (Koka *et al.*, 1995a). gp41 alone produced as much TNF-α as did the full-length env:vaccinia recombinant (vPE16) and heat-inactivated virus. These findings suggest a more important role for gp41 in TNF-α than IL-1 induction. V3 loop is not important in TNF-α production. In fetal cultures, the heat-inactivated macrophage-tropic virus strain induced significantly more TNF-α than did the T-cell-tropic virus strain, but such tropism was not evident in TNF-α induction in neonatal or adult cultures. The heat-inactivated virus and gp41 produced the same amount of TNF-α in all glial cultures when treated separately. Northern blot analysis revealed that the IL-1 and TNF-α were being upregulated in the human glial cells by env proteins at the mRNA level, similar to their rodent counterpart cytokine genes in rat glial cell cultures (Koka *et al.*, 1995b). The levels of IL-1 and TNF-α produced by the cultured primary glial cells are comparable to the elevated levels found to be present in the CSF of patients infected with HIV-1 and suffering from HIV-1-associated cognitive-motor complex (see Koka *et al.*, 1995b).

These results suggest that viral infection is not required and that gp160 epitopes, other than those that bind to CD4, are involved in induction of IL-1 and TNF-α in glial cell cultures. Further, HIV-1 env proteins with closer relevance to their native form, as well as those that are nonglycosylated, could induce proinflammatory cytokines which may be responsible for causing neuropathology in CNS AIDS.

6. ROLE OF NITRIC OXIDE PRODUCTION AND INDUCIBLE NITRIC OXIDE SYNTHASE (iNOS) IN NEUROPATHOLOGY OF HIV-1 INFECTION

During CNS development, death of certain subpopulations of neural cells occurs by necrosis or apoptosis and these are the oligodendrocytes and neurons (Raff, 1992; Merrill *et al.*, 1993; Boje and Arora, 1992; Chao *et al.*, 1992; Cowan *et al.*, 1984). The likely mediators of this cytotoxicity are the brain macrophages and microglia possibly via production of NO (Brosnan *et al.*, 1994; Boje and Arora, 1992; Chao *et al.*, 1992; Merrill *et al.*, 1993). NO possesses multiple roles including as an intercellular messenger and as a toxin to tumor cells and pathogens (Lancaster, 1992). However, NO induced by external stimuli (e.g., viral factors) or as hypothesized to be induced during autoimmune or inflammatory disorders as in HIV-1 infection of CNS can be defensive or deleterious to an individual with such conditions (Milstien *et al.*, 1994; Pietraforte *et al.*, 1994). These NO-mediated consequences in the brain may cause damage to oligodendrocytes and changes in myelin distribution along the axonal tract as well as neuronal injury, seen in neuropathology of CNS AIDS.

The mechanism of gp120-induced production of NO in the brain is discussed by Dawson *et al.* (1994). NO production is induced by a calcium-dependent pathway via activation of nitric oxide synthase (NOS) by calmodulin or by a calcium-independent pathway where the inducing agent of NOS is a cytokine (Dawson *et al.*, 1994; Lancaster, 1992). Cytokines like IL-1 and TNF-α and arachidonic acid metabolites induced by gp120 in brain macrophages and microglia can induce NO by activating the inducible isoform of NOS (iNOS) and human astrocytes have been shown to produce NO in response to cytokines (Brosnan *et al.*, 1994; Dawson *et al.*, 1994; Murphy *et al.*, 1993; Lee *et al.*, 1993a).

Human fetal microglia produce high concentrations of IL-1β which may indirectly cause NO production by stimulation of astrocytes (Lee *et al.*, 1993a,c; Hewett *et al.*, 1993). iNOS has been seen in glial cells in retinas of AIDS patients, suggesting NO as a possible mechanism for CNS damage (Dighiero *et al.*, 1994), and a role for cytokine-induced NO-mediated CNS pathology in AIDS. Other cytokines that can be derived from microglia inhibit NO production, and these include TGF-β, IL-4, and IL-10 (Chao *et al.*, 1993; Simmons *et al.*, 1993; Cunha *et al.*, 1992; Forstermann *et al.*, 1991; Ding *et al.*, 1990). These cytokines also inhibit NO-mediated cytotoxicity to oligodendrocytes and neurons (Chao *et al.*, 1993; Merrill *et al.*, 1993; Gazzinelli *et al.*, 1992). Thus, microglia can be regulatory to NO production via cytokine release which may normally control CNS development, but when the cytokines are overproduced, as in CNS AIDS, it could lead to CNS pathology.

A pediatric patient with advanced AIDS was found to have iNOS mRNA in brain tissue but not in five AIDS patients with early stage disease (Bukrinsky *et al.*, 1995). HIV-1 infection of monocytes increases NO production (Bukrinsky *et al.*, 1995). The cytokine TNF-α further enhances NO production from monocytes and seems to be involved in NO-mediated cytotoxicity of neurons and oligodendrocytes (Bukrinsky *et al.*, 1995; Merrill *et al.*, 1993). Treatment of microglia with antibodies to TNF-α blocks NO production and microglial cytotoxicity of oligodendrocytes (Merrill *et al.*, 1993), although it has not been demonstrated that TNF-α antibodies interfere with microglial cytotoxicity of neurons (Chao *et al.*, 1993). IL-4 may protect neurons from NO-mediated damage because it inhibits TNF-α production (Chao *et al.*, 1993) and also diminishes NO levels in HIV-1-infected monocytes (Bukrinsky *et al.*, 1995). Therefore, inhibition of TNF-α may be a mechanism by which NO production and NO-mediated cytotoxicity are contained.

The severity of HIV-1-induced neurological disease correlated with the presence or absence of iNOS mRNA in AIDS brain tissue (Bukrinsky *et al.*, 1995). The connection between CNS AIDS pathology and NO is probably via HIV-1 induction of cytokines from glial cells. It is proposed that cytokine-induced NO production by astrocytes may be responsible for neurotoxicity in mixed neuronal–glial cultures by the potentiation of NMDA receptors and formation of neurotoxic substances (Hewett and Choi, 1993; Hewett *et al.*, 1994).

7. iNOS SYNTHESIS AND NITRIC OXIDE PRODUCTION IN GLIAL CELLS INDUCED BY HIV-1 ENVELOPE PROTEINS

The finding that gp120 of HIV-1 can induce NO production in certain human brain cells or cultures provides support for the hypothesis that NO may mediate neurological abnormalities associated with HIV-1 cognitive-motor complex and pathology in brains of HIV-1-infected patients. gp120 increased NO production in human monocyte-derived macrophages (Pietraforte *et al.*, 1994). It induced NO-mediated killing of neurons in primary cortical cultures when extracellular glutamate was included (Dawson *et al.*, 1993), and was found to induce iNOS synthesis and NO production in cultured human astrocytoma cells (Mollace *et al.*, 1993). The increase in iNOS activity was calcium independent and the NO production was inhibited by monoclonal antibodies directed against gp120 and also by the iNOS inhibitor, L-NAME (Mollace *et al.*, 1993).

Inhibitors of gp120 mediated neurotoxicity of the constitutive form of NOS (cNOS), activated by stimulation of the NMDA receptor and consequent rise in intracellular calcium (Dawson *et al.*, 1993). In mixed neuronal–glial cultures, superoxide dismutase also inhibits gp120-induced neurotoxicity (Dawson *et al.*, 1993).

Koka *et al.* (1995a) found that fetal glial cells produced more NO_x^- in either GCT or CYTO medium after stimulation with recombinant env proteins compared to medium or HIV-1 p24 core protein controls and supernatants of wild-type WR vaccinia virus. gp160 produced more NO in fetal glial cells cultured in GCT medium but the other proteins were not acted on by CYTO or GCT to produce NO from these glial cells. Env:vaccinia virus recombinants produced less NO than the bacterially derived env proteins. The positive control for NO production used was IFN-γ/IL-1. The V3 loop and amino-terminus of gp120 were not important for NO production. Both gp120 and gp41 induced NO. The production of NO resembled the TNF-α production in response to the envelope proteins. Koka *et al.* (1995a) also demonstrated that the upregulation of NO_x^- production is a consequence of the rise in the level of iNOS mRNA. The induction of iNOS mRNA corroborated the induction of NO in these fetal glial cultures.

8. PRODUCTION OF OTHER gp120-INDUCED SECONDARY NEUROTOXIC FACTORS AND THEIR ROLE IN HIV-1-INDUCED NEUROPATHOGENESIS

In CNS AIDS, it is primarily the macrophages and microglial cells of the brain that are infected with HIV-1. The selective replication of HIV-1 in macrophages and microglia in the nervous system suggests that HIV-1 probably does not directly affect neurons and oligodendrocytes and damage to these cells is via secondary processes. Such processes could occur through secretion of viral antigens from HIV-1 interaction with glial cells as well as events such as production of toxic substances or cytokines. The cytokines, when produced in abnormal concentrations, could dysregulate the normal function of the nervous system. For example, gp120 inhibited the β-adrenergic regulatory functions in astrocytes and microglia possibly mitigating cytokine-mediated defenses against viral and opportunistic infections (Levi *et al.*, 1993).

Using hippocampal structures, Brenneman *et al.* (1988) demonstrated HIV-1 gp120 killing of neural cells. Dreyer *et al.* (1990) have linked gp120 neurotoxicity to the increase in intracellular free calcium in cultures of rodent retinal ganglion cells and hippocampal neurons. In this case, neurons were not infected by HIV-1, but were metabolically altered and eventually died as a result of the binding of HIV-1 proteins to the cell surface. Glowa *et al.* (1992) showed that intracerebral administration of gp120 into adult rats led to cognitive disorders and resulted in impaired memory and learning. Sundar *et al.* (1991) showed that gp120 infusion into rat brains elevated IL-1 and activated the pituitary–adrenal axis. Vasoactive intestinal peptide (VIP) blocked gp120-induced neurotoxicity in culture and a VIP receptor antagonist was neurotoxic in these conditions (Glowa *et al.*, 1992). VIP induced the synthesis of α/β interferon in rat glial cells but not in neurons, possibly protecting the brain from viral infections (Chelbi-Alix *et al.*, 1994). It was reported that a low-molecular-weight heat- and protease-resistant entity from HIV-1-infected macrophages affects neurons *in vitro* (Giulian *et al.*, 1990).

gp120 is known to cause secretion from monocytoid cells of substances that enhance

NMDA receptor-mediated neurotoxicity as well as arachidonic acid and its metabolites and cytokines (Lipton, 1994a,b,c). The enhancement of NMDA receptor-mediated neurotoxicity by substances released by gp120-stimulated macrophages could be either direct or indirect (Lipton *et al.*, 1991; Lipton, 1992).

Some AIDS patients with HIV encephalitis, when treated with zidovudine or 3′-azido-2′,3′-deoxythymidine, showed significant improvement in neurological deficits within a few weeks of treatment (Gray *et al.*, 1994; Portegies *et al.*, 1989, 1991). Such an acute reversal in dementia and ataxia supports the idea that certain abnormal clinical observations are the result of reversible neurological damage related to an indirect effect of the virus on cellular metabolic processes.

9. INVOLVEMENT OF NON-CD4 RECEPTORS IN ENVELOPE PROTEIN INDUCTION OF CYTOKINES, NITRIC OXIDE, AND OTHER SECONDARY SUBSTANCES

Not only the envelope protein but also the tat protein of HIV-1 was found to induce TNF-α, IL-1α/β and IL-6 as well as iNOS mRNA (Philippon *et al.*, 1994). Pentoxifylline reduced IL-1 and iNOS expression as well as the lesions in mouse brain (Philippon *et al.*, 1994). This suggests the importance of non-CD4 receptors causing neuropathological changes in the absence of viral infection. Further, the V3 loop of gp120 appears to be important in the HIV-1 infection of human brain capillary endothelial cells through a CD4- and GalCer-independent receptor, and these cells facilitate the transport of cytokines or other toxic substances from the circulating blood into the brain parenchyma (Moses and Nelson, 1994; Moses *et al.*, 1993). Many examples exist wherein viral epitopes mimic metabolically important ligands and utilize endogenous cell surface molecules to bind or gain entry into cells. The inability of HIV-1 to infect rodent cells but their ability to induce significant and relevant biological consequences *in vitro* and *in vivo* demonstrate (1) a novel brain receptor(s) which is/are not CD4 and (2) viral interaction with brain cells in the absence of infection which lead to pathology. There is evidence to suggest that in the case of neural cells, and even microglia, CD4 may not be the receptor for HIV-1 in the brain to induce pathology (Merrill, 1992). In addition, data from this and other laboratories suggest that HIV-1-induced biological events may occur in the absence of infection and by indirect mechanisms (Merrill *et al.*, 1989; Nakajima *et al.*, 1989; Wahl *et al.*, 1989).

Receptors other than CD4 have been identified for gp120 binding. Antibodies to the lipid galactosylceramide were found to inhibit gp120 binding to it and prevent HIV-1 infection of the neural U373-MG and SK-N-MC cell lines (Bhat *et al.*, 1991). gp120 was shown to bind a 180-kDa receptor protein present on CD4-negative D-54 glioma cells and thereby activate a tyrosine kinase (Schneider-Schaulies *et al.*, 1992). This 180-kDa receptor was not shown to be required for entry of HIV-1 into the glioma cells but its triggering of a signal transduction event could be significant regarding pathogenesis in the human brain in the presence of HIV-1. Further evidence for a non-CD4 receptor is provided by the induction of neurotoxicity by HIV-1 tat peptide analogues via unknown mechanisms, which could also be reduced by blocking NOS and NMDA channels (Hayman *et al.*, 1993). Thus, whether CD4 is the only receptor for infection of human brain cells is in question, although CNS pathology can occur in the absence of viral infection.

10. ANIMAL MODELS TO STUDY HIV ENVELOPE PROTEIN-INDUCED NEUROPATHOGENESIS

Grafting and growth of human brain tissue in animals is a major problem encountered in studying HIV-1-induced pathology in CNS AIDS. Although not the same as human brain and in the absence of infection as well, HIV-1 fortuitously causes pathology when it interacts with rodent brain tissue *in vivo*. Several animal models for retrovirus-induced neuropathogenesis have been developed (reported by Denaro, in Vitkovic *et al.*, 1995). These include the simian immunodeficiency virus causing neuropathogenesis in their respective hosts and the development of HIV-infected human brain implants in severe combined immunodeficient (SCID) mice. Since HIV-1 envelope proteins are capable of causing pathology in rodent brain, gp120-transgenic mice were developed in which neuronal loss was indicated (Toggas *et al.*, 1994). gp120-induced changes in the glial and neuronal cells of these transgenic mice correlated with those occurring in the brains of HIV-1-infected humans. Mice transgenic to IL-6 developed certain neurologic disease indicating that abnormal production of cytokines causes pathology (Campbell *et al.*, 1993). Although not yet performed, it would be interesting to determine if the cytokine levels are elevated in the gp120-transgenic mice. Further, by blocking certain metabolic pathways, the pathology may be reversed or reduced during a condition of constitutive production of gp120-induced cytokines in these transgenic mice.

11. THERAPEUTIC INTERVENTIONS OF NEURONAL INJURY IN HIV-1-INFECTED BRAINS

A positive identification of the nature and metabolic action of the neurotoxic substances produced by microglia would be helpful to design therapeutic strategies to prevent CNS pathology and neuronal injury, the latter damage being irreversible once it has occurred. Voltage-dependent calcium currents may be increased in neurons via the cytokine TNF-α (Soliven and Albert, 1992). IFN-γ can induce production of an NMDA-like agonist and PAF (Heyes *et al.*, 1992; Valone and Epstein, 1988). The cytokines IL-1β and IFN-γ can induce iNOS and NO production in astrocytes (Simmons and Murphy, 1993), which may lead to NMDA receptor-mediated neurotoxicity in mixed neuronal–glial cultures (Hewett *et al.*, 1993, 1994; Hewett and Choi, 1993). In the review articles by Lipton (1994a,b,c), it was suggested that neurotoxin-mediated injury is inhibited by calcium channel and NMDA antagonists and therefore that such reagents be included as part of a regimen to treat CNS AIDS patients. One such inhibitor is pentamidine (Kitamura *et al.*, 1995). Recently, the HIV-1 gp120 was shown to alter Na^+/H^+ transport in astrocytes which was blocked by amiloride or by removal of gp120 leading to neuronal injury (Benos *et al.*, 1994). Proton magnetic resonance spectroscopy is proposed as a useful method to monitor levels of *N*-acetylaspartate (NAA) as an indicator of neuronal loss since lower levels of NAA were found in HIV-infected individuals who were tested and therapeutic interventions to alter NAA levels and consequently decreased neuronal loss may be developed (McConnell *et al.*, 1994). The animal models of CNS AIDS abnormalities are therefore valuable for testing reagents that prevent or reduce neurotoxicity mediated by cytokines or other substances, *in vivo*, in addition to the experiments conducted in *in vitro* culture conditions.

REFERENCES

Achim, C. L., Heyes, M. P., and Wiley, C. A., 1993, Quantitation of human immunodeficiency virus, immune activation factors, and quinolinic acid in AIDS brains, *J. Clin. Invest.* **91**:2769–2775.

Atwood, W. J., Berger, J. R., Kaderman, R., Tornatore, C. S., and Major, E. O., 1993, Human immunodeficiency virus type 1 infection of the brain, *Clin. Microbiol. Rev.* **6**:339–366.

Atwood, W. J., Tornatore, C. S., Traub, R., Conant, K., Drew, P. D., and Major, E. O., 1994, Stimulation of HIV type 1 gene expression and induction of NF-kappaB (p50/p65)-binding activity in tumor necrosis factor alpha-treated human fetal glial cells, *AIDS Res. Hum. Retrovir.* **10**:1207–1211.

Benveniste, E. N., 1994, Cytokine circuits in brain. Implications for AIDS dementia complex, in: *HIV, AIDS, and the Brain*, Volume 72, (R. W. Price and S. W. Perry, eds.) Raven Press, New York, pp. 71–88.

Benos, D. J., Hahn, B. H., Bubien, J. K., Ghosh, S. K., Mashbarn, N. A., Chaikin, M. A., Shaw, G. M., and Benveniste, E. N., 1994, Envelope glycoprotein gp120 of human immunodeficiency virus type 1 alters ion transplant in astrocytes: Implications for AIDS demential complex, *Proc. Natl. Acad. Sci. USA* **91**:494–498.

Bhat, S., Spitalmik, S. L., Gonzalez-Scarano, F., and Silberberg, D. H., 1991, Galactosylceramide or a derivative is an essential component of the neural receptor for human immunodeficiency virus type 1 envelope glycoprotein gp120, *Proc. Natl. Acad. Sci. USA* **88**:7131–7136.

Black, P. H., 1994, Immune system–central nervous system interactions: Effect and immunomodulatory consequences of immune system mediators on the brain, *Antimicrob. Agents Chemother.* **38**:7–12.

Blumberg, B. M., Gelbard, H. A., and Epstein, L. G., 1994, HIV-1 infection of the developing nervous system: Central role of astrocytes in pathogenesis, *Virus Res.* **32**:253–267.

Boje, K. M., and Arora, P. K., 1992, Microglial-produced nitric oxide and reactive nitrogen oxides mediate neuronal cell death, *Brain Res.* **587**:250–256.

Brenneman, D. E., Westbrook, G. L., Fitzgerald, S. P., Ernist, D. L., Elkins, K. L., Rudd, M. R., and Pert, C. B., 1988, Neuronal killing by the envelope protein of HIV and its prevention by vasoactive intestinal peptide, *Nature* **335**:639–642.

Brenneman, D. E., McCune, S. K., Mervis, R. F., and Hill, J. M., 1994, gp120 as an etiologic agent for NeuroAIDS: Neurotoxicity and model systems, *Adv. Neuroimmunol.* **4**:157–165.

Brosnan, C. F., Battistini, L., Raine, C. S., Dickson, D. W., Casadevall, A., and Lee, S. C., 1994, Reactive nitrogen intermediates in human neuropathology: An overview. *Dev. Neurosci.* **16**:152–161.

Budka, H., 1989, Human immunodeficiency virus (HIV) induced disease of the central nervous system: Pathology and implications for pathogenesis, *Acta Neuropathol.* **77**:225–236.

Budka, H., 1991, Neuropathology of human immunodeficiency virus infection, *Brain Pathol.* **1**:163–180.

Bukrinsky, M. E., Nottet, H. S., Schmidtmayerova, H., Dubrovsky, L., Flanagan, C. R., Mullins, M. E., Lipton, S. A., and Gendelman, H. E., 1995, Regulation of nitric oxide synthase activity in human immunodeficiency virus type 1 (HIV-1)-infected monocytes: Implications for HIV-associated neurological disease, *J. Exp. Med.* **181**:735–745.

Campbell, I. L., Cutri, A., Wilkinson, D., Boyd, A. W., and Harrison, L. C., 1989, Intercellular adhesion molecule 1 is induced on isolated endocrine islet cells by cytokines but not by reovirus infection, *Proc. Natl. Acad. Sci. USA* **86**:4282–4286.

Campbell, I. L., Abraham, C. R., Mashih, E., Kemper, P., Inglis, J. D., Oldstone, M. B., and Mucke, L., 1993, Neurologic disease induced in transgenic mice by cerebral overexpression of interleukin 6, *Proc. Natl. Acad. Sci. USA* **90**:10061–10065.

Chao, C. C., Hu, S., Molitor, T. W., Shaskan, E. G., and Peterson, P. K., 1992, Neuroprotective role of IL-4 against activated microglia, *J. Immunol.* **149**:2736–2741.

Chao, C. C., Molitor, T. W., and Hu, S., 1993, Activated microglia mediate neuronal cell injury via a nitric oxide mechanism, *J. Immunol.* **151**:1473–1481.

Chelbi-Alix, M. K., Brouard, A., Boissard, C., Pelaprat, D., Rostene, W., and Thang, M. N., 1994, Induction by vasoactive intestinal peptide of interferon alpha/beta synthesis in glial cells but not in neurons, *J. Cell. Physiol.* **158**:47–54.

Cowan, W. M., Fawcett, J. W., O'Leary, D. D. M., and Stanfield, B. B., 1984, Regressive events in neurogenesis, *Science* **225**:1258–1265.

Cunha, F. Q., Moncada, S., and Liew, F. Y., 1992, Interleukin-10 (IL-10) inhibits the induction of nitric oxide synthase by interferon-gamma in murine macrophages, *Biochem. Biophys. Res. Commun.* **182**:1155–1159.

Dawson, T. M., Dawson, V. L., and Snyder, S. H., 1994, Molecular mechanisms of nitric oxide actions in the brain, *Ann. N.Y. Acad. Sci.* **738**:76–85.

Dawson, V. L., Dawson, T. M., Uhl, G. R., and Snyder, S. H., 1993, Human immunodeficiency virus-1 coat protein neurotoxicity mediated by nitric oxide in primary cortical cultures, *Proc. Natl. Acad. Sci. USA* **90**:3256–3259.

de Cunha, A., Jefferson, J. J., Tyor, W. R., Glass, J. D., Jannotta, F. S., and Vitkovic, L., 1993, Control of astrocytosis by interleukin-1 and transforming growth factor-beta 1 in human brain, *Brain Res.* **631**:39–45.

Dickson, D. W., Belman, A. L., and Park, Y. D., 1989, Central nervous system pathology in pediatric AIDS: An autopsy study, *APMIS Suppl.* **8**:40.

Dighiero, P., Reux, I., Hauw, J.-J., Fillet, A.-M., Courtois, Y., and Gourreau, O., 1994, Expression of nitric oxide synthase in cytomegalovirus infected cells of retinas from AIDS patients, *Neurosci. Lett.* **166**:31–37.

Ding, A., Nathan, C. F., Graycar, J., Derynck, R., Stuehr, D. J., and Srimal, S., 1990, Macrophage deactivating factor and transforming growth factors-beta 1, -beta 2 and -beta 3 inhibit induction of macrophage nitrogen oxide synthesis by IFN-gamma, *J. Immunol.* **145**:940–947.

Dreyer, E. B., Kaiser, P. K., Offermann, J. T., and Lipton, S. A., 1990, HIV-1 coat protein neurotoxicity prevented by calcium channel antagonists, *Science* **248**:364–367.

Dustin, M. L., Sirgen, K. H., Tuck, D. T., and Springer, T. A., 1988, Adhesion of T lymphoblasts to epidermal keratinocytes is regulated by interferon gamma and is mediated by intercellular adhesion molecule 1 (ICAM-1), *J. Exp. Med.* **167**:1323–1340.

Earl, P. L., Koenig, S., and Moss, B., 1991, Biological and immunological properties of human immunodeficiency virus type 1 envelope glycoprotein: Analysis of proteins with truncations and deletions expressed by recombinant vaccinia viruses, *J. Virol.* **65**:31–41.

Ehrenreich, H., Rieckmann, P., Sinowatz, F., Weih, K. A., Arthur, L. O., Goebel, F. D., Burd, P. R., Coligan, J. E., and Clouse, K. A., 1993, Potent stimulation of monocytic endothelin-1 production by HIV-1 glycoprotein 120, *J. Immunol.* **150**:4601–4609.

Elliott, M. J., Vadas, M. A., Cleland, L. G., Gamble, J. R., and Lopez, A. F., 1990, IL-3 and granulocyte–macrophage colony-stimulating factor stimulate two distinct phases of adhesion in human monocytes, *J. Immunol.* **145**:167–176.

Emilie, D., Peuchmaur, M., Maillot, M. C., Crevon, M. C., Brousse, N., Delfraissey, J. F., Dormont, J., and Galanaud, P., 1990, Production of interleukins in human immunodeficiency virus-1-replicating lymph nodes, *J. Clin. Invest.* **86**:148–159.

Epstein, L. G. and Gendelman, H. E., 1993, Human immunodeficiency virus type 1 infection of the nervous system: Pathogenetic mechanism, *Ann. Neurol.* **33**:429–436.

Esiri, M. M., Morris, C. S., and Millard, P. R., 1991, Fate of oligodendrocytes in HIV-1 infection, *AIDS* **5**:1081–1090.

Everall, I., Luthert, P., and Lantos, P., 1993, A review of neuronal damage in human immunodeficiency virus infection: Its assessment, possible mechanism and relationship to dementia, *J. Neuropathol. Exp. Neurol.* **52**:561–566.

Feuerstein, G. Z., Liu, T., and Barone, F. C., 1994, Cytokines, inflammation, and brain injury: Role of tumor necrosis factor-alpha, *Cerebrovasc. Brain Metab. Rev.* **6**:341–360.

Forstermann, U., Schmidt, H. H., Kohlhaas, K. L., and Murad, F., 1992, Induced RAW 264.7 macrophages express soluble and particulate nitric oxide synthase inhibition by transforming growth factor-beta, *J. Pharmacol.* **225**:161–165.

Frendl, G., and Beller, D. I., 1990, Regulation of macrophage activity by IL-3. 1. IL-3 functions as a macrophage-activating factor with unique properties, inducing Ia and lymphocyte function-associated antigen-1 but not cytotoxicity, *J. Immunol.* **144**:3392–3399.

Gazzinelli, R. T., Oswald, I. P., James, S. L., and Sher, A., 1992, IL-10 inhibits parasite killing and nitrogen oxide production by IFN-gamma-activated macrophages, *J. Immunol.* **148**:1792–1796.

Gendelman, H. E., Genis, P., Jett, M., Zhai, Q. H., and Nottet, H. S., 1994, An experimental model system for HIV-1-induced brain injury, *Adv. Neuroimmunol.* **4**:189–193.

Georgsson, G., 1994, Neuropathologic aspects of lentiviral infections, *Ann. N.Y. Acad. Sci.* **724**:50–67.

Giulian, D., Vaca, K., and Noonan, C. A., 1990, Secretion of neurotoxins by mononuclear phagocytes infected with HIV-1, *Science* **250**:1593–1596.

Glass, J. D., Wesselingh, S. L., Selnes, O. A., and McArthur, J. C., 1993, Clinical–neuropathologic correlation in HIV-associated dementia, *Neurology* **43**:2230–2237.

Glowa, J. R., Panlilio, I. V., Brenneman, D. E., Gozer, I., Fridki, M., and Hill, J. M., 1992, Learning impairment following intracerebral administration of the HIV envelope protein gp120 on a VIP antagonist, *Brain Res.* **570**:49–55.

Grau, G. E., Fajardo, L. F., Piguet, P. F., Lambert, P. H., and Vassalli, P., 1987, Tumor necrosis factor (cachetin) as an essential mediator in murine cerebral malaria, *Science* **237**:1210–1212.

Gray, F., Belec, L., Keohane, C., DeTruchis, P., Clair, B., Durigon, M., Sobel, A., and Gherardi, R., 1994, Zidovudine therapy and HIV encephalitis: A 10-year neuropathological survey, *AIDS* **8**:489–493.

Hatch, W. C., Pousada, E., Losev, L., Rashbaum, W. K., and Lyman, W. D., 1994, Neural cell targets of human immunodeficiency virus type 1 in human fetal organotypic cultures, *AIDS Res. Hum. Retrovir.* **10**:1597–1607.

Hayman, M., Arbuthnott, G., Harkiss, G., Brace, H., Filippi, P., Philippon, V., Thomson, D., Vigne, R., and Wright, A., 1993, Neurotoxicity of peptide analogues of the transactivating protein tat from Maedi-Visna virus and human immunodeficiency virus, *Neuroscience* **53**:1–6.

Hery, C., Sebire, G., Peudenier, S., and Tardieu, M., 1995, Adhesion to human neurons and astrocytes of monocytes: The role of interaction of CR3 and ICAM-1 and modulation by cytokines, *J. Neuroimmunol.* **57**:101–109.

Hewett, S. J., and Choi, D. W., 1993, Cytokine-induced nitric oxide production by astroglia potentiates NMDA neurotoxicity in cortical cell cultures, *Soc. Neurosci. Abstr.* **19**:25.

Hewett, S. J., Corbett, J. A., McDaniel, M. L., and Choi, D. W., 1993, Interferon-gamma and interleukin-1 beta induce nitric oxide formation from primary mouse astrocytes, *Neurosci. Lett.* **164**:229–232.

Hewett, S. J., Csernansky, C. A., and Choi, D. W., 1994, Selective potentiation of NMDA-induced neuronal injury following induction of astrocytic iNOS, *Neuron* **13**:487–494.

Heyes, M. P., Saito, K., and Markey, S. P., 1992, Human macrophages convert L-tryptophan to the neurotoxin guinolinic acid, *Biochem. J.* **283**:633–635.

Hill, J. M., Mervis, R. F., Avidor, R., Moody, T. W., and Brenneman, D. E., 1993, HIV envelope protein-induced neuronal damage and retardation of behavioral development in rat neonates, *Brain Res.* **603**:222–233.

Ho, H. N., Hultin, L. E., Mitsuyasn, R. T., Matud, J. L., Hausner, M. A., Bockstoce, D., Chou, C. C., O'Rouke, S., Taylor, J. M., and Giorgi, J. V., 1993, Circulating HIV-specific CD8+ cytotoxic T cells express CD38 and HLA-DR antigens, *J. Immunol.* **150**:3070–3079.

Hofman, F. M., von Harwehr, R. I., Dinarello, C. A., Mizel, S. B., Hinton, D., and Merrill, J. E., 1986, Immunoregulatory molecules and IL2 receptors identified in multiple sclerosis brain, *J. Immunol.* **136**:3239–3245.

Hofman, F. M., Hinton, D. R., Baemayr, J., Weil, M., and Merrill, J. E., 1991, Lymphokines and immunoregulatory molecules in subacute sclerosis panencephalitis, *Clin. Immunol. Immunopathol.* **58**:331–342.

Hurwitz, A. A., Berman, J. W., and Lyman, W. D., 1994, The role of the blood–brain barrier in HIV infection of the central nervous system, *Adv. Neuroimmunol.* **4**:249–256.

Hurwitz, A. A., Lyman, W. D., and Berman, J. W., 1995, Tumor necrosis factor alpha and transforming growth factor beta upregulate astrocyte expression of monocyte chemoattractant protein-1, *J. Immunol.* **57**:193–198.

Hussian, F. A., Coulie, P. G., and van Snick, J., 1989, Distinct roles of IL-1 and IL-6 in human T cell activation, *J. Immunol.* **143**:2520–2524.

Hwang, S. S., Boyl, T. J., Lyerly, H. K., and Cullen, B. R., 1992, Identification of envelope V3 loop as the major determinant of CD4 neutralization sensitivity of HIV-1, *Science* **257**:535–537.

Jurgensen, C. H., Huber, B. E., Zimmerman, T. P., and Wolberg, G., 1990, 3-Deazaadenosine inhibits leukocyte adhesion and ICAM-1 biosynthesis in tumor necrosis factor-stimulated human endothelial cells, *J. Immunol.* **144**:653–661.

Kang, C.-Y., Itaniharan, K., Posner, M. R., and Nara, P., 1993, Identification of a neutralizing epitope conformationally affected by the attachment of CD4 to gp120, *J. Immunol.* **151**:449–457.

Katsuki, H., Nakai, S., Hirai, Y., Akaji, K., Kiso, Y., and Satoh, M., 1990, Interleukin 1β inhibits long-term potentiation in the CA3 region of mouse hippocampal slices, *Eur. J. Pharmacol.* **181**:323–326.

Kitamura, Y., Arima, T., Sato, T., Nakamura, J., and Nomura, Y., 1995, Inhibitory effects of pentamidine on N-methyl-D-aspartate (NMDA) receptor/channels in the rat brain, *Biol. Pharm. Bull.* **18**:234–238.

Koka, P., He, K., Zack, J. A., Kitchen, S., Peacock, W., Fried, I., Tran, T., Yashar, S., and Merrill, J. E., 1995a, HIV-1 envelope proteins induce IL1, TNFα and nitric oxide in glial cultures derived from fetal, neonatal, and adult human brain, *J. Exp. Med.* **182**:941–952.

Koka, P., He, K., Camerini, D., Tran, T., Yashar, S., and Merrill, J. E., 1995b, The mapping of HIV-1 gp160 epitopes required for interleukin-1 and tumor necrosis factor α production in glial cells, *J. Neuroimmunol.* **57**:179–191.

Kure, K., Llena, J. F., Lyman, W. D., Sociro, R., Weidenheim, K. M., Hirano, A., and Dickson, D. W., 1991, Human immunodeficiency virus-1 infection of the nervous system: An autopsy study of 268 adult, pediatric, and fetal brains, *Hum. Pathol.* **22**:700–707.

Kurihara, N., Bertolini, D., Suda, T., Akayama, Y., and Roodman, G. D., 1990, IL-6 stimulates osteoclast-like multinucleated cell formation in long term human marrow cultures by inducing IL-1 release, *J. Immunol.* **144**:4226–4230.

Lancaster, J. R., Jr., 1992, Nitric oxide in cells, *Am. Sci.* **80**:248–259.

Lee, S. C., Dickson, D. W., Liu, W., and Brosnan, C. F., 1993a, Induction of nitric oxide synthase activity in human astrocytes by interleukin-1β and interferon γ, *J. Neuroimmunol.* **46**:19–24.

Lee, S. C., Hatch, W. C., Liu, W., Dress, X., Lyman, W. D., and Dickson, D. W., 1993b, Productive infection of human fetal microglia by HIV-1, *Am. J. Pathol.* **143**:1032–1039.

Lee, S. C., Liu, W., Dickson, D. W., Brosnan, C. F., and Berman, J. W., 1993c, Cytokine production by human fetal microglia and astrocytes, *J. Immunol.* **15**:2659–2667.

Lee, S. C., Liu, W., Brosnan, C. F., and Dickson, D. W., 1994, GM-CSF promotes proliferation of human fetal and adult microglia in primary cultures, *Glia* **12**:309–318.

Levi, G., Patrizio, M., Bernardo, A., Petricci, T. C., and Agresti, C., 1993, Human immunodeficiency virus coat protein gp120 inhibits the beta-adrenergic regulation of astroglial and microglial functions, *Proc. Natl. Acad. Sci. USA* **90**:1541–1545.

Levy, J. A., 1993, Pathogenesis of human immunodeficiency virus infection, *Microbiol. Rev.* **57**:183–210.

Lipton, S. A., 1992, Requirement for macrophages in neuronal injury induced by HIV envelope protein gp120, *Neuroreport* **3**:913–915.

Lipton, S. A., 1994a, AIDS-related dementia and calcium homeostasis, *Ann. N.Y. Acad. Sci.* **747**:205–224.

Lipton, S. A., 1994b, HIV-related neuronal injury. Potential therapeutic intervention with calcium channel antagonists and NMDA antagonists, *Mol. Neurobiol.* **8**:181–196.

Lipton, S. A., 1994c, Neuronal injury associated with HIV-1 and potential treatment with calcium-channel and NMDA antagonists, *Dev. Neurosci.* **16**:145–151.

Lipton, S. A., Sucher, N. J., Kaiser, P. K., and Dryer, E. B., 1991, Synergistic effects of HIV coat protein and NMDA receptor-mediated neurotoxicity, *Neuron* **7**:111–118.

McConnell, J. R., Swindells, S., Ong, C. S., Gmeiner, W. H., Chu, W. K., Brown, D. K., and Gendelman, H. E., 1994, Prospective utility of cerebral proton magnetic resonance spectroscopy in monitoring HIV infection and its associated neurological impairment, *AIDS Res. Hum. Retrovir.* **10**:977–982.

McInnes, A., and Rennick, D. M., 1988, Interleukin 4 induces cultured monocytes/macrophages to form giant multinucleated cells, *J. Exp. Med.* **167**:598–611.

Maggi, E., Gindizi, M. G., Biagidti, R., Annunziato, F., Manetti, R., Piccinni, M. P., Parronchi, P., Sampognaro, S., Giannarini, L., and Zuccati, G., 1994, Th2-like CD8+ T cells showing B cell helper function and reduced cytolytic activity in human immunodeficiency virus type 1 infection, *J. Exp. Med.* **180**:489–495.

Martin, S., Maruta, K., Burkhart, V., Gillis, S., and Kolb, H., 1988, IL-1 and IFN-gamma increase vascular permeability, *Immunology* **74**:301–311.

Masliah, E., Ge, N., Achim, C. L., and Wiley, C. A., 1994, Cytokine receptor alterations during HIV infection in the human central nervous system, *Brain Res.* **663**:1–6.

Merrill, J. E., 1992, Cytokines and retroviruses, *Clin. Immunol. Immunopathol.* **64**:23–27.

Merrill, J. E., and Chen, I. S. Y., 1991, HIV-1, macrophages, glial cells, and cytokines in AIDS nervous system disease, *FASEB J.* **5**:2391–2397.

Merrill, J. E., and Martinez-Maza, O., 1993, Cytokines in AIDS-associated nervous and immune system dysfunction, in: *HIV, AIDS, and the Brain*, Volume 17 (E. B. deSouza, ed.), Academic Press, New York, pp. 243–266.

Merrill, J. E., Koyanagi, Y., and Chen, I. S. Y., 1989, Interleukin-1 and tumor necrosis factor α can be induced from mononuclear phagocytes by human immunodeficiency virus type 1 binding to the CD4 receptor, *J. Virol.* **63**:4404–4408.

Merrill, J. E., Koyanagi, Y., Zack, J., Thomas, L., Martin, F., and Chen, I. S. Y., 1992, Induction of interleukin-1 and tumor necrosis factor alpha in brain cultures by human immunodeficiency virus type 1, *J. Virol.* **66**:2217–2225.

Merrill, J. E., Ignarro, L. J., Sherman, M. P., Melinek, J., and Lane, T. E., 1993, Microglial cell cytotoxicity of oligodendrocytes is mediated through nitric oxide, *J. Immunol.* **151**:2132–2141.

Milstien, S., Sakai, N., Brew, B. J., Krieger, C., Vickers, J. H., Saito, K., and Heyes, M. P., 1994, Cerebrospinal fluid nitrite/nitrate levels in neurologic diseases, *J. Neurochem.* **63**:1178–1180.

Mollace, V., Colasanti, M., Persichini, T., Bagetta, G., Lauro, G. M., and Nistico, G., 1993, HIV gp120 glycoprotein stimulates the inducible isoform of NO synthase in human cultured astrocytoma cells, *Biochem. Biophys. Res. Commun.* **194**:439–445.

Moore, J. P., Thali, M., Jameson, B. A., Vignaux, F., Lewis, G. K., Poon, S.-W., Charles, M., Fung, M. S., Sun, B., Durda, P. J., Akerblom, L., Wahren, B., Ditto, D., Sattentau, Q. J., and Sodroski, J., 1993, Immunochemical analysis of the gp120 surface glycoprotein of human immunodeficiency virus type 1. Probing the structure of the C4 and V4 domains and the interaction of the C5 domain with the V3 loop, *J. Virol.* **67**:4785–4796.

Moore, J. P., Sattentau, Q. J., Waytt, R., and Sodroski, J., 1994, Probing the structure of the human immunodeficiency virus surface glycoprotein gp120 with a panel of monoclonal antibodies, *J. Virol.* **68**:469–475.

Moses, A. V., and Nelson, J. A., 1994, HIV infection of human brain capillary endothelial cells—Implications for AIDS dementia, *Adv. Neuroimmunol.* **4**:239–247.

Moses, A. V., Bloom, F. E., Pauza, C. D., and Nelson, J. A., 1993, Human immunodeficiency virus infection of human brain capillary endothelial cells occurs via a CDR/galactosylceramide-independent mechanism, *Proc. Natl. Acad. Sci. USA* **90**:10474–10478.

Murphy, S., Simmons, M. L., Aqulillo, L., Garcia, A., Feinstein, D. L., Galea, E., Reis, D. J., Minc-Golomb, D., and Schwartz, J. P., 1993, Synthesis of nitric oxide in CNS glial cells, *Trends Neurosci.* **16**:323–328.

Naif, H., Ho-Shon, M., Chang, J., and Cunningham, A. L., 1994, Molecular mechanisms of IL-4 effect on HIV expression in promonocytic cell lines and primary human monocytes, *J. Leuk. Biol.* **56**:335–339.

Nakajima, K., Martinez-Maza, O., Hirano, T., Breen, E. C., Nishanian, P. G., Salazar-Gonzalez, J. F., Fahey, J. L., and Kishimoto, T., 1989, Induction of IL6 (B cell stimulatory factor-2/IFN-β) production by HIV, *J. Immunol.* **142**:531–536.

Perry, V. H., Lawson, L. J., and Reid, D. M., 1994, Biology of the mononuclear phagocyte system of the central nervous system and HIV infection, *J. Leuk. Biol.* **56**:399–406.

Peudenier, S., Itery, C., Montagnier, L., and Tardieu, M., 1993, Human microglial cells characterization in cerebral tissue and in primary culture and study of their susceptibility to HIV-1 infection, *Ann. Neurol.* **29**:152–159.

Philippon, V., Vellutini, C., Gambarelli, D., Harkiss, G., Arbuthnott, G., Metzger, D., Roubin, R., and Filippi, P., 1994, The basic domain of the lentiviral Tat protein is responsible for damages in mouse brain: Involvement of cytokines, *Virology* **205**:519–529.

Pietraforte, D., Tritarelli, E., Testa, U., and Minetti, M., 1994, Gp120 HIV envelope glycoprotein increases the production of nitric oxide in human monocyte derived macrophages, *J. Leuk. Biol.* **55**:175–182.

Poli, G., Bressler, P., Kinter, A., Duh, E., Timmer, W. C., Rabson, A., Justement, J. S., Stanley, S., and Fauci, A. S., 1990, Interleukin 6 induces human immunodeficiency virus expression in infected monocytic cells alone and in synergy with tumor necrosis factor α by transcriptional and post-transcriptional mechanisms, *J. Exp. Med.* **172**:151–160.

Poli, G., Pantaleo, G., and Fauci, A. S., 1993, Immunopathogenesis of human immunodeficiency virus infection, *Clin. Infect. Dis.* **17**:S224–S229.

Portegies, P., deGans, J., Lange, J. M. A., Deux, M. M. A., Speelman, H., Bakker, M., Danner, S. A., and Goudsmit, J., 1989, Declining incidence of AIDS demential complex after induction of zidovudine treatment, *Br. Med. J.* **299**:819–821.

Portegies, P., Algra, P. R., Hollak, C. E., Prins, J. M., Reiss, P., Valk, J., and Lange, J. M., 1991, Response to cytarabine in progressive multifocal leucoencephalopathy in AIDS, *Lancet* **337**:680–681.

Power, C., and Johnson, R. T., 1995, HIV-1 associated dementia: Clinical features and pathogenesis, *Can. J. Neurol. Sci.* **22**:92–100.

Power, C., McArthur, J. C., Johnson, R. T., Griffin, D. E., Glass, J. D., Perrymay, S., and Chesebro, B., 1994, Demented and nondemented patients with AIDS differ in brain-derived human immunodeficiency virus type 1 envelope sequences, *J. Virol.* **68**:4643–4649.

Price, R. N., Brew, B., Sidtis, J., Rosenblum, U., Scheck, A. C., and Cleary, P., 1988, The brain in AIDS: Central nervous system HIV-1 infection and AIDS demential complex, *Science* **939**:586–592.

Pulliam, L., West, D., Haigwood, N., and Swanson, R. A., 1993, HIV-1 envelope gp120 alters astrocytes in human brain cultures, *AIDS Res. Hum. Retrovir.* **9**:439–444.

Pulliam, L., Clarke, J. A., McGuire, D., and McGrath, M. S., 1994, Investigation of HIV-infected macrophage neurotoxin production from patients with AIDS dementia, *Adv. Neuroimmunol.* **4**:195–198.

Raff, M. C., 1992, Social controls on cell survival and cell death, *Nature* **356**:397–400.

Rousset, F., Billaud, M., Blanchard, D., Figdor, C., Lenois, G. M., Spits, H., and De Vries, J. E., 1989, IL-4 induces LFA-1 and LFA-3 expression on Burkitt's lymphoma cell lines. Requirement of additional activation by phorbol myristate acetate for induction of homotypic cell adhesions, *J. Immunol.* **143**:1490–1498.

Schneider-Schaulies, J., Schneider-Schaulies, S., Brinkmann, R., Tas, P., Halbrugge, M., Walter, V., Holmes, H. C., and terMeulen, V., 1992, HIV-1 gp120 receptor on CD4 negative brain cells activates a tyrosine kinase, *Virology* **191**:765–772.

Sharer, L. R., Dowling, P. C., Michaels, J., Cook, J. D., Menonna, J., Blumberg, B. M., and Epstein, L. G., 1990, Spinal cord disease in children with HIV-1 infection: A combined molecular biological and neuropathological study, *Neuropathol. Appl. Neurobiol.* **16**:317–327.

Sharpless, N., Gilbert, D., Vandercam, B., Zhou, J. M., Verdin, E., Ronnett, G., Friedman, E., and Dubois-Dalcq, M., 1992, The restricted nature of HIV-1 tropism for cultured neural cells, *Virology* **191**:813–825.

Simmons, M. L., and Murphy, S., 1993, Cytokines regulate L-arginine-dependent cyclic GMP production in rat glial cells, *Eur. J. Neurosci.* **5**:825–831.

Soliven, B., and Albert, J., 1992, Tumor necrosis factor modulates Ca^{2+} currents in cultured sympathetic neurons, *J. Neurosci.* **12**:2665–2671.

Sundar, S. K., Cierpical, M. A., Kamaraju, L. S., Long, S., Hsieh, S., Lorenz, C., Aaron, M., Richie, J. C., and Weiss, J. M., 1991, Human immunodeficiency virus glycoprotein (gp120) infused into rat brain induced interleukin 1 to elevate pituitary adrenal activity and decrease peripheral cellular immune responses, *Proc. Natl. Acad. Sci. USA* **88**:11246–11250.

Syndulko, K., Singer, E. J., Nogales-Gaete, J., Conrad, A., Schmid, P., and Tourtellotte, W. W., 1994, Laboratory evaluations in HIV-1-associated cognitive/motor complex, *Psychiatr. Clin. North Am.* **17**:91–123.

Talley, A. K., Dewhurst, S., Perry, S. W., Dollard, S. C., Gummuluru, S., Fine, S. M., New, D., Epstein, L. G., Gendelman, H. E., and Gelbard, H. A., 1995, Tumor necrosis factor alpha-induced apoptosis in human neuronal cells: Protected by the antioxidant N-acetylcysteine and the genes bcl-2 and crmA, *Mol. Cell. Biol.* **15**:2359–2366.

Tardieu, M., and Janabi, N., 1994, HIV-1 and the developing human nervous system: In vivo and in vitro aspects, *Dev. Neurosci.* **16**:137–144.

Tardieu, M., Mayaux, M. J., Seibel, N., Funck-Brentano, I., Straub, E., Teglas, J. P., and Blanche, S., 1995, Cognitive assessment of school-age children infected with maternally transmitted human immunodeficiency virus type 1, *J. Pediatr.* **126**:375–379.

Thornhill, M. H., Kyan-Aung, U., and Haskard, D. O., 1990, IL-4 increases human endothelial cell adhesiveness for T cells but not for neutrophils, *J. Immunol.* **144**:3060–3065.

Toggas, S. M., Mashiah, E., Rockenstein, E. M., Rall, G. F., Abraham, C. R., and Mucke, L., 1994, Central nervous system damage produced by expression of the HIV-1 coat protein gp120 in transgenic mice, *Nature* **367**: 188–193.

Tornatore, C., Myers, K., Atwood, W., Conant, K., and Major, E., 1994a, Temporal patterns of human immunodeficiency virus type 1 transcripts in human fetal astrocytes, *J. Virol.* **68**:93–102.

Tornatore, C., Chandra, R., Berger, J. R., and Major, E. O., 1994b, HIV-1 infection of subcortical astrocytes in the pediatric central nervous system, *Neurobiology* **44**:481–487.

Tyor, W. R., Glass, J.-D., Griffin, J. W., Becker, P. S., McArthur, J. C., Begman, L., and Griffin, D. E., 1992, Cytokine expression in the brain during the acquired immunodeficiency syndrome, *Ann. Neurol.* **31**:349–357.

Tyor, W. R., Power, C., Gendelman, H. E., and Markham, R. B., 1993a, A model of human immunodeficiency virus encephalitis in scid mice, *Proc. Natl. Acad. Sci. USA* **90**:8658–8662.

Tyor, W. R., Glass, J. D., Baumrine, N. M., Arthur, J. C., Griffin, J. W., Becker, P. S., and Griffin, D. E., 1993b, Cytokine expression of macrophages in HIV-1 associated vacuolar myelopathy, *Neurology* **43**:1002–1009.

Tyor, W. R., Wesselingh, S. L., Griffin, J. W., McArthur, J. C., and Griffin, D. E., 1995, Unifying hypothesis for the pathogenesis of HIV-associated dementia complex, vacuolar myelopathy, and sensory neuropathy, *J. Acq. Immune Defic. Syndr.* **9**:379–388.

Valentin, A., Lundin, K., Patarroyo, M., and Asjo, B., 1990, The leukocyte adhesion glycoprotein CD18 participates in HIV-1-induced syncytia formation in monocytoid and T cells, *J. Immunol.* **144**:934–937.

Valone, F. H., and Epstein, L. B., 1988, Biphasic platelet-activating factor synthesis by human monocytes stimulated with IL-1β, tumor necrosis factor, or IFN-γ, *J. Immunol.* **141**:3945–3950.

Vazeux, R., Lacroix-Gaudo, C., Blanche, S., Cumont, M.-C., Hemin, D., Gray, F., Boccon-Gibod, L., and Tardieu, M., 1992, Low levels of human immunodeficiency virus replication in the brain tissue of children with severe acquired immunodeficiency syndrome encephalopathy, *Am. J. Pathol.* **140**:149–156.

Vitkovic, L., de Cunha, A., and Tyor, W. R., 1994, Cytokine expression and pathogenesis in AIDS brain, in: *HIV, AIDS, and the Brain*, Volume 72, (R. W. Price and S. W. Perry, eds.) Raven Press, New York, pp. 203–222.

Vitkovic, L., Stover, E., and Koslow, S. H., 1995, Animal models recapitulate aspects of HIV/CNS disease, *AIDS Res. Hum. Retrovir.* **11**:753–759.

Wahl, L. M., Corcoran, M. L., Pyle, S. W., Arthur, L. O., Harel-Bellan, A., and Farrar, W. L., 1989, Human immunodeficiency virus glycoprotein (gp120) induction of monocyte arachidonic acid metabolites and interleukin 1, *Proc. Natl. Acad. Sci. USA* **86:**621–625.

Wahl, S. M., Allen, J. B., McCartney-Francis, N., Morganti-Kossmann, M. C., Kossman, T., Ellingsworth, L., Moi, U. E. H., Mergennagen, S. E., and Orenstein, T. M., 1991, Macrophage and astrocyte derived transforming growth factor β, *J. Exp. Med.* **173:**981–990.

Watkins, B. A., Dorn, H. H., Kelly, W. B., Armstrong, R. C., Potts, B. J., Michaels, F., Kutfta, C. V., and Dubois-Dalcq, M., 1990, Specific tropism of HIV-1 for microglial cells in primary human brain cultures, *Science* **249:** 549–554.

Watret, K. C., Whitetaw, J. A., Froebl, K. S., and Bird, A. G., 1993, Phenotypic characterization of CD8+ T cell populations in HIV disease and in anti-HIV immunity, *Clin. Exp. Immunol.* **92:**93–99.

Weis, S. H., Haug, H., and Budka, H., 1993, Astroglial changes in the cerebral cortex of AIDS brains: A morphometric and immunohistochemical investigation, *Neuropathol. Appl. Neurobiol.* **19:**329–342.

Wesselingh, S. L., Power, V., Glass, J. D., Tyor, W. R., McArthur, J. C., Farber, J.-M., Griffin, J. W., and Griffin, D.-E., 1993, Intracerebral cytokine messenger RNA expression in acquired immunodeficiency syndrome dementia, *Ann. Neurol.* **33:**576–583.

Wesselingh, S. L., Glass, J., McArthur, J. C., Griffin, J. W., and Griffin, D. E., 1994, Cytokine dysregulation in HIV-associated neurological disease, *Adv. Neuroimmunol.* **4:**199–206.

Williams, K., Ulvestad, E., and Antel, J., 1994, Immune regulatory and effector properties of human adult microglia studies in vitro and in situ, *Adv. Neuroimmunol.* **4:**273–281.

Wilt, S. G., Milward, E., Zhou, J. M., Nagasato, K., Patton, H., Rusten, R., Griffin, D. E., O'Connor, M., and Dubois-Dalcq, M., 1995, In vitro evidence for a dual role of tumor necrosis factor-alpha in human immunodeficiency virus type 1 encephalopathy, *Ann. Neurol.* **37:**381–394.

Yeung, M. C., Pulliam, L., and Lau, A. S., 1995, The HIV envelope protein gp120 is toxic to human brain cell cultures through the induction of interleukin-6 and tumor necrosis factor-alpha, *AIDS* **9:**137–143.

CHAPTER 22

IMMUNOPATHOGENESIS OF KAPOSI'S SARCOMA

FELIPE SAMANIEGO and ROBERT C. GALLO

1. INTRODUCTION

Kaposi's sarcoma (KS) is a proliferative disease of vascular origin and is the most frequent tumor of human immunodeficiency virus type 1 (HIV-1)-infected individuals, particularly of homosexual and bisexual men (Friedman-Kien *et al.*, 1981; Havercos *et al.*, 1985; Safai *et al.*, 1985). In patients with acquired immunodeficiency syndrome (AIDS), KS (AIDS-KS) generally has an aggressive and rapid course that is characterized by widely distributed skin lesions, and early dissemination to visceral organs (Safai *et al.*, 1985; Gottlieb and Ackerman, 1982). Other clinical types of KS include classical KS, an indolent disease that affects the lower extremities of elderly men of Mediterranean origin. Iatrogenic KS occurs in 5% of recipients of solid organ transplants, especially those taking glucocorticoids for immune suppression. Endemic KS occurs primarily in men of sub-Saharan Africa origin (Taylor *et al.*, 1972; Slavin *et al.*, 1969).

The early stages of the different clinical types of KS are characterized by the same histopathology: they resemble benign pathology of vascular granulation tissue (Nadji *et al.*, 1981). KS consists of proliferating spindle-shaped cells, termed KS spindle cells, which are the proliferative tumor cell population in these lesions (Ruszczak *et al.*, 1987a; Gottlieb and Ackerman, 1982). Histopathology shows a dense population of endothelial cells that form abnormal vessels, endothelial-lined slit spaces, lymphocyte and mononuclear cell infiltration, and extravasated erythrocytes (Regezi *et al.*, 1993; Gottlieb and Ackerman, 1982). The endothelial and the spindle cells express activation markers and adhesion molecules that bind lymphocytic, monocytic, and dendritic cells (Yang *et al.*, 1994). Thus, immune activation, rather than suppression, is the underlying process in KS. The nodular or late-stage KS lesions are characterized by a predominant spindle cell proliferation and angiogenesis.

Hyperplastic spindle cells derived from KS lesions (AIDS-KS) have been isolated and

FELIPE SAMANIEGO and ROBERT C. GALLO • Institute of Human Virology, Medical Biotechnology Center, University of Maryland, Baltimore, Maryland 21201.

Immunology of HIV Infection, edited by Sudhir Gupta. Plenum Press, New York, 1996.

represent the proliferative cells of early stage KS. Cell lines derived from transformed KS cells (KS Y-1 and KS SLK) have also been established that harbor abnormal chromosomes, are immortalized, and induce lethal tumors in nude mice (Lunardi-Iskandar *et al.*, 1995b; Siegal *et al.*, 1990; Herndier *et al.*, 1994). KS tumors can represent a monoclonal proliferation of cells since a single allele is expressed in tumors from individuals heterozygous for such alleles (Rabkin *et al.*, 1995). Studies in animals reveal that the development of KS tumors is blocked in pregnant mice (Lunardi-Iskandar *et al.*, 1995a,b). The pregnancy hormone human chorionic gonadotropin (hCG) reproduces the antitumor effects associated with pregnancy and induces apoptosis of KS cells (Samaniego *et al.*, 1995a). These findings offer a new perspective on KS pathogenesis and cellular regulation and suggest that hormones can modulate KS cell survival even when cells have clearly acquired a transformed phenotype.

2. CYTOKINES IN KAPOSI'S SARCOMA

2.1. Cytokines in Human Kaposi's Sarcoma Lesions

Homosexual men, the group of HIV-1-infected individuals at highest risk for development of KS, often present with signs of immune system activation (Fan *et al.*, 1993; Janier *et al.*, 1988; Jaffe *et al.*, 1983). They contain in their sera elevated levels of cytokines, such as interleukin-1 (IL-1), IL-6, tumor necrosis factor (TNF) α and β, and interferon-γ (IFN-γ). Serum levels of these cytokines may be elevated in non-HIV-1-infected homosexual males (Fan *et al.*, 1993; Lahdevirta *et al.*, 1988; Lepe-Zanuga *et al.*, 1987). HIV-1-infected individuals also have elevated levels of von Willebrand factor, a product of activated endothelial cells whose release is stimulated by vascular endothelial growth factor (VEGF) (Brock *et al.*, 1991; Janier *et al.*, 1988). Increased inflammatory cytokine levels promote the growth of KS as observed in therapeutic clinical trials of cytokine administration and during acute infections in this patient population (Mitsuyasu, 1994; Aboulafia *et al.*, 1989; Krigel *et al.*, 1985). Normal skin of individuals who have KS contains a significantly higher number of blood vessels, suggesting a systemic defect leading to a generalized vascularization (Ruszczak *et al.*, 1987b). Individuals who have KS and homosexual males at risk for developing KS contain in their bloodstream spindle cells resembling AIDS-KS suggesting a migrating and activated endothelial cell population (Browning *et al.*, 1994b). These spindle cells can also be found associated with lymphoid cells in the normal skin of patients with KS, indicating diffuse skin histopathology (Ruszczak *et al.*, 1987b). Thus, these observations suggest that the high levels of inflammatory cytokines in the setting of a dysregulated immune system are essential to the development of KS.

2.2. Source of Cytokine Production

The stimulus for inflammatory cytokine production in patients with AID-KS is multifactorial. HIV-1-infected individuals are chronically challenged with subclinical and acute infections with viral pathogens, mycoplasma, cytomegalovirus, and other opportunistic organisms. Acute infections coincide with an acceleration of KS disease (Mitsuyasu, 1994). Chronic and repeated infections thus may provide the continuous stimulus for inflammatory cytokine production that contribute to mechanisms in KS lesions (Fig. 1). Few HIV-1-infected cells can be found in KS tissue and normal skin, suggesting a localized

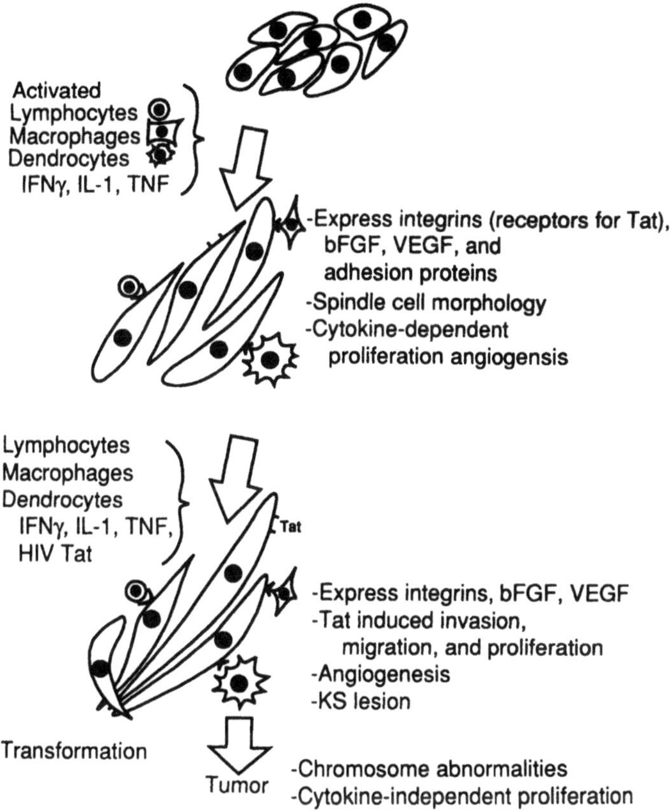

FIGURE 1. A model for the pathogenesis of KS in AIDS. Activated immune cells such as lymphocytes, macrophages, and dendrocytes release inflammatory cytokines (TNF, IL-1, IL-6, IFN-γ) which activate endothelial cells and promote the growth and angiogenic activity of AIDS-KS cells. Few HIV-1-infected dendrocytes can be found in KS tissues and apparently normal skin, suggesting a source for cytokines and HIV-1 Tat. Cytokine-activated endothelial cells adopt new functions including the expression of adhesion molecules (ICAM, VCAM, E-selectin) which bind immune cells, and integrins ($\alpha_5\beta_1$, $\alpha_v\beta_3$) which act as receptors for Tat. Chronic inflammatory cytokine exposure induces a 30-fold increase of bFGF in endothelial cells and induces AIDS-KS cells to secrete VEGF. Both bFGF and VEGF are potent angiogenic cytokines present in KS lesions. The local tissue inflammatory process in turn can activate HIV LTR by inflammatory cytokines (TNF) and promote virus-mediated inflammation and Tat synthesis. AIDS-KS cells respond to inflammatory cytokines by producing an array of cytokines such as bFGF, IL-1, IL-6, IL-8, MCP-1, GM-CSF, and VEGF that magnify the inflammatory response through their autocrine and paracrine pathways. These cytokines of AIDS-KS cells are sufficient to induce KS-like lesions in nude mice. The chronic inflammatory process as well as the continuous oxidizing conditions of inflammation may further contribute to neoplastic transformation. [Figure modified from Ensoli, B., and Gallo, R. C., 1994, Growth factors in AIDS-associated Kaposi's sarcoma: Cytokines and HIV-1 Tat protein, in: *AIDS Updates*, Volume 7 (V. T. DeVita, Jr., S. Hellman, and S. A. Rosenberg, eds.), Lippincott, Philadelphia, p. 1.]

source for inflammation (Mahoney *et al.*, 1991). The recent description of a new virus, herpesvirus 8, in KS lesions and other tumors suggests a link in the pathogenesis of these tumors (Cesarman *et al.*, 1995; Moore and Chang, 1995). The virus, however, has not been detected in the transformed cell lines (KS Y-1 and KS SLK) or in the AIDS-KS 1–14 cell strains, supporting the hypothesis of a bystander role for the virus in KS (results from our laboratory, unpublished). Herpesviruses may exacerbate the course of KS by production of

IFN-γ and other inflammatory cytokines as noted with other infections (Yamamoto *et al.*, 1993) (see below).

Spindle cells of endothelial origin are present in KS lesions and express the same activation markers found in the AIDS-KS spindle cells propagated in culture (Fiorelli *et al.*, 1995; Yang *et al.*, 1994; Regezi *et al.*, 1993). The KS spindle cells appear to represent a functional activated state of endothelial cells (Pober and Cotran, 1990; Nadji *et al.*, 1981). This is in agreement with histological findings indicating that the early stage of KS is characterized by the presence of activated, proliferating endothelial cells that can also be found circulating in the bloodstream (Browning *et al.*, 1994b).

2.3. Effects of Cytokines on Endothelial Cells

The same cytokines that have been found to be elevated in HIV-1-infected homosexual men can induce normal endothelial cells in culture to acquire some of the morphologic characteristics of AIDS-KS spindle cells (Fiorelli *et al.*, 1995; Samaniego *et al.*, 1995c, 1996) which include: the spindle morphology; expression of adhesion molecules that bind inflammatory cells; expression of high levels of membrane integrins which act as receptors for HIV-1 Tat protein; the expression of the angiogenic factors basic fibroblast growth factor (bFGF) and VEGF; and the capacity to form KS-like lesions in nude mice (Table I) (Fiorelli *et al.*, 1995; Samaniego *et al.*, 1995c,d; Ensoli *et al.*, 1989, 1990; Pober and Cotran, 1990). Inflammatory cytokines upregulate the endothelial cell expression of ELAM-1, ICAM-1, and VCAM-1 which are receptors for leukocytes (Yang *et al.*, 1994; Regezi *et al.*, 1993).

2.4. Effects of Cytokines on AIDS-KS Cells

Cultures of KS spindle cells established from KS lesions of HIV-1-infected individuals have been maintained in long-term culture by using conditioned medium (CM) from

TABLE I. Activated T Cells Release Inflammatory Cytokines that Induce Endothelial Cells to Acquire the Phenotypic and Functional Features of AIDS-KS Spindle Cells[a,b]

	Endothelial cells		
Features	Cytokine naive	Cytokine activated	AIDS-KS cells
Spindle-shaped morphology	No	Yes	Yes
Adhesion molecule expression[c] (VCAM, ICAM, LFA)	No	Yes	Yes
Expression of integrin receptors (α5β1 and αvβ3) for Tat	No	Yes	Yes
Expression of bFGF, IL-1, IL-6, GM-CSF	No	Yes[d]	Yes
Expression of IL-8	Yes	Yes	Yes
Proliferation, migration, invasion, and adhesion in response to extracellular HIV-1 Tat	No	Yes	Yes
Induction of KS-like lesions in nude mice	No	Yes	Yes

[a]The supernatant of activated T cells contains inflammatory cytokines that induce endothelial cells to adopt new functions. Endothelial cells treated with CM of T cells or recombinant cytokines contained in CM elicit the phenotype and activities listed.

[b]The results shown are from multiple papers (Samaniego *et al.*, 1995c; Sciacca *et al.*, 1994; Yang *et al.*, 1994; Barillari *et al.*, 1992, 1993; Ensoli *et al.*, 1993; Regezi *et al.*, 1993; Miles *et al.*, 1990; Pober and Cotran, 1990; and our unpublished data).

[c]Adhesion molecules mediate contact with immune cells (ICAM, VCAM, LFA).

[d]A 30-fold elevation of bFGF levels is observed in cytokine-activated endothelial cells.

activated T cells (Nakamura *et al.*, 1988). This CM contains inflammatory cytokines, TNF, IL-1, and IFN-γ, and oncostatin M, which are growth factors for AIDS-KS spindle cells (Miles *et al.*, 1992; Nair *et al.*, 1992). Further, the treatment of AIDS-KS cells, either with this CM or the inflammatory cytokines contained in it, increases the production and release of angiogenic cytokines, the proliferation of endothelial cells induced by KS cells, and ability of cultured spindle cells to induce KS-like lesions after inoculation in nude mice (Samaniego *et al.*, 1995c; Ensoli *et al.*, 1994b). Inflammatory cytokines such as TNF-α, IL-1β, and IFN-γ promote the production and cellular release of bFGF, which functions as an autocrine growth factor (Samaniego *et al.*, 1995c; Ensoli *et al.*, 1989). AIDS-KS cells also produce monocyte chemotactic protein-1 (MCP-1), which recruits leukocytes and induces expression of cell surface adhesion proteins that bind immune cells (Sciacca *et al.*, 1994). The cytokines TNF-α, IL-1β, oncostatin M, and platelet-derived growth factor (PDGF)-BB promote AIDS-KS cells to secrete VEGF, which can mitogenically stimulate endothelial cells (Samaniego *et al.*, 1995d; Werner *et al.*, 1990; Roth *et al.*, 1989). These cytokines induce a synergistic production and release of bFGF and VEGF, two factors with angiogenic and proliferative properties that are coexpressed in the same lesions of AIDS-associated and classical KS (Samaniego *et al.*, 1995d). This suggests that cytokines produced during T-cell activation participate in the progression of KS by stimulating autocrine and paracrine loops of bFGF and VEGF.

3. ANGIOGENESIS IS REGULATED BY CYTOKINES

AIDS-KS spindle cells inoculated into nude mice induce the vascular lesions resembling early KS in humans (Salahuddin *et al.*, 1988). These KS-like lesions are of mouse cell origin, and are characterized by angiogenesis, spindle cell growth, inflammatory cell infiltration, and edema. Thus, KS spindle cells contain the necessary factors sufficient to produce *in vivo* the histological picture of early human KS. AIDS-KS cells produce a variety of cytokines (Table II) that have autocrine functions, form blood vessels, and mediate immune cell binding. They produce bFGF, VEGF, IL-1, IL-6, IL-8, granulocyte–macrophage colony-stimulating factor (GM-CSF), and PDGF, which act on AIDS-KS cells and endothelial cells to promote their growth and further stimulate bFGF production (Miles *et al.*, 1990; Ensoli *et al.*, 1989; Roth *et al.*, 1989). Among these factors, bFGF is an essential

TABLE II. Angiogenic Factors Produced by AIDS-KS Cell Strains[a]

Cytokine	Protein level	Cytokine	Protein level
bFGF	++++	IL-6	++
VEGF	+++	IL-8	++
IL-1α	+	GM-CSF	+
IL-1β	++++	PDGF	++

[a]The results indicate the relative protein levels (low, +; average, ++; high, +++; and highest, ++++) based on Western analysis of cell lysates or ELISA results of cell supernatants or lysates from several reports (Samaniego *et al.*, 1995c,d; Barillari *et al.*, 1992; Miles *et al.*, 1990; Ensoli *et al.*, 1989; Roth *et al.*, 1989; and our unpublished results).

cytokine that acts synergistically with other cytokines to promote vascularization (Pepper *et al.*, 1992). Inoculation of micromolar quantities of bFGF in mice reproduces the histological lesion of KS, suggesting that the inflammatory cytokines promoting the growth of AIDS-KS cells also promote angiogenesis and that both are mediated via bFGF (Ensoli *et al.*, 1994a).

AIDS-KS cells produce and release high levels of bFGF (Samaniego *et al.*, 1995c; Ensoli *et al.*, 1989) as also found in spindle cells in tumors of AIDS-associated and classical KS (Ensoli *et al.*, 1994a; Xerri *et al.*, 1991) (Table II). Inflammatory cytokines mediated their proliferative activity by inducing AIDS-KS cells to produce and release bFGF, a mechanism utilized by cancer cells for vascularization of tumor masses (Samaniego *et al.*, 1995c; Kandel *et al.*, 1991). The proliferation of AIDS-KS cells induced by inflammatory cytokines can be blocked by antibodies to bFGF, indicating disruption of a bFGF autocrine loop (Ensoli *et al.*, 1989). The bFGF that is released from cells is deposited into the extracellular matrix and can be retrieved as active cytokine by heparin, heparinase, and trypsin (Samaniego *et al.*, 1995c; Folkman *et al.*, 1988; Folkman and Klagsbrun, 1987). Antisense oligomers directed to bFGF RNA block KS cell growth and KS lesion formation in nude mice (Ensoli *et al.*, 1994b).

The inflammatory cytokines that promote the proliferation and angiogenic properties of AIDS-KS cells can also induce normal endothelial cells to acquire similar characteristics (Table I). Most importantly, chronic exposure of endothelial cells to TNF-α, IL-1β, and IFN-γ induces 30-fold higher levels of bFGF (Samaniego *et al.*, 1996) and stimulates the cells to release physiologic levels of bFGF, a property shared by tumors with a potent angiogenic response (Kandel *et al.*, 1991). Chronic inflammatory cytokine exposure of endothelial cells at low density promoted production and release of bFGF at physiologic levels that are associated with the capacity to induce angiogenic tumors in mice (Samaniego *et al.*, 1996). This density-dependent bFGF release also operates in cancer cells (Singh *et al.*, 1995). These studies indicate that long-term inflammation endows normal endothelial cells with angiogenic properties that have typically been attributed to cancer cells and suggest that early hyperplastic KS lesions represent preneoplastic growths.

Because of the central role bFGF plays in cell proliferation of KS, many of the antitumor interventions have been targeted against bFGF to block KS cell and tumor growth. Sulfated polysaccharide peptidoglycan and fumagillin inhibit angiogenesis and have antitumor activity (Nakamura *et al.*, 1992; Ingber *et al.*, 1990). IFN-α can reduce the bFGF content of cells and in clinical trials has improved KS disease status (Fidler *et al.*, 1994; Mitsuyasu, 1991; Krown, 1987), indicating that the blocking of bFGF in cell culture and in animal studies also operates in humans. Apolipoprotein E3 blocks bFGF activity in cell culture as well as tumor formation induced by AIDS-KS cells (Browning *et al.*, 1994a).

The florid vascularization and edema of KS indicated to us that other agents were contributing to this histopathology. bFGF by itself causes minimal edema in our animal model system. AIDS-KS cells, as well as KS Y-1 and KS SLK cells, were found to produce VEGF (Table II). In fact, the secretion of VEGF was enhanced by TNF, IL-1, PDGF-BB, and oncostatin M, all factors known to participate in the cytokine cascade of KS lesions (Samaniego *et al.*, 1995d; our unpublished results). AIDS-KS cells produce the 121- and 165-amino-acid isoforms which are two mitogenically active variants of VEGF (Samaniego *et al.*, 1995d). The role of VEGF is underscored by the presence of this angiogenic factor and bFGF in the spindle cells of the same KS lesions. Furthermore, combined VEGF and bFGF lead to synergistic angiogenic activity *in vitro* and *in vivo* (Samaniego *et al.*, 1995d; Pepper *et al.*, 1992).

4. HIV-1 TAT PROTEIN PROMOTES KAPOSI'S SARCOMA CELL PROLIFERATION AND ANGIOGENESIS

4.1. Tat Induces Proliferation, Invasion, and Migration

Classical KS and AIDS-associated KS in their early stage share a similar histologic pattern, but in the setting of AIDS the clinical outcome can be progressive and fatal. The more aggressive course of AIDS-KS appears related in part to the HIV-1 Tat protein. HIV-1 Tat transcriptionally activates viral genes during acute infection and is also released extracellularly as a biologically active protein (Table III) (Ensoli *et al.*, 1993). This released Tat enters other cells (Ensoli *et al.*, 1993) and activates viral and cellular promoters (intercellular transactivation) (Marcuzzi *et al.*, 1992). Tat transactivates cellular genes such as TNF-β through a TAR-like stem loop structure (Buonaguro *et al.*, 1994). Tat induces expression of E-selectin, which is an adhesion protein that binds leukocytes and may contribute to the accumulation of immune cells in KS lesions (Hofman *et al.*, 1993). Tat also induces KS and cytokine-activated endothelial cells to migrate, invade the extracellular matrix, produce collagenase, and proliferate (Ensoli *et al.*, 1994a; Barillari *et al.*, 1992), all steps required for vessel formation. Tat immobilized on plastic surface induces adhesion of both normal vascular cells and KS spindle cells through binding via integrins $\alpha_5\beta_1$ and $\alpha_v\beta_3$ that are upregulated by the cells' prior exposure to inflammatory cytokines and bFGF (Table III) (Barillari *et al.*, 1993). These integrins include the same receptor ($\alpha_v\beta_3$) utilized by endothelial cells in vascular development of tumors (Brooks *et al.*, 1994). Extracellular Tat86 (86 amino acids which contain the RGD amino acid sequence) interacts specifically with integrins in a manner similar to the extracellular matrix proteins fibronectin and vitronectin (Clark and Brugge, 1995; Barillari *et al.*, 1993). Peptides containing an RGD amino acid sequence can block this vascularization by preventing integrin–ligand coupling (Brooks *et al.*, 1994). Transgenic mice with Tat72, which lack the RGD motif, do not develop tumors (O. Prakash, personal communication) while those with Tat86 do develop frequent tumors, suggesting the RGD sequence is necessary for cellular transformation (Vogel *et al.*, 1988). Tat86 transgenic animals show Tat expression in cells surrounding the tumors and not in the tumor cells themselves, implicating the extracellular form of Tat in tumor induction (see below). When Tat protein is inoculated into nude mice, it forms modest histological alterations and coinoculation with subphysiologic concentrations of bFGF can

TABLE III. Effects of HIV-1 Tat Protein on KS Cell and Endothelial Cell Properties[a]

In vitro
1. Induces growth, migration, invasion, and adhesion of spindle cells
2. Induces growth, migration, invasion, tube-formation, and adhesion of cytokine-activated endothelial cells
3. Induces expression of E selectin which mediates leukocyte binding
4. Transcriptionally activates collagenase IV
5. Activated focal adhesion kinase by inducing its phosphorylation
In vivo
6. Potentiates the KS-like lesion formation induced by inoculation of bFGF
7. Promotes the migration of KS Y-1 cells in nude mice
8. Enhances KS Y-1 tumor growth in nude mice

[a]Results from Samaniego *et al.* (1995b), Barillari *et al.* (1992, 1993), Ensoli *et al.* (1990, 1993), Hofman *et al.* (1993), and our *unpublished results*.

induce vascular lesions closely resembling KS (Ensoli *et al.*, 1994a). Because Tat and bFGF coexist in AIDS-KS and only bFGF is present in classical KS (Ensoli *et al.*, 1994a), this suggests that Tat may represent one of the contributing factors responsible for the aggressive clinical course of KS in HIV-1-infected individuals.

4.2. Tat Induces Signal Transduction

In cell culture soluble Tat induces signal transduction by phosphorylating the focal adhesion kinase protein, a regulatory enzyme dependent on integrin–ligand binding for its activation (Clark and Brugge, 1995; Samaniego *et al.*, 1995b; Schlaepfer *et al.*, 1994; Damsky and Werb, 1992). Integrin-mediated signaling confers endothelial cells with the capacity to respond to mitogenic stimuli and this signaling may be the additional stimulus that promotes AIDS-KS cell proliferation over other KS cell types. Normal endothelial cells express low levels of integrin receptor that can be upregulated by inflammatory cytokine treatment and establish the responsiveness to Tat (Barillari *et al.*, 1993). *In vitro*, the proliferative effects of Tat are synergistically augmented by bFGF (Ensoli *et al.*, 1994a). These data may explain why Tat is active on AIDS-KS and cytokine-activated endothelial cells, both of which express high levels of receptors.

The angiogenic and signal transduction activity of Tat can be enhanced by heparin (Samaniego *et al.*, 1995b). Tat contains a highly charged domain similar to the heparin binding domains of growth factors, suggesting that Tat can bind heparin and heparan sulfate of the extracellular matrix. In gel shift assays Tat competes with angiogenic factors for heparin binding, indicating that Tat can potentially displace angiogenic factors occupying heparin binding sites in the extracellular matrix, and ultimately raise angiogenic factor levels (Chang *et al.*, 1995; Folkman *et al.*, 1988; Folkman and Klagsbrun, 1987)

5. MALIGNANT KAPOSI'S SARCOMA CELLS

The progressive and lethal course of KS in the setting of AIDS suggests that KS can progress beyond a cytokine-dependent hyperplasia. In fact, KS has direct involvement in the death of 40% of AIDS patients (Orfanos *et al.*, 1995). In transplant recipients of allogeneic solid organs, KS disease persists in one-half of patients following discontinuation of immunosuppressive drugs. These observations and the common progressive course of late-stage KS, despite chemotherapy, indicate a malignant proliferation. The first malignant KS cell line (KS Y-1) from an AIDS patient was established by Lunardi-Iskandar *et al.* (1995b) in our laboratory. This cell line expresses endothelial cell markers and induces durable metastatic tumors in nude mice (Table IV). KS Y-1 was established from a large volume of pleural effusion that was first depleted of mononuclear cells and selected for adherent cells that survived without exogenous growth factors. A second KS cell line, KS SLK, was isolated from an oral lesion of a kidney transplant patient taking immunosuppressive drugs (Siegal *et al.*, 1990). Both of these cell lines in their early cell passages contain multiple chromosomal rearrangements and marker chromosomes (Table IV) (Lunardi-Iskandar *et al.*, 1995b). Similarly, complex cytogenetic abnormalities were found in early passage cells from KS tumors of HIV-1-infected individuals (Delli Bovi *et al.*, 1986). Interestingly, both the KS Y-1 and KS SLK cell lines contain, in addition to other rearrangements, an identical breakpoint within 3p, suggesting a tumor-specific rearrangement (Lunardi-Iskandar *et al.*, 1995b). In contrast, the AIDS-KS cell strains isolated earlier in our

TABLE IV. AIDS-KS Cell Strains and Malignant KS Cell Lines Express Similar Phenotypic Markers, Are Sensitive to the Cell Kill Effects of hCG, and Induce Tumors in Nude Mice[a]

	Cells		
Features	AIDS-KS 1–14	KS Y-1	KS SLK
CD 34	++	+++	NA[b]
ICAM	++	++	NA
UEA-1 receptor	+++	++	+
CD31	+++	+++	NA
Karyotype	Diploid 46XY	Tetraploid markers	Tetraploid markers
Tumor induction in nude mice	Transient KS-like	Lethal angiogenic	Lethal angiogenic
Cells killed by hCG	Yes	Yes	Yes
Clonal cell	NA	Yes	Yes
Herpesvirus 8 DNA sequences in cells	No	No	No

[a]Results from Fiorelli *et al.* (1995), Lunardi-Iskandar *et al.* (1995a,b), Samaniego *et al.* (1995a), Siegal *et al.* (1990), Nakamura *et al.* (1988), and Salahuddin *et al.* (1988).
[b]NA, not available.

laboratory (AIDS-KS 1–14) contain normal diploid karyotypes (Salahuddin *et al.*, 1988), in agreement with their hyperplastic phenotype. There is no clear etiology for transformation of KS cells. The single underlying force behind AIDS-KS spindle cell proliferation is an inflammatory process and that same process contributes to neoplastic transformation in other active inflammatory disorders such as ulcerative colitis and chronic osteomyelitis (Biasco *et al.*, 1990; Hejna, 1965).

A genetic marker for detection of KS is not available. Because other clinical entities such as hemangioma, bacillary angiomatosis, orf virus infections, and cat scratch disease can result in similar histopathology and require divergent treatments, a diagnostic marker for KS would aid in assigning etiology and appropriate treatment. The identification of a specific genetic marker can also help define the pathogenetic series of events leading to KS. KS may follow the pattern of malignant cell development of Hodgkin's disease where the malignant cells are present at inception of tumor, but are outnumbered and thus obscured by the hyperplastic cell population.

Monoclonal cell expansion in KS has been suggested by Rabkin *et al.* (1995) who examined gene inactivation of paired alleles. A high percentage of women are heterozygous for allelic expression of the androgen receptor and each cell expresses one of two alleles based on random inactivation by DNA methylation. In the small series of cases, late-stage KS tumors expressed only one of two alleles in individuals heterozygous for the androgen receptor (Rabkin *et al.*, 1995). The results in this study suggest that a clonal expansion occurs in late-stage KS and indirectly support the concept that KS is a transformed cell.

6. THE PREGNANCY HORMONE HUMAN CHORIONIC GONADOTROPIN INDUCES APOPTOSIS OF KAPOSI'S SARCOMA CELLS

The establishment of an AIDS-related malignant KS cell line makes available for the first time an *in vivo* model for the testing of therapeutic interventions. All prior investigations for treatment of KS have depended on human trials after very limited preclinical screening. During the characterization of the KS Y-1 cells in animals, some unexpected results were noted: immunodeficient neonatal mice inoculated with KS Y-1 cells routinely developed tumors, but in one particular group none of the females that became pregnant showed tumor development (Lunardi-Iskandar *et al.*, 1995a). This observation led to the hypothesis that the systemic manifestations of pregnancy inhibited KS cell growth. The observation was confirmed. Sera from pregnant mice and humans inhibited colony formation of KS Y-1 and KS SLK cells, suggesting a circulating antitumor factor. During human pregnancy, the serum contains high levels of hormones, hCG, free hCG-α, and free hCG-β. Pregnant mice contain chorionic gonadotropin-like activity in their sera that is maximal during midgestation. It appeared that these hormones or the immunomodulation associated with pregnancy might be mediating antitumor activity. The former was the cause since purified hCG and hCG-β directly inhibited colony formation in clonogenic assays and also prevented tumor formation in mice inoculated with KS Y-1 and KS SLK cells treated *ex vivo* with hCG. hCG-treated tumors stained for DNA termini showed high activity in the dying cell population. Using various methods, such as genomic DNA isolation and confocal microscopy, hCG was shown to induce programmed cell death (Samaniego *et al.*, 1995a). KS lesions stained for hCG receptors contain highly positive staining cells and KS cells in culture contain a candidate receptor that can be cross-linked with radiolabeled hCG and specifically blocked by cold hCG-β (Lunardi-Iskandar *et al.*, 1995a). In culture hCG kills KS Y-1, KS SLK, and AIDS-KS cell strains by inducing apoptosis (Samaniego *et al.*, 1995a).

Clinical trials of intralesional hCG treatment for KS have shown a total response rate (complete and partial response) of greater than 80% without any of the untoward effects commonly associated with conventional combination chemotherapy (our unpublished results). Interestingly, patients receiving hCG had an overall improvement in health status such as an increase in body weight and overall well-being, suggesting that effects beyond antitumor activity are operating.

AIDS-associated, classical, and endemic KS are diseases with a significantly higher incidence in males. In two transgenic models with HIV Tat, the disease is more severe in males (Corallini *et al.*, 1993; Vogel *et al.*, 1988). In women of childbearing age, the hCG-like hormones, follicle-stimulating hormone and luteinizing hormone, are intermittently high during the menstrual cycle. The biological cross-reactivity expressed by these hormones suggests that women may be protected from endothelial and related cell proliferation which may account for the gender-based difference in the prevalence of KS.

ACKNOWLEDGMENTS. We thank our colleagues for providing some of the unpublished data; in particular, B. Ensoli, Y. Lunardi-Iskandar, and J. Bryant.

REFERENCES

Aboulafia, D., Miles, S. A., Saks, S. R., and Mitsuyasu, R. T., 1989, Intravenous recombinant tumor necrosis factor in the treatment of AIDS-related Kaposi's sarcoma, *J. Acq. Immune Defic. Syndr.* **2**:54–58.

Barillari, G., Buonaguro, L., Fiorelli, V., Hoffman, J., Michaels, F., Gallo, R. C., and Ensoli, B., 1992, Effects of cytokines from activated immune cells on vascular cell growth and HIV-1 gene expression: Implications for AIDS-Kaposi's sarcoma pathogenesis, *J. Immunol.* **149**:3727–3734.

Barillari, G., Gendelman, R., Gallo, R. C., and Ensoli, B., 1993, The Tat protein of human immunodeficiency virus type 1, a growth factor for AIDS Kaposi sarcoma and cytokine-activated vascular cells, induces adhesion of the same cell types by using integrin receptors recognizing RGD amino acid sequence, *Proc. Natl. Acad. Sci. USA* **90:**7941–7945.

Biasco, G., Paganelli, G. M., Miglioli, M., Brillanti, S., DiFebo, G., Gizzi, G., Ponz de Leon, M., Campieri, M., and Barbara, L., 1990, Rectal cell proliferation and colon cancer risk in ulcerative colitis, *Cancer Res.* **50:**1156–1159.

Brock, T. A., Dvork H. F., and Senger, D. R., 1991, Tumor-secreted vascular permeability factor increases cytosolic Ca^{2+} and von Willebrand factor release in human endothelial cells, *Am. J. Pathol.* **138:**213–221.

Brooks, P. C., Clark, R. A. F., and Cheresh, D. A., 1994, Requirement of vascular integrin $\alpha v\beta 3$ for angiogenesis, *Science* **264:**569–571.

Browning, P. J., Roberts, D. D., Zabrenetzky, V., Bryant, J., Kaplan, M., Washington, R. H., Panet, A., Gallo, R. C., and Vogel, T., 1994a, Apolipoprotein E (Apo E), a novel heparin-binding protein inhibits the development of Kaposi's sarcoma-like lesions in Balb/c nu/nu mice, *J. Exp. Med.* **180:**1949–1954.

Browning, P. J., Sechler, J. M., Kaplan, M., Washington, R. H., Gendelman, R., Ensoli, B., and Gallo, R. C., 1994b, Identification and culture of Kaposi's sarcoma-like spindle cells from the peripheral blood of human immunodeficiency virus-1-infected individuals and normal controls, *Blood* **84:**2711–2720.

Buonaguro, L., Buonaguro, F. M., Giraldo, G., and Ensoli, B., 1994, The human immunodeficiency virus type 1 Tat protein transactivates tumor necrosis factor beta gene expression through a TAR-like structure, *J. Virol.* **68:** 2677–2682.

Cesarman, E., Chang, Y., Moore, P. S., Said, J. W., and Knowles, D. M., 1995, Kaposi's sarcoma-associated herpesvirus-like DNA sequences in AIDS-related body-cavity-based lymphoma, *N. Engl. J. Med.* **332:**1186–1191.

Chang, H. K., Samaniego, F., Buonaguro, L., Nair, B. C., Gallo, R. C., and Ensoli, B., 1995, Extracellular Tat binds heparan sulfate complexes of the cell surface and extracellular matrix (ECM) through the basic region, *AIDS Res. Hum. Retrovir.* **11:**S116.

Clark, E. A., and Brugge, J. S., 1995, Integrins and signal transduction pathways: The road taken, *Science* **268:** 233–239.

Corallini, A., Altavilla, G., Pozzi, L., Bignozzi, F., Negrini, M., Rimessi, P., Gualandi, F., and Barbanti-Brodano, G., 1993, Systemic expression of HIV-1 *tat* gene in transgenic mice induces endothelial proliferation and tumors of different histotypes, *Cancer Res.* **53:**5569–5575.

Damsky, C. H., and Werb, Z., 1992, Signal transduction by integrin receptors for extracellular matrix: Cooperative processing of extracellular information, *Curr. Opin. Cell Biol.* **4:**772–781.

Delli Bovi, P., Donti, E., Knowles, D. M., Friedman-Kien, A., Luciw, P. A., Dina, D., Dalla-Favera, R., and Basilico, C., 1986, Presence of chromosomal abnormalities and lack of AIDS retrovirus DNA sequences in AIDS-associated Kaposi's sarcoma, *Cancer Res.* **46:**6333–6338.

Ensoli, B., Nakamura, S., Salahuddin, S. Z., Biberfeld, P., Larsson, L., Beaver, B., Wong-Staal, F., and Gallo, R. C., 1989, AIDS-Kaposi's sarcoma-derived cells express cytokines with autocrine and paracrine growth effects, *Science* **243:**223–226.

Ensoli, B., Barillari, G., Salahuddin, S. Z., Gallo, R. C., and Wong-Staal, F., 1990, Tat protein of HIV-1 stimulates growth of AIDS-Kaposi's sarcoma-derived cells, *Nature* **345:**84–86.

Ensoli, B., Buonaguro, L., Barillari, G., Fiorelli, V., Gendelman, R., Morgan, R. A., Wingfeld, P., and Gallo, R. C., 1993, Release, uptake and effects of extracellular human immunodeficiency virus type 1 Tat protein on cell growth and viral transactivation, *J. Virol.* **67:**277–287.

Ensoli, B., Gendelman, R., Markham, P., Fiorelli, V., Colombini, S., Raffeld, M., Cafaro, A., Chang, H. K., Brady, J. N., and Gallo, R. C., 1994a, Synergy between basic fibroblast growth factor and the HIV-1 Tat protein in induction of Kaposi's sarcoma, *Nature* **371:**674–680.

Ensoli, B., Markham, P., Kao, V., Barillari, G., Fiorelli, V., Gendelman, R., Raffeld, M., Zon, G., and Gallo, R. C., 1994b, Block of AIDS-Kaposi's sarcoma (KS) cell growth, angiogenesis and lesion formation in nude mice by antisense oligonucleotides targeting basic fibroblast growth factor: A novel strategy for the therapy of KS, *J. Clin. Invest.* **94:**1736–1746.

Fan, J., Bass, H. Z., and Fahey, J. L., 1993, Elevated IFN-γ and decreased IL-2 gene expression are associated with HIV-1 infection, *J. Immunol.* **151:**5031–5040.

Fidler, I. J., Singh, R. K., Gutman, M., Sanchez, R., and Bucana, C. D., 1994, Interferons α and β downregulate the expression of basic fibroblast growth factor (bFGF) in human carcinomas, *Cancer Res.* **35:**57.

Fiorelli, V., Markham, P., Samaniego, F., Gendelman, R., and Ensoli, B., 1995, Cytokines from activated T cells induce normal endothelial cells to acquire the phenotypic and functional features of AIDS-Kaposi's sarcoma spindle cells, *J. Clin. Invest.* **95:**1723–1734.

Folkman, J., and Klagsbrun, M., 1987, Angiogenic factors, *Science* **235**:442–447.

Folkman, J., Klagsbrun, M., Sasse, J., Wadzinski, M., Ingber, D., and Vlodavsky, I., 1988, A heparin binding angiogenic protein basic fibroblast growth factor is stored within basement membrane, *Am. J. Pathol.* **130**:393–400.

Friedman-Kien, A. E., 1981, Disseminated Kaposi's sarcoma syndrome in young homosexual men, *J. Am. Acad. Dermatol.* **5**:468–471.

Gottlieb, G. J., and Ackerman, A. B., 1982, Kaposi's sarcoma: An extensively disseminated form in young homosexual men, *Hum. Pathol.* **13**:882–886.

Havercos, H. W., Drotman, D. P., and Morgan, M., 1985, Prevalence of Kaposi's sarcoma among patients with AIDS, *N. Engl. J. Med.* **312**:1518–1520.

Hejna, W. F., 1965, Squamous cell carcinoma developing in the chronic draining sinus of osteomyelitis, *Cancer* **18**:128–132.

Herndier, B. G., Werner, A., Arnstein, P., Abbey, N. W., Demartis, F., Cohen, R. L., Shuman, M. A., and Levy, J. A., 1994, Characterization of a human Kaposi's sarcoma cell line that induces angiogenic tumors in animals, *AIDS* **8**:575–581.

Hofman, F. M., Wright, A. D., Dohadwala, M. M., Wong-Staal, F., and Walker, S. M., 1993, Exogenous tat protein activates human endothelial cells, *Blood* **82**:2774–2780.

Ingber, D., Fujita, T., Kishimoto, S., Sudo, K., Kanamaru, T., Brem, H., and Folkman, J., 1990, Synthetic analogues of fumagillin that inhibit angiogenesis and suppress tumour growth, *Nature* **348**:555–557.

Jaffe, H. W., Choi, K., Thomas, P. A., Havercos, H. W., Auerbach, D. M., Guinan, M. E., Rogers, M. F., Spira, T. J., Darrow, W. W., Kramer, M. A., Friedman, S. M., Monroe, J. M., Friedman-Kien, A. E., Laubenstein, L. J., Marmor, M., Safai, B., Dritz, S. K., Crispi, S. J., Fannin, S. L., Orkwis, J. P., Kelter, A., Rushing, W. R., Thacker, S. B., and Curran, J. W., 1983, National case–control study of Kaposi's sarcoma and *Pneumocystis carinii* pneumonia in homosexual men: part 1, epidemiological results, *Ann. Intern. Med.* **99**:145–151.

Janier, M., Flageul, B., Drouet, L., Scobohaci, M. L., Villette, J. M., Palangie, A., and Cottenot, F., 1988, Cutaneous and plasma values of von Willebrand factor in AIDS: A marker of endothelial stimulation? *Invest. Dermatol.* **90**:703–707.

Kandel, J., Bossy-Wetzel, E., Radvanyi, F., Klagsbrun, M., Folkman, J., and Hanahan, D., 1991, Neovascularization is associated with a switch to the export of bFGF in the multistep development of fibrosarcoma, *Cell* **66**:1095–1104.

Krigel, R. L., Odajnyk, C. M., Laubenstein, L. J., Ostreicher, R., Wernz, J., Vilcek, J., Rubinstein, P., and Friedman-Kien, A. E., 1985, Therapeutic trial of interferon-γ in patients with epidemic Kaposi's sarcoma, *J. Biol. Response Modif.* **4**:358–364.

Krown, S. E., 1987, The role of interferon in the therapy of epidemic Kaposi's sarcoma, *Semin. Oncol.* **14**:27–33.

Lahdevirta, J., Maury, C. P. J., Teppo, A. M., and Repo, H., 1988, Elevated levels of circulating cachectin/tumor necrosis factor in patients with acquired immunodeficiency syndrome, *Am. J. Med.* **85**:289–291.

Lepe-Zanuga, J. L., Mansell, P. W. A., and Hersh, E. M., 1987, Idiopathic production of interleukin-1 in acquired immune deficiency syndrome, *J. Clin. Microbiol.* **25**:1695–1699.

Lunardi-Iskandar, Y., Bryant, J. L., Zeman, R. A., Lam, V. H., Samaniego, F., Besnier, J. M., Hermans, P., Thierry, A. R., Gill, P., and Gallo, R. C., 1995a, Tumorigenesis and metastasis of neoplastic Kaposi's sarcoma cell line in immunodeficient mice blocked by a human pregnancy hormone, *Nature* **375**:64–68.

Lunardi-Iskandar, Y., Gill, P., Lam, V. H., Zeman, R. A., Michaels, F., Mann, D. L., Reitz, M. S., Jr., Kaplan, M., Berneman, Z. N., Carter, D., Bryant, J. L., and Gallo, R. C., 1995b, Isolation and characterization of an immortal neoplastic cell line (KS Y-1) from AIDS-associated Kaposi's sarcoma, *J. Natl. Cancer Inst.* **87**:974–981.

Mahoney, S. E., Duvic, M., Nickoloff, B. J., Minshall, M., Smith, L. C., Griffiths, C. E. M., Paddock, S. W., and Lewis, D. E., 1991, Human immunodeficiency virus (HIV) transcripts identified in HIV-related psoriasis and Kaposi's sarcoma lesions, *J. Clin. Invest.* **88**:174–185.

Marcuzzi, A., Weinberger, J., and Weinberger, O. K., 1992, Transcellular activation of the human immunodeficiency virus type 1 long terminal repeat in cocultured lymphocytes, *J. Virol.* **66**:4228–4231.

Miles, S. A., Rezai, A. R., Salazar-Gonzalez, J. F., VanderMeyden, M., Stevens, R. H., Logan, D. M., Mitsuyasu, R. T., Taga, T., Hirano, T., Kishimoto, T., and Martinez-Maza, O., 1990, AIDS Kaposi sarcoma-derived cells produce and respond to interleukin 6, *Proc. Natl. Acad. Sci. USA* **87**:4068–4072.

Miles, S. A., Martinez-Maza, O., Rezai, A., Maypantay, L., Kishimoto, T., Nakamura, S., Radka, S. F., and Linsey, P. S., 1992, Oncostatin M as a potent mitogen for AIDS-KS-derived cells, *Science* **255**:1432–1434.

Mitsuyasu, R. T., 1991, Interferon alpha in the treatment of AIDS-related Kaposi's sarcoma, *Br. J. Haematol.* **79**:69–71.

Mitsuyasu, R. T., 1994, Clinical aspects of AIDS-related Kaposi's sarcoma, in: *Current Review of Oncology* (M. D. Abeloff and J. Klastersky, eds.), Current Science, Baltimore, pp. 835–844.

Moore, P. S., and Chang, Y., 1995, Detection of herpesvirus-like DNA sequences in Kaposi's sarcoma in patients with and those without HIV infection, *N. Engl. J. Med.* **332:**1181–1185.

Nadji, M., Morales, A. R., Ziegles-Weissman, J., and Penneys, N. S., 1981, Kaposi's sarcoma: Immunohistologic evidence for an endothelial origin, *Arch. Pathol. Lab. Med.* **105:**274–275.

Nair, B. C., DeVico, A. L., Nakamura, S., Copeland, T. D., Chen, Y., Patel, A., O'Neil, T., Oroszlan, S., Gallo, R. C., and Sarngadharan, M. G., 1992, Identification of a major growth factor for AIDS-Kaposi's sarcoma cells as oncostatin M, *Science* **255:**1430–1432.

Nakamura, S., Salahuddin, S. Z., Biberfeld, P., Ensoli, B., Markham, P. D., Wong-Staal, F., and Gallo, R. C., 1988, Kaposi's sarcoma cells: Long-term culture with growth factor from retrovirus-infected CD4$^+$ T cells, *Science* **242:**426–430.

Nakamura, S., Sakurada, S., Salahuddin, S. Z., Osada, Y., Tanaka, N. G., Sakamoto, N., Sekiguchi, M., and Gallo, R. C., 1992, Inhibition of development of Kaposi's sarcoma-related lesions by a bacterial cell wall complex, *Science* **255:**1437–1440.

Orfanos, C. E., Husak, R., Wolfer, U., and Garbe, C., 1995, Kaposi's sarcoma: A reevaluation, *Recent Results Cancer Res.* **139:**275–296.

Pepper, M. S., Ferrara, N., Orci, L., and Montesano, R., 1992, Potent synergism between vascular endothelial growth factor and basic fibroblast growth factor in the induction of angiogenesis in vitro, *Biochem. Biophys. Res. Commun.* **189:**824–831.

Pober, J. S., and Cotran, R. S., 1990, Cytokines and endothelial cell biology, *Physiol. Rev.* **70:**427–451.

Rabkin, C. S., Bedi, G., Musaba, E., Sunkutu, R., Mwansa, N., Sidransky, D., and Biggar, R. J., 1995, AIDS-related Kaposi's sarcoma is a clonal neoplasm, *Clin. Cancer Res.* **1:**257–260.

Regezi, J. A., MacPhail, L. A., Daniels, T. E., DeSouza, Y. G., Greenspan, J. S., and Greenspan, D., 1993, Human immunodeficiency virus-associated oral Kaposi's sarcoma: A heterogeneous cell population dominated by spindle-shaped endothelial cells, *Am. J. Pathol.* **43:**240–249.

Roth, W. K., Werner, S., Schirren, C. G., and Hofschneider, P. H., 1989, Depletion of PDGF from serum inhibits growth of AIDS-related and sporadic Kaposi's sarcoma cells in culture, *Oncogene* **4:**483–487.

Ruszczak, Z., Mayer-Da Silva, A., and Orfanos, C. E., 1987a, Kaposi's sarcoma in AIDS: Multicentric angioneoplasia in early skin lesions, *Am. J. Dermatopathol.* **9:**388–398.

Ruszczak, Z., Mayer-Da Silva, A., and Orfanos, C. E., 1987b, Angioproliferative changes in clinically noninvolved, perilesional skin in AIDS-associated Kaposi's sarcoma, *Dermatologica* **175:**270–279.

Safai, B., Johnson, K. G., Myskowski, P. L., Koziner, B., Yang, S. Y., Cunningham-Rundles, S., Godbold, J. H., and Dupont, B., 1985, The natural history of Kaposi's sarcoma in the acquired immunodeficiency syndrome, *Ann. Intern. Med.* **103**:744–750.

Salahuddin, S. Z., Nakamura, S., Biberfeld, P., Kaplan, M. H., Markham, P. D., Larsson, L., and Gallo, R. C., 1988, Angiogenic properties of Kaposi's sarcoma-derived cells after long-term culture *in vitro*, *Science* **242:** 430–433.

Samaniego, F., Bryant, J. L., Lam, V. J., Zeman, R. A., Thierry, A., Judde, J. G., and Gallo, R. C., 1995a, Human chorionic gonadotropin (hCG) prevents development of Kaposi's sarcoma (AIDS-KS Y-1) tumors by inducing apoptosis, *AIDS Res. Hum. Retrovir.* **11:**S76.

Samaniego, F., Chang, H.-K., Gallo, R. C., and Ensoli, B., 1995b, HIV Tat protein induces signal transduction in AIDS-Kaposi's sarcoma and cytokine-activated endothelial cell. Presented at Signal Transductions of Normal and Tumor Cells Meeting, *Cancer Res.* p. A24.

Samaniego, F., Markham, P., Gallo, R. C., and Ensoli, B., 1995c, Inflammatory cytokines induce AIDS-Kaposi's sarcoma-derived spindle cells to produce and release basic fibroblast growth factor and enhance Kaposi's sarcoma-like lesion formation in nude mice, *J. Immunol.* **154:**3582–3592.

Samaniego, F., Markham, P. D., Sturzl, M., Gendelman, R., Ferrara, N., Kao, V., Kowalski, K., Ensoli, B., and Gallo, R. C., 1995d, Vascular endothelial growth factor (VEGF) is expressed by AIDS-Kaposi's sarcoma (KS) cells and synergizes with bFGF to form KS-like lesions in nude mice, *AIDS Res. Hum. Retrovir.* **11:**S95.

Samaniego, F., Markham, P. D., Gendelman, R., Gallo, R. C., and Ensoli, B., 1996, Inflammatory cytokines induce endothelial cells to produce and release basic fibroblast growth factor and to promote Kaposi's sarcoma-like lesions in nude mice, (submitted for publication).

Schlaepfer, D. D., Hanks, S. K., Hunter, T., and van der Geer, P., 1994, Integrin-mediated signal transduction linked to Ras pathway by GRB2 binding to focal adhesion kinase, *Nature* **372:**786–791.

Sciacca, F. L., Sturzl, M., Bussolino, F., Sironi, M., Brandstetter, H., Zietz, C., Zhou, D., Matteucci, C., Peri, G.,

Sozzani, S., Benelli, R., Arese, M., Albini, A., Colotta, F., and Montovani, A., 1994, Expression of adhesion molecules platelet-activating factor, and chemokines by Kaposi's sarcoma cells, *J. Immunol.* **153**:4816–4825.

Siegal, B., Levinton-Kriss, S., Schiffer, A., Sayar, J., Egelberg, I., Vonsover, A., Ramon, Y., and Rubinstein, E., 1990, Kaposi's sarcoma in immunosuppression—Possibly the result of a dual viral infection, *Cancer* **65:** 492–496.

Singh, R. K., Liansa, N., Bucana, C. D., Sanchez, R., and Fidler, I. J., 1995, Cell density-dependent modulation of basic fibroblast growth factor expression by IFN-β, *Proc. Am. Assoc. Cancer Res.* **36**:87.

Slavin, G., Cameron, H. M., and Singh, H., 1969, Kaposi's sarcoma in mainland Tanzania: A report of 117 cases, *Br. J. Cancer* **23**:349–357.

Taylor, J. F., Smith, P. G., Bull, D., and Pike, M. C., 1972, Kaposi's sarcoma in Uganda: Geographic and ethnic distribution, *Br. J. Cancer* **6**:483–497.

Vogel, J., Hinrichs, S. H., Reynolds, R. K., Luciw, P. A., and Jay, G., 1988, HIV-1 *tat* gene induces dermal lesions resembling Kaposi's sarcoma in transgenic mice, *Nature* **335**:606–611.

Werner, S., Hofschneider, P. H., Heldin, C. H., Östman, A., and Roth, W. K., 1990, Cultured Kaposi's sarcoma-derived cells express functional PDGF-A type and B-type receptors, *Exp. Cell Res.* **187**:98–103.

Yamamoto, T., Osaki, T., Yoneda, K., and Ueta, E., 1993, Immunological investigation of adult patients with primary herpes simplex virus-1 infection, *J. Oral Pathol. Med.* **22**:263–267.

Yang, J., Xu, Y., Zhu, C., Hagan, M. K., Lawley, T., and Offermann, M. K., 1994, Regulation of adhesion molecular expression in Kaposi's sarcoma cells, *J. Immunol.* **152**:361–373.

Xerri, L., Haussoun, J., Planche, J., Guigou, V., Grob, J. J., Parc, P., Birnbaum, D., and Delapeyriere, O., 1991, Fibroblast growth factor gene expression in AIDS-Kaposi's sarcoma detected by in situ hybridization, *Am. J. Pathol.* **138**:9–15.

CHAPTER 23

PATHOGENESIS OF HIV-ASSOCIATED LYMPHOMA

VALERIE L. NG and MICHAEL S. McGRATH

1. PREVALENCE OF HIV-ASSOCIATED LYMPHOMAS

1.1. As Index Diagnosis for the Acquired Immunodeficiency Syndrome (AIDS)

The diagnosis of HIV-associated lymphoma was first incorporated in 1985 into the Centers for Disease Control's (CDC) case definition of AIDS (Harnly *et al.*, 1988; Kristal *et al.*, 1988). The incidence of lymphoma in the HIV-1-infected population has been steadily increasing since, and represented 3–4% of AIDS-defining illnesses reported to the CDC in 1991. Except for a surprisingly high incidence of lymphoma observed in one small cohort of HIV-infected individuals (Pluda *et al.*, 1990), there has been no apparent increase in the incidence of lymphoma disproportionate to that for new AIDS diagnoses.

1.2. Impact of Antiretroviral Therapies and Opportunistic Infection Prophylaxis

In the early years of the HIV-1 epidemic, death resulting from opportunistic infections was common. Since then, effective prophylactic regimens for *Pneumocystis carinii*, *Toxoplasma gondii*, and cytomegalovirus infections have dramatically increased the length of survival and quality of life for HIV-1 infected individuals. Whether an increased life span affected the incidence of HIV-associated lymphoma was addressed in a large prospective observational study of a population with advanced HIV infection treated with zidovudine; the results of this study demonstrated a constant 1.6% incidence of HIV-associated lymphomas per year (Moore *et al.*, 1991). It is thus anticipated that more HIV-associated

VALERIE L. NG • Departments of Laboratory Medicine and Medicine, University of California, San Francisco, and San Francisco General Hospital, San Francisco, California 94110. MICHAEL S. McGRATH • Departments of Laboratory Medicine, Medicine, and Pathology, University of California, San Francisco, and San Francisco General Hospital, San Francisco, California 94110.

Immunology of HIV Infection, edited by Sudhir Gupta. Plenum Press, New York, 1996.

lymphomas will arise reflecting the increased longevity of AIDS patients because of effective antiretroviral and opportunistic infection prophylactic regimens. In 1992 it was estimated that 8–27% of approximately 36,000 newly diagnosed cases of lymphoma had arisen in HIV-infected individuals (Gail *et al.*, 1991); it is estimated that 5–10% of all individuals with AIDS will have lymphoma as either their initial or subsequent AIDS-defining condition (Hamilton-Dutoit *et al.*, 1991). Thus, HIV-associated lymphomas represent a significant clinical entity in the differential of HIV-associated diseases.

2. CLINICAL AND LABORATORY FEATURES OF HIV-ASSOCIATED LYMPHOMAS

At least 95% of immune deficiency-associated lymphomas are of B-cell origin (as defined by immunophenotype, immunoglobulin gene rearrangement with or without immunoglobulin production). It was initially thought that, since both groups of patients have defects in cell-mediated immunity (i.e., iatrogenic versus HIV-mediated), HIV-associated B-cell lymphomas might be analogous to those observed in immunosuppressed allograft recipients. As a result, viral or genetic cofactors [e.g., Epstein–Barr virus (EBV), c-*myc* rearrangement] previously linked with B-cell transformation were also sought in HIV-associated lymphomas.

Patients with HIV-associated lymphoma can be subdivided into at least two distinct clinical categories: systemic versus primary central nervous system (CNS) lymphoma on the basis of site of disease, extent of immune function, and response to chemotherapy. Of 2500 cases of HIV-associated lymphomas recently reviewed, approximately 80% were systemic and 20% were primary CNS lymphomas (Beral *et al.*, 1991).

2.1. HIV-Associated Systemic Lymphomas

2.1.1. Clinical Features

Widespread disease involving extranodal sites is the hallmark of HIV-associated systemic lymphoma. In a series of 89 patients diagnosed at New York University (Knowles *et al.*, 1988), 87% had extranodal disease at presentation. Ziegler *et al.* (1984) similarly reported that 95% of patients in their series had evidence of extranodal disease; in addition, 42% of these patients had CNS disease and 33% had bone marrow involvement. At San Francisco General Hospital, two-thirds of patients with HIV-associated lymphoma have presented with stage IV disease and 31% have presented with extranodal disease alone (Kaplan *et al.*, 1989). As observed for other immunosuppressed patients with lymphoma, it is common to have extralymphatic presentations at unusual sites.

Symptoms at the time of presentation can be quite variable and diagnosis may rely on a high index of suspicion. Common sites for presentation include bone marrow, meninges, and liver. Involvement of any part of the gastrointestinal (GI) tract is also frequently observed, with one study demonstrating such involvement in $\leq$ 27% of individuals with HIV-associated lymphoma (Herndier and Friedman, 1992). There are clearly a variety of clinical circumstances in which the diagnosis of lymphoma should be entertained, including presentation with symptoms related to the presence of a mass lesion at any site, chronic GI complaints, hepatic obstruction, unexplained chronic constitutional symptoms, and observation of asymmetric or rapidly progressive lymphadenopathy. Diagnosis is dependent on microscopic examination of tissue obtained from the involved site.

Patients with systemic HIV-associated lymphoma exhibit a wide range of immune function; 75% will have peripheral $CD4^+$ lymphocyte counts of $> 50/\mu l$ at presentation and many will not have had prior opportunistic infections. As an example, in a recent report from a single institution, 49 HIV-1-infected individuals with systemic lymphoma had a median peripheral $CD4^+$ lymphocyte count of $189/\mu l$ (range, 6–987) and only 37% had had a previous opportunistic infection (Levine *et al.*, 1991).

2.1.2. Morphologic Features

Review of 2500 cases of HIV-associated lymphomas revealed that approximately 60% were large cell lymphomas, 20% were Burkitt's (i.e., small noncleaved), and 20% were CNS lymphomas (Beral *et al.*, 1991). Thus, large cell lymphomas comprise the largest morphologic category (i.e., approximately 70–75%) of HIV-associated systemic lymphomas. In this review, the classification of "large cell lymphomas" includes all lymphomas previously classified as large cleaved cell, large noncleaved cell, sclerosing variant large cell, large cell, immunoblastic plasmacytoid, immunoblastic clear cell, polymorphous, immunoblastic, and immunoblastic with epithelial cell component lymphomas (Herndier *et al.*, 1994).

A correlation, albeit imperfect, exists between morphologic and molecular features of HIV-associated lymphomas.

2.1.3. Molecular Features

2.1.3a. Normal Immunoglobulin (Ig) Production. By virtue of their capacity to synthesize immunoglobulins, B cells comprise the secretory component of the immune system. Immunoglobulins are composed of two heavy (H) and two light (L) chains, the synthesis of which results from a distinct sequence of molecular events beginning with rearrangement of specific variable (V), diversity (D), and joining (J) segments to form a continuous V-region gene. The V regions of both the H and L chains interact to form a three-dimensional pocket (i.e., idiotope) which binds the cognate antigen (the antigen is recognized on the basis of shape, which is specified by the primary amino acid sequence that in turn determines its secondary and tertiary structure). Intervening DNA between the V, D, and J genes destined to be "joined" is excised and excluded from the genome. Additional rearrangements to juxtapose constant regions of the H (to produce IgM, IgG, IgA, or IgE) or L chains (to produce kappa or lambda) then occur with the ultimate production of functional Ig. B cells expressing Ig that best "fits" the inciting antigen will be continuously stimulated and clonally proliferate to increase production of its antibody; antibody maturation occurs by further modification of the V regions of both the H and L chains to better modify the antigen binding site such that the expanded clone(s) of B cells produce antibodies with high affinity and avidity.

Since the majority of HIV-associated lymphomas are of B-cell origin, monoclonality has been traditionally defined as detection of Ig gene rearrangement in DNA extracted from the malignant cells. Probes typically used to determine monoclonality are those representative of the entire J_H locus or, because it is the first light chain locus to undergo rearrangement after antigenic stimulus, the constant region of the kappa light chain (i.e., C_{kappa}).

2.1.3b. Interpretation of Ig Gene Rearrangement Studies. Interpretation of Ig gene rearrangement studies in the research laboratory setting has not, unfortunately, been well standardized. Such gene rearrangement studies have been typically performed using a traditional Southern blot approach. In this analysis, detection of hybridization signals at any position other than that present in "normal" tissue lacking clonal B cells (i.e., germline configuration) is evidence of Ig gene rearrangement. The sensitivity of Southern blot analysis has been estimated to be 5% (i.e., a gene rearrangement can be detected if at least 5% of the cells in the population under study are derived from a single clone), yet not all laboratories will include as a control a specimen containing 5% of DNA from a clonal malignancy to reproducibly validate detection of a clone at this level. Southern analysis can also be modified to increase the sensitivity such that Ig gene rearrangements attributable to a clone that comprise less than 5% of the cells present can be detected. Lastly, Southern analysis failing to demonstrate an Ig gene rearrangement (i.e., J_H probe hybridization signal in the germline position at the same or reduced intensity as that of DNA from a nonmalignant control specimen) is interpreted as evidence for polyclonal B-cell population—i.e., multiple B-cell clones, each having different VDJ rearrangements of different sizes that are of insufficient quantity for detection in any single band.

The use of Ig gene rearrangement and other laboratory or molecular studies in the diagnosis of lymphoma varies. At our institution, a diagnosis of lymphoma is based solely on morphologic criteria. In contrast, other institutions may rely on morphologic features in combination with results of immunophenotyping and Ig gene rearrangement studies that are consistent with that expected for a monoclonal process before assigning a diagnosis of lymphoma. This difference in diagnostic approach may partially explain the discrepancies, as discussed below, in the reported clonality results of HIV-associated systemic lymphomas.

2.1.3c. Molecular Features of HIV-Associated Systemic Large Cell Lymphomas. Six large studies (see Table I) have analyzed the molecular features of HIV-associated systemic lymphomas with respect to cofactors traditionally associated with B-cell malignancies—e.g., clonality, presence of EBV (which has been highly associated with endemic Burkitt's lymphoma and B-cell lymphoproliferations in immunosuppressed individuals), and c-*myc* translocations (highly associated with sporadically occurring Burkitt's lymphomas).

Pelicci *et al.* (1986b) were the first to report the molecular features of 11 cases of HIV-associated systemic lymphomas in comparison with those of 22 enlarged but benign hyperplastic lymph nodes obtained from HIV-infected individuals with lymphadenopathy syndrome (LAS). All 11 lymphomas analyzed (7 Burkitt's and 4 large cell lymphomas) were monoclonal as defined by Ig gene rearrangement studies; of interest, monoclonal Ig gene rearrangements were detected in 4 of 22 enlarged benign hyperplastic lymph nodes. c-*myc* translocations were detected in 8 of the 11 lymphomas (all 7 Burkitt's, 1 of the 4 large cell lymphomas) but not in any of the 22 hyperplastic lymph nodes.

Knowles *et al.* (1988) described the experience in New York with 105 cases of HIV-associated lymphomas; molecular analyses were performed on 27 specimens obtained from 26 of these patients (one patient had two different biopsies). Of the 27 specimens, one was a CNS lymphoma (and not further discussed in this section) and the remaining 26 were comprised of 18 Burkitt's and 8 large cell lymphomas. All lymphomas were monoclonal by Ig gene rearrangement studies and expressed cell surface molecules consistent with that expected for B cells; none had evidence of T-cell receptor rearrangements. EBV and c-*myc* translocation studies were not performed.

Shiramizu *et al.* (1992) reported on the molecular features of 40 cases of HIV-

TABLE I. Correlation of Molecular Characteristics of HIV-Associated Systemic Lymphomas with Morphologic Classification[a]

Reference	*n*	Morphology		Clonality	EBV infected	*c-myc* rearranged	p53 mutation	*ras* mutation	RB1 mutation
Pelicci *et al.* (1986b)	11	LCL	4	4M		1			
		Burkitt's	7	7M		7			
Knowles *et al.* (1988)	26	LCL	8	8M					
		Burkitt's	18	18M					
Shiramizu *et al.* (1992)	33	LCL	24	9M	4	5 (2 EBV^+; 3 EBV^-)			
				15P	3	0			
		Burkitt's	9	8M	2	4 (all EBV^-)			
				1P	0	0			
Ballerini *et al.* (1993)	27	LCL	11	11M	5	3	0	1	0
		Burkitt's	16	16M	5	16	10	3	0
Shibata *et al.* (1993)	59	LCL	31		23				
		Burkitt's	28		16				
		LCL	7	7M	5	2 (both EBV^+)			
		Burkitt's	8	8M	6	4 (all EBV^+)			
Delecluse *et al.* (1993)	14	LCL	7	4M	4	2 (both EBV^+)			
				4P	3	0			
		Burkitt's	7	7M	4	6			

[a]Abbreviations: *n*, number reported; LCL, large cell lymphoma; M, monoclonal; P, polyclonal; EBV, Epstein–Barr virus.

associated lymphomas observed in San Francisco, of which 7 were CNS lymphomas (and not further discussed in this section). Of the 33 HIV-associated systemic lymphomas analyzed, 9 were Burkitt's and 24 were large cell lymphomas. Of the 9 Burkitt's lymphomas, 8 were monoclonal and 1 was polyclonal (i.e., no evidence of a rearranged Ig gene). Two of the eight monoclonal Burkitt's tumors contained EBV, and only four (all lacking EBV) had c-*myc* translocations. The single polyclonal Burkitt's lymphoma lacked both EBV and c-*myc* translocations. For the 24 large cell lymphomas, 15 were polyclonal and 9 were monoclonal. Of the 15 polyclonal lymphomas, 3 contained EBV and none had c-*myc* translocations. Of the 9 monoclonal lymphomas, 4 had and 5 lacked EBV (of which additional c-*myc* translocations were detected in 2 and 3 of these respective groups). Immunophenotyping on a subset of the polyclonal tumors verified cell surface expression of markers consistent with that expected of B cells, with half of the tumors containing a significant number (30–80%) of infiltrating T cells.

Ballerini *et al.* (1993) reported yet another series of HIV-associated systemic lymphomas from 27 patients diagnosed in New York (24) and Italy (3). Of the 27 lymphomas, 16 were Burkitt's and 11 were large cell lymphomas. All of the 27 lymphomas were monoclonal, only 10 of 27 had EBV present (5 Burkitt's, 5 large cell lymphomas), and 19 had c-*myc* translocations (all 16 Burkitt's and 3 large cell lymphomas). p53 mutations were detected in only 10 of the 16 Burkitt's lymphomas and were absent in all 11 large cell lymphomas. *Ras* mutations were detected in only a subset of the lymphomas, and RB1 mutations were not present in any.

Shibata *et al.* (1993) reported on two different sets of HIV-associated systemic lymphomas obtained from patients in Los Angeles. Of 59 lymphomas (28 Burkitt's and 31 large cell), 39 (16 Burkitt's and 23 large cell lymphomas) contained EBV; in contrast, EBV was associated with only 2 of 35 non-HIV-associated systemic lymphomas. There was no apparent association of a specific EBV subtype (i.e., type A or type B) with the HIV-associated lymphomas. A subset of 15 lymphomas (8 Burkitt's, 7 large cell) were further analyzed: all 15 had monoclonal Ig gene rearrangements, and none of 8 lymphomas had evidence of T-cell receptor gene rearrangements. Eleven of the fifteen lymphomas (6 Burkitt's, 5 large cell lymphomas) were monoclonally infected with EBV, of which 6 (4 Burkitt's, 2 large cell lymphomas) had additional c-*myc* translocations.

Delecluse *et al.* (1993) reported on 14 cases (7 Burkitt's, 7 large cell) of HIV-associated systemic lymphomas obtained from patients diagnosed in France. All 7 Burkitt's lymphomas were monoclonal, of which 6 had rearranged c-*myc* genes and 4 had EBV present. Of the 7 large cell lymphomas, only 4 were monoclonal, only 2 (both monoclonal) had rearranged c-*myc* genes, and all contained EBV.

With the exception of two studies (Delecluse *et al.*, 1993; Shiramizu *et al.*, 1992), all other HIV-associated systemic lymphomas analyzed have had monoclonal Ig gene rearrangements and EBV present. The occurrence of polyclonal tumors lacking EBV (Delecluse *et al.*, 1993; Shiramizu *et al.*, 1992) was initially controversial but has since been supported by two additional studies. Strigle *et al.* (1993), in a study comparing the diagnostic yield of specimens obtained by fine needle aspiration as compared to biopsy, were unable to show antibody light chain exclusion in more than half of their lymphoma specimens obtained by fine needle aspiration. Similarly, Cherepakhin *et al.* (1992) reported that 11 of 23 HIV-associated lymphomas analyzed failed to demonstrate Ig gene rearrangements. Lastly, an autopsy study (McGrath *et al.*, 1991) of three patients with polyclonal lymphomas who died with widespread lymphoma revealed polyclonal lymphoma occurring as metastatic lesions in the liver, lung, and other organs, suggesting that these lymphomas behaved as aggressively and were clinically indistinguishable from conventional monoclonal lymphomas.

In summary, the molecular features of HIV-associated systemic lymphomas are not uniform. The lymphomas can be monoclonal or polyclonal in origin, EBV is not universally present (and if present, did not correlate with tumor clonality), and c-*myc* translocations are observed in only a subset of the monoclonal lymphomas.

2.1.4. Prognosis

Kaplan *et al.* (1995) demonstrated a variable survival for individuals with HIV-associated systemic lymphomas that was roughly correlated with molecular features. A poor prognosis was associated with monoclonal tumors (median survival of 3.5 months if peripheral $CD4^+$ lymphocytes are $\leqslant 200/\mu l$, 4.9 months if peripheral $CD4^+$ lymphocytes are $\geqslant 200/\mu l$ or with polyclonal tumors occurring in individuals with peripheral $CD4^+$ lymphocytes of $\leqslant 200/\mu l$ (median survival 5.5 months). In contrast, individuals with polyclonal lymphomas but peripheral $CD4^+$ lymphocytes $\geqslant 200/\mu l$ had a markedly longer survival (survival range of 25.9–65.2 months, with more than 50% of subjects still alive at the end of the study period). Multivariate Cox hazards model analysis of this study group revealed that the presence of EBV in the lymphoma increased the risk for poor outcome by 4.95-fold (95% confidence interval, 1.94–12.58).

2.2. HIV-Associated Primary CNS Lymphomas

2.2.1. Clinical Features

Primary CNS lymphomas comprise up to 25% of all HIV-associated lymphomas observed in HIV-infected individuals (Baumgartner *et al.*, 1990; Formenti *et al.*, 1989; Gill *et al.*, 1985). Clinical symptoms at the time of presentation are nonfocal, usually involve subtle changes in cognitive ability, and can include confusion, lethargy, memory loss, and headaches. Other more serious and focal symptoms at presentation can include hemiparesis, aphasia, seizures, and cranial nerve palsies. Computed tomographic (CT) or magnetic resonance (MR) imaging studies of the brain most commonly revealed single or multiple discrete ring-enhancing lesions (Ciricillo and Rosenblum, 1991).

Clinical symptoms and imaging abnormalities observed with HIV-associated primary CNS lymphomas are indistinguishable from those associated with CNS toxoplasmosis which occurs at a similar frequency as that of CNS lymphoma [i.e., 3–10% of AIDS patients in the United States (Luft *et al.*, 1993)]. The number of lesions is not diagnostically useful; although CNS lymphomas tend to be more commonly associated with a single ring-enhancing lesion (as compared to multiple ring-enhancing lesions more commonly associated with CNS toxoplasmosis), half of the HIV-associated CNS lymphomas in one study had multiple ring-enhancing lesions (Ciricillo and Rosenblum, 1991). HIV-associated CNS toxoplasmosis in the United States is believed to be a reactivation disease and only individuals previously exposed to toxoplasma are considered to be a risk to develop CNS toxoplasmosis; serologic tests to detect antitoxoplasma IgG as a marker of previous exposure are, unfortunately, of limited clinical utility since this disease can occur in 10–16% of HIV-infected individuals lacking antitoxoplasma IgG antibodies (Porter and Sande,

1992). Diagnosis of CNS lymphoma is thus dependent on microscopic examination of tissue obtained by brain biopsy. Given the invasiveness of this procedure, the usual clinical approach at our institution to these patients is to treat first with antitoxoplasma agents and to perform brain biopsy to obtain tissue for diagnosis if no clinical response is observed within 7 days.

Patients with primary CNS lymphomas are typically severely immunocompromised (75% will have peripheral $CD4^+$ lymphocyte counts of $\leq 50/\mu l$) and usually have had prior opportunistic infections. In one study, 11 HIV-1-infected individuals with primary CNS lymphoma had a median peripheral $CD4^+$ lymphocyte count of $30/\mu l$ and 73% had a previous AIDS-defining diagnosis (Kristal *et al.*, 1988).

2.2.2. Morphologic Features

The primary CNS lymphomas are generally classified as large cell lymphomas, occur in the brain parenchyma in a perivascular cuffing pattern, and may occur as a single or a small number of parenchymal lesions. In contrast, metastatic systemic lymphoma involving the brain is typically localized to the meninges.

2.2.3. Molecular Features

In contrast to HIV-associated systemic lymphomas, HIV-associated primary CNS lymphomas are a relatively homogeneous molecular subgroup (Shiramizu *et al.*, 1992; Meeker *et al.*, 1991; McMahon *et al.*, 1991). They are monoclonal, as defined by Ig gene rearrangement studies, and are almost universally associated with EBV. [There are only rare cases of HIV-associated primary CNS lymphomas lacking EBV, wherein EBV cannot be detected even with the use of highly sensitive gene amplification-based assays (Gunthel *et al.*, 1994).] c-*myc* rearrangement is not associated with this group of lymphomas (Shiramizu *et al.*, 1992; Meeker *et al.*, 1991).

2.2.4. Prognosis

The prognosis for HIV-associated primary CNS lymphomas is uniformly poor, probably in large part because these lymphomas arise in patients with advanced HIV disease.

2.3. HIV-Associated Body Cavity-Based (BCB) Lymphomas

2.3.1. Clinical Features

A recently described and unusual subset of HIV-associated lymphomas are those that arise in body cavities (i.e., pleural, peritoneal, or pericardial spaces) without evidence of tissue-based lymphoma. Only two series of eight cases each have been reported to date, one originating from New York which focused on molecular features (Cesarman *et al.*, 1995) and one from San Francisco which focused on defining clinical features in common and unique to this subset of lymphomas as well as assessing and correlating their molecular features (Komanduri *et al.*, 1996).

The clinical features of the eight patients in San Francisco who presented with HIV-associated BCB lymphomas revealed that they occurred in individuals with advanced HIV disease (six had had prior opportunistic infections, and all had peripheral $CD4^+$ lymphocytes < 200/μl) and presented clinically with symptoms related to distension of the relevant body cavity. Routine clinical laboratory tests were nondiagnostic, but revealed that all patients were hypoalbuminemic, five were hyponatremic, and five were severely thrombocytopenic (peripheral platelet counts ≤ 50,000/μl).

2.3.2. Morphologic Features

The malignant cells in the BCB lymphomas are large, have moderate to high nucleus-to-cytoplasm ratios and irregularly shaped nuclei, and are hyperchromatic with frequent mitotic figures. Of note, these cells are frequently misclassified as atypical lymphocytes or monocytes when the fluids are examined by clinical laboratory technologists in the routine clinical laboratories.

2.3.3. Molecular Features

Malignant BCB cells are thought to be of B-cell origin based on the following observations. First, monoclonal Ig gene rearrangements in the absence of T-cell receptor gene rearrangements have been demonstrated in most of the reported cases. Second, the malignant cells universally express cell surface CD38 only, a "null" phenotype observed with the malignant cells of multiple myeloma, a B-cell dyscrasia. Thus, although the Ig gene locus frequently rearranges in non-B-cell-derived malignancies and CD38 is expressed on a variety of cells (including hematopoietic stem cells, differentiating myeloid cells, and activated T and B cells), the nonrandom combination of the two findings supports a B-cell origin of the malignant BCB lymphoma cells. There has been no evidence of cytoplasmic or cell surface Ig expression by malignant BCB lymphoma cells to date.

Komanduri *et al.* (in press) demonstrated that IL-6 and IL-10 levels in the malignant fluid effusions were 340- to 16,000-fold higher than in normal plasma. Although similar levels of these two cytokines have been reported in nonmalignant effusions, elevated IL-6 and IL-10 levels in BCB lymphoma fluids may have significance given their ability to induce B-cell proliferation and differentiation.

At least 31 cases of HIV-associated BCB lymphomas have been reported. Cesarman *et al.* (1995) reported eight cases, all of which had monoclonal Ig gene rearrangements, were monoclonally infected with EBV, and had human herpes virus type 8 (HHV-8) gene sequences present. c-*myc* rearrangement was not detected in 5 of the 8 cases so analyzed, Komanduri *et al.* (1996) confirmed the 100% association of HHV-8 gene sequences in their 8 reported cases, but in contrast demonstrated that only half of their BCB lymphomas had monoclonal Ig gene rearrangements, only half (two polyclonal and two monoclonal BCB lymphomas) contained EBV, and only the two monoclonal tumors were monoclonally infected with EBV.

The remaining 13 cases of HIV-associated BCB lymphomas have been reported in conjunction with other HIV-associated nonmalignant effusions, and lacked systematic analysis for clonality, infection with EBV, and presence of HHV-8 gene sequences (Green *et al.*, 1995; Chadburn *et al.*, 1993; Walts *et al.*, 1990; Knowles *et al.*, 1989).

In summary, HIV-associated BCB lymphomas can be monoclonal or polyclonal, do not always contain EBV, but uniformly contain HHV-8 gene sequences.

Of interest, HHV-8 gene sequences were originally discovered in tissue specimens obtained from patients with endemic or HIV-associated Kaposi's sarcoma (KS) (Moore and Chang, 1995; Chang *et al.*, 1994) and initially thought to play a role in its pathogenesis. Of note, 5 of 8 patients in our series, 6 of 8 (Green *et al.*, 1995) and 2 of 12 (Cesarman *et al.*, 1995) in previously reported series lacked clinical evidence of KS. Thus, the observation that HHV-8 is highly associated with KS *and* with BCB lymphomas contradicts a unique association with a single disease entity. HHV-8 gene sequences, in the absence of EBV, have also been reported in a single case of BCB lymphoma occurring in an individual *not* infected with HIV (Nador *et al.*, 1995), further emphasizing the nonrandom association and potential pathogenetic role of this virus in BCB lymphomas regardless of EBV or HIV coinfection.

2.3.4. Prognosis

Given that HIV-associated BCB lymphomas typically arise in patients with advanced HIV disease, it is not surprising that the disease has a uniformly poor prognosis. The median survival for the 8 cases observed in San Francisco was 57 days (range 6–166 days), and previously reported survival times for 8 of 31 reported cases of HIV-associated malignant effusions ranged from 10 days to 14 months (Walts *et al.*, 1990; Knowles *et al.*, 1989; Chadburn *et al.*, 1993; Green *et al.*, 1995; Cesarman *et al.*, 1995). Komanduri and colleagues demonstrated little correlation of molecular features of the BCB lymphoma cells with length of survival, and that the performance status of the individual patient was in fact the best indicator of response to chemotherapy or survival.

2.4. HIV-Associated Hodgkin's Disease

2.4.1. Clinical Features

Six studies (Pelstring *et al.*, 1991; Ames *et al.*, 1991; Ree *et al.*, 1991; Tirelli *et al.*, 1989; Lowenthal *et al.*, 1988; Knowles *et al.*, 1988) have cumulatively reported 114 cases of HIV-associated Hodgkin's disease, and it is apparent that the presentation of HIV-associated Hodgkin's disease has two major differences from its clinical presentation and course in immunocompetent individuals. First, the age at presentation (mean, 32 years, with a large group presenting between 35 and 49 years) does not mimic the usual bimodal age distribution observed for Hodgkin's disease in non-HIV-infected individuals. Second, 50–89% of patients with HIV-associated Hodgkin's disease will present with widespread disease (clinical stages III and IV) with frequent involvement of bone marrow, CNS, GI tract, and skin, whereas only 40% of non-HIV-infected individuals with Hodgkin's disease will present with clinically advanced disease.

2.4.2. Morphologic Features

Of 103 cases of HIV-associated Hodgkin's disease reported in these six independent studies, mixed cellularity was observed in 47% of the cases, nodular sclerosis in 29%, lymphocytes depleted in 10%, and 14% were either not subclassified or had mixed histologic features.

2.4.3. Molecular Features

The Reed–Sternberg cell is considered to be the malignant cell in Hodgkin's disease. Although the cell lineage of origin for Reed–Sternberg cells has not been established with certainty, the universal observation of EBV in Reed–Sternberg cells in virtually all cases of Hodgkin's disease arising in immunocompetent individuals suggested that the malignant cells might originate from B cells. For 11 of 12 cases of HIV-associated Hodgkin's disease, Herndier *et al.* (1993) similarly detected EBV in Reed–Sternberg cells; the single discrepant case lacking EBV was morphologically classified as a nodular lymphocyte predominant subtype, a variant of Hodgkin's disease with morphologic features overlapping that of low-grade B-cell lymphomas and a variant in which EBV has never been detected (Weiss and Chang, 1992; Poppema, 1992).

2.4.4. Prognosis

The clinical behavior of Hodgkin's disease in the setting of HIV disease can be variable. In general, most patients have a clinical response to conventional therapy but succumb to opportunistic infections. Of 41 patients (Tirelli *et al.*, 1989; Lowenthal *et al.*, 1988; Knowles *et al.*, 1988), 21 had complete remissions, 19 partial remissions, and 1 patient died on the first day of therapy; median survival was 15 months. Of note, 7 of 12 patients in another series (Herndier *et al.*, 1993) survived at least 23–98 months after diagnosis.

2.5. HIV-Associated T-Cell Lymphomas

A few HIV-associated peripheral or cutaneous (pseudo-Sezary syndrome) T-cell lymphomas have been reported, and constitute a very small proportion of all HIV-associated lymphomas. No consistent phenotype is expressed by the tumor cells. Prognosis is poor, with survival beyond 9 months unusual.

One HIV-associated T-cell lymphoma had clonally integrated HIV within the tumor genomic DNA, raising the possibility that insertional mutagenesis may have played a role in its pathogenesis (Herndier *et al.*, 1992).

3. PATHOGENESIS OF HIV-ASSOCIATED LYMPHOMAS

The vast majority of HIV-associated lymphomas are of B-cell origin. thus, pathogenetic mechanisms for the origins of these lymphomas must consider events in normal B-cell development as well as cofactors traditionally associated with B-cell immortalization and transformation.

3.1. More on Normal B-Cell Development, Ig Formation, and Maturation

3.1.1. Molecular Events in Immunoglobulin Production and Antibody Maturation

As discussed earlier, the antibody structure can be divided into the N-terminal variable (V) region, the antigen binding site (or idiotype), and C-terminal constant (C) region, the effector portion (e.g., complement binding). The idiotype serves as a unique marker for a B-cell clone and can and has been used as a unique tumor marker for B-cell malignancies producing immunoglobulins.

As discussed earlier, Ig production by B cells involves rearrangement of Ig variable (V), diversity (D), and joining (J) genes to produce heavy (H) and light (L) Ig chains, the pairing of which forms a functional antibody. For humans, it is estimated that the naive antibody repertoire encompassing all possible combinations of heavy and light chain pairings and potential V, D, and J gene rearrangements for both the heavy and light chains is $> 10^{10}$. In other words, at least 10^{10} antibody specificities are theoretically available and genetically encoded in the germline of the antigenically naive host from the simple process of Ig gene rearrangement and H and L chain pairing.

In addition to V-region somatic mutation that increases antibody affinity, the enzyme terminal nucleotidyl transferase adds a variable number of nucleotides ("N" additions) to the VD and DJ junctions, to further modify the binding site of the antibody V gene. The "VDJ" segment of an antibody (i.e., the CDR3 region) thus serves as a "molecular fingerprint" of a specific clone of B cells, since it is highly unlikely that the same combination of V, D, J genes and specific N additions/deletions would have occurred by random chance alone.

As mentioned earlier, the antigen binding site is a three-dimensional "pocket" created by the pairing of the H and L chain variable regions. The variable gene can be further subdivided into three framework regions (Fr1–3) separated by three complementarity determining regions (CDR1–3); the Frs contribute to the structure of the variable region, whereas the CDRs are the regions intimately juxtaposed against the antigen in the antigen binding site.

Longitudinal studies of antibodies produced by mice in response to a chronic antigenic challenge demonstrated initial clonal proliferation of B cells producing antibodies reactive with the inciting antigen. Antibodies produced subsequently were from the same clones of B cells, but contained discrete nucleotide substitutions in the CDR1 and CDR2 regions resulting in amino acid changes that correlated with increased antibody affinity and avidity for the inciting antigen. This process has since been termed *somatic hypermutation* and is the molecular basis for changing the amino acids in contact with the antigen in the antigen binding site to produce antibodies with increased affinity and avidity. Somatic hypermutation, in response to continued antigenic challenge, is thought to favor nucleotide changes in the CDRs over the Frs (Kocks and Rajewsky, 1989; Manser *et al.*, 1987; Shlomchik *et al.*, 1987).

3.1.2. Normal B-Cell Development and B-Cell Lineages

B-cell development has been well defined in mice. Two apparently independent lineages of B cells, B1 and B2, have been functionally and immunophenotypically identified (Haughton *et al.*, 1993; Herzenberg and Herzenberg, 1989). Murine B1 cells can be identified immunophenotypically as $CD5^{+}CD44^{high}CD23^{+}J11d^{high}$ whereas the immunophenotype of murine B2 cells is $CD5^{-}CD44^{high}CD23^{-}J11d^{low}$ (Murphy *et al.*, 1990; Lebrun *et al.*, 1988; Herzenberg *et al.*, 1986; Hayakawa *et al.*, 1986).

The two B-cell lineages differ functionally. B1 cells are a self-renewing population, can present antigen to themselves, typically use Ig V_H genes unmodified from germline, have little or no N additions at the VD and DJ junctions, and produce polyreactive IgMs in a T-cell-independent manner. The mechanism(s) for the apparent lack of somatic hypermutation in immunoglobulins produced by B1 cells remains unclear. In contrast, B2 cells behave as "conventional" B cells, requiring T-cell help to mount an effective immune response, and have a flexible antibody repertoire based on their access to enzymatic mechanisms operative in modification of Ig V_H genes, including somatic hypermutation (i.e., select nucleotide changes resulting in amino acid substitutions from the germline-encoded sequence) and variable amounts of N substitution to the VD and DJ junctions, to produce antibodies with higher affinity and avidity.

The development of human B cells has been postulated to occur in a fashion analogous to that described for mice, although distinct immunophenotypes for the postulated human B1 and B2 subsets have not yet been well defined, and the expression of CD5 as a marker for human B1 cells remains controversial (Haughton *et al.*, 1993).

Of note, the proportion of $CD5^+$ B cells in HIV-infected individuals actually increases with disease progression, although absolute numbers decrease [as a result of increasing lymphopenia and reduced numbers of circulating B cells associated with disease progression (Indraccolo *et al.*, 1993; Moody *et al.*, 1988)].

3.2. Effect of HIV Infection on B Cells

Individuals infected with HIV-1 have a variety of B-cell abnormalities, including polyclonal B-cell activation and aberrant immunoregulation (Yarchoan *et al.*, 1986; Birx *et al.*, 1986; Pahwa *et al.*, 1984; Lane *et al.*, 1983). One of the earliest clinical findings following infection with HIV-1 is hypergammaglobulinemia (Nath *et al.*, 1987), often accompanied by paraproteinemia/oligoclonal bands which display anti-HIV-1 (specifically anti-"gag" and anti-"pol") reactivity (Ng *et al.*, 1988, 1989; Papadopoulos *et al.*, 1988). High levels of circulating HIV-1-containing immune complexes are often present, and autoantibodies can be frequently detected (but usually not manifested as clinically evident autoimmune disease).

B cells of HIV-infected individuals also differ from those obtained from normal healthy donors in *in vitro* assays. B cells from HIV-infected individuals will spontaneously secrete IgG and IgM at high levels, produce cytokines that induce B-cell proliferation and differentiation (i.e., IL-6 and IL-10), and have decreased *in vitro* proliferative responses to recall antigens. Not all of these dysfunctions are corrected by autologous T cells, suggesting that the defects may be intrinsic to B cells themselves.

Despite the B-cell abnormalities associated with HIV infection, HIV-infected individuals can mount specific immune responses and produce antigen-specific antibodies. It is well recognized that anti-HIV antibodies are produced throughout the life of the HIV-infected individual. Of note, in a few well-studied HIV-infected individuals, anti-"gag" (specifically anti-p24) antibodies disappeared with progression of HIV disease whereas anti-"env" antibodies were detectable throughout the course of HIV-associated disease.

One subset of B cells expressing Ig using a particular heavy chain variable region (i.e., the D12 idiotope of the V_H3 gene family) can interact directly with HIV gp120 and thus be directly activated by HIV (Berberian *et al.*, 1991, 1993). Thus, HIV gp120 can act directly as a B-cell superantigen. Population studies have demonstrated initial increases followed by selective clonal depletion of B cells expressing these immunoglobulins in concert with progression of HIV disease and with decreases in levels of serum anti-gp120 antibodies using the D12 idiotope (Berberian *et al.*, 1994).

3.3. Cytokine Perturbations in HIV Infection and HIV-Associated Lymphomas

HIV-infected individuals have elevated levels of serum IL-6 (Birx *et al.*, 1990), and IL-6 and IL-10 as well as their mRNA transcripts have been convincingly demonstrated in the malignant cells of HIV-associated lymphomas (Marsh *et al.*, 1995; Emilie *et al.*, 1992a,b; Benjamin *et al.*, 1992). Since both of these cytokines play a role in B-cell proliferation and differentiation, aberrant control of their production by the malignant B cells themselves may result in an autocrine loop necessary for lymphomagenesis.

3.4. Proposed Models for HIV-Associated Lymphomagenesis

The differing clinical, morphological, and molecular features of the subsets of HIV-associated lymphomas discussed earlier suggest multiple discrete pathogenetic pathways for each subset. Proposed pathogenetic models for each subset are discussed separately.

3.4.1. Pathogenesis of HIV-Associated Systemic Lymphomas

As discussed earlier, approximately 70–75% of all HIV-associated systemic lymphomas are large cell lymphomas, whereas the remainder are Burkitt's lymphomas. The large cell lymphomas are molecularly heterogeneous, whereas the Burkitt's are fairly homogeneous at a molecular level. Proposed pathogenetic mechanisms thus differ and are discussed separately.

3.4.1a. Pathogenesis of HIV-Associated Large Cell Lymphomas. This group constitutes the largest group of HIV-associated lymphomas. They occur in individuals with wide variability in residual immune function, can be polyclonal or monoclonal, and the majority lack EBV and c-*myc* rearrangements.

The most plausible pathogenetic model to account for these varied molecular findings is a multifactorial one. In this model, HIV-associated lymphomas are viewed as a continuum beginning with polyclonal proliferation of B cells in an immunocompromised host lacking sufficient T-cell control of B-cell proliferation, with the continuously proliferating B cells at increased risk for accumulation of additional genetic events and ultimately outgrowth of transformed B-cell clones. EBV or HIV could provide exogenous proliferative stimuli, since HIV is chronically replicating in the infected host, and reactivation of EBV with continuous lytic replication can occur in the immunoincompetent host. The mitogenic potential of EBV for B cells has been well documented, conventional antigenic stimulation by EBV virion-associated proteins could also be occurring, and HIV could provide continuous conventional antigenic or superantigenic (i.e., gp120) stimuli. Additional genetic events presumably leading to transformation are as yet undefined, but genetic lesions typically associated with other malignant processes have not been consistently detected [e.g., p53 and/or *Ras* mutations are observed in only a subset and mutations in the retinoblastoma gene (RB1) have not been detected (Ballerini *et al.*, 1993)]. Given this model, it is conceivable that continuous B-cell proliferation alone, in an immunoincompetent host unable to exert appropriate T-cell control to limit the proliferation, can manifest clinically as a lymphoma.

DNA sequences encoding heavy chain variable regions of the expressed immunoglobulins of a few monoclonal lymphomas lacking EBV and c-*myc* rearrangements support this proposed multifactorial model. Specifically, virtually all expressed HIV-associated lymphoma immunoglobulins examined to date have significant numbers of nucleotide substitutions, with all having <95% nucleotide homology to their germline-encoded counterparts (Ng *et al.*, 1994, 1995). Of note, nucleotide substitutions have not been limited to the CDRs (as would be expected for conventional T-cell-mediated somatic hypermutation), suggesting that unconventional somatic hypermutation may occur. The CDR3s of lymphoma immunoglobulins examined have excessive N additions (such that the germline counterparts cannot be determined), also supporting the hypothesis of chronic B-cell stimulation and subsequent extensive Ig modifications. Of interest, similar findings at the DNA level have been observed with normal anti-HIV immunoglobulins expressed in individuals lacking lymphoma (Andrus *et al.*, 1991), as well as with analysis of random immunoglobulins produced in a hyperplastic lymph node obtained from an HIV-infected individual (Ng *et al.*, 1995). These latter findings in individuals lacking lymphomas suggest that a continuum exists between the population of B cells responding normally to a chronic antigenic stimulus and those destined to become malignant.

Despite the apparent clonal decrease in the subset of B cells expressing the D12 idiotope of V_H3 gene family in the peripheral blood of individuals with progressive HIV-associated disease (Berberian *et al.*, 1991), at least one HIV-associated lymphoma IgM (produced by a monoclonal Burkitt's lymphoma monoclonally infected with EBV but lacking c-*myc* rearrangement) has been demonstrated to use a highly modified (approximately 95% homologous to its most related germline gene) version of this idiotope; this lymphoma Ig retained antigenic specificity for HIV gp160 (Ng *et al.*, 1994). Furthermore, the germline D gene from which the CDR3 was derived could not be identified because of the high degree of N addition and deletion. These findings suggest that this subset of B cells may in fact be localized to sites where HIV replication is continuous and the most active (i.e., lymph nodes), and that this uncontrolled and continuous B-cell proliferation (with subsequent aberrant antibody modifications) can manifest clinically as a lymphoma.

Although EBV and HIV have been implicated as sources for antigenic stimuli in this multifactorial model of lymphomagenesis, host-encoded or "self" antigens that are also chronically present may also play a role. This is supported by studies on a secreted IgM from another monoclonal HIV-associated lymphoma (Burkitt's morphology, no EBV or c-*myc* rearrangement detected) where reactivity with human actin and human IgG, but no HIV-specific proteins, was demonstrated (Ng *et al.*, 1994). The DNA encoding the V_H gene used by this IgM was only 95% homologous to its most related germline gene, and the germline D gene from which its CDR3 arose could not be assigned given the large number of N additions and deletions. Thus, production of autoreactive antibodies may independently permit continuous clonal proliferation and ultimate clinical manifestation as lymphoma.

3.4.1b. Pathogenesis of HIV-Associated Burkitt's Lymphoma. Burkitt's lymphoma in non-HIV-infected individuals occurs in two epidemiological patterns: endemic versus sporadic. Endemic Burkitt's lymphoma is observed in equatorial Africa and New Guinea, and over 95% of cases are associated with EBV. In contrast, only 20–30% of sporadically occurring Burkitt's lymphomas (i.e., those occurring in the United States and Europe) are associated with EBV. The majority of Burkitt's lymphomas (endemic and sporadically occurring) are monoclonal B-cell lymphomas containing c-*myc* translocations. The precise location of the chromosomal breakpoint associated with c-*myc* translocations differs between the two types of Burkitt's lymphoma. In sporadically occurring Burkitt's lymphoma, chromosomal breaks (and subsequent translocation of the telomeric portion) occur within the first exon, first intron, or flanking sequences of the c-*myc* locus (Pelicci *et al.*, 1986a).

HIV-associated Burkitt's lymphomas are most analogous to those occurring sporadically in non-HIV-infected individuals (Magrath, 1990). Specifically, if molecular results are combined for all cases of HIV-associated Burkitt's lymphoma reported in the six major series, only 40% are associated with EBV whereas >75% demonstrate c-*myc* rearrangements.

The high degree of c-*myc* translocations observed in both HIV-associated and sporadically occurring Burkitt's lymphomas suggests a similar pathogenesis. The pathogenetic model for sporadically occurring Burkitt's lymphomas has been attributed to perturbations in normal cellular growth induced by the product of the translocated c-*myc* gene. Specifically, the c-*myc* gene is located on chromosome 8, and translocations to Ig-encoding loci located on chromosomes 2 (kappa), 14 (heavy), and 22 (lambda) are the commonly observed nonrandom cytogenetic abnormalities associated with sporadically occurring Burkitt's lymphomas. The truncated c-*myc* gene, now placed under the transcriptional control of the Ig gene next to which it was juxtaposed, is presumably constitutively expressed and it is this increased expression that induced transformation by pathways not well defined.

3.4.2. Pathogenesis of HIV-Associated Primary CNS Lymphomas

HIV-associated primary CNS lymphomas are a molecularly homogeneous group in that virtually all are monoclonal and infected with EBV. EBV has been proposed to play a pathogenetic role in EBV-associated B-cell lymphomas in the setting of immunodeficiency (i.e., HIV infection, allograft recipients), presumably by conferring a selective growth advantage to a clone of cells infected with EBV. The observation that HIV-associated primary CNS lymphomas occur in individuals with advanced AIDS suggests a pathogenetic model wherein clonal outgrowths of B cells proliferate in response to an opportunistic infection with EBV in the absence of immune regulation. This process is most likely comparable to that proposed for monoclonal EBV-associated B-cell lymphomas arising in all mice with severe combined immunodeficiency disease (SCID) engrafted with peripheral blood lymphocytes obtained from EBV-seropositive donors (Bashir *et al.*, 1991; McCune, 1991), and may use mechanism(s) similar to that by which EBV immortalizes B cells *in vitro*.

3.4.3. Pathogenesis of HIV-Associated BCB Lymphomas

Insight into the pathogenesis of HIV-associated BCB lymphomas is limited by the small number and lack of systematic analysis in the majority of cases reported to date. The only universal finding for this subset of tumors, however, is that HHV-8 gene sequences are present (as contrasted with the inability to detect EBV in a significant number of cases). A pathogenetic model must explain all of the scientific findings of this subset of lymphomas, specifically that the tumors can (1) be monoclonal or polyclonal, (2) lack c-*myc* rearrangements, (3) do not always contain EBV, and (4) occur in body cavities containing excessive levels of IL-6 and IL-10.

It has been proposed that the malignant BCB lymphoma cells are of B-cell lineage based on universal expression of CD38, variable expression of other B-cell surface markers, and evidence of Ig gene rearrangement (Cesarman *et al.*, 1995; Chadburn *et al.*, 1993; Walts *et al.*, 1990; Knowles *et al.*, 1989). If so, perhaps HHV-8 is acting as a B-cell mitogen, analogous to that of EBV, in an environment containing markedly elevated levels of cytokines favoring B-cell proliferation and differentiation in immunoincompetent individuals. Chronic antigenic stimulation by HIV-1 may also contribute to B-cell proliferation.

Continued mitogen- or antigen-driven proliferation could predispose the proliferating cells to additional genetic events leading to the outgrowth of a monoclonal population.

3.4.4. Pathogenesis of Other HIV-Associated Lymphomas

The pathogenesis of conventional Hodgkin's lymphomas is poorly understood; there is a similar lack of insight into the pathogenesis of HIV-associated Hodgkin's lymphomas. Similarly, HIV-associated T-cell or other non-B-cell lymphomas occur so infrequently that systematic molecular analyses have not been performed to gain insight into their pathogenesis.

ACKNOWLEDGMENTS. Supported in part by NIH grant R01CA67381.

REFERENCES

Amadori, A., Gallo, P., Zamarchi, R., Veronese, M. L., De Rossi, A., Wolf, D., and Chieco-Bianchi, L., 1990, IgG oligoclonal bands in sera of HIV-1 infected patients are mainly directed against HIV-1 determinants, *AIDS Res. Hum. Retrovir.* **6:**581–586.

Ames, E. D., Conjalka, M. S., Goldberg, A. F., Hirschman, R., Jain, S., Distenfeld, A., and Metroka, C. E., 1991, Hodgkin's disease and AIDS: Twenty-three new cases and a review of the literature, *Hematol. Oncol. Clin. North Am.* **5:**343–356.

Andrus, J. S., Johnson, S., Zolla-Pazner, S., and Capra, J. D., 1991, Molecular characterization of five human anti-human immunodeficiency virus type 1 antibody heavy chains reveals extensive somatic mutation typical of an antigen-driven immune response, *Proc. Natl. Acad. Sci. USA* **88:**7783–7787.

Ballerini, P., Gaidano, G., Gong, J., Tassi, V., Saglio, G., Knowles, D., and Dalla-Favera, R., 1993, Multiple genetic lesions in acquired immunodeficiency syndrome-related non-Hodgkin's lymphoma, *Blood* **81:**166–176.

Bashir, R., Okano, M., Kleveland, K., Pirrucello, S., Masih, A., Sanger, W., Fordyce-Boyer, R., and Purtilo, D., 1991, SCID/human mouse model of central nervous system lymphoproliferative disease, *Lab. Invest.* **65:** 702–709.

Baumgartner, J., Rachlin, J., Beckstead, J., Meeker, T. C., Levy, R. M., Wara, W. M., and Rosenblum, M. L., 1990, Primary central nervous system lymphomas: Natural history and response to radiation therapy in 55 patients with acquired immunodeficiency syndrome, *J. Neurosurg.* **73:**206–211.

Benjamin, D., Knobloch, T. J., and Dayton, M. A., 1992, Human B cell interleukin 10: B cell lines derived from patients with acquired immunodeficiency syndrome and Burkitt's lymphoma constitutively secrete large quantities of interleukin 10, *Blood* **80:**1289–1298.

Beral, V., Peterman, T., Berkelman, R., and Jaffe, H., 1991, AIDS-associated non-Hodgkin lymphoma, *Lancet* **337:**805–809.

Berberian, L., Valles-Ayoub, Y., Sun, N., Martinez-Maza, O., and Braun, J., 1991, A VH clonal deficit in human immunodeficiency virus-positive individuals reflects a B-cell maturational arrest, *Blood* **78:**175–179.

Berberian, L., Goodglick, L., Kipps, T. J., and Braun, J., 1993, Immunoglobulin VH3 gene products: Natural ligands for HIV gp120, *Science* **261:**1588–1591.

Berberian, L., Shukla, J., Jefferis, R., and Braun, J., 1994, Effects of HIV infection on VH3 (D12 idiotope) B cells in vivo, *J. Acq. Immune Defic. Syndr.* **7:**641–646.

Birx, D. L., Redfield, R. R., and Tosato, G., 1986, Defective regulation of Epstein–Barr virus infection in patients with acquired immunodeficiency syndrome (AIDS) or AIDS-related disorders, *N. Engl. J. Med.* **314:** 874–879.

Birx, D. L., Redfield, R. R., Tencer, K., Fowler, A., Burke, D. S., and Tosato, G., 1990, Induction of interleukin-6 during human immunodeficiency virus infection, *Blood* **76:**2303–2310.

Cesarman, E., Chang, Y., Moore, P. S., Said, J. W., and Knowles, D. M., 1995, Kaposi's sarcoma-associated herpesvirus-like DNA sequences in AIDS-related body-cavity-based lymphomas, *N. Engl. J. Med.* **332:**1186–1191.

Chadburn, A., Cesarman, E., Jagirdar, J., Subar, M., Mir, R. N., and Knowles, D. M., 1993, CD30 (Ki-1) positive anaplastic large cell lymphomas in individuals infected with the human immunodeficiency virus, *Cancer* **72**:3078–3090.

Chang, Y., Cesarman, E., Pessin, M. S., Lee, F., Culpepper, J., Knowles, D. M., and Moore, P. S., 1994, Identification of herpesvirus-like DNA sequences in AIDS-associated Kaposi's sarcoma, *Science* **266**:1865–1869.

Cherepakhin, V., Feigal, E., and Kipps, T. J., 1992, Immunoglobulin heavy chain variable region genes expressed in AIDS-associated monoclonal B-cell lymphomas, *Blood* **80**, No. 10, Suppl. 1:116a (abstract 456).

Ciricillo, S. F., and Rosenblum, M. L., 1991, Imaging of solitary lesions in AIDS, *J. Neurosurg.* **74**:1029.

Delecluse, H. J., Raphael, M., Magaud, J. P., Felman, P., The French Study Group of Pathology for HIV-associated tumors, Abd Alsamad, I., Bornkamm, G. W., and Lenoir, G. M., 1993, Variable morphology of human immunodeficiency virus-associated lymphomas with c-*myc* rearrangements, *Blood* **82**:552–563.

Emilie, D., Coumbaras, J., Raphael, M., Devergne, O., Delecluse, H. J., Gisselbrecht, J. F., Michiels, J. F., Van Damme, J., Taga, T., Kishimoto, T., Crevon, M. D., and Galanaud, P., 1992a, Interleukin-6 production in high-grade B lymphomas: Correlation with the presence of malignant immunoblasts in acquired immunodeficiency syndrome and in human immunodeficiency virus-seronegative patients, *Blood* **80**:498–504.

Emilie, D., Touitou, R., Raphael, M., Peuchmaur, M., Devergne, O., Rea, D., Coumbaras, J., Crevon, M., Edelman, L., Joab, I., and Galanaud, P., 1992b, *In vivo* production of interleukin-10 by malignant cells in AIDS lymphomas, *Eur. J. Immunol.* **22**:2937 –2942.

Formenti, S. C., Gill, P. S., Lean, E., Rarick, M., Meyer, P. R., Boswell, W., Petrovich, Z., Chak, L., and Levine, A. M., 1989, Primary central nervous system lymphoma in AIDS: Results of radiation therapy, *Cancer* **63**:1101–1107.

Gail, M. H., Pluda, J. M., Rabkin, C. S., Biggar, R. J., Goedert, J. J., Horm, J. W., Sondik, E. J., Yarchoan, R., and Broder, S., 1991, Projections of the incidence of non-Hodgkin's lymphoma related to acquired immunodeficiency syndrome, *J. Natl. Cancer Inst.* **83**:;695–701.

Gill, P. S., Levine, A., Meyer, P., Boswell, W. D., Burkes, R. L., Parker, J. W., Hofman, F. M., Dworsky, R. L., and Lukes, R. L., 1985, Primary central nervous system lymphoma in homosexual men, *Am. J. Med.* **78**:742–748.

Green, I., Espiritu, E., Ladanyi, M., Chaponda, R., Wieczorek, R., Gallo, L., and Feiner, H., 1995, Primary lymphomatous effusions in AIDS: A morphological, immunophenotypic, and molecular study, *Mod. Pathol.* **8**:39–45.

Gunthel, C., Ng, V., Herndier, B., McGrath, M. S., and Shiramizu, B., 1994, Epstein–Barr virus subtypes in AIDS-associated central nervous system lymphomas, *Blood* **83**:618.

Hamilton-Dutoit, S. F., Pallesen, G., Franzman, M. B., Karkov, J., Black, F., Skinhoj, P., and Pedersen, C., 1991, AIDS-related lymphoma. Histopathology, immunophenotype and association with Epstein–Barr virus as demonstrated by *in situ* nucleic acid hybridization, *Am. J. Pathol.* **138**:149–163.

Harnly, M. E., Swan, S. H., Holly, E. A., Kelter, A., and Padian, N., 1988, Temporal trends in the incidence of non-Hodgkin's lymphoma and selected malignancies in a population with a high incidence of acquired immunodeficiency syndrome (AIDS), *Am. J. Epidemiol.* **128**:261–267.

Haughton, G., Arnold, L. W., Whitmore, A. C., and Clarke, S. H., 1993, B-1 cells are made, not born, *Immunol. Today* **14**:84–87.

Hayakawa, K., Hardy, R. R., and Herzenberg, L. A., 1986, Peritoneal ly-1 B cells: Genetic control, autoantibody production, increased lambda light chain expression, *Eur. J. Immunol.* **16**:450–456.

Herndier, B. G., and Friedman, S., 1992, Neoplasms of the gastrointestinal tract and hepatobiliary system in acquired immunodeficiency syndrome, *Semin. Liver Dis.* **12**:128–141.

Herndier, B., Shiramizu, B., Jewett, N., Aldape, K., Reyes, G., and McGrath, M. S., 1992, AIDS-associated T cell lymphoma: Evidence for HIV-1 associated T-cell transformation, *Blood* **79**:1768–1774.

Herndier, B. G., Sanchez, H., Chang, K., Chen, Y., and Weiss, L., 1993, High prevalence of Epstein–Barr virus in the Reed–Sternberg cells of HIV-associated Hodgkin's disease, *Am. J. Pathol.* **142**:1073–1079.

Herndier, B. G., Kaplan, L. D., and McGrath, M. S., 1994, Pathogenesis of AIDS lymphomas, *AIDS* **8**:1025–1049.

Herzenberg, L. A., and Herzenberg, L. A., 1989, Toward a layered immune system, *Cell* **59**:953–954.

Herzenberg, L. A., Stall, A. M., Lalor, P. L., Sidman, C., Moore, W. A., Parks, D. R., and Herzenberg, L. A., 1986, The ly-1 B cell lineage, *Immunol. Rev.* **93**:81–102.

Indraccolo, S., Mion, M., Zamarchi, R., Veronesi, A., Veronese, M. L., Panozzo, M., Betterle, C., Barelli, A., Borri, A., Amadori, A., and Chieco-Bianchi, L., 1993, B cell activation and human immunodeficiency virus infection. V. Phenotypic and functional alterations in CD5+ and CD5− B cell subsets, *J. Clin. Immunol.* **13**:381–388.

Kaplan, L. D., Abrams, D. I., Feigal, E., McGrath, M., Kahn, J., Neville, P., Ziegler, J., and Volberding, P., 1989, AIDS-associated non-Hodgkin's lymphoma in San Francisco, *J. Am. Med. Assoc.* **261**:719–724.

Kaplan, L. D., Shiramizu, B., Herndier, B., Kahn, J., Meeker, T. C., Ng, V., Volberding, P. A., and McGrath, M. S., 1995, Influence of molecular characteristics on clinical outcome in human immunodeficiency virus-associated non-Hodgkin's lymphoma: Identification of a subgroup with favorable clinical outcome, *Blood* **85**:1727–1735.

Knowles, D. M., Chamulak, G., Subar, M., Burke, J. S., Dugan, M., Wernz, J., Slywotzky, C., Pelicci, P.-G., Dalla-Favera, R., and Raphael, B., 1988, Lymphoid neoplasia associated with the acquired immunodeficiency syndrome (AIDS). The New York University Medical Center experience with 105 patients, *Ann. Intern. Med.* **108**:744–753.

Knowles, D. M., Inghirami, G., Ubriaco, A., and Dalla Favera, R., 1989, Molecular genetic analysis of three AIDS-associated neoplasms of uncertain lineage demonstrates their B-cell derivation and the possible pathogenetic role of the Epstein–Barr virus, *Blood* **73**:792–799.

Kocks, C., and Rajewsky, K., 1989, Stable expression and somatic hypermutation of antibody V regions in B-cell developmental pathways, *Annu. Rev. Immunol.* **7**:537–559.

Komanduri, K. V., Luce, J. A., McGrath, M. S., Herndier, B. G., and Ng, V. L., Clinical and laboratory features of HIV-associated body cavity based lymphomas, *J. Acq. Immune Defic. Syndr.* (in press).

Kristal, A. R., Nasca, P. C., Burnett, W. S., and Mikl, J., 1988, Changes in the epidemiology of non-Hodgkin's lymphoma associated with epidemic human immunodeficiency virus (HIV) infection, *Am. J. Epidemiol.* **128**:711–718.

Lane, H. C., Masur, H., Edgar, L. C., Whalen, G., Rook, A. H., and Fauci, A. S., 1983, Abnormalities of B cell activation and immunoregulation in patients with the acquired immunodeficiency syndrome, *N. Engl. J. Med.* **309**:453–458.

Lebrun, P., Sidman, C. L., and Spiegelberg, H. L., 1988, IgE formation and Fc receptor-positive lymphocytes in normal, immunodeficient and auto-immune mice infected with *Nippostrongylus brasiliensis*, *J. Immunol.* **141**:249.

Levine, A. M., Sullivan-Halley, J., Pike, M. C., Rarick, M. U., Loureiro, C., Bernstein-Singer, M., Willson, E., Brynes, R., Parker, J., Rasheed, S., and Gill, P. S., 1991, AIDS-related lymphoma: Prognostic factors predictive of survival, *Cancer* **68**:2466–2472.

Lowenthal, D. A., Straus, D. J., Campbell, S. W., Gold, J. W., Clarkson, B. D., and Koziner, B., 1988, AIDS-related lymphoid neoplasias: The Memorial Hospital experience, *Cancer* **61**:2325–2337.

Luft, B. J., Hafner, R., Korzun, A. H., Leport, C., Antoniskis, D., Bosler, E. M., Bourland, D. D., III, Uttamchandani, R., Fuhrer, J., Jackobson, J., Morlat, P., Vilde, J.-L., Remington, J. S., and members of the ACTG 077p/ANRS 009 study team, 1993, Toxoplasmic encephalitis in patients with the acquired immunodeficiency syndrome, *N. Engl. J. Med.* **329**:995–1000.

McCune, J. M., 1991, Epstein–Barr virus associated lymphoproliferative disease in mice and men, *Lab. Invest.* **65**:377–378.

McGrath, M. S., Shiramizu, B., Meeker, T., Kaplan, L., and Herndier, B., 1991, AIDS-associated polyclonal lymphoma: Identification of a new HIV-associated disease process, *J. Acq. Immune Defic. Syndr.* **4**:408–415.

McMahon, E., Glass, J. D., Hayward, S. D., Mann, R. B., Becker, P. S., Charache, P., McArthur, J. C., and Ambinder, R. F., 1991, Epstein–Barr virus in AIDS-related primary central nervous system lymphoma, *Lancet* **338**:969–973.

Magrath, I. T., ed., 1990, *The Non-Hodgkin's Lymphomas*, Williams & Wilkins, Baltimore.

Manser, T., Wysocki, L. J., Margolies, M. N., and Gefter, M. L., 1987, Evolution of antibody variable region structure during the immune response, *Immunol. Rev.* **96**:141–162.

Marsh, J., Herndier, B., Ng, V. L., Shiramizu, B., Abbey, N., Sanchez, H., McGrath, M. S., 1995, Cytokine expression in AIDS associated large cell lymphomas, *I. Interferon and Cytokine Res.* **56**:318–327.

Meeker, T. C., Shiramizu, B., Kaplan, L., Herndier, B., Sanchez, H., Grimaldi, J. C., Baumgartner, J., Rachlin, J., Feigal, E., Rosenblum, M., and McGrath, M. S., 1991, Evidence for molecular subtypes of HIV-associated lymphoma: Division into peripheral monoclonal lymphoma, peripheral polyclonal lymphoma, and central nervous system lymphoma, *AIDS* **5**:669–674.

Moody, D. J., Casavant, C. H., Fulwyler, M. J., McHugh, T. M., and Stites, D. P., 1988, Multiparameter flow cytometric analysis of mononuclear cells from HIV-infected individuals, *Cytometry* (Suppl.) **3**:44–47.

Moore, P. S., and Chang, Y., 1995, Detection of herpesvirus-like DNA sequences in Kaposi's sarcoma in patients with and those without HIV infection, *N. Engl. J. Med.* **332**:1181–1185.

Moore, R. D., Kessler, H., Richman, D. D., Flexner, C., and Chaisson, R. E., 1991, Non-Hodgkin's lymphoma in patients with advanced HIV infection treated with zidovudine, *J. Am. Med. Assoc.* **265**:2208–2211.

Murphy, T. P., Kolber, D. L., and Rothstein, T. L., 1990, Elevated expression of pgp-1 (ly-24) by murine peritoneal lymphocytes, *Eur. J. Immunol.* **20**:1137–1142.

Nador, R. G., Cesarman, E., Knowles, D. M., and Said, J. W., 1995, Herpes-like DNA sequences in a body-cavity-based lymphoma in an HIV-negative patient, *N. Engl. J. Med.* **333**:943.

Nath, N., Wunderlich, C., Darr, F. W., II, Douglas, D. K., and Dodd, R. Y., 1987, Immunoglobulin level in donor blood reactive for antibodies to human immunodeficiency virus, *J. Clin. Microbiol.* **25**:364–369.

Ng, V. L., Hwang, K. M., Reyes, G. R., Kaplan, L. D., Khayam-Bashi, H., Hadley, W. K., and McGrath, M. S., 1988, High titer anti-HIV antibody reactivity associated with a paraprotein spike in a homosexual male with AIDS related complex, *Blood* **71**:1397–1401.

Ng, V. L., Chen, K. H., Hwang, K. M., Khayam-Bashi, H., and McGrath, M. S., 1989, The clinical significance of human immunodeficiency virus type 1-associated paraproteins, *Blood* **74**:2471–2475.

Ng, V. L., Hurt, M. H., Fein, C. L., Khayam-Bashi, H., Marsh, J., Nunes, W., McPhaul, L. W., Feigal, E., Nelson, P., Herndier, B. G., Shiramizu, B. T., Reyes, G. R., Fry, K. E., and McGrath, M. S., 1994, IgMs produced by 2 AIDS lymphoma cell lines: Immunoglobulin binding specificity and V_H gene "putative" somatic mutation analysis, *Blood* **83**:1067–1078.

Ng, V. L., Hurt, M. H., Herndier, B. G., and McGrath, M. S., 1995, V_H gene use by CD5+ AIDS-associated B-cell lymphoproliferations, *Ann. N.Y. Acad. Sci.* **764**:507–509.

Pahwa, S. G., Quilop, M. T. J., Lange, M., Pahwa, R. N., and Grieco, M. H., 1984, Defective B-lymphocyte function in homosexual men in relation to the acquired immunodeficiency syndrome, *Ann. Intern. Med.* **101**:757–763.

Papadopoulos, N. M., Costello, R., and Moutsopoulos, H. M., 1988, Identification of HIV-specific oligoclonal immunoglobulins in serum of carriers of HIV antibody, *Clin. Chem.* (Winston-Salem, NC) **34**:973–975.

Pelicci, P.-G., Knowles, D. M., Magrath, I. T., and Dalla-Favera, R., 1986a, Chromosomal breakpoints and structural alterations of the c-*myc* locus differ in endemic and sporadic forms of Burkitt lymphoma, *Proc. Natl. Acad. Sci. USA* **83**:2984–2988.

Pelicci, P.-G., Knowles, D. M., Zalmen, A. A., Wieczorek, R., Luciw, P., Dina, D., Basilico, C., and Dalla-Favera, R., 1986b, Multiple monoclonal B cell expansions and c-*myc* oncogene rearrangements in acquired immune deficiency syndrome-related lymphoproliferative disorders, *J. Exp. Med.* **164**:2049–2076.

Pelstring, R. J., Zellmer, R. B., Sulak, L. E., Banks, P. M., and Clare, N., 1991, Hodgkin's disease in association with human immunodeficiency virus infection: Pathologic and immunologic features, *Cancer* **67**:1865–1873.

Pluda, J. M., Yarchoan, R., Jaffe, E. S., Feuerstein, I. M., Solomon, D., Steinberg, S. M., Wyvill, K. M., Raubitschek, A., Katz, D., and Broder, S., 1990, Development of non-Hodgkin's lymphoma in a cohort of patients with severe human immunodeficiency virus (HIV) infection on long-term antiretroviral therapy, *Ann. Intern. Med.* **113**:276–282.

Poppema, S., 1992, Lymphocyte-predominance Hodgkin's disease, *Semin. Diagn. Pathol.* **9**:257–264.

Porter, S. B., and Sande, M. A., 1992, Toxoplasmosis of the central nervous system in the acquired immunodeficiency syndrome, *N. Engl. J. Med.* **327**:1643–1648.

Ree, H. J., Strauchen, J. A., Khan, A. A., Gold, J. E., Crowley, J. P., Kahn, H., and Zalusky, R., 1991, Human immunodeficiency virus-associated Hodgkin's disease: Clinicopathologic studies of 24 cases and preponderance of mixed cellular type characterized by the occurrence of fibrohistiocytoid stromal cells, *Cancer* **67**:1614–1621.

Shlomchik, M. J., Aucoin, A. H., Pisetsky, D. S., and Weigert, M. G., 1987, Structure and function of anti-DNA autoantibodies derived from a single autoimmune mouse, *Proc. Natl. Acad. Sci. USA* **84**:9150–9154.

Shibata, D., Weiss, L., Hernandez, A., Nathwani, B., Bernstein, L., and Levine, A. M., 1993, Epstein–Barr virus-associated non-Hodgkin's lymphoma in patients infected with the human immunodeficiency virus, *Blood* **81**:2102–2109.

Shiramizu, B., Herndier, B., Meeker, T., Kaplan, L. D., and McGrath, M. S., 1992, Molecular and immunophenotypic characterization of AIDS-associated EBV-negative polyclonal lymphoma, *J. Clin. Oncol.* **10**:383–389.

Strigle, S., Martin, S., Levine, A. M., and Rarick, M. U., 1993, The use of fine needle aspiration cytology in the management of human immunodeficiency virus-related non-Hodgkin's lymphoma and Hodgkin's disease, *J. Acq. Immune Defic. Syndr.* **6**:1329–1334.

Tirelli, U., Vaccher, E., Rezza, G., Barbui, T., Bernasconi, C., Cajozzo, A., Cargnel, A., de Lalla, F., Dessalvi, P., Fassio, P. G., Gobbi, M., Lambertenghi Deliliers, F. M. G., Lazzarin, A., Luzi, G., Luzzati, R., Mandelli, F., Maserati, R., Piersantelli, N., Puppo, F., Raise, G., Rossi, E., Saliva, G., Scanni, A., Sinicco, A., Foà, R., Gavosto, F., and Monfardini, S., 1989, Hodgkin's disease in association with acquired immunodeficiency syndrome (AIDS): A report on 36 patients, *Acta Oncol.* **28**:637–639.

Walts, A. E., Shintaku, I. P., and Said, J. W., 1990, Diagnosis of malignant lymphoma in effusions from patients with AIDS by gene rearrangement, *J. Clin. Pathol.* **94:**170–175.

Weiss, L., and Chang, K., 1992, Molecular biologic studies of Hodgkin's disease, *Semin. Diagn. Pathol.* **9:** 272–278.

Yarchoan, R., Redfield, R. R., and Broder, S., 1986, Mechanisms of B cell activation in patients with acquired immunodeficiency syndrome and related disorders, *J. Clin. Invest.* **78:**439–447.

Ziegler, J., Beckstead, J., Volberding, P., Abrams, D. I., Levine, A. M., Lukes, R. J., Gill, P. S., Burkes, R. L., Meyer, P. R., Metroka, C. E., Mouradian, J., Moore, A., Riggs, S. A., Butler, J. J., Cabanillas, F. C., Hersh, E., Newell, G. R., Laubenstein, L. J., Knowles, D., Odajnyk, C., Raphael, B., Koziner, B., Urmacher, C., and Clarkson, B. D., 1984, Non-Hodgkin's lymphoma in 90 homosexual men. Relation to generalized lymphadenopathy and the acquired immunodeficiency syndrome, *N. Engl. J. Med.* **311:**565–570.

SECTION III

IMMUNE-BASED THERAPY

CHAPTER 24

THE IMMUNOTHERAPY OF HIV INFECTION WITH DRUGS

JOHN W. HADDEN

1. INTRODUCTION

The history of the effort to treat HIV infection with immunotherapeutic drugs has been a frustrating one. Soon after the onset of this epidemic in 1981, there were extensive efforts to use a long list of drugs being employed in cancer immunotherapy to treat AIDS. As predicted (Hadden, 1985), these attempts failed (Hadden, 1991; Specter and Hadden, 1992). The problem, quite simply, related to the predicted inability of any drug to increase T-cell number by any mechanism other than the inhibition of HIV replication. In approaching this discussion, I recognize that this topic is not in vogue. In fact, in some recent reviews, the subject of immunotherapeutic drugs is not even mentioned (Laurence, 1995; Lederman, 1995). I take a different view (Hadden, 1991). I would contend that the efforts using some of the drugs have taught that not only are they safe but also that they can reduce the development of AIDS-defining clinical events and can often delay the predicted decline in CD4 T lymphocytes. Nevertheless, the efforts have not demonstrated a convincing mechanism of action. The problem remains to be properly phrased: What can immunotherapeutic drugs be expected to do for HIV infection? and How do we measure the effect by other than clinical endpoints?, i.e., how can we prove the mechanism of action? It will be the purpose of this chapter to review the progress of efforts to employ such drugs in HIV infection prior to the development of AIDS and to delineate prospects for better defining and improving such treatment.

2. HISTORICAL REVIEW OF CLINICAL TRIALS

Immunotherapy in AIDS at the end stage of HIV infection has, as noted, been an unsuccessful strategy. Two preparations of interferon-α (IFN-α; Schering and Hoffman–

JOHN W. HADDEN • Department of Internal Medicine, Division of Immunopharmacology, University of South Florida Medical College, Tampa, Florida 33612.

Immunology of HIV Infection, edited by Sudhir Gupta. Plenum Press, New York, 1996.

LaRoche) have been licensed by the Food and Drug Administration (FDA) for treatment of Kaposi's sarcoma. IFN-α is effective alone (20–40% major response rates) and in conjunction with zidovudine (>60% response rate), but it does not reverse the immunodeficiency.

Intravenous immunoglobulin therapy is generally considered to be useful and nontoxic in the treatment of pediatric AIDS patients for the management of bacterial infections. A number of anecdotal reports indicate that such therapy may improve the course of AIDS and AIDS-related complex (ARC) in adult patients and a multicenter trial has been initiated to test this using intravenous immunoglobulin therapy alone and in conjunction with zidovudine.

Initial studies with recombinant IL-2 in AIDS were negative; however, with continuous intravenous infusion of high doses, lymphocytosis was observed. Toxicity was associated with a "flulike" syndrome, fluid accumulation, and increased bacterial infections. Schwartz *et al.* (1991) treated nine patients with the combination of IL-2 and zidovudine; the data indicated that the combination is compatible, that the toxicity levels are acceptable, and that the ability of IL-2 to increase CD4 T-cell counts and cellular cytotoxicity, and to enhance skin test reactivity was not prevented by zidovudine. Kovacs *et al.* (1995) went on to administer intermittent IL-2 and zidovudine to 25 patients. In 6 of 10 patients with initial CD4 cell counts above 200, significant increases in CD4 counts occurred. These results are being pursued (see Fyfe and Lane, this volume).

It is against this background that the immunotherapy of pre-AIDS with drugs is to be viewed.

2.1. Ampligen

Ampligen is a polynucleotide derivative of polyinosinic:polycytidylic acid (poly I:C, a potent IFN inducer) with spaced uridines that serve as RNase cleavage sites. While ampligen is capable of inducing IFN and enhancing NK cell activity, it lacks the toxicity of

TABLE I. Current Status of the Immunotherapy of HIV Infection with Drugs

	Clinical phase	Current status
Ampligen	Phase II	Inactive
Dialyzed leukocyte extracts		
Transfer factor	Phase II	Inactive
ImReg	Phase III	Inactive
H_2 receptor antagonists		
Cimetidine and ranitidine	Phase III	Active
Isoprinosine	Phase III	Inactive
NSAID		
Aspirin	Phase II	Active
Indomethacin	Phase II	Inactive
Soluble CD4	Phase I	Inactive
Thymopentin	Phase III	Active
Miscellaneous agents		
AS-101	Phase I/II	Inactive
Bropirimine (ABPP)	Phase II	Inactive

poly I:C and other related derivatives (Carter *et al.*, 1987), although it does induce flushing, fever, and chills (McMahon *et al.*, 1992). In an initial double-blind multicenter Phase II clinical trial, lack of activity resulted in cessation of the study. However, retrospective examination of the data suggested that the method of drug storage was an important variable in patient response. Patients treated with ampligen stored in glass fared better than those treated with drug stored in plastic containers (Carter *et al.*, 1991). Despite these encouraging results, the clinical development of ampligen has apparently been on hold.

2.2. Dialyzed Leukocyte Extracts

Transfer factor (TF) is a dialyzed extract from peripheral blood leukocytes. This dialysate is believed to contain factors that can transfer both specific immune responses (delayed hypersensitivity) and nonspecific host responses. While the structure of any single transfer factor has not been identified, TF is believed to contain amino acids and possibly inosine (Rozzo and Kirkpatrick, 1992; Wilson *et al.*, 1979). Hadden *et al.* (1986) previously reported that TF has thymomimetic properties, which the author suggests might be attributed to the inosine moiety. TF preparations were used to treat nine anergic HIV-infected patients on a weekly basis for 4 weeks (Carey *et al.*, 1987). Skin test responses returned in six of seven patients, as did *in vitro* mitogen responses, and CD4 lymphocyte counts improved. Kirkpatrick (personal communication) has treated seven patients with TF preparations from leukocytes from several donors or a highly purified preparation derived from *Candida*-sensitized donors. Those treated with the mixed leukocyte preparation had no response, while two AIDS patients with esophageal candidiasis who were treated with the purified TF preparation responded clinically and regained skin test responsiveness to *Candida* antigen. No further clinical work has been performed because of financial constraints.

ImReg-1

ImReg-1 is another dialyzed leukocyte extract shown by Gottlieb (1991) to have immunostimulatory activity. The small peptides Tyr-Gly and Tyr-Gly-Gly are believed to be the active components (Sinha *et al.*, 1988; Sizemore *et al.*, 1991). Intracutaneous injection with tetanus toxoid leads to enhanced dermal skin reactions and *in vitro* treatment of lymphocytes leads to increased lymphokine release. Gottlieb and Trial Investigators (1991) performed a multicenter clinical trial using ImReg-1 to treat 93 ARC patients twice weekly (48 nontreated controls were included). Progression to a clinically defined endpoint (4.3% ImReg versus 25% of control) or to AIDS (3% versus 17%) was significantly reduced. Marginal improvements in CD4 cell counts and clinical symptoms were also recorded. No toxicity was observed. Although FDA protocols for use of ImReg with and without AZT have been approved, no further clinical trials have been performed because of financial constraints.

2.3. Diethyldithiocarbamate (Imuthiol)

One orally active thymomimetic drug that has been examined as an AIDS therapeutic is diethyldithiocarbamate (DTC). This drug is more active and less toxic than its predecessor, levamisole (Renoux and Renoux, 1984). The drug was first shown to be promising in a murine retroviral infection model (Hersh *et al.*, 1991a). Subsequently, clinical trials using DTC (10 mg/kg orally) in HIV-infected patients indicated that the drug could decrease the frequency of ARC symptoms and of conversion from ARC to AIDS (4.5% versus 13% in untreated controls) and could increase CD4 lymphocyte counts (Lang *et al.*, 1988; Reisinger *et al.*, 1990). In a randomized trial of 25 patients with CD4 cell counts greater than 200/mm^3, the group receiving DTC at a dose of 800 mg/m^2 administered twice weekly had a reduction in lymphadenopathy (Kaplan *et al.*, 1989).

These studies were followed by a large multicenter trial of 389 patients (Hersh *et al.*, 1991b), in which a significant (approximately 50%) reduction in opportunistic infections was observed in both the ARC and AIDS patients randomized to receive 400 mg/m^2 of DTC orally once a week. No significant increase in CD4 cells was noted relative to controls. These results suggest that DTC can produce, in *symptomatic* patients, a reduction in symptomatology, lymphadenopathy, opportunistic infections, and progression of disease, while increasing CD4 cell counts. Treatment of *asymptomatic* HIV-infected individuals with DTC in Europe in a study involving 1600 patients was performed and was considered to be negative (HIV-87 Study Group, 1993). Despite the fact that DTC was active in symptomatic patients, development of DTC for HIV infection has been abandoned.

2.4. H_2 Receptor Antagonists: Cimetidine and Ranitidine

The H_2 receptor antagonists are sulfur-containing compounds that would be predicted to have thymomimetic features of their immunopharmacologies similar to levamisole and DTC (Hadden, 1985b) and also immune augmenting effects resulting from the antagonism of histamine-induced suppressor cells (a cyclic AMP-mediated event). Preclinical studies indicate augmentation *in vitro* of lymphoproliferative and NK responses and *in vivo* of DTH responses (Shibata *et al.*, 1992; Turowski and Triozzi, 1994). Interestingly, like imidazole and levamisole, cimetidine augments lymphocyte cyclic GMP levels (Hadden *et al.*, 1975; unpublished). Clinical use of cimetidine in HIV$^+$ individuals was reported to increase CD4 T cells, CD4/CD8 ratio, B cells and immunoglobulins, and DTH reactions and to improve clinical symptoms (Ahuja *et al.*, 1983; Brockmeyer *et al.*, 1988). Clinical use of ranitidine in a similar study was not associated with increased CD4 T cells but did augment NK cell activity (Nielson *et al.*, 1991). Clinical trials with both compounds are in progress (Abrams *et al.*, 1995).

2.5. Isoprinosine

Isoprinosine is an inosine-containing compound with thymomimetic activity (Hadden, 1985a). This compound has been demonstrated to induce T-lymphocyte differentiation and stimulate T-cell function both *in vitro* and *in vivo*. Early controlled trials in HIV-infected patients with CD4 cell counts greater than 500/mm^3 demonstrated increased NK cell activity and increased CD4 counts with a reduction in clinical symptoms and frequency of conversion of ARC to AIDS (Glasky and Gordon, 1986; Bekesi *et al.*, 1987). One study even reported positive effects in AIDS with ACTH (Addo *et al.*, 1989). Disappointing results both clinically and immunologically, however, were obtained in a multicenter trial involving nearly 700 HIV-infected, symptomatic patients with CD4 cell counts of less than 400/mm^3. In contrast, a Scandinavian trial of 866 ARC patients with a mean CD4 count of about 425/mm^3 demonstrated a significant reduction in the conversion of ARC to AIDS (4%

untreated versus 0.5% treated) during a 6-month period (Pederson *et al.*, 1990). In a similar trial conducted in Italy with 553 asymptomatic HIV-infected patients, De Simone *et al.* (1988) found no new opportunistic infections in the isoprinosine-treated patients, while untreated controls had 12 such infections. Several immunologic parameters improved in the treatment group relative to controls. These studies suggest that isoprinosine therapy in pre-AIDS patients with CD4 counts greater than 400/mm^3 provides beneficial effects. Unfortunately, the loss of patent protection by the pharmaceutical company supporting these trials has resulted in failure to apply for licensing of this drug and no further studies have been initiated.

2.6. Nonsteroidal Antiinflammatory Drugs (NSAIDs)

NSAIDs like aspirin and indomethacin block prostaglandin (PG) synthesis by inhibiting cyclooxygenase. Macrophages are one source of PG synthesis and production of PGs by macrophages is well recognized as a downregulator of T-lymphocyte activation (Goodwin and Webb, 1980; Hadden and Coffey, 1990) via increases in cellular cyclic AMP levels.

Indomethacin has been reported to augment T-lymphocyte responses to PHA from HIV-infected donors (Reddy *et al.*, 1985; Siegal *et al.*, 1985; Svedersky *et al.*, 1990). Aspirin has been reported to block the stimulation of p24 and HIV production by PGE and leukotriene LTB *in vitro* in rectal biopsies following *in vitro* treatment (Kotler and Reka, 1990).

2.7. Soluble CD4

Recombinant DNA technology has allowed the preparation of soluble CD4, the cellular receptor for HIV. This molecule will bind to HIV and thus prevent viral attachment to lymphocytes. Phase I/II testing indicated that, with frequent administration, serum CD4 levels of 10–100 ng/ml can be achieved without accompanying toxicity (Kahn *et al.*, 1990; Schooley *et al.*, 1990). These levels are sufficient to inhibit viral replication *in vitro*. Phase I/II trials for HIV-seropositive, asymptomatic individuals with CD4 cell counts between 200 and 500/mm^3 were attempted and failed to show benefit. Development has been abandoned.

There was an attempt using PE-40 bacterial toxin (*Pseudomonas aeruginosa* exotoxin) linked to soluble CD4. The rationale for this approach is based on the binding of soluble CD4 plus PE-40 toxin to gp120 on the surface of HIV-infected cells, with internalization of toxin and selective death of the target cell. Clinical trials with CD4–PE-40 were unsuccessful in showing efficacy and were abandoned (Abrams *et al.*, 1995).

2.8. Thymopentin

Thymopentin is a pentapeptide comprising part of the active site of thymopoietin. Since thymopoietin has not qualified as a thymic hormone, it is considered a drug for this discussion. Thymopentin augments T-lymphocyte proliferation *in vitro* and increases in cyclic GMP and decreases in cyclic AMP levels have been implicated as a mechanistic factor (Sunshine *et al.*, 1978). A dose of 50 mg of thymopentin given subcutaneously three times weekly for 3 weeks resulted in increases in CD4 counts, IgG production, and lymphocyte proliferation in response to pokeweed mitogen in 8 HIV-infected pre-AIDS patients relative to 8 uninfected controls (Barcellini *et al.*, 1987). This trial was extended to 12 months with 29 patients and 11 controls (Silvestris *et al.*, 1989) and similar benefits were again observed. This has been followed by a blinded multicenter trial (Conant *et al.*, 1990) involving 47 thymopentin-treated asymptomatic HIV-seropositive and ARC patients not receiving AZT and 44 placebo-treated controls. Four controls progressed to AIDS, versus none of the thymopentin-treated patients. Treated patients with entry CD4 counts above 400/mm^3 maintained those levels while controls showed reductions in these counts. There was no increase in p24 or β_2-microglobulin levels in thymopentin-treated patients.

Thymopentin was further evaluated with AZT in a double-blind randomized placebo-controlled trial of 352 asymptomatic HIV-infected individuals with CD4 counts of 200–500 at entry (Goldstein *et al.*, 1995). Patients were prestratified as to length of AZT therapy (>6 months; 352 pts: < 6 months; 117 pts). The treatment groups did not differ with respect to CD4 counts or p24 antigen levels. Thymopentin treatment was associated with delayed progression and fewer ARC, AIDS, or death events in both stratum I and II despite positive progression factors (AZT resistance mutation, high viral blood and low CD4 count) (Merigan *et al.*, 1995).

2.9. Miscellaneous Drugs

AS 101 is an ammonium salt of tellurium that can stimulate growth factor production by murine or human lymphocytes (CSF and IL-2) and can augment mitogen-induced lymphoblastogenesis. Phase I/II clinical trials in the United States, testing the efficacy of AS 101 alone or in combination with AZT, showed minor or no effect (LaPorte *et al.*, 1989; Ruiz-Palacios *et al.*, 1988; Falloon *et al.*, 1990) and no trials are active.

Bropirimine (ABPP) is one of a series of 6-aryl-pyrimidinones having oral activity to induce interferon and to augment NK cell activity. Bropirimine also augments T-lymphocyte responses by unknown mechanisms. In a trial of HIV$^+$ individuals with Kaposi's sarcoma, no clinical effects were observed (Chachoua *et al.*, 1988) and the compound has been abandoned for this indication.

Thalidomide and *pentoxifylline* (Abrams *et al.*, 1995) are being employed to counteract the effect of tumor necrosis factor (TNF) in the cachexia of AIDS.

2.10. Summation

The most insightful therapeutic approaches oriented toward improving the function of T lymphocytes in early HIV disease and delaying progression have involved two drugs, DTC and isoprinosine, and two peptides, thymopentin and ImReg-1. No significant side effects with these agents have been noted; thus, they are safe and no incidence of HIV activation has been uncovered.

The total number of reported patients treated with these agents exceeds 2500, which underscores the statistical significance of the findings. Despite these findings, none of the agents have been approved and two have been abandoned. The question remains as to how to improve the approach.

Figure 1 offers a schematic view of this use of immunotherapy, which in this context would be more appropriately termed *postinfection immunoprophylaxis*. The length of the clinical latency period is variable, presumably related to other concomitant immunosuppressive influences.

Conceptually, it will be relevant to introduce immunotherapy at a point before the

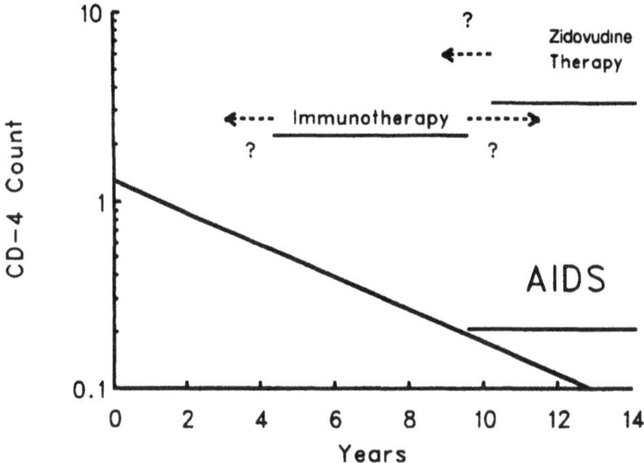

FIGURE 1. Therapy model for HIV infection.

development of poor prognostic indicators in asymptomatic HIV-positive individuals, e.g., p24 antigenemia, elevated neopterin or β_2-microglobulin levels. In early HIV infection before the onset of AIDS, the incidence of infected CD4 lymphocytes in peripheral blood is low (0.1%) (Ho *et al.*, 1989), the degree of immunosuppression in early infection is out of proportion to the frequency of cells affected (Ruegg and Engleman, 1990). When CD4 lymphocyte counts are corrected for *in vitro* tests of lymphoproliferative responses, the degree of functional impairment is also out of proportion to the loss of CD4 cells. Thus, a large number of lymphocytes are dysfunctional. This "pananergy," i.e., a general defect in cellular immune function, presumably results from retrovirus-induced or -produced immunosuppressive factors and/or autoantibodies to T cells. A more detailed analysis of lymphocyte dysfunction in early HIV infection is warranted to determine the effects of soluble serum-borne inhibitors on T-lymphocyte function. Clarification of these factors and their mechanisms is needed.

The molecular strategies to augment T-cell function with thymomimetic agents in pre-AIDS appear to depend on the presence of lymphocytes whose function, when restored, will benefit the host and not result in the activation and spread of virus. Combined use of immunotherapy with zidovudine or other antivirals, based on the experience with isoprinosine, DTC, ImReg-1, and thymopentin, would appear to be appropriate only when CD4 counts are greater than $400/mm^3$. Their combined use with antiviral agents relies on the assumption that the antiviral agents do not inhibit their activity. This remains to be determined.

3. RATIONALE FOR THE USE OF DRUGS IN HIV INFECTION

One cannot expect any existing drug to increase CD4 T-cell numbers through an action to promote directly T-cell maturation and development. In fact, it appears that this process is maximally operant (Pantaleo *et al.*, 1993; Ho *et al.*, 1995). The best one can expect is to improve the function of existing lymphocytes whose function is impaired as a result of

HIV infection and hope that the improvement will benefit the host's more effective resistance mechanisms for holding HIV in check. We admittedly do not know precisely what these resistance mechanisms are.

One fact is that following the initial viremia in early HIV infection, the body is capable of eradicating large amounts of HIV, almost all of the virus by some calculations (see Poli and Fauci, this volume). From what we know about immune responses to viruses in general, both cellular and humoral immunity participate; however, in the absence of humoral immunity, as occurs in Bruton's agammaglobulinemia, the only virus that proves fatal is hepatitis virus. In contrast, in the absence of cellular immune response, the defenses against viral infection are more critically impaired and many different viruses besides HIV can prove fatal. Cellular immune mechanisms seem critical in HIV and recent work by Levy and co-workers (Mackewicz and Levy, 1992; Landay *et al.*, 1993; Blackbourn *et al.*, 1994) and Clerici *et al.* (1994a) point to critical roles for T-cell cytotoxicity and proliferative responses to the HIV virus in defense against infection. Clerici *et al.* (1994a) have shown that peptide epitopes derived from gp160 can induce IL-2 production in HIV-infected individuals and that individuals, exposed to HIV but not infected, frequently have positive responses to these T-cell epitopes. This finding indicates that cell-mediated immune (CMI) responses may be induced without infection and may be protective. Based on these and other findings, Clerici and Shearer (1993, 1994) have suggested that CMI mediated by TH_1 cells is critical to effective defense against HIV and that progression follows a shift from TH_1 to TH_2 responses. This shift of cellular responses involves a shift from IL-2 and IFN-γ cytokine responses to IL-4 and IL-10 cytokine responses. IL-10 is a feedback inhibitor of TH_1 proliferative responses and cytokine responses and elevated levels of IL-10 have been detected in the leukocytes of HIV-infected patients (Clerici *et al.*, 1994a,b). It is of note that, of the many drugs employed in the immunotherapy of HIV infection, the most effective have been those whose actions would be predicted to be on such T-cell responses (Hadden, 1991). It seems logical to emphasize drugs that promote T-lymphocyte responses preferentially, and ideally TH_1 responses in particular.

In the presence of hypergammaglobulinemia and propensity for autoantibody production as occurs in HIV infection, drugs that promote B-lymphocyte function seem inappropriate to use except perhaps in the context of adjuvants for HIV vaccination efforts. An argument can still be made for agents that promote natural defenses (macrophage activators and interferon inducers), yet so far, of these agents, only ampligen has demonstrated any degree of efficacy in HIV infection (Carter *et al.*, 1991).

The idea of promoting the function of T lymphocytes already infected by HIV has little logic and could promote HIV replication as has been observed with IL-2 treatment (Kovacs *et al.*, 1995). The more logical effort would be to promote the impaired responses of normal lymphocytes reactive to T-cell epitopes of HIV-infected cells. What evidence exists to suggest these responses are impaired?

3.1. HIV-Induced Immunosuppression and Its Reversal

Retroviruses, in general, induce suppression of T-lymphocyte-mediated immune responses (Good *et al.*, 1991; Keadle *et al.*, 1996). Such suppression can be perceived as critical to their ability to evade host rejection mechanisms. Much attention has been paid to a protein p15E present in murine and feline retroviruses. A 17-amino-acid active site of this peptide (CKS-17) has been intensely studied for its effects to inhibit T-lymphocyte proliferation and interleukin secretion (Snyderman and Cianciolo, 1984; Good *et al.*, 1991). Recently, it has been shown that this peptide induces IL-10 production and shifts the cytokine secretion pattern from TH_1 to TH_2 (Haraguchi *et al.*, 1995). Increases in cyclic AMP levels were implicated in the mechanism.

Inactivated HIV and gp160 inhibit lymphocyte mitogen responses (Pahwa *et al.*, 1986; Chirmule *et al.*, 1988; Gurley *et al.*, 1989) and both HIV itself and gp160 increase lymphocyte levels of cyclic AMP (Hofmann *et al.*, 1993a,b). The gp41 peptide of HIV is considered to have a segment homologous to CKS-17 (Ruegg *et al.*, 1989) and this peptide fragment has been shown to inhibit proliferation of T lymphocytes and to block calcium influx and protein kinase C (PKC) activation (Ruegg and Strand, 1991). Impaired IL-2 secretion has been implicated in the impaired lymphoproliferative responses to both CKS-17 and gp120 (see Good *et al.*, 1991) and IL-2 augments lymphoproliferative responses of HIV-infected patients (Ciobanu *et al.*, 1983; Kirkpatrick *et al.*, 1985). IL-2 is known to promote transmembrane signaling events associated with mitogen action (calcium influx, PKC activation, and cyclic GMP production) and to inhibit cyclic AMP-promoted events (see Hadden and Coffey, 1990).

Another inhibitor of lymphocyte proliferation and inducer of cyclic AMP increases in lymphocytes which may be increased in HIV infection is prostaglandin E_2 (PGE_2) (Svedersky *et al.*, 1990). Indomethacin, an inhibitor of PG synthesis, augments the impaired lymphoproliferative responses of HIV-infected individuals (Siegal *et al.*, 1985; Hadden *et al.*, 1991) to a greater extent than it affects normals. Data suggest that excessive PG production is occurring in the leukocytes of HIV-infected individuals (Svedersky *et al.*, 1990) and may be serum-induced (Siegal *et al.*, 1985).

In sum, several HIV-derived peptides inhibit normal lymphocyte activation and do so through actions on transmembrane signalling events. An elevation of cyclic AMP levels seems to be a central feature of these actions and elevation of cyclic AMP levels of lymphocytes from patients with HIV infection has been documented (Hofmann *et al.*, 1993a,b). A strong case may be made for immunotherapeutic efforts to interfere with immunosuppression induced by HIV-derived peptides by inhibiting their production, neutralizing them, or blocking their mechanisms of action. From a mechanistic point of view, inhibition of cyclic AMP increases in T lymphocytes may be practical. Additional strategies are needed.

T-lymphocyte proliferative responses of HIV-infected individuals are often measured *in vitro* and are considered to be an important prognostic indicator for HIV progression. Unfortunately, relatively little effort has gone into the analysis of how these functional responses of peripheral blood lymphocytes are impaired, especially since few cells in the peripheral blood are actually infected (Ho *et al.*, 1989). When lymphocytes are prepared for such studies, they are thoroughly washed prior to incubation in media and nonautologous serum. This preparation removes serum inhibitors and may partially reverse serum-derived immunosuppressive influences on the cells themselves. Analysis of HIV serum-borne inhibitors on normal lymphocyte proliferation is critical to elucidate their mechanisms. Testing should include efforts to reestablish the *in vivo* circumstance with use of autologous serum and/or the whole blood (PHA) assay (Park and Good, 1975). Ideally, cytotoxic T-lymphocyte (CTL) responses to HIV-infected targets would be measured as well. If the mechanisms of suppression of proliferation, cytokine secretion (IL-2 and IFN-γ in particular), and cytotoxicity responses of peripheral T lymphocytes of patients with HIV infection were better understood, correction of these responses *in vitro* and subsequently *in vivo* by immunotherapeutic drugs would be more meaningful and would begin to approach the mechanism of action issue.

3.2. Working Hypothesis

In summary, the working hypothesis is that HIV infection is checked by mainly TH_1-mediated CMI responses. This defense mechanism is subverted progressively by immunosuppressive virus-derived peptides like gp120 and gp41 which inhibit these T-cell responses through interfering with transmembrane signaling via the TCR and/or the generation of countersignals via increased intracellular levels of cyclic AMP. Drugs to correct this impairment should augment these responses *in vitro* and *in vivo* and thus promote *in vivo* defenses.

4. A NEW IMMUNORESTORATIVE DRUG FOR USE IN HIV INFECTION: METHYL INOSINE MONOPHOSPHATE

Methyl inosine monophosphate (MIMP) was synthesized to improve on the immunopharmacologic features of isoprinosine, an inosine-containing complex (Hadden *et al.*, 1991, 1992) (Fig. 2). MIMP induces T-cell differentiation *in vitro* and augments T-lymphocyte mitogen and IL-2 responses. It augments PHA responses suppressed by hydrocortisone, interferon, prostaglandin, and aging (J. W. Hadden *et al.*, 1991; E. M. Hadden *et al.*, 1995). *In vivo*, in mice, it augments at low doses (<1 mg/kg) delayed type hypersensitivity more than antibody plaque-forming cell responses (Sosa *et al.*, 1992) and protects against lethal challenges with *Listeria* and *Salmonella* bacteria and influenza virus (Hadden, Semenenko, and Masihi, unpublished).

It reverses the immunosuppression by a 17-amino-acid (#581–597) immunosuppressive peptide of gp41 (Ruegg and Strand, 1991) when mild to moderate, i.e., less than 50% (Hadden *et al.*, 1992) (Fig. 3). It augments the depressed lymphoproliferative responses to PHA of HIV-infected individuals and is additive with the effects of indomethacin and IL-2 to do so (J. W. Hadden *et al.*, 1992; E. M. Hadden *et al.*, 1995) (Fig. 4). MIMP also prolongs life in a murine AIDS model with Friend leukemia virus (FLV) (Hadden *et al.*, 1992) (Fig. 5).

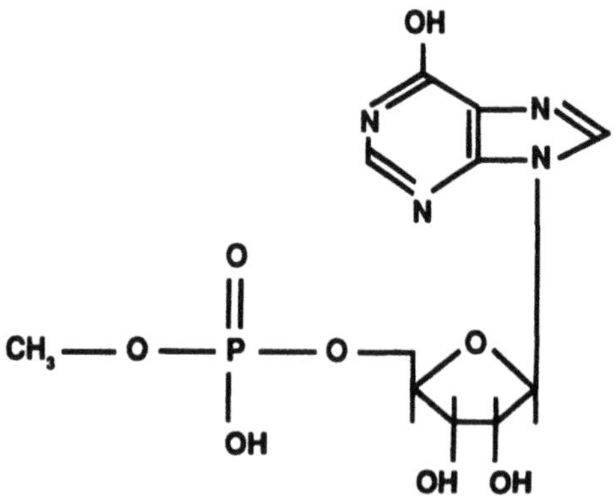

FIGURE 2. Structure of methyl inosine monophosphate (MIMP).

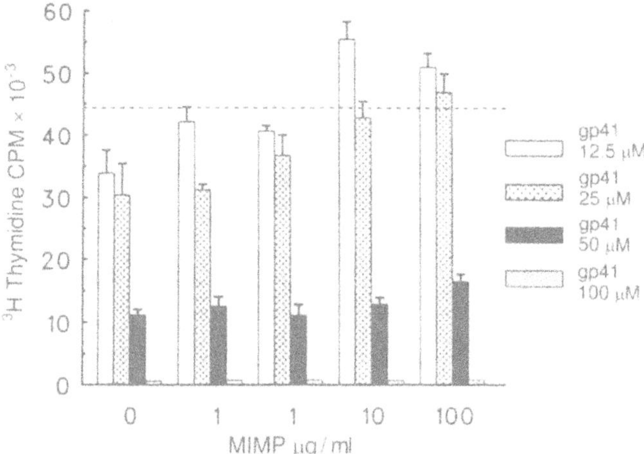

FIGURE 3. Effect of MIMP on suppression of PHA response by gP41 analogue. Proliferation of normal human lymphocytes was measured by [^{3}H]thymidine incorporation (Hadden *et al.*, 1995). Control value is indicated by the dashed line. The response was inhibited by increasing concentrations of a 17-amino-acid fragment of the gP41 of HIV (left-hand columns). Increasing concentrations of MIMP were added to reverse the suppression (right-hand columns). MIMP reverses the suppression at 12.5 and 25 μM peptide but not at higher concentrations of peptide. (Reproduced by permission of the publisher.)

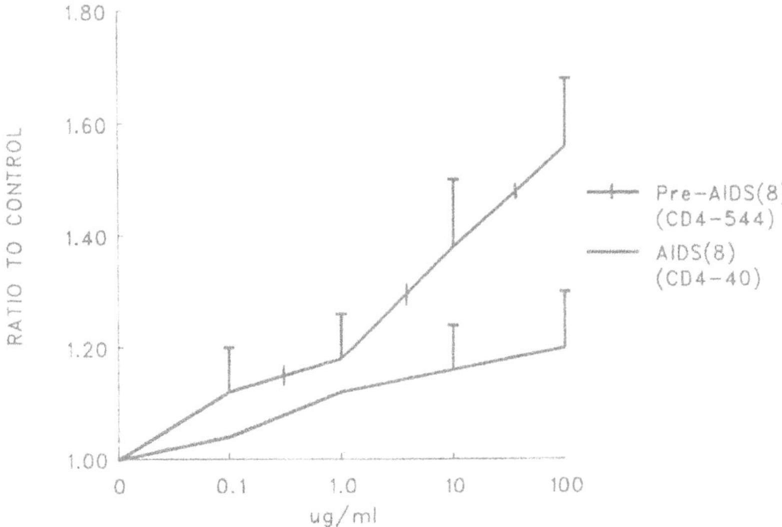

FIGURE 4. The effect of MIMP on the PHA responses of lymphocytes from HIV-infected individuals (Hadden *et al.*, 1992). Lymphocytes from eight patients with pre-AIDS (mean CD4 count 544) and eight patients with AIDS (mean CD4 count 40) were incubated with PHA and varying concentration of MIMP. The data expressed as a ratio to control ± SEM for ARC (35,241 ± 6580 counts/min) or for AIDS (8576 ± 1670 counts/min). (Reproduced by permission of the publisher.)

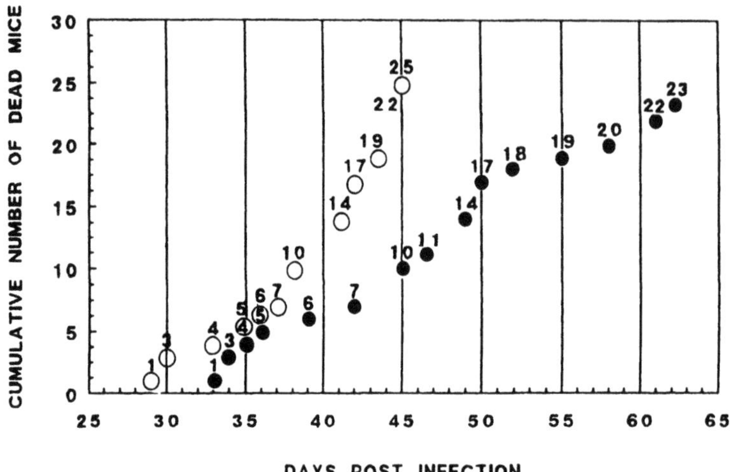

FIGURE 5. The effect of MIMP on survival of mice infected with Friend leukemia virus (FLV) (Hadden *et al.*, 1992). Mice were treated with MIMP (1 mg/kg per day) from day +3 to day +13 after FLV inoculation (solid circles). Mean survival of saline-treated controls (no drug, open circles) was 39 days and of MIMP-treated mice, 46 days ($p < 0.01$).

Based on its immunopharmacology, MIMP is predicted to be a TH_1-active drug and thus appropriate for application to HIV infection prior to the development of the TH_2 shift (Clerici and Shearer, 1993, 1994). Part of its effect to promote TH_1 responses may result from its ability to antagonize IL-10-induced suppression of PHA responses (Fig. 6).

5. COMMENTS ON FUTURE IMMUNOTHERAPY

Our inability to understand fully the relevant resistance mechanisms in the pathogenesis of HIV infection is the greatest impediment to developing effective immunotherapy. The loss of the $CD4^+$ cell population is obvious, but the causes for functional defects must be more clearly identified in order to identify pharmacologic measures necessary to correct the problem. Immune or antiviral therapies that have boosted or maintained $CD4^+$ cell counts have been associated with clinical improvements in the short term. A similar result has not been demonstrated and needs to be for functional improvement of T-cell responses, particularly cytotoxic T-cell responses. Moreover, it is still uncertain what other defects in the immune system contribute to disease progression. Defects in NK cell activity, cytokine production, and others are noted in HIV-infected patients, but their significance remains poorly defined. These gaps in our understanding of HIV infection increase the challenge of finding safe and effective immunotherapeutic approaches.

Vaccine development against HIV is an important strategy for disease management. Vaccines are currently being examined in both HIV-seropositive and HIV-seronegative individuals. The concept of a postexposure vaccine for a virus that has already established latent infection in its target organs is precedented only in rabies immunization. In order to generate an immune response that is protective, it is likely that newer adjuvants (Hadden, 1994) may be necessary, particularly to evoke protective T-cell responses. The clinical

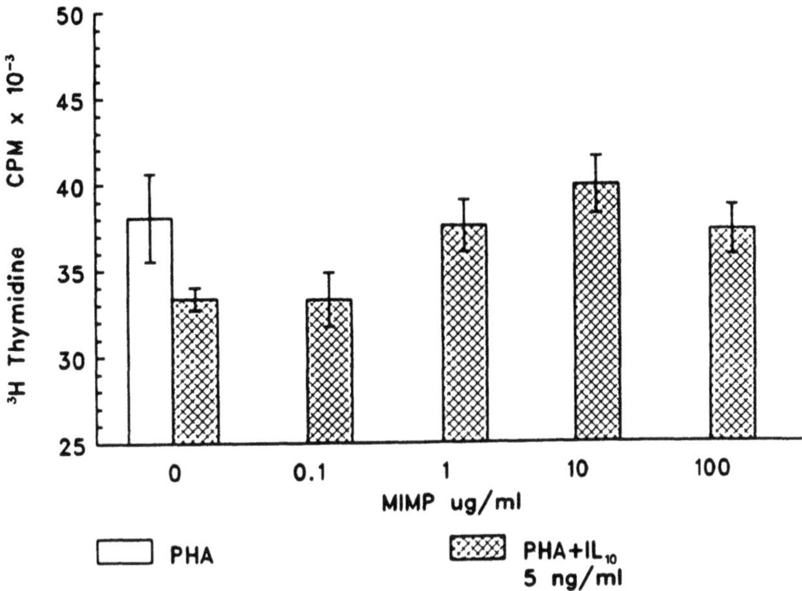

FIGURE 6. The effect of MIMP on PHA responses suppressed by IL-10. Lymphocytes from normals were incubated with PHA (white column) or PHA plus IL-10 (5 ng/ml) ± varying doses of MIMP (cross-hatched columns) and proliferation was measured by [^{3}H]thymidine incorporation (± S.E.M.).

experience with gp120 immunization for seropositive patients (Redfield *et al.*, 1991; Birx and Redfield, 1991) showed that antibody responses could be induced; however, when compared to pediatric immunizations, they were weak and delayed when they occurred. Efficacy of vaccine treatment may depend not only on adjuvant characteristics but also on counteracting virus-induced immune suppression, as discussed, with drugs like MIMP. Ultimately, as the data about the critical resistance mechanisms, particularly those involving T cells, converge with a knowledge about which T-cell epitopes are protective, we will be able to select which drugs, or combination therapy of peptides, will overcome virus-induced immunosuppression and promote the relevant clinical response.

REFERENCES

Abrams, D., Cotton, D., and Mayer, K., eds., 1995, *AIDS/HIV Treatment Directory* Vol. 7, No. 4.

Addo, E., McFarlane, H., and Parsad, K., 1989, ACTH-inosine pranobex in the treatment of AIDS. Encouraging results, *West Indian Med. J.* **38:**142–147.

Ahuja, K., Manvar, D., Reddy, M., Moriarty, M., and Grieco, M. H., 1983, Cimetidine as an immunomodulating agent in the A.I.D. syndrome, *J. Allergy Clin. Immunol.* **71:**132.

Barcellini, W., Meroni, P. L., Frasca, D., Squotti, C., Borghi, M. O., Uberti-Foppa, C., Buzzetti, P., Lazzarin, A., Doria, G., Moroni, M., and Zanussi, C., 1987, Effect of subcutaneous thymopentin treatment in drug addicts with persistent generalized lymphadenopathy, *Clin. Exp. Immunol.* **67:**537–543.

Bekesi, J. G., Tsang, P. H., Wallace, J. I., and Roboz, J. P., 1987, Immunorestorative properties of isoprinosine in the treatment of patients at high risk of developing ARC or AIDS, *J. Clin. Lab. Immunol.* **24:**155–161.

Birx, D. L., and Redfield, R., 1991, HIV vaccine therapy, *Int. J. Immunopharmacol.* **13:**129–132.

Blackbourn, D. J., Mackewicz, C., Barker, E., and Levy, J. A., 1994, Human CD8+ cell non-cytolytic anti-HIV activity mediated by a novel cytokine, *Res. Immunol.* **145**:653–658.

Brockmeyer, N. H., Kreuzfelder, E., Mertins, L., Chalabi, N., Kirch, W., Scheiermann, N., Goos, M., and Ohnhaus, E. E., 1988, Immunomodulatory properties of cimetidine in ARC patients, *Clin. Immunol. Immunopathol.* **48**:50–60.

Carey, J. T., Lederman, M. M., Tossii, Z., Edmonds, K., Hodder, S., Calabrese, L. H., Proffitt, M. R., Johnson, C. E., and Ellner, J. J., 1987, Augmentation of skin test reactivity and lymphocyte blastogenesis in patients with AIDS treated with transfer factor, *J. Am. Med. Assoc.* **257**:651–655.

Carter, W. A., Brodsky, I., Pellegrino, M. G., Henriques, H. F., Parenti, D. M. Schulof, R. S., Robinson, E. W., Volsky, D. J., Paxton, H., Kariko, K., Suhadolnik, R. J., Strayer, D. R., Lewin, M., Einck, L., Simon, G. L., Scheib, R. G., Montefiori, D. C., Mitchell, W. M., Paul, D., Meyer III, W. A., Reichenbach, N., and Gillespie, D. H., 1987, Clinical, immunological and virological effects of ampligen, a mismatched double-stranded RNA in patients with AIDS or AIDS-related complex, *Lancet* **6**:1286–1292.

Carter, W. A., Ventura, D., Shapiro, D. E., Strayer, D. R., Gillespie, D. H., and Hubbell, H. R., 1991, Mismatched double-stranded RNA, ampligen (poly(I):poly(C12U)), demonstrates antiviral and immunostimulatory activities in HIV disease, *Int. J. Immunopharmacol.* **13**:69–76.

Chachoua, A., Hochster, H., Green, M., Ward, C., Gutknecht, G., Chuang-Stein, C., Nicholas, J., and Merritt, J., 1988, Phase II trial of bropirimine in patients with AIDS related Kaposi's sarcoma, *Proc. Am. Soc. Clin. Oncol.* **7**:6 (abstract).

Chirmule, N., Kalynanaraman, V., and Pahwa, S., 1988, Suppression of antigen specific lymphoproliferation by the envelope glycoproteins of the human immunedeficiency virus, *FASEB J.* **46**:A906.

Ciobanu, N., Welte, K., Kruger, G., Ventuta, S., Gold, J., Feldman, S. P., Wang, C. Y., Koziner, B., Moore, M. A. S., Safai, B., and Mertelsmann, R., 1983, Defective T-cell response to PHA and mitogenic monoclonal antibodies in male homosexuals with acquired immunodeficiency syndrome and its in vitro correction by interleukin 2, *J. Clin. Immunol.* **3**:332–340.

Clerici, M., and Shearer, G. M., 1993, A TH1–TH2 switch is a critical step in the etiology of HIV infection, *Immunol. Today* **14**:107–111.

Clerici, M., and Shearer, G. M., 1994, The TH1–TH2 hypothesis of HIV infection: New insights, *Immunol. Today* **15**:575–581.

Clerici, M., Levin, J. M., Kessler, H. A., Harris, A., Berzofsky, J. A., Landay, A. L., and Shearer, G. M., 1994a, HIV-specific T-helper activity in seronegative health care workers exposed to contaminated blood, *J. Am. Med. Assoc.* **271**:42–46.

Clerici, M., Wynn, T. A., Berzofsky, J. A., Blatt, S. P., Hendrix, C. W., Sher, A., Coffman, R. L., and Shearer, G. M., 1994b, Role of IL-2 in T helper cell dysfunction in asymptomatic individuals infected with the human immunodeficiency virus, *J. Clin. Invest.* **93**:768–775.

Conant, M. A., Goldstein, G., Hirsch, R. L., Meyerson, L. A., and Kremer, A. B., 1990, The effect of thymopentin treatment on progression of disease and surrogate markers in HIV-infected patients without AIDS. (UCLA Symposia on Molecular and Cell Biology, San Francisco AIDS Meeting Abstract #L411.) *J. Cell. Biochem.* (Suppl.) **14D**:148.

De Simone, C., Albertini, F., Almaviva, M., Angarano, P., Chiodo, F., Costigliola, P, Delia, S., Ferlini, A., Gritti, F., Mazzarello, G., Milazzo, F., Montroni, M., Narciso, P., Pastore, G., Raise, E., Santini, G., Sorice, F., Terragna, A., Visco, G., and Vullo, V., 1988, Clinical and immunological assessment in HIV+ subjects receiving inosine-pranobex: A randomized, multicentric study, *Med. Oncol. Tumor Pharmacother.* **10**:299–303.

Falloon, J., Ogata-Arakaki, D., Baseler, M., Graziani, A., Armantea, M. A., and Davey, R. T., 1990, Therapy of HIV infection with AS-101 and zidovudine, Abstract, 6th Int. Conf. AIDS.

Glasky, A. J., and Gordon, J., 1986, Inosiplex treatment of acquired immundeficiencies: A clinical model for effective immunomodulation, *Methods Fundam. Exp. Clin. Pharmacol.* **8**:35–40.

Goldstein, G., Conant, M. A., Beall, G., Grossman, H. A., Galpin, J. E., Blick, G., Calabrese, L. H., Hirsch, R. L., Fisher, A., Stampone, P., and Meyerson, L. A., 1995, Safety and efficacy of thymopentin in zidovudine (AZT)-treated asymptomatic HIV-infected subjects with 200–500 CD4 cell/mm^3: A double-blind placebo-controlled trial, *J. Acq. Immune Defic. Syndr. Hum. Retrovirol.* **8**:279–288.

Good, R. A., Haraguchi, S., Lorenz, E., and Day, N. K., 1991, In vitro immunomodulation and in vivo immunotherapy of retrovirus-induced immunosuppression, *Int. J. Immunopharmacol.* **13**:1–8.

Goodwin, J. S., and Webb, D. R., 1980, Regulation of the immune response by prostaglandins, *Clin. Immunol. Immunopathol.* **15**:106–109.

Gottlieb, A. A., 1991, Clinical and immunologic observations in patients with AIDS-related complex treated with IMREG-1, *Int. J. Immunopharmacol.* **13**:29–32.

Gottlieb, A. A., and Trial Investigators, 1988, A phase 3 controlled trial of ImReg 1 in AIDS/ARC patients, 4th Int. Conf. AIDS, Stockholm, June.

Gottlieb, M. S., Zackin, R. A., Fiala, M., Henry, D. H., Marcel, A. J., Combs, K. L., Vieira, J., Liebman, H. A., Cone, L. A., Hillman, B. A., and Gottlieb, A. A., 1991, Response to treatment with the leukocyte-derived immunomodulator IMREG-1 in immunocompromised patients with AIDS-related complex, *Ann. Intern. Med.* **115**:84–91.

Gurley, R. J., Keuchi, K., Byrn, R. A., Anderson, K., and Groopman, J. E., 1989, CD4 lymphocyte function with early human immunodeficiency virus infection, *Proc. Natl. Acad. Sci. USA* **86**:1993–1997.

Hadden, E. M., Wang, Y., Sosa, M., Coffey, R. G., Giner-Sorolla, A., and Hadden, J. W., 1995, Methyl inosine monophosphate (MIMP) augments T lymphocyte mitogen responses and reverses various immunosuppressants, *Int. J. Immunopharmacol.* **17**:763–770.

Hadden, J. W., 1985a, Thymomimetic drugs, in: *Serono Symposium on Immunopharmacology*, Volume 23 (P. A. Miescher, L. Bolis, and M. Ghione, eds.), Raven Press, New York, pp. 183–192.

Hadden, J. W., 1985b, Perspective on the immunotherapy of AIDS, *Ann. N.Y. Acad. Sci.* **437**:76–84.

Hadden, J. W., 1991, Immunotherapy of human immunodeficiency virus (HIV), *Trends Pharmacol. Sci.* **12:** 107–111.

Hadden, J. W., 1994, T-cell adjuvancy, *Int. J. Immunopharmacol.* **16**:703–710.

Hadden, J. W., and Coffey, R. G., 1990, Early biochemical events in the activation of T lymphocytes by mitogenic agents, in: *Immunopharmacology Reviews I* (J. W. Hadden and A. Szentivanyi, eds.), Plenum Press, New York, pp. 273–376.

Hadden, J. W., Coffey, R. G., Hadden, E. M., Lopez-Corrales, E., and Sunshine, G. H., 1975, Effects of levamisole and imidazole on lymphocyte proliferation and cyclic nucleotide levels, *Cell. Immunol.* **20**:98–103.

Hadden, J. W., Specter, S., Galy, A., Touraine, J. L., and Hadden, J. W., 1986, Thymic hormones, interleukins, endotoxins and thymomimetic drugs in T lymphocyte ontogeny, in: *Advances in Immunopharmacology III* (L. Chedid, J. W. Hadden, F. Spreafico, P. Dukor, and D. Willoughby, eds.), Pergamon Press, Elmsford, NY, pp. 487–497.

Hadden, J. W., Giner-Sorolla, A., and Hadden, E. M., 1991, Methyl inosine monophosphate (MIMP), a new purine immunomodulator for HIV infection, *Int. J. Immunopharmacol.* **13**:49–54.

Hadden, J. W., Ongradi, J., Specter, S., Nelson, R., Sosa, M., Strand, M., Giner-Sorolla, A., and Hadden, E. M., 1992, Methyl inosine monophosphate (MIMP): A potential immunotherapeutic for early HIV infection, *Int. J. Immunopharmacol.* **14**:555–563.

Haraguchi, S., Good, R. A., James-Yarish, M., Cianciolo, G. J., and Day, N. K., 1995, Induction of intracellular cAMP by a synthetic retroviral envelope peptide: A possible mechanism of immunopathogenesis in retroviral infections, *Proc. Natl. Acad. Sci. USA* **92**:5568–5571.

Hersh, E. M., Funk, C. Y., Peterson, E. A., and Mosier, D. E., 1991a, Effective therapy of the LP-BM5 murine retroviruse-induced lymphoproliferative disease with diethyldithiocarbamate, *AIDS Res. Hum. Retrovir.* **7**:553–561.

Hersh, E. M., Brewton, G., Abrams, D., Bartlett, J., Galpin, J., Gill, P., Gorter, R., Gottlieb, M., Jonikas, J. J., Landesman, S., Levine, A., Marcel, A., Peterson, E. A., Whiteside, M., Zahradnik, J., Negron, C., Boutitic, F., Caraux, J., Dupuy, J.-M., and Salmi, L. R., 1991b, Ditiocarb sodium (diethyldithiocarbamate) therapy in patients with asymptomatic HIV infection and AIDS. A randomized, double-blind, placebo-controlled, multicenter study, *J. Am. Med. Assoc.* **265**:1538–1544.

The HIV-87 Study Group, 1993, Multicenter, randomized, placebo-controlled study of ditiocarb (Imuthiol) in human immunodeficiency virus-infected asymptomatic and minimally symptomatic patients, *AIDS Res. Hum. Retrovir.* **9**:83–89.

Ho, D. D., Moudgil, T., and Alam, M., 1989, Quantitation of human immunodeficiency virus type I in the blood of infected persons, *N. Engl. J. Med.* **321**:1621–1625.

Ho, D. D., Neumann, A. U., Perelson, A. S., Chen, W., Leonard, J. M., and Markowitz, M., 1995, Rapid turnover of plasma virions and CD4 lymphocytes in HIV-1 infection, *Nature* **373**:123–126.

Hofmann, B., Nishanian, P., Nguyen, T., Liu, M., and Fahey, J. L., 1993a, Restoration of T-cell function in HIV infection by reduction of intracellular cAMP levels with adenosine analogues, *AIDS* **7**:659–664.

Hofmann, B., Nishanian, P., Nguyen, T., Insixiengmay, P., and Fahey, J. L., 1993b, Human immunodeficiency virus proteins induce the inhibitory cAMP/protein kinase A pathway in normal lymphocytes, *Proc. Natl. Acad. Sci. USA* **90**:6676–6680.

Kahn, J. O., Allan, J. D., Hodges, T. L., Kaplan, L. D., Arri, C. J., Fitch, H. F., Izu, A. E., Mordenti, J., Sherwin, S. A., Groopman, J. E., and Volderding, P. A. 1990, The safety and pharmacokinetics of recombinant soluble

CD4 (rCD4) in subjects with the acquired immunodeficiency syndrome (AIDS) and AIDS-related complex, *Ann. Intern. Med.* **112**:254–261.

Kaplan, C. S., Peterson, E. A., Yokum, D., and Hersh, E. M., 1989, A randomized controlled dose response study of intravenous sodium diethyldithiocarbamate in patients with advanced human immunodeficiency virus infection, *Life Sci.* **45**:iii–ix.

Keadle, T. L., Daniel, S., Rouse, B. T., and Horohov, D. W., 1996, Virus induced immunosuppression, in: *Immunopharmacology Reviews*, Vol. 2, pp. 131–156. (J. W. Hadden and A. Szentivanyi, eds.), Plenum Press, New York.

Kirkpatrick, C. H., Davis, K. C., Horsburgh, C. R., Cohn, D. L., Penley, K., and Judson, K. N., 1985, Interleukin 2 production by persons with the generalized lymphadenopathy syndrome or the acquired immune deficiency syndrome, *J. Clin. Immunol.* **5**: 31–37.

Kotler, D. P., and Reka, S., 1990, Modulation of HIV production by rectal mucosa *in vitro*, *Gastroenterology* **98**:457a.

Kovacs, J. A., Baseler, M., Dewar, R. J., Vogel, S., Davey, R. T., Jr., Falloon, J., Polis, M. A., Walker, R. E., Stevens, R., Salzman, N. P., Metcalf, J. A., Masur, H., and Lane, H. C., 1995, Increases in CD4 T lymphocytes with intermittent courses of interleukin-2 in patients with human immunodeficiency virus infection, *N. Engl. J. Med.* **332**: 567–575.

Landay, A. L., Mackewicz, C. E., and Levy, J. A., 1993, An activated CD8+ T cell phenotype correlates with anti-HIV activity and asymptomatic clinical status, *Clin. Immunol. Immunopathol.* **69**:106–116.

Lang, J., Trepo, C., Kirstetter, M., Herrou, L., Retornaz, G., Renoux, G., Musset, M., Touraine, J. L., Choutet, P., Falkenroot, A., Liurdset, J. M., Touraine, F., Renoux, M., Caraux, J., and The AIDS Imuthiol French Study Group, 1988, Randomized and double-blind placebo-controlled trial of ditiocarb sodium (Imuthiol) in human immunodeficiency virus infection, *Lancet* **9**:702–706.

LaPorte, J. P., Gonzalez, C., and Lebas, J., 1989, A new immunomodulating compound (AS101) in the treatment of AIDS, *5th Int. Conf. AIDS, Montreal* p. 399, abstract.

Laurence, J., 1995, Immune reconstitution in HIV/AIDS: Concepts and strategies, *The AIDS Reader* pp. 52–59.

Lederman, M., 1995, Host factor-directed immunotherapies, *The AIDS Reader* pp. 64–68.

Mackewicz, C., and Levy, J. A., 1992, CD8+ cell anti-HIV activity: Nonlytic suppression of virus replication, *AIDS Res. Hum. Retrovir.* **8**:1039–1050.

McMahon, D., Winklestein, A., Huang, X.-L., Armstrong, J., Pazin, G., Rinaldo, C., Tripoli, C., and Ho, M., 1992, Acute reactions associated with the infusion of ampligen, *AIDS* **6**:235–236.

Merigan, T. C., Fisher, A. C., Goldstein, G., Winters, M. A., Meyerson, L. A., and Hirsch, R. L., 1995, Evaluation of codon 215 mutation, viral load, P24 and CD4 as prognostic factors in asymptomatic HIV infected subjects treated with thymopentin, *J. Acq. Immune Defic. Syndr. Hum. Retrovir.* **8**:279–288.

Nielson, H. J., Svenningsen, A., Moesgaard, F., Georgsen, J., Pedersen, C., Mathiesen, L., Dickmeiss, E., Nielsen, J. O., and Kehlet, H., 1991, Ranitidine improves certain cellular immune responses in asymptomatic HIV-infected individuals, *J. Acq. Immune Defic. Syndr.* **4**:577–584.

Pahwa, S., Pahwa, R., Good, R. A., Gallo, R. C., and Saxinger, C., 1986, Stimulatory and inhibitory influences of human immunodeficiency virus on normal B lymphocytes, *Proc. Natl. Acad. Sci. USA* **83**:9124–9128.

Pantaleo, G., Graziosi, C., Demarest, J. F., Butini, L., Montroni, M., Fox, C. H., Orenstein, J. M., Kotler, D. P., and Fauci, A. S., 1993, HIV infection is active and progressive in lymphoid tissue during the clinically latent stage of disease, *Nature* **362**:355–358.

Park, B. Y., and Good, R. A., 1975, Quantitative assessment of thymus-dependent T-cell function in human peripheral blood, *Birth Defects* **11**:10–11.

Pederson, E. C., Sandstrom, E., Peterson, C. S., Norkrans, G., Gerstoft, J., Karlsson, J. O., Jurgenson, H. J., Christianson, K. C., Hakansson, C., Pehrson, P. O., Nielson, H. J., and the Scandinavian Isoprinosine Study Group, 1990, The efficacy of inosine pranobex in preventing the acquired immunodeficiency syndrome in patients with human immunodeficiency virus infection, *N. Engl. J. Med.* **322**:1757–1763.

Reddy, M. M., Manvar, D., Ahuja, K. K., Moriarty, M. L., and Grieco, M. H., 1985, Augmentation of mitogen-induced proliferative responses by in vitro indomethacin in patients with acquired immune deficiency syndrome and AIDS-related complex, *Int. J. Immunopharmacol.* **7**:917–921.

Redfield, R. R., Birx, D. L., Ketter, N., Tramont, E., Polonis, V., Davis, C., Brundage, J. F., Smith, G., Johnson, S., Fowler, A., Wierzba, T., Shafferman, A., Volovitz, F., Oster, C., Burke, D. S., and the Military Medical Consortium for Applied Retroviral Research, 1991, A Phase I evaluation of the safety and immunogenicity of vaccination with recombinant gp160 in patients with early human immunodeficiency virus infection, *N. Engl. J. Med.* **324**:1677–1684.

Reisinger, E. A., Kern, P., Ehrst, M., Bock, P., Flao, H. D., Dietrich, M., and German DTC Study Group, 1990, Inhibition of HIV progression by dithiocarb, *Lancet* **335:**679–682.

Renoux, G., and Renoux, M., 1984, Diethyldithiocarbamate (DTC): A biological augmenting agent specific for T cells, in: *Immune Modulation Agents and Their Mechanisms* (R. L. Fenichel and M. A. Chirigos, eds.), Dekker, New York, p. 7.

Rozzo, S. J., and Kirkpatrick, C. H., 1992, Purification of transfer factors, *Mol. Immunol.* **74:**167–182.

Ruegg, C. L., and Engleman, E. G., 1990, Impaired immunity in AIDS: The mechanisms responsible and their potential reversal by antiviral therapy. *Ann. N.Y. Acad. Sci.* **616**:307–317.

Ruegg, C. L., and Strand, M., 1991, A synthetic peptide with sequence identity to the transmembrane protein PG41 of HIV-1 inhibits distinct lymphocyte activation pathways dependent on protein kinase C and intracellular calcium influx, *Cell. Immunol.* **137:**1–13.

Ruegg, C. L., Monell, C. R., and Strand, M., 1989, Identification, using synthetic peptides, of the minimum amino acid sequence from the retroviral transmembrane protein p15E required for inhibition of lymphoproliferation and its similarity to gp21 of human T lymphotropic virus types I and II, *J. Virol.* **63:**3250–3256.

Ruiz-Palacios, G. M., Ponce de Leon, A., Alacon-Segovia, D., Calva, E., and Vasquez, M., 1988, Tolerance and clinical response to AS101, a new immunomodulator in AIDS patients, *IV Int. Conf. AIDS, Stockholm* p. 229.

Schooley, R. T., Merigan, T. C., Gaut, P., Hirsch, M. S., Holodniy, M., Flynn, T., Liu, S., Byington, R. E., Henochowicz, S., Gubish, E., Spriggs, D., Kufe, D., Schindler, J., Dawson, A., Thomas, D., Hanson, D. G., Letwin, B., Liu, T., Gulinello, J., Kennedy, S., Fisher, R., and Hi, D. D., 1990, Recombinant soluble CD4 therapy in patients with the acquired immunodeficiency syndrome (AIDS) and AIDS-related complex, *Ann. Intern. Med.* **112:**247–253.

Schwartz, D. H., Skowron, G., and Merigan, T. C., 1991, Safety and effects of IL-2 plus zidovudine in a to-matic individuals infected with human immunodeficiency virus, *J. Acq. Immune Defic. Syndr.* **4:**11–23.

Shibata, M., Hoon, D., Okun, E., and Morton, D., 1992, Modulation of histamine type II receptors on CD8+ T cells by interleukin 2 and cimetidine, *Int. Arch. Allergy Appl. Immunol.* **97:**8–16.

Siegal, J. P., Djeu, J., Stocks, N. L., Masur, H., Gelmann, E. P., and Quinnan, G. V., Jr., 1985, Sera from patients with the acquired immunodeficiency syndrome inhibit production of interleukin 2 by normal lymphocytes, *J. Clin. Invest.* **75:**1957–1964.

Silvestris, F., Germone, A., Frassanito, M., and Dammacco, F., 1989, Immunologic effects of long-term thymopentin treatment in patients with HIV-induced lymphadenopathy syndrome, *J. Lab. Clin. Med.* **113:**139–144.

Sinha, S. K., Sizemore, R. C., and Gottlieb, A. A., 1988, Immunomodulatory components present in ImReg-1, an experimental immunosupportive biologic, *Biotechnology* **6:**810–815.

Sizemore, R. C., Dienglewicz, R. L., Pecunia, E., and Gottlieb, A. A., 1991, Modulation of concanavalin A-induced, antigen-nonspecific regulatory cell activity by Leu-enkephalin and related peptides, *Clin. Immunol. Immunopathol.* **60:**310–318.

Snyderman, R., and Cianciolo, G. J., 1984, Immunosuppressive activity of the retroviral envelope protein P15E and its possible relationship to neoplasia, *Immunol. Today* **5:**240–244.

Sosa, M., Saha, A. R., Wang, Y., Wadsworth, T., Coto, J. A., Giner-Sorolla, A., Hadden, E. M., and Hadden, J. W., 1992, Potentiation of immune responses in mice by a new inosine derivative—Methyl inosine monophosphate (MIMP), *Int. J. Immunopharmacol.* **14:**1259–1266.

Specter, S., and Hadden, J. W., 1992, Immunotherapy for acquired immunodeficiency syndrome: Status and prospects, in: *AIDS and Other Manifestations of HIV Infection* (G. Wormser, ed.), Raven Press, New York, pp. 625–632.

Sunshine, G., Basch, R. S., Coffey, R. G., Cohen, K. W., Goldstein, G., and Hadden, J. W., 1978, Thymopoietin enhances the allogenic response and cyclic nucleotide levels of mouse peripheral, thymus-derived lymphocytes, *J. Immunol.* **120:**1594–1599.

Svedersky, L., Roey, S., Scillian, J., Goldyne, M., Moody, D., and Stites, D., 1990, Prostaglandin production is related to decreased lymphocyte responses in HIV-infected individuals, *FASEB J.* **7**(4), ASBMG-AAI Meeting, New Orleans, abstract #3284.

Turowski, R. C., and Triozzi, P. L., 1994, Application of chemical immunomodulators to the treatment of cancer and AIDS, *Cancer Invest.* **12:**620–643.

Wilson, G. B., Paddock, G. V., and Fudenberg, H. H., 1979, The chemical nature of the antigen-specific moiety of transfer factor, *Trans. Assoc. Am. Physicians* **92:**239–256.

CHAPTER 25

BIOLOGIC RESPONSE MODIFIERS (INTERLEUKINS AND INTERFERONS)

GWENDOLYN ANNE FYFE and H. CLIFFORD LANE

1. INTRODUCTION

The first cases of AIDS were described in 1981 and the virus was initially isolated in 1983. Since that time, substantial progress has been made in the prophylaxis and treatment of the opportunistic infections associated with HIV-related immune deficiency and some progress has been made in controlling the persistent viral replication which characterizes HIV infection. Unfortunately, no antiretroviral drug or combination of drugs has yet resulted in complete and lasting suppression of HIV replication and damage and depletion of the immune system continues. Furthermore, the rapid development of antiretroviral resistance limits the utility of even current combination regimens. While the continued development of new antiretroviral agents without overlapping patterns of resistance provides some hope that the progression of HIV disease may be controlled ultimately by a multidrug approach, such as has been successful in tuberculosis, this remains a hypothesis.

Perhaps the most remarkable aspect of HIV infection is the slow progression of immune deficiency, more than a decade in most patients, in spite of the high replicative rate and rapid turnover of HIV. By measuring the kinetics of viral burden decline following the introduction of a novel antiretroviral agent, multiple investigators (Ho *et al.*, 1995; Wei *et al.*, 1995) have demonstrated a rapid rate of viral turnover with a half-life of plasma virus on the order of 1 to 2 days. These results suggest that the apparent latency of HIV for the initial years of infection is most likely attributable to very effective and persistent immunologic mechanisms that limit viral burden. The capacity of the immune system to reduce the acute plasma viremia during primary infection by more than three logs (Daar *et al.*, 1991; Clark *et al.*, 1991) and to delay progression of disease for many years despite rapid viral replication remains an unachieved goal by the best available combination antiretroviral

GWENDOLYN ANNE FYFE • Chiron Corporation, Emeryville, California 94608. H. CLIFFORD LANE • National Institutes of Health, National Institute for Allergy and Infectious Diseases, Bethesda, Maryland 20892.

Immunology of HIV Infection, edited by Sudhir Gupta. Plenum Press, New York, 1996.

regimens. Both relative to the control of HIV replication mediated by the immune system in HIV disease and to standard antimicrobial therapy in most acute infections, current antiretroviral therapy remains at best only partially effective. Given this reality, the current belief that HIV is a viral infection best treated by the exclusive use of antiretroviral therapy seems limited in perspective.

The ability of immune interventions to augment natural immunity and thereby delay HIV progression remains quite hypothetical. In part, experience with immune interventions remains relatively limited because so little of natural or adaptive immunity is understood. A first example is the CD4 count. CD4 number is an important surrogate for overall immune function; for the most part, CD4 count has demonstrated unique utility in signaling the need for prophylaxis for opportunistic infections and overall guidance in patient management. However, CD4 number alone provides only partial information; CD4 function is also important, but has been difficult to measure. The proportion of different CD4 subsets, such as memory versus naive, as well as the diversity of the remaining T-cell repertoire, may also have important clinical implications. Thus, many caveats limit the utility of CD4 and other serologic markers as sole markers of clinical benefit.

A second example is the effector mechanism(s) controlling viral burden. Protection from viral infection has been attributed variously to natural killer (NK) cells which are neither HLA-restricted nor virus-specific, to virus-specific antibodies, to cytotoxic T lymphocytes, and to helper inducer T lymphocytes. The mechanism or mechanisms that predominate in the control of acute as well as chronic HIV viremia have not been established definitively. Cytotoxic T lymphocytes (CTLs) are presumed widely to be the predominant mechanism of reduction in viremia based on the detection of HIV-specific CTL precursors (CTL_p) directed at *gag*, *pol*, or *env* HIV proteins obtained from the blood of patients with symptoms of primary HIV infection. The presence of CTL_p at the time the initial viremia subsides has been taken as proof that CTLs are the primary effector function mediating viral clearance. Ancillary evidence demonstrating that the absence of a diverse CTL response to the virus may be associated with rapid progression of disease also supports this hypothesis (Borrow *et al.*, 1994; Pantaleo *et al.*, 1994). However, the number of acutely infected patients who have been studied is small and the study of patients with clinical symptoms during acute HIV infection represents a substantial selection bias; results from these patients may not reflect HIV disease in the majority of patients. In addition, at least one clinical anecdote suggests that infusion of large numbers of a specific CTL clone can actually increase the rate of progression (Koenig *et al.*, 1995). In sum, the predominant mechanism(s) controlling viral replication and leading to the prolonged course of HIV infection have not been established formally.

For reasons such as these, there is no consensus regarding the primary goals of immune intervention. Is it more important to enhance CD4 cell number and function or improve the effector mechanisms thought to control viral replication? Or should other immune mechanisms, such as NK or macrophage activity, which might compensate in part for T-lymphocyte dysfunction, be targeted? All of these strategies probably have merit in particular clinical situations and, in any case, may be synergistic in approach.

The assays used to measure many immunologic markers complicate this issue further. The majority are cumbersome and expensive, difficult to standardize, and for the most part are measured in blood, where less than 2% of total body lymphocytes reside. It is difficult to correlate improvement in an immunologic parameter with clinical benefit when the outcome cannot be measured reliably.

Thus, HIV immunotherapy remains a field without validated immunologic surrogates for clinical benefit and without validated methodologies. While virologists are agreed that the primary surrogate focus of therapeutic intervention is a decrease in viral burden, the immunotherapy field lacks the primary focus of a prevailing paradigm to direct clinical research.

A second issue that has hampered the development of immunotherapy is the assumption that effective immune therapy should decrease viral burden. Underlying this assumption is the belief that immune reconstitution is a rapid phenomenon akin to viral turnover. However, most clinical examples of immune constitution or reconstitution (e.g., ontogeny, bone marrow transplantation) suggest that the development of immune competence is slow. Recent studies in adults following chemotherapy or bone marrow transplantation suggest that reconstitution of T-cell immunity is a delayed process and lymphocyte counts are subnormal for many years. CD4 counts, especially the CD45RA (naive) subset, are particularly depressed (Storek *et al.*, 1995; Mackall *et al.*, 1995). These examples would predict that rapid improvements in adaptive immunity are unlikely, even in the absence of a rapidly replicating viral infection. In this light, a more reasonable goal for immune intervention might be maintenance of immunity or a delay in progression.

Immune intervention and antiretroviral treatment target different aspects of HIV infection. The remarkable capability of the immune system to control viral replication and the prolonged course of HIV infection in the absence of antiretroviral intervention suggest that augmentation of the immune system is an important and currently underutilized parallel approach to the control of HIV infection. The purpose of this chapter is to review the advances that have been made in active immunotherapy as well as to promote a combination approach to the therapy of HIV disease. Topics covered include the clinical data resulting from the use of IL-2 as an immune modulator in HIV infection, the preliminary data justifying the use of IL-12 in HIV infection, and the use of interferons, particularly in Kaposi's sarcoma (KS).

2. INTERLEUKIN-2 THERAPY

IL-2 is a glycoprotein lymphokine with a molecular weight of approximately 15,000 produced by T cells and large granular lymphocytes. Originally identified in 1975 (Morgan *et al.*, 1976) by its growth-stimulating effects on T lymphocytes, its biologic spectrum of activity includes direct effects on the growth and differentiation of both CD4 and CD8 T lymphocytes, as well as on NK cells, B lymphocytes, lymphokine-activated killer (LAK) cells, macrophages, and even oligodendrocytes. Its direct effects are mediated by binding to the IL-2 receptor, a complex of up to three membrane-associated subunits (IL-2R-α, β, and γ). Each individual chain binds IL-2 with low affinity, but dimers of the β and γ chains and trimers of the α, β, and γ chains bind IL-2 with intermediate or high affinity, respectively. Downstream effects of IL-2 are also mediated by cytokines released by IL-2-activated cells (TNF-α, IL-6, IFN-γ, GM-CSF).

2.1. Rationale for Use in HIV Disease

A wide array of immunologic abnormalities have been described in HIV infection that appear to be IL-2 responsive. The initial rationale for clinical trials was provided by the observation that CMV-specific cytotoxic activity was deficient in AIDS patients and that *in vitro* IL-2 augmented antiviral cytotoxicity (Rook *et al.*, 1983). Since that initial description, multiple other immune parameters have been described that are partially enhanced *in vitro* by exogenous IL-2. These include effects on both T-cell proliferative responses (Ciobanu *et al.*, 1983; Gupta *et al.*, 1984), and effector function such as HIV-specific cell-mediated immunity (Bell *et al.*, 1992), as well as extent of apoptosis of T lymphocytes (Zubiaga *et al.*, 1992; Fei *et al.*, 1994). Local administration of IL-2 induces the immigration of immune cells to the site of injection, increases local expression of MHC class II antigens, and enhances skin antigen reactivity (McElrath *et al.*, 1990). Activation of monocytes is also improved (Murray *et al.*, 1985, 1988). In addition, animal models and *in vitro* data suggest that IL-2 could be a valuable adjunct in the treatment of specific opportunistic infections associated with HIV infection (Benedetto *et al.*, 1991; Jeevan and Asherson, 1988; Reddehause *et al.*, 1987; Bonavida *et al.*, 1986; Toosi *et al.*, 1986; Sheridan *et al.*, 1984).

2.2. Clinical Trials

Clinical trials with IL-2 began in 1983. The initial half-life of partially purified natural IL-2 in humans was defined as 10 min or less with a subsequent clearance of approximately 60–120 min. Subsequent studies with a variety of recombinant products have yielded similar results.

Over the 13 years that IL-2 has been in clinical trials, multiple IL-2 regimens have been assessed. Most studies have been small Phase I or II trials that have examined IL-2's effect on a variety of immunologic parameters including CD4 and CD8 number and function as well as NK number and activity. The varying effect of dose, dose frequency, and duration of therapy relative to rest periods is complex and has not been systematically studied.

Most of the early studies were performed prior to the availability of sensitive assays for HIV RNA. Often the patients treated with IL-2 had clinical symptoms of HIV disease including KS, persistent diarrhea, or a history of a major opportunistic infection. Patients did not receive concurrent antiretroviral therapy and supportive care measures were not as well developed as now. Consequently, data from these studies may not be comparable to those studies performed more recently.

2.3. Early Trials

The earliest trials (Lane *et al.*, 1984; Lotze *et al.*, 1984; Mertelsmann *et al.*, 1984) of IL-2 used natural IL-2 purified from either mitogen-stimulated lymphocytes or tumor cells. The doses delivered were generally lower than those currently in use. Mild toxicities which are now commonly associated with IL-2 were observed including headache, nausea and vomiting, malaise, and fever. Immunologic effects included a recall reaction to a previous tetanus immunization and, at the higher doses given, there were immediate transient declines in CD4 and CD8 cells during therapy. Hypergammaglobulinemia was also noted to decrease in some patients. No clinical improvement in patients with KS or CMV viruria was observed, although Mertelsmann *et al.* reported improvement in retinitis in one patient.

The availability of recombinant IL-2 allowed therapy of patients with higher doses for longer periods of time. In a Phase I trial of recombinant IL-2, Kern *et al.* (1985) delivered increasing doses of intravenous IL-2 by either bolus or 4-hr infusion to a cohort of nine patients with advanced disease. At the higher doses, fatigue, fever, rash, and other common side effects of IL-2 were observed. Lymphocytosis and eosinophilia were observed at the end of therapy; clinically, KS lesions improved but did not resolve and two patients with symptoms of cryptosporidial diarrhea improved. In a subsequent trial, these investigators evaluated the immunologic effect of short infusion therapy and found some improvement in the depressed proliferative response to soluble antigens and alloantigens following systemic therapy, defective NK activity which improved with treatment, minor improvements in DTH, and transient lymphocytosis (Ernst *et al.*, 1986). In a Phase I/II trial, Volberding *et al.* (1987) treated a large cohort of HIV-infected patients with escalating doses of three times weekly bolus IL-2. Doses ranged from 0.006 to 12×10^6 IU/m^2. Most patients treated in this trial had extensive KS and had CD4 counts in the range of 100 cells/μl. At higher IL-2 doses, rigors and transient systolic hypotension were noted. No effect on immunologic parameters was observed, perhaps because IL-2 given by bolus administration results in only transient blood levels. Only three partial remissions were observed among the 55 KS patients treated. In spite of the absence of concurrent antiretroviral therapy, no apparent acceleration in disease course was observed.

2.4. Continuous Infusion IL-2

2.4.1. NIAID Experience

IL-2 has been in clinical trials since 1983; the initial clinical results were not very remarkable and progress was slow. Recent work has been more encouraging. In a recent study (Kovacs *et al.*, 1995a), 23 patients were treated in a dose escalation study with 1.8–24 MIU/day for up to 21 days. The maximum tolerated dose was 12 MIU/day for 21 days and 18 MIU/day when delivered for 5 days. Dose-limiting side effects included capillary leak syndrome, severe flulike symptoms, renal dysfunction, and laboratory abnormalities. There were transient increases in CD4 and CD8 counts at the end of the first week of therapy during the 21-day infusion which returned to baseline in spite of continued therapy. Viral burden, as assessed by p24 and viral coculture, was unchanged.

In the second phase of this study, 10 patients with CD4 > 200 cells/μl and 12 patients with CD4 < 200 cells/μl were treated with repeated courses of 5-day continuous intravenous (CIV) infusions of IL-2 in doses ranging from 6 to 18 MIU/day. Patients received between 4 and 13 courses of IL-2 and follow-up ranged from almost 2 years to more than 3 years. In 6 of the 10 patients with entry CD4 > 200 cells/μl, the CD4 count increased by more than 50%. This increase was sustained over the course of therapy, unlike the transient change in CD4 numbers ("trafficking") commonly observed immediately following many IL-2 regimens. This group of patients also had increased expression of the α chain of the IL-2 receptor on CD4 cells and a decreasing number of $CD8^+DR^+$ and $CD8^+CD38^+$ cells. Overall, CD8 number was not changed during treatment. Patients with CD4 < 200 cells/μl at entry to this trial fared less well with only 2 of the 6 patients with CD4 100–200 cells/μl showing 50% increases in CD4 count and none of the 6 patients with CD4 < 100 cells/μl showing any significant increase. Of concern was the appearance of a transient burst of virus observed at the end of each 5-day infusion in many patients with measurable viral burden. In patients with CD4 > 200 cells/μl this burst was transient, but in patients with CD4 < 200 cells/μl could be sustained.

This same group of investigators (Kovacs *et al.*, 1995b) subsequently performed a randomized trial to assess more precisely the immunologic and virologic effects of a CIV

IL-2 regimen with antiretroviral therapy relative to a regimen of antiretroviral therapy alone over the course of 14 months. In all, 60 patients were randomized, 31 to CIV IL-2 therapy and 29 to antiretroviral therapy. The patients began therapy with CD4 counts in the range of 400 and two-thirds of each group had measurable viral burden as reflected by branched DNA (bDNA) levels prior to therapy. Although patients began treatment at a dose of 18 MIU/day, many were dose reduced quickly and the average dose of IL-2 delivered during the course of the trial was 9 MIU/day. Treatment was delivered on an inpatient basis; the majority of toxicities were secondary to the flulike syndrome associated with IL-2 therapy and these symptoms tended to intensify with duration of therapy. By the end of treatment, the IL-2-treated group had a mean increase in CD4 count of 380 cells/μl versus a loss of 70 cells/μl in the antiretroviral control ($p < 0.001$). No significant changes in CD8 cell number were observed. Viral burden, as assessed by bDNA levels, increased acutely in many patients immediately following an IL-2 infusion, but long-term increases were not observed in the majority of patients. At the end of the study, the mean viral burden in the IL-2-treated group was slightly less than that of the antiretroviral group. In sum, in a single-institution randomized trial, intermittent CIV IL-2 therapy of asymptomatic HIV-infected population resulted in substantial and sustained CD4 increases in the absence of chronic increases in viral burden. These investigators are researching a variety of methods to reduce the toxicity of therapy including subcutaneous delivery and, in collaboration with other investigators, they are studying the immunologic activity of infusions of shorter duration. In addition, agents to block TNF release such as thalidomide or antibodies directed against TNF-α are being evaluated.

2.4.2. Other CIV IL-2 Experiences

A number of other studies have also utilized CIV regimens to ensure sustained blood levels of IL-2. Schwartz *et al.* (1991) treated ten asymptomatic patients with 5 days/week CIV infusions of IL-2 for 1 month in association with ZDV using an intrapatient dose escalation scheme. A total of 27 courses of therapy were given so that most patients received more than 1 course of treatment. Courses at higher doses were delivered approximately 8 weeks after the first if the initial cycle was well-tolerated. Doses ranged from 1.5 to 12 IU/m^2 per day. Dose-limiting side effects included facial angioedema and constitutional symptoms in two patients and two others had significant line complications including a hemothorax following central line placement and septic thrombophlebitis. Immunologic testing at the time of infusion showed a transient increase in circulating CD4 and CD8 cell number at the end of each 5-day infusion of IL-2. NK activity, which was suppressed below baseline by ZDV therapy, increased over the course of IL-2 therapy only at the higher doses. LAK activity was not increased significantly. Long-term evaluation of the patients treated on this trial showed that some patients had sustained increases in their CD4 count (Ramachandran *et al.*, 1994), In this asymptomatic and antiviral-naive population, viral burden, as assessed by proviral DNA measured in PBMC and p24 assay, remained stable over the course of therapy.

CIV IL-2 has also been evaluated in combination with IFN-α (Schnittman *et al.*, 1994). The toxicities were quite significant in the combined regimen with severe flulike symptoms, fever, depression, and liver function abnormalities. For most patients, dose-limiting toxicities constituted a constellation of systemic symptoms rather than a single dose-limiting problem. There was no evidence of synergism with respect to immunologic effects. However, this combination has been used successfully in patients with KS.

Mazza *et al.* (1992) treated 12 patients with HIV lymphoma with repetitive 5-day courses of CIV IL-2 at doses of approximately 6 MIU/m^2 per day in association with ZDV. Many of these patients were given chemotherapy prior to IL-2 therapy, but all but one patient had residual measurable disease. Response to therapy was correlated with CD4 number, with both patients who achieved a complete response having entry CD4 $>$ 100 cells/μl. Three other patients achieved a partial remission. These patients had other evidence of immune benefit as well including transient elevations in CD4 count and improved NK and LAK activity. While these data are preliminary, further studies of IL-2 in HIV lymphoma seem warranted.

2.5. Subcutaneous IL-2

Subcutaneous (SQ) IL-2 has been evaluated by a number of investigators. Davey *et al.* (1994) treated 17 patients with escalating doses of once-daily SQ IL-2 for 5 days every 8 weeks. The maximum tolerated dose on this regimen was 15 MIU/day. The toxicity profile was similar to the CIV IL-2 regimen, although toxicities tended to concentrate 4 to 8 hr postinjection. Occasional patients had significant increases in CD4 counts, but in general, once-daily dosing seemed less active than CIV IL-2. A subsequent amendment to this trial is evaluating twice-daily dosing for 5 days either every 4 or every 8 weeks. McMahon *et al.* (1994) performed a Phase I trial in 16 patients of once-daily SQ IL-2 of either 0.6, 2.1, or 6 MU/m^2 per day for 5 days in association with ZDV therapy. This single course of therapy was associated with increases in CD4, CD8, and CD16 counts which persisted at 10 weeks following treatment as well as increases in NK activity. No changes in viral burden were noted at day 8, as assessed by HIV coculture and p24, but p24 values checked at day 5 of therapy showed transient increases in 2 patients who were previously antigenemic. Deresinski *et al.* (1995) treated 64 patients with twice-daily SQ IL-2 in a five-arm trial which evaluated both the effect of dose and the addition of *ex vivo*-expanded CD8 cells to therapy. Against an antiviral-treated control, IL-2-treated patients had a mean 1.4-fold increase in CD4 cells and patients treated with *ex vivo*-expanded CD8 cells also had significant expansion of $CD8^+CD28^+$ cells. CD4 increases were much more common in this trial, perhaps because of the twice-daily dosing schedule. Relative to entry, there was no increase in viral burden over the course of therapy in any of the treatment arms.

3. PEG IL-2

Polyethylene glycol (PEG)-modified IL-2 (PEG IL-2) is a long-acting formulation of IL-2. By linking PEG molecules to the IL-2 protein via conjugation to primary amino groups, the effective molecular weight of IL-2 is increased and clearance, normally via the kidneys, is decreased. The effective half-life of PEG IL-2 is 10–20 times that of unmodified IL-2; its large size also changes its biodistribution relative to unmodified IL-2 and decreases its affinity for the IL-2 receptor. *In vitro* studies indicate that the effective biologic activity of PEG IL-2 is approximately three- to sixfold less than that of unmodified IL-2.

A number of studies have been performed using PEG IL-2. Intravenous bolus PEG

IL-2 was evaluated by Wood *et al.* (1993) in 19 patients in a Phase I/II trial. Dose-limiting side effects included severe fatigue, hypotension, and a CNS syndrome consistent with a vasculitic process which resolved without therapy. These kinds of CNS episodes have also been described in oncology patients treated with high bolus doses of either intravenous PEG IL-2 or, much less commonly, with intravenous IL-2. Positive immunologic effects observed included increases in CD4 count, NK activity, and HIV-specific cytotoxicity. No evidence of HIV activation was observed using proviral DNA quantification by PCR or by p24 antigen.

Two trials of low-dose SQ PEG IL-2 (Teppler *et al.*, 1993a,b) showed that PEG IL-2 could be delivered with minimal toxicity for extended periods of time. These patients had improved DTH to recall antigens, improved proliferative response to mitogen, and enhanced NK activity. Some of these effects were sustained for several months following cessation of therapy. No clear increase in CD4 cells was observed and no evidence of HIV activation was noted. A Phase I SQ PEG IL-2 trial in 64 patients which included PEG IL-2 doses of up to 1 MIU/week showed some improvement in CD4 cells, mostly in patients with entry CD4 $>$ 200 cells/μl (Waites *et al.*, 1992). An ongoing study in Australia of high-dose PEG IL-2 is currently evaluating whether SQ PEG IL-2 pharmacokinetically modeled to achieve blood levels similar to CIV IL-2 can achieve immunologic effects similar to the CIV IL-2 regimen.

4. CURRENT STATUS

IL-2 and PEG IL-2 have now been evaluated in multiple trials with diverse doses and regimens in a spectrum of HIV-infected patients. Some conclusions are clear. While multiple regimens are immunologically active as reflected by NK activity, transient changes in CD4 and CD8 count, and improved DTH, only a few seem to result in sustained increases in CD4 count over the course of many months. The characteristics of these regimens include alternating cycles of rest and restimulation. A rest period is important since persistent CD4 increases were not observed with prolonged continuous therapy. The optimal duration of the rest period is not known. Sustained blood levels seem important since the CIV IL-2 regimen works best, although twice-daily SQ regimens are still quite active. The optimal dose is not known; it is quite likely that there is a graded response to therapy with lower doses retaining significant immunologic activity.

Further, the ability to achieve a CD4 increase is related to the level of residual immune function as reflected by initial CD4 count. Patients with CD4 counts under 200 cells/μl are less likely to have a CD4 response than patients with CD4 greater than 200 cells/μl. Patients with CD4 greater than 500 cells/μl have the highest rates of response. Other characteristics are also important. High viral burden seems to result in a less sustained IL-2 response. Many factors including previous antiretroviral history as well as access to newer agents make this a complicated relationship.

No answers can be given for other critical questions. Do increases in CD4 count represent a real improvement in immune function? While activation of the virus is clearly undesirable, what is the net effect of a transient increase in viremia? Both of these questions are actually aspects of a more generic question: does IL-2 therapy provide clinical benefit to the patient? The answer to this question can only be provided in a clinical endpoint trial. The laboratory data currently available to address these questions are discussed below. Because the first question is fundamentally directed at the immunologic data and the second at the virologic data, they will be addressed separately.

4.1. IL-2 Effect on Immune Function

Numerous studies have evaluated the ability of IL-2 to modulate immune function in HIV disease. Many beneficial effects on different parameters of immune function have been observed, but it is not yet known whether these improvements will clinically benefit the patient. The immune effects observed vary based on schedule and dose as well as the time of measurement. The time-dependent effect of IL-2 on lymphocyte count during a 5-day infusion is a clinically relevant example. Initially, there is a dose-dependent but transient lymphocytopenia which, in spite of continued therapy, is followed by a marked lymphocytosis with blood lymphocyte counts that often reach two to three times their baseline value. These acute changes in lymphocyte number are commonly referred to as lymphocyte trafficking because they are the result, at least in part, of a redistribution of lymphocytes initially from the circulation, followed by a reciprocal redistribution from other compartments back to the vascular space toward the end of treatment. Increased expression of ICAM-1 by endothelial and mononuclear cells early during IL-2 infusions has been observed consistent with a lymphocyte redistribution phenomenon (Cotran *et al.*, 1987).

Proliferation of lymphocytes outside the vascular space also contributes to the lymphocyte number increase. During the day 5–6 lymphocytosis, as many as 10–15% of circulating cells found in the blood are cycling, and spontaneous blast transformation, a measure of the cells to proliferate in the absence of any stimulus, is markedly increased. However, these profound increases seen following IL-2 therapy are not sustained and lymphocyte count returns to normal over the course of several weeks. Whether the return of PBL number to its baseline values is a reflection of cell death or of redistribution outside the vascular volume is not known.

The acute increase in lymphocyte number does not reflect a uniform improvement in lymphocyte function. Specific lymphocyte function has been measured during this treatment interval and, while NK and LAK activity are increased, measurements of T-lymphocyte function have been variously reported as increased, unchanged, or depressed. Delayed-type hypersensitivity (DTH) has been reported to be both increased and diminished from baseline. Proliferative responses to soluble antigen, alloantigens, and mitogens are also variably reported as increased or decreased (Rosenthal *et al.*, 1988; Lotze *et al.*, 1984). These discrepant results probably reflect differences in the regimen's intensity, time of measurement with respect to therapy duration, and the prior activation of the lymphocytes *in vivo*.

While the trafficking effects discussed above have been noted with most higher-dose IL-2 regimens in a variety of clinical settings, the pronounced increases in CD4 number noted in HIV-infected patients following repetitive 5-day CIV cycles of IL-2 have not been previously described. These increases in CD4 number are distinct from trafficking effects because they persist for months following treatment, because progressive increases in CD4 cell number are seen in responding patients with repetitive cycles of therapy, and because, while trafficking changes are noted for all lymphocyte subsets, only CD4 lymphocytes show persistent increases with this regimen.

In aggregate, functional data suggest that immune function improves over time in responsive patients treated with this regimen. Increases in both memory (CD45RO) and naive (CD45RA) CD4 cell number are observed, although the naive subset appears to be expanded preferentially in most patients. Current knowledge suggests that naive CD4 cells in the adult host have either never encountered their cognate antigen or have done so in the remote past; thus, their importance with respect to protection from opportunistic infections is not certain. Few adults retain functional thymus (Mackall, 1995) and recent data suggest that the T-cell repertoire is maintained, at least in part, by peripheral expansion (Walker *et al.*, 1995) rather than thymic education. Ongoing studies of IL-2 therapy in HIV-infected children will be illuminating with respect to the importance of thymic function in reconstituting immunity.

Evaluation of CD4 expansion using V_β chain T-cell receptor analysis suggests that the CD4 expansion is polyclonal. No evidence of reconstitution of missing V_β subsets has been observed. This observation is consistent with the hypothesis that IL-2 maintains residual immunity rather than reconstituting lost immune responses. By increasing the precursor frequency of certain antigen specificities, IL-2 may protect residual immune function. However, more sensitive techniques of measurement will be necessary to address this issue.

Proliferative response to soluble antigen and alloantigen have been evaluated over multiple courses of treatment in responding patients; proliferative response is often improved in previously responsive patients but only rarely is reconstituted in anergic patients, even those with marked increases in CD4 count. These findings suggest that the overall effect of IL-2 on immune function is salutary, but that the magnitude of benefit is less than the quantitative CD4 increase would suggest.

4.2. IL-2 Effect on HIV Body Burden

Most recent IL-2 studies have evaluated IL-2 in combination with antiretroviral therapy to minimize the risk of IL-2-induced viral replication. This combination approach is based on the known capacity for IL-2 to activate HIV, both in culture and *in vivo*. Both the necessity and the overall effectiveness of this strategy are difficult to demonstrate because of the confounding effects of many variables: patient variability with respect to initial viral burden, the varying effectiveness of different antiretroviral agents, the absence of a sensitive and specific assay for replication-competent virus. However, in some patients, more effective viral blockade with highly active antiretroviral combinations seem to allow a synergistic improvement in CD4 response relative to standard antiretroviral/IL-2 regimens and to convert patients with lower CD4 counts at the time of therapy into a more IL-2-responsive population. A recent randomized Phase II study by Falloon *et al.* (1995) evaluated the utility of a combination of Indinavir (Merck protease inhibitor) with or without IL-2 in a group of patients who had been previously unresponsive to IL-2 or who had CD4 < 300 cells/μl. In this trial, Indinavir alone resulted in a mean increase of 90 cells/μl while the IL-2 combination regimen had a mean increase of 180 cells/μl. No differences were noted in the viral burden decrease seen between the two arms. These observations suggest that IL-2's net effect in any particular patient is a balance between immune activation and viral activation with the outcome influenced greatly by the residual immune function and viral burden of that patient.

However, it is worth noting that earlier studies of IL-2 performed without antiretroviral coverage did not show evidence of progression of disease in patients with preexisting KS or very low CD4 counts. Also, bursts of virus are observed following influenza vaccination (O'Brien *et al.*, 1995), blood transfusions, and acute infections, which would suggest that transient increases in viral burden are not uncommon; in most of these scenarios, patients have returned to the same viral burden present at baseline. In IL-2-treated patients, revaluation of viral quasispecies and resistance patterns in a limited number of patients does not show any deleterious effects. In all, these data suggest that these viral bursts represent only a brief perturbation of an evolving equilibrium rather than a persistent loss of antiviral immunity with prolonged treatment. Further studies in large cohorts of patients with careful evaluation of both baseline immune function and viral burden will be necessary to understand this issue.

5. CONCLUSIONS

IL-2 has pronounced effects on many immune parameters in HIV-infected patients. Intermittent continuous infusion regimens have sustained effects on CD4 number and function. Other regimens are active in increasing NK function and macrophage activity which may become more important as CD4 count wanes. In patients with CD4 > 200 cells/μl, IL-2 transiently activates viral replication. This activation is more sustained in patients with CD4 < 200 cells/μl which may limit the utility of higher-dose IL-2 regimens in this population. Sustained increases in viral burden are not seen in the majority of asymptomatic patients. However, decreases in viral burden associated with increased CD4 number are only rarely observed.

Antiretroviral therapy has been of proven benefit to HIV-infected patients. In most trials, therapy leads to reciprocal changes in CD4 count and viral burden and many clinicians and scientists expect immune therapies to follow the same rules. Thus, an apparent improvement in immune function in the absence of any decrease in viral burden is inconsistent with the viral paradigm of HIV disease. However, IL-2 may be positively affecting residual immunity without affecting an acute change in viral burden. The CD4 increases noted with intermittent IL-2 therapy may reflect a greater reservoir of residual immunity rather than a reconstituted immunity over prolonged treatment. This hypothesis is consistent with the stable viral burden noted over extended therapy. It is also possible that IL-2 therapy, in combination with potent antiviral therapies, may lead to some reconstitution of immunity with prolonged treatment. Ultimately, the benefit of IL-2 therapy can only be answered in controlled trials in HIV-infected patients. However, the ability to address this question in a randomized trial in an asymptomatic patient population remains problematic.

6. INTERLEUKIN-12

IL-12 is a 75-kDa heterodimeric glycoprotein that was originally identified by its ability to activate macrophages, to enhance NK function, and to induce T-cell maturation. Also important, IL-12 is a potent inducer of IFN-γ and TNF-α, which are important mediators of IL-12's biologic activity. Receptors for IL-12 are expressed only on activated T and NK cells and the principal source of IL-12 *in vivo* is activated macrophages and B cells. Multiple *in vitro* and animal models suggest that IL-12 is a critical part of many protective immune responses. IL-12 has been proposed as a cytokine to improve suboptimal immune responses; to augment immunity in infections that have become chronic and that may be immunosuppressive; to augment the immunity of immunocompromised hosts; and as a vaccine adjuvant to promote a cell-mediated immunity rather than an antibody response (Biron and Gazzinelli, 1995).

These general attributes suggest that IL-12 may be useful in HIV disease; in addition, more specific deficits have been noted in HIV-infected patients that suggest that IL-12 may play an important therapeutic role in the management of HIV disease. HIV-infected macrophages do not produce adequate levels of IL-12 (Chouaib *et al.*, 1994; Clerici *et al.*, 1993a; Chehimi *et al.*, 1994). In addition, IL-12 augments NK cytotoxicity and HIV-specific cell-mediated immunity *in vitro* and augments IFN-γ production (Chehimi *et al.*, 1992). However, the most compelling rationale for the use of IL-12 in the management of HIV infection relates to IL-12's ability to promote a Th1 response to infection. Some *in vitro* studies have suggested that there is a progressive imbalance in the T-cell response to antigen in HIV-infected individuals, with a selective defect in Th1-type responses and predominance of Th2 responses (Clerici *et al.*, 1993a). Based on these studies, it has been proposed that a switch from a Th1 to a Th2 cytokine phenotype occurs early in the course of HIV infection and is a critical step in the progression of HIV disease (Clerici and Shearer, 1993).

However, other recent studies have not shown a switch from Th1 to Th2 during the progression of HIV infection (Graziosi *et al.*, 1994; Maggi *et al.*, 1994). Defects in Th1-type responses are present in HIV infection; however, these defects may be related to a decreased number of Th1 cells consistent with HIV-induced CD4 cell depletion, or to a qualitative switch from a Th1 to a Th2 response leading to increased CD4 cell loss.

In multiple animal models, there is a dose-dependent effect of IL-12 administration on disease and both beneficial and detrimental effects in infectious disease models have been observed. In lymphocytic choriomeningitis infection, IL-12 in doses of at least 100 ng/day leads to increased sensitivity to infection while lower doses enhance clearance of virus. Similar dose–response relationships have been noted with IL-2 and it seems likely that the identification of an appropriate IL-12 dose and regimen may be disease specific.

IL-12 has been evaluated in murine acquired immunodeficiency syndrome (MAIDS) and shown to be of benefit even when administered several months after infection. IL-12 inhibited the development of splenomegaly and lymphadenopathy as well as decreasing the hypergammaglobulinemia associated with MAIDS. It also prevented the impairment of IFN-γ production and improved proliferative responses to mitogens. Many of these effects were mediated by IFN-γ production (Gazzinelli *et al.*, 1994).

IL-12 is already in clinical trials, but experience to date in HIV disease is quite limited. However, *in vitro* and preclinical data suggest that IL-12 may be an important cytokine for the treatment of HIV-infected patients. Much work remains to be done in delineating optimal dose and regimen as well as IL-12's utility in association with other treatment modalities.

7. INTERFERONS

Interferons are a group of protein molecules with antiviral, antiproliferative, and immunomodulatory properties (Baron *et al.*, 1991). Interferons can be grouped into two distinct types based on their cell receptors and biological effects. Type I interferons include IFN-α and -β that share a common cellular receptor and are produced by multiple cell types (leukocytes, fibroblasts, and epithelial cells). Type II interferon or IFN-γ is produced by activated T lymphocytes and NK cells and has a cellular receptor distinct from the type I interferons. There are at least 18 different IFN-α genes that encode at least 14 distinct protein products. In contrast, there is only one IFN-β and one IFN-γ gene.

7.1. Interferon-α

Even before the AIDS epidemic, IFN-α was known to exhibit antiretroviral activity. Studies in mice infected with murine leukemia virus indicated that IFN-α can inhibit viral replication *in vitro* by impeding the assembly and maturation of murine leukemia virus (Pitha *et al.*, 1979). With the identification of HIV as the cause of AIDS, several laboratories began to examine the effects of IFN-α on HIV replication. It was initially shown that concentrations of IFN-α in the range of 100 U/ml could suppress HIV replication in tissue culture (Ho *et al.*, 1985). This effect was most pronounced when IFN-α was continually present in the culture media and comparable in magnitude to the level of suppression seen with zidovudine. Subsequent work demonstrated that inhibition of HIV replication was more pronounced with type I interferons than with IFN-γ. In T lymphocytes, IFN-α appears to suppress HIV replication by interfering with the assembly and release of progeny virus (Poli *et al.*, 1989; Francis *et al.*, 1992). In contrast, nucleoside analogues, such as zidovudine, act early in the HIV life cycle by inhibiting reverse transcriptase.

Trials of IFN-α in HIV disease were performed initially in KS. In these first studies, very high doses of IFN-α (25–54 MU/day) were used and significant clinical responses were seen, with response rates of 13–46% (deWit *et al.*, 1988; Lane *et al.*, 1988; Real *et al.*, 1986; Gelmann *et al.*, 1985; Volberding and Mitsuyasu, 1985; Groopman *et al.*, 1984). The probability of a response was correlated highly with CD4 percent or absolute CD4 T-cell number. For example, in one study all of five patients with CD4 counts greater than 400 cells/mm^3 exhibited a partial or complete response of their KS lesions, while none of seven patients with CD4 counts less than 150 cells/mm^3 responded (Lane *et al.*, 1988). These results suggest that the clinical responses seen with IFN-α may be related to multiple activities including its antiproliferative and antiviral effects, and also perhaps by stimulating other immune mechanisms.

Based on these studies, IFN-α was licensed as therapy for patients with HIV-associated KS. Although the package insert describes doses in the range of 35 MU/day, few patients can tolerate this dose because of flulike symptoms, neutropenia, and elevations of hepatic transaminases. Thus, most clinicians will start with lower doses (1–5 MU) and escalate as tolerated on schedules ranging from daily to three times a week (Lane *et al.*, 1988).

Besides the antitumor effect, these studies provided evidence that IFN-α also had an antiretroviral effect. Like the antitumor effect, this anti-HIV effect was strongly correlated with the level of immune competence, again suggesting that IFN-α was acting to enhance the immune response rather than having direct antiviral activity.

To better assess the antiretroviral activity of IFN-α, a randomized, placebo-controlled trial in asymptomatic HIV-infected individuals with CD4 counts greater than 400 cells/mm^3 and positive cultures for HIV was carried out (Lane *et al.*, 1990). Of the 17 patients randomized to IFN-α treatment, 7 (41%) developed persistently negative cultures for HIV, while only 2 of 17 patients randomized to placebo became culture negative. During the treatment period, CD4 percentages remained stable or increased in patients receiving IFN-α and declined slightly in patients receiving placebo. Toxicity associated with IFN-α treatment was substantial as indicated by the fact that 35% of patients randomized to IFN-α withdrew from the study because of toxicity. The most prominent toxicities were flulike symptoms, neutropenia, and elevations of hepatic transaminases. The results of this trial suggest that IFN-α, although associated with considerable toxicity, may exhibit some antiretroviral activity in patients with greater than 400 CD4 cells/mm^3.

IFN-α and zidovudine inhibit HIV replication by different mechanisms and the combination of zidovudine and IFN-α can act synergistically to inhibit HIV replication *in vitro* (Johnson *et al.*, 1990). These considerations, combined with the limited ability of IFN-α to control HIV replication *in vivo*, led to several Phase I/II trials of combination therapy with IFN-α and zidovudine (Edlin *et al.*, 1992; Fischl *et al.*, 1991; Krown *et al.*, 1990; Kovacs *et al.*, 1989). These trials demonstrated that concurrent therapy with IFN-α and zidovudine is associated with a high frequency of certain toxicities (neutropenia, thrombocytopenia, and transaminase elevations) which are dose-limiting. The maximum tolerated dose of IFN-α in these studies was between 4 and 18 MU/day, depending on the zidovudine dose. At these doses of IFN-α, the antitumor effect seen with combination therapy was equivalent to that observed with higher-dose IFN-α monotherapy. The combination of zidovudine and IFN-α also appeared to have significant anti-HIV activity in patients with higher CD4 counts, but it is not clear whether this effect is superior to that of zidovudine alone (Berglund *et al.*, 1991; Lane *et al.*, 1988).

In summary, IFN-α is an important cytokine being evaluated for the therapy of HIV infection. Its well-documented efficacy in the treatment of HIV-associated KS has made it approved therapy for this condition. Both the antitumor and antiviral effects of IFN-α are critically dependent on the level of immune competence, and treatment with this agent is unlikely to be effective in HIV-infected individuals with CD4 counts less than 150 cells/mm^3.

IFN-α can be used in combination with zidovudine but significant toxicity (especially neutropenia) can result. Trials are currently under way comparing the long-term efficacy of IFN-α monotherapy, zidovudine monotherapy, and combination zidovudine plus IFN-α in the treatment of HIV-infected patients with CD4 counts greater than 500 cells/mm^3.

7.2. Interferon-β and -γ

IFN-β is similar to IFN-α in its immunomodulatory effect and *in vitro* activity against HIV (Hartshorn *et al.*, 1987). Results of a single trial in patients with HIV-associated KS suggest that the antiretroviral and anti-KS effects of IFN-β are similar or slightly less than those of IFN-α (Miles *et al.*, 1990).

The *in vitro* activity of IFN-γ against HIV is variable and depends on the tissue culture system that is used. Administration of IFN-γ to patients with HIV-associated KS has shown no apparent clinical benefit (Lane *et al.*, 1989). IFN-γ is a potent macrophage activator and may have a role as adjunctive therapy in the treatment of certain opportunistic infections.

8. SUMMARY

Immune-based therapies for HIV infection are only now being explored. Only a few cytokines have been examined in any depth and only IFN-α in KS has demonstrated clinical benefit. To date, most other therapies have been evaluated in small numbers of patients without a systematic examination of important treatment variables. The history of IL-2 development represents a useful lesson in the development of other immune therapies because of the unique schedule-dependence of its effects. Many patients were treated with diverse doses and regimens prior to the observation of any sustained immune effects. Immune therapies must be explored systematically, as a function both of regimen and of patient characteristics, to ensure that important biologic activities are not missed.

Immunotherapy represents a different approach to the therapy of HIV infection. Expectations must be based on clinical models with biologic similarities. The patterns and timing of immune constitution in infancy and immune reconstitution following bone marrow transplantation suggest that these are slow incremental processes even in the absence of concomitant viral infections. Evaluation of immune-based therapies should be commensurate with these processes.

Because much remains to be learned about both innate and adaptive immunity, it is probable that the initial approaches to immune-based therapies will be only moderately beneficial. The initial antiretroviral therapy of HIV infection utilized zidovudine monotherapy and, years later, it is clear that this monotherapy provided only marginal benefit to patients. However, the persistent pursuit of alternate drugs with different sites of action and a focused program of combination therapy has led recently to regimens that are far more active and that have sustained effects. This same approach must be applied to the field of immune-based therapies in HIV infection. An obvious example is the combination of IL-2 and IL-12. Preclinical data suggest that IL-2 and IL-12 may have synergistic activity in other disease models, but no laboratory or clinical trials of this combination have been performed in HIV infection.

Immune-based therapies are likely to be most effective in combination with antiretroviral therapy. The use of potent protease inhibitors can convert patients who are IL-2-unresponsive into patients with substantial CD4 increases in excess of those seen with protease inhibitors alone. It is likely that the biologic potential of cytokines will only be realized when there is maximum suppression of viral replication. Much remains to be understood in the relationship between viral replication and immune function in HIV infection and biologic compounds such as IL-2 provide a tool to better understand this relationship. This knowledge may provide important direction for new combined evaluations of antiretroviral and immunotherapy to improve and prolong life for the HIV-infected patient.

REFERENCES

Baron, S., Tyring, S. K., Fleischmann, W. R., Coppenhaver, D. H., Niesel, D. W., Klimpel, G. R., Stanton, G. J., and Hughes, T. K., 1991, The interferons. Mechanisms of action and clinical applications. *J. Am. Med. Assoc.* **266**:1375–1383.

Bell, S. J. D., Cooper, D. A., Kemp, B. E., Doherty, R. R., and Penny, R., 1992, Heterogeneous effects of exogenous IL-2 on HIV-specific cell-mediated immunity (CMI), *Clin. Exp. Immunol.* **90**:6–12.

Benedetto, N., Auriault, C., Darcy, F., Lando, D., Watier, H., and Capron, A., 1991, Effect of rIFN-γ and IL-2 treatments in mouse and nude rat infections with *Toxoplasma gondii*, *Eur. Cytokine Network* **2**:107–114.

Berglund, O., Engman, K., Ehrnst, A., Andersson, J., Lidman, K., Åkerlund, B., Sönnerborg, A., and Strannegård, Ö., 1991, combined treatment of symptomatic human immunodeficiency virus type 1 infection with native interferon-alpha and zidovudine, *J. Infect. Dis.* **163**:710–715.

Biron, C. A., and Gazzinelli, R. T., 1995, Effects of IL-12 on immune responses to microbial infections: A key mediator in regulating disease outcome, *Curr. Opin. Immunol.* **7**:485–496.

Bonavida, B., Katz, J., and Gottlieb, M., 1986, Mechanisms of defective NK cell activity in patients with acquired immunodeficiency syndrome (AIDS) and AIDS-related complex. I. Defective trigger on NK cells for NKCF production by target cells and partial restoration by IL-2, *J. Immunol.* **137**:1157–1163.

Borrow, P., Lewicki, H., Hahn, B. H., Shaw, G. M., and Oldstone, M. B., 1994, Virus-specific CD8+ cytotoxic T-lymphocyte activity associated with control of viremia in primary human immunodeficiency virus type 1 infection, *J. Virol.* **68**:6103–6110.

Chehimi, J., Starr, S. E., Frank, I., Rengaraju, M., Jackson, S. J., Llanes, C., Kobayashi, M., Perussia, B., Young, D., Nickbarg, E., Wolf, S. F., and Trinchieri, G., 1992, Natural killer (NK) cell stimulatory factor increases the cytotoxic activity of NK cells from both healthy donors and human immunodeficiency virus-infected patients, *J. Exp. Med.* **175**:789–796.

Chehimi, J., Starr, S. E., Frank, I., D'Andrea, A., Ma, X., MacGregor, R. R., Sennelier, J., and Trinchieri, G., 1994, Impaired interleukin 12 production in human immunodeficiency virus-infected patients, *J. Exp. Med.* **179**:1361–1366.

Chouaib, S., Chehimi, J., Bani, L., Genetet, N., Tursz, T., Gay, F., Trinchieri, G., and Mami-Chouaib, F., 1994, Interleukin 12 induces the differentiation of major histocompatibility complex class I-primed cytotoxic T-lymphocyte precursors into allospecific cytotoxic effectors, *Proc. Natl. Acad. Sci. USA* **91**:12659–12663.

Ciobanu, N., Welte, K., Kruger, G., Venuta, S., Gold, J., Feldman, S. P., Wang, C. Y., Koziner, B., Moore, M. A. S., Safai, B., and Mertelsmann, R., 1983, Defective T-cell response to PHA and mitogenic monoclonal antibodies in male homosexuals with acquired immunodeficiency syndrome and its *in vitro* correction by interleukin 2, *J. Clin. Immunol.* **3**:332–340.

Clark, S. J., Saag, M. S., Decker, W. D., Campbell-Hill, S., Roberson, J. L., Veldkamp P. J., Kappes, J. C., Hahn, B. H., and Shaw, G. M., 1991, High titers of cytopathic virus in plasma of patients with symptomatic primary HIV-1 infection, *N. Engl. J. Med.* **324**:954–960.

Clerici, M., and Shearer, G. M., 1993, A T_H1–T_H2 switch is a critical step in the etiology of HIV infection, *Immunol. Today* **14**:107–111.

Clerici, M., Lucey, D. R., Berzofsky, J. A., Pinto, L. A., Wynn, T. A., Blatt, S. P., Dolan, M. J., Hendrix, C. W., Wolf, S. F., and Shearer, G. M., 1993a, Restoration of HIV-specific cell-mediated immune responses by interleukin-12 in vitro, *Science* **262**:1721–1724.

Clerici, M., Hakim, F. T., Venzon, D. J., Blatt, S., Hendrix, C. W., Wynn, T. A., and Shearer, G. M., 1993b, Changes in interleukin-2 and interleukin-4 production in asymptomatic, human immunodeficiency virus seropositive individuals, *J. Clin. Invest.* **91**:759–765.

Cotran, R. S., Pober, J. S., Gimbrone, M. A., Jr., Springer, T. A., Wiebke, E. A., Gaspari, A. A., Rosenberg, S. A., and Lotze, M. T., 1987, Endothelial activation during interleukin 2 immunotherapy, *J. Immunol.* **139**:1883–1888.

Daar, E. S., Moudgil, T., Meyer, R. D., and Ho, D. D., 1991, Transient high levels of viremia in patients with primary human immunodeficiency virus type 1 infection, *N. Engl. J. Med.* **324**:961–964.

Davey, R. T., Jr., Wells, M. J., Piscitelli, S. C., Kovacs, J. A., Walker, R. E., Polis, M. A., Falloon, J., Masur, H., Metcalf, J. A., Fyfe, G. A., and Lane, H. C., 1994, Subcutaneous administration of interleukin-2 in HIV-1-infected individuals [abstract No. 278], *Infectious Disease Society of America, Orlando, Florida, October 7–9, 1994.*

Deresinski, S. C., Israelski, D. I., Frascino, R. J., Joseph, P., Galpin, J. E., Conant, M. A., Resnick, L., Fyfe, G. A., Alexander, J. M., Moody, D., and Moseley, A., 1995, Randomized multi center comparison of treatment of HIV infected patients: Activated CD8+ cells plus rIL-2 plus antiretroviral (AR) therapy vs rIL2 plus AR therapy vs AR therapy alone [abstract No. 206], *Abstracts of the 2nd National Conference on Human Retroviruses.*

deWit, R., Schattenkerk, J. K. M. E., Boucher, C. A. B., Bakker, P. J. M., Veenhof, K. H. N., and Danner, S. A., 1988, Clinical and virological effects of high-dose recombinant interferon-alpha in disseminated AIDS-related Kaposi's sarcoma, *Lancet* **2**:1214–1217.

Edlin, B. R., Weinstein, R. A., Whaling, S. M., Ou, C.-Y., Connolly, P. J., Moore, J. L., and Bitran, J. D., 1992, Zidovudine–interferon-alpha combination therapy in patients with advanced human immunodeficiency virus type 1 infection: Biphasic response of p24 antigen and quantitative polymerase chain reaction, *J. Infect. Dis.* **165**:793–798.

Ernst, M., Kern, P., Flad, H.-D., and Ulmer, A. J., 1986, Effects of systemic in vivo interleukin-2 (IL-2) reconstitution in patients with acquired immune deficiency syndrome (AIDS) and AIDS-related complex (ARC) on phenotypes and functions of peripheral blood mononuclear cells (PBMC), *J. Clin. Immunol.* **6**: 170–181.

Falloon, J., Owen, C., Kovacs, J., Leavitt, R., Metcalf, J., and Lane, H. C., 1995, MK-639 (Merck HIV Protease

Inhibitor) with interleukin-2 (IL2) in HIV [abstract No. 1176], *ICAAC Abstracts*: 35th Interscience Conference on Antimicrobial Agents and Chemotherapy, San Francisco.

Fei, P. C., Solmone, M., Viora, M., Vanacore, P., Pugliese, O., Giglio, A., Caprilli, F., and Ameglio, F., 1994, Apoptosis in HIV infection: Protective role of IL-2, *J. Biol. Regul. Homeostat. Agents* **8**:60–64.

Fischl, M. A., Uttamchandani, R. B., Resnick, L., Agarwal, R., Fletcher, M. A., Patrone-Reese, J., Dearmas, L., Chickekel, J., McCann, M., and Myers, M., 1991, A phase I study of recombinant human interferon-alpha 2a or human lymphoblastoid interferon-alpha$_{nl}$ and concomitant zidovudine in patients with AIDS-related Kaposi's sarcoma, *J. Acq. Immune Defic. Syndr.* **4**:1–10.

Francis, M. L., Meltzer, M. S., and Gendelman, H. E., 1992, Interferons in the persistence, pathogenesis, and treatment of HIV infection, *AIDS Res. Hum. Retrovir.* **8**:199–207.

Gazzinelli, R. T., Giese, N. A., and Morse, H. C., III, 1994, In vivo treatment with interleukin 12 protects mice from immune abnormalities observed during murine acquired immunodeficiency syndrome (MAIDS), *J. Exp. Med.* **180**:2199–2208.

Gelmann, E. P., Preble, O. T., Steis, R., Lane, H. C., Rook, A. H., Wesley, M., Jacob, J., Fauci, A., Masur, H., and Longo, D., 1985, Human lymphoblastoid interferon treatment of Kaposi's sarcoma in the acquired immune deficiency syndrome. Clinical response and prognostic parameters, *Am. J. Med.* **78**:737–741.

Graziosi, C., Pantaleo, G., Gantt, K. R., Forten, J.-P., Demarest, J. F., Cohen, O. J., Sekaly, R. P., and Fauci, A. S., 1994, Lack of evidence for the dichotomy of T_h1 and T_h2 predominance in HIV-infected individuals, *Science* **265**:248–252.

Groopman, J. E., Gottlieb, M. S., Goodman, J., Mitsuyasu, R. T., Conant, M. A., Prince, H., Fahey, J. L., Derezin, M., Weinstein, W. M., Casavante, C., Rothman, J., Rudnick, S. A., and Volberding, P. A., 1984, Recombinant alpha-2 interferon therapy for Kaposi's sarcoma associated with the acquired immunodeficiency syndrome, *Ann. Intern. Med.* **100**:671–676.

Gupta, S., Gillis, S., Thornton, M., and Goldberg, M., 1984, Autologous mixed lymphocyte reaction in man. XIV. Deficiency of the autologous mixed lymphocyte reaction in acquired immune deficiency syndrome (AIDS) and AIDS-related complex (ARC): In vitro effect of purified interleukin-1 and interleukin-2, *Clin. Exp. Immunol.* **58**:395–401.

Hartshorn, K., Neumeyer, D., Vogt, M., Schooley, R. T., and Hirsch, M. S., 1987, Activity of interferons alpha, beta, and gamma against human immunodeficiency virus replication in vitro, *AIDS Res. Hum. Retrovir.* **3**:125–133.

Ho, D. D., Hartshorn, K. L., Rota, T. R., Andrews, C. A., Kaplan, J. C., Schooley, R. T., and Hirsch, M. S., 1985, Recombinant human interferon alfa-A suppresses HTLV-III replication in vitro, *Lancet* **1**:602–604.

Ho, D. D., Neumann, A. U., Perelson, A. S., Chen, W., Leonard, J. M., and Markowitz, M., 1995, Rapid turnover of plasma virions and CD4 lymphocytes in HIV-1 infection, *Nature* **373**:123–126.

Jeevan, A., and Asherson, G. L., 1988, Recombinant interleukin-2 limits the replication of Mycobacterium lepraemurium and Mycobacterium bovis BCG in mice, *Lymphokine Res.* **7**:129–140.

Johnson, V. A., Barlow, M. A., Merrill, D. P., Chou, T.-C., and Hirsch, M. S., 1990, Three-drug synergistic inhibition of HIV-1 replication in vitro by zidovudine, recombinant soluble CD4, and recombinant interferon-alpha, *J. Infect. Dis.* **161**:1059–1067.

Kern, P., Toy, J., and Dietrich, M., 1985, Preliminary clinical observations with recombinant interleukin-2 in patients with AIDS or LAS, *Blut* **50**:1–6.

Koenig, S., Conley, A. J., Brewah, Y. A., Jones, G. M., Leath, S., Boots, L. J., Davey, V., Pantaleo, G., Demarest, J. F., Carter, C., Wannebo, C., Yannelli, J. R., Rosenberg, S. A., and Lane, H. C., 1995, Transfer of HIV-1-specific cytotoxic T lymphocytes to an AIDS patient leads to selection for mutant HIV variants and subsequent disease progression, *Nature Med.* **1**:330–336.

Kovacs, J. A., Deyton, L., Davey, R., Falloon, J., Zunick, K., Lee, D., Metcalf, J. A., Bigley, J. W., Sawyer, L. A., Zoon, K. C., Masur, H., Fauci, A. S., and Lane, H. C., 1989, Combined zidovudine and interferonalpha therapy in patients with Kaposi's sarcoma and the acquired immunodeficiency syndrome (AIDS), *Ann. Intern. Med.* **111**:280–287.

Kovacs, J. A., Baseler, M., Dewar, R. J., Vogel, S., Davey, R. T., Falloon, J., Polis, M. A., Walker, R. E., Stevens, R., Salzman, N. P., Metcalf, J. A., Masur, H., and Lane, H. C., 1995a, Increases in CD4 T lymphocytes with intermittent courses of interleukin-2 in patients with human immunodeficiency virus infection. A preliminary study, *N. Engl. J. Med.* **332**:567–575.

Kovacs, J. A., Vogel, S., Albert, J., Falloon, J., Davey, R., Walker, R., Polis, M., Metcalf, J., Baseler, M., Foulkes, M., Fyfe, G., Masur, H., and Lane, H. C., 1995b, A randomized trial of intermittent interleukin-2 therapy in HIV-infected patients with CD4 counts >200 cells/mm^3, Abstract presented at the 35th Interscience Conference on Antimicrobial Agents and Chemotherapy, August.

Krown, S. E., Gold, J. W. M., Niedzwiecki, D., Bundow, D., Flomenberg, N., Gansbacher, B., and Brew, B. J., 1990, Interferon-alpha with zidovudine: Safety, tolerance, and clinical and virologic effects in patients with Kaposi sarcoma associated with the acquired immunodeficiency syndrome (AIDS), *Ann. Intern. Med.* **112**:812–821.

Lane, H. C., Siegel, J. P., Rook, A. H., Masur, H., Gelmann, E. P., Quinnan, G. V., and Fauci, A. S., 1984, Use of interleukin-2 in patients with acquired immunodeficiency syndrome, *J. Biol. Response Modif.* **3**:512–516.

Lane, H. C., Kovacs, J. A., Feinberg, J., Herpin, B., Davey, V., Walker, R., Deyton, L., Metcalf, J. A., Baseler, M., Salzman, N., Manischewitz, J., Quinnan, G., Masur, H., and Fauci, A. S., 1988, Anti-retroviral effects of interferon-alpha in AIDS-associated Karposi's sarcoma, *Lancet* **2**:1218–1222.

Lane, H. C., Davey, R. T., Sherwin, S. A., Masur, H., Rook, A. H., Manischewitz, J. F., Quinnan, G. V., Smith, P. D., Easter, M. E., and Fauci, A. S., 1989, Phase I trial of recombinant interferon-gamma in patients with Kaposi's sarcoma and the acquired immunodeficiency syndrome (AIDS), *J. Clin. Immunol.* **9**:351–361.

Lane, H. C., Davey, V., Kovacs, J. A., Feinberg, J., Metcalf, J. A., Herpin, B., Walker, R., Deyton, L., Davey, R. T., Falloon, J., Polis, M. A., Salzman, N. P., Baseler, M., Masur, H., and Fauci, A. S., 1990, Interferon-alpha in patients with asymptomatic human immunodeficiency virus (HIV) infection. A randomized, placebo-controlled trial, *Ann. Intern. Med.* **112**:805–811.

Lotze, M. T., Robb, R. J., Sharrow, S. O., Frana, L. W., and Rosenberg, S. A., 1984, Systemic administration of interleukin-2 in humans, *J. Biol. Response Modif.* **3**:475–482.

McElrath, M. J., Kaplan, G., Burkhardt, R. A., and Cohn, Z. A., 1990, Cutaneous response to recombinant interleukin 2 in human immunodeficiency virus 1-seropositive individuals, *Proc. Natl. Acad. Sci. USA* **87**: 5783–5787.

Mackall, C. L., Fleisher, T. A., Brown, M. R., Andrich, M. P., Chen, C. C., Feuerstein, I. M., Horowitz, M. E., Magrath, I. T., Shad, A. T., Steinberg, S. M., Wexler, L. H., and Gress, R. E., 1995, Age, thymopoiesis, and CD4+ T-lymphocyte regeneration after intensive chemotherapy, *N. Engl. J. Med.* **332**:143–149.

McMahon, D. K., Armstrong, J. A., Huang, X. L., Rinaldo, C. R., Jr., Gupta, P., Whiteside, T. L., Pazin, G. J., Tripli, C., and Ho, M., 1994, A phase I study of subcutaneous recombinant interleukin-2 in patients with advanced HIV disease while on zidovudine, *AIDS* **8**:59–66.

Maggi, E., Mazzetti, M., Ravina, A., Annunziato, F., De Carli, M., Piccinni, M. P., Manetti, R., Carbonari, M., Pesce, A. M., Del Prete, G., and Romagnani, S., 1994, Ability of HIV to promote a T_H1 to T_H0 shift and to replicate preferentially in T_H2 and T_H0 cells, *Science* **265**:244–248.

Mazza, P., Bocchia, M., Tumietto, F., Costigliola, P., Coronado, O., Bandini, G., Conte, R., Ricchi, E., Vianelli, N., Raise, E., Fondacaro, A., Re, M. D., Vignoli, M., Chiodo, F., and Tura, S., 1992, Recombinant interleukin-2 (rIL-2) in acquired immune deficiency syndrome (AIDS): Preliminary report in patients with lymphoma associated with HIV infection, *Eur. J. Haematol.* **49**:1–6.

Mertelsmann, R., Welte, K., Sternberg, C., O'Reilly, R., Moore, M. A. S., Clarkson, B. D., and Oettgen, H. F., 1984, Treatment of immunodeficiency with interleukin-2: Initial exploration, *J. Biol. Response Modif.* **4**:483–490.

Miles, S. A., Wang, H. J., Cortes, E., Carden, J., Marcus, S., and Mitsuyasu, R. T., 1990, Beta-interferon therapy in patients with poor-prognosis Kaposi sarcoma related to the acquired immunodeficiency syndrome (AIDS). A phase II trial with preliminary evidence of antiviral activity and low incidence of opportunistic infections, *Ann. Intern. Med.* **112**:582–589.

Morgan, D. A., Ruscetti, F. W., and Gallo, R., 1976, Selective in vitro growth of T lymphocytes from normal bone marrows, *Science* **193**:1007–1008.

Murray, H. W., Welte, K., Jacobs, J. L., Rubin, B. Y., Mertelsmann, R., and Roberts, R. B., 1985, Production of and in vitro response to interleukin 2 in the acquired immunodeficiency syndrome, *J. Clin. Invest.* **76**:1959–1964.

Murray, H. W., DePamphilis, J., Schooley, R. T., and Hirsch, M. S., 1988, Circulating interferon gamma in AIDS patients treated with interleukin-2, *N. Engl. J. Med.* **318**:1538–1539.

O'Brien, W. A., Grovit-Ferbas, K., Namazi, A., Ovcak-Derzic, S., Wang, H.-J., Park, J., Yeramian, C., Mao, S.-H., and Zack, J. A., 1995, Human immunodeficiency virus-type 1 replication can be increased in peripheral blood of seropositive patients after influenza vaccination, *Blood* **86**:1082–1089.

Pantaleo, G., Demarest, J. F., Soudeyns, H., Graziosi, C., Denis, F., Adelsberger, J. W., Borrow, P., Saag, M. S., Shaw, G. M., Sekaly, R. P., and Fauci, A. S., 1994, Major expansion of CD8+ T cells with a predominant Vβ usage during the primary immune response to HIV, *Nature* **370**:463–467.

Pitha, P. M., Wivel, N. A., Fernie, B. F., and Harper, H. P., 1979, Effect of interferon and murine leukaemia virus infection. IV. Formation of non-infectious virus in chronically infected cells, *J. Gen. Virol.* **42**:467–480.

Poli, G., Orenstein, J. M., Kinter, A., Folks, T. M., and Fauci, A. S., 1989, Interferon-alpha but not AZT suppresses HIV expression in chronically infected cell lines, *Science* **244**:575–577.

Ramachandran, R. V., Katzenstein, D., and Merigan, T. C., 1994, Long-term effects of interleukin-2 on CD4 cell counts in human immunodeficiency virus-infected patients, *J. Infect. Dis.* **170**:1044–1046.

Real, F. X., Oettgen, H. F., and Krown, S. E., 1986, Kaposi's sarcoma and the acquired immunodeficiency syndrome: Treatment with high and low doses of recombinant leukocyte A interferon, *J. Clin. Oncol.* **4**: 544–551.

Reddehause, M. J., Mutter, W., and Koszinowski, U. H., 1987, In vivo application of recombinant interleukin 2 in the immunotherapy of established cytomegalovirus infection, *J. Exp. Med.* **165**:650–656.

Rook, A. H., Masur, H., Lane, H. C., Frederick, W., Kasahara, T., Macher, A. M., Djeu, J. Y., Manischewitz, J. F., Jackson, L., Fauci, A. S., and Quinnan, G. V., Jr., 1983, Interleukin-2 enhances the depressed natural killer and cytomegalovirus-specific cytotoxic activities of lymphocytes from patients with the acquired immune deficiency syndrome, *J. Clin. Invest.* **72**:398–403.

Rosenthal, N. S., Hank, J. A., Kohler, P. C., Minkoff, D. Z., Moore, K. H., Bechhofer, R., Hong, R., Storer, B., and Sondel, P. M., 1988, The in vitro function of lymphocytes from 25 cancer patients receiving four to seven consecutive days of recombinant IL-2, *J. Biol. Response Modif.* **7**:123–139.

Schnittman, S. M., Vogel, S., Baseler, M., Lane, H. C., and Davey, R. T., Jr., 1994, A phase I study of interferon-α2b in combination with interleukin-2 in patients with human immunodeficiency virus infection, *J. Infect. Dis.* **169**:981–989.

Schwartz, D. H., Skowron, G., and Merigan, T. C., 1991, Safety and effects of interleukin-2 plus zidovudine in asymptomatic individuals infected with human immunodeficiency virus, *J. Acq. Immune Defic. Syndr.* **4**: 11–23.

Sheridan, J. F., Aurelian, L., Donnenberg, A. D., and Quinn, T. C., 1984, Cell-mediated immunity to cytomegalovirus (CMV) and herpes simplex virus (HSV) antigens in the acquired immune deficiency syndrome: Interleukin-1 and interleukin-2 modify *in vitro* responses, *J. Clin. Immunol.* **4**:304.

Storek, J., Witherspoon, R. P., and Storb, R., 1995, T cell reconstitution after bone marrow transplantation into adult patients does not resemble T cell development in early life, *Bone Marrow Transplant.* **16**:413–425.

Teppler, H., Kaplan, G., Smith, K. A., Montana, A. L., Meyn, P., and Cohn, Z. A., 1993a, Prolonged immunostimulatory effect of low-dose polyethylene glycol interleukin 2 in patients with human immunodeficiency virus type 1 infection, *J. Exp. Med.* **177**:483–492.

Teppler, H., Kaplan, G., Smith, K., Cameron, P., Montana, A., Meyn, P., and Cohn, Z., 1993b, Efficacy of low doses of the polyethylene glycol derivative of interleukin-2 in modulating the immune response of patients with human immunodeficiency virus type 1 infection, *J. Infect. Dis.* **167**:291–298.

Toosi, Z., Kleinhenz, M. E., and Ellner, J. J., 1986, Defective interleukin 2 production and responsiveness in human pulmonary tuberculosis, *J. Exp. Med.* **163**:1162–1172.

Volberding, P. A., and Mitsuyasu, R., 1985, Recombinant interferon-alpha in the treatment of acquired immune deficiency syndrome related Kaposi's sarcoma, *Semin. Oncol.* **12**:2–6.

Volberding, P., Moody, D. J., Beardslee, D., Bradley, E. C., and Wofsy, C. B., 1987, Therapy of acquired immune deficiency syndrome with recombinant interleukin-2, *AIDS Res. Hum. Retrovir.* **3**:115–124.

Waites, L., Fyfe, G., Senechek, D., and Vollmer, C., 1992, Polyethylene glycol modified interleukin-2 (PEG IL-2) therapy in HIV seropositive individuals [abstract No. PuB 7580], *Program and Abstracts: VIII International Conference on AIDS*, Amsterdam, Congrex Holland BV.

Walker, R. E., Carter, C. S., Muul, L., Natarajan, V., Herpin, B. R., Leitman, S. F., Klein, H. G., Falloon, J., Davey, R. T., Kovacs, J. A., Polis, M. A., Masur, H., Blaese, R. M., and Lane, H. C., 1995, Survival and distribution of genetically modified cells in identical twins discordant for HIV-1 infection, *AIDS Res. Hum. Retrovir.* **11(Suppl. 1)**:S166.

Wei, X., Ghosh, S. K., Taylor, M. E., Johnson, V. A., Emini, E. A., Deutsch, P., Lifson, J. D., Bonhoeffer, S., Nowak, M. A., Hahn, B. H., Saag, M. S., and Shaw, G. M., 1995, Viral dynamics in human immunodeficiency virus type 1 infection, *Nature* **373**:117–122.

Wood, R., Montoya, J. G., Kundu, S. K., Schwartz, D. H., and Merigan, T. C., 1993, Safety and efficacy of polyethylene glycol-modified interleukin-2 and zidovudine in human immunodeficiency virus type 1 infection: A phase I/II study, *J. Infect. Dis.* **167**:519–525.

Zubiaga, A. M., Munoz, E., and Huber, B. T., 1992, IL-4 and IL-2 selectively rescue Th cell subsets from glucocorticoid-induced apoptosis, *J. Immunol.* **149**:107–112.

CHAPTER 26

THYMIC HORMONES IN THE TREATMENT OF AIDS AND OTHER INFECTIOUS DISEASES

ALLAN L. GOLDSTEIN, PREM S. SARIN,
and ENRICO GARACI

1. INTRODUCTION

The role of the thymus in the modulation of T-cell function and in the release of various hormonelike factors (thymic hormones) has been the subject of major studies in a number of laboratories (Bach, 1983; Goldstein, 1993; Goldstein *et al.*, 1982; Goldstein and White, 1971; Miller, 1961; Oates and Goldstein, 1991; Schulof *et al.*, 1986, 1988; Stutman, 1983; Trainin *et al.*, 1979). It is well known that the thymus undergoes a gradual age-dependent involution during which the thymic parenchymal tissue is infiltrated with fat and adipose cells (Hammar, 1971). The thymus reaches its maximum size just before puberty and then gradually decreases in size and weight. The loss of hormone-producing epithelial cells begins early in life and by the second decade in humans, there is a substantial decrease in the number of hormone-containing medullary thymic epithelial cells. The number of hormone-containing thymic cortical epithelial cells also gradually decreases, although these cells can still be observed in the fifth decade of life (Hirokawa *et al.*, 1982). The age-associated decrease in thymic hormone-like activity correlates with the decrease in hormone-containing thymic epithelial cells in both humans (Bach and Dardenne, 1972; Iwata *et al.*, 1981; Lewis *et al.*, 1978; Twomey *et al.*, 1979; Wara and Amman, 1976) and animals (Dardenne *et al.*, 1974; Hammar, 1971; Savino *et al.*, 1983).

Several thymic hormones (TF), which are members of a large family of immune modulators now better known as biological response modifiers (BRMs), have been identified and chemically characterized and still others await further characterization. The well-

---

ALLAN L. GOLDSTEIN and PREM S. SARIN • Department of Biochemistry and Molecular Biology, The George Washington University Medical Center, Washington, D.C. 20037. ENRICO GARACI • Department of Experimental Medicine and Biochemical Sciences, University of Rome "Tor Vergata," 00173 Rome, Italy.
Immunology of HIV Infection, edited by Sudhir Gupta. Plenum Press, New York, 1996.

studied thymic preparations include thymosin fraction 5 (TF5); thymosin alpha 1 (Tα_1); thymosin beta 4 (Tβ_4); thymostimulin (TS); thymulin (FTS-Zn); thymopoietin (TP); thymopentin, a synthetic pentapeptide of thymopoietin (TP-5); thymic humoral factor (THF-γ2); and thymic factor X (TFX) (Table I). The primary structure of Tα_1, one of the most thoroughly studied of the TF, is shown in Fig. 1. The proposed role of Tα, and several other TF on T-cell maturation is illustrated in Fig. 2. Despite the difficulty in assigning a unique biological activity to each of these factors in well-defined biological assays, a number of them have been employed in the treatment of patients with different diseases including cancer, immunodeficiency disorders, and AIDS.

2. BACKGROUND STUDIES WITH THYMIC HORMONES (TF) IN INFECTIOUS DISEASES

The potential importance of TF in preventing infections in immunocompromised patients was first suggested by studies in immunosuppressed animals. Early studies demonstrated an increased survival rate of immunosuppressed mice infected with BCG (Collins and Morrison, 1979), *Candida*, or *Cryptococcus* when these animals were treated with TF5 and Tα_1. The administration of TF5 or Tα_1 also stimulated an increase in the production of interferon (IFN) in mice infected with Newcastle disease virus (Huang *et al.*, 1981). In other studies, injection of TF5 or Tα_1 in mice increased resistance to infection with *Candida albicans* (Bistoni *et al.*, 1982; Salvin and Neta, 1983). The increased resistance to infection with an infectious agent after administration of TF5 has been attributed to an increase in the release of MIF and IFN-γ (Neta and Salvin, 1983). Injection of TF5 and Tα_1 has been shown to protect 5-fluorouracil (5-FU)- or morphine-immunosuppressed mice against opportunistic infections with *C. albicans*, *Listeria monocytogenes*, *Pseudomonas aeruginosa*, and *Serratia marcescens* (Ishitsuka *et al.*, 1983; Di Francesco *et al.*, 1994). The efficacy of Tα_1 administered in combination with the antiviral drug Amantadine and α/β IFN was also demonstrated in mice infected with influenza A PR8 virus. This new chemoimmunotherapy protocol has been found to significantly increase the long term survival, to reduce viral titer in the lungs, and to restore the immunological parameters tested (natural killer cell activity, cytotoxic T-lymphocyte responses, CD4+/CD8+ lymphocyte subset) (D'Agostini *et al.*, 1996).

Clinical studies in humans using various TF preparations (THF-γ2, TFX, TP-1) have

TABLE I. Characteristics of Thymic Hormones (TF)

TF	Properties	Molecular weight(s)
Thymosin fracton 5 (TF5)	Heat-stable, mixture of 40 peptides	1000–15000
Thymosin α_1 (Tα_1)	Acetylated N-terminus, 28 amino acids, pI 4.2	3108
Thymosin β_4 (Tβ_4)	Acetylated N-terminus, 43 amino acids, pI 5.1	4982
Thymopoietin (TP)	49 amino acids	5562
Thymopentin (TP5)	Pentapeptide of TP (aa 32–36)	
Thymic humoral factor (THF-γ2)	Octapeptide	918
Thymulin (FTS-Zn)	Nonapeptide, heat-labile, pI 7.3	847
Thymostimulin (TP-1)	Mixture of peptides	
Thymic factor X (TFX)	Mixture of peptides	Active peptide 4200

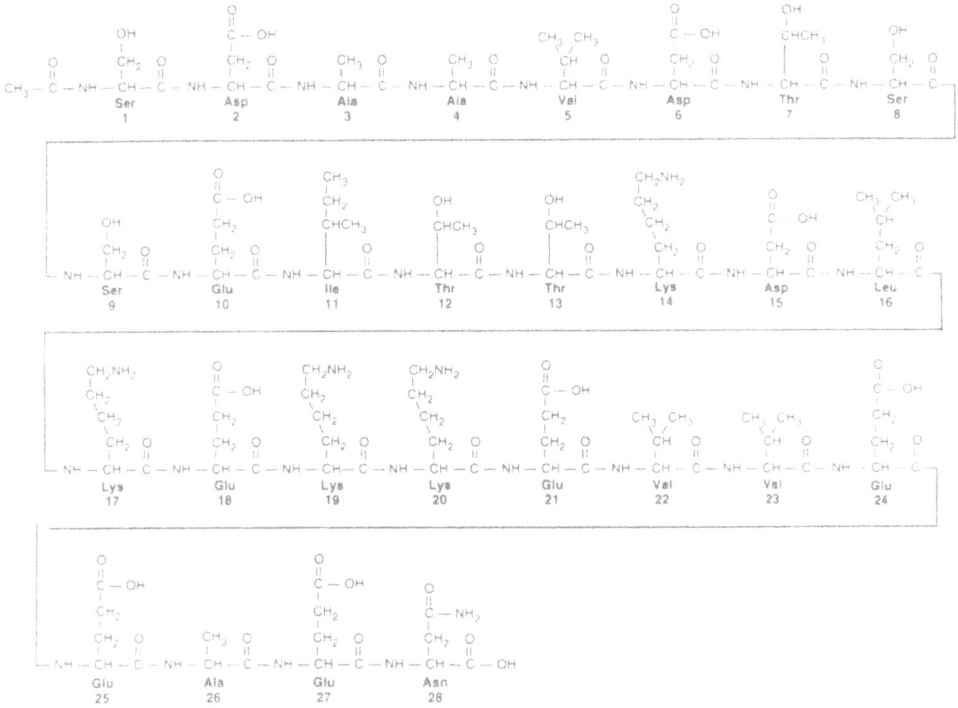

FIGURE 1. Structure of thymosin α_1.

shown that the administration of thymic factors can shorten the course of viral infections (e.g., herpes zoster, herpes simplex, adenovirus, hepatitis, and cytomegalovirus) and increase the restoration of T-cell immunity in these patients (Aiuti *et al.*, 1984; Businco and Rezza, 1981; DeMartino *et al.*, 1984; Schulof and Goldstein, 1983; Trainin *et al.*, 1981). In placebo-controlled studies, TP-1 decreased the number or recurrences of herpes simplex labialis infections in immunosuppressed patients (Aiuti *et al.*, 1984) and decreased the incidence of respiratory infections in children (DeMartino *et al.*, 1984). These studies suggest that TF may be useful in preventing or attenuating infections in immunocompromised hosts.

3. TF IN THE TREATMENT OF IMMUNODEFICIENCY DISEASES

TF have been utilized in clinical trials in patients with primary and secondary immunodeficiencies.

3.1. Primary Immunodeficiencies

A number of syndromes related to congenital defects of the immune system are included in this category. These may include T-cell, B-cell or both lymphocyte populations. An *in vitro* increase in the percentage and numbers of E-rosette-forming cells after

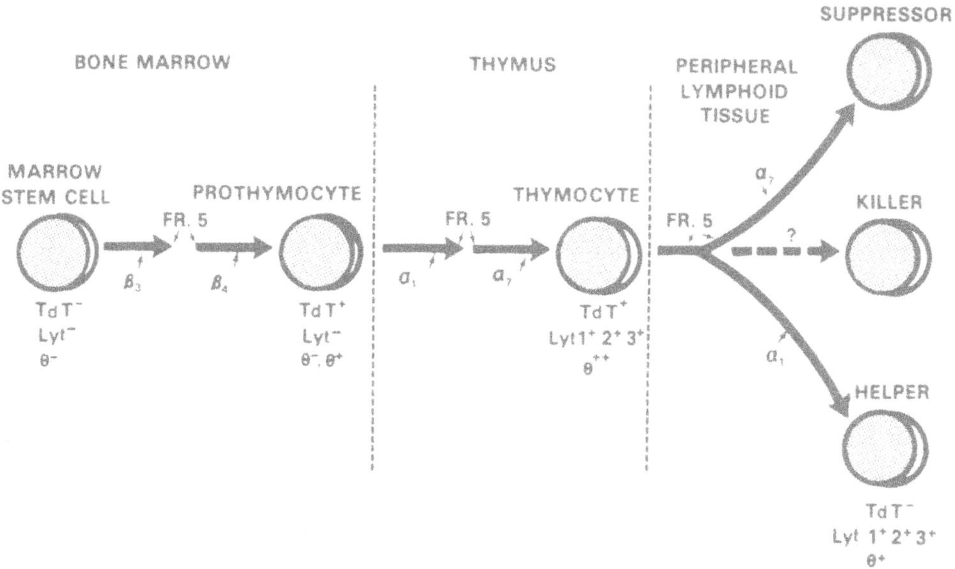

FIGURE 2. Proposed role of thymosin peptides in T-cell maturation.

incubation with thymic factors (TF5, THF-γ2, TP, TP-5, and thymulin) has been reported (Schulof and Goldstein, 1983). Several of the factors (TF5, TP-1, TP-5, thymulin, THF-γ2, and TFX) have been studied in clinical trials in children with primary immunodeficiency diseases (Aiuti and Businco, 1983; Bach and Dardenne, 1984; Davies and Levinsky, 1984; Goldstein, 1993, 1994; Schulof and Goldstein, 1983; Skotnicki *et al.*, 1984; Wara *et al.*, 1984).

By far the best results have been achieved in children with DiGeorge syndrome (Wara *et al.*, 1984). Improvement in T-cell functions of these patients have been reported with TF5 (Wara *et al.*, 1984), TP-1 and TP-5 (Aiuti and Businco, 1983), and thymulin (Bach and Dardenne, 1984). Clinical trials in patients with ataxia telangiectasia (AT) using thymulin (Wara *et al.*, 1984) or THF-γ2 (Aiuti and Businco, 1983) and in patients with Wiskott–Aldrich syndrome treated with TF5 (Wara *et al.*, 1984) have shown clinical improvement. These studies indicate that thymic factors are useful in reconstituting cellular immune responses and improving clinical status in these patients.

3.2. Secondary Immunodeficiencies

Clinical conditions including severe burns, viral infections, and chronic renal failure generally result in secondary immunodeficiencies. Thymic factors appear to improve immune status in animals affected by several of these conditions. Patients with severe burns, viral infections, and uremia have been reported to show improvement in their immune status (Schulof and Goldstein, 1983). In patients with chronic renal failure, reconstitution of $CD4^+$ cells to their normal levels has been reported without any change in the percentage of $CD8^+$ T cells (Abiko and Sekino, 1984).

4. AIDS

$T\alpha_1$ and TF5

A number of studies have been carried out to determine the usefulness of thymic factors in the treatment of AIDS. The first such studies in the treatment of AIDS were carried out by Schulof *et al.* (1986) using $T\alpha_1$ and TF5 in four consecutive studies carried out on 42 HIV-1-infected patients. $T\alpha_1$ (600 μg) or TF5 (30, 60, or 120 mg) was administered daily for 10 weeks followed by twice weekly injections for 4 weeks. $T\alpha_1$ was well tolerated by the patients and no local systemic or laboratory toxicities were observed. Some of the patients receiving TF5, however, had mild erythema and skin reactions. The clinical trial, although demonstrating imunomodulation, did not change viremia and was not of sufficient size and duration to establish the efficacy of single-agent treatment of these patients. The conclusion from this study was that TF would probably not be effective in treating AIDS unless given in conjunction with an antiviral agent. A similar conclusion was reported in the case of experimental infection with influenza virus in mice (D'Agostini *et al.*, 1996).

5. COMBINATION THERAPIES WITH TF IN THE TREATMENT OF AIDS

5.1. $T\alpha_1$

In a pilot study Garaci *et al.* (1993, 1994) have reported on the effect of combination of $T\alpha_1$ with natural lymphoblastoid IFN-α and AZT on HIV-infected asymptomatic patients with CD4 counts between 200 and 500 mm/c. Patients were treated with: AZT alone, AZT plus IFN-α, and AZT plus IFN-α and $T\alpha_1$. The doses for three drugs were AZT, 500 mg/day; IFN-α, 2 MU s.c. twice weekly; and $T\alpha_1$, 1 mg s.c. twice weekly. After 12 months of therapy, the combination of $T\alpha_1$ with IFN-α and AZT was well tolerated, and resulted in a substantial increase in the number and function of $CD4^+$ T cells compared with groups receiving AZT alone or AZT plus IFN-α. The group receiving combination therapy with $T\alpha_1$, IFN, and AZT had a significantly lower level of virus load as measured by PCR analysis after 12-month treatment. Based on these promising results, a large multicenter randomized open study of 100 HIV-infected asymptomatic patients was initiated by the Italian researchers. Accrual was completed in January, 1996. Preliminary analysis of this ongoing study is quite promising and confirms the advantage of combination therapy with $T\alpha_1$, AZT, and IFN-α in terms of CD4 counts, p24 antigenemia, and HIV viremia (E. Garaci, personal communication).

5.2. Thymostimulin

The usefulness of treating HIV-infected patients with another thymic hormone, thymostimulin (TP-1), has been reported by Carco and Guazzotti (1993). They selected 70 HIV-infected patients with lymphadenopathy for treatment with TP-1. The treatment protocol included administration of TP-1 at a dose of 50 mg/day (i.m.) for 30 days followed by 50 mg three times a week for the next 3 months. This treatment schedule was followed by administration of TP-1 at a dose of 50 mg once a week for the next 2 months. Sixty patients completed the study and were observed for a period of 12 months.

Of the treated patients, 66.7% showed an improvement in skin reaction to Multitest

(CMI) antigens, whereas 30% of the patients showed no improvement. An increase in the total lymphocyte counts was observed at 6 months and remained stable at 9- and 12-month observation periods. A significant increase in CD4 lymphocytes was observed at 6 months along with CD4/CD8 ratio close to normal which remained stable up to the 12-month observation point. None of the treated patients developed any opportunistic infections during the course of treatment. These studies point to the potential of TP-1 either alone or in combination with AZT or other antiviral agents in the treatment of AIDS.

In another study, Frega *et al.* (1994) used a combination of TP-1 and IFN-β in the treatment of HIV-infected women with human papilloma virus vulvoperineal infection. Nineteen women were enrolled in this study (age 19-32 years). All of the women were smokers and 58% were intravenous drug users with a mean period of drug addiction of 5 years. None of the patients were on AZT treatment. All patients received IFN-β (3 MU/day for 7 days, i.m.) and subsequently on alternate days for 2 weeks along with TP-1 (70 mg, i.m.) administered on alternate days for a period of 30 days. Of the treated patients, 37% showed a complete recovery at the end of follow-up, 26% showed a partial response, and 37% showed no response to therapy. These studies indicate the potential of TP-1 immunotherapy in the treatment of HIV-infected patients carrying other viral infections.

5.3. Thymopentin

In an early double-blind placebo-controlled study, TP-5 was evaluated in 91 HIV-infected patients (52 asymptomatic and 39 symptomatic) who had not developed AIDS (Conant *et al.*, 1992). Patients were stratified into asymptomatic and symptomatic groups and given TP-5 (50 mg three times a week) or placebo for 24 or 52 weeks.

TP-5-treated asymptomatic patients had more $CD4^+$ cells with a shorter median time to a 20% increase in percentage of $CD4^+$ cells in both 24- and 52-week observation periods. No differences in the number of $CD4^+$ cells or progression to AIDS were observed in symptomatic patients receiving TP-5 or the placebo group. None of the treated asymptomatic patients progressed to AIDS during this period. Based on these results, it was suggested that TP-5 could slow or arrest the immune decline and disease progression in HIV-infected asymptomatic patients by maintaining the level of $CD4^+$ cells.

More recently, a safety and efficacy study of TP-5 in AZT-treated asymptomatic HIV-infected subjects with 200–500 $CD4^+$ cells was reported by G. Goldstein *et al.* (1995). Subjects ($N = 352$) were prestratified by prior AZT use into group 1 (235 subjects > 6 months' AZT at entry) and group 2 (117 subjects $<$ months' AZT at entry). TP-5 was administered in addition to AZT at a dose of 50 mg three times a week (s.c.) and the patients were evaluated for 48 weeks. In group 1 (mean 16 months' AZT at entry), 2 AIDS or death events occurred in the TP-5-treated group and 10 in the placebo group. There were 3 AIDS-related complex (ARC), AIDS, or death events in the TP-5-treated group and 18 in the placebo group. In group 2 (mean 3 months' AZT at entry), 4 ARC, AIDS, or death events occurred in the TP-5 group and 2 in the placebo group. The treatment groups did not show significant differences in CD4 counts or p24 antigen levels. TP-5 was well tolerated by the treated patients. These results indicate that TP-5 treatment can reduce the progression of the disease in AZT-treated patients whereas patients with low prior exposure to AZT did not significantly differ in their disease progression outcome. Further studies with a combination of AZT and TP-5 may shed more light on the usefulness of TP-5 and other TF in the treatment of AIDS.

5.4. Thymic Humoral Factor (THF-γ2)

Kouttab *et al.* (1992) evaluated 14 HIV-infected subjects with CD4 counts of 100–500/ mm^3 who were taking AZT by administering THF-γ2 (5, 10, or 25 mg/kg per day, i.m.) on a 2 weeks on/1 week off cycle for a period of 12 weeks. Treatment of these patients with THF-γ2 produced an overall increase in mitogen-dependent cellular responses as well as natural killer (NK) cell activity and DTH responses. In another trial, Maggliolo *et al.* (1994) have treated 12 patients in a double-blind placebo-controlled trial using AZT (500 mg/day) and THF-γ2 4 g, THF-γ2 240 g, or placebo given twice a week for a period of 6 months. Analysis of the results of the double-blind study is in progress. Other clinical trials utilizing THF-γ2 in combination with antiretroviral agents are also in progress (Abrams *et al.*, 1995). The results of these studies will determine if combination therapy with THF-γ2 is beneficial in the treatment of patients with AIDS.

6. TF IN THE TREATMENT OF HEPATITIS

Early studies with Tα_1 in a woodchuck hepatitis virus model indicated that Tα_1 significantly inhibited the serum virus titers in the Tα_1-treated animals compared to the untreated animals (Korba *et al.*, 1990). The woodchuck hepatitis virus model has been used as a model for human chronic hepatitis B virus.

Evaluation of the safety and efficacy of TF5 and Tα_1 in a placebo-controlled Phase III trial in 12 patients with chronic hepatitis B was carried out by Mutchnick *et al.* (1991). The patients entered in this trial had active liver disease for at least 6 months before treatment and were positive for serum hepatitis B DNA and HBsAg. Seventy-five percent of the thymosin-treated patients and twenty-five percent of the patients receiving placebo cleared hepatitis B DNA from serum (Table II). Thymosin was well tolerated by these patients and thymosin treatment resulted in a significant increase in $CD4^+$ counts and in production of IFN-γ. In a follow-up study of the same patients, Mutchnick *et al.* (1992) reported that 78% of the patients treated with Tα_1 responded to treatment and were in remission for at least 6 months after the termination of treatment. Sixty-six percent of the thymosin-treated responders remained in remission for a period of 3½ years. More recently, a Phase III

TABLE II. Metaanalysis of Thymosin α_1 Clinical Trials for Hepatitis B[a,b]

	Treated group			Control group		
Study	Total	Responder	%	Total	Responder	%
U.S. Phase II	12	9	75	8	2	25
U.S. Phase III	49	12	25	48	6	13
Taiwan Phase III[c] 6-month treatment	17	6	35	16	3	19
Total	78	27	35	72	11	15

[a]David Horwitz, SciClone Pharmaceuticals, Inc. (personal communication).
[b]$p = 0.018$ (Mantel–Haenszel Chi Square Test)—metaanalysis. $p = 0.009$ (Fisher's Exact Test)—group totals.
[c]Interim results.

multicenter trial has been carried out with approximately 100 patients enrolled in the study. Metaanalysis of the Phase III trial (which did not reach statistical significance) and an ongoing study in Taiwan suggest that $T\alpha_1$ may be useful in the treatment of chronic hepatitis B (see Table II). Ongoing studies suggest that $T\alpha_1$ acts via a different mechanism than nucleoside analogues or IFN-α, and has a significant advantage over these treatments because of its lack of toxic side effects (Table III). Studies in progress in Italy using $T\alpha_1$ in combination with IFN-α suggest that $T\alpha_1$ may lower the side effects (toxicity) of IFN-α, and also may allow IFN-α to be used at lower doses. In two clinical trials, the first in chronic hepatitis B, and the second in chronic hepatitis C, patients were treated for six months with $T\alpha_1$ and low doses of IFN-α. Eleven of fifteen patients in the hepatitis B trial had previously failed standard IFN therapy. Nine (60%) of the fifteen patients (including six (55%) of the eleven patients failing previous IFN-α treatment) responded by losing hepatitis B virus DNA and normalizing ALT values. Seven of the nine responders seroconverted to HBeAg(−) status while two patients remained HBeAg(+). Six (67%) of the nine responders became HBsAg(−) and anti-HBs(+) (Rasi *et al.* 1996). Fifteen patients with chronic hepatitis C were treated for one year with a combination of thymosin α_1 and lymphoblastoid interferon α. All patients were positive for serum HCV RNA and thirteen were for serotype 1b. Six months after initiation of treatment seven (47%) patients had negative serum HCV RNA and at completion of the 12-month course of therapy eleven (73%) patients, including two failing previous standard IFN treatment, had lost serum HCV RNA. Six months following treatment completion, six (40%) patients, including five with HCV type 1b, showed a sustained response (Rasi *et al.* 1995). These two studies suggest that a combination of $T\alpha_1$ with IFN-α may overcome two major IFN-related problems, i.e. toxicity and unresponsiveness.

In other studies, elderly uremic patients who were nonresponders to hepatitis vaccine showed an improvement in response to a new vaccination after administration of TP-5 (Ervo *et al.*, 1992; Melappioni *et al.*, 1992). Similar results have been obtained by administration of TP-1 to nonresponder patients before revaccination (Sapio *et al.*, 1992).

TABLE III. Comparison of Nucleoside Analogues, Interferon, and Thymosin α_1 in the Treatment of Hepatitis B

	Nucleoside analogues	Interferon	Thymosin α_1
Mechanism of action	Inhibit DNA and RNA replication	Increases MHC adhesion molecule expression, enhances effector cell function	Increases effector cell number and enhances function
Site of action	Ribosome and nucleus	Nucleus	Pre-T cell, thymocyte
Timing	Days	Days to weeks	Weeks to months
Toxicity	Nucleoside analogue specific; mild to lethal	Hematologic, CNS; mild to lethal	None
Side effects	Neuropathies to liver function abnormalities; mild to severe	Nausea, flulike symptoms; mild to severe	Virtually none
Efficacy	Rapid decrease of circulating HBV DNA levels; integrated HBV DNA present; nondurable response	Varied clearance of HBV DNA and HBeAg; durable response	Varied clearance of HBV DNA and HBeAg; durable response

7. TF IN THE TREATMENT OF INFLUENZA

Influenza is a major cause of death in the elderly and children under 2 years of age and is related to diminution of the immune system in the elderly and lack of full development of the thymus-dependent immune system in children. It is estimated that in the United States there are around 20,000 influenza virus infection-associated deaths in the elderly during a typical influenza epidemic. A number of studies have been carried out to examine the effect of $T\alpha_1$ in improving the response in the elderly to influenza vaccination.

In a study conducted at The Cornell Medical Center, $T\alpha_1$ was administered to elderly patients who also received influenza vaccine (see Gravenstein *et al.*, 1989). Of the subjects who received $T\alpha_1$, 66% demonstrated a greater than fourfold increase in production of influenza virus antibodies whereas only 16% of the individuals who did not receive $T\alpha_1$ demonstrated a similar fourfold increase in antibody production as a result of vaccination. In a study carried out at the University of Wisconsin on elderly patients (64 and older) (Gravenstein *et al.*, 1989), 68% of the patients receiving $T\alpha_1$ showed increased antibody responses compared to 46% of the individuals receiving placebo. In a study carried out at The George Washington University (McConnell *et al.*, 1989) on 330 elderly patients living at the U.S. Soldier's and Airmen's Home, subjects receiving eight injections of $T\alpha_1$ along with influenza vaccine had higher antibody titers than the placebo group. In a similar study carried out at the University of Maryland (Shen *et al.*, 1990) on hemodialysis patients, 71% of the patients treated with $T\alpha_1$ developed a greater than fourfold increase in antibodies compared to 43% of the placebo group. These studies with influenza virus vaccine immunization in the presence of $T\alpha_1$ suggest that $T\alpha_1$ could be very useful in improving the immune response of the elderly to the influenza vaccine.

8. FUTURE PERSPECTIVE

Investigations on TF have reached a stage where a great deal is known about their chemistry, structure, and mechanism of action (Table III). Several TF have been utilized in clinical trials for the treatment of patients with cancer, immunodeficiency disorders including AIDS, chronic hepatitis B, and influenza viruses. These studies have established the potential usefulness of TF as modulators of the immune system in controlling the course of infection and disease progression. Future studies on the biologic function of thymic hormones as immune modulators will provide a better understanding of the mechanism of action of this family of polypeptides. Clinical studies in different diseases including cancer, AIDS, chronic hepatitis B, and influenza will establish the usefulness of TF in the treatment of these diseases in humans.

REFERENCES

Abiko, T., and Sekino, H., 1984, Deacetyl-thymosin β_4: Synthesis and effect on the impaired peripheral T-cell subsets in patients with chronic renal failure, *Chem. Pharm. Bull.* **32:**4497.

Abrams, D., Cotton, D., and Mayer, K., 1995, AIDS/HIV Treatment Directory **7:**59.

Aiuti, F., and Businco, L., 1983, Effects of thymic hormones on immunodeficiency, in: *Clinics in Immunology and Allergy*, Volume 3 (J. F. Bach, ed.), Saunders, Philadelphia, p. 187.

Aiuti, F., Sirianni, M. C., Fiorilli, M., Paganelli, R., Stella, A., and Turbessi, G. A., 1984, A placebo controlled trial of thymic hormone treatment of recurrent herpes simplex labialis infection in immunodeficient host: Results after a 1 year follow up, *Clin. Immunol. Immunopathol.* **30:**11.

Bach, J. F., ed., 1983, Thymic hormones, *Clin. Immunol. Allergy* **3**.

Bach, J. F., and Dardenne, M., 1972, Thymic dependency of rosette forming cells: Evidence of a circulating thymic hormone, *Transplant. Proc.* **4**:345.

Bach, J. F., and Dardenne, M., 1984, Clinical aspects of thymulin (FTS), in: *Thymic Hormones and Lymphokines* (A. L. Goldstein, ed.), Plenum Press, New York, p. 593.

Bistoni, F., Marconi, P., Frati, L., Bonmassar, E., and Garaci, E., 1982, Increase of mouse resistance to *Candida albicans* infection by Thymosin α1. *Infect. Immun.* **36(2)**:609–614.

Businco, L., and Rezza, E., 1981, Therapy of viral disease in immunosuppressed patients with TP-1, in: *Thymic Hormones and T-lymphocytes* (A. F. Wigzel, ed.), Academic Press, New York, p. 295.

Carco, F., and Guazzotti, G., 1993, Therapeutic use of thymostimulin in HIV seropositive subjects and with lymphadenopathy syndrome, *Recent Prog. Med.* **84**:756–764.

Collins, F. M., and Morrison, N. E., 1979, Restoration of T-cell responsiveness by thymosin: Expression of antituberculosis immunity in mouse lungs, *Infect. Immun.* **23**:330.

Conant, M. A., Calabrese, L. H., Thompson, S. E., Poeisz, B. J., Rasheed, S., Hirsch, R. L., Meyerson, L. A., A. B., Wang, C. C., and Goldstein, G., 1992, Maintenance of CD4 cells by thymopentin in asymptomatic HIV-infected subjects: Results of a double blind placebo controlled study, *AIDS* **6**:1335–1339.

D'Agostini, C., Favalli, C., Palamara, A. T., Sivilia, M., Febbraro, G., Buò, C., and Garaci, E., 1996, Efficacy of combination therapy with amantadine, Tα1 and α/β IFN in mice infected with influenza A virus, *Int. J. Immunopharmacol.* in press.

Dardenne, M., Papiernik, M., and Bach, J. F., 1974, Studies on thymus products. III. Epithelial origin of the serum thymic factor, *J. Immunol.* **27**:299.

Davies, E. G., and Levinsky, R. J., 1984, Experience in the use of thymic hormones for immunodeficiency disorders, in: *Thymic Factor Therapy*, Volume 16 (N. A. Byron and J. R. Hobbs, eds.), Serono Symposium Publications, Raven Press, New York. p. 156.

DeMartino, M., Ross, M. E., Muccioli, A. T., and Vierucci, A., 1984, T-lymphocytes in children with respiratory infections: Effect of the use of thymostimulin on the alteration of T-cell subsets, *Int. J. Tissue React.* **6**:223.

Di Francesco, P., Graziano, R., Casalinuovo, I. A., Belogi, L., Palamara, A. T., Favalli, C., and Garaci, E., 1994, Combined effect of fluconazole and thymosin α1 on systemic candidiasis in mice immunosuppressed by morphine treatments, *Clin. Exp. Immunol.* **97**:347–352.

Ervo, R., Faletti, P., Magni, S., and Cavatorta, F., 1992, Evaluation of treatments for the vaccination against hepatitis B plus thymopentine, *Nephron* **61**:371–372.

Frega, A., di-Renzi, F., Stentella, P., and Pachi, A., 1994, The management of human papilloma virus vulvo-perineal infection with systemic beta-interferon and thymostimulin in HIV-positive patients, *Int. J. Gynaecol. Obstet.* **44**:255–258.

Garaci, E., Rocchi, G., Perroni, L., D'Agostini, C., Soscia, F., Mastino, A., Grelli, S., Perno, C. F., and Favalli, C., 1993, Combined therapy with zidovudine, thymosin α_1 and α-interferon in the treatment of HIV-infected patients, in: *Combination Therapies 2* (E. Garaci and A. L. Goldstein, eds.), Plenum Press, New York, p. 33.

Garaci, E., Rocchi, G., Perroni, L., D'Agostini, C., Soscia, F., Grelli, S., Mastino, A., and Favalli, C., 1994, Combination treatment with zidovudine, thymosin α_1 and interferon-α in human immunodeficiency virus infection, *Int. J. Clin. Lab. Res.* **24**:23–28.

Goldstein, A. L., 1993, Thymosin alpha-1: Chemistry, mechanism of action and clinical applications, in: *Combination Therapies 2* (E. Garaci and A. L. Goldstein, eds.), Plenum Press, New York, pp. 39–48.

Goldstein, A. L., 1994, Clinical applications of thymosin alpha-1, *Cancer Invest.* **12**:545–547.

Goldstein, A. L., and White, A., 1971, The thymus gland: Experimental and clinical studies of its role in the development and expression of immune functions, in: *Advances in Metabolic Disorders*, Volume 5, Academic Press, New York, p. 149.

Goldstein, A. L., Low, T. L. K., Thurman, G. B., Zatz, M., Hall, N. R., McClure, J. E., Hun, S., and Schulof, R. S., 1982, Thymosins and other hormone like factors of the thymus gland, in: *Immunological Approaches to Cancer Therapeutics* (E. Mihich, ed.), Wiley, New York, p. 137.

Goldstein, G., Conant, M. A., Beall, G., Grossman, H. A., Galpin, J. E., Blick, G., Calabrese, L. H., Hirsch, R. L., Fisher, A., Stampone, P., and Meyerson, L. A., 1995, Safety and efficacy of thymopentin in zidovudine (AZT) treated asymptomatic HIV-infected subjects with 200–500 CD4 cells/mm^3. A double blind placebo controlled trial, *J. Acq. Immune Defic. Syndr. Hum. Retrovirol.* **8**:279–288.

Gravenstein, S., Duthie, E. H., Miller, B. A., and Roecker, E., 1989, Augmentation of influenza antibody response in elderly men by thymosin alpha-1, a double blind placebo controlled clinical study, *J. Am. Gerontol. Soc.* **37**:1–8.

Hammar, J. A., 1971, The new views as to the morphology of the thymus gland and their bearings on the problem of the function of the thymus, *Endocrinology* **5**:543, 731.

Hirokawa, K., McClure, J. E., and Goldstein, A. L., 1982, Age related changes in localization of thymosin in the human thymus, *Thymus* **4**:19.

Huang, K., Kind, P. D., Jagoda, E. M., and Goldstein, A. L., 1981, Thymosin treatment modulates production of interferon, *J. Interferon Res.* **1**:411.

Ishitsuka, A., Umeda, Y., Nakamura, J., and Yagi, Y., 1983, Protective activity of thymosin against opportunistic infections in animal models, *Cancer Immunol. Immunother.* **14**:145.

Iwata, T., Incefy, G., and Cunningham-Rundles, S., 1981, Circulating thymic hormone activity in patients with primary and secondary immunodeficiency diseases, *Am. J. Med.* **71**:385.

Korba, B. E., Tennant, B. C., Cote, P. J., Mutchnick, M., and Gerin, J. L., 1990, Treatment of chronic woodchuck hepatitis virus infection with thymosin alpha-1, *Hepatology* **12**:880.

Kouttab, N., Acetta, G., Calabresi, P., and Skowron, G., 1992, Phase I trial of intramuscular (i.m.) thymic humoral factor (THF) in combination with zidovudine (ZDV) in HIV-infected individuals, *VIII Int. Conf. AIDS, Amsterdam*, Abstr. PoB 3447.

Lewis, V., Twomey, J. J., and Bealmear, P. N., 1978, Age, thymic involution and circulating thymic hormone activity, *J. Clin. Endocrinol. Metab.* **47**:45.

McConnell, L. T., Gravenstein, S., Roecker, E., Spencer, S. J., Simon, G. L., and Ershler, W. B., 1989, Augmentation of influenza antibody levels and reduction in attack rates in elderly subjects by thymosin alpha-1 (TA-1), *Gerontologist* **29**:188A.

Maggliolo, F., 1994, AZT and THF therapy in HIV positive patients, *34th ICAAC, Orlando*, Abstr. 118.

Melappioni, M., Baldassari, M., Baldini, S., Radicioni, R., Panichi, N., and Baldini, S., 1992, Use of immunomodulators (thymopentine) in hepatitis B vaccine in elderly patients undergoing chronic hemodialysis, *Nephron* **61**:358–359.

Miller, J. F. A. P., 1961, Immunologic function of the thymus, *Lancet* **2**:748–749.

Mutchnick, M. G., Appleman, H. D., Chung, H. T., Aragona, E., Gupta, T. P., Cummings, G. D., Eaggoner, J. G., Hoofnagle, J. H., and Shafritz, D. A., 1991, Thymosin treatment of chronic hepatitis B: A placebo controlled pilot trial, *Hepatology* **14**:409–415.

Mutchnick, M. G., Jaureavi, J. I., and Shafritz, D. A., 1993, Sustained response to thymosin therapy in patients with chronic active hepatitis B (CAHB), *2nd Int. Symp. Combination Therapies*, p. 36.

Neta, R., and Salvin, S. B., 1983, Resistance and susceptibility to infections in inbred murine strains. II. Variations in the effect of treatment with thymosin fraction 5 on the release of lymphokines in vivo, *Cell. Immunol.* **75**:173.

Oates, K., and Goldstein, A. L., 1991, Thymosin, in: *Biological Therapy of Cancer* (V. T. DeVita, S. Hellman, and S. A. Rosenberg, eds.), Lippincott, Philadelphia, pp. 705–718.

Rasi, G., Mutchnick, M. G., Di Virgilio, D., Pierimarchi, P., Sinibaldi-Vallebona, P., Colella, F., Favalli, C., and Garaci, E., 1996, Combination low-dose lymphoblastoid interferon (L-IFN) and thymosin $\alpha 1$ (T$\alpha 1$) therapy in the treatment of chronic hepatitis, *B. J. Vir. Hepatitis* (in press).

Rasi, G., Mutchnick, M. G., Di Virgilio, D., Pierimarchi, P., Sinibaldi-Vallebona, P., Colella, F., and Garaci, E., 1995, Combination thymosin $\alpha 1$ (T$\alpha 1$) and lymphoblastoid interferon (L-IFN) and therapy in chronic hepatitis C (CHC), *Gastroenterology,* **108(4)**:1153.

Salvin, S. B., and Neta, R., 1983, Resistance and susceptibility to infection in inbred murine strains. I. Variations in the response to thymic hormones in mice infected with Candida albicans, *Cell. Immunol.* **75**:160.

Sapio, C., Bonifati, A., Confessore, A., Gatti, M., Maimone, I., Minella, M. P., Scarpino, L., and D'Alessandro, C., 1992, Primary prevention: HBV vaccination in hemodialysis unit, *Nephron* **61**:360–361.

Savino, W., Dardenne, M., and Bach, J. F., 1983, Thymic hormone-containing cells. II. Evolution of cells containing the serum factor (FTS or thymulin) in normal and autoimmune mice, as revealed by anti-FTS monoclonal antibodies. Relationship with IA bearing cells, *Clin. Exp. Immunol.* **52**:1.

Schulof, R. S., and Goldstein, A. L., 1983, Clinical applications of thymosin and other thymic hormones, in: *Recent Advances in Clinical Immunology* (R. A. Thompson and N. R. Rose, eds.), Churchill Livingstone, Edinburgh, p. 243.

Schulof, R. S., Simon, G. L., Sztein, M. B., Parenti, D. M., Digioa, R. A., Courtless, J. W., Orenstein, J. M., Kessler, C. M., Kind, P. D., Schlessman, S., Paxton, H. M., Robet-Guroff, M., and Goldstein, A. L., 1986, Phase I/II trial of thymosin fraction 5 and thymosin alpha-1 in HTLV-III seropositive subjects, *J. Biol. Resp. Modif.* **3**:429–443.

Schulof, R. S., Sztein, M. B., and Goldstein, A. L., 1988, Thymic factors, in: *Biological Response Modifiers and Cancer Therapy*, (J. W. Chiao, ed.) Dekker, New York, pp. 267–316.

Shen, S. Y., Corteza, Q. B., Josselson, J., Gravenstein, S., Ershler, W. B., Sadler, J. H., and Chretien, P. B., 1990, Age dependent enhancement of influenza vaccine responses by thymosin in chronic hemodialysis patients, in: *Biomedical Advances in Aging*, (A. L. Goldstein, ed.), Plenum Press, New York, pp. 523–530.

Skotnicki, A. B., Dabrowska-Bernstein, B. K., Dabrowski, M. P., Gorsky, A. J., Czarneck, J., and Aleksandrowicz, J., 1984, Biological properties and clinical use of calf thymus extract TFX-Polfa, in: *Thymic Hormones and Lymphokines* (A. L. Goldstein, ed.), Plenum Press, New York, p. 545.

Stutman, O., 1983, Role of thymic hormones in T-cell differentiation, *Clin. Immunol. Allergy* **3**:9.

Trainin, N., Rotter, V., and Yakir, Y., 1979, Biochemical and biological properties of THF in animal and human models, *Ann. N.Y. Acad. Sci.* **332**:9.

Trainin, N., Handzel, Z. T., Pecht, M., Netzer, L., Elmalek, M., and Zaizow, R., 1981, The role of THF, a thymic hormone, as a regulator of T-cell differentiation in umans, in: *Current Concepts in Human Immunology and Cancer Immunomodulation* (B. Serrpu, C. Rosefeld, J. C. Daniels, and J. P. Saunders, eds.), Elsevier Biomedical, New York, p. 295.

Twomey, J. J., Lewis, V. M., Patten, B. M., Goldstein, G., and Good, R. A., 1979, Myasthenia gravis, thymectomy and serum thymic hormone activity, *Am. J. Med.* **66**:639.

Wara, D. W., and Ammann, A. J., 1976, Thymic cells and humoral factors as therapeutic agents, *Pediatrics* **57**: 641–648.

Wara, D. W., Cowan, M. J., and Ammann, A. J., 1984, Thymosin fraction 5 therapy in patients with primary immunodeficiency disorders, in: *Thymic Factor Therapy*, Volume 16 (N. A. Byron and J. R. Hobbs, eds.), Serono Symposia Publications, Raven Press, New York, p. 123.

CHAPTER 27

GROWTH FACTORS IN THE TREATMENT OF HIV DISEASE

DAVID T. SCADDEN and DAVID W. GOLDE

Cytokines have been portrayed as both sinner and saint in HIV disease as they play a role in both the pathogenesis of disease progression as well as its treatment. The contribution of cytokine dysregulation to the evolution of clinical decline following HIV infection has been suspected as an explanation for escape from latency as well as the wasting syndrome in advanced disease. More recently, cytokines have been implicated pathogenically in associated conditions such as Kaposi's sarcoma and non-Hodgkin's lymphoma (Masood *et al.*, 1995; Wang *et al.*, 1995; Pluda *et al.*, 1993). While some cytokines are believed to be involved in the disease process, others have attracted attention for possible positive therapeutic manipulation of the immune response. The use of interleukin (IL)-2, IL-12, and others with potential in this setting are reviewed elsewhere in this volume.

Cytokines primarily regulating blood cell production have been tested extensively in the clinical care of patients with HIV disease. Specifically, recombinant human erythropoietin, granulocyte colony-stimulating factor (G-CSF), granulocyte–macrophage colony-stimulating factor (GM-CSF), and IL-3 have been evaluated as therapies to ameliorate the low blood cell counts accompanying AIDS. Reviewing the background and experience with these cytokines is the focus of this chapter.

1. BACKGROUND

Peripheral blood cytopenia is one of the hallmarks of HIV infection with a decline in blood cell counts accompanying the gradual deterioration of immune function. $CD4^+$ lymphocytes, while central to the pathophysiologic process, are just one of the cell types to decrease in number during HIV disease progression. Anemia is reported in 10–20% of

DAVID T. SCADDEN • Massachusetts General Hospital and Harvard Medical School, Boston, Massachusetts 02114. DAVID W. GOLDE • Memorial Sloan-Kettering Cancer Center, New York, New York, and Cornell University Medical College, New York, New York 10021.

Immunology of HIV Infection, edited by Sudhir Gupta. Plenum Press, New York, 1996.

patients at the time of presentation and eventually occurs in 70–80%. The decline in hemoglobin concentration has been noted to have prognostic value as it parallels the deterioration of overall clinical status. Thrombocytopenia is reported to occur in 40% and neutropenia in 50% of patients with AIDS. Although decreases in cell numbers are generally considered markers of more advanced HIV disease, thrombocytopenia may occur at any time during HIV infection (Miles, 1995; Harbol *et al.*, 1994; Scadden *et al.*, 1989).

The association of thrombocytopenia with HIV occurred early in the AIDS epidemic with the first report antedating the full recognition of HIV in the hemophiliac population (Ratnoff *et al.*, 1983). It has since been noted in virtually every subset of HIV transmittal type, often occurring before any other clinical manifestation of HIV infection (Sloand *et al.*, 1992). The clinical picture resembles that of immune thrombocytopenic purpura (ITP) with adequate megakaryocytes in the bone marrow and often detectable antibody on the platelet surface. However, frequently there is splenic enlargement, the antibody composition on the platelet surface differs from that generally seen in ITP, and more precise analysis of platelet kinetics has revealed decreased platelet production as well as increased consumption in this setting (Ballem *et al.*, 1992; Bettaieb *et al.*, 1992; Karpatkin and Nardi, 1992).

The cytopenias of more advanced HIV disease are also of complex etiology with a number of interacting processes contributing to the clinical picture. Disturbed regulation of antibody production leads to hypergammaglobulinemia in virtually all patients with advanced HIV infection. The antibodies produced appear to be oligoclonal, often with anti-HIV specificity, and at times are autoreactive (Bettaieb *et al.*, 1992; Karpatkin and Nardi, 1992). Immune complexes and occasionally specific antibodies have been detected on the surface of red cells, neutrophils, and platelets (Harbol *et al.*, 1994; Murphy *et al.*, 1987; McGinnis *et al.*, 1986). The presence of antibody may contribute to the increased clearance of these cells; however, the presence of cell surface-associated antibody is not predictive of decreased cell counts. Rather, the cytopenias appear to largely relate to hematopoietic defects. The specific nature of these defects remains controversial and is often multifactorial. Certainly blood cell production may be compromised by the complex pharmacologic intervention with multiple agents used to treat HIV disease and its complications. Most myelosuppressive among the commonly used agents are zidovudine (AZT), ganciclovir, trimethoprim/sulfamethoxazole, pyramethamine/sulfadiazine, and interferon-α. The newer antiretrovirals, dideoxyinosine (ddI), dideoxycytidine (ddC), and stavudine (d4T), are not associated with significant myelosuppression. In addition, hematopoietic compromise related to involvement of the marrow with infectious or neoplastic processes occurs commonly. In particular, mycobacterial infection frequently accompanies advanced AIDS, suppresses hematopoiesis, and may be diagnosed by bone marrow examination. Fungal disease similarly causes impairment in blood cell production with morphologic evidence of direct bone marrow infiltration. Less obvious pathologically are the defects induced by cytomegalovirus (CMV) infection which is accompanied by no specific histologic appearance of the bone marrow. Parvovirus may induce predominantly red cell abnormalities with giant pronormoblasts evident in the bone marrow aspirate, but a generalized aplasia may also occur. Lymphoma, particularly that of the small, noncleaved cell histologic subset, has a predilection for marrow infiltration. The most common morphologic abnormalities seen on examination of the bone marrow, however, are not those associated with known secondary agents.

Dysplastic, megaloblastoid changes with normal to increased cellularity are common, as are increased reticulin, atypical lymphoid aggregates, increased plasma cells, and loosely organized granulomata (Treacy *et al.*, 1987; Castella *et al.*, 1985). Specific evaluation for acid-fast or fungal forms as well as a full panel of microbiologic evaluations should routinely be performed to assess secondary causes of hematopoietic failure. How HIV itself participates in the process of bone marrow dysfunction remains ill-defined. The bulk of evidence suggests that HIV does not directly infect primitive blood progenitor cells or, if it does so, it infects with very low frequency (Kaczmarski *et al.*, 1992; Louache *et al.*, 1992; Davis *et al.*, 1991; Kitano *et al.*, 1991; Steinberg *et al.*, 1991; Molina *et al.*, 1990; von Lear *et al.*, 1990). The virus may alter the function of these cells, however, possibly through interaction with surface CD4 and the subsequent induction of programmed cell death (Zauli *et al.*, 1994; Bagnara *et al.*, 1990). In addition, there are data suggesting that the bone marrow microenvironment may be altered by HIV infection of accessory cells (Scadden *et al.*, 1990). To what extent the infection of these cells leads to altered hematopoietic support remains in question. HIV has been documented, however, to perturb the production of the hematopoietic cytokine erythropoietin by a posttranslational mechanism (Wang *et al.*, 1993).

Given the frequency of cytopenias observed in HIV disease and the need for multiple drug regimens with myelosuppressive potential, hematopoietic growth factor use has become common practice. Clinical trial data provide some guidance as to the appropriate use of cytokines in these patients.

2. ERYTHROPOIETIN

The most extensively studied growth factor in HIV disease is recombinant human erythropoietin (Epo). Epo has been evaluated in four randomized, placebo-controlled trials of patients experiencing anemia while receiving AZT (Henry *et al.*, 1992a). In a subset of patients administered Epo 100–200 U/kg three times per week, a statistically significant improvement in hematocrit and decreased transfusion requirement were observed with little associated toxicity. Importantly, however, the benefit was restricted to those patients with a pretreatment serum Epo level of < 500 IU/liter. The group with Epo serum concentrations greater than this threshold comprised approximately one-third of the patients and they derived no appreciable benefit from the use of Epo.

A small randomized trial of anemic AIDS patients not receiving AZT demonstrated a trend toward similar improvements (Henry *et al.*, 1992b). In a large open-label study of anemic AIDS patients with serum Epo concentrations < 500 IU/liter treated with Epo 4000 U/day 6 days a week, transfusion-requiring patients were reduced from 40% at baseline to 18% (Phair *et al.*, 1993).

Recombinant Epo therapy may therefore provide an alternative to AZT dose reduction and may be an important supportive measure in patients requiring frequent transfusions. Pretreatment serum Epo levels are necessary to guide this treatment choice. The complications of Epo therapy observed in other treatment populations (such as hypertension and seizures) have not been associated with Epo use in AIDS. The patient's iron status needs to be monitored since Epo treatment will be ineffective in the face of iron deficiency. Theoretical benefits of Epo over transfusion are the absence of immune alterations associated with transfused blood in other settings and more even modulation of hemoglobin levels, avoiding the symptoms commonly experienced before and after blood transfusion. These may be offset by the discomfort of frequent self-injection and the often reduced, but not eliminated, requirement for transfusion. Cost differences have not been systematically studied; however, it has been reported that selection of growth factors instead of alternative antiretroviral therapy in patients intolerant of AZT can result in a 77% increase in cost (Bozzette *et al.*, 1994).

3. NEUTROPHIL GROWTH FACTORS

Neutropenia is a frequently encountered laboratory abnormality in HIV disease that has led to a range of physician responses from prompt use of growth factors to simple observation. There has been little information regarding the risk of neutropenia in this population compared with the neutropenia accompanying cancer chemotherapy. Preliminary reports suggest that bacterial infection risk is increased with neutrophil counts below 1000 cells/ml (relative risk 2.33) and below 500 cells/ml (relative risk 7.92) as might be expected (Moore *et al.*, 1995). The frequency of such infections, however, appears low enough (3–5 infections per 100 patient years) that routine use of growth factors may not be cost effective. More definitive evaluation of this issue is the subject of ongoing clinical trials. Data regarding the activity of neutrophil growth factors in HIV-infected individuals and the experience with them in specific clinical settings are presented below.

GM-CSF was first tested clinically in AIDS patients and has since undergone extensive evaluation in this patient population (Groopman *et al.*, 1987). It has been demonstrated to mitigate the neutropenia seen in HIV-associated bone marrow failure (Groopman *et al.*, 1987) or in settings associated with drug-induced neutropenia accompanying AZT (Levine *et al.*, 1991) or AZT combined with interferon-α therapy (Scadden *et al.*, 1991; Davey *et al.*, 1991; Krown *et al.*, 1992). Generally, patients respond promptly to the GM-CSF with neutrophil counts increasing by 24–48 hr postadministration at relatively low doses of GM-CSF (125 mg/m^2 per day or less when using the now commercially available yeast-derived product). Eosinophilia commonly accompanies GM-CSF therapy irrespective of the product origin (yeast or *E. coli*), but at usual dose levels no adverse clinical sequelae have been associated with this laboratory abnormality.

Two Phase III studies have evaluated GM-CSF in conjunction with either ganciclovir for CMV retinitis (Hardy, 1991) or CHOP chemotherapy for AIDS-related non-Hodgkin's lymphoma (Kaplan *et al.*, 1991). The CMV trial was conducted by the U.S. National Institute of Allergy and Infectious Diseases' AIDS Clinical Trials Group to determine if GM-CSF could alter the neutropenic complications of intravenous ganciclovir therapy for CMV retinitis. Fifty-one patients were randomized to receive ganciclovir alone or ganciclovir plus *E. coli*-derived GM-CSF for 16 weeks following which AZT was added to the regimen and patients were permitted GM-CSF on an as needed basis regardless of the original treatment arm. Patients receiving ganciclovir plus GM-CSF did experience fewer days with an absolute neutrophil count (ANC) < 750 cells/ml and a trend, which did not achieve statistical significance, toward improved ganciclovir drug delivery and reduced incidence of retinitis relapse ($p = 0.05$, 0.12, and 0.29, respectively) (Hardy, 1991). Because of the small number of patients evaluated in this trial, it is difficult to conclude definitively whether growth factors can alter the clinical outcome for patients treated with ganciclovir. However, given the association of better CMV control with full dose ganciclovir and the reduced incidence of neutropenia in association with growth factor use, cytokine support has become common clinical practice. Performing a larger trial designed to have the statistical power to define this issue is currently not feasible.

The Phase III non-Hodgkin's lymphoma trial also evaluated a small number of patients, but more conclusively showed benefit in the GM-CSF recipient group (Kaplan *et al.*, 1991). Patients were randomized to receive either CHOP chemotherapy or CHOP chemotherapy plus GM-CSF. Those patients receiving GM-CSF beginning 3 days post-administration of chemotherapy at a dose of 10 mg/kg per day subcutaneously for 10 days had a reduced incidence of fever, neutropenia, and days of hospitalization ($p < 0.05$ for each). Any impact on survival or relapse could not be assessed in this small trial ($n = 30$).

G-CSF has enjoyed widespread clinical use with very limited investigation as to its impact in HIV disease. The effects of G-CSF on AIDS bone marrow failure or combined G-CSF/Epo on bone marrow failure with AZT administration were evaluated in one report (Miles *et al.*, 1991b). An improvement in neutrophil counts was documented with G-CSF with minimal toxicity. Addition of Epo resulted in an increase in hemoglobin as well with no adverse effect on the neutrophil series. AZT could then be added to the growth factor regimen without significant hematologic toxicity. These data support a widespread clinical impression that G-CSF induces a rapid rise in neutrophil counts in patients with HIV infection in a range of clinical contexts. Other than occasional patients with bone pain following injection, toxic complications are rare with this growth factor.

IL-3 was recently tested in a Phase I/II trial of cytopenic HIV-infected individuals not being treated with myelosuppressive medications (Scadden *et al.*, 1995). Four dose level cohorts of three patients each received daily subcutaneous injections of 0.5, 1.0, 2.5, or 5.0 mg/kg per day. The hematologic effects were minor with changes in neutrophil (up to 2.6-fold increase) and eosinophil counts (mean 17-fold increase) seen in all patients. Occasional patients were observed to have changes in hemoglobin levels or platelet counts, but there were no overall increases in either of these parameters. Lymphocyte subsets were similarly unaffected.

The side effect profiles of G-CSF or GM-CSF have been similar to other patient groups and patients receiving long-term administration of GM-CSF were not found to develop either tachyphylaxis or anti-GM-CSF antibodies (Scadden and Agosti, 1993). One patient receiving IL-3 did experience a transient prominent reaction at the injection site which was pathologically consistent with a leukocytoclastic vasculitis (Scadden *et al.*, 1995). An ongoing concern is the effect of the growth factors on HIV replication.

4. EFFECTS OF GROWTH FACTORS ON HIV

In vitro data have generally shown that HIV replication in monocytes/macrophages may be augmented by GM-CSF and IL-3, but not by G-CSF (Koyanagi *et al.*, 1988). However, some investigators have not observed this effect of GM-CSF, suggesting that culture conditions or virus stocks could play a role in the variability of *in vitro* results (Hammer *et al.*, 1986). Similar variability is found in the clinical studies that have evaluated this issue. Two trials have demonstrated increased HIV p24 antigen blood concentrations (Kaplan *et al.*, 1991; Pluda *et al.*, 1990) while two others have not (Hardy, 1991; Scadden *et al.*, 1991). The clinical data regarding this issue, however, generally antedate the availability of sensitive measures of circulating virus. The sole parameter of virus activity generally used in these studies was an ELISA assay for serum HIV p24 antigen, not acid-dissociated p24 antigen, quantitative microculture, or quantitative nucleic acid amplification techniques (QC-PCR or branched chain analysis). In trials employing quantitative virus culture or quantitative virus culture plus polymerase chain reaction techniques, G-CSF/Epo or IL-3, respectively, was shown to have no consistent impact on virus levels (Scadden *et al.*, 1995; Miles *et al.*, 1991b).

A related issue is the observation *in vitro* that GM-CSF enhances intracellular uptake and phosphorylation of AZT in monocytes/macrophages (Perno *et al.*, 1989, 1992). GM-CSF upregulated the specific activity of thymidine kinase resulting in increased intracellular pools of the triphosphorylated form of AZT (Dhawan *et al.*, 1990). This produced a 1–2 log shift in the dose–response curve for AZT resulting in improved antiretroviral activity (Perno *et al.*, 1989, 1992). Notably, the phenomenon was restricted to AZT and another thymidine analogue, d4T, but was not observed when either ddI or ddC was used. In the presence of the latter reverse transcriptase inhibitors, GM-CSF induced an increase in viral replicative activity. Using GM-CSF to modulate AZT's ability to suppress HIV *in vivo* has been suggested as a possible therapy, particularly for those patients in whom relative resistance to AZT has developed and who are intolerant of other nucleoside analogues. A trial testing this issue has recently been completed with data analysis pending.

5. FUTURE DIRECTIONS

Growth factors have been employed primarily as supportive care in AIDS as well as other clinical settings. The growth factors with the most selective effects on hematopoiesis, Epo and G-CSF, have been used most extensively in these supportive care roles. In the context of HIV disease, cytokines with more pleiotropic effects, such as GM-CSF, have been hypothesized to have other potential therapeutic benefits. For example, GM-CSF's ability to alter the pharmacodynamics of AZT in specific cell types suggests one such alternative use which is being tested clinically. In addition, immunomodulatory characteristics of GM-CSF have been noted *in vitro* and in animal models with effects suggesting therapeutic potential. GM-CSF has been reported to improve the ability of peripheral blood mononuclear cells to kill Mycobacterium avium complex (MAC) organisms and to improve the survival of mice challenged with MAC (Kemper *et al.*, 1995; Bermudez *et al.*, 1994; Bermudez and Young, 1990; Blanchard *et al.*, 1991). GM-CSF has also been demonstrated to augment clearance of *Candida*, *Cryptococcus*, *Histoplasma* and to improve neutrophil activity against *Pneumocystis carinii* (Calderone and Sturtevant, 1994; Chen *et al.*, 1994; Lechner *et al.*, 1994; Nassar *et al.*, 1994; Laursen *et al.*, 1993; Collins and Bancroft, 1992; Richardson *et al.*, 1992; Levitz, 1991; Robin *et al.*, 1991; Taylor and Easmon, 1991; Djeu, 1990; Smith *et al.*, 1990). In tumor models, GM-CSF produced by transduced tumor cells can improve immunologic control of tumor growth (Dranoff *et al.*, 1993), perhaps providing the physiologic basis for the intriguing observation of intralesional GM-CSF inducing the regression of AIDS-related Kaposi's sarcoma in a case report (Boente *et al.*, 1993). Finally, both G-CSF and GM-CSF have been demonstrated to correct the deficits of neutrophil function seen in some patients with HIV disease (Baldwin *et al.*, 1988, 1989). Translating these effects into meaningful therapies is the subject of a number of active areas of clinical investigation.

Growth factors with activity earlier in the hematopoietic cascade, particularly at the level of the stem cell or on primitive lymphoid precursors, are of potential importance in HIV disease (Scadden *et al.*, 1994; Miles *et al.*, 1991a). Supporting the production of lymphoid cells central to the pathophysiologic basis for AIDS is a highly desirable target for the clinical development of these growth factors. Finally, alternative dosing regimens for growth factors in AIDS are beginning to be explored with some reports indicating hematologic effectiveness even with alternate day or twice weekly schedules (Balbiano *et al.*, 1994; Jacobson *et al.*, 1992). These data will have profound cost implications as well as affect patient acceptance of therapy. Cost analyses need to be further pursued and benefits more precisely determined to refine guidelines for use of these agents. The ability of growth factors to positively impact the care of patients with HIV disease is evident and anticipated to extend beyond that of supportive care as further research unfolds. Modulation of impaired host defense through manipulation of cytokines continues to offer an approach of considerable therapeutic potential in HIV disease.

REFERENCES

Bagnara, G. P., Zauli, G., Giovannini, M., Re, M. C., Furlini, G., and La Placa, M., 1990, Early loss of circulating hematopoietic progenitors in HIV-1 infected subjects, *Exp. Hematol.* **18**:426–430.

Balbiano, R., Degioanni, M., Valle, M., 1994, Prevention of severe neutropenia in AIDS patients with intermittent, low-dose G-CSF (filgrastim), *Int. Conf. AIDS* **10**:223.

Baldwin, G. C., Gasson, J. C., Quan, S. G., Fleischmann, J., Weisbart, R., Oette, D., Mitsuyasu, R. T., and Golde, D. W., 1988, Granulocyte–macrophage colony-stimulating factor enhances neutrophil function in acquired immunodeficiency syndrome patients, *Proc. Natl. Acad. Sci. USA* **85**:2763–2766.

Baldwin, G. C., Fuller, N. D., Roberts, R. L., Ho, D. D., and Golde, D. W., 1989, Granulocyte-and-granulocyte–macrophage colony-stimulating factors enhance neutrophil cytotoxicity toward HIV-infected cells, *Blood* **74**:1673–1677.

Ballem, P. J., Belzberg, A., Devine, D. V., Lyster, D., Spruston, B., Chambers, H., Doubroff, P., and Mikulash, K., 1992, Kinetic studies of the mechanism of thrombocytopenia in patients with human immunodeficiency virus infection, *N. Engl. J. Med.* **327**:1779–1784.

Bermudez, L. E. M., and Young, L. S., 1990, Recombinant granulocyte–macrophage colony-stimulating factor activates human macrophages to inhibit growth or kill *Mycobacterium avium* complex, *J. Leuk. Biol.* **48**: 67–73.

Bermudez, L. E., Martinelli, J., Petrofsky, M., Kolonoski, P., and Young, L. S., 1994, Recombinant granulocyte–macrophage colony-stimulating factor enhances the effects of antibiotics against *Mycobacterium avium* complex infection in the beige mouse model, *J. Infect. Dis.* **169**:575–580.

Bettaieb, A., Fromont, P., Louache, F., Oksenhendler, E., Vainchenker, W., Duedari, N., and Bierling, P., 1992, Presence of cross-reactive antibody between human immunodeficiency virus (HIV) and platelet glycoproteins in HIV-related immune thrombocytopenic purpura, *Blood* **80**:162–169.

Blanchard, D. K., Michelini-Norris, M. B., Pearson, C. A., McMillen, S., and Djeu, J. Y., 1991, Production of granulocyte–macrophage colony-stimulating factor (GM-CSF) by monocytes and large granular lymphocytes stimulated with *Mycobacterium avium–M. intracellulare*: Activation of bactericidal activity by GM-CSF, *Infect. Immun.* **59**:2396–2402.

Boente, P., Sampaio, C., Brandao, M. A., Moreira, E. D., Badaro, R., and Jones, T. C., 1993, Local peri-lesional therapy with rhGM-CSF for Kaposi's sarcoma, *Lancet* **341**:1154.

Bozzette, S. A., Parker, R., and Hay, J., 1994, A cost analysis of approved antiretroviral strategies in persons with advanced human immunodeficiency virus disease and zidovudine intolerance, *J. Acq. Immune Defic. Syndr.* **7**:355–362.

Calderone, R., and Sturtevant, J., 1994, Macrophage interactions with Candida, *Immunol. Ser.* **60**:505–515.

Castella, A., Croxson, T., and Mildvan, D., 1985, The bone marrow in AIDS: A histologic, hematologic, and microbiologic study. *Am. J. Clin. Pathol.* **84**:425–432.

Chen, G. H., Curtis, J. L., Mody, C. H., Christensen, P. J., Armstrong, L. R., and Toews, G. B., 1994, Effect of granulocyte–macrophage colony-stimulating factor on rat alveolar macrophage anticryptococcal activity in vitro, *J. Immunol.* **152**:724–734.

Collins, H. L., and Bancroft, G. J., 1992, Cytokine enhancement of complement-dependent phagocytosis by macrophages: Synergy of tumor necrosis factor-alpha and granulocyte–macrophage colony-stimulating factor for phagocytosis of *Cryptococcus neoformans*, *Eur. J. Immunol.* **22**:1447–1454.

Davey, R. T., Davey, V. J., Metcalf, J. A., Zurlo, J. J., Kovacs, J. A., Falloon, J., Polis, M. A., Zunich, K. M., Masur, H., and Lane, H. C., 1991, A Phase I/II trial of zidovudine, interferon-α, and granulocyte–macrophage colony-stimulating factor in the treatment of human immunodeficiency virus type 1 infection, *J. Infect. Dis.* **164:** 43–52.

Davis, B. R., Marx, J. C., Johnson, C. E., Berry, J. M., Lyding, J., Zander, A., Merigan, T. C., and Schwartz J., 1991, Absent or rare HIV infection of bone marrow stem/progenitor cells in vivo, *J. Virol.* **65:**1985–1990.

Dhawan, R. K., Kharbanda, S., Nakamura, M., Ohno, T., and Kufe, D., 1990, Effects of granulocyte–macrophage colony-stimulating factor on 3′-azido-3′-deoxythymidine uptake, phosphorylation and nucleotide retention in human U-937 cells, *Biochem. Pharmacol.* **40:**2695–2700.

Djeu, J.Y., 1990, Role of tumor necrosis factor and colony-stimulating factors in phagocyte function against candida albicans, *Diagn. Microbiol. Infect. Dis.* **13:**383–386.

Dranoff, G., Jaffee, E., Lazenby, A., Golumbek, P., Levitsky, H., Brose, K., Jackson, V., Hamada, H., Pardoll, D., and Mulligan, R.C., 1993, Vaccination with irradiated tumor cells engineered to secrete murine granulocyte–macrophage colony-stimulating factor stimulates potent, specific, and long-lasting anti-tumor immunity, *Proc. Natl. Acad. Sci. USA* **90:**3539–3543.

Groopman, J. E., Mitsuyasu, R. T., DeLeo, M. J., Oette, D. H., and Golde, D. W., 1987, Effect of recombinant human granulocyte–macrophage colony-stimulating factor on myelopoiesis in the acquired immunodeficiency syndrome, *N. Engl. J. Med.* **317:**593–598.

Hammer, S. M., Gillis, J. M., Groopman, J. E., and Rose, R. M., 1986, *In vitro* modification of human immunodeficiency virus infection by granulocyte–macrophage colony-stimulating factor and α interferon, *Proc. Natl. Acad. Sci. USA* **83:**8734–8738.

Harbol, A. W., Liesveld, J. L., Simpson-Haidaris, P. J., and Abboud, C. N., 1994, Mechanisms of cytopenia in human immunodeficiency virus infection, *Blood Rev.* **8:**241–251.

Hardy, W. D., 1991, Combined anciclovir and recombinant granulocyte–macrophage colony-stimulating factor in the treatment of cytomegalovirus retinitis in AIDS patients, *J. Acq. Immune Defic. Syndr.* **4:**S22.

Henry, D. H., Beall, G. N., Benson, C. A., Carey, J., Cone, L. A., Eron, L. J., Fiala, M. Fischl, M. A., Gavin, S. J., and Gottlieb, M. S., 1992a, Recombinant human erythropoietin in the treatment of anemia associated with human immunodeficiency virus (HIV) infection and zidovudine therapy. Overview of four clinical trials, *Ann. Intern. Med.* **117:**739–748.

Henry, D. H., Jemsek, J. G., Levin, A. S., Levine, J. D., Levine, R. L., Abels, R. I., Nelson, R. A., Thompson, D., and Rudnick, S. A., 1992b, Recombinant human erythropoietin and the treatment of anemia in patients with AIDS or advanced ARC not receiving ZDV, *J. Acq. Immun. Defic Syndr.* **5:**847–852.

Jacobson, M. A., Stanley, H. D., and Heard, S. E., 1992, Ganciclovir with recombinant methionyl human granulocyte colony-stimulating factor for treatment of cytomegalovirus disease in AIDS patients [letter], *AIDS* **6:**515–517.

Kaczmarski, R. S., Davison, F., Blair, E., Sutherland, S., Moxham, J., McManus, T., and Mufti, G. J., 1992, Detection of HIV in hematopoietic progenitors, *Br. J. Hematol.* **82:**764–769.

Kaplan, L. D., Kahn, J. O., Crowe, S., Northfelt, D., Neville, P., Grossberg, H., Abrams, D. I., Tracey, J., Mills, J., and Volberding, P. A., 1991, Clinical and virologic effects of recombinant human granulocyte–macrophage colony-stimulating factor in patients receiving chemotherapy for human immunodeficiency virus-associated non-Hodgkin's lymphoma: Results of a randomized trial, *J. Clin. Oncol.* **9:**929–940.

Karpatkin, S., and Nardi, M., 1992, Autoimmune anti-HIV-1gp120 antibody with antiidiotype-like activity in sera and immune complexes of HIV-1-related immunologic thrombocytopenia, *J. Clin. Invest.* **89:**356–364.

Kemper, C. A., Bermudez, L., Agosti, J., and Deresinski, S., 1995, Immunomodulatory therapy of mycobacterium avium (MAC) bacteremia in AIDS with rhGM-CSF, *Proceedings, 35th Interscience Conference on Antimicrobial Agents and Chemotherapy, San Francisco* p. 177.

Kitano, K., Abboud, C. N., Ryan, D. H., Quan, S. G., Baldwin, G. C., and Golde, D. W., 1991, Macrophage-active colony-stimulating factors enhance human immunodeficiency virus type 1 infection in bone marrow stem cells, *Blood* **77:**1699–1705.

Koyanagi, Y., O'Brien, W. A., Zhao, J. Q., Golde, D. W., Gasson, J. C., and Chen, I. S. Y., 1988, Cytokines alter production of HIV-1 from primary mononuclear phagocytes, *Science* **241:**1673–1675.

Krown, S. E., Paredes, J., Bundow, D., Polsky, B., Gold, J. W., and Flomenberg, N., 1992, Interferon-α, zidovudine, and granulocyte–macrophage colony-stimulating factor: A Phase I AIDS Clinical Trials Group study in patients with Kaposi's sarcoma associated with AIDS, *J. Clin, Invest.* **10:**1344–1351.

Laursen, A. L., Obel, N., Rungby, J., and Andersen, P. L., 1993, Phagocytosis and stimulation of the respiratory burst in neutrophils by Pneumocystis carinii, *J. Infect. Dis.* **168:**1466–1471.

Lechner, A. J., Lamprech, K. E., Potthoff, L. H., Tredway, T. L., and Matuschak, G. M., 1994, Recombinant GM-CSF reduces lung injury and mortality during neutropenic candida sepsis, *Am. J. Physiol.* **266:**L561–L568.

Levine, J. D., Allan, J. D., Tessitore, J. H., Falcone, N., Galasso, F., Israel, R. J., and Groopman, J. E., 1991, Recombinant human granulocyte–macrophage colony-stimulating factor ameliorates zidovudine-induced neutropenia in patients with acquired immunodeficiency syndrome (AIDS)/AIDS-related complexes, *Blood* **78:**3148–3154.

Levitz, S. M., 1991, Activation of human peripheral blood mononuclear cells by interleukin-2 and granulocyte–macrophage colony-stimulating factor to inhibit *Cryptococcus neoformans*, *Infect. Immun.* **59:**3393–3397.

Louache, F., Henri, A., Bettaieb, A., Oksenhendler, E., Raguin, G., Tulliez, M., and Vainchenker, W., 1992, Role of human immunodeficiency virus replication in defective in vitro growth of hematopoietic progenitors, *Blood* **80:**2991–2999.

McGinniss, M., Macher, A., and Rook, A., 1986, Red cell autoantibodies in patients with acquired immune deficiency syndrome. *Transfusion* **26:**405–409.

Masood, R., Zhang, Y., Bond, M. W., Scadden, D. T., Moudgil, T., Law, R. E., Kaplan, M. H., Jung, B., Espina, B. M., Lunardi-Iskandar, Y., Levine, A. M., and Gill, P. S., 1995, Interleukin-10 is an autocrine growth factor for acquired immunodeficiency syndrome-related B-cell lymphoma, *Blood* **85:**3423–3430.

Miles, S., 1995, The use of hematopoietic growth factors in treating HIV infection, *Curr. Sci.* **2:**227–233.

Miles, S. A., Lee, K., Hutlin, L., Zsebo, K. M., and Mitsuyasu, R. T., 1991a, Potential use of human stem cell factor as adjunctive therapy for human immunodeficiency virus-related cytopenias, *Blood* **78:**3200–3208.

Miles, S. A., Mitsuyasu, R. T., Moreno, J., Baldwin, G., Alton, N. K., Souza, L., and Glaspy, J. A., 1991b, Combined therapy with recombinant granulocyte colony-stimulating factor and erythropoietin decreases hematologic toxicity from zidovudine, *Blood* **77:**2109–2117.

Molina, J. M., Scadden, D. T., Molina, J. M., Groopman, J. E., Sakaguchi, M., Fuller, B., and Woon, A., 1990, Lack of evidence for infection of or effect on growth of hematopoietic progenitor cells after *in vivo* or *in vitro* exposure to human immunodeficiency virus, *Blood* **76:**2476–2482.

Moore, R. D., Keruly, J. C., and Chaisson, R. E., 1995, Neutropenia and bacterial infection in AIDS, *Proceedings, 35th Interscience Conference on Antimicrobial Agents and Chemotherapy*, San Francisco (abstract) p. 250.

Murphy, M., Metcalf, P., and Waters, A., 1987, Incidence and mechanism of neutropenia and thrombocytopenia in patients with human immunodeficiency virus infection, *Br. J. Haematol.* **66:**337–340.

Nassar, F., Brummer, E., and Stevens, D. A., 1994, Effect of in vivo macrophage colony-stimulating factor on fungistasis of bronchoalveolar and peritoneal macrophages against *Cryptococcus neoformans*, *Antimicrob. Agents Chemother.* **38:**2162–2164.

Perno, C. F., Yarchoan, R., Cooney, D. A., Hartman, N. R., Webb, D. S., Hao, Z., Mitsuya, H., Johns, D. G., and Broder, S., 1989, Replication of human immunodeficiency virus in monocytes. Granulocyte/macrophage colony-stimulating factor (GM-CSF) potentiates viral production yet enhances the antiviral effect mediated by 3′-azido-2′3′-dideoxythymidine (AZT) and other dideoxynucleoside congeners of thymidine, *J. Exp. Med.* **169:**933–951.

Perno, C. F., Cooney, D. A., Gao, W. Y., Hao, Z., Johns, D. G., Foli, A., Hartman, N. R., Calio, R., Broder, S., and Yarchoan, R., 1992, Effects of bone marrow stimulatory cytokines on human immunodeficiency virus replication and the antiviral activity of dideoxynucleosides in cultures of monocyte/macrophages, *Blood* **80:**995–1003.

Phair, J. P., Abels, R. I., McNeill, M. V., and Sullivan, D. J., 1993, Recombinant human erythropoietin treatment: Investigational new drug protocol for the anemia of the acquired immunodeficiency syndrome, *Arch. Intern. Med.* **153:**2669.

Pluda, J. M., Yarchoan, Y.R., and Smith, P. D., 1990, Subcutaneous recombinant granulocyte–macrophage colony-stimulating factor used as a single agent and in an alternative regimen with azidothymidine in leukopenia patients with severe human immunodeficiency virus infection, *Blood* **76:**2303.

Pluda, J. M., Venzon, D. J., Tosato, G., Lietzau, J., Wyvill, K., Nelson, D. L., Jaffe, E. S., Karp, J. E., Broder, S., and Yarchoan, R., 1993, Parameters affecting the development of non-Hodgkin's lymphoma in patients with severe human immunodeficiency virus infection receiving antiretroviral therapy, *J. Clin. Oncol.* **11:**1099–1107.

Ratnoff, O. D., Menitove, J. E., Aster, R. H., and Lederman, M. M., 1983, Coincident classic hemophilia and "idiopathic" thrombocytopenic purpura in patients under treatment with concentrates of anti-hemophilic factor (Factor VIII), *N. Engl. J. Med.* **308:**439–442.

Richardson, M. D., Brownlie, C. E., and Shankland, G. S., 1992, Enhanced phagocytosis and intracellular killing of candida albicans by GM-CSF-activated human neutrophils, *J. Med. Vet. Mycol.* **30:**433–441.

Robin, G., Markovich, S., Athamna, A., and Keisari, Y., 1991, Human recombinant granulocyte–macrophage colony-stimulating factor augments viability and cytotoxic activities of human monocyte-derived macrophages in long-term cultures, *Lymphokine Cytokine Res.* **10:**257–263.

Scadden, D. T., and Agosti, J., 1993, No antibodies to granulocyte macrophage colony-stimulating factor with prolonged use in AIDS [letter], *AIDS* **7:**438.

Scadden, D. T., Zon, L. I., and Groopman, J. E., 1989, Pathophysiology and management of HIV-associated hematologic disorders, *Blood* **74:**1455.

Scadden, D. T., Zeira, M., Woon, A., Wang, Z., Schieve, L., Ikeuchi, K., Lim, B., and Groopman, J. E., 1990, HIV infection of human bone marrow stromal fibroblasts, *Blood* **76:**317–322.

Scadden, D. T., Bering, H. A., Levine, J. D., Bresnahan, J., Evans, L., Epstein, C., and Groopman, J. E., 1991, Granulocyte–macrophage colony-stimulation factor mitigates the neutropenia of combined interferon alfa and zidovudine treatment of acquired immune deficiency syndrome-associated Kaposi's sarcoma, *J. Clin. Oncol.* **9:**802–808.

Scadden, D. T., Levine, J. D., Bresnahan, J., Gere, J., McGrath, J., Wang, Z., Resta, D. J., Young, D., and Hammer, S. M., 1995, In vivo effects of interleukin-3 in HIV-1 infected patients with cytopenia, *AIDS Res. Hum. Retrovir.* **11:**731–740.

Scadden, D. T., Wang, A., Zsebo, K. M., and Groopman, J. E., 1994, In vitro effects of stem cell factor or interleukin-3 on myelosuppression associated with AIDS, *AIDS* **8:**193–196.

Sloand, E. M., Klein, H. G., Banks, S. M., Vareldzis, B., Merritt, S., and Pierce, P., 1992, Epidemiology of thrombocytopenia in HIV infection, *Eur. J. Haematol.* **48:**168–172.

Smith, P. D., Lamerson, C. L., Banks, S. M., Saini, S. S., Wahl, L. M., Calderone, R. A., and Wahl, S. M., 1990, Granulocyte–macrophage colony-stimulating factor augments human monocyte fungicidal activity for Candida albicans, *J. Infect. Dis.* **161:**999–1005.

Steinberg, H. N., Crumpacker, C. S., and Chatis, P. A., 1991, In vitro suppression of normal human bone marrow progenitor cells by human immunodeficiency virus, *J. Virol.* **65:**1765–1769.

Taylor, M. B., and Easmon, C. S. F., 1991, The neutrophil chemiluminescence response to *Pneumocystis carinii* is stimulated by GM-CSF and gamma interferon, *FEMS Microbiol. Immunol.* **89:**41–44.

Treacy, M., Lai, I., Costello, C., and Clark, A., 1987, Peripheral blood and bone marrow abnormalities in patients with HIV related disorders, *Br. J. Haematol.* **65:**289–294.

von Lear, D., Hufert, F. T., Fenner, T. E., Schwander, S., Dietrich, M., Schmitz, H., and Kern, P., 1990, CD34+ hematopoietic progenitor cells are not a major reservoir of the human immunodeficiency virus, *Blood* **76:** 1281–1286.

Wang, C-Y. E., Schroeter, A. L., and Su, W. P. D., 1995, Acquired immunodeficiency syndrome-related Kaposi's sarcoma, *Mayo Clin. Proc.* **70:**869–879.

Wang, Z., Goldberg, M., and Scadden, D. T., 1993, HIV-1 suppresses erythropoietin production in vitro, *Exp. Hematol.* **21:**683–688.

Zauli, G., Furlini, G., Vitale, M., Re, M. C., Gibellini, D., Zamai, L., Visani, G., Borgatti, P., Capitani, S., and La Placa, M., 1994, A subset of human CD34+ hematopoietic progenitors express low levels of CD4, the high-affinity receptor for human immunodeficiency virus-type 1, *Blood* **84:**1896–1905.

CHAPTER 28

T-CELL VACCINATION FOR HIV-SEROPOSITIVE PATIENTS

HENRI ATLAN and IRUN R. COHEN

1. INTRODUCTION

T-cell vaccination is a way to induce the immune system to downregulate the pathogenic activities of autoimmune T cells (Cohen, 1991). The concept of T-cell vaccination, in principle, is simple: a sample of the specific autoimmune T cells is separated physically from the individual's total pool of T cells, these autoimmune T cells are activated *in vitro* and attenuated so as to abolish their potential to cause harm. The individual at risk or suffering from the disease is then immunized with their own autoimmune T cells as an autologous vaccine. Vaccination with such activated and attenuated autoimmune T cells has been found to prevent or arrest the specific autoimmune process by activating an immune response within the treated individual directed specifically against the T cells comprising the vaccine and similar T cells in the body (Zhang and Raus, 1995).

The potential usefulness of T-cell vaccination in persons infected with HIV would depend on several conditions: first, that the pathogenesis of the immune suppression resulting from HIV infection is caused, at least in part, by host T cells; second, that the pathogenic host T cells can be identified, separated from the nonpathogenic T cells, and rendered into a T-cell vaccine; third, that the immune system of the patient is capable of mobilizing an effective response to the T-cell vaccine; and fourth, that the response to such vaccination benefits the patient without toxicity.

The aims of this chapter are to review what is known about T-cell vaccination in experimental animals and humans, to review briefly the immunology of HIV infection and what is known about the role of autoimmunity in AIDS, and to consider how T-cell vaccination might be done advantageously.

HENRI ATLAN • Human Biology Research Center/Department of Biophysics, Hadassah University Hospital, Jerusalem, Israel, and Medical Center Broussais-Hôtel Dieu, University of Paris VI, Paris, France; *present address*: Service de Biophysique, Hôpital de l'Hôtel Dieu, 75014 Paris, France. IRUN R. COHEN • Department of Immunology, Weizmann Institute of Sciences, Rehovot, Israel.

Immunology of HIV Infection, edited by Sudhir Gupta. Plenum Press, New York, 1996.

The term *T-cell vaccination* (TCV) was coined more than 10 years ago to denote the use of attenuated autoimmune T cells as vaccines to prevent experimental autoimmune diseases (Ben-Nun *et al.*, 1981a). TCV is not a vaccination in the classical sense of a procedure aimed at preventing an infection. Rather, TCV is a form of *active immunotherapy* aimed at arresting or reversing pathogenic autoimmune disorders, whether "spontaneous" in predisposed individuals, or triggered by some specific intercurrent infection. When applied to HIV infection, and viral infection in general, the concept of TCV is opposite to the idea of adoptive *transfer cell immunotherapy* (Riddell and Greenberg, 1995; Whiteside *et al.*, 1993; Ho *et al.*, 1993), which tries to strengthen antiviral cell-mediated immunity (CMI) by injection of protective cytotoxic lymphocytes (CTL) after their activation and expansion *in vitro*. In TCV, the cells to be injected after activation and expansion serve as a vaccine to *induce a response against their activities*. Rather than being protective, the T cells to be used for TCV are effectors of a pathogenic autoreactivity directed against self-antigens, either directly or through cross-reactivity with bacterial or viral antigens. That is why, as in usual vaccinations, the T cells are injected in an attentuated form, after X-ray irradiation or fixation by cross-linking agents that kill them or otherwise attenuate their virulence while retaining the immunogenic properties of the T cells. The work on TCV was initiated by Cohen and colleagues in animal models of autoimmune diseases and showed that it was possible to modulate autoimmunity by developing a specific T-cell anti-T-cell immune response (Zhang and Raus, 1995; Cohen, 1991; Cohen and Young, 1991; Lohse *et al.*, 1989; Cohen *et al.*, 1985; Holoshitz *et al.*, 1983). Applications to human autoimmune diseases seem to reproduce these results under the conditions of Phase I clinical trials (Zhang and Raus, 1995; van Laar *et al.*, 1993; Zhang *et al.*, 1993; Hafler *et al.*, 1992).

Work on TCV has led to the development of new concepts of natural autoimmunity and on network regulation (Horton, 1993; Cohen, 1989a,b, 1992a,b; Cohen and Atlan, 1989). Contrary to what was thought in the context of the classical clonal selection theory, it has been established that specific effector T cells and antibodies against self-antigens are found under normal conditions in healthy individuals. In the absence of diseasè, these effector cells are normally inactivated by a regulatory network of interconnected, antigen-specific and antiidiotypic, helper, and suppressor T-cell populations.

According to this view, the occurrence of autoimmune pathology is related to a change in the state of the network from suppression to activation. Such a transition can be experimentally induced by an excess of self-antigen, an excess of activated effector cells, or by a mechanism particularly relevant to the topic of autoimmunity associated with microbial or viral infection, namely by antigens from foreign pathogens that mimic self-antigens. Conversely, the state of the network can be altered from activation to suppression by TCV.

Experimental allergic encephalomyelitis (EAE) (Lider *et al.*, 1988), adjuvant arthritis (Holoshitz *et al.*, 1983b), experimental autoimmune thyroiditis (EAT) (Roubaty *et al.*, 1990), or collagen-induced arthritis (CIA) (Chiocchia *et al.*, 1993; Kakimoto *et al.*, 1988) could be inhibited by vaccination with the respective antigen-specific T-cell clones or lines. Furthermore, it was demonstrated, both in EAE (Owhashi and Heber-Katz, 1989) and in EAT (Texier *et al.*, 1992), that anticlonotypic antibodies specific for the TCR of vaccinating T-cell clones can, similarly to the T-cell clone, inhibit the autoimmune disorder.

In humans, clinical trials initiated to explore the use of TCV did not show any evidence of toxicity (Zhang *et al.*, 1993; van Laar *et al.*, 1993; Hafler *et al.*, 1992). In patients treated for multiple sclerosis, it is still too early to make any assessment of possible clinical improvement because of the slow evolution of the disease. However, as expected from animal studies in EAE (Lohse *et al.*, 1989; Lider *et al.*, 1988), an antiidiotypic response has been observed after TCV with myelin basic protein-specific T-cell clones (Zhang *et al.*, 1993). A similar procedure was achieved by a different group (van Laar *et al.*, 1993) on patients suffering from rheumatoid arthritis with variable disease duration. On the average, a slight decrease in disease activity was observed, with an indication of a clearer improvement in patients with recent onset of the disease.

Abundant literature is available on the physiopathology of AIDS supporting the likelihood of one or several autoimmune or immunopathic autoimmunelike components related to different kinds of immune activation (Hoffman *et al.*, 1991; Ascher and Sheppard, 1988, 1990; Bacchetti and Moss, 1989; Kowalski *et al.*, 1989; Schnittman *et al.*1989; Isaksson *et al.*, 1988; Kaplan *et al.*, 1988; Kopelman and Zolla-Pazner, 1988; Schattner, 1988; Martinez *et al.*, 1988; Procaccia *et al.*, 1987; Stricker *et al.*, 1987; Shearer, 1986; Klatzmann and Gluckman, 1986; Klatzmann and Montagnier, 1986; Ziegler and Stites, 1986; Andrieu *et al.*, 1986). Recently, several reviews have been published (Via and Sarwari, this volume, Silvestris *et al.*, 1995; Atlan *et al.*, 1994; Frost and McLean, 1994; Morrow *et al.*, 1991). However, little has been published on possible preventive or therapeutic measures that might be taken to counteract, attenuate, or even cure this pathologic autoimmune activity. The idea of treating HIV-seropositive patients with nonspecific immunosuppressors such as cyclosporine (Andrieu *et al.*, 1986, 1988; Klatzmann and Montagnier, 1986) or glucocorticoids (Andrieu *et al.*, 1995) may be dangerous because such treatment could suppress the protective effects of the immune response together with its pathogenic components. However, it is possible that suppression of immune activation might be beneficial before progression into AIDS has already advanced to a stage of severe immunosuppression. For a discussion of conflicting reports see Fauci (1993). More recently, we suggested applying TCV to immunotherapy of HIV-seropositive patients aimed at preventing or stopping progression into immunodeficiency (Atlan *et al.*, 1993; Atlan, 1992).

The purpose of this chapter is to discuss different strategies of TCV for AIDS depending on possible mechanisms of HIV-induced autoreactive immune activity.

2. IMMUNOPATHOLOGY IN THE PATHOGENESIS OF AIDS

The central immunological defect induced by infection with HIV is the decline in $CD4^+$ T lymphocytes which precedes the progression from asymptomatic infection to the immunodeficiency syndrome. The duration of this process can be greater than a decade and exhibits a wide range of individual variations.

During the asymptomatic phase of the infection, two main processes have been identified and correlated with the progression into immunological and clinical AIDS:

1. Progressive loss of $CD4^+$ circulating T cells associated initially with low virus numbers and replicating activity in the peripheral blood (Embretson *et al.*, 1993) until the patient enters the preterminal, high viremia phase of the disease.
2. High viral burden and intense viral proliferation in lymphoid organs associated with the progressive destruction of lymph node follicular dendritic cells (FDC) and the disruption of their normal network architecture (Pantaleo *et al.*, 1993a,b).

Although rapid progression into AIDS is obviously correlated with the intensity and activity of the HIV infection, most of the progressive loss of $CD4^+$ T cells leading to immunodeficiency is not likely to be due only to direct killing of infected cells by replicating virions, despite recent findings on high turnover of virus actively stimulating $CD4^+$ cells. These data were documented in patients whose $CD4^+$ cell counts were maintained at a steady state thanks to active antiviral treatment (Wei *et al.*, 1995; Ho *et al.*, 1995). The fall in $CD4^+$ counts that followed interruption of treatment made it possible to estimate the high turnover rate of $CD4^+$ cells, which compensated for the viral replication at least until the terminal phase of the disease. However, these data are mostly relevant to HIV-infected patients who have already progressed into AIDS with high viremia and large numbers of infected virus-producing cells. During the asymptomatic phase, the latently infected cells far outnumber the actively replicating virus-producing cells.

The observed correlation between the intense replicating activity of the virus and the massive destruction of $CD4^+$ cells temporarily compensated by rapid cell turnover, provides evidence for the direct killing of the infected cells but does not explain how latently infected and noninfected cells are killed. The main result of these studies is that the fall in $CD4^+$ cell counts during advanced HIV-1 infection is related to the loss of actively reproducing cells rather than to a defect in cell regeneration. However, the results also indicate that rapid turnover of HIV is likely to take place in the lymphoid organs even during early phases of infection, being a source for the continuous generation of viral diversity and the infection of new cells passing through these organs. Ho *et al.* (1995) reported that their findings "strongly support the view that AIDS is primarily a consequence of continuous high level replication of HIV-1, leading to virus- and immune-mediated killing of CD4 lymphocytes." An example of a possible mechanism for an immune-mediated killing of $CD4^+$ T cells is based on the finding that some $CD8^+$ T cells expressing the ligand to the membrane marker CD30 enhance the multiplication of HIV in infected $CD4^+$ T cells (Del Prete *et al.*, 1995). This mechanism implies that killing of infected $CD4^+$ T cells by CMI, usually assumed to be a protective antiviral immune response, might be accompanied instead by amplification of the infection.

Moreover, recent reports support the notion of indirect killing of CD4 cells associated with intense viral activity in the lymph nodes during the asymptomatic phase (Finkel *et al.*, 1995). Looking for *in situ* markers of cellular death by apoptosis (DNA fragmentation) and of viral activity and replication (viral RNA quantitation by *in situ* PCR), the authors found very little overlap between the two, indicating that most cells dying by apoptosis were not infected with HIV. On the other hand, in confirmation of previous reports (Frost and McLean, 1994; Pantaleo *et al.*, 1993a; Embretson *et al.*, 1993), most of the virions were found either trapped in immune complexes at the surface of the cellular processes of the FDC network or in infected $CD4^+$ cells. This finding does not exclude the possibility of a direct cytopathic effect of the virus and killing of $CD4^+$ cells by cytolytic mechanisms different from apoptosis. However, the results clearly indicate that at least some indirect killing of uninfected cells contributes significantly to the cellular destruction (of both $CD4^+$ T cells and FDC) which takes place in the lymph nodes during the asymptomatic phase and leads, more or less rapidly, to progression into AIDS.

A number of immunopathic mechanisms with features of autoimmunity have been proposed as contributing to the development of AIDS. Circulating CTL capable of lysing uninfected $CD4^+$ cells were found in HIV-infected humans but not in chimpanzees (Zarling *et al.*, 1990). Since these animals do not develop AIDS in spite of being chronically infected by HIV, this finding supports the idea that CTL might be pathogenic *in vivo* and contribute to the development of the disease in humans.

Apoptosis, a mechanism of cell death at work in intrathymic negative selection and in a variety of normal developmental and pathological processes (for reviews see Berke, 1995; J. J. Cohen, 1995; Ameisen, 1994; Carson and Ribeiro, 1993), has been demonstrated in both $CD4^+$ and $CD8^+$ T cells of HIV-seropositive individuals (Finkel *et al.*, 1995; Lewis *et al.*, 1994; Groux *et al.*, 1992; Terai *et al.*, 1991; Ameisen and Capron, 1991). Again, this phenomenon was not observed in HIV-infected chimpanzees as far as $CD4^+$ cells were concerned, nor in African green monkeys which remain healthy in spite of infection by simian immunodeficiency virus (SIV), while apoptosis of $CD4^+$ cells was observed indeed in SIV-infected rhesus macaques which do develop the disease (Estaquier *et al.*, 1994; Ameisen, 1994). As a possible mechanism for this abnormal autoreactivity triggered by HIV, it has been suggested that the binding of gp120 to CD4 induces a state of anergy followed by apoptosis when the cell is subsequently activated (Banda *et al.*, 1992). Similarly, cross-linking of CD4 induces apoptosis in $CD4^+$ T cells when performed in unfractionated PBMC (Oyaizu *et al.*, 1993). In addition, the Fas protein, a cell surface receptor that mediates TCR-activation-induced apoptosis (Dhein *et al.*, 1995; Brunner *et al.*, 1995; Ju *et al.*, 1995), is one of the many membrane proteins of the immune system that exhibit molecular mimicry with gp120 (Silvestris *et al.*, 1995). Binding of gp120 to uninfected $CD4^+$ cells is very likely to occur *in vivo* in view of the high degree of gp120 shedding (Schneider *et al.*, 1986; Gelderblom *et al.*, 1985) and the detection of free gp120 in the sera of HIV-seropositive individuals (Oh *et al.*, 1992). Lysis of uninfected $CD4^+$ T cells coated with gp120 by gp120-specific cytotoxic cells (Weinhold *et al.*, 1989) and by antibody-dependent cell cytotoxicity (ADCC) (Lyerly *et al.*, 1987a,b) have been observed. ADCC was not found in HIV-infected chimpanzees (Ferrari *et al.*, 1994), and again, this observation was mentioned as supporting the pathogenic effect of anti-gp120 ADCC in humans.

Several mechanisms to explain elimination of uninfected T4 cells *in vivo* by immune responses directed against HIV antigens were supported by the identification in HIV-seropositive patients of cytotoxic cells directed against HIV-infected and noninfected $CD4^+$ T cells *in vitro* (Grant *et al.*, 1993, 1994; Israël-Biet *et al.*, 1990; Hoffenbach *et al.*, 1989; Sethi *et al.*, 1988). HIV-specific $CD8^+$ CTL have been isolated from seronegative donors (Hoffenbach *et al.*, 1989) suggesting that HIV antigens are mimicked by other foreign antigens, or even by self-antigens.

$CD4^+$ CTL producing lysis of uninfected CD4 lymphocytes coated with gp120 were isolated in individuals vaccinated with env vaccine (Hammond *et al.*, 1992). In a previous work (Orentas *et al.*, 1990), different clones of $CD4^+$ CTL were isolated following such vaccination. While some of them killed specifically HIV-infected $CD4^+$ cells that synthesized the viral envelope endogenously, some others lysed uninfected $CD4^+$ cells that had taken up and processed exogenous gp120 released by infected cells. These findings indicate that "therapeutic vaccination" of seropositive patients with HIV envelope immunogens might be dangerous as was already noted (Weiss, 1993; Lanzavecchia, 1989).

Cytotoxic $CD4^+$ T-cell clones were isolated from seronegative donors and shown to kill noninfected $CD4^+$ T cells pulsed with gp120 (Siliciano *et al.*, 1988). $CD4^+$ T cells were found capable to present gp120 as a target to their own surface molecules (Lanzavecchia *et al.*, 1988). More recently, the CD4 molecule in $CD4^+$ cells pulsed with gp120 was shown to be recognized as an autoantigen because of exposure of normally hidden antigenic determinants (Salemi *et al.*, 1995).

Other suggested mechanisms include: virus-induced T-cell-mediated immunopathology similar to those observed in human hepatitis B and mouse lymphocytic choriomeningitis (Zinkernagel and Hengartner, 1994); graft-versus-host-like disease induced by cross-reactivity between MHC and HIV proteins (Habeshaw *et al.*, 1992; Andrieu *et al.*, 1986); infection by macrophage-tropic HIV leading to a permanent source of infectious virus and/or permanent exposure of viral proteins and activation of many generations of T cells passing through lymphoid organs (Mosier and Sieburg, 1994; Gartner *et al.*, 1986; Koenig *et al.*, 1986); defective antigen presentation and loss of memory T lymphocytes (Helbert *et al.*, 1993); activation of natural killer cells (Berke, 1995); HIV superantigens producing chronic activation of the immune system (Koup and Ho, 1994; Janeway, 1991; Imberti *et al.*, 1991); suppressive effects of HIV or HIV proteins on uninfected $CD4^+$ cells (Manca *et al.*, 1990; Gurley *et al.*, 1989; Hoffmann *et al.*, 1989; Amadori *et al.*, 1988), release of suppressive factors inhibiting proliferation of $CD4^+$ cells (Israël-Biet *et al.*, 1988) or lytic activity of antigen-specific and nonspecific killer cells (Sadat-Sowti *et al.*, 1991) which may be either protective or detrimental or both, and patterns of cytokine production (Clerici and Shearer, 1994; Salk *et al.*, 1993), including increased production of interferon-α favoring resistance of the virus (Künzi *et al.*, 1995), or increased production of soluble CD30 favoring viral multiplication (Del Prete *et al.*, 1995). (For recent reviews see Pantaleo and Fauci, 1995; Frost and McLean, 1994; Fauci, 1993; Weiss, 1993; Levy, 1993.)

Thus, on the one hand, immune response to HIV infection obviously can be protective through destruction of infected cells and neutralization of free virus (Detels *et al.*, 1994; Venet *et al.*, 1993; Plata, 1989). This classical appreciation of the protective role of antiviral immunity is strengthened by clinical and biological studies of long-term nonprogressors (LTNP) (Cao *et al.*, 1995; Pantaleo *et al.*, 1995; Kirchhoff *et al.*, 1995). High titers of neutralizing antibodies and HIV-specific, HLA-restricted, $CD8^+$ CTL were found in the blood of these patients who do not show any sign of the disease and have kept normal $CD4^+$ cell counts after more than 10 years of infection. This finding is significant by comparison with the typical disappearance of such $CD8^+$ CTL usually observed toward the entry into the final stages of the disease. The reason for this unusual increased efficiency in antiviral humoral and cellular responses is not clear and may reflect atypical peculiar circumstances. In some cases, attenuated or even defective HIV-1 isolates were identified (Cao *et al.*, 1995; Kirchhoff *et al.*, 1995). In different, earlier studies, genetic predisposition seemed to be involved (Giorgi *et al.*, 1994; Itescu *et al.*, 1994; Louie *et al.*, 1991; Simmonds *et al.*, 1991).

On the other hand, however, some aspects of the immune response might be autoimmune and contribute to the development of immunodeficiency through destruction of infected and uninfected T4 cells, and/or of FDC in the lymph nodes. The rate of CD4-cell decline and HIV disease progression might thus reflect, in part, the balance between immunoprotective and autoimmunopathic facets of the anti-HIV immune response (McLean, 1993; Weiss, 1993). However, as mentioned in a recent review (Pantaleo and Fauci, 1995), each of the many components of the immune response may have a dual effect, protective and pathogenic. Among these components, one can mention initial localization of HIV infection in lymphoid organs, persistence of viral antigens, complement-binding antibodies, ADCC, HIV-specific CTL, nonspecific natural killer cells, cytokine activities, and apoptosis of different kinds. In addition, it is likely that the overall effect leading to disease or prevention of disease progression depends on other factors such as genetic restrictions (Giorgi *et al.*, 1994; Itescu *et al.*, 1994; Louie *et al.*, 1991; Puppo *et al.*, 1991; Simmonds *et al.*, 1991; Jeannet *et al.*, 1989; Steel *et al.*, 1988), strains of HIV with different virulence and antigenic diversity (Weiss, 1993), and previous and concurrent exposures to other pathogens (Bentwich *et al.*, 1995; Lusso and Gallo, 1994; Montagnier and Blanchard, 1993). As a result, it is not surprising to find a high degree of individual variation in the intensity and pattern of immune responses observed in different HIV-seropositive patients and in the same patient at different times. For example, an oligoclonal expansion of subpopulations of $CD8^+$ T cells expressing certain Vβ families seems to play a decisive protective role in the specific primary immune response to HIV leading to the observed decrease in viremia following acute infection. On the other hand, however, the nature and intensity of this primary response may determine the subsequent evolution into a rapidly or slowly progressing disease. A strong expansion of a too limited repertoire may facilitate the development of viral variants that escape the initial response and maintain chronic infection (Pantaleo *et al.*, 1994; Kalams *et al.*, 1994; Koup and Ho, 1994). This hypothesis is supported by the observation of a case of precipitated disease progression following adoptive transfer of an expanded clone of HIV-1-specific autologous CTL and associated with selection for viral variants (Koenig *et al.*, 1995). These data indicate that the primary immune response shows already a large qualitative and quantitative heterogeneity among different individuals which is not taken into account in the usual studies of cytotoxic activity and other parameters as indicators of the CMI response. "It is conceivable that the immune response (i.e. stimulation of different TCR combination) may be significantly diverse in individuals who have similar or even identical genetic backgrounds, but who have been infected with genotypically and phenotypically different virus isolates. Alternatively, the immune response may be diverse in individuals with different genetic background but who are infected with genotypically and phenotypically similar virus isolates" (Pantaleo and Fauci, 1995).

3. POSSIBLE MECHANISMS OF AUTOIMMUNE AND AUTOIMMUNELIKE ACTIVITY IN HIV INFECTION: PROSPECTS FOR THERAPEUTIC INTERVENTIONS

Granted that host T cells may contribute to the pathology of AIDS (the first condition for considering TCV), if TCV is going to be helpful it must be adapted to the kind of pathogenic effects actually involved in the evolution of a given patient. This amounts to the need for a proper definition and identification of the effector cells to be looked for and prepared as a vaccine. This is the second condition mentioned at the outset.

Schematically, pathogenic autoimmunity triggered by HIV can be divided into two, nonexclusive categories: (1) natural autoimmunity against $CD4^+$ T cells completely or partially suppressed under normal conditions in noninfected people and activated out of control by HIV infection; (2) immune reactivity against self-antigens in cells of different kinds involved in various responses to HIV infection, because of molecular mimicry with HIV antigens.

The first category implies a direct destruction of $CD4^+$ T cells by specific anti-CD4 CTL or antibodies normally present in noninfected people (Hoffenbach *et al.*, 1989; Siliciano *et al.*, 1988), or mediated through $CD4^+$ memory cells cross-reactive with HIV proteins, such as p24 and gp41, also present in noninfected people (Vyakarnam *et al.*, 1991; Davis *et al.*, 1990), but kept under control by a proper functioning of a regulatory network. HIV infection could trigger a dysregulated state of activity in several different ways related to the activation of different regulatory cell populations in the network by several possible viral antigens. For example, direct autoimmunity may be activated, either by the CD4 molecule itself, possibly induced by its interaction with gp120 as mentioned above (Salemi *et al.*, 1995), or by a different self-antigen borne by CD4$^+$ T cells and cross-reacting with gp120. A different but related possibility involves increased expression of the surface molecule CD30 by CD4$^+$ T cells in HIV-infected individuals and HIV multiplication triggered in those cells by some CD8$^+$ T cells which thus contribute to the infection and death of more CD4$^+$ T cells (Del Prete *et al.*, 1995). In any case, the end product would be the same, the activation of some specific effector T cells killing infected and uninfected CD4$^+$ T cells coated or not with gp120 (Atlan *et al.*, 1994). One must note that the antigenic determinant may be part either of a surface molecule of CD4$^+$ cells (CD4 itself or else) or of the gp120 molecule. In other words, as was stressed by Lanzavecchia (1989), anti-gp120 CTL found in the plasma of seropositives may indeed be detrimental rather than protective. Therefore, the putative effector cells may be anti-CD4 or anti-gp120. The main task for effective TCV, in this case, would be to identify those pathogenic effector T cells in order to activate and expand them *in vitro* before killing them and using them as a vaccine.

The second category of autoreactive activity would imply a more complicated strategy for vaccination, adapted, in principle, to T cells specific for different autoantigens that are mimicked by HIV determinants. A variety of possible self-antigen targets for anti-HIV CTL can be considered. For example, apart from direct specific activity against CD4$^+$ T cells, a large number of homologies have been detected between HIV antigens (especially, but not only, gp120) and normal cell membrane components (Silvestris *et al.*, 1995; Zagury *et al.*, 1993; Morrow *et al.*, 1991; Bjork, 1991; Young, 1988; Golding *et al.*, 1988; Beretta *et al.*, 1987). This situation, as well as priming of the host, before HIV infection, by ubiquitous immunodominant antigens from viral or parasitic origins (Vyakarnam *et al.*, 1991; Davis *et al.*, 1990), can result in more indirect effects such as cross-reactive recognition of self-MHC, defective antigen presentation, exposure of cryptic determinants sustained by vicious circles of pathogenic cytokine production (Lehmann *et al.*, 1993), and activation of non-specific natural killers.

Another distinction must be made between immunopathic effects leading directly or indirectly to destruction of uninfected CD4$^+$ T cells, and those where CD4$^+$ cell loss is mediated by a destruction of lymph node FDC and is due mostly to failure to trap and contain the HIV infection within the lymph nodes (Finkel *et al.*, 1995; Embretson *et al.*, 1993; Pantaleo *et al.*, 1993a). In the latter case, the main target for autoreactivity is not CD4$^+$ T cells but FDC and the effector cells should be looked for in the large number of CTL infiltrating the infected lymph nodes during the asymptomatic period (Finkel *et al.*, 1995; Pantaleo *et al.*, 1993a,b; Devergne *et al.*, 1991; Tenner-Racz *et al.*, 1987; Klatzmann and Gluckman, 1986).

Finally, typical expressions of standard autoimmunity appear to be associated with AIDS/ARC syndromes. A large variety of known pathological autoantibodies have been found in HIV-seropositive patients and autoimmune disorders resembling known autoimmune diseases are observed in these patients (see for a recent review Silvestris *et al.*, 1995). Conspicuous examples are provided by neurological impairments associated with HIV-1 infection, most likely related to macrophage-tropic strains of virus (Nottet and Gendelman, 1995).

Evidence can be found in the literature for all of these kinds of autoimmune and autoimmunelike activities in HIV-infected people. Since we do not know which one, if any, is relevant to the actual progression of a given HIV-seropositive individual into the disease, several strategies should be attempted within the constraints imposed by feasibility and toxicity. As has been the case for experimental autoimmune diseases, the changes produced by TCV on the state of the immune system must be studied by careful clinical and immunological follow-up to teach us about the relevance of the different hypothetical mechanisms. Thus, TCV, apart from its expected protective effect, would serve as a probe for pathogenesis.

4. T-CELL VACCINATION AND REGULATORY NETWORKS OF AUTOIMMUNE ACTIVITY

Based on accumulated experience in the study of experimental autoimmune diseases, the mechanisms of T-cell vaccination can be understood as follows.

In spite of intrathymic negative selection, persistent autoimmunity against some immunodominant self-antigens is "natural" (Horton, 1993) and can be observed under normal, nonpathological circumstances. Such self-antigens serve as a potential target for effector cytotoxic cells and/or autoantibodies normally present in healthy organisms. However, for a given antigen, the state of activity of these effectors is controlled by a relatively small network of regulatory T-cell populations (and possibly cytokines, B cells, antibodies) with helper and suppressor properties. Some of these T cells are directly activated by the self-antigen, others are indirectly activated by idiotypic determinants of the former and of autoreactive cells and antibodies. Less specific effects, produced by other cell populations and cytokines with activating or suppressive effects, can be superimposed and modulate the state of the network. Under normal circumstances, this regulatory network prevents the existing effectors from being activated.

The balance between stimulating and suppressive effects depends on the connection structure of the network, the nature and the strength of the interactions between the network elements. Depending on that structure, the network stabilizes in a normal or pathological state, where the effector cells directly responsible for the disease are activated or inactivated, respectively. However, the connections between the elements can be modified by external antigenic stimuli or internal regulatory signals produced by the network's own temporal evolution. Thus, such a network, like neural networks in the central nervous system, is endowed with "cognitive" properties, i.e., self-organizing learning and adaptive capacities (Cohen, 1992a,b; Atlan and Cohen, 1992; Atlan and Hoffer-Snyder, 1989).

Contrary to the global theories of the idiotypic network initiated by the pioneering work of Jerne (1974), this network theory of autoimmunity is a local description of interactions between identified cell populations involved in specific autoimmune diseases (Cohen and Atlan, 1989; Cohen, 1989a). It is based on the evidence that effector cells with specificity for self-antigens normally exist *in vivo* (Cohen and Young, 1991; Burns *et al.*, 1983; Guilbert *et al.*, 1982). Such effector cells are either prevented or not from exerting autoimmune effects. This depends on the state of activity of other, regulatory, helper, and suppressor cell populations, mainly (but not solely) antigen-specific and idiotypic-specific (Roubaty *et al.*, 1990; Lohse *et al.*, 1989; Kakimoto *et al.*, 1988; Lider *et al.*, 1987, 1988; Holoshitz *et al.*, 1983a,b; Ben-Nun *et al.*, 1981a). When this finely tuned regulatory system is perturbed by the introduction of a foreign antigen, cross-reactive with a given self-antigen or interfering with antigen presentation, the ensuing stimuli delivered to the various component cells of the network change the steady state of the network in such a way that expression, rather than suppression, of pathogenic autoimmunity occurs.

Conversely, the regulatory network is enhanced or strengthened with respect to its ability to suppress autoimmunity by exposure to a nonpathogenic form of the relevant effector cells. Such enhancement is learned and "memorized" in the structure of the network, so that subsequent exposure either to the pathogenic effector cells or to the potentially immunopathogenic antigen does not produce autoimmunity. This concept is particularly relevant to studies of TCV as a prophylactic and therapeutic procedure against autoimmune diseases (Hafler *et al.*, 1992; Atlan and Cohen, 1992; Cohen, 1986, 1989b, 1991; Beraud, 1991; Elias *et al.*, 1991; Cohen and Young, 1991; Roubaty *et al.*, 1990; Atlan and Hoffer-Snyder, 1989; Cohen *et al.*, 1985; Ben-Nun *et al.*, 1981a).

Studies of experimental autoimmune diseases have provided most of the data underlying the network theory of autoimmunity. The best studied model has been experimental autoimmune encephalomyelitis (EAE). This disease, characterized by the acute onset of paralysis in genetically susceptible animals following appropriate inductive stimuli, has been shown to be mediated by $CD4^+$ effector cells specific for myelin basic protein (MBP) (Ben-Nun *et al.*, 1981b). Spontaneous recovery may occur and is associated with the appearance of suppressor cells which react specifically with idiotypic determinants present on the anti-MBP $CD4^+$ cells (Ellerman *et al.*, 1988; Ben-Nun and Cohen, 1982), or with antigenic determinants on MBP (Ben-Nun *et al.*, 1981b). These and other observations (Lohse *et al.*, 1989; Lider *et al.*, 1988) have led to the formulation of a model in which the onset, remissions, and relapses of EAE, and other autoimmune diseases, can be explained by changes in the interactions among an effector cell and two pairs of regulatory elements: (1) antigen-specific helper and suppressor cells; (2) idiotype-specific helper and suppressor cells (Cohen and Atlan, 1989). According to this model, once a state of autoimmunity has resulted from a change in the normal balance among the various elements of the regulatory network that has previously served to suppress an antiself response, the autoimmune state may be stable and persist even after the agent that precipitated the change is no longer present. Alternatively, if the host response to a foreign antigen induces the *de novo* formation of a regulatory network leading to autoimmunity, then the continued presence of cross-reactive self-epitopes may perpetuate the autoimmunopathic state of the network even after the precipitating antigen has been cleared.

Other experimental models of autoimmune disease suggest the existence of further levels of complexity in the regulation of autoimmunity. For example, adjuvant arthritis (AA) is an autoimmune disease that may be experimentally induced by injection of killed *Mycobacterium tuberculosis*, which contains an antigenic protein cross-reactive with a joint cartilage proteoglycan (van Eden *et al.*, 1985). The disease may also be induced by inoculating cells from an anti-*M. tuberculosis* T4 cell clone which also recognize the proteoglycan (van Eden *et al.*, 1985, 1988). Recent investigation into the nature and dynamics of the regulatory network in AA suggests that at least one additional component may be involved. The onset and severity of the autoimmune disease triggered by *M. tuberculosis* has been correlated with the presence of a population of nonspecific $CD8^+$ suppressor cells that downregulate the antiidiotypic regulatory cells to a greater extent than they do the cytolytic effector cells. According to the proposed network model (Atlan and Cohen, 1992), this results in a net increase in effector activity. This contrasuppressive, pathogenic response is partially nonspecific (Lohse *et al.*, 1989), being directed not only against the specific antiidiotypic regulatory cells, but also against other anticlonotypic regulatory cells. The latter include cells that control responses to different epitopes of the self-antigen and others that are involved in the regulation of unrelated autoimmune diseases, such as EAE. It is thus conceivable that partially nonspecific suppressor cells might exert contrasuppressive effects and facilitate the expression of autoimmunopathic responses in other diseases. This is reminiscent of the suppressive effects associated with HIV infection and mediated by a subpopulation of CD8$^+$ suppressor cells acting via release of a soluble inhibitory factor (Joly *et al.*, 1989; Sadat-Sowti *et al.*, 1991).

The pathogenesis of experimental autoimmune thyroiditis (EAT) provides another example of additional network complexity. This disorder, which can be produced experimentally by inoculation of cells from a thyroglobulin-specific cytotoxic T-cell clone, may entail dysfunction of an immune regulatory network containing humoral as well as cellular components (Roubaty *et al.*, 1990). In this regard, given the homologies that have been described between the HIV envelope glycoprotein (gp120) and immunoglobulins (Bjork, 1991), it is possible that anti-HIV responses, cross-reactive with self-immunoglobulins, might nonspecifically perturb the humoral arm of a bipartite cellular/humoral regulatory system and thereby contribute to the immunopathogenesis of AIDS.

Although the detailed mechanisms of network regulation of autoimmunity may be more complicated than presently understood, an appreciation of the dynamic aspect of regulatory networks is useful when considering TCV as a means to perturb the system intentionally so as to strenghten or to restore the development of a nonimmunopathic state. An interesting feature of the behavior of such regulatory networks is that the same state of activity (or suppression) can be induced by different perturbations acting in opposite directions which would be expected, intuitively, to produce opposite outcomes, unless it is appreciated that the effects are mediated by several interacting units in the network. For example, the spontaneous autoimmune process that produces diabetes in NOD strain mice can be cured by TCV using as a vaccine a T-cell clone that recognizes a peptide epitope, the p277 peptide, of the 60-kDa heat-shock protein (Elias *et al.*, 1991); but the disease can also be cured by vaccination with the p277 target peptide itself (Elias and Cohen, 1994).

In any case, experimental data and network models suggest that vaccination with autoimmune effector cells (in a form in which the cells are not capable of exerting pathogenic effects) should elicit antiidiotypic and other regulatory cells that can suppress an autoimmune effector cell response, thereby preventing or ameliorating the autoimmune disease. An example of such a model involves a network of effector cells and five populations of regulatory cells that account for complicated and paradoxical data on adjuvant arthritis (Atlan and Cohen, 1992). This example is particularly relevant since it involves the participation of a foreign pathogen (*M. tuberculosis*) working as an adjuvant in the triggering of autoimmunity. In the framework of the proposed hypothesis on AIDS, the role of HIV could be similar.

Figure 1 shows a simplified representation of some of the interactions between cell populations known to take place in lymph nodes during HIV infection. Despite its oversimplification (several subpopulations being pooled into a single network unit), this representation makes possible a semiquantitative computation of the steady states of the network resulting from its connection structure. As explained in the legend, one can understand how the diversity of direct and indirect cellular immune responses to HIV infection can produce a large variability in the resulting steady states ranging from a relatively healthy state, where all of the units are maintained in activity, to a severe terminal immunodepressed state, where all of the units representing CD4$^+$ T cells and antigen-presenting cells are inactivated. In between, several more or less pathological states are produced by different connections representing different kinds of cellular interactions. According to this analysis, TCV could

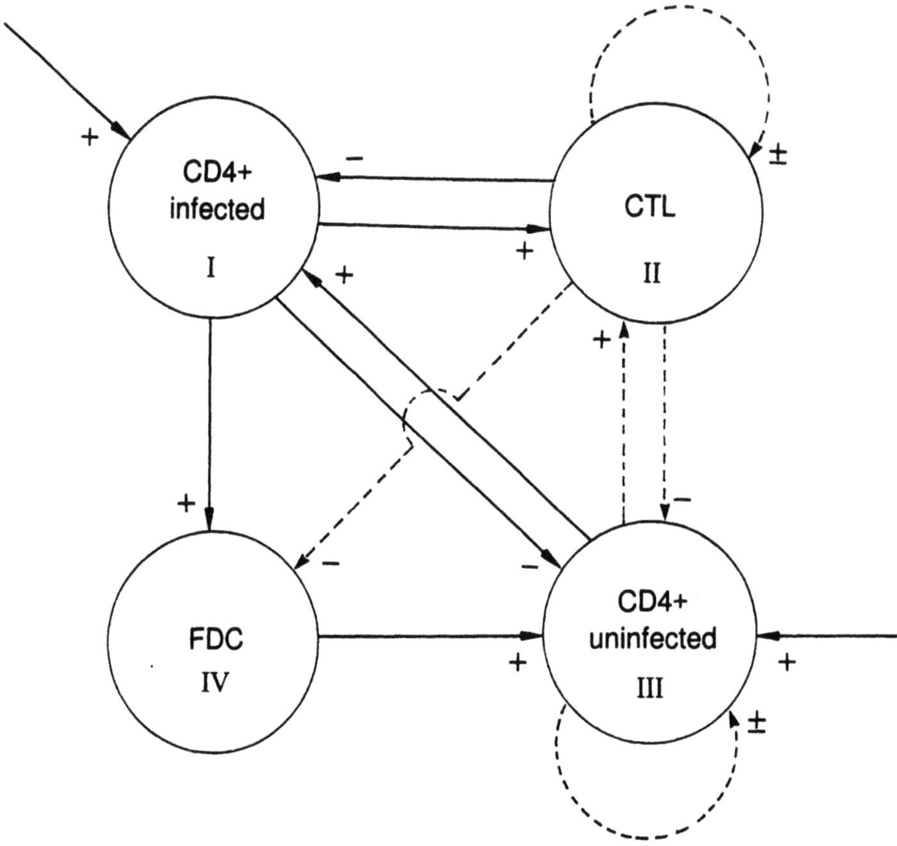

FIGURE 1. Neural network computation of local interactions between cell populations in HIV-infected lymph nodes. The connections (positive or negative arrows) between the four automata of the network represent assumed interactions (activation or suppression) between cell populations in lymph nodes, for which experimental evidence has been reported at some stage of the evolution of HIV infection, in a simplified way that allows for semiquantitative analysis (Cohen and Atlan, 1989). The automata represent cell populations which can be in any of three states: 0—inactivated or dead; 1—moderately activated; and 2—actively proliferative. Units I and III represent HIV-infected and uninfected CD4+ T cells, respectively. II represents CTL where several subpopulations have been pooled into a single automaton because the respective contributions of their effects on other cells are not known. Automaton IV represents FDC and other antigen-presenting cells.

The connections in dashed lines indicate interactions that have been described under some but not all circumstances. For example, connections between II and III stand for cytolysis of uninfected CD4+ T cells following activation of CTL; those between II and IV for killing of FDC and other APCs by CTL. The connections of II and III back on themselves represent apoptosis of CD4+ and CD8+ T cells, respectively. These circular connections are programmed to produce an output equal to the state of the unit when it is 0 or 1, and equal to −1 when the unit is fully activated in state 2. (All other connections are programmed to produce an output equal to the state of the unit from which they originate, with a + or − sign according to their sign.) We can assume that interactions between cell populations within the small limited compartment of a lymph node take place simultaneously. Therefore, the states of the network were computed in parallel. [For a discussion of the effects of different possible orders in the computation of the states of the units, see Cohen and Atlan (1989) and Atlan and Snyder (1993).] We propose that the "healthy" baseline of immune reactivity to HIV can be represented by the solid lines of connection. The dashed lines, whose effects we add in stages to the network, can be viewed as representing aspects of the observed pathogenic evolution of the disease in some people. Variations in the addition of dashed connections may characterize individuals differences.

The results of the computations are the following. Early in the disease, when the dashed connections are not be effective in various possible ways, provided that at least some of the subpopulations responsible for detrimental connections would be suppressed.

5. EFFECTORS OF DIFFERENTIAL RESPONSES: PREPARATION OF THE CELL VACCINE

As was mentioned above, cellular immune responses to HIV infection have shown a high degree of variability from patient to patient and in the same patient at different times. Although the responses are sometimes very intense and show relatively high frequencies of circulating CTL or CTL precursors, the high degree of antigenic polymorphism and the variability in the mechanisms of cytotoxicity observed *in vitro*, indicate that CTL as identified by *in vitro* techniques alone cannot be considered as a functionally homogeneous cell population. Moreover, the question remains regarding the relevance of these different cytotoxic activities to the actual *in vivo* processes responsible for disease progression. That is why the preparation of a vaccine for TCV should take into account the heterogeneity of CTL activities in order to vaccinate only against the pathogenic T cells. Therefore, the ideal goal for each patient should be to identify and separate active autologous pathogenic cells from protective ones. Then, only the former would be used as a killed vaccine and to trigger an immune response against them on reinjection into the patient, without decreasing significantly the potentially protective activity of the latter.

This requirement has implications regarding the timing and the techniques for the preparation of the vaccine.

5.1. Timing

Not every stage in the evolution of the infection is likely to be optimal for TCV of HIV-seropositive individuals. In general, circulating CTL tend to disappear at advanced stages of the disease. More specifically, non-MHC-restricted cytolytic activity against *in vitro* activated infected and uninfected autologous and heterologous $CD4^+$ T cells seems to be correlated with the degree of advancement of the disease (Grant *et al.*, 1994). These authors reported such cytotoxic activity from CTLs of HIV-seropositives but not from seronegatives. However, they noticed a tendency for this cytotoxic activity to be lost when autologous but not heterologous $CD4^+$ cells were used as targets. This may be a bad prognostic sign, indicating the disappearance of target $CD4^+$ cells from patients with severely progressive disease. This suggests that identification of cytotoxic effector cells to be used as

---

functional, the network stabilizes either in state 1111 or in a limit cycle where the states of the units rapidly oscillate with III being most of the time in state 2 or 1. Thus, all of the cell populations are still active and manage to coexist with the virus. Later in the evolution of the disease, when all of the dashed connections are functional, the network stabilizes by cycling through states 2201, 1010, 0000, 0100. This cycle represents a preterminal state where units III and IV are most of the time in state 0. When some of the dashed connections are functional, the network stabilizes in different limit cycles. They indicate oscillations in the state of the network which goes more frequently through pathological states (with III in state 0) when more of the dashed connections are functional. A detailed analysis of the consequences of each of the computed states of the system will be presented elsewhere. At present, one should note that the network analysis transforms into a variable dynamic evolutionary process a static accumulation of discrete observations reported in the literature.

vaccines may not be possible at advanced stages of the disease, at least using these techniques.

On the other hand, seropositive individuals with stable cell counts and no signs of disease progression may be LTNP who have succeeded in mounting an efficient protective immune response and do not need TCV treatment. Therefore, seropositive patients at early stages of disease progression, with detectable active cellular immunity but showing a progressive decrease in $CD4^+$ cell counts, seem to be the preferred candidates for TCV.

5.2. Preparation and Identification of Effector Cell Populations

As is evident from the literature quoted above, the nature of the effector cells and their assumed mechanisms of action are likely to be different from patient to patient ($CD4^+$ or $CD8^+$, MHC-restricted or nonrestricted cytolysis, TCR-activated or non-TCR-activated apoptosis, ADCC, direct or cytokine-mediated suppression of proliferation, and so forth). Therefore, for any given patient, screening procedures must be used for the preparation and identification of the effector cells to be used as a vaccine.

The preparation of the cell vaccine involves two stages, each of which contributes to the selection and identification of CTL populations most likely to be pathogenic: (1) selective activation and expansion of populations of lymphocytes from the patient PBMC; (2) *in vitro* functionality testing for cytotoxic or suppressive or other activities of the expanded population to establish the specificity of the prospective vaccine.

5.2.1. Preparation of Effector T Cells by Selective Activation

The *vaccine precursors* will be isolated from the PBMC or as $CD4^+$ cells and $CD8^+$ cells separated by positive selection or by depletion of $CD8^+$ or $CD4^+$ cells, respectively.

PBMC would be advantageous in that they represent a natural cell population. However, the stimulation of whole PBMC by mitogens or relevant antigens may be difficult in HIV-infected patients, especially those who begin to enter into immune deficiency.

Positive or negative selection of $CD4^+$ and $CD8^+$ cells has advantages and disadvantages related to the respective techniques involved: positive selection is more efficient but it involves cell adhesion on beads which might alter the physiological state of the cells.

Selective activation will be achieved more or less specifically by exposure to single antigens, to mixtures of antigens, or to standard mitogens such as phytohemagglutinin (PHA) or concanavalin A (Con A).

Stimulation by a mitogen alone and expansion by IL-2 is the less specific but the easiest to achieve since specific responses to antigens may be difficult to produce in HIV-infected patients. In cases where mitogenic stimulation by PHA or Con A is the only way to grow lymphocytes from such patients, TCV is still possible if the expanded cells still show some specific properties, since it was shown in animal models of autoimmune diseases that Con A produced a selective stimulation of memory cells and could be used to prepare effective T-cell vaccines in the absence of stimulation by specific antigens (Mor *et al.*, 1990). Stimulation by autologous $CD4^+$ cells and/or a mixture of viral antigens as obtained for example in supernatants of HIV culture, would be more specific. However, mitogenic stimulation of precursors from HIV-seropositives and not from seronegatives was found to be effective in producing CTL able to lyse uninfected $CD4^+$ cells but not B-lymphoblastoid cell lines (BLCL) from the same donor (Grant *et al.*, 1993, 1994; Zarling *et al.*, 1990). This showed that stimulated and expanded cells from seropositives only were cytotoxic to uninfected $CD4^+$ cells from normal donors and that they were not conventional alloreactive CTL directed against HLA class I or II antigens which are present on BLCL also. However, different data were reported using different CTL populations expanded by mitogens (Israël-Biet *et al.*, 1990). These cells produced lysis of EBV-transformed B cells as well as blast $CD4^+$ and $CD8^+$ cells, and though the cells were $CD3^+$, they were only occasionally found to be $CD8^+$ or $CD4^+$. In any case, these results are indicative of at least some degree of specificity in the CTL population of HIV-infected patients stimulated by mitogens only.

However, whenever possible, the method of choice is certainly to activate a population of lymphocytes using a specific antigen likely to be responsible for a pathogenic response *in vivo*. In view of the arguments mentioned above and developed elsewhere (Atlan *et al.*, 1994), the most likely candidate antigens are the gp120 and CD4 molecules. Autologous APC pulsed with gp120 or CD4 and irradiated may be used to stimulate the T cells. To enhance specificity, one could use autologous APC pulsed with peptides from gp120 or CD4 known to be presented by the class I HLA molecules of the patient. If successful, this would select a population of CTL, MHC-restricted against gp120 or CD4. Addition to the growth medium of cytokines like IL-12 may facilitate a proliferative response of precursor CTL from HIV-infected individuals, by restoring their defective type 1 function (Clerici *et al.*, 1993). A schematic protocol following this idea is summarized in Table I.

5.2.2. Target Cells and *in Vitro* Functionality Testing for the Cell Vaccine

Different assays can be used as functional tests for the pathogenic properties of T cells against different target cells: MHC-restricted (Zarling *et al.*, 1990) and non-MHC-restricted cytotoxicity (Grant *et al.*, 1993, 1994; Israël-Biet *et al.*, 1990), induction of apoptosis of different kinds (Ameisen, 1994; Schwartz and Osborne, 1993; Cohen, J. J. 1995), suppression of proliferation (Zagury *et al.*, 1992; Israël-Biet *et al.*, 1988), and various impairments of cytokine release.

TABLE I. Outline of a T-Cell Vaccination Protocol Based on the Hypothesis of Immunopathogenic Responses to HIV Infection Directed against CD4 or gp120

A. Patients
   1. HIV-seropositive subjects
   2. Minimal immunosuppression
   3. Evidence of declining $CD4^+$ cell numbers
B. Preparation of T-cell vaccine
   1. Culture of peripheral blood T cells responding to CD4 or to gp120
   2. Assay of antigen specificity
   3. Expansion of the cell number
   4. Chemical fixation of the cells
   5. Vaccination with autologous T cells ($5–10 \times 10^7$)
C. Follow-up
   1. $CD4^+$ cell count
   2. Immune response to vaccine cells
   3. Maintenance of immune function
   4. Effects on viral load

The target cells for these assays must be chosen according to the assumed mechanisms of immunopathogenicity discussed above. *Autologous noninfected CD4$^+$ cells* are the obvious targets to be tested. In patients where the viral load in circulating PBL is still low, one can assume that most of the circulating autologous CD4$^+$ cells are not infected. The finding of T cells targeted specifically against the autologous CD4$^+$ cells disproportionate with a low percentage of infection of such cells would be evidence for the pathogenic character of the selected effector T cells.

As mentioned above, *heterologous CD4$^+$* cells from noninfected people can be used also to look for a non-MHC-restricted cytotoxic effect. *Addition of gp120* to CD4$^+$ cells could be used to detect gp120-dependent triggering of an immunopathogenic response.

Finally, *follicular dendritic cells* (FDC) grown from lymph nodes after biopsies should also be considered as possible targets to detect the pathogenic T cells. Additional ethical problems are involved here because of the need for such biopsies. However, the accumulated evidence indicating the likely role of lymph node FDC destruction in the pathogenesis of progression into the disease recommends developing such an approach. Experiments in animal models such as SIV-infected rhesus macaques, following the work of Finkel *et al.* (1995), are needed to gather more information on the role of CTL populations infiltrating the lymph nodes.

To summarize the above, it would be important to choose for the vaccine a sample of the specific T cells responsible for the pathogenic features of AIDS that are inflicted on the host by his or her own immune system. The most specific would be likely to constitute the safest and most effective vaccine, a vaccine leaving intact the anti-HIV response to contain or eliminate the virus while regulating the harmful autoimmunity induced by the infection. Host T cells that respond to the CD4 molecule are probably pathogenic and vaccines composed of specific anti-CD4 T cells, or T cells specific for other self-antigens, would be reasonable candidates for vaccines. T cells specific for gp120 also may be pathogenic and might be considered for use as vaccines, particularly if they could be shown to harm uninfected CD4$^+$ T cells.

In vitro assays of specificity and pathogenicity would include lysis or induction of apoptosis in uninfected CD4$^+$ cells or production of suppressor or proinflammatory cytokines triggered by self-antigens.

Preparation of T-cell vaccines would be made easier by the development of culture techniques for the rapid expansion of antigen-specific T cells.

Effective TCV has been done using cells that have undergone fixation with glutaraldehyde or paraformaldehyde (Cohen, 1991; Lider *et al.*, 1987), and it would be advisable to fix the cells of HIV-infected persons to inactivate any virus as well as to prevent the autoimmune T cells from causing any direct harm.

The number of cells needed to be injected for effective vaccination in humans is not known, but can be extrapolated by surface area from the animal studies. If 5 to 10 $\times 10^6$ are effective in mice and rats, then a reasonable dose of fixed T cells for humans would be 5 to 10 $\times 10^7$. Several booster vaccinations should be considered. The problem of optimal dose and scheduling of repeated doses is important. Theoretical considerations of network relationships, confirmed by experimentation, indicate that the use of too many cells can reduce effectiveness of TCV (Segel *et al.*, 1995). Another problem is the lack of a specific marker to ascertain the effect of the vaccination on the patients. Stabilization of CD4$^+$ T-cell counts is a logical follow-up, but more useful would be a direct measure of the patient's antiidiotypic or regulatory response to the vaccine. Perhaps a decrease in anti-CD4 or anti-gp120 activity in the peripheral blood, or an improvement in lymph node pathology might be predictive markers.

6. CONCLUSION

In experimental autoimmune diseases, it has been possible to use TCR peptides or anti-TCR antibodies instead of whole autologous cells because of common TCR V-region usage in some instances, conserved even across species (Texier *et al.*, 1992; Cohen, 1991; Offner *et al.*, 1991; Burns *et al.*, 1989; Howell *et al.*, 1989; Owhashi and Heber-Katz, 1989; Vandenbark *et al.*, 1989). However, in the response to HIV, the expansion of subpopulations of CTL varies from patient to patient, which makes the feasibility of this technique highly questionable. Nevertheless, it is still conceivable that some common TCR regions could be correlated with patterns of disease evolution. In such a case, for example if some TCR V_β families would appear to be correlated with rapidly progressing disease, the use of vaccination with an appropriate TCR peptide could be attempted. This would obviously make the TCV technique much more convenient since it would relieve the burden of tailoring autologous cells to each patient.

At the outset, we enumerated four conditions that would support the use of TCV in AIDS. The first condition is that host T cells have some pathogenic role in the progression of the disease. There now seems to be ample evidence that this is the case, despite the original expectation that all features of the immunosuppression could be attributed to the virus itself. The virus apparently induces or unleashes pathogenic autoimmune behavior and therefore TCV is proposed for consideration as autoimmune therapy.

The second condition is that we can isolate the pathogenic T cells and separate them from the healthy T cells to prepare a specific vaccine. The problem in fulfilling this condition is that we are not certain which T cells to select, although we can argue for the use of anti-CD4 or anti-gp120 T cells. Assays of the pathologic effects of these T cells also have to be developed. We must also improve the methods used for growing T cells from HIV-infected persons.

The third condition is that the patient should be able to respond to vaccination. This means that we should use TCV before the onset of severe immune deficiency and that we should have follow-up markers of effectiveness. Such markers have not been developed.

The fourth condition is that TCV will benefit the patient. This last requirement can only be tested by trying the procedure.

ACKNOWLEDGMENTS. We thank Jeanine Chareire, Joelle Nataf, and Alain Venet for helpful comments and discussions during the preparation of the manuscript. H.A. is director of the Human Biology Research Center and Ishaiah Horowitz scholar in residence at Hadassah University Hospital in Jerusalem. I.R.C. is the Mauerberger professor of immunology and the director of the Robert Koch-Minerva Center for research in autoimmune diseases at the Weizmann Institute of Sciences.

REFERENCES

Amadori, A., Faulkner-Valle, G. P., De Rossi, A., Zanovello, P., Collavo, D., and Chieco-Bianchi, L., 1988, HIV-mediated immunodepression: In vitro inhibition of T-lymphocyte proliferative response by ultraviolet-inactivated virus, *Clin. Immunol. Immunopathol.* **46:**37–54.

Ameisen, J. C., 1994, Programmed cell death (apoptosis) and cell survival regulation: Relevance to AIDS and cancer, *AIDS* **8:**1197–1213.

Ameisen, J. C., and Capron, A., 1991, Cell dysfunction and depletion in AIDS: The programmed cell death hypothesis, *Immunol. Today* **12:**102–105.

Andrieu, J. M., Even, P., and Venet, A., 1986, AIDS and related syndromes as a viral-induced autoimmune disease of the immune system: An anti-MHC II disorder. Therapeutic Implications, *AIDS Res.* **2**:163–174.

Andrieu, J. M., Even, P., Venet, A., Tourani, J.-M., Stern, M., Lowenstein, W., Audroin, C., Eme, D., Masson, D., Sors, H., Israël-Biet, D., and Beldjord, K., 1988, Effects of cyclosporin on T-cell subsets in human immunodeficiency virus disease, *Clin. Immunol. Immunopathol.* **46**:181–198.

Andrieu, J. M., Lu, W., and Jevy, R., 1995, Sustained increases in CD4 cell counts in asymptomatic human immunodeficiency virus type 1-seropositive patients treated with prednisolone for 1 year, *J. Infect. Dis.* **171**:523–530.

Ascher, M. S., and Sheppard, H. W., 1988, AIDS as immune system activation: A model for pathogenesis, *Clin. Exp. Immunol.* **73**:165–167.

Ascher, M. S., and Sheppard, H. W., 1990, AIDS as immune system activation. II. The panergic imnesia hypothesis, *J. Acq. Immune Defic. Syndr.* **3**:177–191.

Atlan, H., 1992, T cell vaccination of HIV-seropositives: A therapeutic test for the autoimmune component of AIDS, in: *7th Cent Gardes Meeting* (M. Girard and L. Valette, eds.), Pasteur-Mérieux, Paris, pp. 315–319.

Atlan, H., and Cohen, I. R., 1992, Paradoxical effects of suppressor T cells in the onset of adjuvant arthritis: Neural network analysis, in: *Theoretical and Experimental Insights into Immunology* (A. S. Perelson and G. Weisbuch, eds.), Springer-Verlag, Berlin, NATO ASI Series H., Volume 66, pp. 379–395.

Atlan, H., and Hoffer-Snyder, S., 1989, Simulation of the immune cellular response by small neural networks, in: *Theories of Immune Networks* (H. Atlan and I. R. Cohen, eds.), Springer-Verlag, Berlin, pp. 85–98.

Atlan, H., and Snyder, S. H., 1993, Invariance under the order of updating in automata networks, *Network* **4(1)**: 117–130.

Atlan, H., Gersten, M. J., Salk, P. L., and Salk, J., 1993, Can AIDS be prevented by T-cell vaccination? *Immunol. Today* **14**:200–202.

Atlan, H., Gersten, M. J., Salk, P. L., and Salk, J., 1994, Mechanisms of autoimmunity and AIDS: Prospects for therapeutic intervention, *Res. Immunol.* **145**:165–183.

Bacchetti, P., and Moss, A. R., 1989, Incubation period of AIDS in San Francisco, *Nature* **338**:251–253.

Banda, N. K., Bernier, J., Kurahara, D. K., Kurrle, R., Haigwood, N., Sekaly, R. P., and Finkel, T. H., 1992, Crosslinking CD4 by human immunodeficiency virus gp120 primes T cells for activation-induced apoptosis, *J. Exp. Med.* **176**:1099–1106.

Ben-Nun, A., and Cohen, I. R., 1982, Spontaneous remission and acquired resistance to autoimmune encephalomyelitis (EAE) are associated with suppression of T cell reactivity: Suppressed EAE effector T cells recovered as T cell lines, *J. Immunol.* **128**:1450–1457.

Ben-Nun, A., Wekerle, H., and Cohen, I. R., 1981a, Vaccination against autoimmune encephalitis with T-lymphocyte line cells reactive against myelin basic protein, *Nature* **292**:60–61.

Ben-Nun, A., Wekerle, H., and Cohen, I. R., 1981b, The rapid isolation of clonable antigen-specific T lymphocyte lines capable of mediating autoimmune encephalomyelitis, *Eur. J. Immunol.* **11**:195–199.

Bentwich, Z., Kalinkovich, A., and Weisman, Z., 1995, Immune activation is a dominant factor in the pathogenesis of African AIDS, *Immunol. Today* **16**:187–191.

Beraud, E., 1991, T cell vaccination in autoimmune diseases, *Ann. N.Y. Acad. Sci.* **636**:124–134.

Beretta, A., Grassi, F., Pelagi, M., Clivio, A., Parravicini, C., Giovinazzo, G., Andronico, F., Lopalco, L., Verani, P., Butto, S., Titti, F., Rossi, G. B., Viale, G., Ginelli, E., and Siccardi, A. G., 1987, HIV *env* glycoprotein shares a cross-reacting epitope with a surface protein present on activated human monocytes and involved in antigen presentation, *Eur. J. Immunol.* **17**:1793–1798.

Berke, G., 1995, Unlocking the secrets of CTL and NK cells, *Immunol. Today* **16**:343–346.

Bjork, R. L., Jr., 1991, HIV-1: Seven facets of functional molecular mimicry, *Immunol. Lett.* **28**:91–95.

Brunner, T., Mogil, R. J., LaFace, D., Yoo, N. J., Mahboubi, A., Echeverri, F., Martin, S. J., Force, W. R., Lynch, D. H., Ware, C. F., and Green, D. R., 1995, Cell-autonomous Fas(CD95)/Fas-ligand interaction mediates activation-induced apoptosis in T-cell hybridomas, *Nature* **373**:441–444.

Burns, F., Li, X., Shen, N., Offener, K., Chou, Y. K., Vanderbark, A. A., and Heber-Katz, E., 1989, Both rat and mouse T cell receptors specific for the encephalitogenic determinant of myelin basic protein use similar V_α and V_β chain genes even though the major histocompatibility complex and encephalitogenic determinants being recognized are different, *J. Exp. Med.* **169**:27–39.

Burns, J., Rosenzweig, A., Zweiman, B., and Lisak, R. P., 1983, Isolation of myelin basic protein-reactive T-cell lines from normal human blood, *Cell Immunol.* **81**:435–440.

Cao, Y., Qin, L., Zhang, L., Safrit, J., and Ho, D. D., 1995, Virologic and immunologic characterization of long-term survivors of human immunodeficiency virus type 1 infection, *N. Engl. J. Med.* **332**:201–208.

Carson, D. A., and Ribeiro, J. M., 1993, Apoptosis and disease, *Lancet* **341**:1251–1254.

Chiocchia, G., Boisser, M. C., Manoury, B., and Fournier, C., 1993, T-cell regulation of induced arthritis in mice: Immunomodulation of arthritis by cytotoxic T-cell hybridomas specific for type II collagen, *Eur. J. Immunol.* **23**:327–332.

Clerici, M., and Shearer, G. M., 1994, The Th1–Th2 hypothesis of HIV infection: New insights, *Immunol. Today* **15**:575–581.

Clerici, M., Lucey, D. R., Berzofsky, J. A., Pinto, L. A., Wynn, T. A., Blatt, S. P., Dolan, M. J., Hendrix, C. W., Wolf, S. F., and Shearer, G. M., 1993, Restoration of HIV-specific cell-mediated immune responses by interleukin-12 in vitro, *Science* **262**:1721–1724.

Cohen, I. R., 1986, Regulation of autoimmune disease: Physiological and therapeutic, *Immunol. Rev.* **94**:5–21.

Cohen, I. R., 1989a, Natural id–anti-id networks and the immunological homunculus, in: *Theories of Immune Networks* (H. Atlan and I. R. Cohen, eds.), Springer-Verlag, Berlin, pp. 6–12.

Cohen, I. R., 1989b, Physiological basis of T-cell vaccination against autoimmune disease, *Cold Spring Harbor Symp. Quant. Biol.* **54**:879–884.

Cohen, I. R., 1991, T-cell vaccination in immunological disease, *J. Intern. Med.* **230**:471–477.

Cohen, I. R., 1992a, The cognitive principle challenges clonal selection, *Immunol. Today* **13**:441–444.

Cohen, I. R., 1992b, the cognitive paradigm and the immunological homunculus, *Immunol. Today* **13**:490–494.

Cohen, I. R., and Atlan, H., 1989, Network regulation of autoimmunity: An automaton model, *J. Autoimmun.* **2**:613–625.

Cohen, I. R., and Young, D. B., 1991, Autoimmunity, microbial immunity and the immunological homunculus, *Immunol. Today* **12**:105–110.

Cohen, I. R., Holoshitz, J., van Eden, W., and Frenkel, A., 1985, T lymphocyte clones illuminate pathogenesis and affect therapy of experimental arthritis, *Arthritis Rheum.* **28**:841–845.

Cohen, J. J., 1995, Exponential growth in apoptosis, *Immunol. Today* **16**:346–348.

Davis, D., Chaudhri, B., Stephens, D. M., Carne, C. A., Willers, C., and Lachmann, P. J., 1990, The immunodominance of epitopes within the transmembrane protein (gp41) of human immunodeficiency virus type 1 may be determined by the host's previous exposure to similar epitopes on unrelated antigens, *J. Gen. Virol.* **71**:1975–1983.

Del Prete, G., Maggi, E., Pizzolo, G., and Romagnani, S., 1995, CD30, Th2 cytokines and HIV infection: A complex and fascinating link, *Immunol. Today* **16**:76–80.

Detels, R., Liu, Z., Hennessey, K., Kan, J., Visscher, B. R., Taylor, J. M. G., Hoover, D. R., Rinaldo, C. R., Jr., Phair, J. P., Saah, A. J., and Giorgi, J. V., for the Multicenter AIDS Cohort Study, 1994, Resistance to HIV-1 infection, *J. Acq. Immune Defic. Syndr.* **7**:1263–1269.

Devergne, O., Peuchmaur, M., Crevon, M. C., Trapani, J. A., Maillot, M. C., Galanaud, P., and Emilie, D., 1991, Activation of cytotoxic cells in hyperplastic lymph nodes from HIV-infected patients, *AIDS* **5**(9):1071–1079.

Dhein, J., Walczak, H., Bäumler, C., Debatin, K.-M., and Krammer, P. H., 1995, Autocrine T-cell suicide mediated by APO-1/(Fas/CD95), *Nature* **373**:438–440.

Elias, D., and Cohen, I. R., 1994, Peptide therapy for diabetes in NOD mice, *Lancet* **343**:704–706.

Elias, D., Reshef, T., Birk, O. S., van der Zee, R., Walker, M. D., and Cohen, I. R., 1991, Vaccination against autoimmune mouse diabetes with a T-cell epitope of the human 65-kDa heat shock protein, *Proc. Natl. Acad. Sci. USA* **88**:3088–3091.

Ellerman, K. E., Powers, J. M., and Brostoff, S. W., 1988, A suppressor T-lymphocyte cell line for autoimmune encephalomyelitis, *Nature* **331**:265–267.

Embretson, J., Zupancic, M., Ribas, J. L., Burke, A., Racz, P., Tenner-Racz, K., and Haase, A. T., 1993, Massive covert infection of helper T lymphocytes and macrophages by HIV during the incubation period of AIDS, *Nature* **362**:359–362.

Estaquier, J., Idziorek, T., DeBels, F., Barre Sinoussi, F., Hurtrel, B., Aubertin, A. M., Venet, A., Mehtali, M., Muchmore, R., Michel, P., Mouton, Y., Girard, M., and Ameisen, J. C., 1994, Programmed cell death and AIDS: The significance of T-cell apoptosis in pathogenic and non pathogenic primate models of lentiviral infection, *Proc. Natl. Acad. Sci. USA* **91**:9431–9435.

Fauci, A. S., 1993, Multifactorial nature of human immunodeficiency virus disease: Implications for therapy, *Science* **262**:1011–1018.

Ferrari, G., Place, C. A., Ahearne, P. M., Nigida, S. M., Jr., Arthur, L. O., Bolognesi, D. P., and Weinhold, K. J., 1994, Comparison of anti-HIV-1 ADCC reactivities in infected humans and chimpanzees, *J. Acq. Immune Defic. Syndr.* **7**:325–331.

Finkel, T. H., Tudor-Williams, G., Banda, N. K., Cotton, M. F., Curiel, T., Monks, C., Baba, T. W., Ruprecht, R. M., and Kupfer, A., 1995, Apoptosis occurs predominantly in bystander cells and not in productively infected cells of HIV- and SIV-infected lymph nodes, *Nature Med.* **1**:129–134.

Frost, S. D. W., and McLean, A. R., 1994, Germinal center destruction as a major pathway of HIV pathogenesis, *J. Acq. Immune Defic. Syndr.* **7**:236–244.

Gartner, S., Markovitz, P., Markovitz, D. M., Kaplan, M. H., Gallo, R. C. and Popovic, M., 1986, The role of mononuclear phagocytes in HTLV-III/LAC infection, *Science* **233**:215–219.

Gelderblom, H. R., Reupke, H., and Pauli, G., 1985, Loss of envelope antigens of HTLV-III/LAV, a factor in AIDS pathogenesis? *Lancet* **2**:1016–1017.

Giorgi, J. V., Ho, H.-N., Hirji, K., Chou, C.-C., Hultin, L. E., O'Rourke, S., Park, L., Margolick, J. B., Ferbas, J., Phair, J. P., and the Multicenter AIDS Cohort Study Group, 1994, CD8+ lymphocyte activation at human immunodeficiency virus type 1 seroconversion: Development of HLA-DR+ CD38− CD8+ cells is associated with subsequent stable CD4+ cell levels, J. Infect. Dis. **170**:775–781.

Golding, H., Robey, F. A., Gates, F. T., III, Linder, W., Beining, P. R., Hoffman, T., and Golding, B., 1988, Identification of homologous regions in human immunodeficiency virus I gp 41 and human MHC class II B1 domain, *J. Exp. Med.* **167**:914–923.

Grant, M. D., Smaill, F. M., and Rosenthal, K. L., 1993, Lysis of CD4+ lymphocytes by non-HLA-restricted cytotoxic T lymphocytes from HIV-infected individuals, *Clin. Exp. Immunol.* **93**:356–362.

Grant, M. D., Smaill, F. M., and Rosenthal, K. L., 1994, Cytotoxic T-lymphocytes that kill autologous CD4+ lymphocytes are associated with CD4+ lymphocyte depletion in HIV-1 infection, *J. Acq. Immune Defic. Syndr.* **7**:571–579.

Groux, H., Torpier, G., Monté, D., Mouton, Y., Capron, A., and Ameisen, J. C., 1992, Activation-induced death by apoptosis in CD4+ T cells from human immunodeficiency virus-infected asymptomatic individuals, *J. Exp. Med.* **175**:331–340.

Guilbert, B., Dighiero, G., and Avrameas, S., 1982, Naturally occurring antibodies against nine common antigens in human sera. I. Detection, isolation, and characterization, *J. Immunol.* **128**:2779–2787.

Gurley, R. J., Ikeuchi, K., Byrn, R. A., Anderson, K., and Groopman, J. E., 1989, CD4+ lymphocyte function with early human immunodeficiency virus infection, *Proc. Natl. Acad. Sci. USA* **86**:1993–1997.

Habeshaw, J., Hounsell, E., and Dalgleish, A., 1992, Does the HIV envelope induce a chronic graft-versus-host-like disease? *Immunol. Today* **13**:207–210.

Hafler, D. A., Cohen, I., Benjamin, D. S., and Weiner, H. L., 1992, T cell vaccination in multiple sclerosis: A preliminary report, *Clin. Immunol. Immunopathol.* **62**:307–313.

Hammond, S. A., Bollinger, R. C., Stanhope, P. E., Quinn, T. C., Schwartz, D., Clements, M. L., and Siliciano, R. F., 1992, Comparative clonal analysis of human immunodeficiency virus type 1 (HIV-1)-specific $CD4^+$ and $CD8^+$ cytolytic T lymphocytes isolated from seronegative humans immunized with candidate HIV-1 vaccines, *J. Exp. Med.* **176**:1531–1542.

Helbert, M. R., L'age-Stehr, J., and Mitchison, N. A., 1993, Antigen presentation, loss of immunological memory and AIDS, *Immunol. Today* **14**:340–344.

Ho, D. D., Neumann, A. U., Perelson, A. S., Chen, W., Leonard, J. M., and Markowitz, M., 1995, Rapid turnover of plasma virions and CD4 lymphocytes in HIV-1 infection, *Nature* **373**:123–126.

Ho, M., Armstrong, G., McMahon, D., Pazin, G., Huang, X., Rinaldo, C., Whiteside, T., Tripoli, C., Levine, G., Moody, D., Okarma, T., Elder, E., Gupta, P., Tauxe, N., Torpey, D., and Heberman, R., 1993, A phase 1 study of adoptive transfer of autologous CD8+ T lymphocytes in patients with (AIDS)-related complex or AIDS, *Blood* **81**:2093–2101.

Hoffenbach, A., Langlade-Demoyen, P., Dadaglio, G., Vilmer, E., Michel, F., Mayaud, C., Autran, B., and Plata, F., 1989, Unusually high frequencies of HIV-specific cytotoxic T lymphocytes in humans, *J. Immunol.* **142**:452–462.

Hoffman, G. W., Kion, T. A., and Grant, M. D., 1991, An idiotypic network model of AIDS immunopathogenesis, *Proc. Natl. Acad. Sci. USA* **88**:3060–3064.

Hoffmann, B., Langhoff, E., Lindhardt, B. O., Odum, N., Hyldig-Nielsen, J. J., Ryder, L. P., Platz, P., Jakobsen, B. K., Bendtzen, K., Jacobsen, N., Lerche, B., Schaffer-Nielsen, C., Dickmeiss, E., Ulrich, K., and Svejgaard, A., 1989, Investigation of immunosuppressive properties of inactivated human immunodeficiency virus and possible neutralization of this effect by some patient sera, *Cell, Immunol.* **121**:336–348.

Holoshitz, J., Frenkel, A., Ben-Nun, A., and Cohen, I. R., 1983a, Autoimmune EAE mediated or prevented by T-lymphocyte lines directed against antigenic determinants of myelin base protein. Vaccination is determinant-specific, *J. Immunol.* **131**:2810–2813.

Holoshitz, J., Naparstek, Y., Ben-Nun, A., and Cohen, I. R., 1983b, Lines of T lymphocytes induce or vaccinate against autoimmune arthritis, *Science* **219**:56–58.

Horton, R., 1993, Natural autoimmunity, *Lancet* **341:**932–933.

Howell, M. D., Winters, S. T., Olee, T., Powell, H. C., Carlo, D. J., and Brostoff, S. W., 1989, Vaccination against experimental allergic encephalomyelitis with T-cell receptor peptides, *Science* **246:**668–670.

Imberti, L., Sottini, A., Bettinardi, A., Puoti, M., and Primi, D., 1991, Selective depletion in HIV infection of T cells that bear specific T cell receptor V_{β} sequences, *Science* **254:**860–862.

Isaksson, B., Albert, J., Chiodi, F., Furucrona, A., Krook, A., and Putkonen, P., 1988, AIDS two months after primary human immunodeficiency virus infection, *J. Infect. Dis.* **158:**866–868.

Israël-Biet, D., Ekwalanga, M., Venet, A., Even, P., and Andrieu, J. M., 1988, Serum suppressive activity of HIV seropositive patients, *Clin. Exp. Immunol.* **74:**185–189.

Israël-Biet, D., Venet, A., Beldjord, K., Andrieu, J. M., and Even, P., 1990, Autoreactive cytotoxicity in HIV-infected individuals, *Clin. Exp. Immunol.* **81:**18–24.

Itescu, S., Rose, S., Dwyer, E., and Winchester, R., 1994, Certain HLA-DR5 and -DR6 major histocompatibility complex class II alleles are associated with a CD8 lymphocytic host response to human immunodeficiency virus type 1 characterized by low lymphocyte viral strain heterogeneity and slow disease progression, *Proc. Natl. Acad. Sci. USA* **91:**11472–11476.

Janeway, C., 1991, Mls (minor lymphocyte stimulating): makes a little sense, *Nature* **349:**459–461.

Jeannet, M., Sztajzel, R., Carpentier, N., Hirschel, B., and Tiercy, J.-M., 1989, HLA antigens are risk factors for development of AIDS, *J. Acq. Immune Defic. Syndr.* **2:**28–32.

Jerne, N. K., 1974, Towards a network theory of the immune system, *Ann. Immunol. Inst. Pasteur* **124C:** 373–389.

Joly, P., Guillon, J.-M., Mayaud, C., Plata, F., Theodorou, I., Denis, M., Debré, P., and Autran, B., 1989, Cell-mediated suppression of HIV-specific cytotoxic T lymphocytes, *J. Immunol.* **143:**2193–2201.

Ju, S. T., Panka, D. J., Cui, H., Ettinger, R., El-Khatib, N. M., Sherr, D. H., Stanger, B. Z., and Marshak-Rothstein, A., 1995, Fas(CD95)/FasL interactions required for programmed cell death after T-cell activation, *Nature* **373:**444–448.

Kakimoto, K., Katsuki, M., Hirofuji, T., Iwata, H., and Koga, T., 1988, Isolation of T-cell line capable of protecting mice against collagen-induced arthritis, *J. Immunol.* **140:**78–83.

Kalams, S. A., Johnson, R. P., Trocha, A. K., Dynan, M. J., Ngo, H. S., D'Aquila, R. T., Kurnick, J. T., and Walker, B. D., 1994, Longitudinal analysis of T cell receptor (TCR) gene usage by human immunodeficiency virus 1 envelope-specific cytotoxic T lymphocyte clones reveals a limited TCR repertoire, *J. Exp. Med.* **179:**1261–1271.

Kaplan, J. E., Spira, T. J., Fishbein, D. B., Bozeman, L. H., Pinsky, P. F., and Schonberger, L. B., 1988, A six-year follow-up of HIV-infected homosexual men with lymphadenopathy: Evidence for an increased risk for developing AIDS after the third year of lymphadenopathy, *J. Am. Med. Assoc.* **260:**2694–2697.

Kirchhoff, F., Greenough, T. C., Brettler, D. B., Sullivan, J. L., and Desrosiers, R. C., 1995, Brief report: Absence of intact *nef* sequences in a long-term survivor with non progressive HIV-1 infection, *N. Engl. J. Med.* **332:** 228–232.

Klatzmann, D., and Gluckman, J. C., 1986, HIV infection: Facts and hypothesis, *Immunol. Today* **7:**291–296.

Klatzmann, D., and Montagnier, L., 1986, Approaches to AIDS therapy, *Nature* **319:**10–11.

Koenig, S. Gendelman, H. E., Orenstein, J. M., DalCanto, M. C., Pezeshkpour, G. H., Yungbluth, M., Fanotta, F., Aksamit, A., Martin, M. A. and Fauci, A. S., 1986, Detection of AIDS virus in macrophages in brain tissue from AIDS patients with encephalopathy. *Science,* **233:**1089–1093.

Koenig, S., Conley, A. J., Brewah, Y. A., Jones, G. M., Leath, S., Boots, L. J., Davey, V., Pantaleo, G., Demarest, J. F., Carter, C., Wannebo, C., Yannelli, J. R., Rosenberg, S. A., and Lane, H. C., 1995, Transfer of HIV-1-specific cytotoxic T lymphocytes to an AIDS patient leads to selection for mutant HIV variants and subsequent disease progression, *Nature Med.* **1:**330–336.

Kopelman, R. G., and Zolla-Pazner, S., 1988, Association of human immunodeficiency virus infection and autoimmune phenomena, *Am. J. Med.* **84:**82–88.

Koup, R. A. and Ho, D. D., 1994, Shutting down HIV, *Nature* **370:**416.

Kowalski, M., Ardman, B., Basiripour, L., Lu, Y., Blohm, D., Haseltine, W., and Sodroski, J., 1989, Antibodies to CD4 in individuals infected with human immunodeficiency virus type 1, *Proc. Natl. Acad. Sci. USA* **86:**3346–3350.

Künzi, M. S., Farzadegan, H., Margolick, J. B., Vlahov, D., and Pitha, P. M., 1995, Identification of human immunodeficiency virus primary isolates resistant to interferon-α and correlation of prevalence to disease progression, *J. Infect. Dis.* **171:**822–828.

Lanzavecchia, A., 1989, Harming and protecting responses to HIV, *Res. Immunol.* **140:**99–103.

Lanzavecchia, A., Roosnek, E., Gregory, T., Berman, P., and Abrignani, S., 1988, T cells can present antigens such as HIV gp120 targeted to their own surface molecules, *Nature* **334**:530–532.
Lehmann, P. V., Sercaz, E. E., Forsthuber, T., Dayan, C. M., and Gamon, G., 1993, Determinant spreading and the dynamics of the autoimmune T-cell repertoire, *Immunol. Today* **14**:203–208.
Levy, J. A., 1993, Pathogenesis of human immunodeficiency virus infection, *Microbiol. Rev.* **57**:183–289.
Levy, J. J., 1993, Apoptosis, *Immunol. Today* **14**:126–130.
Lewis, D. E., NgTang, G. S., Adu-Oppong, A., Schober, W., and Rodgers, J. R., 1994, Anergy and apoptosis in CD8+ T cells from HIV-infected persons, *J. Immunol.* **153**:412–420.
Lider, O., Karin, N., Shinitzky, M., and Cohen, I. R., 1987, Therapeutic vaccination against adjuvant arthritis using autoimmune T-lymphocytes treated with hydrostatic pressure, *Proc. Natl. Acad. Sci. USA* **84**:4577–4580.
Lider, O., Reshef, T., Beraud, E., Ben-Nun, A., and Cohen, I. R., 1988, Anti-idiotypic network induced by T cell vaccination against experimental autoimmune encephalomyelitis, *Science* **239**:181–183.
Lohse, A. W., Mor, F., Karin, N., and Cohen, I. R., 1989, Control of experimental autoimmune encephalomyelitis by T cells responding to activated T cells, *Science* **244**:820–822.
Louie, L. G., Newman, B., and King, M.-C., 1991, Influence of host genotype on progression to AIDS among HIV-infected men, *J. Acq. Immune Defic. Syndr.* **4**:814–818.
Lusso, P., and Gallo, R. C., 1994, Human herpes virus 6 in AIDS, *Lancet* **343**:555–556.
Lyerly, H. K., Matthews, T. H., Langlois, A. J., Bolognesi, D. P., and Weinhold, K. J., 1987a, Human T-cell lymphotropic virus III_R glycoprotein (gp120) bound to CD4 determinants on normal lymphocytes and expressed by infected cells serves as target for immune attack, *Proc. Natl. Acad. Sci. USA* **84**:4601–4605.
Lyerly, H. K., Reed, D. L., Matthews, T. J., Langlois, A. J., Ahearne, P. A., Petteway, S. R., Jr., and Weinhold, K. J., 1987b, Anti-GP antibodies from HIV seropositive individuals mediate broadly reactive anti-HIV ADCC, *AIDS Res. Hum. Retrovir.* **3**:409–422.
McLean, A. R., 1993, The balance of power between HIV and the immune system, *Trends Microbiol.* **1**:9–13.
Manca, F., Habeshaw, J. A., and Dalgleish, A. G., 1990, HIV envelope glycoprotein, antigen specific T-cell responses, and soluble CD4, *Lancet* **335**:811–815.
Martinez, A. C., Marcos, M. A. R., de la Hera, A., Marquez, C., Alonso, J. M., Toribio, M. L., and Coutinho, A., 1988, Immunological consequences of HIV infection: Advantage of being low responder casts doubts on vaccine development, *Lancet* **1**:454–457.
Montagnier, L., and Blanchard, A., 1993, Mycoplasmas as cofactors in infection due to the human immunodeficiency virus, *Clin. Infect. Dis.* **1**:S309–S315.
Mor, F., Lohse, A. W., Karin, N., and Cohen, I. R., 1990, Clinical modeling of T cell vaccination against autoimmune disease in rats, *J. Clin. Invest.* **85**:1594–1598.
Morrow, W. J., Isenberg, D. A., Sobol, R. E., Stricker, R. B., and Kieber-Emmons, T., 1991, AIDS virus infection and autoimmunity: A perspective of the clinical, immunological, and molecular origins of the autoallergic pathologies associated with HIV disease, *Clin. Immunol. Immunopathol.* **58**:163–180.
Mosier, D., and Sieburg, H., 1994, Macrophage-tropic HIV: Critical for AIDS pathogenesis? *Immunol. Today* **15**:332–338.
Nottet, H. S. L. M., and Gendelman, H. E., 1995, Unraveling the neuroimmune mechanisms for the VIV-1-associated cognitive/motor complex, *Immunol. Today* **16**:441–448.
Offner, H., Hashim, G. A., and Vandenbark, A. A., 1991, T-cell receptor peptide therapy triggers autoregulation of experimental encephalomyelitis, *Science* **251**:430–432.
Oh, S.-K., Cruikshank, W. W., Raina, J., Blanchard, G. C., Alder, W. H., Walker, J., and Kornfeld, H., 1992, Identification of HIV-1 envelope glycoprotein in the serum of AIDS and ARC patients, *J. Acq. Immune Defic. Syndr.* **5**:251–256.
Orentas, R. J., Hildreth, J. E. K., Obah, E., Polydefkis, M., Smith, G., Clements, M. L., and Siliciano, R. F., 1990, Induction of CD4+ human cytolytic T cells specific for HIV-infected cells by a gp160 subunit vaccine, *Science* **248**:1234–1237.
Owhashi, M., and Heber-Katz, E., 1989, Protection from experimental allergic encephalomyelitis conferred by a monoclonal antibody directed against a shared idiotype on rat T-cell receptors specific for myelin basic protein, *J. Exp. Med.* **169**:27–35.
Oyaizu, N., McCloskey, T. W., Coronesi, M., Chirmule, N., Kalyanaraman, V. S., and Pahwa, S., 1993, Accelerated apoptosis in peripheral blood mononuclear cells (PBMCs) from human immunodeficiency virus type-1 infected patients and in CD4 cross-linked PBMCs from normal individuals, *Blood* **82**:3392–3400.
Pantaleo, G., and Fauci, A. S., 1995, New concepts in the immunopathogenesis of HIV infection, *Annu. Rev. Immunol.* **13**:487–512.

Pantaleo, G., Graziosi, C., Demarest, J. F., Butini, L., Montroni, M., Fox, C. H., Orenstein, J. M., Kotler, D. P., and Fauci, A. S., 1993a, HIV infection is active and progressive in lymphoid tissue during the clinically latent stage of disease, *Nature* **362**:355–358.

Pantaleo, G., Graziosi, C., and Fauci, A. S., 1993b, The immunopathogenesis of human immunodeficiency virus infection, *N. Engl. J. Med.* **328**:327–335.

Pantaleo, G., Demarest, J. F., Soudeyns, H., Graziosi, C., Denis, F., Adelsberger, J. W., Borrow, P., Saag, M. S., Shaw, G. M., Sekaly, R. P., and Fauci, A. S., 1994, Major expansion of CD8+ T cells with a predominant Vβ usage during the primary immune response to HIV, *Nature* **370**:463–467.

Pantaleo, G., Menzo, S., Vaccareza, M., Graziosi, C., Cohen, O. J., Demarest, J. F., Montefiori, D., Orenstein, J. M., Fox, C., Schrager, L. K., Margolick, J. B., Buchbinder, S., Giorgi, J. V., and Fauci, A. S., 1995, Studies in subjects with long-term nonprogressive human immunodeficiency virus infection, *N. Engl. J. Med.* **332**: 209–216.

Plata, F., ed., 1989, HIV-specific cytotoxic T lymphocytes, *Res. Immunol.* **140**:89–95.

Procaccia, S., Lazzarin, A., Colucci, A., Gasparini, A., Forcellini, P., Lanzanova, D., Uberti Foppa, C., Novati, R., and Zanussi, C., 1987, IgM, IgG and IgA rheumatoid factors and circulating immune complexes in patients with AIDS and AIDS-related complex with serological abnormalities, *Clin. Exp. Immunol.* **67**:236–244.

Puppo, F., Ruzzenenti, R., Brenci, S., Lanza, L., Scudeletti, M., and Indiveri, F., 1991, Major histocompatibility gene products and human immunodeficiency virus infection, *J. Lab. Clin. Med.* **117**:91–100.

Riddell, S. R., and Greenberg, P. D., 1995, Principles for adoptive T cell therapy of human viral diseases, *Annu. Rev. Immunol.* **13**:545–586.

Roubaty, C., Bedin, C., and Charreire, J., 1990, Prevention of experimental autoimmune thyroiditis through the anti-idiotypic network, *J. Immunol.* **144**:2167–2172.

Sadat-Sowti, B., Debré, P., Idziorek, T., Guillon, J.-M., Hadida, F., Okzenhendler, E., Katlama, C., Mayaud, C., and Autran, B., 1991, A lectin-binding soluble factor released by CD8+CD57+ lymphocytes from AIDS patients inhibits T cell cytotoxicity, *Eur. J. Immunol.* **21**:737–741.

Salemi, S., Caporossi, A. P., Boffa, L., Longobardi, M. G., and Barnaba, V., 1995, HIV gp120 activates autoreactive CD4-specific T cell responses by unveiling of hidden CD4 peptides during processing, *J. Exp. Med.* **181**: 2253–2257.

Salk, J., Bretscher, P. A., Salk, P. L., Clerici, M., and Shearer, G. M., 1993, A strategy for prophylactic vaccination against HIV, *Science* **260**:1270–1272.

Schattner, A., 1988, Human immunodeficiency virus infection and autoimmune phenomena, *Am. J. Med.* **85**: 463–464.

Schneider, J., Kaaden, P., Copeland, T. D., Oroszlan, S., and Hunsmann, G., 1986, Shedding and interspecies type sero-reactivity of the envelope glycopolypeptide gp120 of the human immunodeficiency virus, *J. Gen. Virol.* **67**:2533–2538.

Schnittman, S. M., Psallidopoulos, M. C., Lane, H. C., Thompson, L., Baseler, M., Massari, F., Fox, C. H., Salzman, N. P., and Fauci, A., 1989, The reservoir for HIV-1 in human peripheral blood is a T cell that maintains expression of CD4. *Science* **245**:305–308.

Schwartz, L. M., and Osborne, B. A., 1993, Programmed death, apoptosis, and killer genes, *Immunol. Today* **14**:582–590.

Segel, L. A., Jager, E., Elias, D., and Cohen, I. R., 1995, A quantitative model of autoimmune disease and T-cell vaccination: Does more mean less? *Immunol. Today* **16**:80–84.

Sethi, K. K., Naher, H., and Stroehmann, I., 1988, Phenotypic heterogeneity of cerebro-spinal fluid-derived HIV-specific and HLA-restricted cytotoxic T-cell clones, *Nature* **335**:178–181.

Shearer, G. M., 1986, AIDS: An autoimmune pathologic model for the destruction of a subset of helper T lymphocytes, *Mt. Sinai J. Med.* **53**:609–615.

Siliciano, R. F., Lawton, T., Knall, C., Karr, R. W., Berman, P., Gregory, T., and Reinherz, E. L., 1988, Analysis of host–virus interactions in AIDS with anti-gp120 T cell clones: Effect of HIV sequence variation and a mechanism for CD4+ cell depletion, *Cell* **54**:561–575.

Silvestris, F., Williams, R. C., and Dammacco, F., 1995, Autoreactivity in HIV-1 infection: The role of molecular mimicry, *Clin. Immunol. Immunopathol.* **75**:197–205.

Simmonds, P., Beatson, D., Cuthbert, R. J. G., Watson, H., Reynolds, B., Peutherer, J. F., Parry, J. V., Ludlam, C. A., and Steel, C. M., 1991, Determinants of HIV disease progression: Six year longitudinal study in the Edinburgh haemophilia/HIV cohorts, *Lancet* **338**:1159–1163.

Steel, C. M., Beatson, D., Cuthbert, R. J. G., Morrison, H., Ludlam, C. A., Peutherer, J. F., Simmonds, P., and Jones, M., 1988, HLA haplotype A1 B8 DR3 as a risk factor for HIV-related disease, *Lancet* **332**:1185–1188.

Stricker, R. B., McHugh, T. M., Moody, D. J., Morrow, W. J. W., Stites, D. P., Shuman, M. A., and Levy, J. A., 1987, An AIDS-related cytotoxic autoantibody reacts with a specific antigen on stimulated CD4+ T cells, *Nature* **327**:710–713.

Tenner-Racz, K., Racz, P., Dietrich, M., Kern, P., Janossy, G., Veronese-Dimarzo, F., Klatzmann, D., Gluckman, J.-C., and Popovic, M., 1987, Monoclonal antibodies to human immunodeficiency virus: Their relation to the patterns of lymph nodes changes in persistent generalized lymphadenopathy and AIDS, *AIDS* **1**:95–104.

Terai, C., Kornbluth, R. S., Pauza, C. D., Richman, D. D., and Carson, D. A., 1991, Apoptosis as a mechanism of cell death in cultured T lymphoblasts acutely infected with HIV-1, *J. Clin. Invest.* **87**:1710–1715.

Texier, B., Bedin, C., Roubaty, C., Brezin, C., and Charreire, J., 1992, Protection from experimental autoimmune thyroiditis conferred by a monoclonal antibody to T-cell receptor from a cytotoxic hybridoma specific for thyroglobulin, *J. Immunol.* **148**:439–444.

Vandenbark, A. A., Hashim, G. A., and Offner, H., 1989, Immunization with a synthetic T-cell receptor V-region peptide protects against experimental autoimmune encephalomyelitis, *Nature* **341**:541–544.

van Eden, W., Holoshitz, J., Nevo, Z., Frenkel, A., Klajman, A., and Cohen, I. R., 1985, Arthritis induced by a T-lymphocyte clone that responds to *Mycobacterium tuberculosis* and to cartilage proteoglycans, *Proc. Natl. Acad. Sci. USA* **82**:5117–5120.

van Eden, W., Thole, J. E. R., van der Zee, R., Noordzij, A., van Embden, J. D. A., Hensen, E. J., and Cohen, I. R., 1988, Cloning of the mycobacterial epitope recognized by T lymphocytes in adjuvant arthritis, *Nature* **331**: 171–173.

van Laar, J. M., Miltenburg, A. M. M., Verdonk, M. J. A., Leow, A., Elferink, B. G., Daha, M. R., Cohen, I. R., deVries, R. R. P., and Breedveld, F. C., 1993, Effects of inoculation with attenuated autologous T cells in patients with rheumatoid arthritis, *J. Autoimmun.* **6**:159–167.

Venet, A., Gomard, E., and Levy, J.-P., 1993, Human T-cell responses to HIV, in: *Viruses and the Cellular Immune Response* (D. B. Thomas, ed.), Dekker, New York, pp. 165–200.

Vyakarnam, A., Matear, P. M., Cranenburg, C., Michie, C., Beverley, P. C. L., Wahren, B., Gill, S. K., and Weller, I., 1991, T cell responses to peptides covering the gag p24 region of HIV-1 occur in HIV-1 seronegative individuals *Int. Immunol.* **3**:939–947.

Wei, X., Ghosh, S. K., Taylor, M. E., Johnson, V. A., Emini, E. A., Deutsch, P., Lifson, J. D., Bonhoeffer, S., Nowak, M. A., Hahn, B. H., Saag, M. S., and Shaw, G. M., 1995, Viral dynamics in human immunodeficiency virus type 1 infection, *Nature* **373**:117–122.

Weinhold, K. J., Lyerly, H. K., Matthews, T. J., Tyler, D. S., Ahearne, M., Stine, K. C., Langlois, A. J., Durack, D. T., and Bolognesi, D. P., 1988, Cellular anti-gp120 cytolytic reactivities in HIV-1 seropositive individuals, *Lancet* **1**:902–905.

Weinhold, K. J., Lyerly, H. K., Stanley, S. D., Austin, A. A., Matthews, T. J., and Bolognesi, D. P., 1989, HIV-1 gp120-mediated immune suppression and lymphocyte destruction in the absence of viral infection, *J. Immunol.* **142**:3091–3097.

Weiss, R. A., 1993, How does HIV cause AIDS? *Science* **260**:1273–1279.

Whiteside, T. L., Elder, E. M., Moody, D., Armstrong, J., Ho, M., Rinaldo, C., Huang, X., Torpey, D., Gupta, P., McMahon, D., Okarma, T., and Heberman, R. B., 1993, Generation and characterization of ex vivo propagated autologous CD8+ cells used for adoptive immunotherpy of patients infected with human immunodeficiency virus, *Blood* **81**:2085–2092.

Young, A. T., 1988, HIV and HLA similarity, *Nature* **333**:215.

Zagury, D., Bernard, J., Halbreich, A., Bizzini, B., Carelli, C., Achour, A., Defer, M. C., Bertho, J. M., Lanneval, K., Zagury, J. F., Salaun, J. J., Lurhuma, Z., Mbayo, K., Aboud-Pirak, E., Lowell, G., Lebon, P., Burny, A., and Picard, O., 1992, One-year follow-up of vaccine therapy in HIV-infected immune-deficient individuals, *J. Acq. Immune Defic. Syndr.* **5**:676–681.

Zagury, J. F., Bernard, J., Achour, A., Asigen, A., Lachgar, A., Fall, L., Carelli, C., Issing, W., Mbika, J. P., Picard, O., Carlotti, M., Callebaut, I., Mornon, J. P., Burny, A., Feldman, M., Bizzini, B., and Zagury, D., 1993, Identification of CD4 and major histocompatibility complex functional peptide sites and their homology with oligopeptides from human immunodeficiency virus type 1 glycoprotein gp120: Role in AIDS pathogenesis, *Proc. Natl. Acad. Sci. USA* **90**:7573–7577.

Zarling, J. M., Ledbetter, J. A., Sias, J., Fultz, P., Eichberg, J., Gjerset, G., and Moran, P. A., 1990, HIV-infected humans, but not chimpanzees, have circulating cytotoxic T lymphocytes that lyse uninfected CD4+ cells, *J. Immunol.* **144**:2992–2998.

Zhang, J., and Raus, J., eds., 1995, *T Cell Vaccination and Autoimmune Disease*, Medical Intelligence Unit Series, R. G. G. Landes Co., Austin.

Zhang, J., Medaer, R., Stinissen, P., Hafler, D., and Raus, J., 1993, MHC-restricted depletion of human myelin basic protein-reactive T cells by T cell vaccination, *Science* **261:**1451–1454.

Ziegler, J. L., and Stites, D. P., 1986, Hypothesis: AIDS is an autoimmune disease directed at the immune system and triggered by a lymphocytic retrovirus, *Clin. Immunol. Immunopathol.* **41:**305–313.

Zinkernagel, R. M., and Hengartner, H., 1994, T-cell mediated immunopathology *versus* direct cytolysis by virus: Implications for HIV and AIDS, *Immunol. Today* **15:**262–268.

CHAPTER 29

HIV VACCINES

DANI P. BOLOGNESI

1. INTRODUCTION

The spread of HIV-1 infection that exploded on the scene in the 1980s continues in pandemic proportions and is having a major impact on public health worldwide. Although the rate of new infections in some parts of the world such as North America and Europe has stabilized, it is rising dramatically in parts of Asia, Latin America, and Africa. An effective prophylactic vaccine that can protect HIV-exposed individuals from infection and disease offers the best hope for combating this pandemic and is a global public health priority. More than 10 years has passed since the identification of HIV-1 as the cause of AIDS and despite intensive research, a path toward a vaccine remains cluttered with obstacles, disappointments, and knowledge gaps. Much of this dilemma stems from the unique features of the virus, particularly its genomic diversification, its multiple routes of infection, and its mechanisms of pathogenesis.

In most instances viral entry into the host occurs via free virions or infected cells following sexual intercourse. Virus is also transmitted at a high rate from mother to infant, and by direct entry into the bloodstream in drug addicts exchanging contaminated needles. Other modes of transmission, such as those found in doctor/patient relationships or in laboratory accidents, occur much less frequently. In aggregate, each of these presents different challenges for eventual application of vaccines or other prophylactic approaches.

Very little is known about the events that are associated with HIV entry and subsequent dissemination from the initial site of infection in a host. Such information may be crucial for vaccine strategies. Studies in the macaque model using simian immunodeficiency viruses (SIV) applied intravaginally (Miller *et al.*, 1989, 1994) provide the best insights to identify the initial target cells and tissues infected by the virus as well as its movement from the cervicovaginal mucosa to the blood (Spira *et al.*, 1996).

By contrast, extensive information about the primary viral syndrome that occurs after

---

DANI P. BOLOGNESI • Center for AIDS Research, Duke University Medical Center, Durham, North Carolina 27708.

Immunology of HIV Infection, edited by Sudhir Gupta. Plenum Press, New York, 1996.

exposure and entry has been obtained in HIV-infected humans. From studies performed with small cohorts of largely symptomatic patients, it appears that primary infection is characterized by extensive viral replication and dissemination resulting in high levels of plasma viremia (Albert *et al.*, 1987; Clark *et al.*, 1991; Daar *et al.*, 1991), and is often associated with an acute clinical viral syndrome (Tindall and Cooper, 1991). Within days to a few weeks, infected individuals mount vigorous humoral and cellular antiviral immune responses that are accompanied by dramatic decreases in plasma viremia and resolution of the acute clinical syndrome. Yet HIV-1 is neither eliminated from the body nor driven into complete latency as both a cell-free and a cell-associated viral burden persists. Following the acute phase, HIV-1 disease is usually characterized by an asymptomatic phase of variable duration with a mean time from HIV-1 infection to progression to AIDS of about 10 years (Pantaleo *et al.*, 1993a).

One of the more intriguing aspects of primary HIV infection relates to the dynamics of viral replication. Recent studies using quantitative analysis of viral RNA in plasma suggest that there is indeed a correlation between the steady-state levels of virus achieved within the first years of infection and the rate of disease progression (Mellors *et al.*, 1995). This "set point" may reflect the efficiency with which HIV was able to establish a pool of infected cells actively replicating the virus. The best evidence to date indicates that this probably occurs in secondary lymphoid organs rather than in blood (Pantaleo *et al.*, 1993b,c; Embretson *et al.*, 1993). During this early phase, the virus is remarkably homogeneous and this has implications for both vaccine and treatment strategies. Recent reports have in fact suggested that early treatment with nucleoside analogues may be effective (Loes *et al.*, 1995), possibly because drug resistance is more easily avoided (Ho, 1995).

The multicomponent responses appearing in association with acute infection are believed to play central roles in the initial suppression of viremia and the steady state in viral replication that is eventually achieved. It is likely that the subsequent course of disease is dictated by the balance between viral replication and the effectiveness of the host responses in suppressing or clearing the virus. Initial studies of the early immune responses have been documented (Albert *et al.*, 1990; Koup *et al.*, 1994) and while it remains unclear what mechanisms are at play for suppressing the viremic peak, the dramatic decline in plasma viremia from peak levels to the set point eventually established is pronounced and in some cases exceeds the suppression achieved by the most potent antivirals. At the same time the host immune response to the virus could also facilitate dissemination of virus by a number of possible mechanisms such as providing a more favorable milieu for viral replication resulting from immune activation (Fauci, 1993). Certain immune responses may also promote redistribution of virus from one compartment to another (e.g., from plasma to secondary lymphoid organs) (Montefiori *et al.*, 1994). Finally, immune pressure could also contribute toward selection of viral variants that are potentially more successful in propagating the infection and eventually the disease.

2. HISTORICAL PRINCIPLES OF VACCINE DEVELOPMENT

Many features of HIV are absent in viruses against which effective vaccines have been developed (Fig. 1). Antiviral vaccines have been successful against agents that exhibit a simple pathogenic profile and do not present complicating characteristics such as antigenic variation, latency, and immunopathogenicity that are characteristic of HIV. It follows that

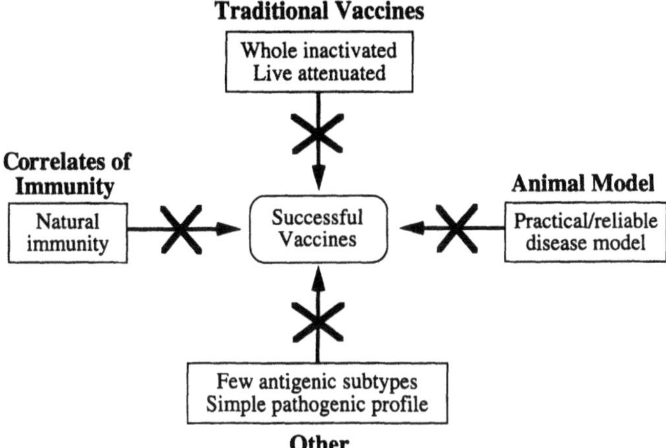

FIGURE 1. For most existing viral vaccines, the existence of natural immunity enabled correlates of immunity to be established and the rationale to use whole inactivated or live attenuated preparations. Simple pathogenic profiles and only limited antigenic diversity significantly reduced the complexity of vaccine development. Though not always critical, good animal models facilitated development of some vaccines. None of these principles have been successfully applied to HIV vaccine development to date (X).

most of the vaccines developed have been live attenuated or inactivated forms of the organism. If the host recovers from such an infection, lifelong immunity to subsequent exposures to the pathogen generally results. This natural immunity provides the rationale for developing vaccines since it signals that the pathogen harbors targets against which successful immune defenses can be mounted. Like the pathogen itself, the vaccine organisms would also be eliminated from the host after establishment of protective immunity, thus providing an important measure of safety. Such vaccines function not by preventing infection completely but rather the inducing antibodies that blunt the viremic phase and prevent the virus from reaching the target tissue in significant amounts. The limited infection that occurs is then cleared, most likely by the cellular arm of the immune system, and a long-term immunologic memory is established similar to that following host recovery from primary natural infection. In this group are viruses such as polio, measles, mumps, and rubella. Important breakthroughs such as development of methods to culture virus and identification of correlates of protection greatly accelerated the development of effective viral vaccines.

In the absence of natural immunity, one faces several serious obstacles: (1) correlates of protection become difficult to establish, (2) the rationale for live attenuated or whole inactivated vaccines is weakened because of concerns for safety, (3) the specter that all immune responses to the pathogen may not be beneficial must be resolved, and (4) the need to better understand virulence and how to overcome it becomes paramount. These issues are further complicated by several properties of HIV outlined above that have thwarted vaccine development against other organisms. Thus, empiricism that historically has been so dominant in vaccine development against viruses, gives way to a concerted effort to understand the fine details of infection and pathogenesis and how this is correlated with the ensuing host responses.

3. ANIMAL MODELS FOR HIV VACCINE DEVELOPMENT

When faced with such obstacles, vaccine developers have sometimes turned to animal models, especially in the search of immune correlates such as is the case with HIV. However, extensive vaccine studies in animal models with lentiviruses have been unable to provide uniform guiding principles or correlates of protection against infection. Vaccine studies have been performed in several animal species using feline (FIV), simian (SIV), and human (HIV-1 and HIV-2) immunodeficiency viruses. FIV and SIV induce disease in cats and several species of small monkeys while HIV infects chimpanzees, but with no disease sequelae. HIV-2 infects some macaques without disease, but studies in pigtailed macaques (*M. nemestrina*) and baboons surprisingly produced an AIDS-like fatal disease (McClure *et al.*, 1994; Barnett *et al.*, 1995). There are also models with chimeric viruses where the envelope of HIV-1 replaces that of SIV (SHIV) which grow in macaques and can be used to test the efficacy of HIV-1 envelope vaccine approaches (Li *et al.*, 1992; Shibata *et al.*, 1991). Finally, there are two models in SCID/Hu mice where infection with HIV-1 is possible and vaccine responses can be monitored by adoptive transfer of antibodies or cellular components (McCune *et al.*, 1988; Mosier *et al.*, 1993). Although some degree of HIV-1 infection of macaques (*M. nemestrina*) has been reported, this model has yet to be exploited in vaccine studies (Agy *et al.*, 1992).

Among these models, by far the most utilized are the SIV, HIV-1, and HIV-2 systems. However, the requirements for protection in each of these have been uneven, which has led to questions of their value for HIV vaccine development. This issue bears closer scrutiny. The differences between the models and the vaccine outcomes may reflect the respective virulence of the virus in a particular host (Fig. 2). Acute disease models induced by strains such as the SIVmac251 isolate are refractory to most vaccination attempts with the exception of live attenuated viruses and, to a lesser extent, whole inactivated virus approaches (Daniel *et al.*, 1992). On the other hand, a more moderate but nonetheless lethal

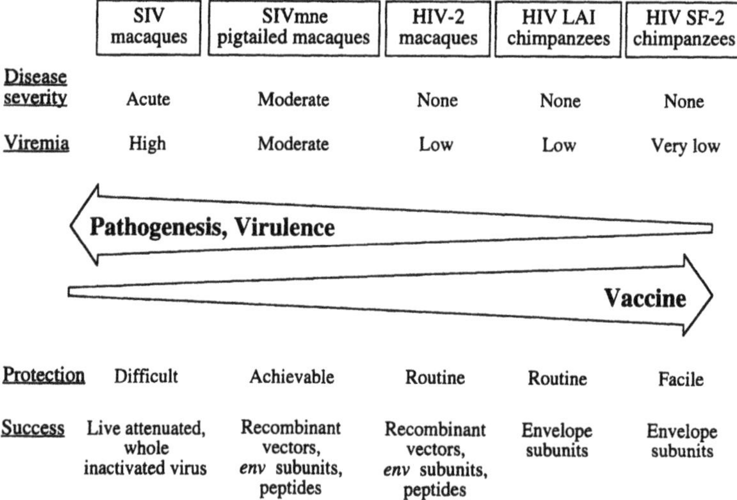

FIGURE 2. Relative vaccine efficacy in non-human primates infected with SIV, HIV-2, and HIV-1 suggests that viral pathogenesis/virulence correlates inversely with ease of vaccination.

disease course occurs in pigtailed macaques and HIV-1 infection in chimpanzees, neither of which has produced disease. All of this may reflect the measure of host control on the virus; the more effective this is, the more likely it is that a vaccine will be efficacious.

In aggregate, these observations may be related to the question of natural immunity in that even degrees of host control that fall short of complete clearance of the virus appear to be important. The overriding issue to be resolved is which, if any, of these models are the most representative of HIV infection and disease in humans and how best to utilize them. Possibly each one represents a segment of the overall spectrum of HIV infection in people roughly defined as rapid progressors (e.g., SIVmac251), intermediate progressors (SIVmne), and long-term nonprogressors (most macaque/HIV-1 models, chimpanzees/HIV-1).

4. THE FIRST WAVE OF HIV VACCINE CANDIDATES

Against this backdrop of uncertainty, vaccine manufacturers initially selected the HIV-1 chimpanzee model on which to base their vaccine development strategies. The principal reasons for this were that (1) chimpanzees could be infected with HIV-1, (2) the chimpanzee is phylogenetically similar to humans, and (3) there have been several indications of success with experimental vaccines, not necessarily based on live attenuated and whole inactivated virus approaches, but rather concepts such as viral subunits that were more practical, particularly from the standpoint of safety. There were, however, several limitations associated with this model. Principal among these is the absence of disease but also practical issues such as availability of animals and (until recently) the fact that only one HIV isolate was available for challenge.

Between 1985 and 1989 a number of vaccine-related studies were conducted in chimpanzees using a variety of immunogens but with little success in protection against virus challenge (for review see Girard and Eichberg, 1990). Much better results were obtained when immunogens were used that raised substantial levels of neutralizing antibodies (Berman *et al.*, 1990; Girard *et al.*, 1991). In these successful studies the titer of neutralizing antibodies, particularly antibodies directed to the third variable domain of the HIV *env* (the V3 loop), appeared to be the best correlate of protection. In an effort to demonstrate that *in vitro* neutralization is also important *in vivo*, Emini *et al.* (1992) used monoclonal antibodies to the V3 domain to obtain complete protection against infection of chimpanzees. Thus, a certain threshold of neutralizing antibodies to this region was sufficient for protection against parenteral infection with the homologous virus.

The combination of successful vaccine experiments against HIV-1 infection in chimpanzees using simple and safe approaches based on the HIV envelope with a potential correlate of protection in the form of neutralizing antibodies made plausible the hypothesis that such approaches could protect people against some HIV infections. This led to the development of several envelope products for testing in humans. The experimental trials conducted thus far have had as their major aim the assessment of safety and immunogenicity of such vaccines (Walker and Fast, 1994). They have included volunteers at low risk for HIV infection (Phase I) as well as individuals at higher risk (Phase II).

With currently more than 1600 subjects evaluated, the envelope products have been well tolerated and have accrued a remarkable record of safety, exhibiting no evidence of overt immunosuppression or any other form of immune impairment or autoimmune symptoms based on standard clinical and immunologic evaluations. However, the observations thus far do not exclude long-term side effects and continued monitoring of immunized individuals is important. When an immunized individual meets the virus is the next point where safety becomes an issue. This relates to the question of whether vaccine-induced responses could facilitate infection and accelerate disease. Whereas there are now over a dozen individuals who have become infected in HIV vaccine trials (Belshe *et al.*, 1993), it is too early to tell whether or not vaccination has influenced the course of infection in any way. Infections in vaccinees are important not only to determine issues related to safety but also to provide an opportunity to answer several important scientific questions that will be addressed later.

The immunogenicity profile of the various vaccine candidates has been studied in considerable depth. A wide variety of immunologic assays have been used to track vaccine

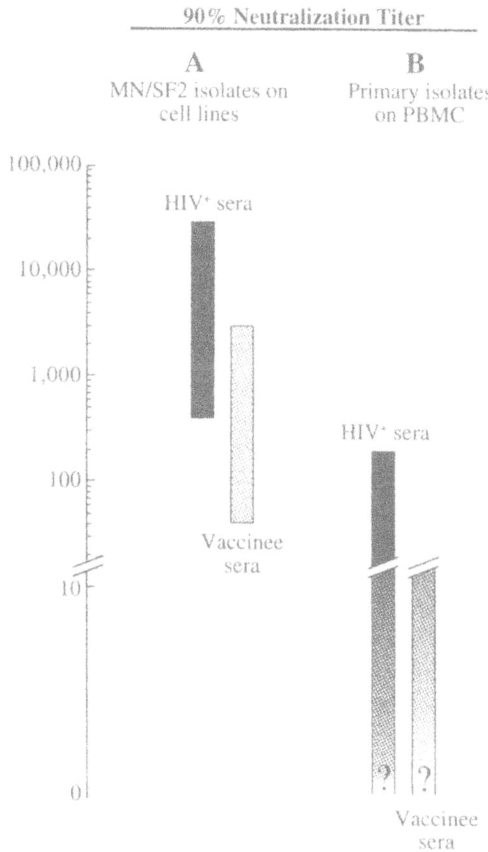

FIGURE 3. Neutralization of laboratory strains versus primary isolates. The bars indicate the range of neutralization titers of sera from HIV-1-infected individuals and uninfected volunteers who have been vaccinated with MN and SF-2 envelope glycoproteins on (A) laboratory isolates grown on T-cell lines (MN, SF-2) and (B) primary isolates (panel of 10) representative of clade B (origin of MN and SF-2) passaged only on peripheral blood mononuclear cells (PBMC). Note that sensitivity of neutralization of primary isolates drops dramatically with both sets of sera but that while a fraction of sera from HIV-1-infected individuals can still neutralize some of the isolates, none of the vaccinee sera tested register positive readings.

responses in human volunteers, with special attention on functional responses such as neutralizing antibodies and cytotoxic T cells. Recombinant envelope subunits have been the most extensively studied vaccines and have induced a broad range of neutralizing antibodies. By far the best responses have been achieved with products derived from mammalian expression systems that produce envelope products that approximate the native molecule (Walker and Fast, 1994). Such vaccines induce good levels of neutralizing antibodies when tested on the homologous virus grown on T-cell lines. The range of neutralizing antibodies in vaccinees receiving such immunogens overlaps that of infected individuals, though the mean titers are approximately one order of magnitude lower (Belshe *et al.*, 1993, 1994; Graham *et al.*, 1993). While there is some cross neutralization of other laboratory isolates belonging to the same virus genetic subtype or clade, the titers are between one and two orders of magnitude lower, indicating that the predominant response is, in the main, isolate specific.

The concept that neutralizing antibodies might represent a correlate of immunity against HIV infection remained a plausible hypothesis that was worthy of further clinical testing. Two vaccine products representing recombinant gp120 envelope subunits were moved forward to a placebo-controlled Phase II trial involving nearly 300 volunteers at high risk of HIV infection. Recruitment and execution of this trial were highly successful and the performance of the vaccines was similar to that in Phase I studies (McElrath *et al.*, 1994).

It was at this point that the question arose of proceeding to large definitive trials to evaluate efficacy of these vaccines. An issue that remained outstanding, however, was how well they matched the target viruses in the population virologically, immunologically, and genetically. The initial approach used to determine this was to evaluate their ability to induce antibodies capable of neutralizing fresh patient isolates using peripheral blood mononuclear cells (PBMC) as targets (Fig. 3). Although quite effective in their ability to induce neutralizing antibodies to HIV isolates that were adapted to T-cell lines, which actually overlapped with those found in HIV-infected individuals as noted earlier, the immune responses elicited by these vaccines have failed to neutralize fresh patient isolates on PBMC (Matthews, 1994; Hanson, 1994). The inability to demonstrate neutralizing activity against viruses circulating in the target population has prevented these vaccines from entering efficacy trials in the United States, at least until a better explanation for this phenomenon could be obtained.

5. THE DILEMMA OF POOR NEUTRALIZATION OF PRIMARY ISOLATES

That primary isolates might exhibit a radically different neutralization phenotype than viruses selected for growth in T-cell lines is surprising and was not considered in the strategies that generated the first wave of HIV vaccine candidates. Such a phenomenon is also unprecedented as a bottleneck for development of vaccines against other viruses. On the other hand, one might have forecast the relative neutralization resistance of primary isolates from their low susceptibility to soluble recombinant CD4 when compared to T-cell-line-adapted viruses (Daar *et al.*, 1990). The lack of therapeutic efficacy of recombinant CD4 observed *in vivo* thus portends for ineffectiveness of nonneutralizing or weakly neutralizing antibodies.

One of the first questions that these observations raise is whether or not primary isolates are inherently neutralization resistant. Indeed, it is not only vaccine-induced antibodies that neutralize these isolates poorly but also sera from HIV-infected individuals (Table I). However, good neutralization is occasionally observed with some HIV$^+$ sera and especially with monoclonal antibodies derived from HIV-infected individuals (Muster *et al.*, 1994; Burton *et al.*, 1994). The neutralization observed with monoclonal antibodies can completely block infectivity with as little as 0.1 μg of antibody. Moreover, certain monoclonal antibodies are able to neutralize a significant proportion of different primary isolates (T. Matthews and P. D'Souza, personal communication). Nonetheless, the sensitivity of T-cell-line-adapted viruses to neutralization by these monoclonal antibodies remains one to two orders of magnitude greater.

To what feature(s) of primary and T-cell-line-adapted viruses might one ascribe these differences? Among several possible explanations are the following:

1. Assay conditions are not comparable
2. Genomic diversity of the target virus
3. Structural differences in the viral envelopes

The major issue concerning the assay relates to the use of activated PBMC as target cells. Treatment of the cells with phytohemagglutinin (PHA) or other activating agents results in expression of adhesion molecules at the cell surface and viral stocks prepared in activated PBMC also incorporate such molecules during virion morphogenesis. It is believed that such molecules may play important roles in viral attachment to the target cell surface and thereby in infection. Conversely, neutralization of viruses bearing adhesion molecules by antibodies might be much less efficient. Two lines of evidence supporting these notions have been reported: (1) monoclonal antibodies to certain adhesion molecules facilitate neutralization by anti-HIV antibodies (Gomez and Hidreth, 1995) and (2) neutralization assays performed with primary viruses in resting PBMC are more sensitive than the corresponding assays in activated PBMC (Zolla-Pazner and Sharpe, 1995).

Virus heterogeneity may also be an important contributing factor. By and large, T-cell-line-adapted viruses are much more homogeneous than primary isolates, apparently representing a subpopulation that selectively grow in T-cell lines. The degree of heterogeneity is also an important factor particularly in relationship to how well it is matched with the antibodies present in the test serum. Much like development of resistance to antiviral agents, HIV diversification could result in virus that would not be susceptible to neutralization by a particular antibody population. If such are present even as a minority in a viral population, they would grow through in the presence of neutralizing antibodies. Neutralization escape variants have been documented in serum prophylaxis studies in chimpanzees (Emini *et al.*,

TABLE I. Neutralization Sensitivity of HIV Isolates

Target virus	HIV$^+$ sera[a]	Hu mAb[b]	Vaccine Ab[c]
T-cell-line-adapted	~10,000 (>80%)	~0.1 μg/ml (many)	~500
Primary isolates	~50 (10%)	~10 μg/ml (few)	0

[a]Representative 90% neutralization titers and percent sera positive.
[b]Relative amount of antibody required for 90% neutralization.
[c]Representative 90% neutralization titer in sera from human volunteers receiving subunit envelope vaccines.

1990) and in natural infections in chimpanzees (Rimsky-Clarke *et al.*, submitted for publication) and humans (M. Greenberg, personal communication).

Finally, there is also considerable information supporting the notion that several features of the envelopes of primary viruses are distinct from those of T-cell-line-adapted viruses. These are best reflected by different degrees of binding of monoclonal antibodies to the native oligomeric form of the envelope as displayed on the cell surface (Sattentau and Moore, 1995). As noted earlier, the apparent different features of the respective envelopes are also reflected in the differential susceptibility to blockade of infection by recombinant CD4 (Daar *et al.*, 1990). These observations have suggested that immunization with the native oligomeric envelope of a primary virus would be more effective that the monomeric subunits of T-cell-line-adapted viruses used this far. However, one must consider that the neutralizing antibodies found in HIV-infected individuals that probably arise in response to the native envelope are relatively ineffective except in rare instances.

Although there are other features that sharply distinguish primary isolates from T-cell-line-adapted viruses (Table II), the *in vivo* relevance of these differences is not known. To illustrate this point, a study was performed in chimpanzees with the two gp120 envelope vaccines mentioned earlier using a challenge virus (SF-2) that had never been grown in T-cell lines. Although this virus was not neutralized by the antibodies induced by the two envelope vaccines, protection was nevertheless achieved in two separate studies (El-Amad *et al.*, 1996; Berman *et al.*, 1996). While these studies have been criticized because of the lack of vigor of this challenge virus in chimpanzees, they nonetheless raise important cautions about the predictive value of *in vitro* tests.

6. CELLULAR RESPONSES AGAINST HIV INFECTION

There is ample rationale for an important role of cellular immunity in protection against HIV infection. Cellular responses to HIV, including cytotoxic lymphocytes (CTL), have been documented in individuals exposed to HIV but who did not seroconvert or become infected (Rowland-Jones *et al.*, 1995). Parallel observations of CTL activity in the absence of antibodies or infection have been reported in newborns (Rowland-Jones *et al.*, 1993). When compared to neutralizing activity against the autologous virus, CTL activity

TABLE II. Features of Primary and T-Cell-Line-Adapted Viruses

	T cell	Primary
Growth on T-cell lines	Yes	No
Growth on PBMC	Yes	Yes
Growth on monocytes	No	Yes
SI phenotype[a]	Yes	No
NSI phenotype[b]	No	Yes
Efficient neutralization by sCD4[c]	Yes	No
Efficient neutralization by Ab	Yes	No

[a]SI, syncytium-inducing.
[b]NSI, non-syncytium-inducing.
[c]Soluble recombinant CD4 receptor for HIV-1.

is a much better temporal correlate for the decline of the viremic peak typical of primary HIV infection (Koup *et al.*, 1994). Neutralizing antibodies are detectable sporadically and well after the acute viremic phase is resolved (Koup *et al.*, 1994). It has also long been recognized that anti-HIV CTL activity correlates with slower progression to disease (Walker and Plata, 1991) and is pronounced in long-term nonprogressors (Ferbas *et al.*, 1995).

HIV vaccine candidates that induce CTL activity include live recombinant vector strategies, DNA vaccines, and approaches based on synthetic peptides bearing CTL epitopes (Walker and Fast, 1994). By far the most extensive experience in human volunteers has been with live recombinant poxvirus vectors including vaccinia and canarypox. In strategies where vectors bearing the HIV envelope gene were used to prime the immune response and followed by boosting with recombinant envelope subunits, both CTL and neutralizing antibodies (still only to T-cell-line-adapted viruses) were induced (Cooney *et al.*, 1993). To date, the best CTL responses have occurred with the canarypox *env* construct (Egan *et al.*, 1995). They have appeared in roughly a quarter of the vaccinated volunteers and have reached levels of cytotoxicity of 75% at a 50:1 ratio of effector to target cells and some have persisted for over 200 days (Fig. 4) which is a good indication of immune memory (K. Weinhold, personal communication). Second- and third-generation vectors into which multiple HIV genes (*env*, *pol*, *gag*, *nef*) have been inserted should be capable of a much broader CTL response and such constructs have already or are about to enter clinical trials.

As for neutralizing antibodies, the challenges for CTL activity as a correlate of protection are many. To date, most of the assays used to study CTL employ B-cell lines infected by the recombinant vectors (Cooney *et al.*, 1993; Egan *et al.*, 1995). Very few studies have been done with HIV-infected cells, and none using primary isolates or CD4$^+$ T cells as targets. Such studies are needed to ascertain the effect of vaccine-induced CTL in a

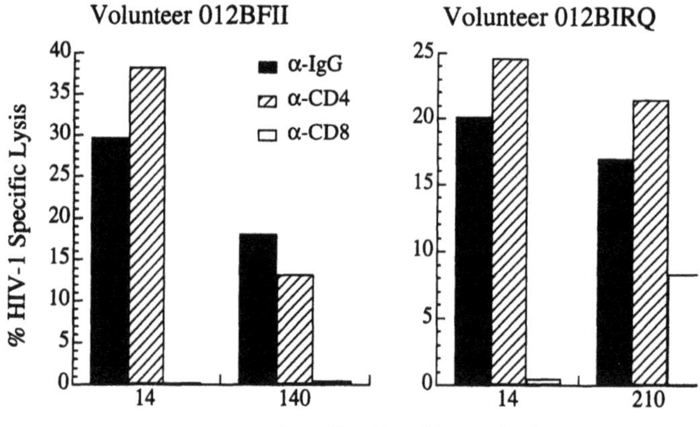

FIGURE 4. Persistence of anti-*env* CTL activity. HIV-specific CTL in human volunteers immunized with a recombinant avipox vector bearing the envelope gene of HIV. Depletion studies with anti-CD4, anti-CD8, and control (anti-IgG) reagents demonstrate the presence of CD8 CTL that persist for significant periods of time. (Studies performed by K. Weinhold in association with the AIDS Vaccine Evaluation Group of the National Institute of Allergy and Infectious Disease, National Institutes of Health.)

more relevant setting where virus-expressed antigens processed by cells infected by HIV *in vivo* become the targets of CTL activity. Also important is a measure of the frequency of CTL precursors and whether or not these are circulating or residing in tissues.

Not much is known about the role of other cellular responses, such as noncytolytic CD8 cells, that are able to suppress HIV replication (Walker *et al.*, 1986). Neither is it known what the proper balance should be between TH1 and TH2 responses. Mechanisms that involve both cellular and humoral reactivities such as antibody-dependent cellular cytotoxicity may also play important roles in protection against HIV infection.

7. GOALS OF VACCINATION AGAINST HIV

There are two major goals to be considered for an HIV vaccine:

1. To prevent infection
2. To attenuate viral infection so as to prevent disease

Prevention of the establishment of infection or induction of immunity able to clear infection are the most desirable goals. However, they are also the most difficult to achieve and may be out of reach for current vaccine strategies. On the other hand, attenuation of infection not only is a worthwhile goal for prevention of disease but by exerting a better control on viral replication, the degree of transmission may also be significantly reduced.

Attenuation of infection is also being recognized as an important objective as a result of natural history studies indicating that early steady-state levels of "set point" of virus load are predictive of the rate of progression to disease (Mellors *et al.*, 1995). Virus load might then represent a surrogate marker of vaccine efficacy even if infection occurs. More and more, studies in animal models support this concept. Even in the SIV acute disease models, several vaccine approaches that are ineffective at preventing infection have significantly impacted on the degree of viral replication and the onset of disease (Israel *et al.*, 1994; Hirsch *et al.*, 1994; Mossman *et al.*, 1996). Thus, if the goal of attenuation of viral replication is applied to the animal models, existing vaccine candidates are effective and possibly predictive of a similar outcome in people.

8. CONCLUDING REMARKS

With no clear path toward a vaccine in sight, it may be useful to reflect in hindsight on the experience over the past 10 years (Table III). For this discussion four general areas will be considered: (1) vaccine goals, (2) correlates of immunity, (3) animal models, and (4) clinical trials.

Until recently much of the focus of vaccination against HIV has been to block infection. This is based on the premise that allowing any degree of infection with this virus would eventually result in disease. Otherwise stated, once infection becomes established, host defenses would be unable to control the evolution of the viral quasispecies toward producing disease. With the realization that a subset of HIV-infected individuals, termed long-term nonprogressors, appear to be able to control the virus and can be spared of its pathogenic effects, the possibility that vaccination might bring about a similar outcome is becoming a focus of considerable attention. Thus, the extent of viral replication that can

TABLE III. What Has Been Learned from 10 Years of HIV Vaccine Research

	Past focus	New focus
Vaccine goals	Prevention of infection	Attenuation of infection
Correlates of protection	Virus neutralization	Other host defense mechanisms • Cellular • Humoral • Mucosal
Animal models	Empiric/convenient	Systematic • Model HIV infection in humans • Derive immune correlates • Tailor to vaccine goals

now be quantitated by sensitive PCR techniques and is a surrogate marker for disease progression, may indeed become an important indicator of eventual vaccine efficacy. While prevention of infection should remain a primary goal of vaccination, attenuation of infection can be a favorable outcome, but its ramifications, particularly long-term effects on the host and impact on transmission, must be carefully studied. Animal models using SIV (disease) but also HIV and SHIV (viral replication) can be vigorously exercised to test this concept.

To date, the major focus to establish correlates of protection has been in the role of neutralizing antibodies. This has roots in historical precedents that an effective antibody response is required to initially blunt infection wherever other host responses, notably the cellular arm of the immune system, are able to clear the residual infection. In this chapter the difficulties in harnessing neutralizing antibodies against HIV infection have been discussed, but the perspective that other immune responses play more important roles in controlling HIV is only beginning to be fully appreciated. Notable among these are the cellular responses, particularly cytotoxic T cells and CD8 cells that suppress HIV replication. Host responses that are able to both prevent infection and control viral replication that cannot be defined by classical effector mechanisms may be indicative of a unique balance of cytokines known to affect HIV replication (Fauci, 1993). Other forms of humoral and cellular responses should also be considered such as antibodies that promote attachment of the virus to complement or Fc receptors on cell surfaces. Such mechanisms may play important roles in viral clearance, on the one hand, but possibly also viral dissemination on the other (Montefiori *et al.*, 1994). The role of antibody-dependent cellular cytotoxicity (ADCC) to HIV, one of the earliest responses detectable during primary infection, may also be an important defense mechanism (K. Weinhold, personal communication). Finally, what is perhaps the initial barrier to the majority of HIV infection, the mucosal immune responses, loom as a primary target for vaccination and strategies toward this end, though still at the research stage, are receiving more and more attention (for review see Chapter 20).

Animal model studies will play an important role toward identifying promising vaccine approaches. However, as noted in the introductory comments, animal models have suffered from the lack of standardization from the perspective of primary (disease) or secondary endpoints (viremia). Comparison of results using models with different degrees of virulence have been difficult. This has perhaps exacerbated the frustrating search for correlates of protection and has certainly lessened the important role of the animal models as a guide for selection of vaccines for studies in people. Appreciation of this dilemma and efforts to make better use of the animal model toward these ends are critical elements for future progress in HIV vaccine development.

The ultimate tests for vaccine safety, immunogenicity, and efficacy require evaluation in human volunteers. Such studies are costly, labor-intensive, and employ elaborate infrastructures. Selection of vaccine candidates for entry into clinical trials necessitates that appropriate criteria be established such that the most promising approaches take precedence. Unless and until the animal model studies are established as good predictors for HIV vaccines, clinical trials in high-risk volunteers can provide important information for vaccine performance. Trial designs for testing a vaccine concept and facilitating decisions for movement of a vaccine toward definitive efficacy trials are being developed (Hoff and Lawrence, 1996).

An overall strategy one might follow for a vaccine approach is shown in Fig. 5. From concepts and principles derived from basic studies, the vaccine would proceed to animal model testing for efficacy, including both prevention and attenuation of infection. In such studies, attempts to derive correlates of protection would be made. Promising vaccines would then move to human trials initially for safety and immunogenicity assessment and then to a placebo-controlled "test of concept" study in high-risk volunteers. Appropriately designed, such a trial could either reject or accept a vaccine for further testing in a definitive efficacy trial or indicate, with less certainty, that additional studies might be warranted. Such trials might also provide valuable information for surrogate markers of disease progression (e.g., virus load) or immune correlates of protection. Definitive trials to prove ultimate efficacy of vaccines would validate markers of disease progression and correlates of protection that could then be used to more easily evaluate future generations of vaccine candidates.

The essential ingredients of such a path are (1) an effective discovery engine in academia and industry to uncover basic information and develop novel vaccine concepts, (2) an appropriate infrastructure to conduct preclinical testing of vaccine approaches in animal models, (3) a development program to produce and eventually market vaccine candidates for humans, and (4) an infrastructure elaborate for conducting all phases of clinical trial testing of vaccine candidates.

It follows that a close and effective partnership between government, academia, and industry must exist in order to maintain the impetus to create an effective HIV vaccine.

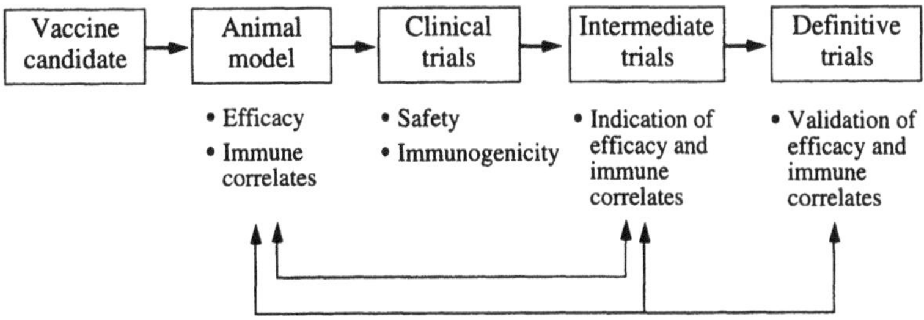

FIGURE 5. HIV vaccine development pathway. Animal models can best be used to identify promising vaccines and indications of immune correlates. Proof of concept (intermediate) trials would serve to accept or reject vaccines for further testing and to provide preliminary indication of correlates of protection. Definitive trial with vaccines would validate efficacy and correlates of protection.

One is now witnessing a waning interest of the private sector in maintaining HIV vaccine research and development programs. One can thus foresee the need for an enhanced role of government and academia, particularly in the discovery phase, along with sustained efforts to encourage industry to participate by developing the most promising candidates.

REFERENCES

Agy, M. B., Frumkin, L. R., Corey, L., Coombs, R. W., Wolinsky, S. M., Koehler, J., Morton, W. R., and Katz, M. G., 1992, Infection of Macaca nemestrina by human immunodeficiency virus type-1, *Science* **257**:103–106.

Albert, J., Gaines, H., Sonnerborg, A., Nystrom, G., Pehrson, P. O., Chiodi, F., von Sydow, M., Moberg, L., Lidman, K., and Christensson, B., 1987, Isolation of human immunodeficiency virus (HIV) from plasma during primary HIV infection, *J. Med. Virol.* **23**:67–73.

Albert, J., Abrahamsson, B., Nagy, K., Aurelius, E., Gaines, H., Nystrom, G., and Fenyo, E. M., 1990, Rapid development of isolate-specific neutralizing antibodies after primary HIV-1 infection and consequent emergence of virus variants which resist neutralization by autologous sera, *AIDS* **4**:107–112.

Barnett, S. W., Murthy, K. M., Herndier, B. G., and Levy, J. A., 1995, An AIDS-like condition is induced in baboons by HIV-2, *Science* **266**:642–646.

Belshe, R. B., Clements, M. L., and Dolin, R., 1993, Safety and immunogenicity of a fully glycosylated recombinant gp160 HIV-1 vaccine in low risk volunteers, *J. Infect. Dis.* **168**:1387–1395.

Belshe, R. B., Graham, B. S., and Keefer, M. C., 1994, Neutralizing antibody to HIV-1 in seronegative volunteers immunized with recombinant gp120 from the MN strain of HIV-1, *J. Am. Med. Assoc.* **272**:475–480.

Berman, P. W., Gregory, T. J., Riddle, L., Nakamure, G. R., Champe, M. A., Porter, J. P., Wurm, F. M., Hershberg, R. D., Cobb, E. K., and Eichberg, J. W., 1990, Protection of chimpanzees from infection by HIV-1 after vaccination with recombinant glycoprotein gp120 but not gp160, *Nature* **345**:622.

Berman, P. W., Murthy, K. K., Wrin, T., Vennari, J. C., Cobb, E. K., Eastman, D. J., Champe, M., Nakamura, G. R., Davison, D., Powell, M. F., Bussiere, J., Francis, D. P., Mathews, T., Gregory, T. J., and Obijeski, J. F., 1996, Protection of MN-rgp120–immunized chimpanzees from heterologous infection with a primary isolate of human immunodeficiency virus type 1, *J. Infect. Dis.* **173**:52–59.

Burton, D. R., Pyati, J., Koduri, R., Thornton, G. B., Sawyer, L. S. W., Hendry, R. M., Dunlop, N., Nara, P. L., Lamacchia, M., Garratty, E., Stiehm, E. R., Bryson, Y. J., Moore, J. P., Ho, D. D., and Barbas, C. F., III, 1994, Efficient neutralization of primary isolates of HIV-1 by a recombinant human monoclonal antibody, *Science* **266**:1024–1027.

Clark, S. J., Saag, M. S. Decker, W. D., Campbell-Hill, S., Roberson, J. L., Veldkamp, P. J., Kappes, J. C., Hahn, B. H., and Shaw, G. M., 1991, High titers of cytopathic virus in plasma of patients with symptomatic primary HIV-1 infection, *N. Engl. J. Med.* **324**:954–960.

Cooney, E. L., McElrath, M. J., Corey, L., Ju, S.-L., Collier, A. C., Arditti, D., Hoffman, M., Coombs, R. W., Smith, G. E., and Greenberg, P. D., 1993, Enhanced immunity to human immunodeficiency virus (HIV) envelope elicited by a combined vaccine regimen consisting of priming with a vaccinia recombinant expressing HIV envelope and boosting with gp160 protein, *Proc. Natl. Acad. Sci. USA* **90**:1882.

Daar, E. S., Li, X. L., Moudgil, T., and Ho, D. D., 1990, High concentrations of recombinant soluble CD4 are required to neutralize primary human immunodeficiency virus type 1 isolates, *Proc. Natl. Acad. Sci. USA* **87**:6674.

Daar, E. S., Moudgil, T., Meyer, R. D., and Ho, D. D., 1991, Transient high levels of viremia in patients with primary human immunodeficiency virus type 1 infection, *N. Engl. J. Med.* **324**:961–964.

Daniel, M. D., Kirchhoff, F., Czajak, S. C., Sehgal, P. K., and Desrosiers, R. C., 1992, Protective effects of a live attenuated SIV vaccine with a deletion in the nef gene, *Science* **258**:1938.

Egan, M. A., Pavlat, W. A., Tartaglia, J., Paoletti, E., Weinhold, K. J., Clements, M. L., and Siliciano, R. F., 1995, Induction of human immunodeficiency virus type 1 (HIV-1)-specific cytolytic T lymphocyte responses in seronegative adults by a nonreplication, host-range-restricted canarypox vector (ALVAC) carrying the HIV-MN *env* gene, *J. Infect. Dis.* **171**:1623–1627.

El-Amad, Z., Murthy, K. K., Higgins, K., Cobb, E. K., Haigwood, N. L., Levy, J. A., and Steimer, K. S., 1996, Resistance of chimpanzees immunized with recombinant $gp120_{SF2}$ to challenge by $HIV\text{-}1_{SF2}$, *AIDS 1995*, **9**:1313–1322.

Embretson, J., Zupancic, M., Ribas, J. L., Burke, A., Racz, P., Tenner-Racz, K., and Haase, A. T., 1993, Massive covert infection of helper T lymphocytes and macrophages by HIV during the incubation period of AIDS, *Nature* **362**:359–362.

Emini, E. A., Nara, P. L., and Scheif, W. A., 1990, Antibody-mediated *in vitro* neutralization of human immunodeficiency virus type 1 abolished infectivity for chimpanzees, *J. Virol.* **64**:3674–3678.

Emini, E. A., Schleif, W. A., Nunberg, J. H., Conley, A. J., Eda, Y., Tokiyoshi, S., Putney, S. D., Matsushita, S., Cobb, K. E., Jett, C. M., Eichberg, J. W., and Murthy, K. K., 1992, Prevention of HIV-1 infection in chimpanzees by gp120 V3 domain-specific monoclonal antibody, *Nature* **355**:728.

Fauci, A. S., 1993, Multifactorial nature of human immunodeficiency virus disease: Implications for therapy, *Science* **262**:1011–1018.

Ferbas, J., Kaplan, A. H., Hausner, M. A., Hultin, L. E., Matud, J. L., Liu, Z., Panicali, D. L., Nerng-Ho, H., Detels, R., and Giorgi, J. V., 1995, Virus burden in long-term survivors of human immunodeficiency virus (HIV) infection is a determinant of anti-HIV CD8+ lymphocyte activity, *J. Infect. Dis.* **172**:329–339.

Girard, M. P., and Eichberg, J. W., 1990, Progress in the development of SIV vaccines, *AIDS* **4**:S143.

Girard, M., Kieny, M. P., Pinter, A., Barre-Sinoussi, F., Nara, P., Kolbe, H., Kusumi, K., Chaput, A., Reinhart, T., and Muchmore, E., 1991, Immunization of chimpanzees confers protection against challenge with human immunodeficiency virus, *Proc. Natl. Acad. Sci. USA* **88**:542.

Gomez, M. P., and Hildreth, J. E. K., 1995, Antibody to adhesion molecule LFA-1 enhances plasma neutralization of HIV-1, *J. Virol.* **69**:4628–4632.

Graham, B. S., Matthews, T. J., and Belshe, R. B., 1993, augmentation of human immunodeficiency virus type 1 neutralizing antibody by priming with gp160 recombinant vaccinia and boosting with rgp160 in vaccinia-naive adults. The NIAID AIDS Vaccine Clinical Trials Network, *J. Infect. Dis.* **167**:533–537.

Hanson, C. V., 1994, Measuring vaccine-induced HIV neutralization: Report of a workshop, *AIDS Res. Hum. Retrovir.* **10**:645–648.

Hirsch, V. M., Goldstein, S., Elkins, W. R., London, W. T., Zack, P. M., Montefiori, D. C., and Johnson, P. R., 1994, Prolonged clinical latency and survival of macaques given a whole inactivated simian immunodeficiency virus vaccine, *J. Infect. Dis.* **170**:51–59.

Ho, D. D., 1995, Time to hit HIV, early and hard, *N. Engl. J. Med.* **333**:450–451.

Hoff, R., and Lawrence, D. N., 1996, Preparation for vaccine trials, in: *Development and Applications of Vaccines and Gene Therapy in AIDS Antibiotics and Chemotherapy*, Volume 48 (G. Giraldo, ed.) S. Karger A.G., Basel, Switzerland.

Israel, Z. R., Edmonson, P. F., Maul, D. H., O'Neil, S. P., Mossman, S. P., Thiriart, C., Fabry, L., van Opstal, O., Bruck, C., Bex, F., Burny, A., Fultz, P. N., Mullins, J. I., and Hoover, E. A., 1994, Incomplete protection, but suppression of virus burden, elicited by subunit simian immunodeficiency virus vaccines, *J. Virol.* **68**:1843–1853.

Koup, R. A., Safrit, J. T., Cao, Y., Andrews, C. A., McLeod, G., Borkowsky, W., Farthing, C., and Ho, D. D., 1994, Temporal association of cellular immune responses with the initial control of viremia in primary human immunodeficiency virus type I syndrome, *J. Virol.* **68**:4650–4655.

Li, J., Lord, C. I., Haseltine, W., Letvin, N. L., and Sodroski, J., 1992, Infection of cynomolgus macaques with a chimeric HIV-1/SIV mac virus that expresses the HIV-1 envelope glycoprotein, *J. Acq. Immune Defic. Syndr.* **5**:639–646.

Loes, S. K. L., Hirschell, B. J., Hoen, B., and Cooper, D. A., 1995, A controlled trial of zidovudine in primary human immunodeficiency virus infection, *N. Engl. J. Med.* **333**:408.

McClure, J., Scheibel, M., Anderson, D., Steele, J., Misher, L., Morton, W., and Hu, S.-L., 1994, Pathogenicity and infectivity of HIV-1 in macaques, in: *Abstract Book* Volume 1, Tenth International Conference on STB, Yokohama, Japan, p. 60, Abstract #193A.

McCune, J. M., Namikawa, R., Kaneshima, H., Shultz, L. D., Lieberman, M., and Weissman, I. L., 1988, The SCID-hu mouse: Murine model for the analysis of human hematolymphoid differentiation and function, *Science* **241**:1632–1639.

McElrath, M. J., Corey, L., Clements, M. L., Belshe, R., Keefer, M., Graham, B., Fast, P., Matthews, T., Duliege, A. M., Francis, D., and the NIAID AVEG, 1994, A phase II HIV vaccine trial in seronegative subjects: Safety, immunogenicity and future direction, in: *Abstract Book* Volume 1, Tenth International Conference on STB, Yokohama, Japan, p. 91, Abstract #317A.

Matthews, T. J., 1994, Dilemma of neutralization resistance of HIV-1 field isolates and vaccine development, *AIDS Res. Hum. Retrovir.* **10**:631–632.

Mellors, J. W., Kingsley, L. A., Rinaldo, C. R., Todd, J. A., Hoo, B. S., Kokka, R. P., and Gupta, P., 1995,

Quantitation of HIV-1 RNA in plasma predicts outcome after seroconversion, *Ann. Intern. Med.* **122:** 573–579.

Miller, C. J., Alexander, N. J., Sutjipto, S., Lackner, A. A., Gettie, A., Hendrickx, A. G., Lowenstine, L. J., Jennings, M., and Marx, P. A., 1989, Genital mucosal transmission of simian immunodeficiency virus, *J. Virol.* **63:**4277–4284.

Miller, C. J., Marthas, M., Torten, J., Alexander, N. J., Moore, J. P., Doncel, G., and Hendrickx, A., 1994, Intravaginal inoculation of rhesus macaques with cell free simian immunodeficiency virus results in persistent or transient viremia, *J. Virol.* **68:**6391–6400.

Montefiori, D. C., Graham, B. S., Zhou, J. Y., Zhou, J. T., and Ahearn, J. M., 1994, Binding of human immunodeficiency virus type 1 to the C3b/C4b receptor, CR1 (CD35), and red blood cells in the presence of envelope-specific antibodies and complement, *J. Infect. Dis.* **170:**429–432.

Mosier, D. E., Culizia, R. J., Macisaac, P. D., Corey, L., and Greenberg, P. D., 1993, Resistance to human immunodeficiency virus I infection of SCID mice reconstituted with peripheral blood leukocytes from donors vaccinated with vaccinia gp160 and recombinant gp160, *Proc. Natl. Acad. Sci. USA* **90:**2443–2447.

Mossman, S. P., Bex, F., Berglund, P., Arthos, J., O'Neil, S. P., Riley, D., Maul, D. H., Bruck, C., Momin, P., Burny, A., Fultz, P. N., Mullins, J. L., Liljestrom, P., and Hoover, E. A., 1996, Protection against lethal SIVsmmPBj14 disease by recombinant Semliki Forest virus gp160 vaccine and by a gp120 subunit vaccine, *J. Virol.* **70**:1953–1960.

Muster, T., Guinea, R., Trkola, A., Purtscher, M., Steindl, F., Palese, P., and Katinger, H., 1994, Cross-neutralizing activity against divergent human immunodeficiency virus type 1 isolates induced by the gp41 sequence ELDKWAS, *J. Virol.* **68:**4031–4034.

Pantaleo, G., Graziosi, C., and Fauci, A. S., 1993a, Mechanisms of disease: The immunopathogenesis of human immunodeficiency virus infection, *N. Engl. J. Med.* **328:**324–335.

Pantaleo, G., Graziosi, C., Demarest, J. F., Butini, L., Montroni, M., Fox, C. H., Orenstein, J. M., Kotler, D. P., Fauci, A. S., 1993b, HIV infection is active and progressive in lymphoid tissue during the clinically latent stage of disease, *Nature* **362:**355–358.

Pantaleo, G., Graziosi, C., Demarest, J. F., Butini, L., Montroni, M., Fox, C. H., Orenstein, J. M., Kotler, D. P., and Fauci, A. S., 1993c, HIV infection is active and progressive in lymphoid tissue during the clinically latent stage of disease, *Nature* **362:**355–358.

Rimsky-Clarke, L., Weinhold, K. J., Arthur, L. O., Hassler, L. E., Kosloff, B., Wakefield, D., Bolognesi, D. P., and Matthews, T. J., 1996, HIV-1 evasion from immune response: Dynamic evolution in a chimpanzee of both virus and anti-HIV-1 humoral immune response, *J. Virol.* (submitted for publication).

Rowland-Jones, S. L., Nixon, D. F., Aldhous, M. C., Gotch, F., Ariyoshi, K., Hallam, N., Kroll, J. S., Froebel, K., and McMichael, A. J., 1993, HIV-specific CTL activity in an HIV-exposed but uninfected infant, *Lancet* **341:**860–861.

Rowland-Jones, S. L., Sutton, J., Ariyoshi, K., Dong, T., Gotch, F., McAdam, S., Whitby, D., Sabally S., Gallimore, A., Corrah, T., Takiguchi, M., Schultz, T., McMichael, A. J., and Whittle, H., 1995, HIV-specific cytotoxic T cells in HIV-exposed but uninfected Gambian women, *Nature Med.* **1:**59–64.

Sattentau, Q. J., and Moore, J. P., 1995, HIV-1 neutralization is determined by epitope exposure on the gp120 oligomer, *J. Exp. Med.* **182:**185–196.

Shibata, R., Kawamura, M., Sakai, H., Hayami, M., Ishimoto, A., and Adachi, A., 1991, Generation of a chimeric human and simian immunodeficiency virus infectious to monkey peripheral blood mononuclear cells, *J. Virol.* **65:**3514–3520.

Spira, A. I., Marx, P. A., Patterson, B. K., Mahoney, J., Koup, R. A., Wolinsky, S. M., and Ho, D. D., 1995, Cellular targets of infection and route of viral dissemination following an intravaginal inoculation of SIV into rhesus macaques, *J. Exp. Med.* **183:**215–225.

Tindall, B., and Cooper, D. A., 1991, Primary HIV infection: Host responses and intervention strategies, *AIDS* **5:** 1–14.

Walker, B. D., and Plata, F., 1991, Cytotoxic T lymphocytes against HIV, *AIDS* **4:**177–184.

Walker, C. M., Moody, D. J., Stites, D. P., and Levy, J. A., 1986, CD8+ lymphocytes can control HIV infection *in vitro* by suppressing virus replication, *Science* **234:**1563–1566.

Walker, M. C., and Fast, P. E., 1994, Clinical trials of candidate AIDS vaccines, *AIDS* **8(Suppl. 1):**213–236.

Zolla-Pazner, S., and Sharpe, S., 1995, A resting cell assay for improved detection of antibody-mediated neutralization, *AIDS Res. Hum. Retrovir.* **11:**1449–1458.

CHAPTER 30

GENE THERAPY

RICHARD A. MORGAN

1. INTRODUCTION

Therapeutic strategies for intervening in HIV disease currently include antiretroviral therapy, treatment and prophylaxis of opportunistic infections, antitumor therapy, immunomodulator therapy, and immunologic restoration using the immune-based therapies described in this book. There are, however, some significant practical and theoretical difficulties with available antiretroviral agents. Although mortality and frequency of opportunistic infections are reduced in patients taking zidovudine, a complete and sustained improvement in immune status has not been achieved (Fischl *et al.*, 1989). In addition, frequent toxic effects prevent many individuals from tolerating these drugs for extended periods (Richman *et al.*, 1987). Recent *in vitro* evidence of retroviral resistance has also been presented, although the clinical importance of this is as yet unknown (Larder *et al.*, 1989). In hopes of increasing efficacy and reducing toxicity, studies are now under way examining the potential role of combination therapies for HIV infection (Fauci, 1992). Such approaches include combined therapy with two or more agents from the same class [e.g., reverse transcriptase (RT) inhibitors] or from distinct classes with different mechanisms of action (e.g., RT inhibitors plus immunomodulators). Despite the major advances in treating HIV disease that have occurred in the past 5 years, it is clear that the need is still great for more efficacious, less toxic therapies with novel mechanisms of action. It is therefore important to explore and develop new modalities for the treatment of this deadly disease. Gene therapy, defined as the introduction of new genetic material into cells of an individual with resulting therapeutic benefit to the individual, may be an effective treatment for a variety of disorders (Anderson, 1984; Morgan and Anderson, 1993). Since HIV integrates itself into the host's genome, AIDS can be considered an "acquired genetic disease" and thus potentially amenable to treatment using gene therapy.

Gene therapy for HIV requires the introduction of anti-HIV genes into cells, to prevent

RICHARD A. MORGAN • Clinical Gene Therapy Branch, National Center for Human Genome Research, National Institutes of Health, Bethesda, Maryland 20892.

Immunology of HIV Infection, edited by Sudhir Gupta. Plenum Press, New York, 1996.

or inhibit HIV gene expression or function and consequently to limit HIV replication and AIDS pathogenesis. This concept was termed *intracellular immunization* by David Baltimore and has been the subject of recent reviews (Gilboa and Smith, 1994; Vanden-Driessche *et al.*, 1994; Yu *et al.*, 1994). Anti-HIV gene therapy offers new opportunities for the intervention of HIV replication at the molecular level, such as the possibility to target conserved *cis*-acting regulatory sequences or essential HIV proteins. A combination of different anti-HIV genes can be simultaneously introduced into cells to target multiple stages in the viral life cycle. Anti-HIV gene therapy can also be used to downregulate HIV gene expression. Interest in decreasing HIV gene expression is receiving increasing emphasis because of results suggesting virus-independent pathology associated with Tat, Env, and Vpr proteins (Banda *et al.*, 1992; Ensoli *et al.*, 1990; Jowett *et al.*, 1995). This chapter will describe (1) technologies used to transfer genetic material, (2) cells that are potential targets for engineering, (3) potential anti-HIV gene therapy strategies, and (4) the presently approved HIV gene therapy clinical trials.

2. GENE TRANSFER METHODS

In order for gene therapy to be effective, it is vital to efficiently deliver genes to the target cells. A variety of gene delivery systems including viral vectors based on retrovirus, adenovirus, and adeno-associated virus, as well as non-virus-based gene transfer techniques are currently being evaluated for their effectiveness for gene delivery (Mulligan, 1993; Morgan and Anderson, 1993). Of the many different virus-mediated gene transfer systems under development, only two are likely to be useful in anti-HIV gene therapy protocols because of their potential to stably introduce therapeutic gene; these are retroviral vectors and adeno-associated viral vectors. While the initial emphasis in gene therapy research has been on viral transfer systems, nonviral gene transfer methods are receiving increasing study as alternatives to viral vectors.

2.1. Nonviral Transfer Methods

Non-virus-mediated gene transfer systems include liposomes, molecular conjugates, receptor ligands, direct injection of naked DNA, and particle-mediated gene transfer (Ledley, 1995). The main advantage of these systems over viral vectors is that there is no cotransfer of unwanted viral genetic material to the cell, and they lend themselves more readily to large-scale manufacturing conditions. These gene transfer methods are effective in situations where transient expression of the gene product is desired. To date, direct DNA injection, lipid-mediated gene transfer, and particle-mediated gene transfer have been approved for clinical experimentation.

Gene transfer via cationic lipid (commonly, but incorrectly referred to as liposomes) DNA complexes has been shown to be capable of mediating high-level *in vitro* gene transfer ($>$ 90% for some cells) and direct *in vivo* gene transfer has been accomplished and appears to be associated with minimal toxicity (Felgner *et al.*, 1987; Stewart *et al.*, 1992; Nabel *et al.*, 1992; Lin *et al.*, 1990). While in standard lipid–DNA preparations there is no specificity to the gene transfer process, localized *in vivo* uptake and expression has been reported in blood vessel walls and tumor deposits following direct *in situ* administration. Although various lipid combinations have been shown to have quantitatively different gene transfer efficiencies (in different cell types), there is no consensus as to the optimal features for lipid-mediated gene delivery. Further, the main disadvantage of lipid-mediated gene transfer, as well as for most nonviral transfer techniques, is that stable/long-term gene transfer has not been accomplished and thus repeated administrations would be necessary to effect continued gene expression.

Particle-mediated gene transfer is performed by coating DNA onto submicroscopic particles (usually made of gold) and accelerating them at a speed sufficient to "shoot" them into cells. One major advantage of particle bombardment is the very large number of plasmid DNA molecules that can be coated onto the surface of individual beads. Thus, for any given cell that receives a gold particle, the number of transferred transgenes is very high (in the thousands). Particle bombardment technology has recently been utilized to deliver the Rev M10 *trans*-dominant negative protein to human $CD4^+$ lymphocytes (Woffendin *et al.*, 1994). The efficacy of particle-mediated gene transfer was equal to retrovirus-mediated gene transfer, with the initial levels of gene transfer ranging between 0.1 and 10%. While the majority of the gene expression resulting from particle bombardment was transient, long-term gene transfer can be obtained at reduced efficiencies. This experiment demonstrates the potential for the use of particle-mediated gene transfer in HIV gene therapy.

2.2. Retrovirus-Mediated Gene Transfer

Retrovirus-based gene transfer vectors are currently one of the most widely used and highly effective gene transfer systems available. Sophisticated molecular biology techniques have led to the development of a family of vectors that utilize the effective replication and integration mechanisms of retroviruses to stably transfer genes into a wide variety of cell types, such as hepatocytes and peripheral blood lymphocytes (Miller, 1992; Morgan, 1994; Mulligan, 1993). In retrovirus-mediated gene transfer, the inherent separation of the protein coding domains from the *cis*-acting regulatory elements is taken advantage of to create an efficient gene transfer system. The first retroviral vectors were produced by inserting intact genes into naturally occurring deleted retrovirus genomes. These defective viruses are rescued with replication-competent helper virus. Because these vectors require helper virus for infection, their use was limited. The elucidation that retroviruses have a defined packaging element within the 5′ region of their RNAs prompted a greatly expanded effort by many laboratories to develop designs for retroviral vectors (Mann *et al.*, 1983; Armentano *et al.*, 1987; Adam and Miller, 1988).

Current vectors can routinely generate titer between 10^6 and 10^7 cfu/ml and can be used to transduce many kinds of primary cells. The main limitation to the existing retroviral vectors is that they cannot transduce nondividing cells. A wide variety of retroviral designs now exist from simple one-gene LTR-driven vectors to complex multigene vectors that use internal promoters. No one design has been shown to be consistently better than any other and it is usually helpful to construct a few different designs and evaluate them before committing to a specific vector.

Retrovirus packaging cell lines provided all of the proteins required to assemble a functional retroviral vector. The development of packaging cell lines has progressed through three generations, with each generation becoming more complex. The first-generation packaging cell lines were constructed by deletion of the retrovirus packaging elements from the replication-competent retroviral genome (Mann *et al.*, 1983). The principle behind these cell lines was that the virus genome synthesized all of the native proteins, but the genomic RNA was inefficiently packaged into virions, while the recombinant retroviral vector genome, containing the packaging elements, would efficiently be packaged into virions. Further retroviral genome modifications led to the second-generation packaging cell lines. The new packaging cell lines contained multiple deletions in the 5′ and 3′ regulatory elements in addition to the deletion of the packaging elements. An example of the second-generation packaging cell line is PA317 (Miller and Buttimore, 1986). The third generation of packaging cell lines utilize two modified genomes in combination to provide the necessary viral proteins. The packaging cell lines Psi-CRIP, GP&E86, and PG13 are examples of third-generation cell lines in which the *gag/pol* and *env* protein coding regions are supplied on different plasmids (Danos and Mulligan, 1988; Markowitz *et al.*, 1988; Miller *et al.*, 1991). The principle behind these new generation cell lines is that they will require multiple recombination events in order to produce a replication-competent retrovirus.

One of the essential principles behind the development of packaging cell lines is the capability to pseudotype vector-derived virus with envelope components of retroviruses that have a specific host range. The retrovirus envelope protein is the major determinant in viral tropism (host range). In a study designed to improve gene transfer into human lymphocytes, we demonstrated that a packing cell line based on the Gibbon ape leukemia virus affords high-efficiency gene transfer into human lymphocytes (Bunnell *et al.*, 1995). Most recently, it has been shown that nonretroviral envelopes, such as VSV-G, can also be used to construct retrovirus packaging cell lines (Burns *et al.*, 1993; Yang *et al.*, 1995).

2.3. Adeno-Associated Virus Vectors

The only other viral gene transfer system that has the potential to undergo efficient stable gene transfer is based on adeno-associated virus (AAV). AAV is a small single-stranded DNA parvovirus of length 4.7 kb. The AAV genome consists of two proteins Cap (which produces the structural capsid proteins) and Rep (which makes the proteins associated with replication and chromosomal integration). AAV is a defective virus and requires coinfection with a helper virus (usually adenovirus but herpesvirus can also provide helper function) in order to complete an infectious cycle. While vectors based on AAV can only accept small inserts (< 4.2 kb), it has a theoretical advantage of being able to undergo specific integration into a small region of human chromosome 19 (Muzyczka, 1992; Samulski, 1994). Site-specific integration is a unique and highly desirable event for a gene transfer vector, but while it occurs at a reasonable frequency in wild-type AAV infections, it has not yet been shown to occur with AAV vectors.

To make recombinant AAV vectors, the Cap and Rep proteins are removed, leaving the inverted terminal repeat (ITR) sequences (the ITRs are necessary for replication and integration). A promoter and gene of interest are then inserted in place of the Rep and Cap. To produce recombinant AAV vector particles, the AAV vector is transfected into a human cell line along with a second plasmid that independently expresses the Rep and Cap proteins. The transfected cells must next be infected with the helper virus (adenovirus). Amplification of the AAV vector occurs over the next 1–2 days. The cells are then lysed, adenovirus is destroyed by heat inactivation, and recombinant AAV vector particles purified (usually by CsCl gradient centrifugation). Packaging cell lines necessary to simplify the process of AAV vector production are under development but are hampered by the toxicity of the Rep protein. The use of AAV vectors in human gene therapy experimentation is increasing but their utility remains to be established. Conflicting reports concerning the ability of the recombinant vectors to integrate into targets cells have appeared (Halbert *et al.*, 1995; Alexander *et al.*, 1994). It appears that AAV can remain episomal in nondividing cells and that true stable integrated gene transfer does not occur at high efficiency.

3. TARGET CELLS

3.1. Hematopoietic Stem Cells

The dominant sites of HIV infection and replication are cells of lymphoid and myeloid origin. In order for HIV gene therapy to be effective, it is vital that cells derived from these lineages be utilized as recipients for anti-HIV gene therapeutics. The pluripotent hematopoietic stem cells (HSCs) generate all cells of lymphoid and myeloid origin; therefore, these cells are the ideal candidates for use in gene therapy. In theory, permanent protection from HIV infection could be achieved through the introduction of anti-HIV genes into HSCs because these cells are self-regenerating. It is not currently possible to isolate pure HSC populations, but several enrichment techniques based on selection for $CD34^+$ cells have been developed. The $CD34^+$ enriched cells isolated from bone marrow, mobilized peripheral blood cells, or umbilical cord blood have been used for *in vivo* analysis (Rill *et al.*, 1992; Van Beusechem *et al.*, 1992; Kohn *et al.*, 1994). Unfortunately, the level of gene transfer into these cells is very low (1 to 10%) and the cells that express the introduced gene may eventually extinguish expression by silencing the promoter contained in the expression vector (Apperly *et al.*, 1991; Challita and Kohn, 1994). Improvements in gene transfer technology may eventually make HSCs viable candidates for use in gene therapy.

3.2. Lymphocytes

Because of the inefficiency of gene transfer into HSCs, investigators have turned to the major host cell of HIV, the mature $CD4^+$ T cell, as an alternative target for gene therapy. The $CD4^+$ lymphocytes are more desirable because of their ease of isolation from the peripheral blood, ease of enrichment for $CD4^+$ cells by depletion of $CD8^+$ cells, high levels of transduction can be achieved, and the cells can be expanded in tissue culture prior to reinfusion into a patient (Bunnell *et al.*, 1995). The questions surrounding the use of $CD4^+$ lymphocytes for gene therapy deal with the *in vivo* growth potential and life span of the cells. Early investigations using nonhuman primates revealed that a small number of transduced autologous T cells could be recovered from the peripheral blood of rhesus monkeys 2 years after a single injection of gene-marked cells (Culver *et al.*, 1990). Human studies using gene-marked tumor-infiltrating lymphocytes (TIL) demonstrated that reinfused transduced TIL cells survived several weeks (Rosenberg *et al.*, 1990). Recent primate studies using autologous $CD4^+$ lymphocytes indicate that vector-transduced lymphocytes survive for several months in the peripheral blood and lymph nodes of rhesus monkeys (Bunnell *et al.*, unpublished observations). A gene-making clinical protocol involving identical twins suggests that the *NeoR*-marked lymphocytes survive at low levels for up to 44 weeks in HIV-infected individuals (see below).

Further results from the adenosine deaminase (ADA-SCID) human gene therapy trial indicate that the infused lymphocytes survive and divide for up to 4 years after infusion of the cells (Blaese *et al.*, 1995). Two patients with severe combined immunodeficiency (SCID) related to adenosine deaminase deficiency have been treated with infusions of autologous lymphocytes transduced with the ADA gene via a retroviral vector. To date, no significant side effects have occurred and immunologic benefit has been observed. Continuous circulation of modified cells for the 51 months of observation has been seen in the first patient enrolled on the protocol, including a 28-month period when this patient received no additional infusions of cells. ADA levels in the circulating T cells have increased from initially undetectable levels to approximately 50% of those measured in the carrier parents. The studies of these children with SCID demonstrate that significant reconstitution of T-cell function can be achieved in immunodeficient patients with infusions of autologous genetically engineered polyclonal T cells. Since enhanced immune function has been observed in children with inherently defective T cells, it is possible that infusion of anti-HIV engineered T cells may be helpful in reconstituting immune function in HIV-infected individuals.

4. ANTI-HIV GENE THERAPY STRATEGIES

Many molecular strategies have been developed to inhibit HIV *in vitro*. The strategies described below are examples of those approaches in clinical trial or those proposed for clinical experimentation.

4.1. RNA Decoys

This technique disrupts the normal interaction of HIV regulatory proteins with their *cis*-acting regulatory elements through the overexpression of short RNA molecules that compete with the viral RNAs for binding of proteins that are required for viral replication. The TAR (transactivation response) and RRE (Rev-response element) are two such viral regulatory elements (binding the Tat and Rev proteins, respectively). The antiviral activity of the TAR element decoys was examined by retrovirus-mediated gene transfer into CEM-SS cell lines *in vitro*. Overexpression of the TAR decoys inhibited Tat-mediated transcriptional activation and markedly reduced HIV replication for up to 30 days after challenge with laboratory HIV isolates (Sullenger *et al.*, 1991). Expression of a polymeric TAR decoy containing up to 50 TAR repeats has been demonstrated to effectively inhibit HIV replication in T-cell lines and primary lymphocytes (Lisziewicz *et al.*, 1993). It is clear that the overexpression of TAR and RRE decoys has strong antiviral activity, but there is some question as to the effect that the presence of the RNA decoys will have on the normal function of the cell. Both TAR and RRE bind cellular factors, in addition to viral proteins. The overexpression of the decoys may also lead to sequestration of proteins required for normal functioning of the cell and thus have negative effects on cell viability or function. To eliminate this potential problem, an RRE decoy of 13 nucleotides that retained the *rev*-binding domain but could not bind cellular factors was tested for antiviral activity. This minimal RRE decoy was shown to suppress HIV replication *in vitro* (Lee *et al.*, 1994).

4.2. Antisense DNA and RNA

Antisense nucleic acids utilize Watson–Crick nucleic acid base pairing to block gene expression in a sequence-specific fashion. Antisense transcripts can be designed to target various regions of the HIV genome. Although the mechanism of antisense-mediated inhibition of gene expression is not completely understood, it is hypothesized that RNA duplexes (antisense RNA and target RNA) are degraded by RNase H or by blocking subsequent translation of the mRNA. Stable intracellular expression of antisense HIV sequences is currently the most efficient method by which antisense technology can be used for the long-term inhibition of HIV gene expression. The use of antisense sequences has been thoroughly investigated, but the success has been limited to *in vitro* studies. Preliminary studies demonstrated limited antiviral activity with antisense transcripts to the viral genes *tat*, *rev*, *vpu*, *gag*, as well as the primer binding site (Kinchington *et al.*, 1992; Morvan *et al.*, 1993).

A major limitation to the use of stable expression of antisense sequences as a therapy for HIV infection is that long-term high levels of antisense expression are required in order to effectively inhibit viral replication. The mechanism through which antisense moieties inhibit gene expression requires that one antisense molecule efficiently bind to one target molecule. The stoichiometry of antisense sequences to target sequences must be a minimum 1:1 antisense to target, but ratios of 5:1 or greater lead to more effective inhibition of viral replication. Thus, the antisense gene expression must be much higher than the levels of HIV expression for an antisense gene therapy strategy to be effective. Standard retroviral vectors containing *pol* II promoters often do not produce sufficient levels of antisense sequence to inhibit viral replication. To subvert this problem, retroviral vectors containing alternative promoter systems have been developed. A retroviral vector containing a *pol* III promoter in the context of a double-copy expression cassette (the *pol* III promoter and antisense gene of interest are contained within each of the retroviral vector LTRs) potentially could achieve high levels of expression (Sullenger *et al.*, 1991). We have shown that such a *pol* III double-copy vector producing antisense to the TAR sequence is a more potent inhibitor of HIV replication than either antisense to the Tat or Tat/Rev open reading frames (Chuah *et al.*, 1994; VandenDriessche *et al.*, 1995).

4.3. Ribozymes

Ribozymes are antisense RNA molecules that have catalytic activity. Ribozymes function by binding to the target moiety through antisense sequence-specific hybridization and inactivate it by cleaving the phosphodiester backbone at a specific site. A distinct advantage of ribozymes is that they are not consumed during the target cleavage reaction and, therefore, a single ribozyme can inactivate multiple targets. Because of their unique catalytic properties, ribozymes have the potential to be highly efficient inhibitors of gene expression, even at low concentrations. Ribozymes also have greater sequence specificity than antisense RNA because the target must have the correct sequence to allow binding, and the cleavage site must be present in the right position.

The first investigation into ribozymes designed to inhibit HIV was performed by transfecting a hammerhead ribozyme targeted to the viral *gag* sequence into $CD4^+$ HeLa cells (Sarver *et al.*, 1990). On challenge with HIV, the cells were demonstrated to express reduced levels of full-length *gag* RNA molecules and markedly reduced levels of the *gag*-derived protein p24. A hairpin ribozyme targeted to the leader sequence was demonstrated to efficiently inhibit viral replication, but also to inactivate incoming viral RNAs prior to integration into the genome thereby inhibiting the establishment of infection (Wong-Staal *et al.*, 1994; Leavitt *et al.*, 1994). This ribozyme has further been demonstrated to provide protection from HIV infection in human PBL *in vitro* (Leavitt *et al.*, 1994).

A potential drawback to the use of ribozymes for HIV gene therapy is that they are inherently limited in effectiveness because of the high rate of mutation associated with HIV replication. Any disruption within the binding or cleavage sites within the target sequence required by the ribozyme for activity could render the ribozyme totally inactive. Ribozyme transcriptional units are small enough that several ribozymes could be incorporated into a single vector, and thus ribozymes targeted to several regions of the HIV genome can be delivered within the same cell. Multitarget ribozymes have also been developed in which a single ribozyme cleaves at multiple highly conserved targets within the HIV genome (Chen *et al.*, 1992). These approaches may circumvent the problem of target site mutagenesis.

4.4. DNA Vaccines

An additional use of nucleic acid-based approaches to gene therapy is to attempt to elicit an immune response to native HIV proteins encoded by transfer of genes into cells. This approach is being actively investigated as a technique to optimize HIV vaccination strategies. The rationale behind these gene vaccines is to generate an HIV-specific cytotoxic T-cell response via the MHC class I antigen presentation pathway. Introduction of the HIV-IIIB *env* gene into cells led to the formation of highly specific humoral and cellular immune responses in mice (Warner *et al.*, 1991; Jolly *et al.*, 1992). Recently, expression vectors encoding the HIV-NL4-3 envelope glycoprotein or a noninfectious NL4-3 particle were shown to produce transient antibody to anti-Env IgG and the defective genome expression vector raised persistent cytotoxic activity to the p24 protein (Lu *et al.*, 1995). These studies elucidate the potential formation of strong HIV-directed immune response, but the ability of such an immune response to persist and protect against polymorphic HIV strains is under study.

4.5. Single-Chain Antibodies

Single-chain antibodies (also called intrabodies) consist of an immunoglobulin heavy-chain leader sequence to target the intrabody to the endoplasmic reticulum (ER) and rearranged heavy- and light-chain variable regions that are connected by a flexible inter-chain linker (Marasco *et al.*, 1993). Since the single-chain antibody cannot be secreted without the other chain, it is efficiently retained within the ER through its interaction with the ER-specific BiP protein. Intrabodies are utilized to sequester viral proteins in inappropriate cellular compartments such that the viral life cycle is disrupted. Expression of an intrabody specific for the CD4 binding region of the HIV gp120 markedly reduced the HIV replication by trapping the gp160 in the ER and preventing its maturation by cleavage into the gp120/gp41 proteins (Marasco *et al.*, 1993). Intrabodies developed to the Rev protein trapped Rev in a cytoplasmic compartment and blocked HIV expression by inhibiting the export of HIV RNAs from the nucleus (Duan *et al.*, 1994). Recently, intrabodies containing an SV40 nuclear localization signal sequence were developed to Tat (Mhashilkar *et al.*, 1995). The anti-Tat single-chain antibody blocked Tat-mediated transactivation of the HIV LTR and rendered T-cell lines resistant to HIV infection. The potential of single-chain antibodies to act as therapeutic agents *in vivo* has been proposed.

4.6. *trans*-Dominant Negative Proteins

trans-Dominant negative proteins (TNPs) are mutated versions of HIV proteins that can inhibit HIV replication. HIV regulatory (Tat and Rev) and structural proteins (Env and

Gag) are potential targets for the development of TNPs. TNPs are defined as mutants that lack a wild-type function and inhibit the normal function of the wild-type counterpart in *trans* (Herskowitz, 1987; Feinberg and Trono, 1992). TNPs block the wild-type activity by direct competition for a cofactor or substrate that is available in limited quantities, or by the formation of a mixed multimer which is inactive because of the presence of the TNP.

The most thoroughly investigated TNP is a mutant Rev protein denoted Rev M10 (Malim *et al.*, 1989). The Rev protein is rendered a TNP through a series of mutations introduced into a well-conserved leucine-rich carboxy-terminal domain. The leucine-rich motif is absolutely required for wild-type Rev function. The Rev M10 protein contains two amino acid substitutions in this leucine-rich domain (position 78 L to D, position 79 E to L). Cell lines stably expressing Rev M10 are protected from HIV infection in long-term assays (Bahner *et al.*, 1993). Transduction of Rev M10 into T-cell lines and primary PBL delays viral replication without any negative effects on the cells (Woffendin *et al.*, 1994). Recently, it has been demonstrated that Rev M10 inhibits HIV replication in chronically infected T cells (Esaich *et al.*, 1995). Another TNP Rev protein developed by our group contains a single point mutation at leucine 78 and can effectively inhibit HIV replication in T-cell lines and PBL challenged with both laboratory and clinical HIV isolates (Ragheb *et al.*, 1995; VandenDriessche *et al.*, 1995). Two Phase I clinical trials based on Rev TNPs have been approved.

5. HIV-DIRECTED CLINICAL TRIALS

Eleven anti-HIV gene transfer or gene therapy protocols have been reviewed and approved by the National Institutes of Health Recombinant DNA Advisory Committee (RAC) (as of September, 1995). The following is a brief description of these clinical protocols describing the technologies involved and preliminary data that have been presented at relevant meetings.

5.1. Gene Marking of Syngeneic T Cells

Three of the approved HIV gene therapy protocols are being conducted at the NIH using a unique patient population. This patient population is HIV-discordant identical twins. All three protocols call for the manipulation of different subsets of lymphocytes from the uninfected twin followed by infusion into the infected recipient. The availability of healthy T cells from the uninfected donor permits rigorous expansion under conditions that can be difficult with T cells from infected patients.

The first of these studies involves gene marking of syngeneic T lymphocytes. This study aims to determine the survival of genetically marked syngeneic lymphocytes in HIV-discordant identical twins. The protocol is designed to evaluate the potential value of genetically modified T lymphocytes ($CD4^+$ and $CD8^+$) on the functional immune status of the infected twin, and will provide baseline data on the fate of activated $CD4^+$ and $CD8^+$ cells after reinfusion of HIV-infected individuals. By monitoring functional immune status, measure of viral burden, and physiological markers, it may be possible to determine whether this potential therapeutic approach is feasible and safe.

To date, six twin pairs have undergone the protocol (Walker, 1993). At study entry, three patients had CD4 counts above 200 cells/mm^3 and three were below 200 cells/mm^3. T lymphocytes from each seronegative twin were obtained by apheresis, and polyclonal T-cell proliferation was induced with anti-CD3 and rIL-2 stimulation. Once the cells begin dividing, they are genetically marked by transduction with a *NeoR* gene-containing retroviral vector and expanded 10- to 100-fold. The vector contains unique sequences allowing discrimination by PCR. The marked T cells were subsequently infused into the seropositive twins. Efficacy evaluation includes assessment of the survival of the uniquely marked T-cell populations by serial quantitative determination of the *NeoR* gene in PBL by vector-specific PCR, serial determination of $CD4^+$ and $CD8^+$ counts and percentages, T-cell proliferative responses and cytotoxicity, serial p24 antigen levels and serial quantitative determination of HIV viremia.

Results indicate that gene-marked T cells (both $CD4^+$ and $CD8^+$) could be detected in the circulation from all six infused patients for 4–12 weeks following infusion. The first patient remained vector-positive out to 20 weeks postinfusion of the *NeoR* gene-marked T cells. All patients have tolerated the therapy well and no side effects related to the gene transfer procedure have been observed. Transient increases in T-cell counts appeared in most recipients within 2 weeks posttransfer. These increases have generally waned during the subsequent few weeks. Sampling of lymph nodes at later time points (14–25 weeks postinfusion) demonstrated that gene-marked cells traffic to lymphoid tissues and are found in percentages equivalent to peripheral blood. A major finding suggested by the persistence of the gene-marked cells is that the $CD4^+$ T-cell pool may be maintained by division of mature T cells in adults. Thus, differentiation and subsequent expansion of prethymic T-precursor cells may not be a major contributing source to the mature T-cell pool in adults. This also implies that the immunological repertoire of the mature T-cell population may be limited to the currently existing cell population.

5.2. Marking of Cytotoxic T Cells

A second protocol involves gene-marking of HIV Gag-specific $CD8^+$ T cells from HIV-infected individuals (Riddell *et al.*, 1992). The objectives of this trial are threefold: (1) to evaluate the safety of administering increasing doses of autologous $CD8^+$ HIV-specific cytotoxic T-cell clones, (2) to determine the survival of adoptively transferred HIV-specific T-cell clones, and (3) to evaluate markers of HIV disease activity in these recipients. The adoptive immunotherapy using *in vitro*-expanded CMV-specific clones has proven effective for reconstituting CMV-specific T-cell responses following BMT (Reusser *et al.*, 1991). In this trial, HIV Gag-specific CTL clones were marked with a retroviral vector that expresses a hybrid fusion protein of the hygromycin resistance gene (*HygR*) and the herpes simplex virus thymidine kinase (HSV-TK) gene (*HyTK*). The advantage of using the *HyTK* fusion protein is that while it serves as a unique marker to follow the infused CTL clones, *HyTK* is also a conditionally lethal (suicide) gene. Thus, engineered cells can be ablated *in vivo* by administration of ganciclovir to the CTL recipient if unwanted CTL growth or response is observed.

Six patients with $CD4^+$ cell counts between 200 and 500 cells/mm^3 were given four doses of increasing amounts of gene-marked cells at 2-week intervals. Assessment of the clinical data includes determination of survival of the infused CTL clones by PCR and/or Southern analysis, characterization of HIV-specific CTL generation and HIV status (such as quantitation of serum p24 antigen levels). Analysis of the *in vivo* data indicated that the CTL clones could be detected after the first and second infusions at low levels (between 1 in 1,000 and 1 in 100,000 cells). This and other studies (see Section 5.4) utilizing $CD8^+$ cells suggest that *ex vivo*-cultured $CD8^+$ CTL life span may be adversely affected by the decline in $CD4^+$ cell function during AIDS progression. It is possible that CD4 cell help is needed to sustain an effective CTL response.

The gradual loss of detectable HIV-specific CTL correlates with increases in plasma viremia, reduction in $CD4^+$ T-cell counts, and the development of clinical AIDS (Pantaleo *et al.*, 1990; Walker and Plata, 1990; Fauci *et al.*, 1991). It may be possible to overcome these limitations by the development of helper-independent CTL clones, potentially by engineering the CD8 cells to secrete IL-2 in an autocrine fashion. A potentially unique and problematic finding of this report was the demonstration of an immune response to the *HyTk* transgene (both *HyTk*- and *Tk*-specific CTL were measured) (Riddell *et al.*, 1996). This immune response to the transgene may be responsible for the lack of the ability to detect significant levels of gene-marked cells following the third and fourth infusions. Similar immune responses have not been detected in gene therapy trials using the *Neo* gene as a marker.

5.3. Gene Vaccines

Almost all HIV-infected persons develop HIV-specific antibodies, but such antibodies appear to be unable to clear HIV infection. There is suggestive evidence that a CTL response may play an important role in controlling HIV infection (Pantaleo *et al.*, 1990; Walker and Plata, 1990; Fauci *et al.*, 1991; Carmichael *et al.*, 1993). An augmented CTL response may have a beneficial clinical effect in HIV-infected patients. It has been speculated that retroviral vector-mediated immunization or "genetic vaccination" for HIV may deliver intracellular HIV-derived antigenic peptides to the endogenous MHC class I antigen presentation pathway leading to CTL activation.

Three related clinical protocols have been approved by the RAC/FDA to test the safety and potential efficacy of genetic vaccination in HIV-infected individuals. In one protocol, HIV-infected patients have their fibroblasts removed for *ex vivo* transduction with a retroviral vector encoding the HIV Env/Rev proteins (designated as HIV-IT), and in another protocol HIV-IT retroviral vector is injected intramuscularly into the HIV-infected patient to achieve *in situ* transduction. The *ex vivo* genetic vaccination Phase I clinical protocol involves three successive doses of HIV-IT-transduced autologous fibroblasts. The direct *in vivo* injection protocol is a placebo-controlled clinical trial involving the administration of the HIV-IT vector or a diluent control to HIV-infected, seropositive, asymptomatic individuals not currently receiving antiretroviral treatment. Direct vector treatment consists of a series of three monthly intramuscular injections. Treated individuals are evaluated for acute toxicity and for normal clinical parameters, CD4 levels, HIV-specific T-cell responses, and viral load prior to, during, and following treatment. Preliminary clinical data suggest that HIV-infected patients treated with vector-transduced autologous fibroblasts show augmented HIV IIIB Env-specific $CD8^+$ CTL responses. It is hoped that the retroviral vector-mediated immunization will induce HIV-specific CTL and antibody responses that may help to eliminate HIV-infected cells and virus from an HIV-infected individual.

5.4. Universal Chimeric T-Cell Receptor

As described in Section 5.2 on gene-marker studies of HIV-specific $CD8^+$ CTL, these cells may have potential as an immunotherapy for HIV-infected individuals. Investigators at Cell Genesys, Inc. have designed a universal, MHC class I-unrestricted chimeric T-cell receptor that can redirect the antigenic specificity of peripheral blood mononuclear cell-derived $CD8^+$ T-cell populations to recognize the HIV envelope protein gp120 on the surface of the infected cells. This anti-HIV chimeric universal receptor (UR) is composed of the extracellular domain of the human CD4 receptor that recognizes the gp120 moiety of the HIV *env*, fused to the cytoplasmic domain of the IL-2R zeta chain, that can mediate signal transduction in T cells. It is hoped that on binding to gp120, these $CD4^-$ URs may initiate T-cell activation, resulting in induction of effector functions including cytolysis of the virus-infected cell. Hence, this strategy using CTLs engineered to express gp120-specific $CD4^-$ URs can have potentially therapeutic benefit in HIV-infected individuals.

The protocol using this approach is similar in design to the identical twin marker study (Walker, 1993), but in this case $CD8^+$ CTL will be transduced with a retroviral vector encoding the universal, MHC class I-unrestricted chimeric $CD4^-$ zeta receptor. This study is divided into two treatment periods. In the initial period, single doses of genetically unmodified T lymphocytes or single, escalating doses of genetically modified T lymphocytes will be administered. In the second period, multiple doses of the maximum tolerated cell dose will be administered. The objective of this protocol is to evaluate the distribution and survival, tolerance, safety, and efficacy of infusions of these genetically engineered universal CTL obtained from HIV-seronegative identical twins, on the functional immune status of HIV-infected twin recipients.

5.5. *trans*-Dominant Rev

Based on the extensive preclinical data obtained with the Rev M10 *trans*-dominant mutant (see Section 2.1), a clinical protocol has been initiated where $CD4^+$ T lymphocytes from an HIV-infected individual are engineered with Rev M10 expression vectors and reinfused into the patient. In this study, the efficacy of intracellular inhibition of HIV infection by the M10 *trans*-dominant mutant Rev protein will be evaluated. The major aim of this study is to determine whether expression of M10 can prolong the survival of PBL in AIDS patients, by conferring protection against HIV-mediated cell death. $CD4^+$ T lymphocytes will be genetically modified in patients using either particle-mediated gene transfer or retrovirus-mediated gene transfer. In each case, a control vector identical to the Rev M10 but with a frameshift that inactivates gene expression will be used to transduce a parallel population of $CD4^+$ cells. Retroviral transductions and particle-mediated transfections are initiated following stimulation of $CD4^+$-enriched cells with IL-2 and either anti-CD3 or anti-CD28 antibodies. During *in vitro* lymphocyte expansion, activation of endogenous HIV is inhibited by addition of reverse transcriptase inhibitors plus an HIV-specific toxin gene (CD4-PE40). The engineered and expanded cells are reinfused into the patient, and the survival of the cells in each group compared by limiting dilution PCR. One set of PCR primers is used to amplify both the control and therapeutic vectors. The effect of Rev M10 on HIV status and immunological parameters is being evaluated. Preliminary data using gold particle-mediated gene transfer show a small percentage of vector-engineered cells in the circulation of six patients treated for the first few weeks following reinfusion.

5.6. Anti-HIV Ribozyme

As described above, ribozymes are catalytic RNA molecules that hybridize specifically to a complementary RNA target analogous to conventional antisense molecules but in addition functionally inactivate it by cleaving the phosphodiester backbone at a specified location. A clinical protocol for AIDS gene therapy using the HIV leader-specific hairpin ribozyme has been proposed by Wong-Staal and co-workers. In this Phase I clinical trial, the safety and efficacy of ribozyme gene therapy will be evaluated in HIV-infected patients (CD4 counts between 250 and 500 cells/mm^3) by reinfusing autologous $CD4^+$ T cells that have been transduced *ex vivo* with a retroviral vector that expresses the HIV leader sequence ribozyme. Transduction of HIV-infected cells *in vitro* will require culture conditions that inhibit the spread of endogenous HIV as discussed for the transdominant Rev protocol (e.g., using nevirapine plus CD4-PE40). The *in vivo* kinetics and survival of ribozyme-transduced cells will be compared by limiting dilution PCR with those of a separate aliquot of cells transduced with a control vector (identical except for the ribozyme cassette). The level and persistence of ribozyme expression will also be assessed. The results will determine whether this ribozyme can protect $CD4^+$ T cells in patients with HIV infection and will aid design of future trials of hematopoietic stem cell gene therapy for AIDS.

5.7. *trans*-Dominant Rev in Combination with Antisense-*TAR*

To specifically inhibit the function of Rev, we have generated a new *trans*-dominant Rev mutant (*RevTD*) based on the previously described Rev M10 mutant, and showed that the presence of just one point mutation in the activator domain (Leu-78 to Asp-78) was sufficient to confer a dominant negative phenotype. To inhibit Tat function, we developed an antisense strategy targeted at the HIV transactivation response (*TAR*) element. To evaluate the efficacy of both *RevTD* and antisense-*TAR* in conditions relevant for clinical anti-HIV gene therapy, primary patient HIV isolates, including AZT-resistant strains, were used to challenge $CD4^+$ T lymphocytes that were transduced with retroviral vectors expressing *RevTD*, antisense-*TAR*, or a combination of both elements in the same vector. We demonstrated effective protection against the primary patient isolates with all of the vectors tested but greater inhibition of HIV was observed with *RevTD* plus antisense-*TAR* (Vanden-Driessche *et al.*, 1995). These preclinical data support the use of *RevTD* and antisense-*TAR* as a gene therapy strategy for inhibiting HIV in infected persons. We have proposed a clinical protocol for AIDS gene therapy using retrovirus-mediated gene transfer to deliver antisense-*TAR* and *RevTD* genes to syngeneic lymphocytes in identical twins discordant for HIV infection.

This study is based on these preclinical data with the antisense-*TAR* and *RevTD* retroviral vectors and on the adoptive transfer of *NeoR*-marked syngeneic $CD4^+$ T cells in HIV-discordant identical twins described above (Walker, 1993). In this clinical trial we will evaluate the safety, survival, and potential efficacy of the adoptive transfer of genetically engineered syngeneic lymphocytes obtained from HIV-seronegative identical twins on the functional immune status of HIV-infected twin recipients. T cells from each seronegative twin will be obtained by periodic apheresis, enriched for $CD4^+$ T cells by immunomagnetic depletion of $CD8^+$ T cells, induced to polyclonal proliferation with anti-CD3 and rIL-2 stimulation, divided into aliquots which will then be transduced with a control *NeoR* retroviral vector and up to two additional retroviral vectors containing the potentially therapeutic antisense-*TAR* and/or *RevTD* genes. These engineered T-cell populations will be expanded 10- to 100-fold in numbers prior to infusion into the seropositive twin. The relative survival of the uniquely engineered T-cell populations will be analyzed by vector-specific PCR, while the recipients' immune condition and HIV status will be monitored.

5.8. Intracellular Antibodies

As described above, intracellular antibodies can be constructed that target a variety of HIV proteins. A protocol by Marasco and colleagues proposes to use the antienvelope intracellular antibody sFv105 in an anti-HIV gene therapy trial. The choice of the HIV envelope as a target for attack is supported by the potential detrimental role of gp160 in syncytium formation, single cell killing, and potential virus-independent cytopathology. This study plan is to enroll six patients with $CD4^+$ cell counts < 250 cells/mm^3 who will undergo lymphopheresis from which $CD4^+$-enriched PBMC will be obtained. Again, as in the other protocol using HIV-infected cells, the anti-HIV drugs nevarapine and CD4-PE40 will be used to inhibit *in vitro* HIV expansion.

Two identical aliquots of lymphocytes will then be transduced either with the sFv105-expressing retroviral vector or with a control *Neo* gene-containing vector. Following transduction, it is proposed to enrich for gene-engineered cells by selection for the *Neo* gene by growth in G418-containing medium. Large numbers of transduced and culture-expanded cells (between 3.5 and 7.0×10^{10}) cells are proposed to be returned to the patient. Patients will subsequently be monitored by limiting dilution PCR to quantitate transduced cells in the circulation, to evaluate *in vivo* expression of the sFv105 transgene in transduced lymphocytes, and to make preliminary observations on the effects of gene therapy on HIV viral burden and $CD4^+$ lymphocyte levels.

6. CONCLUSIONS

A large variety of anti-HIV-1 gene therapy strategies have been developed that effectively inhibit HIV-1 *in vitro*. Based on these preclinical findings, several anti-HIV gene therapy strategies have received RAC/FDA approval for testing in HIV-1-infected individuals. These clinical trials may be able to address the question of whether rendering a cell resistant to HIV-1 infection by gene therapy will have a therapeutic benefit to the patient. These proposed protocols should also help in the design of future trials to test whether resistance to HIV-1 can ultimately be transferred to the entire lymphohematopoietic system by gene transfer into hematopoietic precursor/stem cells. Some gene transfer/therapy protocols should also help to further understand the mechanisms of immunopathogenesis leading to AIDS. The T-cell gene-marking trial in HIV-discordant twins has already provided data suggesting that T cells may have longer *in vivo* half lives than recently suggested. The gene vaccine protocols and the adoptive transfer of gene-marked CTL should contribute to further evaluate the potential importance of CTL in limiting HIV-1 infection. Ultimately, if these techniques prove beneficial, it will be necessary to develop alternative gene-delivery systems to minimize *ex vivo* manipulation of patients' cells and to make gene therapy accessible on a wider scale.

REFERENCES

Adam, M. A., and Miller, A. D., 1988, Identification of a signal in a murine retrovirus that is sufficient for packaging of nonretroviral RNA into virions, *J. Virol.* **62:**3802–3806.

Alexander, I. E., Russell, D. W., and Miller, A. D., 1994, DNA-damaging agents greatly increase the transduction of nondividing cells by adeno-associated virus vectors, *J. Virol.* **68:**8282–8287.

Anderson, W. F., 1984, Prospects toward human gene therapy, *Science* **226**:401–409.

Apperly, J. F., Luskey, B. D., and Williams, D. A., 1991, Retroviral gene transfer of human adenosine deaminase in murine hematopoietic cells: Effect of selectable marker sequences on long-term expression, *Blood* **78**:310–317.

Armentano, D., Yu, S. F., Kantoff, P. W., von Ruden, T., Anderson, W. F., and Gilboa, E., 1987, Effects of internal viral sequences on the utility of recombinant retroviral vectors, *J. Virol.* **61**:1647.

Bahner, I., Zhou, C., Yu, X. J., Guatelli, J. C., and Kohn, D. B., 1993, Comparison of trans-dominant inhibitory mutant human immunodeficiency virus type 1 genes expressed by retroviral vectors in human T lymphocytes, *J. Virol.* **67**:3199–3207.

Banda, N. K., Bernier, J., Kurahara, D. K., Kurrle, R., Haigwood, N., Sekaly, R. P., and Finkel, T. H., 1992, Crosslinking CD4 by human immunodeficiency virus gp120 primes T cells for activation-induced apoptosis, *J. Exp. Med.* **176**:1099–1106.

Blaese, R. M., Culver, K. W., Miller, A. D., Carter, C. S., Fleisher, T., Clerici, M., Shearer, G., Chang, L., Chiang, Y., Tolstoshev, P., Greenblatt, J. J., Rosenberg, S. A., Klein, H., Berger, M., Mullen, C. A., Ramsey, W. J., Muul, L., Morgan, R. A., and Anderson, W. F., 1995, T lymphocyte directed gene therapy for ADA deficiency (SCID): Results of the initial trial with 4 years of observation, *Science* **270**:475–480.

Bunnell, B. A., Muul, L. M., Donahue, R. E., Blaese, R. M., and Morgan, R. A., 1995, High-efficiency retroviral-mediated gene transfer into human and nonhuman primate peripheral blood lymphocytes, *Proc. Natl. Acad. Sci. USA* **92**:7739–7743.

Burns, J. C., Friedmann, T., Driever, W., Burrascano, M., and Yee, J. K., 1993, Vesicular stomatitis virus G glycoprotein pseudotyped retroviral vectors: Concentration to very high titer and efficient gene transfer into mammalian and non-mammalian cells, *Proc. Natl. Acad. Sci. USA* **90**:8033–8037.

Carmichael, A., Jin, X., Sissons, P., and Borysiewicz, L., 1993, Quantitative analysis of the human immunodeficiency virus type 1 (HIV-1)-specific cytotoxic T lymphocyte (CTL) response at different stages of HIV-1 infection: Differential CTL responses to HIV-1 and Epstein–Barr virus in late disease, *J. Exp. Med.* **177**:249–256.

Challita, P.-M., and Kohn, D. B., 1994, Lack of expression from a retroviral vector after transduction of murine hematopoietic stem cells is associated with methylation in vivo, *Proc. Natl. Acad. Sci. USA* **91**:2567–2571.

Chen, C. J., Banerjea, A. C., Hamison, G. G., Hagland, K., and Schubert, M., 1992, Multitarget-ribozyme directed to cleave at up to nine highly conserved HIV-1 env RNA regions inhibits HIV-1 replication-potential effectiveness against most presently sequenced HIV-1 isolates, *Nucleic Acids Res.* **20**:4581–4589.

Chuah, M. K. L., VandenDriessche, T., Chang, H., Ensoli, B., and Morgan, R. A., 1994, Inhibition of human immunodeficiency virus type-1 by retroviral vectors expressing antisense TAR, *Hum. Gene Ther.* **5**:1467–1475.

Culver, K. C., Morgan, R. A., Osborne, W. R. A., Lee, T., Lenscow, D., Able, C., Cornetta, K., Anderson, W. F., and Blaese, R. M., 1990, In vivo expression and survival of gene-modified T lymphocytes in rhesus monkeys, *Hum. Gene Ther.* **1**:399–409.

Danos, O., and Mulligan, R. C., 1988, Safe and efficient generation of recombinant retroviruses with amphotropic and ecotropic host ranges, *Proc. Natl. Acad. Sci. USA* **85**:6460–6464.

Duan, L., Bagasra, O., Laughlin, M. A., Oakes, J. W., and Pomerantz, R. J., 1994, Potent inhibition of human immunodeficiency virus type 1 by an intracellular anti-Rev single-chain antibody, *Proc. Natl. Acad. Sci. USA* **91**:5075–5079.

Ensoli, B., Barillari, G., Salahuddin, S. Z., Gallo, R. C., and Wong-Staal, F., 1990, Tat protein of HIV-1 stimulates growth of cells derived from Kaposi's sarcoma lesions of AIDS patients, *Nature* **344**:84–86.

Esaich, S., Kalfoglou, C., Plavec, I., Kaushal, S., Mosca, J. D., and Bohnlein, E., 1995, RevM10-mediated inhibition of HIV-1 replication in chronically infected T-cells, *Hum. Gene Ther.* **6**:625–634.

Fauci, A. S., 1992, Combination therapy for HIV infection: Getting closer, *Ann. Intern. Med.* **116**:85–86.

Fauci, A. S., Schnittman, S. M., Poli, G., Koenig, S., and Pantaleo, G., 1991, Immunopathogenic mechanisms in human immunodeficiency virus (HIV) infection, *Ann. Intern. Med.* **114**:678–693.

Feinberg, M. B., and Trono, D., 1992, Intracellular immunization: Trans-dominant mutants of HIV gene products as tools for the study and interruption of viral replication, *AIDS Res. Hum. Retrovir.* **8**:1013–1022.

Felgner, P. L., Gadek, T. R., Holm, M., Roman, R., Chan, H. W., Wenz, M., Northrop, J. P., Ringold, G. M., and Danielsen, M., 1987, Lipofection: A highly efficient, lipid-mediated DNA-transfection procedure, *Proc. Natl. Acad. Sci. USA* **84**:7413–7417.

Fischl, M. A., Richman, D. D., Causey, D. M., Grieco, M. H., Bryson, Y., Mildvan, D., Laskin, O. L., Groopman, J. E., Volberding, P. A., Schooley, R. T., Jackson, G. G., Durack, D. T., Andrews, J. C., Nusinoff-Lehrman, S., Barry, D. W., and the AZT Collaborative Working Group, 1989, Prolonged zidovudine therapy in patients with AIDS and advanced AIDS-related complex. AZT Collaborative Working Group, *J. Am. Med. Assoc.* **262**:2405–2410.

Gilboa, E., and Smith, C., 1994, Gene therapy for infectious diseases: The AIDS Model, *Trends Genet.* **10:**139–144.

Halbert, C. L., Alexander, I. E., Wolgamot, G. M., and Miller, A. D., 1995, Adeno-associated virus vectors transduce primary cells much less efficiently than immortalized cells, *J. Virol.* **69:**1473–1479.

Herskowitz, I., 1987, Functional inactivation of genes by dominant negative mutations, *Nature* **329:**219–222.

Jolly, D., Chada, S., Townsend, K., De Jesus, C., Chang, S., Weinhold, K., Anderson, C.-G., Lynn, A., Bodner, M., Barber, J., and Warner, J., 1992, CTL cross reactivity between HIV strains, *AIDS Res. Hum. Retrovir.* **8:**1369–1371.

Jowett, J. B., Planelles, V., Poon, B., Shah, N. P., Chen, M. L., and Chen, I. S. Y., 1995, The human immunodeficiency virus type 1 vpr gene arrests infected T cells in the G2$^+$ M phase of the cell cycle, *J. Virol.* **69:**6304–6313.

Kinchington, D., Galpin, S., Jaroszewski, J., Ghosh, K., Sabasinghe, C., and Cohen, J. S., 1992, A comparison of gag, pol and rev antisense oligodeoxynucleotides as inhibitors of HIV-1, *Antiviral Res.* **17:**53–62.

Kohn, D. B., Weinberg, K. I., Parkman, R., Lenarsky, C., Crooks, G. M., Shaw, K., Hanley, M. E., Lawrence, K., Annett, G., Brooks, J. S., Wara, D., Elder, M., Bowen, T., Hershfield, M. S., Berenson, R. I., Moen, R. C., Mullen, C. A., and Blaese, R. M., 1994, Gene therapy for neonates with ADA-deficient SCID by retroviral-mediated transfer of the human ADA cDNA into umbilical cord CD34+ cells, *J. Cell. Biochem. Suppl.* **18A:**238.

Larder, B. A., Darby, G., and Richman, D. D., 1989, HIV with reduced sensitivity to zidovudine (AZT) isolated during prolonged therapy, *Science* **243:**1731–1734.

Leavitt, M. C., Yu, M., Yamada, O., Kraus, G., Looney, D., Poeschla, E., and Wong-Staal, F., 1994, Transfer of an anti-HIV-1 ribozyme gene into primary human lymphocytes, *Hum. Gene Ther.* **5:**1115–1120.

Ledley, F. D., 1995, Nonviral Gene Therapy: The promise of genes as pharmaceutical products, *Hum. Gene Ther.* **6:**1129–1144.

Lee, S. W., Gallardo, H. F., Gilboa, E., and Smith, C., 1994, Inhibition of human immunodeficiency virus type 1 in human T cells by a potent Rev response element decoy consisting of the 13-nucleotide minimal Rev-binding domain, *J. Virol.* **68:**8254–8264.

Lin, H., Parmacek, M. S., Marle, G., Bolling, S., and Leiden, J. M., 1990, Expression of recombinant genes in myocardium in vivo after direct injection of DNA, *Circulation* **82:**2217–2221.

Lisziewicz, J., Sun, D., Smythe, J., Lusso, P., Loni, F., Louie, A., Markham, P., Rossi, J., Reitz, M., and Gallo, R. C., 1993, Inhibition of human immunodeficiency virus type 1 replication by regulated expression of a polymeric Tat activation response RNA decoy as a strategy for gene therapy for AIDS, *Proc. Natl. Acad. Sci. USA* **90:**8000–8004.

Lu, S., Santoro, J. S., Fuller, D. H., Hayes, J. R., and Robinson, H. L., 1995, Use of DNAs expressing HIV-1 env and noninfectious HIV-1 particles to raise antibody-responses in mice, *Virology* **209:**147–154.

Malim, M. H., Bohnlein, S., Hauber, J., and Cullen, B. R., 1989, Functional dissection of the HIV-1 Rev trans-activator: Derivation of a transdominant repressor of rev function, *Cell* **58:**205–214.

Mann, R., Mulligan, R. C., and Baltimore, D., 1983, Construction of a retrovirus packaging mutant and its use to produce helper-free defective retrovirus, *Cell* **33:**153–159.

Marasco, W. A., Haseltine, W. A., and Chen, S. Y., 1993, Design intracellular expression, and activity of a human anti-human immunodeficiency virus type 1 gp120 single-chain antibody, *Proc. Natl. Acad. Sci. USA* **90:**7889–7893.

Markowitz, D., Goff, S., and Bank, A., 1988, A safe packaging cell line for gene transfer: Separating viral genes on two different plasmids, *J. Virol.* **62:**1120–1124.

Mhashilkar, A. M., Bagley, J., Chen, S. Y., Szilvoy, A. M., Helland, D. G., and Marasco, W. A., 1995, Inhibition of HIV-1 Tat-mediated LTR transactivation and HIV-1 infection by anti-Tat single chain intrabodies, *EMBO J.* **14:**1542–1551.

Miller, A. D., 1992, Retroviral vectors, *Curr. Top Microbiol. Immunol.* **158:**1–24.

Miller, A. D., and Buttimore, C., 1986, Redesign of retrovirus packaging cell lines to avoid recombination leading to helper virus production, *Mol. Cell. Biol.* **6:**2895.

Miller, A. D., Garcia, J. V., von Suhr, N., Lynch, M., Wilson, C., and Eden, M. V., 1991, Construction and properties of retrovirus packaging cells based on gibbon ape leukemia virus, *J. Virol.* **65:**2220–2224.

Morgan, R. A., 1994, Retroviral vectors in human gene therapy, in: *Human Viruses in Gene Therapy* (J.-M. H. Vos, ed.), Academic Pres, San Diego, pp. 77–107.

Morgan, R. A., and Anderson, W. F., 1993, Human gene therapy, *Annu. Rev. Biochem.* **62:**191–217.

Morvan, F., Porumb, H., Degols, G., Lefebvre, I., Pompon, A., Sproat, B. S., Rayner, B., McIvy, C., Lebl, B., and Imbach, J. L., 1993, Comparative evaluation of seven oligonucleotide analogues as potential antisense agents, *J. Med. Chem.* **36:**280–287.

Mulligan, R. C., 1993, The basic science of gene therapy, *Science* **260:**926–932.

Muzyczka, N., 1992, Use of adeno-associated virus as a general transduction vector for mammalian cells, *Curr. Top. Microbiol. Immunol.* **158:**97–129.

Nabel, E. G., Gordon, D., Yang, Z.-Y., Xu, L., San, H., Plautz, G. E., Wu, B. Y., Gao, K., Huang, L., and Nabel, G. J., 1992, Gene transfer in vivo with DNA–liposome complexes: Lack of autoimmunity and gonadal localization, *Hum. Gene. Ther.* **3:**649–656.

Pantaleo, G., Koenig, S., Baseler, M., Lane, H. C., and Fauci, A. S., 1990, Defective clonogenic potential of CD8+ lymphocytes in patients with AIDS: Expansion in vivo of a nonclonogenic CD3+ CD8+ DR+ CD25− T cell population, *J. Immunol.* **144:**1696–1704.

Ragheb, J. A., Bressler, P., Daucher, M., Chiang, L., Chuah, M. K. L., VandenDriessche, T., and Morgan, R. A., 1996, Analysis of transdominant mutants of the HIV-1 rev protein for their ability to inhibit Rev function, HIV-1 replication, and their use as anti-HIV gene therapeutics, *AIDS Res. Hum. Retrovir.* **11:**1343–1353.

Reusser, P., Riddell, S. R., Meyers, J. D., and Greenberg, P. D., 1991, Cytotoxic T-lymphocyte response to cytomegalovirus after human allogeneic bone marrow transplantation: Pattern of recovery and correlation with cytomegalovirus infection and disease, *Blood* **78:**1373–1380.

Richman, D. D., Fischl, M. A., Grieco, M. H., Gottlieb, M. S., Volberding, P. A., Laskin, O. L., Leedom, J. M., Groopman, J. E., Mildvan, D., Hirsch, M. S., Jackson, G. G., Durack, D. T., Nusinoff-Lehrman, S., and the AZT Collaborative Working Group, 1987, The toxicity of azidothymidine (AZT) in the treatment of patients with AIDS and AIDS-related complex: A double-blind, placebo-controlled trial, *N. Engl. J. Med.* **317:**192–197.

Riddell, S. R., Greenberg, P. D., Overell, R. W., Loughran, T. P., Gilbert, M. J., Lupton, S. O., Agosti, J., Scheeler, S., Coombs, R. W., and Corey, L., 1992, Phase I study of cellular adoptive immunotherapy using genetically modified CD8+ HIV-specific T-cells for HIV seropositive patients undergoing allogeneic bone marrow transplant, *Hum. Gene Ther.* **3:**319–338.

Riddell, S. R., Elliott, M., Lewinsohn, D. A., Gilbert, M. J., Wilson, L., Manley, S. A., Lupton, S. D., Overell, R. W., Reynolds, T. C., Corey, L., and Greenberg, P. D., 1996, T-cell mediated rejection of gene-modified HIV-specific cytotoxic T lymphocytes in HIV-infected patients, *Nature Medicine* **2:**216– 223.

Rill, D. R., Moen, R. C., Buschle, M., Bartholomew, C., Foreman, N. K., Mirro, J., Jr., Krance, R. A., Ihle, J. N., and Brenner, M. K., 1992, An approach for the analysis of relapse and marrow reconstitution after autologous marrow transplantation using retrovirus-mediated gene transfer, *Blood* **79:**2694–2700.

Rosenberg, S. A., Aebersold, P. M., Cornetta, K., Kasid, A., Morgan, R. A., Moen, R., Karson, E. M., Lotze, M. T., Yang, J. C., Topalien, S. L., Merino, M. J., Culver, K., Miller, A. D., Blaese, R. M., and Anderson, W. F., 1990, Gene transfer into humans: Immunotherapy of patients with advanced melanoma using tumor infiltrating lymphocytes modified by retroviral gene transduction, *N. Engl. J. Med.* **323:**570–578.

Samulski, R. J., 1994, Parvoviruses, in: *Human Viruses in Gene Therapy* (J.-M. H. Vos, ed.), Academic Press, San Diego, pp. 53–76.

Sarver, N., Cantin, E. M., Chang, P. S., Zaia, J. A., Ladne, P. A., Stephens, D. A., and Rossi, J. J., 1990, Ribozymes as potential anti-HIV-1 therapeutic agents, *Science* **247:**1222–1225.

Stewart, M. J., Plautz, G. E., Yang, Z.-Y., Xu, L., Gao, X., Huang, L., Nabel, E. G., and Nabel, G. J., 1992, Gene transfer in vivo with DNA–liposome complexes: Safety and acute toxicity in mice, *Hum. Gene. Ther.* **3:** 267–275.

Sullenger, B. A., Gallardo, H. F., Ungers, G. E., and Gilboa, E., 1991, Analysis of trans-acting response decoy RNA-mediated inhibition of human immunodeficiency virus type 1 transactivation, *J. Virol.* **65:**6811–6816.

Van Beusechem, V. W., Kukler, A., Heidt, P. J., and Valerio, D., 1992, Long-term expression of human adenosine deaminase in rhesus monkeys transplanted with retrovirus-infected bone-marrow cells, *Proc. Natl. Acad. Sci. USA* **89:**7640–7644.

VandenDriessche, T., Chuah, M. K. L., and Morgan, R. A., 1994, Gene therapy for acquired immune deficiency syndrome, in: *AIDS Updates* Volume 7(4) (V. T. DeVita, S. Hellman, and S. A. Rosenberg, eds.), Lippincott, Philadelphia, pp. 1–14.

VandenDriessche, T., Chuah, M. K. L., Chiang, L., Chang, H. K., Ensoli, B., and Morgan, R. A., 1995, Inhibition of clinical HIV-1 isolates in primary CD4+ T lymphocytes by retroviral vectors expressing anti-HIV genes, *J. Virol.* **69:**4045–4052.

Walker, B. D., and Plata, F., 1990, Cytotoxic T lymphocytes against HIV, *AIDS* **4:**177–184.

Walker, R., 1993, A study of the safety and survival of the adoptive transfer of genetically marked syngeneic lymphocytes in HIV-infected identical twins, *Hum. Gene Ther.* **4:**659–680.

Warner, J. F., Anderson, C.-G., Laube, I., Jolly, D. J., Townsend, K., Chada, S., and St. Louis, D., 1991, Induction of HIV-specific CTL and antibody responses in mice using retroviral vector-transduced cells, *AIDS Res. Hum. Retrovir.* **7:**645–655.

Woffendin, C., Yang, Z.-Y., Udaykumar, Xu, L., Yang, N. S., Sheehy, M. J., and Nabel, G. J., 1994, Nonviral and viral delivery of a human immunodeficiency virus protective gene into primary human T cells, *Proc. Natl. Acad. Sci. USA* **91**:11581–11585.

Wong-Staal, F., Yu, M., Yamada, O., *et al.*, 1994, Development of ribozyme gene therapy against HIV, *J. Cell. Biochem. Suppl.* **18A**:221.

Yang, Y., Vanin, E. F., Whitt, M. A., Fornerod, M., Zwart, R., Schneiderman, R. D., Grosveld, G., and Nienhuis, A. W., 1995, Inducible high-level production of infectious murine leukemia retroviral vector particles psuedotyped with vesicular stomatitis virus G envelope protein, *Hum. Gene Ther.* **6**:1203–1213.

Yu, M. Poeschla, E., and Wong-Staal, F., 1994, Progress towards gene therapy for HIV infection, *Gene Ther.* **1**: 13–26.

INDEX

The letter *f* following a page number indicates that the term involved can be found in a figure; the letter *t* following a page number indicates that the term involved can be found in a table.

GPSR Compliance
The European Union's (EU) General Product Safety Regulation (GPSR) is a set of rules that requires consumer products to be safe and our obligations to ensure this.

If you have any concerns about our products, you can contact us on

ProductSafety@springernature.com

In case Publisher is established outside the EU, the EU authorized representative is:

Springer Nature Customer Service Center GmbH
Europaplatz 3
69115 Heidelberg, Germany

www.ingramcontent.com/pod-product-compliance
Ingram Content Group UK Ltd.
Pitfield, Milton Keynes, MK11 3LW, UK
UKHW051132260726
13967UKWH00010B/2993

* 9 7 8 1 4 8 9 9 0 1 9 2 7 *